Clinical Sports Medicine

Clinical Sports Medicine

Edited by

Darren L. Johnson MD
Professor and Chair
Department of Orthopaedic Surgery
Director of Sports Medicine
University of Kentucky School of Medicine
Lexington, KY

Scott D. Mair MD
Associate Professor
Department of Orthopaedic Surgery
University of Kentucky
Lexington, KY

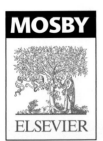

MOSBY
ELSEVIER

1600 John F. Kennedy Blvd.
Ste 1800
Philadelphia, PA 19103-2899

Notice

Knowledge and best practice in Medicine are constantly changing. As new research and experience broaden our knowledge, changes in practice, treatment and drug therapy may become necessary or appropriate. Readers are advised to check the most current information provided (i) on procedures featured or (ii) by the manufacturer of each product to be administered, to verify the recommended dose or formula, the method and duration of administration, and contraindications. It is the responsibility of the practitioner, relying on their own experience and knowledge of the patient, to make diagnoses, to determine dosages and the best treatment for each individual patient, and to take all appropriate safety precautions. To the fullest extent of the law, neither the Publisher nor the Editors assume any liability for any injury and/or damage to persons or property arising out or related to any use of the material contained in this book.

Printed in China.

Last digit is the print number: 9 8 7 6 5 4 3 2 1

Contributors

J. Winslow Alford MD
West Bay Orthopaedics, Warwick, RI.
Rotator Cuff Disorders

Answorth A. Allen MD
Hospital for Special Surgery, New York, NY.
Knee: Graft Choices in Ligament Surgery

David R. Anderson MD
Orthopedic Surgeon, Minnesota Sports Medicine,
   Minneapolis, MN.
Superior Labrum Anterior to Posterior Lesions

Robert B. Anderson MD
Chief, Foot and Ankle Service, Department of
   Orthopaedic Surgery, Carolinas Medical Center;
   Co-Director, Foot and Ankle Fellowship
   OrthoCarolina, Charlotte, NC.
Ankle Ligament Injury and Instability

Thomas D. Armsey MD
Associate Professor; Director Sports Medicine
   Fellowship, Palmetto Health Family Practice
   Center, Columbia, SC.
On-Field Emergencies and Preparedness

Bernard R. Bach, Jr. MD
The Claude Lambert-Susan Thomson Professor of
   Orthopedic Surgery; Rush University Medical
   Center, Chicago, IL.
*Complex Issues in Anterior Cruciate Ligament
   Reconstruction*

Champ L. Baker, Jr. MD
Clinical Assistant Professor, Department of
   Orthopaedics, Medical College of Georgia,
   Augusta; Chair, Sports Medicine Fellowship
   Program, The Hughston Clinic, Columbus,
   GA.
Elbow: Physical Examination and Evaluation

George K. Bal MD, FACS
Assistant Professor, Sports Medicine and Shoulder
   Reconstructive Surgery, Department of
   Orthopaedics, West Virginia University,
   Morgantown, WV.
Clavicle Fractures and Sternoclavicular Injuries

R. Shane Barton MD
Assistant Professor, Department of Orthopaedic
   Surgery, Louisiana State University Health
   Sciences Center; Medical Director, Sports
   Medicine, Willis Knighton Hospital System,
   Shreveport, LA.
Shoulder: Nerve Injuries

Carl J. Basamania MD, FACS
Division of Orthopaedic Surgery, Duke University
   Medical Center, Durham, NC.
Clavicle Fractures and Sternoclavicular Injuries

Frank H. Bassett III MD
Sports Medicine Service, Duke University Medical
   Center, Durham, NC.
The Role of the Team Physician

Todd C. Battaglia MD, MS
Clinical Instructor, Department of Orthopaedics,
   Tufts University School of Medicine;
   Fellow, Sports Medicine and Arthroscopic
   Surgery, New England Baptist Hospital, Boston,
   MA.
Posterior Cruciate Ligament

Nathalee S. Belser MPA
Department of Orthopaedic Surgery, University of
   Louisville School of Medicine, Louisville, KY.
Pediatric Knee

Philip E. Blazar MD
Assistant Professor of Orthopaedic Surgery, Harvard
   Medical School; Assistant Professor of Orthopaedic
   Surgery, Brigham and Women's Hospital, Boston,
   MA.
Wrist Soft-Tissue Injuries

Michael R. Boland MBChB, FRCS, FRACS
Assistant Professor, University of Kentucky; Chief,
   Orthopaedic Hand and Upper Extremity Surgery,
   University of Kentucky Medical Center, Veterans
   Administration Hospital, Lexington, KY.
*Wrist and Hand: Physical Examination and
   Evaluation*

Craig R. Bottoni LTC, MD
Chief, Sports Medicine, Orthopaedic Surgery Service,
   Tripler Army Medical Center; Assistant Clinical
   Professor, Department of Surgery, John A. Burns
   School of Medicine, University of Hawaii,
   Honolulu HI; Assistant Professor of Surgery,
   Department of Surgery, F. E. Edward Hébert
   School of Medicine, Uniformed Services University
   of the Health Sciences, Bethesda, MD.
Shoulder: Anterior Instability

Jeff C. Brand, Jr. MD
Alexandria Orthopaedics and Sports Medicine,
   Alexandria, MN.
Knee: Tendon Ruptures

Stephen F. Brockmeier MD
Chief Resident, Department of Orthopaedics,
   Georgetown University, Washington, DC.
Knee: Overuse Injuries

Amy Bullens-Borrow MD
Georgia Sports Orthopedic Specialists, Gainesville,
   GA.
Elbow: Instability and Arthroscopy

J.W. Thomas Byrd MD
Nashville Sports Medicine and Orthopaedic Center,
   Nashville, TN.
Hip Joint

E. Lyle Cain, Jr. MD
Fellowship Director, American Sports Medicine
   Institute; Orthopaedic Surgeon, Alabama Sports
   Medicine and Orthopaedic Center, Birmingham,
   AL.
Internal Impingement

Kenneth Cayce IV
Cincinnati Sports Medicine and Orthopaedics Center,
   Cincinnati, OH.
The Preparticipation Physical Examination

Constantine Charoglu MD
Southern Bone and Joint Specialists, PA, Hattiesburg,
   MS.
Hand and Wrist Rehabilitation

Kevin Charron MD
Chief Resident, Department of Orthopaedic Surgery,
   Boston University Medical Center, Boston, MA.
Patellofemoral Instability

Michael J. Coen MD
Department of Orthopaedic Surgery, Loma Linda
   University, East Campus, Loma Linda, CA.
Thigh and Leg

Brian J. Cole MD
Associate Professor, Department of Orthopaedic
   Surgery, Section Head, Cartilage Restoration Center,
   Rush University Medical Center, Chicago, IL.
Knee: Articular Cartilage

Adam C. Crowl MD
Attending Physician, Orthopedic Spine Surgery,
   Advanced Orthopedic Centers, Richmond,
   VA.
Cervical Spine

Lisa T. DeGnore MD
Volunteer Faculty, Department of Orthopaedic
   Surgery, University of Kentucky, Lexington,
   KY.
Forefoot and Toes

Christopher C. Dodson MD
Resident, Department of Orthopaedic Surgery,
   Hospital for Special Surgery, New York, NY.
Traumatic Shoulder Muscle Ruptures

Jeffrey R. Dugas MD
Fellowship Director, American Sports Medicine
   Institute, Birmingham, AL.
Elbow: Instability and Arthroscopy

R. Matthew Dumigan MD
Fellow, Steadman-Hawkins Clinic, Vail, CO.
Ankle Intra-articular Injury

T. Bradley Edwards MD
Clinical Instructor, Department of Orthopedic
   Surgery, University of Texas at Houston; Shoulder
   Surgeon, Fondren Orthopedic Group, Texas
   Orthopedic Hospital, Houston, TX.
Pediatric Shoulder

Hussein Elkousy MD
Volunteer Faculty, University of Texas Health Sciences
   Center, Houston, TX.
Principles of Shoulder Arthroscopy

Ivan Encalada-Diaz MD
Associate Clinical Professor of Orthopedic Surgery,
   National Autonomous University of Mexico;
   Attending Orthopedic Surgeon, Arthroscopy and
   Sports Medicine Service, Institute of Orthopedics,
   National Center for Rehabilitation, Mexico City,
   Mexico.
Meniscal Injury

Kyle R. Flik MD
Attending Surgeon, Sports Medicine, Northeast
   Orthopaedics, LLP, Albany, NY.
Knee: Articular Cartilage

Philip C. Forno MD
Orthopaedic Resident, University of South Cardina,
   Columbia, SC.
Shoulder: Overuse Injuries

Stephen French MD
Big Thunder Orthopedics, Thunder Bay, Ontario,
   Canada.
Knee: Arthritis in the Athlete

Freddie H. Fu MD
Department of Orthopaedic Surgery, University of
   Pittsburgh School of Medicine; Chief, Department
   of Orthopaedic Surgery, UPMC Presbyterian
   Hospitals, Pittsburgh, PA.
Anterior Cruciate Ligament

James R. Gardiner MD
Pacific Sports Medicine at Multicare, Tacoma, WA.
Multiligament Knee Injuries

Gary Gartsman MD
Clinical Professor, Department of Orthopaedics,
   University of Texas Health Sciences Center; Texas
   Orthopedic Hospital, Houston, TX.
Principles of Shoulder Arthroscopy

C. David Geier, Jr. MD
Assistant Professor, Orthopaedic Surgery; Chief,
Sports Medicine Service, Medical University of
South Carolina, Charleston, SC.
Pediatric Elbow

Thomas J. Gill MD
Assistant Professor of Orthopaedic Surgery, Harvard
Medical School; Sports Medicine Service,
Department of Orthopedic Surgery, Massachusetts
General Hospital, Boston, MA.
Shoulder: Nerve Injuries

Jennifer A. Graham MD
Resident, Harvard Combined Orthopaedic Surgery
Program, Boston, MA.
Wrist Soft-Tissue Injuries

Letha Y. Griffin MD, PhD
Team Physician, Adjunct Professor, Department of
Kinesiology and Health, Georgia State University;
Partner, Peachtree Orthopaedic Clinic, Atlanta,
GA.
The Female Athlete

Kevin M. Guskiewicz PhD, ATC
Professor and Chair, Department of Exercise and Sport
Science; Professor, Department of Orthopaedics,
University of North Carolina, Chapel Hill, NC.
Head Injuries

Jeffrey A. Guy MD
Assistant Professor, Director, Sports Medicine Center,
Medical Director, University of South Carolina;
Orthopedic Surgeon, Palmetto Health Richland,
Columbia, SC.
Shoulder: Overuse Injuries

Christopher D. Harner MD
Blue Cross of Western Pennsylvania Professor,
University of Pittsburgh; Medical Director,
UPMC Center for Sports Medicine, Pittsburgh,
PA.
Safety Issues for Musculoskeletal Allografts; The Stiff Knee

Richard J. Hawkins MD
Attending Physician, Steadman-Hawkins Clinic of the
Carolinas, Spartanburg, SC.
Shoulder: Physical Examination and Evaluation

Robert Hosey MD
Associate Professor, Department of Family Medicine
and Orthopaedics, Director, Primary Care Sports
Medicine Fellowship, University of Kentucky,
Lexington, KY.
The Preparticipation Physical Examination

Joel Hurt MD
Orthopedic Surgeon, Texas Bone and Joint Sports
Medicine Institute, Austin, TX.
Ankle and Foot: Physical Examination and Evaluation

Peter Indelicato MD
Professor, Shands Healthcare, University of Florida,
Gainesville, FL.
Knee: Medial Collateral Ligament

William M. Isbell MD
Raleigh Orthopaedic Clinic, Raleigh, NC.
Elbow: Tendon Ruptures

Darren L. Johnson MD
Professor and Chair, Department of Orthopaedic
Surgery; Director of Sports Medicine,
University of Kentucky School of Medicine,
Lexington, KY.
Multiligament Knee Injuries

Grant L. Jones MD
Assistant Professor, Department of Orthopaedic
Surgery, Ohio State University College of
Medicine; Vice Chair, Department of
Orthopaedics, Ohio State University Medical
Center, Main Campus; Ohio State University
Hospital East, Columbus, OH.
Elbow: Physical Examination and Evaluation

James D. Kang MD
Associate Professor of Orthopaedic and Neurological
Surgery, University of Pittsburgh School of
Medicine; University of Pittsburgh Medical Center,
Pittsburgh, PA.
Cervical Spine

Richard W. Kang BS
Research Coordinator, Rush University Medical
Center, Chicago, IL.
Knee: Articular Cartilage

Spero G. Karas MD
Assistant Professor of Orthopaedic Surgery, Emory
University School of Medicine, Atlanta, GA.
Shoulder: Multidirectional Instability

James Kercher MD
Department of Orthopaedics, Emory University
School of Medicine, Atlanta, GA.
The Female Athlete

John J. Klimkiewicz MD
Assistant Professor, Department of Orthopedic
Surgery, Georgetown University Hospital–
MEDSTAR Health; Head Team Physician,
Georgetown Hoyas, Washington, DC.
Knee: Overuse Injuries

Mininder Kocher MD, MPH
Assistant Professor, Department of Orthopaedic
Surgery, Harvard Medical School; Associate
Director, Division of Sports Medicine, Children's
Hospital, Boston, MA.
The Pediatric Athlete

Sumant G. Krishnan MD
Clinical Assistant Professor, Department of
Orthopaedic Surgery, University of Texas
Southwestern; Attending Orthopedic Surgeon,
Shoulder and Elbow Service, The Carrell Clinic,
Dallas, TX.
Shoulder: Physical Examination and Evaluation

John E. Kuhn MS, MD
Associate Professor, Department of Orthopaedics
and Rehabilitation, Vanderbilt University Medical
School; Chief of Shoulder Surgery, Team Physician,
Vanderbilt University and Nashville Sounds
Baseball Club, Vanderbilt Sports Medicine,
Nashville, TN.
Scapulothoracic Disorders

Laurence Laudicina MD
Orthopaedic Surgeon, Steadmans-Hawkins Fellow,
Florida Sports Medicine Institute, St. Augustine, FL.
*Elbow: Overuse Injuries, Tendinosis, and Nerve
Compression*

Steven J. Lawrence MD
Head, Foot and Ankle Section, University of
Kentucky; Associate Professor of Orthopedics, A.B.
Chandler Medical Center, University of Kentucky,
Lexington, KY.
Midfoot and Hindfoot

Jeffrey N. Lawton MD
Hand and Upper Extremity Surgeon, Department of
Orthopaedic Surgery, Cleveland Clinic Foundation,
Cleveland, OH.
Carpal Fractures

Paul Lewis MS
Rush University Medical Center, Chicago, IL.
Knee: Articular Cartilage

Robert Litchfield MD, FRCS(C)
Associate Professor, Department of Surgery, Fowler
Kennedy Sports Medicine Center, University of
Western Ontario, London, Ontario, Canada.
Knee: Arthritis in the Athlete

Daniel S. Lorenz PT, ATC, CSCS
Department of Sports Medicine, Duke University,
Durham, NC.
Knee: Posterolateral Corner

Walter R. Lowe MD
Associate Professor, Baylor College of Medicine;
Chief, Sports Medicine Section, Department of
Orthopedic Surgery, Baylor College of Medicine,
Houston, TX.
Superior Labrum Anterior to Posterior Lesions

Scott D. Mair MD
Associate Professor, Department of Orthopaedic
Surgery; University of Kentucky, Lexington, KY.
Shoulder: Posterior Instability

Terry Malone PT, EdD, ATC
Professor of Physical Therapy, University of Kentucky,
Lexington, KY.
Knee Rehabilitation

Todd C. Malvey DO, CAQSM
Physician, Moncrief Army Community Hospital, Fort
Jackson, SC.
On-Field Emergencies and Preparedness

Bert R. Mandelbaum MD
Santa Monica Orthopaedic Surgery and Sports
Medicine Group, Orange, CA.
Abdomen and Pelvis

Steven D. Maschke MD
Department of Orthopaedic Surgery, Cleveland
Clinic Foundation, Cleveland, OH.
Carpal Fractures

Elizabeth G. Matzkin MD
Foundry Sports Medicine, Providence, RI.
Clavicle Fractures and Sternoclavicular Injuries

Craig S. Mauro MD
Resident, Department of Orthopaedic Surgery,
University of Pittsburgh Medical Center, Pittsburgh,
PA.
*Safety Issues for Musculoskeletal Allografts; The Stiff
Knee*

David Mayman MD
Department of Orthopedic Surgery, Hospital for
Special Surgery, New York, NY.
Shoulder: Nerve Injuries

L. Pearce McCarty III MD
Sports and Orthopaedic Specialists, P.A., Edina, MN.
*Complex Issues in Anterior Cruciate Ligament
Reconstruction*

Ryan C. Meis MD
Center for Neurosciences, Orthopaedics, and Spine,
Dakota Dunes, SD.
Internal Impingement

William C. Meyers MD
Professor and Chairman, Department of Surgery;
Senior Associate Dean for Clinical Affairs, Drexel
University College of Medicine, Philadelphia, PA.
Abdomen and Pelvis

Mark D. Miller MD
Professor of Orthopedic Surgery, Head of Division of
Sports Medicine, University of Virginia,
Charlottesville; Team Physician, James Madison
University, Harrisonburg, VA.
Posterior Cruciate Ligament

Peter J. Millet MD
Steadman-Hawkins Clinic, Vail, CO.
Shoulder: Nerve Injuries

Amir R. Moinfar MD
Chesapeake Orthopedics, Glen Burnie, MD.
Knee: Posterolateral Corner

Claude T. Moorman III MD
Associate Professor, Department of Orthopaedic
Surgery; Director, Sports Medicine, Duke Medical
Center; Head Team Physician, Duke Athletics;
Durham, NC.
*The Role of the Team Physician; Knee: Posterolateral
Corner*

Steve A. Mora MD
Active Staff, Orthopedic Department, St. Joseph
Hospital, Orange, CA.
Abdomen and Pelvis

Kevin J. Mulhall MB, MCh, FRCSI
Consultant Orthopaedic Surgeon, Department of
Orthopaedic Surgery, Dublin, Ireland.
Posterior Cruciate Ligament

Gregory Nicholson MD
Department of Orthopedics, Division of Shoulder
and Sports Medicine, Rush University, Chicago, IL.
Rotator Cuff Disorders

Thomas Noonan MD
Partner, Steadman-Hawkins Clinic–Denver,
Greenwood Village; Medical Director, Colorado
Rockies Baseball Club, Denver, CO.
*Elbow: Overuse Injuries, Tendinosis, and Nerve
Compression*

James Nunley MD
J. Leonard Goldner Professor of Surgery; Chief of
Orthopedics, Duke University Medical Center,
Durham, NC.
Ankle Tendon Disorders and Ruptures

John Nyland EdD, PT, SCS, ATC, CSCS, FACSM
Assistant Professor, Department of Orthopaedic
Sugery, Division of Sports Medicine, University of
Louisville; Consultant, Sports Health Program,
Norton Hospital, Louisville, KY.
Foot and Ankle Rehabilitation

Adam C. Olsen MPT, ATC
Rehabilitation Coordinator, St. Louis Cardinals,
St. Louis, MO.
Principles of Rehabilitation

George A. Paletta, Jr. MD
Orthopedic Center of St. Louis, St. Louis, MO.
Pediatric Elbow

Kyle Parish MD
Assistant Professor, Departments of Family and
Community Medicine and Sports Medicine,
University of Kentucky, Lexington, KY.
Environmental Stressors

Andrew D. Pearle MD
Instructor of Orthopedic Surgery, Cornell University
New York Hospital; Assistant Attending
Orthopedic Surgeon, Hospital for Special Surgery,
New York, NY.
Knee: Graft Choices in Ligament Surgery

George C. Phillips MD
Clinical Assistant Professor of Pediatrics, Children's
Hospital of Iowa, University of Iowa Carver
College of Medicine, Iowa City, IA.
Medications, Supplements, and Ergogenic Drugs

James C. Puffer MD
Professor, Department of Family and Community
Medicine, University of Kentucky School of
Medicine; President and Chief Executive Office,
American Board of Family Medicine, Lexington, KY.
Cardiac Problems and Sudden Death

Matthew Alan Rappé MD
Resident Physician, University of Florida, Gainesville,
FL.
Knee: Medial Collateral Ligament

Fred Reifsteck MD
Clinical Assistant Professor, Medical College of
Georgia, Augusta; Head Team Physician, University
of Georgia, Athens, GA.
The Female Athlete

Michael M. Reinold PT, DPT
Adjunct Faculty, Department of Physical Therapy,
Northeastern University; Assistant Athletic Trainer,
Boston Red Sox, Boston, MA.
Principles of Rehabilitation

Arthur C. Rettig MD
Clinical Instructor, Orthopedic Surgery, Wishard
Memorial Hospital; Clinical Assistant Professor,
Orthopedic Surgery, Indiana University Medical
Center; Adjunct Professor, Butler University,
Indianapolis; Adjunct Professor, Purdue University,
West Lafayette; Orthopedic Surgeon and Partner,
Methodist Sports Medicine Center, Indianapolis,
IN.
Hand Injuries

Lance A. Rettig MD
Volunteer Clinical Assistant Professor of Orthopedics,
Indiana University; Staff Orthopedic Surgeon,
Methodist Sports Medicine Center, Indianapolis,
IN.
Hand Injuries

John C. Richmond MD
Professor, Orthopedic Surgery, Tufts University
School of Medicine; Chair, Department of
Orthopaedic Surgery, New England Baptist
Hospital, Boston, MA.
Meniscal Injury

Jeffrey A. Rihn MD
Resident Physician, Department of Orthopaedic
Surgery, University of Pittsburgh Medical Center,
Pittsburgh, PA.
Safety Issues for Musculoskeletal Allografts

Craig S. Roberts MD
Professor, Residency Program Director,
Department of Orthopaedic Surgery, School
of Medicine, University of Louisville, Louisville,
KY.
Pediatric Knee

Richard Rodenberg MD
Assistant Professor, Department of Family Medicine,
Program Director, Sports Medicine Fellowship,
Grant Medical Center, Columbus, OH; Assistant
Professor, Department of Family Medicine,
Lexington, KY.
Environmental Stressors

Mark W. Rodosky MD
Center for Sports Medicine, University of Pittsburgh
Medical Center, Pittsburgh, PA.
Biceps Tendon Disorders

Anthony R. Romeo MD
Department of Orthopedics, Division of Shoulder
and Sports Medicine, Rush University, Chicago,
IL.
Rotator Cuff Disorders

Greg Sassmannshausen MD
Clinical Faculty, Fort Wayne Medical Education
Program Fort Wayne, IN.
The Older Athlete

Anthony Schepsis MD
Professor, Department of Orthopaedic Surgery;
Director, Department of Sports Medicine, Boston
University Medical Center, Boston, MA.
Patellofemoral Instability

Theodore F. Schlegel MD
Assistant Professor, Department of Orthopaedic
Surgery, University of Colorado–Denver; Team
Physician, Denver Broncos and Colorado Rockies;
Consultant, Steadman-Hawkins Clinic–Denver,
Denver CO.
Disorders of the Acromioclavicular Joint

Jeffrey B. Selby MD
University of Kentucky; VA Medical Center,
Lexington, KY.
Ankle Fractures and Syndesmosis Injuries

Patrick Siparsky BS
University of Colorado Health Sciences Center,
Denver, CO.
*Disorders of the Acromioclavicular Joint; The Pediatric
Athlete*

Dale S. Snead MD
Partner, Methodist Sports Medicine Center,
Indianapolis, IN.
Hand Injuries

Jeffrey T. Spang MD
Chief Resident, Department of Orthopaedics,
University of North Carolina, Chapel Hill,
NC.
Shoulder: Multidirectional Instability

Tracy Spigelman Med, ATC
Doctoral Student and Graduate Assistant, University
of Kentucky, Lexington, KY.
Shoulder Rehabilitation

J. Richard Steadman MD
Steadman-Hawkins Clinic; Steadman-Hawkins
Research Foundation, Vail, CO.
Psychological Aspects of Healing the Injured Athlete

William I. Sterett MD
Steadman-Hawkins Clinic; Steadman-Hawkins
Research Foundation, Vail, CO.
Ankle Intra-articular Injury

Steven J. Svoboda MD
Orthopedic Surgery Service, Brooke Army Medical
Center, Fort Sam Houston, TX.
Muscle Injuries

Dean C. Taylor MD
Department of Orthopaedic Surgery, University of
Minnesota, Minneapolis, MN.
Muscle Injuries

John M. Tokish MD, USAF MC
Head Team Physician, U.S. Airforce Academy,
Colorado Springs, CO.
Physical Examination and Evaluation

Rachael Tucker MBChB, BHB
Research Assistant, Clinical Effectiveness Unit,
Children's Hospital, Boston, MA.
The Pediatric Athlete

Tim Uhl PhD, ATC, PTC
Associate Professor, Department of Rehabilitation
Sciences, Division of Athletic Training; Director of
Musculoskeletal Laboratory, University of Kentucky,
Lexington, KY.
Shoulder Rehabilitation

William P. Urban MD
Clinical Associate Professor; Chair, Orthopaedics and
Rehabilitation, SUNY Downstate Medical Center,
Brooklyn, NY.
Principles of Knee Arthroscopy

Armando F. Vidal MD
Blue Sky Orthopedics and Sports Medicine, Brighton,
CO.
Anterior Cruciate Ligament

K. Mathew Warnock MD
Fondren Orthopedic Group; Texas Orthopedic
Hospital, Houston, TX.
Pediatric Shoulder

Robert G. Watkins MD
Professor of Clinical Orthopaedic Surgery, University
of Southern California; Orthopaedic Surgeon; Los
Angeles Spine Surgery Institute at St. Vincent
Medical Center, Los Angeles, CA.
Lumbar Spine

Daniel E. Weiland MD
Orthopaedic and Sports Medicine Center, Trumball,
CT.
Biceps Tendon Disorders

Kevin E. Wilk PT, DPT
Clinical Director, Champion Sports Medicine and
Rehabilitation Center; Vice President of Education,
Benchmark Medical, Birmingham, AL.
Principles of Rehabilitation

Jeffrey D. Willers MD
Staff, Orthopaedic Surgery, Baptist Hospital and
   St. Thomas Hospital, Nashville, TN.
Ankle Ligament Injury and Instability

Riley J. Williams III MD
Associate Professor, Weill Cornell Medical College;
   Attending Orthopaedic Surgeon, Hospital for
   Special Surgery, New York, NY.
Traumatic Shoulder Muscle Ruptures

Sharrona Williams MD
Southern Orthopaedic Specialists, Atlanta, GA.
Ankle Tendon Disorders and Ruptures

Timothy C. Wilson MD
Central Kentucky Orthopaedics, Georgetown,
   KY.
Knee: Physical Examination and Evaluation

Preface

"It's what you learn after you know it all that counts."—
John Wooden

Sports medicine is an ever-expanding and changing field, but the primary goal remains the same as it was decades ago—to allow the injured athlete to return safely to participation and perform to the best of his or her ability. *Clinical Sports Medicine* presents, in a concise manner, the latest techniques for achieving this goal. Emphasis is placed on summary boxes, illustrations, and algorithms in order to provide an easy reference to commonly seen medical problems and injuries. All chapters are written with the treatment of the athlete in mind. The resultant text is a useful reference to all members of the sports medicine team—trainers, therapists, physicians, and even coaches and parents. The authors were selected based on their specific areas of expertise, and were asked to cover essential material and pearls based on their personal experience.

The first 15 chapters cover general principles and medical issues. The remainder of the book is divided by anatomic areas. Emphasis is placed on physical examination and evaluation of the injured athlete because the key to proper treatment almost always starts with an accurate diagnosis. Also emphasized is appropriate rehabilitation, with five chapters devoted solely to this topic, and further mention made in each chapter addressing specific types of injuries. Surgery is addressed, not with the goal of presenting step-by-step instructions, but rather the rationale for surgical intervention, general principles, and tips based on experiences, good and bad.

Athletes seem to be getting both younger and older at the same time. As children strive to become the next Michael Jordan or Mia Hamm, the number of pediatric injuries (particularly those related to overuse) has risen dramatically. Four chapters are devoted to prevention and treatment of pediatric injuries. On the other end of the spectrum, "weekend warriors" participate into their retirement years, and chapters addressing the older athlete and arthritis in the athlete are included.

Chapters are organized for easy reference. Each starts with a section titled "In This Chapter" to emphasize what is covered. This is followed by an introductory summary box of the most important concepts. The general outline follows with clinical features and evaluation, relevant anatomy, treatment options, surgery, rehabilitation, criteria for return to sports, results and outcomes, and potential complications. We hope that the text is an easy-to-read reference that helps those who treat athletes to achieve the preceding goals. We wish to thank all of the authors for all of their work in organizing the material in a concise and interesting format.

Scott D. Mair

Darren L. Johnson

Foreword

It has been several years since a comprehensive book on the medical aspects of clinical sports medicine has been published. In the early 1990s, books by The Hughston Clinic, Drs. Fu and Stone, and Drs. Drez and DeLee made important contributions to the sports medicine literature. Since that time, the sports medicine subspecialty has come a long way.

The American Board of Orthopaedic Surgery has recognized sports medicine as a clinical subspecialty. A test leading to a certificate of subspecialization in sports medicine is presently being written and will be offered in 2007. Indeed, we have come a long way from the old concept of "orthopaedics for people with numbers."

Clinical Sports Medicine is an excellent representation of where sports medicine is in the early 21st century. Chapters dealing with the role of the team physician; preparticipation physicals; on-field emergencies and preparedness; as well as specialized chapters on the pediatric, female, and older athlete, ensure full coverage of the ever-widening spectrum of sports medicine. There is even a chapter on the psychology of the injured athlete that deals with how injury affects the athlete's well-being.

The remainder of the book is broken down into sections dealing with various anatomic regions. Each chapter is written by an expert in the field, often with assistance from their younger partners. Each chapter has a well-identified introduction. Tables throughout the book are easily readable and are quite helpful as short, quick studies for the chapter.

The authors are orthopaedic surgeons, family physicians, internists, physical therapists, and athletic trainers. Their combined experience is overwhelming, and their writing style is very compatible.

Sports medicine has a separate specialized core curriculum, and this book encompasses the aspects of that curriculum. It should be included in the library of all residency and fellowship programs and should be valued as a reference for practicing orthopaedists regardless of their training level or expertise. Drs. Johnson and Mair should be commended for their success in gathering together so many well-respected physicians to share their knowledge in this exciting book on sports medicine.

Congratulations to you both.

Champ L. Baker, Jr., MD

Contents

Clinical Sports Medicine

Overview

SECTION

I Overview

The Role of the Team Physician

Claude T. Moorman III and Frank H. Bassett III

In This Chapter

Responsibilities of the team physician
   Preparticipation clearance
   In-season coverage
   Game coverage

INTRODUCTION

- The defining role for physicians in sports medicine is to serve as team physician.

- The role of the physician in a sports medicine environment may at times require responsibility for the surgical, medical, emotional, and even spiritual well-being of the athlete.

- Specific responsibilities for the team physician can be broken down into roles that evolve over the course of the athlete's season. At different times in the year, the physician will be responsible for preparticipation clearance, practice and game injury evaluation, treatment of practice and game injuries, coordination and implementation of postseason medical and surgical treatment, and the continuing education of both him- or herself and the rest of the health care team.

RESPONSIBILITIES OF THE TEAM PHYSICIAN

The responsibilities facing the team physician are considerable, and all of them have ethical and legal ramifications. This creates some potential conflicts that need to be resolved in order to care safely and effectively for the athlete. The intention of this chapter is to outline the specific roles and responsibilities of the team physician. We also discuss potential sociopolitical conflicts and strategies for managing these conflicts.[1] Several of the great team physicians of the past generation are featured in an attempt to further understand the role of the team physician and the many subtleties that exemplify a successful sports medicine team.

Preparticipation Clearance
The team physician is responsible for the overall process through which athletes are cleared to play. This requires coordination of the various subspecialists who often assist in these evaluations as well as determining the setting and facility requirements to implement this important portion of the athlete's evaluation (Box 1-1).[2] At different levels of participation, the requirements vary, as does the sophistication of the testing measures instituted. In the high school environment, the evaluations are often carried out in the school gymnasium, usually with a relatively

minimal number of subspecialty providers available. The various different governing bodies in sports medicine, including the American Orthopaedic Society for Sports Medicine (AOSSM), the American Academy of Family Physicians, the American Academy of Pediatrics, the American College of Sports Medicine, the American Medical Society for Sports Medicine, and the American Osteopathic Academy of Sports Medicine have come together with a consensus document for what is required for preparticipation physical examinations (John Bergfeld, personal communication, 1996).

At the collegiate and professional levels, oftentimes more sophisticated measures and a more comprehensive array of consulting physicians are available to assist with the screening. In many scenarios, electrocardiograms and echocardiograms are a common part of the screening. The goal is to rule out conditions such as hypertrophic cardiomyopathy, which may predispose the participating athlete to significant risk or even death. The team physician's responsibility to the athlete generally begins with this preparticipation clearance. (Please see Chapter 2 for additional detail.)

In-Season Coverage
During the athlete's season, the physician's role varies considerably depending on the sport and the setting. The majority of team physicians are involved, at some point in time, in coverage of contact sports, particularly football. The majority of the following discussion centers on football with the realization that lower risk sports will generally require less frequent on-site presence of the team physician. In the majority of situations, the physicians are involved in game coverage with a more limited role in the practice setting. At our institution, the standard has been to cover both home and away games, with training room presence of the attending team physician at the heavy contact practice during the week as well. In the collegiate environment, Tuesday practice tends to be the heaviest contact day, and this is the day that we have selected as the most important for physician presence. In our setting, this translates into the physician arriving toward the end of the practice setting with involvement in running a clinic in the training room following that practice. We have found this to be the highest yield in terms of determining the significant injuries that require physician attention.

It is also important to make a distinction between a true team physician and the "office arthroscopist."[3] With the increasing financial pressures in the health care market today, there is increasing pressure for the team physician to play a decreasing role in the true environment of the athlete. This represents a substantive threat to the team physician's persona as it has been reflected through the ages. Now more than ever before, the team physician needs to recognize work in the training room as a true "labor of love" as there is seldom any opportunity to financially benefit from this activity. There is clearly a large distinction between the physicians who are willing to make the sacrifices to become an integral part of the athletic environment and those who simply manage an office practice with a very limited on-site role for the athlete. This distinction, while obvious, has important ramifications for the quality of care that we deliver to the athlete. There is no question that a physician who is familiar with the athlete and his or her environment and who takes the time to get to know the players, managers, trainers, and administrators involved in the milieu that makes up the athlete's world, will be a much more effective physician when called on to manage injury and illness. The physicians highlighted in the next section have all demonstrated an excellent understanding of this concept. There is no way that the labor of love that is required to be effective in this role can ever be justified on a financial basis. Few physicians even at the professional level are financially rewarded for their role.

Game Coverage

The team physician needs to be present on the game day for contact sports such as football. There are several different logistical arrangements, depending on the level (Box 1-2). At our institution, the team physician arrives 90 minutes prior to the posted kick-off time. Final evaluations are made at this time and any concerns addressed. Under some circumstances, it may be appropriate for athletes with soft-tissue injuries to receive intramuscular ketorolac (Toradol) injections 1 hour prior to the kickoff, which may help to minimize their pain. Additionally, it is occasionally appropriate to consider a local anesthetic injection for a limited number of conditions. In our practice, it has been safe and effective to consider Marcaine injections for grade 1 acromiodavicular (AC) separations, hip pointers, and bruised ribs. These are the only three conditions for which pregame local anesthetics are considered to be both safe and effective. We do discourage the use of local anesthetics for any joint, muscular, and/or bony lesion that does not fall into these three categories. While the skill and expertise of the individual physician may allow for additional indications, this intervention must be very carefully balanced with risks and carefully agreed to by the athlete with full informed consent. Few areas of the physician-athlete relationship generate more controversy or concern on the part of the general public.

It is important for the physician to understand the subtleties of game flow to position him- or herself effectively on the sideline. In most scenarios, this requires the physician to be on the sideline on the end of the field in which the ball is in play. This

will allow ready access to injured players while staying out of the way of the coaches and players as they orchestrate the game. Each staff member must determine the appropriateness of the initial on-field evaluations. At our institution, the trainers make the initial evaluations; they call for the physician, should this be necessary. In the majority of cases, the trainers evaluate the players on the field and escort them off without the physician needing to be involved directly until the player reaches the sideline. We do have an examination table set up on the sideline for evaluations. In most scenarios, it is best to get the player off of the field as soon as it is safely possible following an injury and to do the more detailed evaluations on the sideline. This allows the game to continue and minimizes the crowd's focus on management of the athlete's injury. Obviously, when a player has a significant cervical spine or head injury, this scenario is considerably different (see Chapter 15 on cervical spine injury). For injuries that may represent fracture or significant joint injury, radiographs are oftentimes appropriate. It is important to have a scenario whereby imaging studies can be obtained when necessary. At our institution, we have a radiology technician on the sideline and imaging apparatus within 100 yards of the playing field. Many institutions and stadiums have portable fluoroscopy machines available that may serve the same purpose. Additional personnel who can be quite helpful are a paramedic or emergency medical team with medical evacuation equipment if transfer of the athlete is necessary. Some health care teams have anesthesiologists and neurosurgeons available depending on the sport and the setting.

Postgame evaluations are done in the training room with careful attention to any injuries that may require further evaluation. A true team approach with trainers, primary care team physicians, and orthopaedic surgeons is helpful to provide a comprehensive approach to the myriad of injuries from muscle strains to concussions that are seen in contact athletics. Neuropsychological testing is used at our institution for mild traumatic brain injuries; the testing is performed following the game with comparison to baseline testing performed during the preparticipation examinations.

An injury clinic is commonly held on the day following the game. This allows further identification of potential and real injury problems that may not have been obvious to the athlete or physician on the day of the game. It has also been our experience that following a victory, many of the athletes who actually have seemingly smaller injuries do not report for postgame evaluation and are better assessed on the day following the game. This provides a less harried environment after the excitement of the game has passed to get a true handle on the extent of injuries and to provide a plan for timely imaging and other treatments. This training room clinic generally sets the tone for the week to come and prepares the coaches and players for the availability or lack thereof of key players.

LIABILITY

Team physicians have come under increasing scrutiny in recent years, an extension of what has become commonplace in the medicolegal environment in the rest of medicine. As recently as 2003, there were 18 active lawsuits against National Football League team physicians. This is reflective of the general attitude in society of persons seeking financial compensation through the legal system in the case of injury. In many environments, it is common for professional athletes who have not been able to fit into the plans of the various franchises to seek remuneration through the medicolegal pathway. This creates additional strain on the doctor-patient relationship for team physicians and exposes the team physicians to significant financial risk. While there is no way to eliminate this concern completely, there are some steps that can be taken to attempt to minimize the risk. First, the physician needs to maintain the tradition of honor, service, integrity, and dedication required in our role of protecting the well-being of the athlete. Second, the team physician should maintain a very active pursuit of continuing medical education to stay up with modern techniques and treatment options so that the athletes receive the very best care possible. Third, it is imperative that the team physician be a true on-site provider with good relationships with the coaches, trainers, and players rather than serving in a remote setting as an "office arthroscopist." Fourth, it is important for the team physician to understand his or her options in relation to his or her role in a professional sports setting. Oftentimes, the physician can be indemnified as a member of the organization and, therefore, at decreased risk. Another option is to consider additional riders on malpractice policies to cover the potentially exorbitant awards that may be made in the setting of a perceived medicolegal injury. Fifth, it is imperative to review very carefully the service contract as it relates to high school and collegiate relationships. It is not uncommon for some institutional malpractice coverage to contain exclusions for community service. The unsuspecting team physician may be caught in a bind if these matters are not carefully analyzed ahead of time. While these measures will not prevent exposure from an egregious plaintiff's bar, they may well head off many of the problems that increase liability exposure.

REPRESENTATIVE TEAM PHYSICIANS

While it is possible to summarize the tasks that a team physician carries out, simple descriptions cannot adequately portray the passion involved in truly caring for athletes. With this in mind, a summary of the careers of five pioneers in the field of sports medicine provide the best definition of what it means to be a team physician.

Dr. Jack Hughston

The recent passing of Dr. Jack Hughston has been difficult for many of us who believe that he was the consummate team physician. Dr. Hughston, a brilliant man with many attributes that placed him way ahead of his time, is often considered to be the "father of sports medicine."[4] He started the Hughston Clinic, P.C., in Columbus, GA, more than 50 years ago as a site not only for elite athletes but also for the "young boy or girl playing school or neighborhood sports, the weekend golf or tennis player, and the employee in the work place or industrial setting."[5] Dr. Hughston received his undergraduate education at Auburn University and did his orthopaedic residency at Duke University. Dr. Hughston was active in the care of recreational, high school, collegiate, and professional athletes. He seldom missed a game of his beloved Auburn Tigers (Fig. 1-1). He emphasized the truly multidisciplinary team approach among health care professionals including physicians, physical therapists, athletic trainers, and administrators and insisted that each work toward the common goal of serving the athlete.[5]

Dr. Hughston was also an innovator in the field of education and started one of the first sports medicine fellowship programs in 1970 to train orthopedic residents in the subtleties of sports

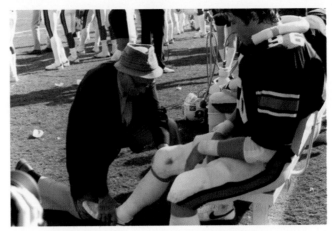

Figure 1-1 Dr. Jack Hughston as many of us remember him—in his role as a dedicated team physician for the Auburn Tigers.

medicine, preparing them for service at the highest level. He was a founding member of the AOSSM in the early 1970s and also served a term as society president. He founded the *American Journal of Sports Medicine*, which he edited until 1990. Many of us consider the *American Journal of Sports Medicine* to be his most important contribution, because the *Journal* serves today as the most important vehicle for disseminating new information in the field. For his many accomplishments, he was named Mr. Sports Medicine by the AOSSM and inducted into its Hall of Fame. He has also received the distinguished Southern Orthopaedist Award and many other honors too numerous to mention (see Fig. 1-1).

Dr. John Bergfeld

Dr. Bergfeld distinguished himself on the playing fields and developed his love of sports medicine while an offensive lineman at Bucknell University. He did his internship and residency at the Cleveland Clinic Foundation and subsequently served as the team physician at the Naval Academy where he honed his skills along with another well-known sports medicine team physician, Dr. Bill Clancy. He subsequently served for more than 25 years as the Cleveland Browns team physician (Fig. 1-2) and was very active in helping set up the medical staff for the Baltimore Ravens during the mid-1990s. He has been one of the top mentors for young orthopedists in the history of the AOSSM. For these efforts and general excellence in the field of sports medicine education, he received the George D. Rovere Award in 1996. His fellowship group, The Warthog Society, is perhaps the most active alumni group of any of the fellowship programs in North America. Dr. Bergfeld, known to many of us as "Bergie," is a beloved figure as an educator, researcher, and team physician. He has had a particular interest in the posterior cruciate ligament and has been responsible for the popularity of the inlay technique and for better understanding which injuries may be managed nonoperatively. Perhaps his greatest contribution has been the integration of the primary care sports medicine team physicians into the active care of the athletes. He has worked hard to break down the sociopolitical barriers and "turf" concerns that had impeded this progress previously. His only concern has been that the athlete is cared for and is the focus of a truly multidisciplinary approach. His many colorful aphorisms have been widely quoted throughout his alumni group and

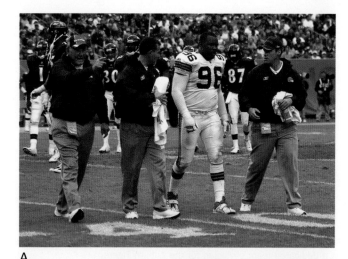

A

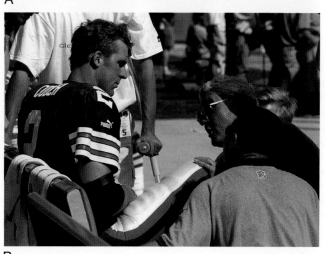

B

Figure 1-2 A and **B,** Dr. John Bergfeld served as the head team physician for the Cleveland Browns for more than 25 years.

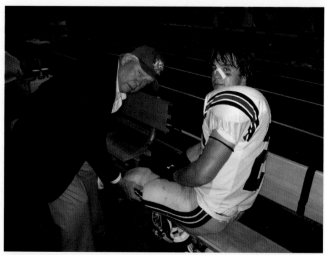

Figure 1-3 Dr. James Andrews is perhaps best known for his care of professional athletes in many sports. He also has a love for participation in collegiate and high school sports as well. Here he is seen attending to a local high school athlete in Birmingham.

those of us who have been directly and indirectly influenced by him. His insistence that you "do what you do best" has been a mantra for young physicians confused over particular techniques of management.

For many years, Dr. Bergfeld has also been an innovator in running the safety committee of the National Football League Team Physician Society. He has been a trusted confidant of both management council and the National Football League Players Association in traversing very difficult sociopolitical issues related to the care of the professional athlete. He has been responsible for distributing millions of dollars of grant funding for National Football League charities and has never lost sight of the big picture as it relates to integrity and dedication in the care of the athlete at every level (see Fig. 1-2).

Dr. James Andrews

Dr. Andrews is perhaps the best known of all the sports medicine team physicians in our era. Dr. Andrews graduated from Louisiana State University in 1963 where he was a southeastern conference indoor and outdoor pole vault champion. He did his orthopedic residency at Tulane Medical School and had sports medicine fellowships at the University of Virginia and at the University of Lyon, France. He joined the staff at the Hughston Clinic where he served for many years prior to starting the

Alabama Sports Medicine and Orthopaedic Center in Birmingham in 1986. He has been involved in the care of athletes at all levels from high schools in the Birmingham area (Fig. 1-3) and management of Division I-AA programs such as Troy State, to Auburn, AL, and many of the professional teams, including the Washington Redskins.

Dr. Andrews has also been a tremendous gentleman in terms of helping young physicians to become successful in their practice. He developed one of the top fellowship programs in the world, and many of his fellows have become high-level team physicians, many with careers in academic sports medicine. He has also been a true favorite among the agents caring for the athletes due to his tremendous technical skills and capability in managing the sociopolitical aspects and his considerable attention to detail. In spite of his schedule, which is tremendously busy, he has also maintained a role as an excellent communicator and facilitator of information in consultation with other physicians in the care of their athletes.

Dr. Andrews's specific contributions are many, and he has been a leader in both the AOSSM and the Arthroscopy Association of North America, having served on the board of directors of both societies. He is known for his marked technical proficiency and has built one of the most impressive surgical setups in the world at the American Sports Medicine Institute. He is also known for his colorful aphorisms and his insistence that the team physician be careful to avoid being the one to make the "big statement." He is referring to the tendency for some of us to state that the athlete will "never play again" or that he will be ready to play by a "certain date" or other ways in which we box ourselves in with statements that may come back to haunt us and perhaps to have a negative impact on the athlete's situation. His wisdom and mentorship are evidenced by the fact that his fellowship has trained the largest number of fellows of any of the major programs over the past decade (see Fig. 1-3).

Dr. Russell F. Warren

Many consider Dr. Russell F. Warren to be the epitome of the physician/scientist. Few if any physicians have achieved the same balance of scientific innovation and true clinical excellence as Dr. Warren. Dr. Warren was a standout running back at Columbia in the early 1960s. He had a tryout and made it to the last cut with the New York Giants as a professional player. He subsequently did his orthopedic training at the Hospital for Special Surgery and initially went into private practice in Lynchburg, VA, for 4 years before going back to do a shoulder fellowship at Columbia. He subsequently joined the staff at the Hospital for Special Surgery where he served as surgeon-in-chief until July 2004. He has served as the head team physician for the New York Giants since 1984 (Fig. 1-4). Dr. Warren is perhaps the most decorated academic surgeon in history having won the O'Donoghue Award for the outstanding clinical contribution to the AOSSM three times and also having won the Neer Award three times for making the most outstanding contribution in shoulder surgery. He was named Mr. Sports Medicine by the AOSSM in 2003 and has a list of scientific publications that is perhaps unsurpassed in the history of academic sports medicine.

Dr. Warren is known to have a completely open mind and is willing to learn from anyone around him. This is in contrast to the majority of us who, over the ages, become narrower in our focus and less willing to learn from others. His fellowship training program has been very heavy in basic science, and he has led the field in innovations regarding cellular level research.

Dr. Warren has also been very altruistic in the use of funding as it comes from his innovations. In many instances, he has directed the royalties from product innovations in the laboratory to support general orthopedic sports medicine research. This research has not only led to many innovations but has also had a substantive impact on education of the next generation of leaders in the field of orthopedic sports medicine. Dr. Warren's fellowship alumni group occupies more team physician positions at the professional level than any other institution. He has also been a tremendous innovator in operative technique and has helped to create many of the techniques and approaches that we use in both shoulder and knee surgery today. He has further created an environment at the Hospital for Special Surgery where fellowship training can and does involve active basic science research with a rigorous clinic exposure. He has created a fellowship program that has provided many of the innovators who represent our generation's best physicians.

In spite of his capabilities in the laboratory and in the operating room, he is perhaps best known for his familiarity on the sideline and in the training rooms with the New York Giants. During my (CTM III) fellowship with Dr. Warren, his happiest moments were on the Wednesday afternoons when we were headed out to the Giants training room at the Meadowlands or on the sidelines at Giants games on Sundays. His relationship with Ronnie Barnes, the head athletic trainer for the New York Giants, has been legendary and a model for those of us who aspire to develop a quality interdisciplinary sports medicine team (see Fig. 1-4).

Dr. Frank H. Bassett III

To those of us who trained in the Duke program, the ultimate example of the team physician has always been Dr. Frank H. Bassett III. Dr. Bassett played for Coach Paul "Bear" Bryant at the University of Kentucky before being drafted into the military and serving in the Korean conflict. He was the first infantry soldier to try out the new body armor and this ultimately saved his life when he was shot but sustained only bruises rather than a through and through gunshot wound that would have occurred without the protective body armor. He was awarded the Purple Heart for this incident. He subsequently did his training at Duke under Lenox Baker and became the head team physician at Duke University in 1966. Dr. Bassett cared for the athletic teams at Duke for over 30 years and was the epitome of the true team physician (Fig. 1-5). In his honor, the Bassett Society has been created to provide scholarship support for Duke lettermen who enter medical and dental school.

In addition to his role as a professor in orthopedics, he was also a faculty member in the Department of Anatomy. Many of his research papers focused on identification of new structures and a further delineation of the pathoanatomy of orthopedic entities. Dr. Bassett has also served as a mentor for many physicians who have pursued careers in sports medicine. He has been the "godfather" for the AOSSM Traveling Fellowship and has received many research honors including the O'Donoghue Award. He has been president of the AOSSM and has been

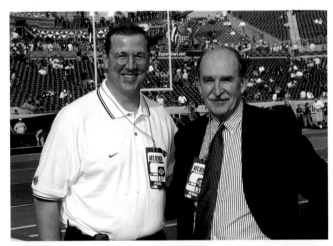

Figure 1-4 Dr. Russell F. Warren on the sidelines with author Dr. C. T. Moorman III prior to the Giants-Ravens game in the Super Bowl XXXV. Dr. Warren has been the Giants team physician for more than 20 years.

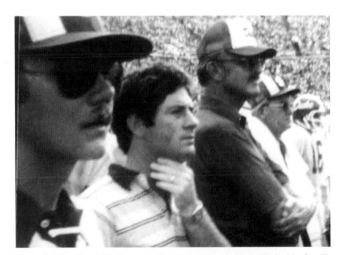

Figure 1-5 Dr. Frank H. Bassett III *(right center [with hat])*, in his familiar surroundings on the sidelines of a Duke football game. He is standing by Dr. William E. Garrett, Jr., at the time a Duke orthopedic resident. Dr. Garrett is immediate past president of the American Orthopaedic Society for Sports Medicine and has a career in the care of collegiate, Olympic, and professional soccer athletes.

honored as Mr. Sports Medicine and also named to the AOSSM Hall of Fame.

Dr. Bassett's greatest contributions have been in caring for the athletes and mentoring the next generation of sports medicine physicians. He has been particularly innovative in furthering the art of sideline and training room management of the athlete. His love for Duke University has more recently placed him in a position to successfully build endowment support for the athletic department and a considerable upgrade to the facilities. He has been one of the favorites among the coaches to assist in recruiting athletes, particularly those interested in a career in medicine (see Fig. 1-5).

FUTURE OF THE TEAM PHYSICIAN'S ROLE

In spite of the many challenges, particularly involving financial and liability pressures, we do believe that the future is bright for the team physician. The blessings that come from caring for the athlete at all levels will continue to be tremendously rewarding for the team physician and motivate the next generation of physicians to continue to serve in this role. It will be increasingly important to "dot the Is and cross the Ts" regarding contracts and to be increasingly vigilant regarding the pitfalls of the liability situation. Furthermore, we believe that it will be very important for the physician to run counter to some of the financial pressures that may limit our involvement in the training room and to play an active role in on-site management of our athletes. This will be increasingly important to maintain good relationships with the coaches, administration, and the training staff as well as the athletes themselves. It is important for the team physician to remember that this is a "labor of love."

The additional burden of the regulatory process as it relates to resident and fellow involvement in the care of athletes also needs careful attention. The Accreditation Council for Graduate Medical Education (ACGME) and other governing bodies are placing additional administrative demands on the supervising team physicians in terms of understanding the role of supervision in the training process. This requires additional documentation and in some instances a restructuring in terms of making sure that supervision requirements are met. This requires considerable case-by-case evaluation. These requirements need to be carefully reviewed and the contractual side of those attended to in order to avoid pitfalls in these areas. At our institution, contractual agreements are required with each of the high schools and collegiate relationships that we serve.

We believe that today's team physician is better educated and more likely to be part of a coordinated multidisciplinary relationship that allows the best care of our athletes than ever before. We must be mindful of the liability and confidentiality issues that face us today that were not present in the past. Though the team physician's role has evolved in these areas, we do think that it will always be a tremendous honor to serve in what we consider to be the defining role for the sports medicine doctor, that of the team physician.

CONCLUSIONS

As a result of the dedication and excellence of the team physicians who have gone before us, some of whom are highlighted in this chapter, we believe that today's team physician is better educated and more likely to be skilled in managing the issues that athletes of all levels face. It is imperative that we always keep care of the athlete as a central focus of our efforts. We must be mindful of the liability and confidentiality issues that face us today but not allow this to interfere in a negative way with our relationship with the athletes for whom we care. The team physician's role and responsibilities will continue to evolve. We should never lose sight of what a tremendous honor that it is to serve in the defining role for the sports medicine doctor, that of team physician.

REFERENCES

1. Rubin A: Team physician or athlete's doctor? Physician Sportsmedicine 1998;26:27–29.
2. Madden CC, Walsh WM, Mellion MB: The team physician: The preparticipation examination and on-field emergencies. In DeLee JD, Drez DD, Miller MM (eds): Orthopaedic Sports Medicine: Principles and Practice, 2nd ed. Philadelphia, Saunders, 2003, pp 737–768.
3. American Academy of Family Physicians, American Academy of Pediatrics, American College of Sports Medicine, American Medical Society for Sports Medicine, American Orthopaedic Society for Sports Medicine, American Osteopathic Academy of Sports Medicine: Preparticipation Physical Evaluation, 3rd ed. Overland Park, KS, American Medical Society for Sports Medicine, 2005, pp 93–98.
4. Jacobson KE: Jack C. Hughston, MD—Orthopaedist and pioneer of sports medicine. Am J Sports Med 2004;32:1816–1817.
5. Johnston L: From orthopaedics to sports medicine—One man's vision. M.D. News, Western Georgia Edition 2003;3:6–10.

The Preparticipation Physical Examination

Robert Hosey and Kenneth Cayce IV

In This Chapter

INTRODUCTION

- The preparticipation sports examination is a tool to detect medical and orthopedic conditions that may be problematic for safe participation in athletics.

- The origins of the preparticipation examination date back about 35 years when the American Medical Association Committee on Medical Aspects of Sports drafted the first guidelines for a preparticipation examination.[1] Since then, there have been many alterations and changes to the way in which physicians complete the examination.

- It is now an annual event that sports medicine physicians conduct to clear athletes to participate in sports.

In 1992, the first standardized preparticipation examination form was introduced to the sports medicine community.[2] Despite the availability of standardized examination forms, there has not been widespread use of a common form. Ninety-seven percent of colleges and universities require the preparticipation examination process, and all 50 states and the District of Columbia require a preparticipation examination to be completed for high school athletes.[3,4] When preparticipation examinations are used in colleges and universities, only 51% required it to be done annually. These examinations have often been performed by various health care providers, including athletic trainers and nurse practitioners.[5]

The primary objectives of the preparticipation examination are to screen for conditions that may be life threatening or disabling or that may predispose to injury or illness and to meet administrative requirements. Secondary objectives include determining general health, serving as an entry point to the health care system for adolescents, and providing opportunity to discuss health-related topics.[6] Recently, a consensus panel made up of practitioners from the American Academy of Family Physicians, American Academy of Pediatrics, American Medical Society of Sports Medicine, American College of Sports Medicine, American Orthopaedic Society for Sports Medicine, and American Osteopathic Academy of Sports Medicine has evaluated and updated the preparticipation sports examination.[6] The resulting monograph, published in 2004, was designed to help physicians identify specific and relative contraindications to participate in certain sports and to attempt to produce a standardized preparticipation examination.

TIMING AND FREQUENCY

The preparticipation examination should be done at least 6 weeks prior to beginning the sport season to allow time for rehabilitation of old injuries, improvement of flexibility and strength, and further evaluation of any illness or injury that may restrict participation. A complete preparticipation examination should be done upon entry to junior high, high school, and college. Screening history and blood pressure monitoring should be done in subsequent years. In addition, a more detailed examination on identified areas of illness and injury that occurred during the previous year should also be performed. This is the process that is endorsed by the National Collegiate Athletic Association, but few states have seen fit to follow.[7]

For those athletes older than the age of 35, the American Heart Association recommends exercise testing in men older than 40 years of age and women older than 50 who have one or more cardiac risk factors and/or symptoms of chest pain, palpitations, or syncope. Athletes who are 65 years or older and athletes with a history of coronary artery disease with or without symptoms should have an exercise stress test regardless of risk factors.[8] When athletes are not allowed to participate in their sport, recommendations should be made for activity that is appropriate.

METHODS OF CONDUCTING PREPARTICIPATION EXAMINATIONS

Preparticipation examinations may be performed in the office or at a mass screening venue. An office examination gives the physician and the athlete time to build rapport and discuss health issues at length. When a mass screening format is employed, a station-based preparticipation examination is often used. In this setting, a single physician may do the entire medical portion of the examination or it may be divided among a number of physicians. In the station-based examination, information gathering is typically divided between several different stations. An example of a station format for a preparticipation examination is outlined in Table 2-1. Additional stations for evaluation of body composition, flexibility, nutrition, strength, speed, agility,

Table 2-1 Representative Stations for a Mass Screening Preparticipation Examination
1. Fill out history form
2. Sign in, height, and weight
3. Visual acuity
4. Blood pressure screening
5. Medical examination
6. Orthopedic examination
7. Checkout (review forms, determination of clearance)

power, endurance, and balance may also be incorporated. With the use of these formats, an excellent preparticipation examination can be completed in 30 to 60 minutes.

HISTORY

A complete and accurate medical history is the cornerstone of a good preparticipation examination. Approximately 75% of problems can be discovered by history alone in the preparticipation examination.[9] In younger athletes, emphasis is placed on fitness evaluation, obesity, maturity assessment, and identification of medical, orthopedic, and psychosocial situations.[10] In older athletes, emphasis is placed on the detection of previous injuries and ongoing problems. In both age groups, one should ask about any recent illnesses, allergic reactions, cardiac/pulmonary complications, previous head injuries or other neurologic deficits, skin problems, loss of organs, history of heat illness, medications and substance/supplement abuse, blood-borne pathogens, and immunizations.[7]

In a recent study, female athlete participation had grown to 1 in 2.5 of high school athletes and 43% of all college athletes in the United States.[11] Recent findings of six medical societies have found that questions relating to eating, amenorrhea, and osteopenia/osteoporosis need to be emphasized. The combination of all three symptoms has been termed the female athlete triad.[12] Some things that should be screened for include dry skin and mucous membranes, history of fractures, menstrual history, and hair loss.

Most of the history and physical examination is dedicated to the cardiovascular and musculoskeletal portions. A thorough cardiovascular history should include questions to determine

1. prior occurrence of exertional chest pain/discomfort or syncope/near-syncope as well as excessive, unexpected, and unexplained shortness of breath or fatigue associated with exercise
2. previous detection of a heart murmur or increased systemic blood pressure
3. family history of premature death or significant disability from cardiovascular disease in close relatives younger than 50 years old or specific knowledge of the occurrence of certain conditions (cardiomyopathy, Marfan syndrome, arrhythmia).

Screening for medications or drug abuse is also important due to the potential side effect of arrhythmia.[8] If the athletes answer affirmatively any portion of the history, then detailed evaluation of these areas in the physical examination is necessary.

PHYSICAL EXAMINATION

The physical examination should include measurement of height and weight. Significant, unexpected changes should warn physicians of the potential of eating disorder or steroid use. General assessment of the head, ears, eyes, nose, and throat is performed. If the athlete has corrected vision less than 20/40, one eye, or history of eye trauma or surgery, then eye protection is required. Anisocoria, astigmatism, strabismus, refractive errors, and poor visual acuity should also be evaluated in athletes and noted in the chart for possible assessment of head injuries in the future.[7]

For the physical examination of the cardiovascular system, the American Heart Association recommends checking blood pressure, auscultating for murmurs, palpating peripheral pulses to determine for coarctation, and assessing for Marfan syndrome.[9] The heart should be auscultated with the athlete in the standing and supine positions. Murmurs that need further evaluation by a cardiologist include 3/6 or higher systolic murmur, any diastolic murmur, and any murmur that increases with standing or with Valsalva maneuver.

Sudden cardiac death is the most common cause of non-traumatic death in young athletes and occurs in approximately one in 200,000 with a few cases each year.[9] Many cases occur in individuals with pre-existing heart disease.[4] In the United States, most cases are due to hypertrophic cardiomyopathy (26.4%), followed by commotio cordis (19.9%), and coronary artery anomalies (13.7%).[13] The American Heart Association and 26th Bethesda Conference have developed various guidelines and recommendations for athletic screening and participation[14] (Table 2-2).

Abnormal cardiovascular examinations are uncommon in athletes younger than the age of 35. In one study of high school athletes, it was found that 0.37% of the participants had either severe hypertension or syncope that prompted further evaluation.[15] Many studies have been conducted on the effectiveness and cost efficiency of electrocardiography in risk stratifying athletes who need further evaluation by a cardiologist. Today, there is no consensus on the use of electrocardiography in the preparticipation examination. Another tool for sports medicine physicians to evaluate athletes at risk for sudden cardiac death is echocardiography. It has been proposed, because of its low positive predictive value and cost, that echocardiography should only be used as a follow-up examination in selected patients and not as a primary screening tool.[10] Noninvasive screening tests may be developed in the future to help sports medicine physicians diagnose athletes who are at significant risk of cardiac sudden death. This may potentially include a portable echocardiography machine and genetic screening for coronary disease.[10]

The athlete must be further evaluated if chest tightness, shortness of breath, cough, or wheezing within the first 10 minutes after exercise is noted. The lungs should be auscultated for any wheezes, crackles, or rubs. If the athlete is found to have any of the features, they must be suspected of having exercise-induced bronchospasm, especially if the athlete has a history of asthma.[7] It is now recommended that all elite athletes in swimming, cycling, rowing, snow skiing, cross-country skiing, scuba diving, and figure skating have a bronchial provocation test prior to competition to exclude exercise-induced bronchospasm.[16] The eucapnic voluntary hyperpnea challenge test is recom-

Table 2-2 26th Bethesda Conference Guidelines for Athletic Participation for Selected Cardiovascular Abnormalities	
Hypertrophic cardiomyopathy	Exclusion from most competitive/noncompetitive sports, with possible exception of low-intensity sports, regardless of medical treatment, absence of symptoms, or implantation of defibrillator.
Coronary artery abnormalities	Exclusion from all competitive sports. Participation may be considered 6 months after surgical correction and after exercise stress testing.
ARVD	Exclusion from all competitive sports.
Mitral valve prolapse	Exclusion if history of syncope is associated with arrhythmia, family history of mitral valve prolapse and sudden death, documented arrhythmia, or moderate to severe mitral regurgitation.
Ebstein's anomaly	Severe disease precludes participation in all sports. After surgical repair, low-intensity sports are permitted if tricuspid regurgitation is absent or mild, heart size is normal, and no arrhythmias are present on Holter monitoring and stress testing.
Marfan syndrome	Exclusion from contact sports. Patients with aortic regurgitation and marked dilation of aorta are excluded from all competitive sports. Others may participate in low-intensity sports, with biannual echocardiography.
Long QT syndrome	Exclusion from all competitive sports.
Myocarditis	Athletes with history of myocarditis in previous 6 months are excluded from all competitive sports.
Wolff-Parkinson-White syndrome	Patients with normal exercise testing ± electrophysiologic study may be eligible for participation in all sports.
Coronary artery disease	Individual risk assessment based on ejection fraction, exercise tolerance, presence of inducible ischemia or arrhythmias, and presence of hemodynamically significant coronary stenoses on angiography.

ARVD, arrhythmogenic right ventricular dysplasia.
Reprinted from American College of Sports Medicine and American College of Cardiology: 26th Bethesda Conference. Recommendations for determining eligibility for competition in athletes with cardiovascular abnormalities. Med Sci Sport Exerc 1994;26:5223–5283, with permission from the American College of Cardiology Foundation.

mended by the International Olympic Committee (IOC) for elite athletes. This test has two different protocols: stepped and single stepped. The stepped protocol is indicated for athletes with severe or unstable airway disease and involves increasing the athlete's ventilation over three stages. The single-stepped protocol is indicated for athletes with asthma or exercise-induced bronchospasm and involves a single level of ventilation for 6 minutes. Each protocol measures lung function and a decrease of more than 10% from baseline indicates exercise-induced bronchospasm.[17] The type of test to perform for confirmation of exercise-induced bronchospasm is determined by what is most readily available.

For the abdominal examination, one should pay particular attention to abdominal distention and tenderness, organomegaly, rigidity, or masses. A hernia by itself is not a disqualifying factor but needs further evaluation and possible treatment prior to play. Female athletes should be questioned about the possibility of pregnancy. If there is a possibility of pregnancy, pain, or enlargement of the abdomen, a pelvic examination should be performed in a private setting prior to participation.[7]

In the past, physicians have provided a male testicular examination during the preparticipation examination. Today, the evidence has shown that counseling, describing the examination, and having athletes do the examination at home allows the athlete to learn more about testicular cancer and its symptoms.[17] The sports medicine physician should ask about history of undescended testes, masses, loss of a testicle, and inguinal hernias, and, if positive, then a testicular examination may be warranted. Tanner staging is no longer recommended as part of the preparticipation examination. Its use is mainly for evaluating musculoskeletal injuries in the physically immature.

The musculoskeletal examination should be done in an orderly manner with attention to identifying potential abnormalities in musculature and bone structure. An example that is evidence based is the 14-point examination[6] (Table 2-3; Figs.

2-1 through 2-3), as outlined in the consensus monograph, with additions to measure supraspinatus strength and a dynamic strength test (balancing on one foot).[18] This examination is good for most athletes, but a more detailed examination should be performed for certain populations (e.g., professional athletes).[19] If an athlete has a history of an injury (e.g., fracture, joint pain) or answers yes to any musculoskeletal question in the original history form, then that athlete should be evaluated further with a detailed examination of that bone or joint. A major goal of the orthopedic examination is that full rehabilitation of injuries is accomplished prior to participation in the sport. Some sports medicine physicians have included measurements of endurance, strength, and flexibility with the preparticipation examination, but these measurements add significant time to the overall process.

Neurologic examination should be done while performing the musculoskeletal examination. Any neurologic deficits (e.g., loss of strength, paresthesias) should be explored, as should a history of stingers/burners or head injury. The athlete must be without signs or symptoms of neurologic deficit prior to starting sports. The preparticipation examination may give the sports medicine physician the opportunity to assess baseline neuropsychological function. This can be a helpful tool for guiding return to play decisions in the concussed athlete.[20]

Any skin problems (e.g., rashes, infections, abrasions, blisters) should be assessed during the examination. By addressing these skin reactions early and prior to the start of the season, the athlete can be treated and participate in sports. Skin infections need to be treated prior to participating in sports involving body contact.

THE SPECIAL-NEEDS ATHLETE

Special-needs athletes include athletes with cerebral palsy, blindness, paralysis, mental retardation, amputation, arthritis,

Table 2-3 The 14-Point Musculoskeletal Screening Examination[6]	
Examination	Assessment
1. Inspection, athlete standing, facing examiner	Symmetry of trunk, upper extremities
2. Forward flexion, extension, rotation, lateral flexion of neck	Cervical spine range of motion
3. Resisted shoulder shrug	Trapezius strength
4. Resisted shoulder abduction	Deltoid strength
5. Internal and external rotation of shoulder	Glenohumeral joint range of motion
6. Extension and flexion of elbow	Elbow range of motion
7. Pronation and supination of forearm	Wrist range of motion
8. Clench fist, spread fingers	Hand and fingers range of motion
9. Inspection, athlete facing away from examiner	Symmetry of truck, upper extremities
10. Back extension, knees straight	Spondylolysis, spondylolisthesis
11. Back flexion with knees straight (see Fig. 2-1)	Spine range of motion, scoliosis, hamstring flexibility
12. Inspection of lower extremities, quadriceps contraction	Alignment, symmetry
13. "Duck walk" four steps (see Fig. 2-2)	Hip, knee, ankle motion, strength/balance
14. Standing on toes, then heels (see Fig. 2-3)	Symmetry, calf strength, balance

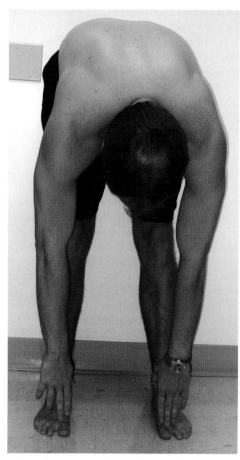

Figure 2-1 Assessment of back flexion with knees straight.

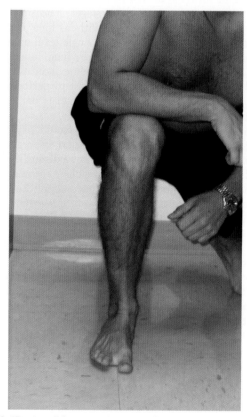

Figure 2-2 "Duck walk" to assess range of motion, strength, and balance.

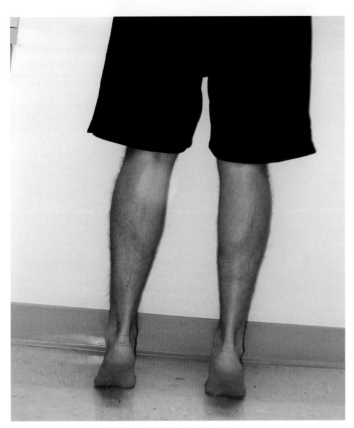

Figure 2-3 Standing on toes.

Table 2-4 Sample History Questions for the Special-Needs Athlete

Does the athlete have any history of any of the following:
   Seizures
   Hearing loss
   Vision loss
   Cardiopulmonary disease
   Renal disease or a unilateral kidney
   Atlantoaxial instability
   Pressure sores or ulcers
   Heat stroke or heat exhaustion
   Fractures or dislocations
   Autonomic dysreflexia

Are seizures controlled and with what medications?
What prosthetic devices or special equipment are required?
Is there an indwelling urinary catheter or requirement of intermittent catheterization? What levels has the athlete participated in previously?
What is the level of independence?
Is a special diet required?

muscular dystrophy, and multiple sclerosis. The benefits of exercise for the special-needs athlete are the same as those for other athletes. Additionally, special-needs athletes have fewer pressure ulcers, fewer infections, improved proprioception, increased proficiency using prosthetic devices, and decreased hospitalizations. The Special Olympics and the United States Paralympics require a preparticipation examination to be done within 12 months of competition. An office-based examination is preferred for these athletes. Questions on which the physician should focus are listed in Table 2-4. These questions should be asked and appropriate consultations made if needed. Special attention should be given to the vision, cardiovascular, neurologic, dermatologic, genitourinary, and musculoskeletal portions of the examination. The functional assessment with sport-specific tasks should be done on all athletes with special needs. Diagnostic imaging should be done on all athletes at risk of atlantoaxial instability, including athletes with Down syndrome wanting to compete in judo, equestrian sports, gymnastics, diving, pentathlon, swimming (butterfly stroke and diving starts), high jump, Alpine skiing, snowboarding, squat lift, and soccer.[21]

DETERMINATION OF CLEARANCE

Clearance for the athlete is the most important decision to be made at the completion of the preparticipation examination. Fortunately, only approximately 11.9% of athletes who have a preparticipation examination will require further evaluation and about 1.9% are not allowed to participate in their sport.[22]

The American Academy of Pediatrics Committee on Sports Medicine and Fitness has developed a guideline for clearance for athletes[23] (Table 2-5). For each athlete, one must determine whether participation in that sport will put the athlete, teammate, or competitors at risk of injury. It must be determined whether there is treatment for the athlete, such as medicines or protective gear, that will allow the athlete to compete safely. The answers to these questions make it easier for the sports medicine physician to decide whether the athlete is cleared without restriction, cleared after completing further evaluation, cleared after completing rehabilitation for a particular injury/illness, or not cleared for participation.[2] These decisions should be discussed with the athlete, parents, trainer, and coach.

Many medical conditions must be evaluated prior to starting any type of sport. In some cases, an athlete is not allowed to participate in one sport but may be allowed to participate in a less strenuous type of activity. The American Academy of Pediatrics Committee on Sports Medicine and Fitness has classified individual sports based on the amount of contact and strenuousness[23] (Tables 2-6 and 2-7). Although there are many guidelines that assist the sports medicine physician in determining eligibility, each athlete should be considered individually. It should be noted that only a few athletes are not allowed to participate after completion of the preparticipation examination. If there is any disagreement between the athlete and the physician, it may be wise for the physician to obtain written consent or a legal waiver signed by the athlete and the parent. A second opinion may also be obtained. If there is still disagreement between the athlete and the physician, legal counsel may be useful in providing information regarding issues related to athletic participation or disqualification.[2]

FUTURE OF THE PREPARTICIPATION EXAMINATION

The future of the preparticipation examination is headed to the computer age. Today, there are institutions that use electronic

Table 2-5 Medical Conditions and Sports Participation*	
Condition	*May Participate*
Atlantoaxial instability (instability of the joint between cervical vertebrae 1 and 2) Explanation: Athlete needs evaluation to assess risk of spinal cord injury during sports participation.	Qualified yes
Bleeding disorder[†] Explanation: Athlete needs evaluation.	Qualified yes
Cardiovascular disease	
Carditis (inflammation of the heart) Explanation: Carditis may result in sudden death with exertion.	No
Hypertension (high blood pressure) Explanation: Those with significant essential (unexplained) hypertension should avoid weight and power lifting, body building, and strength training. Those with secondary hypertension (hypertension caused by a previously identified disease) or severe essential hypertension need evaluation. The National High Blood Pressure Education Working group defined significant and severe hypertension.	Qualified yes
Congenital heart disease (structural heart defects present at birth) Explanation: Those with mild forms may participate fully; those with moderate or severe forms or who have undergone surgery need evaluation. The 26th Bethesda Conference defined mild, moderate, and severe disease for common cardiac lesions.	Qualified yes
Dysrhythmia (irregular heart rhythm) Explanation: Those with symptoms (chest pain, syncope, dizziness, shortness of breath, or other symptoms of possible dysrhythmia) or evidence of mitral regurgitation (leaking) on physical examination need evaluation. All others may participate fully.	Qualified yes
Heart murmur Explanation: If the murmur is innocent (does not indicate heart disease), full participation is permitted. Otherwise, the athlete needs evaluation (see "Congenital heart disease" above).	Qualified yes
Cerebral palsy[†] Explanation: Athlete needs evaluation.	Qualified yes
Diabetes mellitus Explanation: All sports can be played with proper attention to diet, blood glucose concentration, hydration, and insulin therapy. Blood glucose concentration should be monitored every 30 minutes during continuous exercise and 15 minutes after completion of exercise.	Yes
Diarrhea Explanation: Unless disease is mild, no participation is permitted because diarrhea may increase the risk of dehydration and heat illness. See "Fever" below.	Qualified no

Eating disorders
   Anorexia nervosa, bulimia nervosa
   Explanation: Patients with these disorders need medical and psychiatric assessment before participation.
	Qualified yes

Eyes
   Functionally one-eyed athlete, loss of an eye, detached retina, previous eye surgery, or serious eye injury
   Explanation: A functionally one-eyed athlete has a best-corrected visual acuity of less than 20/40 in the eye with worse acuity. These athletes would suffer significant disability if the better eye were seriously injured, as would those with loss of an eye. Some athletes who previously have undergone eye surgery or had a serious eye injury may have an increased risk of injury because of weakened eye tissue. Availability of eye guards approved by the American Society for Testing and Materials and other protective equipment may allow participation in most sports, but this must be judged on an individual basis.
	Qualified yes

Fever Explanation: Fever can increase cardiopulmonary effort, reduce maximum exercise capacity, make heat illness more likely, and increase orthostatic hypertension during exercise. Fever may rarely accompany myocarditis or other infections that may make exercise dangerous.	No
Heat illness, history of Explanation: Because of the increased likelihood of recurrence, the athlete needs individual assessment to determine the presence of predisposing conditions and to arrange a prevention strategy.	Qualified yes
Hepatitis Explanation: Because of the apparent minimal risk to others, all sports may be played that the athlete's state of health allows. In all athletes, skin lesions should be covered properly, and athletic personnel should use universal precautions when handling blood or body fluids with visible blood.	Yes
Human immunodeficiency virus infection Explanation: Because of the apparent minimal risk to others, all sports may be played that the athlete's state of health allows. In all athletes, skin lesions should be covered properly, and athletic personnel should use universal precautions when handling blood or body fluids with visible blood.	Yes
Kidney, absence of one Explanation: Athlete needs individual assessment for contact, collision, and limited-contact sports.	Qualified yes

Condition	May Participate
Liver, enlarged Explanation: If the liver is acutely enlarged, participation should be avoided because of risk of rupture. If the liver is enlarged, individual assessment is needed before collision, contact, or limited-contact sports are played.	Qualified yes
Malignant neoplasm[†] Explanation: Athlete needs individual assessment.	Qualified yes
Musculoskeletal disorders Explanation: Athlete needs individual assessment.	Qualified yes

Neurologic disorders
   History of serious head or spinal trauma, severe or repeated concussions, or craniotomy
      Explanation: Athlete needs individual assessment for collision, contact, or limited-contact sports and also for noncontact sports if deficits in judgment or cognition are present. Research supports a conservative approach to management of concussion.
	Qualified yes

Seizure disorder, well controlled Explanation: Risk of seizure during participation is minimal.	Yes
Seizure disorder, poorly controlled Explanation: Athlete needs individual assessment for collision, contact, or limited-contact sports. The following noncontact sports should be avoided: archery, riflery, swimming, weight or power lifting, strength training, or sports involving heights. In these sports, occurrence of a seizure may pose a risk to self or others.	Qualified yes
Obesity Explanation: Because of the risk of heat illness, obese persons need careful acclimatization and hydration.	Qualified yes
Organ transplant recipient[†] Explanation: Athlete needs individual assessment.	Qualified yes
Ovary, absence of one Explanation: Risk of severe injury to the remaining ovary is minimal.	Yes

Respiratory conditions
   Pulmonary compromise, including cystic fibrosis
      Explanation: Athlete needs individual assessment, but generally, all sports may be played if oxygenation remains satisfactory during a graded exercise test. Patients with cystic fibrosis need acclimatization and good hydration to reduce the risk of heat illness.
	Qualified yes

Asthma Explanation: With proper medication and education, only athletes with the most severe asthma will need to modify their participation.	Yes
Acute upper respiratory infection Explanation: Upper respiratory obstruction may affect pulmonary function. Athlete needs individual assessment for all but mild disease. See "Fever."	Qualified yes
Sickle cell disease Explanation: Athlete needs individual assessment. In general, if status of the illness permits, all but high exertion, collision, and contact sports may be played. Overheating, dehydration, and chilling must be avoided.	Qualified yes
Sickle cell trait Explanation: It is unlikely that persons with sickle cell trait have an increased risk of sudden death or other medical problems during athletic participation, except under the most extreme conditions of heat, humidity, and, possibly, increased altitude. These persons, like all athletes, should be carefully conditioned, acclimatized, and hydrated to reduce any possible risk.	Yes
Skin disorders (boils, herpes simplex, impetigo, scabies, molluscum contagiosum) Explanation: While the patient is contagious, participation in gymnastics with mats, martial arts, wrestling, or other collision, contact, or limited-contact sports is not allowed.	Qualified yes
Spleen, enlarged Explanation: A patient with an acutely enlarged spleen should avoid all sports because of risk of rupture. A patient with a chronically enlarged spleen needs individual assessment before playing collision, contact, or limited-contact sports.	Qualified yes
Testicle, undescended or absence of one Explanation: Certain sports may require a protective cup.	Yes

*This table is designed for use by medical and nonmedical personnel. "Needs evaluation" means that a physician with appropriate knowledge and experience should assess the safety of a given sport for an athlete with the listed medical condition.

†Not discussed in the text of the monograph.

Reproduced with permission from American Academy of Pediatrics Committee on Sports Medicine and Fitness: Medical conditions affecting sports participation. Pediatrics 2001;107:1205–1209.

Table 2-6 Classification of Sports by Contact		
Contact or Collision	*Limited Contact*	*Noncontact*
Basketball	Baseball	Archery
Boxing*	Bicycling	Badminton
Diving	Cheerleading	Body building
Field hockey	Canoeing or kayaking	Bowling
Football, tackle	(white water)	Canoeing or kayaking
Ice hockey†	Fencing	(flat water)
Lacrosse	Field events	Crew or rowing
Martial arts	High jump	Curling
Rodeo	Pole vault	Dancing§
Rugby	Floor hockey	Ballet
Ski jumping	Football, flag	Modern
Soccer	Gymnastics	Jazz
Team handball	Handball	Field events
Water polo	Horseback riding	Discus
Wrestling	Racquetball	Javelin
	Skating	Shot put
	Ice	Golf
	In-line	Orienteering¶
	Roller	Power lifting
	Skiing	Race walking
	Cross-country	Riflery
	Downhill	Rope jumping
	Water	Running
	Skateboarding	Sailing
	Snowboarding†	Scuba diving
	Softball	Swimming
	Squash	Table tennis
	Ultimate frisbee	Tennis
	Volleyball	Track
	Windsurfing or surfing	Weight lifting

*Participation not recommended by the American Academy of Pediatrics.
†The American Academy of Pediatrics recommends limiting the amount of body checking allowed for hockey players 15 years and younger to reduce injuries.
†Snowboarding has been added since previous statement was published.
§Dancing has been further classified into ballet, modern, and jazz since the previous monograph was published.
¶A race in which competitors use a map and compass to find their way through unfamiliar territory.
Reproduced with permission from American Academy of Pediatrics Committee on Sports Medicine and Fitness: Medical conditions affecting sports participation. Pediatrics 2001;107:1205–1209.

Table 2-7 Classification of Sports by Strenuousness		
High to Moderate Intensity		
High to Moderate Dynamic and Static Demands	*High to Moderate Dynamic and Low Static Demands*	*High to Moderate Static and Low Dynamic Demands*
Boxing*	Badminton	Archery
Crew or rowing	Baseball	Auto racing
Cross-country skiing	Basketball	Diving
Cycling	Field hockey	Horseback riding (jumping)
Downhill skiing	Lacrosse	Field events (throwing)
Fencing	Orienteering	Gymnastics
Football	Race walking	Karate or judo
Ice Hockey	Racquetball	Motorcycling
Rugby	Soccer	Rodeo
Running (sprint)	Squash	Sailing
Speed skating	Swimming	Ski jumping
Water polo	Table tennis	Waterskiing
Wrestling	Tennis	Weight lifting
	Volleyball	
Low Intensity		
Low Dynamic and Low Static Demands		
Bowling		
Cricket		
Curling		
Golf		
Riflery		

*Participation not recommended by the American Academy of Pediatrics.
Reproduced with permission from American Academy of Pediatrics Committee on Sports Medicine and Fitness: Medical conditions affecting sports participation. Pediatrics 2001;107:1205–1209.

medical records as a tool for obtaining a history and physical examination to screen athletes for participation in sports. In addition, a Web-based preparticipation examination questionnaire has been used. The questionnaire is provided to athletes and answered prior to the physical examination. When the athlete comes for his or her physical examination, the physician is provided with the history. In 1998, Stanford University started using the Web-based preparticipation examination history. They posted the questionnaire on a Web site, which allowed access for the athletes to answer questions about their history prior to the physical examination. The sports medicine physicians reported that they were allowed more time to spend with the athlete to counsel athletes on health issues. The Web-based preparticipation examination was found to be 97% sensitive in detecting medical issues that needed further evaluation. Athletes reported that the Web-based preparticipation examination was easy to use and allowed the overall time for the examination to be reduced.[24]

There are many variations of the preparticipation examination, which in some cases tailor the examination and screening tests to specific populations (e.g., females, adolescents). The use of an electronic medical record or the Web-based preparticipation examination will perhaps aid sports medicine physicians come to a consensus on a common preparticipation examination for athletes of all sports.[1]

REFERENCES

1. Best TM: The preparticipation evaluation, an opportunity for change and consensus. Clin J Sport Med 2004;14:107–108.
2. Armsey TD, Hosey RG: Medical aspects of sports: Epidemiology of injuries, preparticipation physical examination, and drugs in sports. Clin Sports Med 2004;23:255–279.
3. Glover DW, Maron BJ: Profile of preparticipation cardiovascular screening for high school athletes. JAMA 1998;279:1817–1819.
4. Gomez JE, Lantry BR, Saathoff KN: Current use of adequate preparticipation examination history forms for heart disease screening of high school athletes. Arch Pediatr Adolesc Med 1999;153:723–726.
5. Pfister GC, Puffer JC, Maron BJ. Preparticipation cardiovascular screening for US collegiate of student athletes. JAMA 2000;283:1597–1599.

6. American Academy of Family Physicians, American Academy of Pediatrics, American Medical Society of Sports Medicine, American Orthopaedic Society for Sports Medicine, American Osteopathic Academy of Sports Medicine: Preparticipation Physical Examination, 3rd ed. Minneapolis, The Physician and Sportsmedicine, 2004.

7. Madden CC, Walsh MW, Mellion MB: The Team Physician: The Preparticipation Examination and On-Field Emergencies. Orthopaedic Sports Medicine, Principals and Practice, 2nd ed. Philadelphia, WB Saunders, 2003.

8. Beckerman J, Wang P, Hlatky M: Cardiovascular screening of athletes. Clin J Sport Med 2004;14:127–132.

9. Maron BJ, Thompson PD, Puffer JC, et al: Cardiovascular preparticipation screening of competitive athletes. Circulation 1996;94:850–856.

10. Wingfield K, Matheson GO, Meeuwisse WH: Preparticipation evaluation, an evidence based review. Clin J Sport Med 2004;14:109–122.

11. The National Coalition for Women and Girls in Education: Title XI at 30: Report card on gender equity. Washington, DC, 2002. Available at www.scwge.org/

12. Otis CL, Drinkwater B, Johnson M, et al: American College of Sports Medicine position stand: The female athlete triad. Med Sci Sports Exerc 1997;29:i–ix.

13. Maron BJ, Araujo CG, Thompson PD, et al: Recommendations for pre-participation screening and the assessment of cardiovascular disease in masters athletics: An advisory for healthcare professionals for the working groups of the World Heart Federation, the International Federation of Sports Medicine, and the American Heart Association on exercise, cardiac rehabilitation and prevention. Circulation 2001;103:327–334.

14. American College of Sports Medicine, American College of Cardiology: 26th Bethesda Conference. Recommendations for determining eligibility for competition in athletes with cardiovascular abnormalities. Med Sci Sport Exerc 1994;26:5223–5283.

15. Smith J, Laskowski ER: The Preparticipation physical examination: Mayo Clinic experience with 2,739 examinations. Mayo Clin Proc 1998;5:419–429.

16. Holzer K, Brukner P: Screening of athletes for exercise-induced bronchoconstriction. Clin J Sports Med 2004;14:134–137.

17. United States Preventative Services Task Force (USPSTF) Web site: Available at www.ahcpr.gov/clinic/uspstfix.htm/

18. Gomez JE, Landry GL, Bernhardt DT: Critical evaluation of the 2-minute orthopaedic screening examination. Sports Med 1993;147:1109–1113.

19. Garrick JG: Preparticipation orthopedic screening evaluation. Clin J Sport Med 2004;14:123–126.

20. McCrory P: Preparticipation assessment for head injury. Clin J Sports Med 2004;14:139–144.

21. Boyajian-O'Neill, Cardone D, Dexter W, et al: The preparticipation examination for the athlete with special needs. Physician Sportsmedicine 2004;32:13–19.

22. Corrado D, Basso C, Schiavon M, et al: Screening for hypertrophic cardiomyopathy in young athletes. N Engl J Med 1998;339:364–369.

23. American Academy of Pediatrics Committee on Sports Medicine and Fitness: Medical conditions affecting sports participation. Pediatrics 1994;94:757–760.

24. Peltz JE, Haskell WL, Matheson GO: A comprehensive and cost-effective preparticipation exam implemented on the World Wide Web. Med Sci Sports Exerc 1999;31:1727–1740.

In This Chapter

INTRODUCTION

- Life-threatening emergencies in athletics are rare, but the potential causes of an on-field emergency are numerous.

- Adequate preparation and management of an on-field emergency is key to a successful outcome.

- Initial management of an on-field emergency includes a primary survey using the ABCDE (airway, breathing, circulation, disability/neurologic status, exposure) method and cervical immobilization. When appropriate, immediate use of cardiopulmonary resuscitation, an automated external defibrillator, and artificial ventilation improves the chances of survival.

- Special considerations must be followed when caring for an athlete with a suspected head or spinal cord injury as well as an athlete wearing a helmet and face mask.

- A major goal of the sports medicine team's preseason planning is to develop and implement an emergency response plan.

- By maintaining a sideline "medical bag" and emergency equipment, the sports medicine team can provide rapid and appropriate treatment to an athlete in an emergency situation.

Emergencies at sporting events are usually caused by trauma, aggravation of a known medical problem, presentation of a previously unknown medical problem, or an environmental cause/catastrophe. The list of potential causes of on-field emergencies is numerous and still expanding (Table 3-1). Some of the potential causes of on-field emergencies are immediately life threatening (cardiac arrhythmia, airway compromise), while others may rapidly become life threatening if medical care is not administered quickly (cervical spine injury, traumatic brain injury). The team physician and other medical personnel should be able to acutely assess, manage, and triage both traumatic injuries and numerous medical conditions.

When reaching an athlete that is injured, a primary survey should be made using the ABCDE method (airway, breathing, circulation, disability/neurologic status, exposure). Cervical immobilization should be started immediately, especially if the athlete has neurologic deficits, pain, or altered mental status. Immobilization of the cervical spine should be maintained until spinal cord and brain injury is ruled out.

Evidence of airway compromise includes labored and/or unequal breath sounds. Noisy respirations may be an indication of a partial airway obstruction, and clearing the airway of the obstruction should be attempted by sweeping a gloved finger into the oropharynx and/or by suction. The athlete's circulatory status can be affirmed by palpation of a carotid artery pulse. Any bleeding should be identified and controlled by applying a pressure dressing.

If spontaneous respirations and/or a pulse are absent, then cardiopulmonary resuscitation should be started immediately. The athlete is artificially ventilated with either mouth-to-mouth, mouth-to-mask, bag-valve mask, or oropharyngeal airway (unconscious athletes only) respirations, cricothyrotomy, or endotracheal intubation. Chest compressions should be started, and an automated external defibrillator should be attached to the athlete as soon as possible. It has been shown that early defibrillation helps to save lives by converting ventricular fibrillation, the most common lethal arrhythmia, to a normal rhythm.

HEAD AND SPINAL CORD INJURY

One of the more common emergency conditions encountered during coverage of athletic events are head and neck injuries. Any athlete that has altered mental status, neck pain, or neurologic complaints should be considered to have a spinal cord or brain injury. By properly managing head and neck injuries, the medical team can lessen the chance of complications and expedite emergency transportation.

The first step in managing a cervical spinal injury is cervical immobilization. This immobilization should be maintained until a spinal cord or brain injury is ruled out by a thorough examination and/or radiographic studies at an emergency facility. Cervical immobilization is typically achieved by one of the responders. Care needs to be taken to keep the head in a neutral position in line with the spine and to avoid flexion and extension of the cervical spine. If the athlete is lying prone, the log roll maneuver is used to turn the athlete to the supine position. Once the athlete has been placed in a cervical collar and attached to a spine board, he or she is transported by paramedics to a previously determined emergency facility for a more detailed evaluation.

**TABLE 3-1 Potential Causes of On-Field Emergencies
in the Athlete[5,6]**

Trauma	Medical
Head injury	Coronary artery disease
Spinal cord injury	Arrhythmia
Flail chest	Congenital abnormality
Hemothorax	Hypertrophic cardiomyopathy
Tension pneumothorax	Hyperthermia
Laryngeal fracture	Hypothermia
Cardiac tamponade	Cerebrovascular accident
Cardiac contusion	Hypoglycemia
Commotio cordis	Hyponatremia
Ruptured viscus	Asthma
Multiple fractures, e.g., femur, pelvis	Spontaneous pnuemothorax
Blood loss	Pulmonary embolism
Pulmonary contusion	Allergic anaphylaxis
	Drugs, e.g., cocaine, morphine
	Other, e.g., vasovagal, postural hypotension
	Blood pooling postexercise, hyperventilation, hysteria
	Lightning

Athletes with a Helmet and Face Mask

Particular attention needs to be given to emergency conditions occurring in the athlete wearing a helmet and face mask. Unless there are special circumstances such as respiratory distress coupled with an inability to access the airway, the helmet should never be removed during the prehospital care of the athlete with a potential head or neck injury.[1] The helmet and shoulder pads hold the cervical spine in relative alignment, and removal of them would cause movement of the cervical spine that could trigger neurologic complications. Table 3-2 lists the only exceptions to the guideline of never removing the helmet in the prehospital setting. Leaving the helmet in place does not inhibit assessment of the athlete's airway, breathing, circulatory, and neurologic status. Prior to transport, care should be given to stabilizing the head and neck to the spine board by strapping, taping, and/or using lightweight bolsters. Once at an emergency care facility, satisfactory radiographs can usually be obtained with the helmet in place.[1]

**TABLE 3-2 Only Exceptions to Guideline of Never
Removing Helmet of an Athlete with a Suspected
Head or Neck Injury in the Prehospital Setting[1]**

1. Helmet does not hold the head securely, such that immobilization of the helmet does not immobilize the head.
2. Even after removal of the face mask, the airway cannot be controlled or ventilation provided.
3. After a reasonable period of time, the face mask cannot be removed.
4. Helmet prevents immobilization for transportation in an appropriate position.

TABLE 3-3 Protocol for Helmet Removal[2]

1. Manually stabilize the head, neck, and helmet throughout the procedure.
2. Cut the chin strap.
3. Remove the cheek pads by slipping the flat blade of a screwdriver or bandage scissor under the pad snaps and above the inner surface of the shell.
4. If an air cell padding system is present, deflate it by releasing the air at the external port with an inflation needle or large-gauge hypodermic needle.
5. Rotate the helmet slightly forward; it should now slide off the occiput.
6. Slight traction can be applied to the helmet as it is carefully rocked anteriorly and posteriorly without moving the head/neck unit.
7. Do not spread apart the helmet by the ear holes because this will tighten the helmet on the forehead and occiput regions.

While in most circumstances the helmet should not be removed, the face mask should be taken off soon after the primary survey. The face mask should be removed to monitor breathing, care for facial injury, or prior to transport regardless of respiratory status.[1] This can be done by unscrewing or cutting the loops that attach the mask to the helmet. A PVC pipe cutter, garden shears, screwdriver, or pocketknife will all work. It is essential that the medical team readily have the proper tools for face mask removal and should practice face mask removal prior to the season.[2]

If the helmet needs to be removed to initiate life-saving treatment, ensure cervical immobilization, or obtain special radiographic studies, a specific protocol needs to be followed (Table 3-3).[1] Both on-field medical personnel and medical staff in emergency care facilities should be trained to remove athletic helmets in a safe and efficient manner. All staff who participate in a helmet removal should perform the maneuver with caution and coordination of every move in the protocol.[1]

LIGHTNING SAFETY

Nature itself can cause an emergency situation on an athletic field. Lightning is the most common weather hazard that affects athletics.[3] The National Severe Storms Laboratory estimates that 100 fatalities and 400 to 500 injuries requiring medical treatment occur from lightning strikes in the United States each year.[1] A lightning strike should be considered a life-threatening emergency situation. While the probability of being struck by lightning is extremely low, the odds are significantly greater when a storm is in the area and proper safety precautions are not followed.[1] The National Collegiate Athletic Association and National Severe Storms Laboratory have developed lightning safety guidelines to diminish the lightning hazard at an athletic event (Table 3-4).[1]

The most important aspect to monitor is how far away the lightning is occurring and how fast the storm is approaching, relative to the distance of shelter.[1] The flash-to-bang method is the easiest and most convenient way to estimate how far away lightning is occurring.[1] To use the flash-to-bang method, count the seconds from the time the lightning is sighted to when the clap of thunder is heard. Divide this number by five to obtain how

TABLE 3-4 Lightning Safety Guidelines Developed by the National Collegiate Athletic Association and National Severe Storms Laboratory[1]
1. Designate a chain of command as to who monitors the weather and who makes the decision to remove a team or individuals from an athletic site or event.
2. Obtain a weather report each day before a practice or event.
3. It does not have to be raining for lightning to strike.
4. Be aware of National Weather Service–issued thunderstorm "watches" and "warnings" and the signs of thunderstorms developing nearby.
5. By the time a monitor obtains a flash-to-bang count of 30 seconds (equivalent to 6 miles), all individuals should have left the athletic site and reached a safe structure or location.
6. Know where the closest safe structure or location is and how long it takes to get there. A safe structure or location is defined as: (a) Any building normally occupied or frequently used by people. Avoid using shower facilities for shelter and do not use showers or plumbing facilities during a thunderstorm. (b) Any vehicle with a hard metal roof and rolled-up windows. Do not touch the sides of the vehicle.
7. If no safe structure or location is within a reasonable distance, find a thick grove of trees surrounded by taller trees or a dry ditch. Assume a crouched position on the ground with only the balls of the feet touching the ground, wrap your arms around your knees, and lower your head. Minimize contact with the ground and do not lie flat. Stay away from the tallest trees or objects, individual trees, standing pools of water, and open fields. Avoid being the highest object in a field.
8. A person who feels his or her hair stand on end or skin tingle should immediately crouch as described above.
9. Avoid using the telephone, except in emergency situations. A cellular phone or portable remote phone is a safe alternative if the person and antenna are located within a safe structure or location.
10. Athletic activity can be resumed after waiting for 30 minutes after the last flash of lightning or sound of thunder.
11. People who have been struck by lightning do not carry an electrical charge, and cardiopulmonary resuscitation is safe for the responder. If possible, the injured person should be moved to a safer location before starting cardiopulmonary resuscitation.

far away (in miles) the lightning is occurring. When the flash-to-bang count is less than 30 seconds (6 miles), all individuals should leave the athletic field and move to shelter.[1] Everyone can return to the athletic field 30 minutes after the last flash of lightning or sound of thunder.[1]

PREPAREDNESS

The key to managing on-field emergencies is thorough preparation. To accomplish this goal, the sports medicine physician should assist in developing an integrated medical system that includes extensive preparation and evaluation in the off-season, as well as game-day planning.[4]

Preseason Planning

Preseason planning is the most important facet of sideline preparedness. It should promote safety and minimize routine prob-

lems associated with athletic participation as well as emergency situations. All personnel who have the potential to be involved with the medical care of athletes (e.g., athletic trainers, coaches) should use this time to maintain their training in cardiopulmonary resuscitation and basic first aid as a minimum requirement. Additional training in advanced cardiac life support and advanced trauma life support is strongly recommended for team physicians. The goals of the sports medicine team's preseason planning should include the following[2]:

- All athletes complete a preparticipation evaluation by a licensed physician
- Development of a chain of command that establishes and defines the responsibilities of all parties involved
- Establishment of an emergency response plan for practice and competition
- Compliance with Occupational Safety and Health Administration standards relevant to the medical care of the athlete
- Establishment of a policy to assess environmental concerns and playing conditions for modification or suspension of practice or competition
- Compliance with all local, state, and federal regulations regarding storing and dispensing pharmaceuticals
- Establishment of a plan to provide for proper documentation and medical record keeping
- Regular rehearsal of the emergency response plan
- Establishment of a network with other health care providers, including medical specialists, athletic trainers, and allied health professionals
- Establishment of a policy that includes the team physician in the dissemination of any information regarding the athlete's health
- Preparation of a letter of understanding between the team physician and the administration that defines the obligations and responsibilities of the team physician

Emergency Planning

A major objective of the sports medicine team's preseason planning is to develop and implement an emergency plan. Professional and legal requirements mandate that organizations or institutions sponsoring athletic activities have a written emergency plan.[5] Limb-threatening or life-threatening emergencies on the athletic field are unpredictable and therefore have the potential to cause chaos and an ineffective response if medical personnel are not well prepared for these situations. A well-designed and rehearsed emergency plan can provide the medical team with an organized approach to handle an emergency. Preparation for response to emergencies includes education and training, maintenance of emergency equipment and supplies, appropriate use of personnel, and the formation and implementation of an emergency plan.[3] In addition, medical personnel have a legal duty to provide high-quality care to athletic participants and failure to have an emergency response plan could be considered negligence.[3] Table 3-5 highlights some recommended guidelines to use when establishing an emergency response plan.

For an emergency response plan to be effective, careful planning and organization should be given to personnel, equipment, communication, transportation, the referring emergency care facility, and documentation. All personnel associated with practices, competitions, skills instruction, and strength and conditioning activities should have training in automatic external defibrillation and current certification in cardiopulmonary resus-

TABLE 3-5 Recommendations to Establish an Effective Emergency Response Plan[3,4]

1. Each institution or organization that sponsors athletic activities must have a written emergency plan that is comprehensive, practical, and flexible.

2. It should be distributed to athletic trainers, team physicians, institutional and organizational safety personnel and administrators, and coaches.

3. It should be developed with local emergency receiving facility and emergency medical services personnel.

4. It must identify the personnel involved in carrying out the emergency plan and outline the qualifications of those executing the plan.

5. Sports medicine professionals, officials, and coaches should be trained in automatic external defibrillation, cardiopulmonary resuscitation, first aid, and prevention of disease transmission.

6. It should specify the equipment needed and the location of the emergency equipment.

7. It should establish a clear mechanism for communication to appropriate emergency care service providers and identify the mode of transportation for the injured participant.

8. The plan should be specific to the activity venue.

9. Emergency receiving facilities should be notified in advance of scheduled events and contests.

10. It should include an inclement weather policy with specific provisions for decision making and evacuation plans.

11. It should identify who is responsible for documenting actions taken during the emergency, evaluation of the emergency response, and institutional personnel training.

12. The plan should be reviewed and rehearsed at least annually.

13. The plan should be reviewed by the administration and legal counsel of the sponsoring organization or institution.

citation, first aid, and the prevention of disease transmission.[3,4] The emergency plan should also specifically name who is responsible for summoning help and clearing the noninjured athletes from the field.

It is recommended that an emergency plan follow the most recent American Heart Association guidelines for cardiopulmonary resuscitation and emergency cardiovascular care.

The American Heart Association guidelines state that defibrillation is considered a component of basic life support and call for the availability and use of automated external defibrillators.[3] Also, the guidelines emphasize the use of a bag-valve mask, oxygen, and advanced airways in emergency care.[3] Therefore, all personnel on the medical team should receive appropriate training for these devices. All necessary supplemental equipment should be at the site of the athletic event and quickly accessible. In addition, all equipment should be checked on a regular basis to ensure that it is in proper working order.

The medical team has numerous communication options including land-line phones, cell phones, or walkie-talkies as their primary communication system in the emergency plan. However, access to a working telephone, whether fixed or mobile, should always be ensured.[3] Verifying that the communication system is operational prior to each practice or competition is essential. A list of emergency numbers should be prominently posted as well as the street address and directions to the athletic venue.

In an emergency situation, the athlete should be transported by ambulance to the most appropriate receiving facility.[3] When determining on-site medical coverage of athletic events, it is important to consider emergency medical services response time and the level of transportation service that is available.[3] It is recommended to have an ambulance on-site at high-risk events (Table 3-6).[3,4] When an ambulance is on-site, a location should be designated with rapid access to the site and a cleared route for entering and exiting the venue.[5]

Access to an emergency care facility is part of the emergency plan. When choosing an emergency care facility, consideration should be given to its location with respect to the athletic venue and the level of service available.[3] This will help to ensure rapid and effective care of athletes. Also, steps should be taken to notify the emergency care facility in advance of athletic events. The facilities administration and medical staff should review the emergency response plan to address any care issues from their perspective.

The primary documentation will be the written emergency response plan itself. The emergency plan will be separate and specific to each athletic venue. Each emergency plan should name a person or group to be responsible for documenting the events of the emergency situation.[3] Also, documentation of regular rehearsal of the emergency plan, personnel training, and equip-

TABLE 3-6 National Collegiate Athlete Association Guidelines for Recommended On-Site Medical Coverage of Sport Activities[4]

Minimum qualifications: certification in cardiopulmonary resuscitation, first aid, and prevention of disease transmission

High-risk sports: certified athletic trainer physically present during all practices and competitions
  Basketball (men)
  Football
  Skiing
  Gymnastics
  Ice hockey
  Wrestling

Moderate-risk sports: certified athletic trainer (ATC), or other designated person with the minimal qualifications physically present, or ATC must be able to respond within 4 minutes
  Basketball (women)
  Diving
  Soccer
  Indoor track
  Lacrosse
  Volleyball
  Field hockey

Low-risk sports: Any individual who possesses the minimum qualifications
  Baseball
  Outdoor track
  Water polo
  Golf
  Tennis
  Fencing
  Swimming
  Cross country
  Crew
  Softball
  Strength/conditioning, individual skill sessions, and voluntary summer workouts

ment maintenance is recommended to ensure high-quality medical care.[3]

Once the emergency response plan has been developed, the plan must be implemented. The first step to implement the emergency response plan is to have the plan committed to writing to provide a clear response mechanism and to allow for continuity among emergency team members.[3] Typically, this is accomplished by using a flow sheet or organizational chart. Table 3-7 shows an example for a venue-specific emergency response plan. The written plan will need to have the ability to be mod-

ified depending on the athletic venue and for practices versus games.

The second step in implementing an emergency response plan is educating the members of the medical team.[3] All personnel should be given a written copy of the emergency response plan to review. The emergency plan should provide team members with a description of their roles and responsibilities during an emergency situation. Also, a copy of the emergency response plan specific to each venue should be posted in a prominent area, such as by an available telephone.[3]

The third and final step to ensure proper implementation of the emergency response plan is rehearsal.[3] By rehearsing the emergency plan and procedures, the medical team can continue to improve their emergency skills. In addition, this allows medical and emergency medical services personnel to communicate and modify the plan if needed. A minimum of an annual in-service meeting/rehearsal is recommended to achieve these goals.

The sports medicine team should strive to provide improved medical care to its athletes each season. The team physician should coordinate a postseason meeting with appropriate team personnel and administration to review the injuries and illnesses that occurred during the season.[2] This postseason meeting would be a good time to review and modify the existing medical and administrative protocols as well as implement new strategies to improve sideline preparedness for the upcoming season. Postseason evaluation of the sports medicine team's sideline coverage will promote improvement of medical services for future seasons and optimize the medical care of injured or ill athletes.[4]

GAME-DAY PLANNING

Game-day planning will optimize the medical care for an athlete on the day of the event. The duties of the team physician on a game day are numerous and were covered in Chapter 1. However, essential duties of the team physician on game day to prevent, prepare for, or manage an emergency situation are shown in Box 3-1.[2]

TABLE 3-7 Sample Venue–Specific Emergency Protocol[3]
University Sports Medicine Football Emergency Protocol
1. Call 911 or other emergency number consistent with organizational policies.
2. Instruct emergency medical services (EMS) personnel to "report to _____ and meet _____ at _____ as we have an injured student athlete in need of emergency medical treatment."   University Football Practice Complex: _____ Street entrance (gate across street from _____) cross street: _____ Street   University Stadium: Gate _____ entrance off _____ Road
3. Provide necessary information to EMS personnel: a. Name, address, telephone number of caller   b. Number of victims, condition of victims   c. First-aid treatment initiated   d. Specific directions as needed to locate scene   e. Other information as requested by dispatcher
4. Provide appropriate emergency care until arrival of EMS personnel; on arrival of EMS personnel, provide pertinent information (method of injury, vital signs, treatment rendered, medical history) and assist with emergency care as needed.
Note
1. Sports medicine staff member should accompany student athlete to hospital.
2. Notify other sports medicine staff immediately.
3. Parents should be contacted by sports medicine staff.
4. Inform coach(es) and administration.
5. Obtain medical history and insurance information.
6. Appropriate injury reports should be completed.
Emergency Telephone Numbers
_____ Hospital _____-_____
_____ Emergency department _____-_____
University Health Center _____-_____
Campus Police _____-_____
Emergency Signals
Physician: arm extended overhead with clenched fist
Paramedics: point to location in end zone by home locker room and wave onto field
Spine board: arms held horizontally
Stretcher: supinated hands in front of body or waist level
Splints: hand to lower leg or thigh

Box 3-1 Game-day Planning
• Determination of final clearance or return-to-play status of injured or ill athletes   • Preparation of sideline "medical bag" (Table 3-8) and check of sideline medical equipment (Table 3-9) to ensure all is in working order   • Close observation of the game from an appropriate location   • Assessment of environmental concerns and playing conditions   • Presence of medical personnel at the competition site with sufficient time for all pregame preparations   • Planning with the medical staff of the opposing team for medical care of the athletes   • Introductions of the medical team to game officials   • Review of the emergency medical response plan with all personnel who are responsible for carrying out the plan   • Checking and confirming communication equipment   • Identification of examination and treatment sites

TABLE 3-8 Description of What to Include in Sideline "Medical Bag"[2,5,6]
• Alcohol swabs and providone iodine swabs
• Bandage scissors
• Bandages, sterile/nonsterile, Band-Aids
• 50% dextrose water solution
• Disinfectant
• Gloves, sterile/nonsterile
• Large-bore Angiocath for tension pneumothorax (14–16 gauge)
• Local anesthetic/syringes/needles
• Sharps box and red bag
• Suture set/Steri-Strips
• Wound irrigation materials (e.g., sterile normal saline, 10–50 mL syringe)
• Oral airway
• Blood pressure cuff
• Cricothyrotomy kit
• Epinephrine, 1:1000 in a prepackaged unit
• Mouth-to-mouth mask
• Short-acting beta agonist inhaler
• Stethoscope
• Dental kit (e.g., cyanoacrylate, Hank's solution)
• Eye kit (e.g., blue light, fluorescein stain strips, eye patch pads, cotton tip applicators, ocular anesthetic and antibiotics, contact remover, mirror)
• Flashlight
• Pin or other sharp object for sensory testing
• Reflex hammer
• Rectal thermometer
• Benzoin
• Blister care materials
• Contact lens case and solution
• 30% ferric subsulfate solution (e.g., Monsel's solution)
• Injury and illness care instruction sheets for the patient
• List of emergency phone numbers
• Nail clippers
• Nasal packing material
• Oto-ophthalmoscope
• Paper bags for treatment of hyperventilation
• Prescription pad
• Razor and shaving cream
• Scalpel
• Skin lubricant
• Skin staple applicator
• Small mirror
• Supplemental and parenteral
• Tongue depressors
• Topical antibiotics

MEDICAL BAG

The team physician needs to be prepared to treat a wide variety of traumatic and medical conditions. By maintaining a sideline "medical bag," the team physician can provide rapid and appropriate treatment to an athlete, especially in an emergency situation. Table 3-8 provides a list of suggested items to carry in the team physician's bag for contact/collision and high-risk sports. The contents of this bag may vary somewhat depending on the type of sport, the availability of medical supplies provided by the athletic trainer or event site, and the physician's own preferences.[2,5,6]

Sideline Medical Supplies

There are several sideline medical supplies that may be needed in an emergency situation (Table 3-9). Many of these items are too bulky to be carried in the team physician's bag, so care should be taken to ensure that these supplies are provided by the athletic trainer, athletic venue, or on-site paramedics.[2,5,6] The most essential of these supplies would be items used for cardiopulmonary resuscitation and airway management, such as an automated external defibrillator, advanced cardiac life support drugs, and a bag-valve mask with an oxygen supply. Once again, the type of sport, level of competition, and available medical resources must all be considered when determining the on-site sideline medical supplies.

TABLE 3-9 Recommended Sideline Medical Supplies[2,5,6]
• Automated external defibrillator
• Advanced cardiac life support drugs and equipment (crash cart)
• IV fluids and administration set
• Tourniquet
• Access to a phone
• Extremity splints
• Ice
• Oral fluid replacement
• Plastic bags
• Sling
• Blanket
• Crutches
• Mouth guards
• Sling psychrometer and temperature/humidity activity risk chart
• Tape cutter
• Sideline concussion assessment protocol
• Face mask removal tool
• Semirigid cervical collar
• Spine board and attachments

REFERENCES

1. Klossner D, Schluep C, Allen B (eds): NCAA Sports Medicine Handbook, 16th ed. Indianapolis, National Collegiate Athletic Association, 2003.
2. The American Academy of Family Physicians, American Academy of Orthopedic Surgeons, American College of Sports Medicine, American Medical Society for Sports Medicine, American Orthopaedic Society for Sports Medicine, American Osteopathic Society for Sports Medicine. Sideline preparedness for the team physician: A consensus statement, 2000. Available at: www.amssm.org/SidelinePrepare.html.
3. Anderson JC, Courson RW, Kleiner DM, et al: National Athletic Trainers' Association position statement: Emergency planning in athletics. J Athletic Train 2002;37:99–104.
4. The National Athletic Trainers' Association Recommendations and Guidelines for Appropriate Medical Coverage of Intercollegiate Athletics, 2003. Available at: www.nata.org/publicinformation/files/amciarecsandguidesrevised.pdf.
5. Brukner P, Khan K: Clinical Sports Medicine, 2nd ed. New York, McGraw-Hill, 2002, pp 713–725.
6. Delee JC, Drez D, Miller MD: Orthopaedic Sports Medicine Principles and Practice, 2nd ed. Philadelphia, Elsevier, 2003, pp 737–768.

Cardiac Problems and Sudden Death

James C. Puffer

In This Chapter

INTRODUCTION

- Sudden cardiac death (SCD) in young athletes occurs infrequently, but most occurrences are highly publicized and renew questions about screening and prevention.

- Approximately 85% of deaths in young athletes are cardiovascular in nature.

- Hypertrophic cardiomyopathy and congenital coronary artery abnormalities are the most common causes of SCD.

- The rate of SCD has been estimated between 0.46 and 1.6 per 100,000 athletes annually.

- Premonitory symptoms in athletes, such as syncope and chest pain, deserve aggressive investigation.

- The current American Heart Association recommendation for screening of athletes is a careful history and physical examination with specific attention to 13 recommended items.

Perhaps nothing is more sobering than to pick up the newspaper and learn of the sudden and tragic death of a promising young athlete. While many of these unfortunate events are traumatic in nature, some are due to structural or acquired heart disease. Even though sudden death due to cardiac disease is a relatively infrequent event in athletes, a single occurrence is almost always highly publicized and renews questions about the screening of young athletes and the ability of such screening to prevent these rare, but highly visible events. In this chapter, we explore the common causes of SCD in athletes and review the clinical assessment of these disorders. We contrast these pathologic conditions with the normal physiologic changes that occur in the heart in response to athletic training. Finally, we critically assess the utility of the cardiac preparticipation examination as a screening tool and the extent to which it can prevent SCD in athletes.

ETIOLOGY

Sudden death in young athletes is usually associated with physical exertion, and unsuspected congenital cardiac abnormalities are usually found postmortem in young athletes. For the purposes of this chapter, we limit our discussion of SCD to the younger athlete (those younger than 35 years of age), since in the older athlete, this issue is relatively straightforward; the overwhelming majority of sudden deaths are caused by atherosclerotic coronary artery disease.

The etiology of SCD in young athletes has been well documented. Maron et al[1] analyzed 158 sudden deaths in athletes in the United States from 1985 to 1995. Eighty-five percent of deaths were cardiovascular in nature, and hypertrophic cardiomyopathy (HCM) and congenital coronary artery abnormalities were the most common causes of sudden death. Basketball and football players accounted for 68% of deaths, this in large part due to the greater number of athletes participating in these two sports at all levels. The common causes of SCD in young athletes are listed in Table 4-1.

EPIDEMIOLOGY

SCD occurs infrequently in young athletes. Using mandatory catastrophic insurance program data for high school athletes in Minnesota, Maron et al[2] calculated prevalence rates of SCD during the 12-year period from 1985 to 1997 for athletes in grades 10 through 12. A total of 651,695 athletes competed in 27 sports for a total of 1,453,280 overall participations. Three deaths occurred, one from anomalous origin of the left main coronary artery from the right sinus of Valsalva, one from congenital aortic stenosis, and one from myocarditis. The calculated risk of sudden death was 1 per 500,000 participations. The annual rate of sudden death was 0.46 per 100,000 participants.

Somewhat similar findings have been reported by Waller et al.[3] Using data over 6 years from 44,481 necropsies in Marion County, they found that 18 athletic deaths had occurred for an overall incidence of 0.04%. Eighty-eight percent of deaths were cardiac in origin.

As would be expected, the incidence of SCD varied annually, ranging from a low of 0% in 1989 to a high of .09% in 1988.

It might be instructive to look at the epidemiologic aspects of SCD in a country where aggressive screening strategies are mandated by law for comparison. Thiene et al[4] assessed the prevalence of sudden death in young athletes in the Veneto region of Italy and found an annual SCD rate of 0.75 per 100,000 in nonathletes compared to an annual rate of 1.6 per 100,000 athletes. Unlike the United States, arrhythmogenic right ventricular cardiomyopathy (ARVC) was found to be the

Table 4-1 Causes of Sudden Cardiac Death in Young Athletes

Hypertrophic cardiomyopathy
Possible hypertrophic cardiomyopathy
Coronary artery abnormalities
Ruptured aortic aneurysm
Myocarditis
Aortic stenosis
Arrhythmogenic right ventricular dysplasia

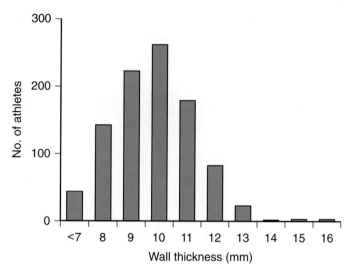

Figure 4-1 Left ventricular dimensions in the athletic heart.

leading cause of death, followed by atherosclerotic coronary artery disease and coronary artery abnormalities as the second and third leading causes, respectively.

ATHLETIC HEART

Before reviewing in detail the specific causes of sudden cardiac death in athletes, it is important to review the normal adaptations that occur in the athlete's heart in response to training. These adaptations result in changes in heart morphology, increased parasympathetic activity, and down-regulation of sympathetic drive, with characteristic findings on the electrocardiogram (ECG) and echocardiogram. Collectively, this constellation of findings has been described as the athletic heart syndrome; it has been well described in the medical literature.[5] It is important to contrast these normal physiologic adaptations to training with the pathologic conditions that are described later in this chapter, and for purposes of discussion in this chapter, we focus primarily on the morphologic changes that occur in the heart in response to athletic training.

Historical Perspective

For more than a century, it has been well known that athletes benefit from hearts that are larger. Indeed, Sir William Osler appropriately recognized the importance of both genetic endowment and physical training in creating a heart that conferred advantage in athletic competition when he opined in 1892: "In the process of training, the getting of wind as it is called, is largely a gradual increase in the capability of the heart . . . . The large heart of athletes may be due to the prolonged use of their muscles, but no man becomes a great runner or oarsman who has not naturally a capable if not large heart." Unfortunately, at the turn of the past century, many believed that the cardiac changes that resulted from vigorous exercise were potentially deleterious to the athlete's health.

These misconceptions were eventually dispelled, and work in the early 20th century by Deutsch and Kauf[6] helped ground our understanding of the athletic heart. They systematically studied the radiographic dimensions of thousands of hearts of athletes of all ages at the Vienna Heart Station by measuring the transverse diameter of the hearts of male and female competitors in 16 sports and compared them to published norms. Not surprisingly, the average heart size for male competitors exceeded norms by 30% to 40%, and the average heart size for female competitors exceeded norms by 4% to 12%. Older athletes and those who had trained longer had the largest transverse diameters.

Changes in Cardiac Morphology

Grasping a few basic concepts of cardiac physiology will help explain the changes in cardiac dimensions that occur in specific

groups of athletes. It is important to remember that the heart maintains its ability to function adequately as a pump by altering heart rate and contractility when a sudden demand is placed on it. However, when chronic demand is imposed on the heart, pump function is maintained by means of dilation and hypertrophy. Therefore, we would expect that athletes who participate primarily in activities that place chronic volume demands on the heart (e.g., runners, swimmers) would increase end-diastolic diameter with resultant increases in wall thickness to normalize wall tension. On the other hand, athletes who participate in sports that place chronic pressure demands on the heart (e.g., weight lifters) would be expected to increase wall thickness without corresponding changes in end-diastolic diameter.

These expected changes have been confirmed by numerous authors using noninvasive imaging. Perhaps the earliest work in this regard was that of Morganroth et al,[7] who used echocardiography to assess left ventricular (LV) dimensions in 56 athletes. They found LV end-diastolic volume and mass increased in isotonic athletes (those who place volume demands on the heart) compared to controls. On the other hand, isometric athletes (those who place pressure demands on the heart) had increased LV mass but normal end-diastolic volume. Wall thickness was greater in the isometric athletes. These changes can be quite impressive as demonstrated by the work of Pelliccia et al.[8] If we consider that 10 mm is usually considered the upper limit of normal for the thickness of the LV free wall and 11 to 13 mm is considered the "gray zone" into which many athletes' LV dimensions may fall, they found 16 of 947 elite athletes studied with echocardiography to have measurements greater than 13 mm. Fifteen of the athletes with the greatest wall thicknesses were rowers or canoeists, and the highest measured LV free wall was 16 mm (Fig. 4-1). It will be important to keep these findings in mind as we discuss some of the pathologic conditions that can cause SCD in athletes, particularly hypertrophic cardiomyopathy.

SPECIFIC CAUSES OF SUDDEN DEATH

Hypertrophic Cardiomyopathy
Pathology
HCM is a condition characterized by marked LV hypertrophy (LVH) with asymmetrical hypertrophy of the interventricular septum when compared to the posterior free wall. In approxi-

Table 4-2 Pathologic Features of Hypertrophic Cardiomyopathy
Left ventricular hypertrophy
Asymmetrical septal hypertrophy
Systolic anterior motion of the septal leaflet of the mitral valve
Myofibrillar disarray

Table 4-3 Historical Features Deserving Aggressive Evaluation
Family history of sudden death at an early age
Family history of heart disease
History of a heart murmur
Syncope with exertion
Presyncope with exertion
Chest pain with exertion
Palpitations with exertion

mately 20% to 25% of individuals, this asymmetrical hypertrophy will cause obstruction of the LV outflow tract. Significant variability in hypertrophy of the left ventricle can be seen; this is the result of the unique genetic mutations that cause this disease as described later. For the most part, higher mortality is associated with greater degrees of hypertrophy. Paradoxical anterior motion of the septal leaflet of the mitral valve can be seen during systole. Microscopically, myofibrillar disarray and fibrosis can be demonstrated and is a hallmark of this disorder. This disarray provides the underlying substrate for electrical instability and the lethal arrhythmias that lead to SCD in athletes. A summary of the salient pathologic features of HCM can be found in Table 4-2.

Genetics
The genetics of this disorder are well understood. Half of all cases result from inherited mutations, while the other half are the result of sporadic mutations. Fifty percent of these mutations occur in the beta cardiac myosin heavy chain on chromosome 14. Watkins et al[9] screened beta cardiac myosin heavy chain genes for mutations in 25 unrelated families with HCM. Seven missense mutations were uncovered in 12 families. Six of these mutations resulted in a change in the electrical charge of the altered amino acid, and these were found to be associated with a shorter life expectancy. Patients with the mutation that did not produce a change in charge had almost normal survival.

Mutations have also been discovered in other myocardial contractile elements, including troponin T, tropomyosin, and myosin-binding protein C. Further evidence of the variability in the lethality of specific mutations has been shown in these contractile elements. Watkins et al[10] assessed mutations in the troponin T and tropomyosin genes in 27 families with familial HCM. Troponin T mutations accounted for 15% of the cases; while these mutations were characterized by mild to subclinical hypertrophy, they were uncharacteristically associated with a high incidence of sudden death.

Clinical Evaluation
The majority of patients with HCM will not have symptoms nor will they have a positive family history for the disease. Therefore, careful attention must be paid to any of the historical features noted in Table 4-3, and an aggressive workup should be pursued in any athlete for whom such a history can be elicited. The physical examination also may provide little information to support the diagnosis of HCM. Only 20% of patients will demonstrate the auscultatory features suggestive of this disorder. These characteristic findings include a late systolic, harsh, crescendo/decrescendo murmur that can be accentuated with a Valsalva maneuver, and an accompanying S4 gallop. Those with pronounced LV hypertrophy will have a sustained and displaced LV impulse on palpation.

Diagnostic Studies
While ECG and a chest radiograph may be abnormal in those athletes with HCM, it is important to note that the findings typically demonstrated in these studies are not specific for the disease. The electrocardiogram is abnormal in approximately 90% of those with HCM. While the tracings in those with this disorder may be quite bizarre, typical findings include evidence of ventricular hypertrophy and associated ST segment and T-wave changes. On the other hand, the majority of those with HCM will not have an abnormal chest radiograph. Those athletes with positive radiographs will demonstrate an enlarged cardiac silhouette with evidence of LV hypertrophy. Given the poor specificity of these two studies, a more sensitive and specific test must be used to assess those athletes in whom the diagnosis of HCM is being considered. Echocardiography is a highly sensitive and specific test for HCM, and the characteristic findings of asymmetrical septal hypertrophy and paradoxical systolic anterior motion of the septal leaflet of the mitral valve are pathognomonic for this disease.

Differentiating Hypertrophic Cardiomyopathy from the Athletic Heart
Occasionally, differentiating HCM from the athletic heart can be challenging. In fact, considering the data presented earlier in this section with regard to the magnitude of LV hypertrophy that can be seen in the elite athlete's heart, it is obvious that when considering this feature alone, considerable overlap can exist between those LV dimensions seen in HCM and those seen in the athletic heart. This concept can best be appreciated by viewing the Venn diagram in Figure 4-2.

Several distinguishing features may help separate these two clinical entities. First, the hypertrophy seen in the athletic heart is usually concentric. While HCM can also present with concentric LVH, it usually is asymmetrical. Second, the internal dimension of the left ventricle is usually large in the athletic heart (>55 mm) and diminished in HCM (<45 mm). In HCM, an enlarged left atrium is usually seen in conjunction with the

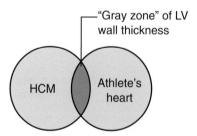

Figure 4-2 Overlap of left ventricular hypertrophy in hypertrophic cardiomyopathy (HCM) and the athlete's heart.

Table 4-4 Most Common Coronary Artery Abnormalities in Athletes
Anomalous origin of the left coronary artery from the right sinus of Valsalva
Tunneled or intramural coronary arteries
Anomalous origin of the left coronary artery from the pulmonary artery
Anomalous origin of the right coronary artery from the left sinus of Valsalva
Hypoplastic coronary arteries

hypertrophied left ventricle, and LV filling is abnormal. Finally, the bizarre electrocardiographic patterns sometimes seen with HCM are not seen in the athletic heart. However, it is important to note that occasionally none of these distinguishing features are present, and the clinician may be left with LV wall thicknesses that fall into the "gray zone." In these instances, a period of deconditioning may be useful in differentiating these two entities. The athlete with an athletic heart will demonstrate regression of hypertrophy after a period of detraining, while one with HCM will have no change in LV hypertrophy.

Coronary Artery Abnormalities
Incidence
Coronary artery abnormalities are rare. Davis et al[11] examined proximal coronary artery anatomy in 2388 pediatric and adolescent patients referred for echocardiography over a 3-year period and found four children with anomalous origin of either the left or right proximal coronary artery for an incidence of 0.17%.

Pathology
While these congenital conditions are rare and may have a benign course, they are a frequent cause of sudden death in athletes. A number of coronary artery abnormalities have been reported in athletes who have died suddenly, and these are listed in Table 4-4. The most common abnormality is the anomalous origin of the left main coronary artery from the right sinus of Valsalva rather than its normal origin from the left sinus. As seen in Figure 4-3, after originating from the right sinus, the anom-

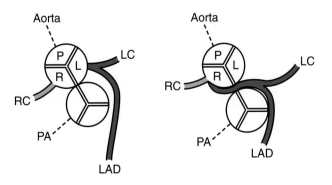

Normal anatomy   Anomalous origin of the left main coronary artery

Figure 4-3 Comparison of normal origin of the left main coronary artery with anomalous origin of the left main coronary artery from the right sinus of Valsalva. LAD, left anterior descending artery; LC, left circumflex artery; PA, pulmonary artery; RC, right coronary artery.

alous artery must make an acute turn and pass between the aorta and pulmonary artery to provide distribution to the anterior heart. The acute angle that the anomalous artery makes before it turns between the two great vessels can lead to significant ischemia during exercise. This resultant ischemia may lead to the development of malignant arrhythmias, which can be fatal.

This pathophysiology has been demonstrated during noninvasive studies. In the previously cited study of Davis et al,[11] the four patients with anomalies detected on echocardiography were studied further. All were asymptomatic at the time of the investigation. One patient with anomalous origin of the right coronary artery had decreased perfusion in the distribution of the right coronary artery and ventricular ectopy on ECG at rest. One patient with an anomalous origin of the left main coronary artery had atrial tachycardia with inferior and lateral ischemia with exercise on ECG.

Clinical Investigation
Detection of coronary abnormalities can be challenging. Most of these abnormalities are detected postmortem after an athlete dies suddenly. However, some athletes may manifest premonitory symptoms and careful attention to these may be life saving. A recent study by Basso et al[12] underscores this important point. These authors reviewed two registries, collected in Italy and the United States, of athletes who died suddenly. Twenty-seven deaths were attributed to anomalous coronary arteries and identified solely at autopsy. Twenty-five athletes died during and two immediately after intense exercise. Twenty-three were found to have anomalous origin of the left main coronary artery and four had anomalous origin of the right coronary artery . Fifteen (55%) athletes had no cardiac manifestations or studies during life, but the remaining 12 had clinical data recorded in their medical records before the SCD that was subsequently collected premortem. Premonitory symptoms occurred in 10 athletes, including syncope in four and chest pain in five. Premonitory symptoms occurred 3 to 24 months before death. All cardiovascular tests were within normal limits including ECG in nine athletes, maximal exercise tests in six, and two-dimensional echocardiography in two athletes.

It is important to discuss the role of two-dimensional echocardiography in the evaluation of athletes with suspected coronary artery abnormalities. Zeppilli et al[13] used two-dimensional echocardiography to study the ostia and first tracts of coronary arteries in 3650 athletes. Clear visualization of them was obtained in 90% of the studies. Three asymptomatic athletes (0.09%) had abnormalities; angiography confirmed anomalous origin of the right coronary artery in two and the other had anomalous origin of the left main coronary artery.

These data are very instructive. They reinforce the notion that any symptoms previously noted in Table 4-3 must be investigated aggressively and suggest that invasive studies may need to be performed in those athletes presenting with such symptoms in order to exclude coronary artery abnormalities as the cause of their symptoms. Therefore, while the initial evaluation of athletes with premonitory symptoms should include a careful history, physical examination, and ECG, it is important to emphasize that these may be not be revealing. Stress echocardiography and, if necessary, coronary angiography should be performed to either confirm or exclude the diagnosis of anomalous coronary arteries in these athletes.

Arrhythmogenic Right Ventricular Cardiomyopathy

Pathology

ARVC, formerly termed arrhythmogenic right ventricular dysplasia, is an inherited disorder characterized by patchy fibrofatty replacement of the right ventricular myocardium. The diagnosis of ARVC is most likely underestimated due to the subtle morphologic and histologic changes seen in some cases and the lack of a single, confirmatory diagnostic test. ARVC is a genetically heterogeneous disorder, linked to several chromosomal loci, and, as previously mentioned, has been found with greatest prevalence in certain regions of Italy.[4] Many believe that myocarditis may play a key role as a contributing or precipitating etiologic factor.

Clinical Manifestations

Athletes with this disorder usually are diagnosed during adolescence or young adulthood. They may present with palpitations, shortness of breath, or dyspnea on exertion. The physical examination may be unremarkable. ECG will usually demonstrate depolarization and repolarization changes localized to the right precordial leads, and echocardiography may reveal right ventricular dilation with global and/or regional wall motion abnormalities. Continuous electrocardiographic monitoring can reveal arrhythmias of right ventricular origin. Magnetic resonance imaging may be useful in demonstrating telltale fibrofatty infiltration and structural alteration of the right ventricle.

Clinical Evaluation

Based on the preceding discussion, the clinical evaluation of the athlete with suspected ARVC should be straightforward. A detailed history, with particular focus on family history, should be performed, followed by physical examination of the athlete with special emphasis placed on the cardiac examination. Initial noninvasive studies should include ECG, two-dimensional echocardiography, and magnetic resonance imaging. In those individuals in whom the diagnosis is still in doubt after completion of the preliminary diagnostic studies, an endomyocardial biopsy may be necessary to confirm the diagnosis.

SCREENING

Considerable interest has centered on the ability of the cardiovascular preparticipation examination to prevent SCD in athletes. Because of the nonstandardization of most preparticipation examinations conducted in the United States and controversy surrounding the specific elements that should be included in those examinations, an expert panel was convened by the American Heart Association in 1995 to study these issues. After thoroughly reviewing the evidence concerning cardiovascular evaluation of athletes available at that time, they published a consensus statement the following year with specific recommendations to guide clinicians in their cardiovascular assessment of athletes.[14] The statement endorsed the notion that the most cost-effective method of conducting cardiovascular preparticipation examinations in the United States was by performing a careful history and physical examination with specific attention to 13 recommended items that should be routinely assessed (Table 4-5). Despite the widespread publication of these recommendations, subsequent work has demonstrated that cardiovascular preparticipation screening still leaves much to be desired at both the interscholastic[15] and intercollegiate levels,[16] with many of the recommended elements absent in a

Table 4-5 Recommended Elements of the Cardiovascular Preparticipation Examination
Family History
Premature sudden death
Heart disease in surviving relatives
Personal History with Parental Verification
Heart murmur
Systemic hypertension
Excessive fatigability
Syncope
Exertional dyspnea
Exertional chest pain
Physical Examination
Blood pressure
Femoral pulses
Heart murmur
Stigmata of Marfan syndrome
Auscultation in the supine or sitting and standing positions to detect murmurs consistent with left ventricular outflow tract obstruction

majority of formats used by state high school jurisdictions or intercollegiate institutions to evaluate their athletes before athletic participation.

Recently, both the International Olympic Committee and the European Society of Cardiology recommended that preparticipation cardiovascular screening of athletes should routinely include ECG.[17,18] In large part, these recommendations were based on Italy's 25-year history of aggressively screening competitive athletes as mandated by Italian law; these evaluations include the routine performance of an ECG.

An excellent study that highlights the results of this vigorous approach was that of Corrado et al,[19] which prospectively studied sudden death in athletes and nonathletes younger than 35 years of age followed for 17 years in the Veneto region of Italy. Cardiovascular reasons for disqualification from sport and follow-up of 33,735 athletes screened with history, physical examination, and ECG during the same period in Padua were also investigated. Of the 269 sudden deaths in young people in the Veneto region, 49 occurred in athletes. Arrhythmogenic right ventricular dysplasia (22.4%), atherosclerotic coronary artery disease (18.4%), and anomalous origin of coronary arteries (12.2%) were the most common causes of sudden death. HCM resulted in 16 sudden deaths in the nonathletes, but only one in the athletes. In Padua, HCM was detected in 22 athletes and accounted for 3.5% of the disqualifications during the same period of time.

None of the athletes with HCM who were disqualified died during a mean follow-up period of 8.2 (±5) years. The calculated sudden death rate in this study was 1.6 per 100,000 athletes.

Based on this evidence as well as other studies emanating from Italy, the European group believes that the standard 12-lead ECG may be more sensitive than echocardiography in detecting HCM. Furthermore, they state "These findings indicate that the Italian screening modality has 77% greater power for detecting HCM and is expected to result in a corresponding additional number of lives saved."[18] Interestingly, a similar argument has been made with respect to the use of the ECG as the sole screening modality for the cardiac preparticipation evaluation of high school athletes in the United States.[20] Echocardiography has been advocated as a more sensitive and specific screening modality by others.[21,22] Despite these findings, significant issues with regard to the cost-effectiveness of this approach in the United States remain. For purposes of appreciating the magnitude of this problem, we can conservatively calculate the number of false-positive findings that would need to be investigated if we screened six million middle school, high school, and intercollegiate athletes with a hypothetical test that had 100% sensitivity and 98% specificity for detecting a condition that placed an athlete at risk of sudden death. Appreciate that this hypothetical test is far better than any currently available noninvasive test that could be conveniently used for screening. Given the current prevalence of sudden death reported in the literature, we would end up with 30 true-positive tests and 60,000 false-positive tests that would require follow-up. Even with this highly sensitive and specific hypothetical test, the cost to pursue further evaluation of these false positives would be staggering.

Fuller has studied the cost-effectiveness of three different screening strategies in the cardiac preparticipation evaluation of high school athletes.[23] Using the American Heart Association recommended history and physical examination, ECG, or two-dimensional echocardiography as screening options, he found ECG to be the most cost-effective strategy for screening athletes for SCD, with an approximate cost of $44,000 per year of life saved. Using the American Heart Association history and physical examination resulted in a cost of $84,000 per year of life saved, while the cost per year of life saved for echocardiography was $200,000. Significant methodologic problems exist with this study. The cost of further cardiac evaluation is probably underestimated as is the number of abnormal electrocardiograms that would require further investigation. Nevertheless, this is the only study that has attempted to analyze this critical issue. Further investigation into the fiscal impact of screening for SCD is desperately needed to guide public policy on cardiac preparticipation screening.

SUMMARY

SCD in athletes is a relatively infrequent phenomenon. However, the high visibility afforded its unfortunate occurrence in young athletes has compelled the medical community to attempt to design screening programs to reduce the likelihood of its occurrence. The most common causes of SCD in the United States are HCM and coronary artery abnormalities. ARVC probably accounts for more SCD than currently estimated, given the lack of a specific test to confirm the diagnosis. Athletes with symptoms suggestive of underlying cardiac disease deserve a rigorous and aggressive evaluation to exclude potentially lethal conditions that can cause SCD. Currently, a thorough cardiac history and physical examination that adhere to the 1996 American Heart Association recommendations remain the strategy of choice to screen athletes for causes of SCD. Further research on the cost-effectiveness of cardiac preparticipation evaluation for SCD is required to formulate sound recommendations for future screening strategies.

REFERENCES

1. Maron BJ, Shirani J, Poliac LC, et al: Sudden death in young competitive athletes: Clinical, demographic and pathological profiles. JAMA 1996;276:199–204.
2. Maron BJ, Gohman TE, Aeppli D: Prevalence of sudden cardiac death during competitive sports activities in Minnesota high school athletes. J Am Coll Cardiol 1998;32:1881–1884.
3. Waller BF, Hawley DA, Clark MA, et al: Incidence of sudden deaths between 1985 and 1990 in Marion County, Indiana. Clin Cardiol 1992;15:851–858.
4. Thiene G, Basso C, Corrado D: Is prevention of sudden death in young athletes feasible? Cardiologia 1999;44:497–505.
5. Huston TP, Puffer JC, Rodney WM: The athletic heart syndrome. N Engl J Med 1985;313:24–32.
6. Deutsch E, Kauf E: Heart and Athletics [Warfield LM, trans.]. St. Louis, CV Mosby, 1927, pp 17–103.
7. Morganroth J, Maron BJ, Henry WL, et al: Comparative left ventricular dimensions in trained athletes. Ann Intern Med 1975;82:521–524.
8. Pelliccia A, Maron BJ, Culasso F, et al: The upper limit of physiologic cardiac hypertrophy in highly trained elite athletes. N Engl J Med 1991;324:295–301.
9. Watkins H, Rosenzweig A, Hwang D-S, et al: Characteristics and prognostic implications of myosin missense mutations in familial hypertrophic cardiomyopathy. N Engl J Med 1992;326:1108–1114.
10. Watkins H, McKenna WJ, Thierfelder L, et al: Mutations in the genes for cardiac troponin T and alpha-tropomyosin in hypertrophic cardiomyopathy. N Engl J Med 1995;332:1058–1064.
11. Davis JA, Cecchin F, Jones TK, et al: Major coronary artery anomalies in a pediatric population: Incidence and clinical importance. J Am Coll Cardiol 2001;37:593–597.
12. Basso C, Maron BJ, Corrado D, et al: Clinical profile of congenital coronary artery anomalies with origin from the wrong aortic sinus leading to sudden death in young competitive athletes. J Am Coll Cardiol 2000;35:1493–1501.
13. Zeppilli P, dello Russo A, Santini C, et al: In vivo detection of coronary artery anomalies in asymptomatic athletes by echocardiographic screening. Chest 1998;114:89–93.
14. Maron BJ, Thompson PD, Puffer JC, et al: Cardiovascular screening of competitive athletes: A statement for health professionals from the sudden death committee (clinical cardiology) and congenital cardiac defects committee (cardiovascular disease in the young), American Heart Association. Circulation 1996;94:850–856.
15. Glover DW, Maron BJ: Profile of preparticipation cardiovascular screening for high school athletes. JAMA 1998;279:1817–1819.
16. Pfister GC, Puffer JC, Maron BJ: Preparticipation cardiovascular screening for US collegiate student-athletes. JAMA 2000;283:1597–1599.
17. International Olympic Committee Medical Commission: Sudden cardiovascular death in sport: Lausanne recommendations, 2004.
18. Study Group of Sport Cardiology of the Working Group of Cardiac Rehabilitation and Exercise Physiology and the Working Group of Myocardial and Pericardial Diseases of the European Society of Cardiology: Cardiovascular preparticipation screening of young competitive athletes for prevention of sudden death: Proposals for a common European protocol. Eur Heart J 2005;26:516–524.
19. Corrado D, Basso C, Sachiavon M, et al: Screening for hypertrophic cardiomyopathy in young athletes. N Engl J Med 1998;339:364–369.
20. Fuller CM, McNulty CM, Spring A, et al: Prospective screening of 5615 high school athletes for risk of sudden cardiac death. Med Sci Sports Exerc 1997;29:1131–1138.

21. Feinstein RA, Colvin E, Oh MK: Echocardiographic screening as a part of a preparticipation examination. Clin J Sports Med 1993;3:149–152.

22. Weidenbener EJ, Krauss BF, Waller BF, et al: Incorporation of screening echocardiography in the preparticipation exam. Clin J Sports Med 1995;5:86–89.

23. Fuller CM: Cost effectiveness analysis of screening of high school athletes for risk of sudden cardiac death. Med Sci Sports Exerc 2000;32:887–890.

Medications, Supplements, and Ergogenic Drugs

George C. Phillips

In This Chapter

INTRODUCTION

- Athletes often take medications for treatment of medical conditions, requiring the physician to have an understanding of side effects and impacts on sports performance.

- Dietary supplements are popular among athletes of all ages. Physicians should inquire as to supplement use in order to provide counseling regarding risks and benefits.

- Anabolic steroids are used by 4% to 12% of high school students. These ergogenic drugs are known to affect multiple organ systems.

- Inappropriate use of medications, supplements, and other drugs has become increasingly common, placing both fair competition and the health of athletes in jeopardy.

The ability to manage sports-related injuries, through both surgical and nonsurgical interventions, has blossomed due to the efforts of the growing field of sports medicine practitioners. While our efforts and interests often focus on musculoskeletal conditions, athletes also require treatment for other medical conditions; these conditions may affect their sports performance as significantly as injury. Athletes turn to sports medicine professionals to maximize their ability to compete, and the pressures that athletes face may drive them to search for other means of performance enhancement. Unfortunately, these other means may include inappropriate and illegal use of various substances.

MEDICATIONS

Many forces affect the use of medications in sports medicine. The impact of specific medical conditions on athletic participation requires physicians to understand not only side effects of standard treatment but any potential effects of treatment on sport performance as well. Direct marketing of various over-the-counter and prescription medications to the general public also brings a unique pressure to bear on the physician caring for athletes at all skill levels. The recent emphasis on lifelong physical activity for prevention and management of various conditions, such as hypertension and obesity, has expanded the population served by the field of sports medicine as well. This section reviews several different medications that may be used by recreational and elite athletes for one or more of the reasons previously stated and is organized by the condition treated.

Hypertension

Hypertension remains one of the most prevalent medical conditions treated in primary care and has been cited as the most common medical indication for disqualification or mandatory follow-up in athletic medicine.[1] Although multiple classes of medications have been introduced over the years to treat hypertension, the most recent expert guidelines on management of hypertension continue to support primary treatment with diuretics, with possible early addition of a β-blocker or angiotensin-converting enzyme inhibitor (ACEI; Table 5-1).[2]

Diuretics

The Antihypertensive and Lipid-Lowering Treatment to Prevent Heart Attack Trial (ALLHAT) study, which involved approximately 33,000 patients older than 55 years of age with hypertension plus one cardiovascular risk factor, rated diuretic therapy as superior to either calcium channel blockers or ACEI with regard to risk of heart attack, stroke, or congestive heart failure; diuretics were also less expensive.[3] Diuretics can result in decreased plasma volume, cardiac output, and peripheral vascular resistance, although these effects are more prominent in loop diuretics as opposed to thiazide diuretics. This effect on volume may predispose athletes using these medications to heat-related illness, varying from muscle cramps to the extremes of heat stroke. For casual athletes, the benefit of diuretic therapy with moderate exercise likely outweighs any concerns of this treatment, provided these same athletes carefully monitor their hydration status. For elite athletes, diuretic use is rendered moot as it is banned by many regulatory agencies.[4] For events regulated according to weight class, diuretic use imparts an obvious direct effect. Diuretic use is also banned for its employment as a masking agent for other drugs by increasing urine output and diluting other doping agents, although this method is generally ineffective for evading detection.[5]

β-Blockers

As second-line drugs, β-blockers, ACEIs, and calcium channel blockers tend to have similar efficacies. β-Blockers have direct

Table 5-1 Antihypertensive Medications

Class of Medication	Characteristics
Diuretics	Age >55, lower risk of cardiovascular complications Less expensive Can lower plasma volume, cardiac output, peripheral vascular resistance Banned in elite athletes
β-Blockers	Decrease cardiac output May decrease exercise tolerance Can cause hypoglycemia Banned in some Olympic sports
ACE inhibitors	Can decrease heart rate and total peripheral resistance Prevent kidney remodeling effects of chronic hypertension Often cause cough Risk of hyperkalemia
Calcium channel blockers	Result in generalized vasodilation Concerns regarding side effects and cardiovascular risks

ACE, angiotensin-converting enzyme.

effects on exercise parameters by decreasing cardiac output. β-Blockers have been suggested to increase perceived effort with exercise, which may lead to decreased exercise tolerance. β-Blockers may also cause hypoglycemia after exercise due to inhibition of glycolysis and glycogenolysis.[6] The use of combination α- and β-blockers has been proposed in hopes of limiting the impairment of skeletal blood flow and oxygen uptake due to the β-blocker effects of decreased cardiac output.[4] However, there are concerns for α-blockers, discussed later, which may preclude the use of such combination agents.

More recently, abnormal recovery of heart rate after exercise has been linked with increased risk of cardiovascular and all-cause mortality. The negative chronotropic effects of β-blockers can decrease heart rate recovery following exercise, and the risk of using this medication in an already at-risk population with hypertension is unclear. Desai et al[7] argue that heart rate recovery is not a separate variable but a reflection of a patient's chronotropic response to exercise. However, this does not remove the potential risk associated with the negative chronotropic effects of β-blockers, and this risk must be weighed against the benefit of blood pressure control on an individual basis.

β-Blockers have also been shown to increase the likelihood that an exercise treadmill test will be nondiagnostic. While a negative exercise treadmill test did not lose predictive value in the face of β-blocker use, as many as 20% of patients on β-blockers with a nondiagnostic exercise treadmill test were subsequently found to have significant coronary artery disease.[8] Following a myocardial infarction, patients on long-acting β-blockers for 3 months experienced increased exercise capacity. This finding runs counter to the general association of decreased exercise tolerance with β-blockers, as mentioned previously. In patients who have had a heart attack, this difference in long-acting β-blocker effects may be explained by improved left ventricular filling during diastole with improved subendocardial perfusion and subsequently less ischemia.[9]

β-Blockers are banned in certain Olympic sports, although this is more for their calming or anxiolytic effect. In fact, β-blockers are generally accepted as ergolytic with regard to endurance activities.[5]

Angiotensin-Converting Enzyme Inhibitors

ACEIs can cause slight decreases in heart rate and total peripheral resistance along with an increase in stroke volume. ACEIs have not been shown to impair energy metabolism, maximal oxygen uptake, or training capacity.[4] ACEIs have special utility in preventing kidney remodeling effects due to chronic hypertension. As this utility especially applies to African-American patients and patients with diabetes mellitus, ACEIs may be superior to β-blockers for these patients.[10] It has also been suggested that ACEIs are most effective in combination with diuretics and that the renoprotective effect of ACEIs counterbalances the increase in creatinine that can be seen with diuretic use. The antihypertensive effects of ACEIs may be blocked by use of nonsteroidal anti-inflammatory drugs (NSAIDs).[11]

ACEIs are notorious for causing significant cough. For patients who experience cough, consideration may be given to switch to an angiotensin-receptor blocker. Angiotensin-receptor blockers also prevent proteinuria, which is beneficial for diabetic patients with renal disease.[11] As compared to β-blockers, angiotensin-receptor blockers improve the risk of stroke and equally protect against high blood pressure and all-cause mortality.[12] Also among the medications affecting the renin-angiotensin-aldosterone axis are aldosterone-receptor antagonists. These medications are relatively new and do not have large amount of study data to support effects on morbidity and mortality. They also carry significant risks of hyperkalemia and interaction with medications metabolized by cytochrome P-450.[2] The general utility of aldosterone-receptor antagonists remains unclear.

Calcium Channel Blockers

Calcium channel blockers (CCBs) result in generalized vasodilation, but they do not have effects on energy metabolism or oxygen uptake.[4] While previously popular, newer evidence based on side effect profiles and cardiovascular risks discourages early use of short-acting calcium channel blockers, with consideration for the use of other CCBs only if ACEIs or β-blockers are ineffective.[13]

α-Blockers

α-Blockers decrease systemic vascular resistance without changes in heart rate or cardiac output, and they do not change energy metabolism or oxygen uptake. Their use may also result in centrally mediated side effects such as dry mouth, drowsiness, and decreased sexual function.[4] The use of α-blockers was discontinued in the ALLHAT study due to an associated increased risk of congestive heart failure and stroke.[14]

Hypercholesterolemia
Statins

Hypercholesterolemia contributes significantly to overall cardiovascular morbidity and mortality. Statins are the number one class of anticholesterol medications. They are well known for side effects of gastrointestinal disturbance, headache, and rash. For athletes, myalgias and, rarely, rhabdomyolysis are possible complications of significant import. Baseline creatine kinase levels prior to onset of statin therapy may be useful in case these complications arise.[15] Most changes in creatine kinase levels with statin use and/or exercise are asymptomatic. Rhabdomyolysis appears to be more likely to occur due to a combination of statin use, exercise, and another medication metabolized by cytochrome P-450.[16] In an experimental trial of over-the-counter use of statins, 17% of users experienced a drug-related adverse event, and 12% of users discontinued statin therapy due to an adverse event.[17] Most studies of statins and exercise involve patients with some form of vascular disease. In patients with claudication due to peripheral artery disease, statin use improved total treadmill time and walking distance.[18,19] In patients with significant coronary artery disease, statin use significantly decreased myocardial ischemia due to exercise without affecting peak heart rate, systolic blood pressure, or diastolic blood pressure.[20]

Exercise-Induced Asthma

The prevalence of exercise-induced asthma ranges from 9% to 50%, depending on the sport cited.[21] The acute release of bronchoconstricting agents and the chronic inflammatory airway changes, both of which are complexly intertwined, suggest two pathways to target for prevention of exercise-induced asthma attacks. A recent Cochrane review confirms that albuterol, a short-acting beta agonist, is the number one treatment for exercise-induced asthma episodes. The bronchodilating effects of albuterol are superior in the acute setting to the anti-inflammatory effects of cromolyn (a mast cell stabilizer) or the anticholinergic effects of ipratropium.[22] Appropriate use of albuterol must consider tolerance, timing of use, and ergogenic effects.

Beta Agonists

Daily use of short-acting beta agonists has been linked with increased frequency of bronchoconstriction during exercise and suboptimal efficacy of rescue.[23] While no ergogenic effects of short-acting beta agonists have been demonstrated at therapeutic doses, increased use among Olympic athletes has been documented.[24] Long-acting beta agonists are equally effective, can have similarly quick time to onset, and often result in longer periods of protection.[25,26] Long-acting beta agonists have also not been shown to possess ergogenic benefits.[27]

Anti-inflammatory Medications

Inhaled corticosteroids are standard therapy for patients with persistent asthma. While not well studied in exercise, the pulmonary delivery of inhaled corticosteroids has not shown any evidence of ergogenic or anabolic effects, and they are approved by the International Olympic Committee (IOC) via medical waiver for athletes with asthma.[21] Leukotriene inhibitors are a new class of oral anti-inflammatory medications for asthmatics. While considered to be less effective than inhaled corticosteroids, the oral delivery of leukotriene inhibitors may provide better compliance for some asthmatics. They can prevent acute episodes of exercise-induced asthma,[28–30] but optimal protection requires them to be used 12 hours prior to exercise.[28] Studies in children and adults have shown protective benefits after a brief period of 5 to 7 days of use.[29,30] Minimal studies in adults have shown no change in time to anaerobic threshold with leukotriene inhibitor use, but there was a decrease in ratings of perceived exertion.[30] Further studies of potential ergogenic effects of leukotriene inhibitors would be helpful.

Psychiatric Conditions
Antidepressants and Anxiolytics

Primary care physicians commonly treat patients with depression and anxiety, and athletes with these conditions compete at all skill levels. However, very little research exists studying the interaction of medications for these conditions and exercise. In a study of patients with major depressive disorder, decreases in isokinetic quadriceps and hamstring strength were shown to improve significantly after 3 months of treatment with a selective serotonin reuptake inhibitor.[31] However, selective serotonin reuptake inhibitors have also been linked with significant weight gain after 6 to 12 months of use[32] and possible episodes of heat-related illness and hyponatremia.[33,34] In a small trial of patients, use of loprazolam, a benzodiazepine that can be used for anxiety, did not affect hand-eye coordination, 30-m sprint time, $\dot{V}O_{2max}$, or time to exhaustion. However, use of loprazolam was associated with prolonged reaction time and a significant hangover effect.[35] In a smaller study with midazolam, subjects experienced significant changes in heart rate variability and had significant orthostatic changes in blood pressure.[36] No large, double-blind, randomized, controlled trials exist for either class of medication. Accordingly, no contraindications exist for the appropriate treatment of depression or anxiety. The only performance concerns might relate to a possible advantage from the anxiolytic effects of these medications (especially benzodiazepines) in shooting events such as the biathlon.

Stimulant Therapy for Attention Deficit Disorder

Attention-deficit disorder (ADD) affects an estimated 5% of the school-age population,[37] with a growing trend toward the identification of impairment due to ADD among adults. Methylphenidate is the standard treatment for ADD with either hyperactive, inattentive, or mixed predominance of symptoms. Methylphenidate is also a stimulant with properties and side effects similar to those of other drugs in the amphetamine class, including an ergogenic effect mediated by delayed fatigue. Methylphenidate is banned by the IOC and the National Collegiate Athletic Association. However, the National Collegiate Athletic Association has recognized the utility of methylphenidate in helping student athletes with ADD to succeed academically. Therefore, a therapeutic use exemption exists for National Collegiate Athletic Association athletes with documented ADD and appropriate methylphenidate therapy.[38]

ADD is known to affect athletic participation in a number of ways, including lessened motivation to participate, impaired motor skills, and decreased performance success.[39,40] Methylphenidate has been shown to improve the attention of youths with ADD during baseball games, as reflected in higher rates of on-task behavior while on the field and better knowledge of their current game-specific situation.[41] Methylphenidate has also been demonstrated to improve visual tracking by athletes with ADD during table tennis by maintaining their gaze on the ball in flight for significantly longer periods of time.[42] Athletes with ADD who use methylphenidate should be aware of a possible increased risk of heat-related illness due to the stimulant's cardiovascular properties. However, methylphenidate may not only help athletes with ADD to succeed at work or school, but it may help them to more fully participate in athletics, thereby receiving a boost in self-esteem that many patients with ADD need.

Pain Relievers/Osteoarthritis
Acetaminophen

Acetaminophen is a well-known pain reliever, yet it is often thought of as secondary to NSAIDs because it is thought to not possess anti-inflammatory effects (Table 5-2). However, acetaminophen has been shown to affect prostaglandin production in

Table 5-2 Pain Relievers/Osteoarthritis Medications	
Medication	Characteristics
Acetaminophen	Better side effect profile, especially for gastrointestinal effects No anti-inflammatory effects? Less pain relief?
NSAIDs	Analgesic, anti-inflammatory Impaired healing of muscle, tendon, and bone?
COX-2 inhibitors	Decreased gastrointestinal side effects Increased risk of thrombotic events?
Glucosamine	Good safety profile Efficacy less proven?

COX, cyclooxygenase; NSAIDs, nonsteroidal anti-inflammatory drugs.

exercised muscle, which may be linked to decreasing the building of new muscle after exercise.[43] In low back pain, acetaminophen has been shown to be equally beneficial as compared to NSAIDs.[44] Acetaminophen also has a role in first-line pharmaceutical management of osteoarthritis,[45] with studies suggesting benefit equal to that of NSAIDs in pain relief with a better side effect profile, especially for gastrointestinal effects.[46] More recent research has suggested that acetaminophen provides less pain relief without side effect benefits as compared to cyclooxygenase (COX)-2 inhibitors such as celecoxib.[47] Yet given the newer concerns for COX-2 inhibitors and their prothrombotic potential, acetaminophen remains for most patients a more appropriate first-line choice for analgesia based on side effect profiles.

Nonsteroidal Anti-inflammatory Drugs

NSAIDs make up a popular class of over-the-counter and prescription pain relievers. Advertisements for NSAIDs are often targeted at athletes of all levels for their anti-inflammatory effects, which differentiate this class from other pain relievers such as acetaminophen. Such directed marketing is apparently effective, as one study found that at least 20% of high school football players surveyed used NSAIDs on a daily basis in season. These athletes used NSAIDs with expectations of improved athletic performance and prevention of pain that might occur during practice or competition.[48] NSAIDs are not thought to have stand-alone ergogenic properties. Their analgesic effect may allow increased training and/or performance, but the masking of pain by use of NSAIDs interrupts a natural defense mechanism for preventing further injury. Additionally, as inflammation is a part of the healing process for most injuries, the anti-inflammatory effect of NSAIDs may be detrimental to recovery from injury.

Several studies, using animal and human models, have examined the impact of various NSAIDs on the healing of injuries to soft tissue and bone. In the case of muscle injury, NSAIDs may provide an initial protective effect in the first several days, but over time their use has been associated with impaired rates of healing in both macrotrauma and microtrauma.[49,50] One human subject study showed that naproxen did improve recovery from delayed-onset muscle soreness, but the study did not examine the drug's effects on muscle structure or objective strength.[51] In animal studies of medial collateral ligament injuries, use of NSAIDs was again associated with a brief initial improvement,[52]

yet no benefit to ligament strength was shown 3 to 4 weeks after the injury.[52,53] In human subject testing, the Kapooka Ankle Sprain Study is perhaps the best investigation of the effects of NSAIDs on ligamentous injury. Following treatment with piroxicam, the military recruits in the study noted better pain relief and a faster return to physical training compared to placebo. However, the authors noted "some evidence of local abnormalities such as instability and reduced range of movement" with NSAID therapy.[54]

For tendon injuries, a review of nine studies of treatment with NSAIDs documented significant pain relief compared to placebo in only five of the studies.[55] In a separate study of Achilles' tendon injury, no benefit to either range of motion or strength was seen following piroxicam therapy.[56] It should be noted that none of these studies involved biopsy of the tendons involved, possibly reflecting the different characteristics of tendonopathy versus tendonitis. For injuries to bone, use of NSAIDs is of concern for two reasons. NSAIDs likely inhibit the production of prostaglandin E_2, a prostaglandin with a known role in bone healing. NSAIDs also inhibit pain, which is a useful marker in recovery from injury, especially stress fracture. One study from the United Kingdom showed that regular use of NSAIDs was associated with a 47% increase in the rate of nonvertebral fractures.[57]

In comparison with acetaminophen, a Cochrane review demonstrated no evidence that NSAIDs are more effective for low back pain.[44] A recent meta-analysis of studies involving patients with osteoarthritis showed NSAIDs were superior to acetaminophen in terms of pain relief, but the better analgesia came at the cost of a significant increase in side effects, with gastrointestinal effects being most common.[58] Therefore, NSAIDs may benefit minor muscle injury, but they appear equivocal at best for ligament and tendon injuries and may hinder healing of more severe muscle and bone injuries. While effective at pain relief, the analgesia of NSAIDs may block an important defense mechanism to further injury and be accompanied by significant side effects.

Cyclooxygenase-2 Inhibitors

The cyclooxygenase-2 (COX-2) enzyme mediates production of prostaglandins involved in tissue inflammation, while prostaglandins that protect the mucosal lining of the gastrointestinal tract are made via COX-1 pathways. NSAIDs are nonspecific in their inhibition of COX-1 and COX-2. Therefore, a new class of medication, COX-2 inhibitors, was designed to specifically target the COX-2 enzyme and improve the side effect profile of earlier NSAIDs. Two studies of ankle sprains in human subjects showed no difference between the COX-2 inhibitor celecoxib and ibuprofen or naproxen with regard to reports of pain or activity levels; celecoxib did outperform placebo therapy. As expected, the gastrointestinal side effects were significantly reduced with COX-2 inhibitor therapy.[59,60]

COX-2 inhibitors have been more prominent in the news in recent months due to an associated risk of thrombotic events with use of rofecoxib. In reviewing the data surrounding this controversy, it is important to remember that COX-2 inhibitors were initially designed for use in patients with rheumatoid arthritis and that studies reflect their use in that population. It has yet to be determined whether the results are generalizable to younger athletes or how this association might affect adults without rheumatoid arthritis but who have significant cardiovascular risk factors and attempt to exercise regularly.

The Vioxx Gastrointestinal Outcomes Research study compared treatment with rofecoxib versus naproxen in patients with rheumatoid arthritis. Rofecoxib successfully decreased serious gastrointestinal events by one half (4% incidence to 2%). However, the incidence of myocardial infarction in users of rofecoxib was 500% higher than among naproxen users.[61] It was initially argued that the difference seen might be attributed to the relatively small number of cardiac events and/or a possible protective effect of naproxen, as COX-1 inhibition can prevent platelet aggregation. More recently, the APPROVe (Adenomatous Polyp Prevention on Vioxx) study was stopped early because an 84% increase in heart attacks and a 390% increase in serious thrombotic events were observed among rofecoxib users.[62] Some researchers believe that this association is due to the inhibition of prostaglandin I_2, which normally blocks platelet aggregation and protects the endothelial surface of blood vessels. Prostaglandin I_2 production was previously believed to be mediated by COX-1, but new research has determined that prostaglandin I_2 is regulated by COX-2. Also concerning was the fact that the APPROVe study was not aimed at patients with rheumatoid arthritis, but was rather a more general study of adult patients. Therefore, this prothrombotic effect may be more generalizable than previously believed, as well as a class effect of COX-2 inhibitors and not specific to rofecoxib.

The Celecoxib Long Term Arthritis Safety study published data showing no increase in cardiovascular risks after 6 months of celecoxib therapy. However, after 12 months of use, a trend toward increased risk of thrombotic events was noted, although the study was not specifically designed to detect this specific risk. Additionally, celecoxib appeared to lose its effectiveness in preventing gastrointestinal side effects in those patients on daily aspirin therapy.[62] Therefore, COX-2 inhibitors possess similar analgesic properties as compared to general NSAIDs, and the improvement in side effect profile of the COX-2 inhibitors seems tenuous when the prothrombotic risks associated with rofecoxib are considered.

Glucosamine

Glucosamine is a popular over-the-counter supplement for osteoarthritis. Most studies support glucosamine as effective in both symptom improvement and prevention of joint space loss.[63-65] One additional study suggests no improvement compared with placebo, but this was an Internet-based survey using only subjective measures of symptoms and function.[66] All the studies cited agree on the relative safety of glucosamine use, at least in the short term. Little can be said for long-term effectiveness or safety of glucosamine beyond 3 years of use. Interestingly, there is some evidence that glucosamine may not prevent flare-ups of osteoarthritis symptoms even after previous improvement with glucosamine.[67] These differences between studies, as well as differences between patients, may exist based on rates of cartilage turnover. Research exists suggesting that high rates of cartilage turnover support a favorable response to glucosamine therapy.[68] Overall, glucosamine appears safe and effective for many with osteoarthritis, and based on population studies, it is considered cost-effective for improving the quality of life of these patients.[69]

SUPPLEMENTS

Dietary supplements grew in popularity in the late 20th century out of a confluence of various motivations, including nutritional improvement, weight control, and performance enhancement.

Many dietary supplements contained ingredients found in other foods and/or medications, yet their production alone or in certain combinations placed them outside of both of these well-regulated categories. In 1994, the U.S. Congress passed the Dietary Supplement Health and Education Act, creating separate regulatory control for the multibillion dollar industry of dietary supplement manufacturing. Unfortunately, as evidenced by the 7-year process that culminated in the 2004 ban on products containing ephedra, the Dietary Supplement Health and Education Act lacks effective means for enforcing production standards and protecting consumers' health.[70] Nevertheless, dietary supplements remain immensely popular among athletes of all ages and skill levels. Physicians should actively inquire as to the use of supplements by their patients and provide appropriate counseling for informed decision making.

Creatine

Creatine is one of the most common nutritional supplements employed for possible ergogenic benefits. The Metzl et al[71] survey of high school students reported use by as many as 44% of high school senior athletes, which parallels estimates of collegiate use. Creatine has become generally accepted to provide benefit in short, maximally anaerobic events, likely through enhancement of adenosine triphosphate regeneration.[72] There is also some evidence suggesting a possible direct effect of creatine on muscle development through increased expression of mRNA and growth factors specific to muscle.[73] Whether by direct effect or through increased capacity for resistance training, creatine has been linked with increases in muscle mass, including by direct measurements such as ultrasonography.[74]

As to the effects of creatine on actual strength and sports performance, the supplement has had mixed results at best. Some authors have demonstrated improvement in short-duration events like repeated sprints,[75] although this has not been reproduced in other trials.[76] Other investigators have shown improvement in specific soccer drills,[77] but again this has not held for studies with athletes from other sports such as rugby or softball.[78,79] Kilduff et al[80] noted that subjects with the largest increases in body mass had the greatest increases in strength, suggesting that there are some athletes who are "responders" to creatine while others are not.

Overall, creatine may have some benefit for short-term bursts of exercise, yet this benefit is highly variable and may not apply to all athletes. Creatine has been linked anecdotally to reports of heat-related illness and renal dysfunction. However, with the brief use of 6 to 12 weeks documented in most trials, creatine has appeared to be relatively safe. With its popularity among young athletes, concern should be given to the possible effects of increased muscle mass on open growth plates, as well as the lack of studies involving long-term use among children and adolescents.

Prohormones

Prohormones such as DHEA (dehydroepiandrosterone) and androstenedione reached a peak in popularity during the 1990s as their use by high-profile athletes became common knowledge. In a survey conducted by the Department of Health and Human Services in 2002, an estimated 2% to 2.5% of high school students reported using androstenedione.[81] Unfortunately, the perceived success of athletes known to use these products has been interpreted by many youths as a cause-and-effect relationship, when medical evidence runs to the contrary.

In his review of the literature, Ahrendt[82] found no published studies that reported ergogenic benefits of DHEA use. In one study, DHEA did increase androgen levels, but there were no increases in strength or lean body mass measurements following resistance training.[83] Similarly, Tokish et al[72] reviewed the literature and found no evidence of ergogenic benefits of androstenedione. In fact, there may be an increased risk of cardiovascular disease with androstenedione use due to decreased high-density lipoprotein levels. Other studies have demonstrated no effect of androstenedione on testosterone levels while increasing estrogen levels in males.[84,85] Conversely, androstenedione has also been linked to elevating testosterone levels in females,[86] suggesting a gender-specific metabolism of these products. Based on the clear estrogenic and androgenic effects of these products in the absence of any reasonable benefits, the U.S. Food and Drug Administration in 2004 issued a summary of the negative effects of androstenedione and a warning to its manufacturers that such products are in violation of the 1994 Dietary Supplement Health and Education Act, and that their production and marketing should cease.[81,87]

Beta-hydroxy-beta-methylbutyrate

Beta-hydroxy-beta-methylbutyrate (HMB) is a relatively new product marketed as an "anti-catabolic" compound. Use of HMB has been associated with increased lean muscle mass and decreased CPK levels after exercise, but the mechanism of these effects is unclear.[72] In a separate study, brief use of HMB did not prevent common effects of exercise such as muscle soreness or swelling.[88] Other studies have shown HMB does not have an androgenic effect nor does it have a significant impact beyond resistance training alone on strength and body composition among athletes.[89–91] Used either alone or with creatine, HMB has not shown ergogenic effects on either aerobic or anaerobic exercise, although one isolated study did demonstrate an increased time to peak lactate production with its use.[92,93] Again, no clear mechanism exists to explain this effect. No major risks have been associated with HMB use. In fact, HMB may impart favorable cardiovascular effects via lipid metabolism.[94] In summary, no clear performance advantage or positive health benefit has been attributed to HMB.

Alpha Agonists

Phenylpropanolamine and pseudoephedrine, both alpha agonists, are commonly found in over-the-counter medications and known for their stimulant effects. In fact, since the U.S. Food and Drug Administration banned dietary supplements containing ephedrine, many manufacturers have replaced ephedrine with a variety of alpha agonist compounds. Numerous studies of the effects of phenylpropanolamine and pseudoephedrine on aerobic and anaerobic exercise have failed to show ergogenic benefits, with no significant benefits to power, work, VO_{2max}, or perceived exhaustion.[95–100] These studies have tended to demonstrate a relatively safe cardiovascular profile, which would parallel the safety of these compounds in over-the-counter medications.[96,98] However, one study has suggested increased heart rate at submaximal exercise levels and prolonged time to heart rate recovery with a common nonprescription dose of pseudoephedrine.[100] An older trial also demonstrated an increased incidence of sinus arrhythmias without complication at maximal over-the-counter dose of pseudoephedrine.[101] Cardiovascular side effects at supratherapeutic doses have not been studied, although these risks persist in theory. However, even at therapeutic doses, phenylpropanolamine and pseudoephedrine are easily detected with blood and urine testing.[99]

Caffeine

Caffeine is perhaps the most popular stimulant used by the general population. Prior to the U.S. Food and Drug Administration ban on products containing ephedrine, products combining caffeine and ephedrine were among the most purchased dietary supplements and weight-control compounds. Accordingly, much of the research into the ergogenic properties of caffeine actually studies combinations of caffeine and ephedrine. With regard to caffeine alone, caffeine is thought to be most beneficial for performance in endurance events, perhaps to enable the "kick" at the end of such an event.[102] The meta-analysis of Doherty and Smith[103] demonstrated caffeine's ergogenic benefits, primarily in studies of endurance exercise and time-to-exhaustion measurements.

The IOC threshold for caffeine, the equivalent of five to six cups of coffee, recognizes that dietary caffeine intake is ubiquitous. A commonly studied dose of 5 mg/kg 1 to 2 hours before exercise falls well below the IOC threshold for caffeine.[102] However, that dose has been shown to decrease ratings of perceived exertion, increase power, and increase time to exhaustion.[104–107] Effects appear to last for as long as 6 hours, but the effects are not enhanced by a second dose.[105] The ergogenic effects are more pronounced in those who do not normally use caffeine,[106] and similar results have been reproduced following as short as 6 days of abstinence from caffeine.[107] Users should consider a recent study suggesting that heavy coffee consumption increased the short-term risk of heart attack and sudden cardiac death regardless of other cardiovascular risk factors.[108] Yet at appropriate doses, caffeine appears to be a relatively safe ergogenic aid for endurance events.

ERGOGENIC DRUGS

Clearly, athletes employ the supplements discussed previously in hopes of gaining an ergogenic benefit. However, this section focuses on drugs with clear ergogenic effects, as well as some that may result in ergolytic effects with long-term use. These drugs are banned by most sports-governing bodies, and most are illegal to obtain except for specific therapeutic purposes. However, these drugs remain relatively easy to procure, they pose significant health risks, and their use jeopardizes fair competition in sports.

Anabolic-Androgenic Steroids

Anabolic-androgenic steroids (AASs) have well-known ergogenic effects, resulting in increased muscle mass and strength. Estimated gains in strength with AAS use range from 5% to 20%, but the doses of AAS used in studies may not match doses of abuse.[109] More recent research has focused on the side effects of AAS use as well as strategies to prevent the use and abuse of AASs, especially among adolescents.

AAS use is known to affect multiple organ systems. Negative effects on lipid profiles, especially decreases in high-density lipoprotein, have been known since the mid-1980s.[110] While cardiac hypertrophy is commonly associated with steroid use, a recent review of the literature provided mixed results regarding this relationship.[111] However, other research suggests that steroids may also cause abnormal left ventricular wall motion in an additive effect to resistance exercise.[112] Steroids also affect red blood cell mass via erythropoietin production, as well as bone metabolism.[109] Research has also explored the effects of AAS use on mental health. While AAS use has been linked with increased levels of aggression and manic behavior, these effects appear to vary greatly among individuals at controlled doses of AASs.[113]

In their survey published in 1998, Faigenbaum et al[114] estimated that nearly 3% of junior high school students had used AASs, with the average user participating in three to four sports.[114] With the frightening thought of the long-term repercussions of AAS use prior to or during puberty, research explored avenues of preventing AAS use among adolescents. The ATLAS study demonstrated rates of AAS use among high school students at 4% to 12%. During the intervention phase, adolescents were less likely to use or intend to use AASs. However, one year after the intervention, rates of actual use did not decline, demonstrating the difficulties in diverting adolescents from using "performance enhancers" such as AASs.[115]

The effects of AASs appear to be dose dependent as well as proportional to the duration of use.[72] Therefore, testing not only plays a role in maintaining fair competition, but it also plays a preventive health role for these athletes. Traditional testing has analyzed the testosterone-to-epitestosterone ratio, with the cutoff ratio of 6 being two to six times greater than normal.[72] However, the emergence of compounds such as tetrahydrogestrinone illustrates the sophistication of doping in sports. Tetrahydrogestrinone was identified thanks to the provision of a sample by a U.S. track coach in 2003. Tetrahydrogestrinone was a completely new compound, as opposed to an older steroid or veterinary medication.[116] In vitro testing showed tetrahydrogestrinone to be highly androgenic but with no estrogenic activity.[117] Tetrahydrogestrinone is a prime example of the need for cooperation among athletes, coaches, and medical professionals to not only police sport but to protect the health of athletes as well.

Human Growth Hormone

Human growth hormone (HGH) has been approved for treatment of persons with endogenous HGH deficiency or short stature secondary to chronic renal failure. Additionally, HGH is used off label for patients with Turner's syndrome and children born small for gestational age who have not had sufficient catch-up growth.[118] However, because of its success in treating these conditions, the abuse of HGH as an ergogenic aid has become widespread as well. In a survey of high school sophomores, Rickert et al[119] found 5% of respondents had used HGH, with a significant association with AAS use as well.

HGH is known to increase uptake of glucose and amino acids by skeletal muscle, increase protein synthesis, increase lipid breakdown, and increase rate of bone growth. At therapeutic doses of HGH, no studies have reported improvement in exercise performance parameters, including work capacity and strength.[118] However, athletes abusing HGH are likely to use doses that surpass the therapeutic range. Known side effects of excess HGH include acromegaly, in which skeletal muscles are weaker. This myopathic effect likely explains the lack of performance enhancement at therapeutic doses. Other side effects of HGH abuse include insulin resistance and cardiomyopathy.[72] Healy et al[120] studied the use of HGH at doses similar to those in anecdotal reports of HGH abusers. While some "positive" effects such as increased protein synthesis and increased lean body mass were demonstrated, adverse effects were also found, including increased fasting insulin levels and increased insulin resistance. Additionally, no changes in body fat or performance parameters were seen after 4 weeks of HGH use.

In addition to the negative health effects of HGH abuse by athletes, Conrad and Potter[121] excellently summarize the ethical dilemma of HGH use for purported antiaging effects and for idiopathic short stature. Consider the potential impact of using HGH for otherwise healthy pediatric patients at the third percentile for growth, resulting in a vicious cycle as the third percentile would then shift higher and higher with time. Equally disturbing would be the treatment of the 5 foot 10 inch high school basketball player in the hopes of reaching 6 feet and the perceived benefits of that difference. These possibilities highlight the need for testing for HGH abuse. Although difficulties in direct testing may exist due to similarities between endogenous and exogenous HGH, research has shown dose-dependent changes in markers of bone turnover that may be used for detection of HGH abuse.[122] Sports-governing bodies must support further efforts to protect the health of their athletes as well as the integrity of their sport.

Erythropoietin

Aerobic performance obviously requires oxygen delivery, and athletes have employed many methods to enhance oxygen delivery. Training at high altitudes to increase oxygen carrying capacity has become commonplace for elite athletes. Blood doping using autologous transfusions is a common illegal practice that continues to be employed, although it is more easily discovered with testing techniques for red blood cell age and requires equipment for storage, processing, and reinfusion.[123]

Erythropoietin (EPO) is the hormone responsible for red blood cell production in the human body. In the late 1980s, recombinant EPO (rEPO) was developed for patients with anemia secondary to chronic renal failure. Subsequently, the use of rEPO has been expanded to include patients with cancer and patients with human immunodeficiency virus.[123] rEPO has been shown to increase hematocrit concentration in as little as 4 weeks, accompanied by significant increases in $\dot{V}O_{2max}$[124,125] and time to exhaustion.[126] However, the mechanism of rEPO's benefits relies on polycythemia with the potential for hyperviscosity.[127] Therefore, the potential side effects of rEPO abuse include heart attack, stroke, and pulmonary embolus. While not linked conclusively, rEPO has been implicated in the deaths of several elite athletes.

Testing for rEPO abuse initially focused on testing serum hematocrit levels, as well as levels of other blood cells that may reflect rEPO use.[128] While generally effective, this method can be avoided by serum dilution with saline infusion. rEPO can be detected by urine or blood electrophoresis, but only if the testing occurs within a few days of rEPO administration.[129] New research suggests that increases in the levels of soluble transferrin receptor occur with rEPO abuse and that this may be used for testing purposes.[124]

Alcohol

Alcohol is the most popular mind-altering substance used. Athletes may use alcohol for an ergogenic benefit, believing that its anxiolytic effects can enhance self-confidence and thereby improve athletic performance.[130] For certain sports, this anxiolytic effect may improve performance by decreasing tremor. Accordingly, the IOC has banned alcohol for fencing and shooting sports. Beyond these sports, however, alcohol tends to have negative impacts on performance, otherwise known as ergolytic effects. The American College of Sports Medicine released a position statement on alcohol use in 1982 citing detrimental psychomotor effects, no benefit to the work of skeletal muscle, decreased ability to control body temperature in cold temperatures, and no positive benefits to cardiopulmonary variables including $\dot{V}O_{2max}$.[131] Since then, further studies have shown actual declines in performance due to acute alcohol ingestion as measured by decreased time to exhaustion,[132] slower distance run times,[133] and slower times on short and middle distance run.[134] The hangover effect of alcohol has also been estimated to decrease aerobic performance by 11%.[135]

Long-term concerns for alcohol use by athletes have centered on the profile of athletes as risk takers. Rates of alcohol abuse by athletes in one survey were 21%, and alcohol abuse was correlated with depression and other mental health symptoms. In a separate survey, drinking to cope with stress had the strongest link with negative consequences of alcohol use, including repercussions on athletes' education, health, legal problems, and involvement in violent acts.[136] A European survey showed that young adults who drank alcohol had a significantly higher risk of sports injury compared to nondrinkers.[137]

Marijuana

Marijuana is the number one illegal drug used in the United States. Its legal status remains controversial, with viewpoints polarized between critics who view marijuana as a possible gateway drug and advocates for its medicinal use for patients undergoing chemotherapy or with acquired immunodeficiency syndrome.[138] For athletes, concern again rises for possible marijuana use among a population of risk takers. In a survey of U.S. high school students, Ewing[139] found that male athletes used marijuana more than their nonathlete peers, but that female athletes used marijuana less than their nonathlete peers. Interestingly, a French study suggests that elite athletic participation by adolescents and young adults has a protective effect against marijuana use.[140]

Marijuana might provide a performance benefit at low doses through relaxation and a possible improvement in auditory and visual perception.[130] However, persistent use of marijuana, which is often accompanied by increased use or abuse due to tolerance, has definite ergolytic effects. THC (delta-9-tetrahydrocannabinol), the active compound in marijuana, causes significant increases in heart rate with either no change or a reduction in stroke volume, as well as an inappropriate chronotropic response to exercise.[141] Decreases in $\dot{V}O_{2max}$ and maximal exercise tolerance have also been demonstrated with long-term marijuana use.[142] Long-term use or abuse of marijuana can lead to an "amotivational syndrome,"[130] from which loss of ambition, poor academic performance, and impaired social relationships can negatively affect athletic, academic, and professional success for athletes at all levels.

Cocaine

Reaching its peak in popularity during the 1980s, the use of cocaine declined during the 1990s. The cardiac risks of cocaine use are well-known, especially following the sudden deaths of high-profile athletes. Yet cocaine continues to be used by an estimated 2% of young adults.[130] While cocaine enhances a sense of euphoria, it has been shown to be definitively ergolytic in animal studies. Cocaine use leads to faster depletion of muscle glycogen stores and lactate accumulation, along with decreased time to exhaustion.[143] Interestingly, South Americans who routinely chew coca leaves were found to have increased plasma levels of free fatty acids, which might allow longer periods of submaximal exercise. However, these persons did not have any increase in maximal exercise capacity or efficiency with chewing coca leaves.[144] Chronic use of crack cocaine has been linked in nonathletes with decreased aerobic capacity and decreased maximal heart rate.[145]

Methamphetamine

Methamphetamine may have replaced cocaine in popularity as an illegal stimulant and euphoric. Methamphetamine is the number one controlled substance produced clandestinely since 1997. Methamphetamine should be considered ergogenic in the same manner as the class of amphetamines and other stimulants, with delayed time to exhaustion and improved ratings of perceived exertion. Its short-term effects include decreased appetite and increased energy, along with increases in heart rate and body temperature. However, long-term use of methamphetamine is directly linked with poor nutrition, fatigue, mental health disturbance, and lasting impairment in cognitive function. As mentioned before with alcohol, use of methamphetamine is also linked to coping with various stressors. Women tend to use methamphetamine for issues such as family/social dysfunction, emotional problems, and weight control. For men, parental use of methamphetamine or other drugs appears to have the strongest gender-specific influence on personal use. Most importantly, methamphetamine's ease of acquisition is the number one factor in its use by all abusers.[146] Athletes should be educated about the long-term debilitating effects of methamphetamine, and drug testing in sports should continue to include screening for amphetamine abuse.

CONCLUSIONS

The lines between treating illness, maximizing health, and sports performance enhancement have been blurred by well-intentioned medical advances and societal pressures that lead athletes of all levels to seek a competitive edge. Unfortunately, for many athletes the inappropriate use of medications, supplements, and other drugs not only damage the image of their sport but also cause significant health consequences that extend well beyond the field of competition. Sports medicine professionals must remain educated regarding the impact of medications, supplements, and ergogenic drugs on both sport performance and, more importantly, the health of the patients whom they serve.

REFERENCES

1. Lively MW: Preparticipation physical examinations: A collegiate experience. Clin J Sport Med 1999;9:3–8.
2. Magill MK, Gunning K, Saffel-Shrier S, Gay C: New developments in the management of hypertension. Am Fam Physician 2003;68:853–858.
3. ALLHAT Officers and Coordinators for the ALLHAT Collaborative Research Group. The Antihypertensive and Lipid-Lowering Treatment to Prevent Heart Attack Trial: Major outcomes in high-risk hypertensive patients randomized to angiotensin-converting enzyme inhibitor or calcium channel blocker vs diuretic: The Antihypertensive and Lipid-Lowering Treatment to Prevent Heart Attack Trial (ALLHAT). JAMA 2002;288:2981–2997. [Published errata in JAMA 2003;289:178 and JAMA 2004;291:2196.]
4. Niedfeldt MW: Managing hypertension in athletes and physically active patients. Am Fam Physician 2002;66:445–452, 457–458.

5. Knopp WD, Wang TW, Bach BR Jr: Ergogenic drugs in sports. Clin Sports Med 1997;16:375–392.

6. Chick TW, Halperin AK, Gacek EM: The effect of antihypertensive medications on exercise performance: A review. Med Sci Sports Exerc 1988;20:447–454.

7. Desai MY, De la Pena-Almaguer E, Mannting F: Abnormal heart rate recovery after exercise as a reflection of an abnormal chronotropic response. Am J Cardiol 2001;87:1164–1169.

8. Diercks DB, Kirk JD, Turnipseed SD, Amsterdam EA: Utility of immediate exercise treadmill testing in patients taking beta blockers or calcium channel blockers. Am J Cardiol 2002;90:882–885.

9. Poulsen SH, Jensen SE, Egstrup K: Improvement of exercise capacity and left ventricular diastolic function with metoprolol XL after acute myocardial infarction. Am Heart J 2000;140:6–11.

10. Wright JT Jr, Bakris G, Greene T, et al, for the African American Study of Kidney Disease and Hypertension Study Group: Effect of blood pressure lowering and antihypertensive drug class on progression of hypertensive kidney disease: Results from the AASK trial. JAMA 2002;288:2421–2431.

11. Thurman JM, Schrier RW: Comparative effects of angiotensin-converting enzyme inhibitors and angiotensin receptor blockers on blood pressure and the kidney. Am J Med 2003;114:588–598.

12. Dahlof B, Devereux RB, Kjeldsen SE, et al: Cardiovascular morbidity and mortality in the Losartan Intervention for Endpoint reduction in hypertension study (LIFE): A randomised trial against atenolol. Lancet 2002;359:995–1003.

13. Opie LH, Schall R. Evidence-based evaluation of calcium channel blockers for hypertension: Equality of mortality and cardiovascular risk relative to conventional therapy. J Am Coll Cardiol 2002;39:315–322. [Published erratum in J Am Coll Cardiol 2002;39:1409–1410.]

14. ALLHAT Collaborative Research Group: Major cardiovascular events in hypertensive patients randomized to doxazosin vs chlorthalidone: The Antihypertensive and Lipid-Lowering Treatment to Prevent Heart Attack Trial (ALLHAT). JAMA 2000;283:1967–1975. [Published erratum in JAMA 2002;288:2976.]

15. Safeer RS, Lacivita CL: Choosing drug therapy for patients with hyperlipidemia. Am Fam Physician 2000;61:3371–3382.

16. Durstine JL, Thompson PD: Exercise in the treatment of lipid disorders. Cardiol Clin 2001;19:471–488.

17. Melin JM, Struble WE, Tipping RW, et al: A Consumer Use Study of Over-the-Counter Lovastatin (CUSTOM). Am J Cardiol 2004;94:1243–1248.

18. Aronow WS, Nayak D, Woodworth S, Ahn C: Effect of simvastatin versus placebo on treadmill exercise time until the onset of intermittent claudication in older patients with peripheral arterial disease at six months and at one year after treatment. Am J Cardiol 2003;92:711–712.

19. Mondillo S, Ballo P, Barbati R, et al: Effects of simvastatin on walking performance and symptoms of intermittent claudication in hypercholesterolemic patients with peripheral vascular disease. Am J Med 2003;114:359–364.

20. Ramires JAF, Sposito AC, Mansur AP, et al: Cholesterol lowering with statins reduces exercise-induced myocardial ischemia in hypercholesterolemic patients with coronary artery disease. Am J Cardiol 2001;88:1134–1138.

21. Storms WW: Review of exercise-induced asthma. Med Sci Sports Exerc 2003;35:1464–1470.

22. Spooner CH, Spooner GR, Rowe BH: Mast-cell stabilising agents to prevent exercise-induced bronchoconstriction. Cochrane Database of Systematic Reviews 2003;4:CD002307.

23. Hancox RJ, Subbarao P, Kamada D, et al: β2-agonist tolerance and exercise-induced bronchospasm. Am J Respir Crit Care Med 2002;165:1068–1070.

24. McKenzie DC, Stewart IB, Fitch KD: The asthmatic athlete, inhaled beta agonists, and performance. Clin J Sport Med 2002;12:225–228.

25. Shapiro GS, Yegen U, Xiang J, et al: A randomized, double-blind, single-dose, crossover clinical trial of the onset and duration of protection from exercise-induced bronchoconstriction by formoterol and albuterol. Clin Ther 2002;24:2077–2087.

26. Richter K, Janicki S, Jorres RA, Magnussen H: Acute protection against exercise-induced bronchoconstriction by formoterol, salmeterol, and terbutaline. Eur Respir J 2002;19:865–871.

27. Stewart IB, Labreche JM, McKenzie DC: Acute formoterol administration has no ergogenic effect in nonasthmatic athletes. Med Sci Sports Exerc 2002;34:213–217.

28. Peroni DG, Piacentini GL, Ress M, et al: Time efficacy of a single dose of montelukast on exercise-induced asthma in children. Pediatr Allergy Immunol 2002;13:434–437.

29. Melo RE, Sole D, Naspitz CK: Exercise-induced bronchoconstriction in children: Montelukast attenuates the immediate-phase and late-phase responses. J Allergy Clin Immunol 2003;111:301–307.

30. Steinshamm S, Sandsund M, Sue-Chu M, Bjermer L: Effects of montelukast on physical performance and exercise economy in adult asthmatics with exercise-induced bronchoconstriction. Scand J Med Sci Sports 2002;12:211–217.

31. Bilici M, Koroglu MA, Cakirbay H, et al: Isokinetic muscle performance in major depressive disorder: Alterations by antidepressant therapy. Int J Neurosci 2001;109:149–164.

32. Masand PS: Weight gain associated with psychotropic drugs. Expert Opin Pharmacother 2000;1:377–389.

33. Coris EE, Ramirez AM, Van Durme DJ: Heat illness in athletes: The dangerous combination of heat, humidity, and exercise. Sports Med 2004;34:9–16.

34. Palmer BF, Gates JR, Lader M: Causes and management of hyponatremia. Ann Pharmacother 2003;37:1694–1702.

35. Grobler LA, Schwellnus MP, Trichard C, et al: Comparative effects of zopiclone and loprazolam on psychomotor and physical performance in active individuals. Clin J Sport Med 2000;10:123–128.

36. Lindqvist A, Jalonen J, Laitinen LA, et al: The effects of midazolam and ephedrine on post-exercise autonomic chronotropic control of the heart in normal subjects. Clin Auton Res 1996;6:343–349.

37. American Psychiatric Association: Diagnostic and Statistical Manual of Mental Disorders, 4th ed. Washington, DC, American Psychiatric Association, 1994.

38. Mazur AF: ADHD exception available. The NCAA News April 12, 2004. Available at www.ncaa.org/news/2004/20040412/active/4108n36.html/.

39. Pascual-Castroviejo I: Attention deficit hyperactivity syndrome and the capacity to practice sports. Rev Neurol 2004;38:1001–1005.

40. Karatekin C, Markiewicz SW, Siegel MA: A preliminary study of motor problems in children with attention-deficit/hyperactivity disorder. Percept Mot Skills 2003;97:1267–1280.

41. Pelham WE Jr, McBurnett K, Harper GW, et al: Methylphenidate and baseball playing in ADHD children: Who's on first? J Consult Clin Psychol 1990;58:130–133.

42. Vickers JN, Rodrigues ST, Brown LN: Gaze pursuit and arm control of adolescent males diagnosed with attention deficit hyperactivity disorder (ADHD) and normal controls: Evidence of a dissociation in processing visual information of short and long duration. J Sports Sci 2002;20:201–216.

43. Trappe TA, Fluckey JD, White F, et al: Skeletal muscle PGF2a and PGE2 in response to eccentric resistance exercise: Influence of ibuprofen and acetaminophen. J Clin Endocrinol Metab 2001;86:5067–5070.

44. Harwood MI, Chang SI: Clinical inquiries. What is the most effective treatment for acute low back pain? J Fam Pract 2002;51:118.

45. Brandt KD: The role of analgesics in the management of osteoarthritis pain. Am J Ther 2000;7:75–90.

46. Bradley JD, Brandt KD, Katz BP, et al: Comparison of an antiinflammatory dose of ibuprofen, an analgesic dose of ibuprofen, and acetaminophen in the treatment of patients with osteoarthritis of the knee. N Engl J Med 1991;325:87–91.

47. Pincus T, Koch G, Lei H, et al: Patient Preference for Placebo, Acetaminophen (Paracetamol) or Celecoxib Efficacy Studies (PACES): Two randomised, double blind, placebo controlled, crossover clinical trials in patients with knee or hip osteoarthritis. Ann Rheum Dis 2004;63:931–939.

48. Warner DC, Schnepf G, Barrett MS, et al: Prevalence, attitudes, and behaviors related to the use of nonsteroidal anti-inflammatory drugs (NSAIDs) in student athletes. J Adolesc Health 2002;30:150–153.

49. Almekinders LC, Gilbert JA: Healing of experimental muscle strains and the effects of nonsteroidal antiinflammatory medication. Am J Sports Med 1986;14:303–308.

50. Mishra DK, Friden J, Schmitz MC, Lieber RL: Anti-inflammatory medication after muscle injury. A treatment resulting in short-term improvement but subsequent loss of muscle function. J Bone Joint Surg Am 1995;77:1510–1519.

51. Dudley GA, Czerkawski J, Meinrod A, et al: Efficacy of naproxen sodium for exercise-induced dysfunction muscle injury and soreness. Clin J Sport Med 1997;7:3–10.

52. Dahners LE, Gilbert JA, Lester GE, et al: The effect of a nonsteroidal antiinflammatory drug on the healing of ligaments. Am J Sports Med 1988;16:641–646.

53. Moorman CT III, Kukreti U, Fenton DC, Belkoff SM: The early effect of ibuprofen on the mechanical properties of healing medial collateral ligament. Am J Sports Med 1999;27:738–741.

54. Slatyer MA, Hensley MJ, Lopert R: A randomized controlled trial of piroxicam in the management of acute ankle sprain in Australian Regular Army recruits. The Kapooka Ankle Sprain Study. Am J Sports Med 1997;25:544–553.

55. Almekinders LC, Temple JD: Etiology, diagnosis, and treatment of tendonitis: An analysis of the literature. Med Sci Sports Exerc 1998;30:1183–1190.

56. Astrom M, Westlin N: No effect of piroxicam on Achilles tendinopathy. A randomized study of 70 patients. Acta Orthop Scand 1992;63:631–634.

57. van Staa TP, Leufkens HG, Cooper C: Use of nonsteroidal anti-inflammatory drugs and risk of fractures. Bone 2000;27:563–568.

58. Zhang W, Jones A, Doherty M: Does paracetamol (acetaminophen) reduce the pain of osteoarthritis? A meta-analysis of randomised controlled trials. Ann Rheum Dis 2004;63:901–907.

59. Ekman EF, Fiechtner JJ, Levy S, Fort JG: Efficacy of celecoxib versus ibuprofen in the treatment of acute pain: A multicenter, double-blind, randomized controlled trial in acute ankle sprain. Am J Orthop 2002;31:445–451.

60. Petrella R, Ekman EF, Schuller R, Fort JG: Efficacy of celecoxib, a COX-2-specific inhibitor, and naproxen in the management of acute ankle sprain: Results of a double-blind, randomized controlled trial. Clin J Sport Med 2004;14:225–231.

61. Bombardier C, Laine L, Reicin A, et al: Comparison of upper gastrointestinal toxicity of rofecoxib and naproxen in patients with rheumatoid arthritis. VIGOR Study Group. N Engl J Med 2000;343:1520–1528.

62. Fitzgerald GA: Coxibs and cardiovascular disease. N Engl J Med 2004;351:1709–1711.

63. Reginster JY, Deroisy R, Rovati LC, et al: Long-term effects of glucosamine sulphate on osteoarthritis progression: A randomised, placebo-controlled clinical trial. Lancet 2001;357:251–256.

64. Pavelka K, Gatterova J, Olejarova M, et al: Glucosamine sulfate use and delay of progression of knee osteoarthritis: A 3-year, randomized, placebo-controlled, double-blind study. Arch Intern Med 2002;162:2113–2123.

65. Bruyere O, Pavelka K, Rovati LC, et al: Glucosamine sulfate reduces osteoarthritis progression in postmenopausal women with knee osteoarthritis: Evidence from two 3-year studies. Menopause 2004;11:138–143.

66. McAlindon T, Formica M, LaValley M, et al: Effectiveness of glucosamine for symptoms of knee osteoarthritis: Results from an Internet-based randomized double-blind controlled trial. Am J Med 2004;117:643–649.

67. Cibere J, Kopec JA, Thorne A, et al: Randomized, double-blind, placebo-controlled glucosamine discontinuation trial in knee osteoarthritis. Arthritis Rheum 2004;51:738–745.

68. Christgau S, Henrotin Y, Tanko LB, et al: Osteoarthritic patients with high cartilage turnover show increased responsiveness to the cartilage protecting effects of glucosamine sulphate. Clin Exp Rheumatol 2004;22:36–42.

69. Segal L, Day SE, Chapman AB, Osborne RH: Can we reduce disease burden from osteoarthritis? Med J Aust 2004;180:S11–S17.

70. Phillips GC: Medicolegal issues and ergogenic AIDS: Trade, tragedy, and public safety, the example of ephedra and the dietary supplement health and education act. Curr Sports Med Rep 2004;3:224–228.

71. Metzl JD, Small E, Levine SR, Gershel JC: Creatine use among young athletes. Pediatrics 2001;108:421–425.

72. Tokish JM, Kocher MS, Hawkins RJ: Ergogenic aids: A review of basic science, performance, side effects, and status in sports. Am J Sports Med 2004;32:1543–1553.

73. Willoughby DS, Rosene JM: Effects of oral creatine and resistance training on myogenic regulatory factor expression. Med Sci Sports Exerc 2003;35:923–929.

74. Chilibeck PD, Stride D, Farthing JP, Burke DG: Effect of creatine ingestion after exercise on muscle thickness in males and females. Med Sci Sports Exerc 2004;36:1781–1788.

75. Mujika I, Padilla S, Ibanez J, et al: Creatine supplementation and sprint performance in soccer players. Med Sci Sports Exerc 2000;32:518–525.

76. Redondo DR, Dowling EA, Graham BL, et al: The effect of oral creatine monohydrate supplementation on running velocity. Int J Sport Nutr 1996;6:213–221.

77. Ostojic SM: Creatine supplementation in young soccer players. Int J Sport Nutr Exerc Metab 2004;14:95–103.

78. Ahmun RP, Tong RJ, Grimshaw PN: The effects of acute creatine supplementation on multiple sprint cycling and running performance in rugby players. J Strength Cond Res 2005;19:92–97.

79. Ayoama R, Hiruma E, Sasaki H: Effects of creatine loading on muscular strength and endurance of female softball players. J Sports Med Phys Fitness 2003;43:481–487.

80. Kilduff LP, Pitsiladis YP, Tasker L, et al: Effects of creatine on body composition and strength gains after 4 weeks of resistance training in previously nonresistance-trained humans. Int J Sport Nutr Exerc Metab 2003;13:504–520.

81. HHS launches crackdown on products containing andro: FDA warns manufacturers to stop distributing such products. U.S. Dept. of Health and Human Services, March 11, 2004. Available at www.fda.gov/bbs/topics/news/2004/hhs_031104.html/.

82. Ahrendt DM: Ergogenic aids: Counseling the athlete. Am Fam Physician 2001;63:913–922.

83. Brown GA, Vukovich MD, Sharp RL, et al: Effect of oral DHEA on serum testosterone and adaptations to resistance training in young men. J Appl Physiol 1999;87:2274–2283.

84. King DS, Sharp RL, Vukovich MD, et al: Effect of oral androstenedione on serum testosterone and adaptations to resistance training in young men: A randomized controlled trial. JAMA 1999;281:2020–2028.

85. Leder BZ, Longcope C, Catlin DH, et al: Oral androstenedione administration and serum testosterone concentrations in young men. JAMA 2000;283:779–782.

86. Leder BZ, Leblanc KM, Longcope C, et al: Effects of oral androstenedione administration on serum testosterone and estradiol levels in postmenopausal women. J Clin Endocrinol Metab 2002;87:5449–5454.

87. FDA White Paper: Health Effects of Androstenedione. U.S. Food and Drug Administration, March 11, 2004. Available at www.fda.gov/oc/whitepapers/andro.html/.

88. Paddon-Jones D, Keech A, Jenkins D: Short-term beta-hydroxy-beta-methylbutyrate supplementation does not reduce symptoms of eccentric muscle damage. Int J Sport Nutr Exerc Metab 2001;11:442–450.

89. Slater GJ, Logan PA, Boston T, et al: Beta-hydroxy beta-methylbutyrate (HMB) supplementation does not influence the urinary testosterone: Epitestosterone ratio in healthy males. J Sci Med Sport 2000;3:79–83.

90. Ransone J, Neighbors K, Lefavi R, Chromiak J: The effect of beta-hydroxy beta-methylbutyrate on muscular strength and body composition in collegiate football players. J Strength Cond Res 2003;17:34–39.

91. Slater G, Jenkins D, Logan P, et al: Beta-hydroxy-beta-methylbutyrate (HMB) supplementation does not affect changes in strength or body composition during resistance training in trained men. Int J Sport Nutr Exerc Metab 2001;11:384–396.

92. O'Connor DM, Crowe MJ: Effects of beta-hydroxy-beta-methylbutyrate and creatine monohydrate supplementation on the aerobic and anaerobic capacity of highly trained athletes. J Sports Med Phys Fitness 2003;43:64–68.

93. Vukovich MD, Dreifort GD: Effect of beta-hydroxy beta-methylbutyrate on the onset of blood lactate accumulation and VO2 peak in endurance-trained cyclists. J Strength Cond Res 2001;15:491–497.

94. Nissen S, Sharp RL, Panton L, et al: β-Hydroxy-β-methylbutyrate (HMB) supplementation in humans is safe and may decrease cardiovascular risk factors. J Nutr 2000;130:1937–1945.

95. Hodges AN, Lynn BM, Bula JE, et al: Effects of pseudoephedrine on maximal cycling power and submaximal cycling efficiency. Med Sci Sports Exerc 2003;35:1316–1319.

96. Chester N, Reilly T, Mottram DR: Physiological, subjective and performance effects of pseudoephedrine and phenylpropanolamine during endurance running exercise. Int J Sports Med 2003;24:3–8.

97. Chu KS, Doherty TJ, Parise G, et al: A moderate dose of pseudoephedrine does not alter muscle contraction strength or anaerobic power. Clin J Sport Med 2002;12:387–390.

98. Swain RA, Harsha DM, Baenziger J, Saywell RM Jr: Do pseudoephedrine or phenylpropanolamine improve maximum oxygen uptake and time to exhaustion? Clin J Sport Med 1997;7:168–173.

99. Gillies H, Derman WE, Noakes TD, et al:. Pseudoephedrine is without ergogenic effects during prolonged exercise. J Appl Physiol 1996;81:2611–2617.

100. Clemons JM, Crosby SL: Cardiopulmonary and subjective effects of a 60 mg dose of pseudoephedrine on graded treadmill exercise. J Sports Med Phys Fitness 1993;33:405–412.

101. Bright TP, Sandage BW Jr, Fletcher HP: Selected cardiac and metabolic responses to pseudoephedrine with exercise. Clin Pharmacol 1981;21:488–492.

102. Schwenk TL, Costley CD: When food becomes a drug: Nonanabolic nutritional supplement use in athletes. Am J Sports Med 2002;30:907–916.

103. Doherty M, Smith PM: Effects of caffeine ingestion on exercise testing: A meta-analysis. Int J Sport Nutr Exerc Metab 2004;14:626–646.

104. Doherty M, Smith P, Hughes M, Davison R: Caffeine lowers perceptual response and increases power output during high-intensity cycling. J Sports Sci 2004;22:637–643.

105. Bell DG, McLellan TM: Effect of repeated caffeine ingestion on repeated exhaustive exercise endurance. Med Sci Sports Exerc 2003;35:1348–1354.

106. Bell DG, McLellan TM: Exercise endurance 1, 3, and 6 h after caffeine ingestion in caffeine users and nonusers. J Appl Physiol 2002;93:1227–1234.

107. Doherty M, Smith PM, Davison RC, Hughes MG: Caffeine is ergogenic after supplementation of oral creatine monohydrate. Med Sci Sports Exerc 2002;34:1785–1792.

108. Happonen P, Voutilainen S, Salonen JT: Coffee drinking is dose-dependently related to the risk of acute coronary events in middle-aged men. J Nutr 2004;134:2381–2386.

109. Hartgens F, Kuipers H: Effects of androgenic-anabolic steroids in athletes. Sports Med 2004;34:513–554.

110. Hurley BF, Seals DR, Hagberg JM, et al: High-density-lipoprotein cholesterol in bodybuilders v powerlifters. Negative effects of androgen use. JAMA 1984;252:507–513.

111. Joyner MJ: Designer doping. Exerc Sport Sci Rev 2004;32:81–82.

112. Climstein M, O'Shea P, Adams KJ, DeBeliso M: The effects of anabolic-androgenic steroids upon resting and peak exercise left ventricular heart wall motion kinetics in male strength and power athletes. J Sci Med Sport 2003;6:387–397.

113. Pope HG Jr, Kouri EM, Hudson JI: Effects of supraphysiologic doses of testosterone on mood and aggression in normal men: A randomized controlled trial. Arch Gen Psychiatry 2000;57:133–140.

114. Faigenbaum AD, Zaichkowsky LD, Gardner DE, Micheli LJ: Anabolic steroid use by male and female middle school students. Pediatrics 1998;101:E6.

115. Goldberg L, MacKinnon DP, Elliot DL, et al: The adolescents training and learning to avoid steroids program: Preventing drug use and promoting health behaviors. Arch Pediatr Adolesc Med 2000;154:332–338.

116. Catlin DH, Sekera MH, Ahrens BD, et al: Tetrahydrogestrinone: Discovery, synthesis, and detection in urine. Rapid Commun Mass Spectrom 2004;18:1245–1249.

117. Death AK, McGrath KC, Kazlauskas R, Handelsman DJ: Tetrahydrogestrinone is a potent androgen and progestin. J Clin Endocrinol Metab 2004;89:2498–2500.

118. Stacy JJ, Terrell TR, Armsey TD: Ergogenic AIDS: Human growth hormone. Curr Sports Med Rep 2004;3:229–233.

119. Rickert VI, Pawlak-Morello C, Sheppard V, Jay MS: Human growth hormone: A new substance of abuse among adolescents? Clin Pediatr (Phila) 1992;31:723–726.

120. Healy ML, Gibney J, Russell-Jones DL, et al: High dose growth hormone exerts an anabolic effect at rest and during exercise in endurance-trained athletes. J Clin Endocrinol Metab 2003;88:5221–5226.

121. Conrad P, Potter D: Human growth hormone and the temptations of biomedical enhancement. Soc Health Illn 2004;26:184–215.

122. Longobardi S, Keay N, Ehrnborg C, et al: Growth hormone (GH) effects on bone and collagen turnover in healthy adults and its potential as a marker of GH abuse in sports: A double blind, placebo-controlled study. The GH-2000 Study Group. J Clin Endocrinol Metab 2000;85:1505–1512.

123. Scott J, Phillips GC: Erythropoietin in sports: A new look at an old problem. Curr Sports Med Rep 2005;4:224–226.

124. Birkeland KI, Stray-Gundersen J, Hemmersbach P, et al: Effect of rhEPO administration on serum levels of sTfR and cycling performance. Med Sci Sports Exerc 2000;32:1238–1243.

125. Lundin AP, Akerman MJ, Chesler RM, et al: Exercise in hemodialysis patients after treatment with recombinant human erythropoietin. Nephron 1991;58:315–319.

126. Ekblom B, Berglund B: Effect of erythropoietin administration on maximal aerobic power. Scand J Med Sci Sports 1991;1:88–93.

127. Denker B: Erythropoietin: From bench to bedside. Nephrol Rounds 2004;2.3 www.nephrologyrounds.org/

128. Pascual JA, Belalcazar V, de Bolos C, et al: Recombinant erythropoietin and analogues: A challenge for doping control. Ther Drug Monit 2004;26:175–179.

129. Wide L, Bengtsson C, Berglund B, Ekblom B: Detection in blood and urine of recombinant erythropoietin administered to healthy men. Med Sci Sports Exerc 1995;27:1569–1576.

130. Iven VG: Recreational drugs. Clin Sports Med 1998;17:245–259.

131. The use of alcohol in sports. American College of Sports Medicine Position Stand. Med Sci Sports Exerc 1982;14:ix–xi.

132. Bond V, Franks BD, Howley ET: Effects of small and moderate doses of alcohol on submaximal cardiorespiratory function, perceived exertion and endurance performance in abstainers and moderate drinkers. J Sports Med Phys Fitness 1983;23:221–228.

133. Houmard JA, Langenfeld ME, Wiley RL, Siefert J: Effects of the acute ingestion of small amounts of alcohol upon 5-mile run times. J Sports Med Phys Fitness 1987;27:253–257.

134. McNaughton L, Preece D: Alcohol and its effects on sprint and middle distance running. Br J Sports Med 1986;20:56–59.

135. O'Brien CP: Alcohol and sport. Impact of social drinking on recreational and competitive sports performance. Sports Med 1993;15:71–77.

136. Martens MP, Cox RH, Beck NC: Negative consequences of intercollegiate athlete drinking: The role of drinking motives. J Stud Alcohol 2003;64:825–828.

137. O'Brien CP, Lyons F: Alcohol and the athlete. Sports Med 2000;29:295–300.

138. Campos DR, Yonamine M, de Moraes Moreau RL: Marijuana as doping in sports. Sports Med 2003;33:395–399.

139. Ewing BT: High school athletes and marijuana use. J Drug Educ 1998;28:147–157.

140. Peretti-Watel P, Guagliardo V, Verger P, et al: Sporting activity and drug use: Alcohol, cigarette and cannabis use among elite student athletes. Addiction 2003;98:1249–1256.

141. Sidney S: Cardiovascular consequences of marijuana use. J Clin Pharmacol 2002;42(11 suppl):64S–70S.

142. Renaud AM, Cormier Y: Acute effects of marihuana smoking on maximal exercise performance. Med Sci Sports Exerc 1986;18:685–689.

143. Braiden RW, Fellingham GW, Conlee RK: Effects of cocaine on glycogen metabolism and endurance during high intensity exercise. Med Sci Sports Exerc 1994;26:695–700.

144. Spielvogel H, Caceres E, Koubi H, et al: Effects of coca chewing on metabolic and hormonal changes during graded incremental exercise to maximum. J Appl Physiol 1996;80:643–649.

145. Marques-Magallanes JA, Koyal SN, Cooper CB, et al: Impact of habitual cocaine smoking on the physiologic response to maximum exercise. Chest 1997;112:1008–1016.

146. Cretzmeyer M, Sarrazin MV, Huber DL, et al: Treatment of methamphetamine abuse: Research findings and clinical directions. J Subst Abuse Treat 2003;24:267–277.

Environmental Stressors

Richard Rodenberg and Kyle Parish

In This Chapter

INTRODUCTION

- As the new breed of endurance athletes and adventure seekers push the limits of human endurance in extreme environments and competitions, health care professionals must strive to better understand the demands placed on human physiology by these extreme conditions.

- Early recognition and treatment of heatstroke is imperative.

- The best treatment for heat illness is prevention.

- Hypothermia may be treated with passive or active rewarming.

- Recommendation for rewarming of frostbite injury is a water bath at 40° to 42°C.

- High-altitude illnesses include acute mountain sickness, high-altitude pulmonary edema, and high-altitude cerebral edema.

HEAT ILLNESS

Every summer the topic of heat illness gains increased press in the news headlines. Much of this press is related to the fact that heatstroke is the third most common cause of exercise-related death in U.S. high schools, following head injuries and cardiac disorders.[1]

With the increasing popularity of endurance and ultra-endurance competitions (marathons, ultra-marathons, and triathlons), our understanding of exercise-associated collapse (EAC) falls into question. No longer can an athlete who collapses during endurance competitions, in heat-related conditions, be simply diagnosed as a casualty of heat-related exertion. The mechanisms of collapse can be very different when comparing this new endurance athlete and the classic high school or collegiate competitor. Treatment of athletic populations that exercise in heat-related conditions requires medical personnel to have a thorough understanding of thermoregulatory physiology, dehydration in athletics, populations at risk of heat illness,

and treatment of the various heat-related illnesses. At the same time, one must be able to keenly and astutely recognize and treat the athlete affected by other conditions surrounding EAC.[2]

Thermoregulation is normally a highly efficient process. Normal core body temperature, as regulated by the hypothalamus, varies based on environmental climate and internal metabolic function associated with work-related activity. It is estimated that there is only a 1°C change in core temperature for every 25° to 30°C change in ambient temperature.[3,4] It is thought that for every 0.6°C increase in core temperature, there is a 10% elevation in the basal metabolic rate.[3] Muscle contraction is an inefficient process, allowing only 20% to 25% of the energy sources converted to muscle activity to be converted into work.[1,5] The hypothalamus regulates the parasympathetic nervous system, which controls sweating, and the sympathetic nervous system, which regulates skin blood flow and vasodilatation for heat dissipation.[3,4] There are many conditions, including chronic disease states and pre-existing conditions, medications, and poor physical conditioning, that can impair the body's normal mechanisms for dissipating ambient temperature (Table 6-1). Ambient temperature is related to environmental factors such as clothing, temperature, and humidity.[3]

In addition to the previously mentioned conditions for impaired heat dissipation, there are known differences in heat dissipation between children, adults, and elderly and between females and males. It is known that children are at a greater disadvantage when exercising in the heat compared to adults secondary to the following factors: (1) children produce more heat relative to body mass for the same exercise,[1,3,5,6] (2) children are less efficient in dissipating heat secondary to a larger body surface area,[1,3,5,6] (3) children have a lower sweating rate,[1,5,6] (4) the sweating threshold is increased in children,[6] (5) composition of sweat is different in children compared to adolescents,[6] (6) children develop higher body temperatures with the same amount of dehydration,[1,3,5,6] and (7) overall cardiac output per unit of oxygen uptake is lower in children.[6] The practical implication is that children have a slower rate of acclimation to heat (2 weeks in children compared to 1 week in young adults).[1,3,5,6] Transition to an adult pattern of sweating and sweat composition occurs in early puberty.[6] It is also known that elderly individuals, like children, have a lower sweat rate compared to young adults.[7] Elderly individuals are afflicted with more chronic medical conditions that impair the body's ability to dissipate heat. These chronic medical conditions are often also treated with many of the medications that decrease the body's ability to dissipate heat.[3]

There are four mechanisms by which the body regulates excessive heat accumulation. These same four mechanisms of heat dispersion are at work during activity in the cold environ-

Table 6-1 Predisposing Conditions and Medications for Heat Illness
Conditions
Recent or current illness
Febrile state
Chronic illnesses   DM, CHF, CF, sweating inefficiency syndromes
Mental retardation
Anorexia/Bulemia
Previous episode of heat illness
Poorly conditioned athlete
Certain medications
Age
Medications

Sympathomimetics
  Amphetamines
  Epinephrine
  Ephedrine
  Cocaine
  Norepinephrine

Anticholinergics
  Atropine sulfate
  Scopolamine
  Bentropine
  Belladona and synthetic alkaloids
  Antihistamines

Diuretics
  Furosemide
  Hydrochlorothiazide
  Bumetanide

Phenothiazines
  Prochloroperazine
  Chlorpromazine
  Promethazine

Butyrophenones   Haloperidol

Cyclic antidepressants
  Amitriptyline
  Imipramine
  Nortriptyline
  Protriptyline

Monoamine oxidase inhibitors
  Phenelzine
  Tranlcypromine sulfate

Alcohol
Lysergic acid diethlamide
Lithium
Multiple supplement medications (i.e., herbal)

Dehydration interferes with the evaporative process, resulting in decreased blood volume, stroke volume, and cardiac output. The body responds to this assault with protective mechanisms. The body's first response is with vasoconstriction, preferentially shunting blood to vital organs and away from the muscles (where it picks up heat), skin, and sweat glands (where it is dissipated by the previously mentioned mechanisms). The body is then overwhelmed with decreased sweat production in the face of a rising body temperature.[9] This adaptive response is particularly applicable when explaining the contribution dehydration makes in at-risk and/or unacclimated populations. However, some researchers believe that evidence-based medicine does not support the assumption that dehydration is the sole underlying cause of heat illness or EAC in acclimated and endurance trained athletes. The study of Wyndham and Strydom[10] in 1969 forced the athletic community to recognize the dangers of dehydration, but may have led to the popular belief that everyone who collapses in heat, during exercise, must have dehydration-induced heat illness.[9-11] Noakes points out that dehydration is just one factor contributing to increased body temperature; metabolic rate is the major determinant during exercise in endurance athletes.[9,11] Through his own research, Noakes stresses that no published data show that an acclimated endurance athlete afflicted with heat illness is more dehydrated than those who complete the same race with normal body temperature.[11] In a study looking at impaired high-intensity cycling performance time at low levels of dehydration, Walsh et al[12] were able to show that fluid ingestion may enhance performance time to exhaustion by changes in unexplained psychological factors, as opposed to measurable differences in physiologic factors (rectal or skin temperature, heart rate, oxygen consumption, plasma electrolyte concentrations, plasma volume changes, sweat rate, or leg muscle power). Also, dehydration was not found to affect leg muscle power, correlating with previous studies documenting dehydration causing up to a 7% decrease in body mass does not impair strength or muscular force generation. This study supports replacement of fluid losses, in exercise lasting longer than 60 minutes, to prevent impairment of exercise performance, not prevention of heat illness in endurance athletes.[12]

Heat cramps are painful muscle spasms that commonly affect abdominal or calf muscles.[2,3] Historically, it has been thought that since this condition is usually associated with physically fit individuals exercising in excessive heat, the condition was secondary to severe dehydration, large sodium chloride losses, and muscle fatigue.[2,11]

There are few data to support the belief that heat cramps are caused by dehydration or excessive electrolyte losses during exercise. In fact, cramps can occur at rest or during or after exercise in a variety of environmental conditions.[11] Clinicians have advocated many methods for treating and preventing heat cramps including salt replacement, IV fluid administration, muscle massage and stretching, and even use of IV benzodiazepines. Keep in mind that most of the information on preventing heat cramps is more anecdotal than scientific and based on the experience of individual practitioners.[2,13] Until further research distinguishes the inherent mechanism of muscle cramping during exercise, recommendations for prevention of cramps include stretching, adequate hydration, and maintaining a high level of physical fitness.[2]

The classic definition of heat exhaustion is a core body temperature greater than 38°C (100.4°F) but below the cutoff for heatstroke (40°C or 104°F), associated with tachycardia and

ment. The mechanisms consist of conduction (heat transfer by direct contact), convection (heat transfer by movement such as air current over the body), radiation/infrared dissipation (heat transfer to the environment), and evaporation (heat transfer through the loss of water vapor from the skin and airway).[3,8] Evaporation plays the major role in the body's ability to dissipate heat when the ambient temperature is above 20°C (68°F).[3]

postural hypotension. Signs and symptoms of heat exhaustion include nausea/vomiting, headache, malaise, myalgia, lightheadedness, irritability, or confusion. Many believe that heat exhaustion is a more mild form or precursor to heatstroke, which mani-fests as the core body temperature elevates above 40°C (104°F) with more severe manifestations of shock and cognitive dysfunction (delirium, obtundation, coma, or seizures). Popular thought has upheld the notion that heat exhaustion can precede heatstroke.[2,3,11,13] As in heat cramps, dehydration has been traditionally reported as the underlying mechanism for the development of heat exhaustion and heatstroke. However, studies have shown that rectal temperatures are not abnormally elevated in all individuals with symptoms of heat exhaustion, nor is there published evidence supporting the notion that individuals with heat exhaustion will progress to heatstroke if left untreated. Based on experience in treating collapsed athletes in endurance running events, there has been no evidence that collapsed athletes are more dehydrated or hyperthermic compared to their well counterparts.[2,11,14,15] In fact, rectal temperatures in excess of 40°C (104°F) are commonly found in asymptomatic subjects performing exercise of moderate to high intensity.[15]

Based on the preceding discrepancies, the term heat exhaustion has been called into question. The term heat exhaustion and the traditional association with dehydration and hyperthermia may be more appropriately applied to unacclimated individuals, children, elderly, and individuals with pre-existing medical conditions that may predispose themselves to heat illness. A more appropriate term, when discussing the new breed of endurance athlete, would be EAC. EAC does not include cardiovascular collapse, chest pain, insulin reaction/hypoglycemia, seizures, or other readily identifiable medical conditions.[2,16] EAC is not a diagnosis but instead describes a main complaint characterized by the inability to stand or walk unaided as a result of lightheadedness, faintness, dizziness, or syncope in association with a constellation of symptoms such as exhaustion, nausea, cramps, and normal, low, or high body temperatures.[2,15,17] The cause of EAC has yet to be determined. Recent thought points to postural blood pressure changes as the main cause of EAC. Cessation of exercise causes inactivation of the muscle pump resulting in pooling of large amounts of blood volume in the lower extremities and pelvis leading to circulatory collapse and syncope.[15] A number of other factors, such as a lack of a readily available energy source, temporary dysfunction of the central nervous system or temperature-regulating system, excessive racing effort, mild dehydration, and training-induced reduction in the vasoconstrictor response to any hypotensive stress may contribute to EAC.[2,15,16]

It is important to recognize the two categories of heatstroke: classic and exertional. Classic heatstroke affects individuals at the extremes of age or with chronic medical conditions in hot conditions. The triad of classic heatstroke consists of hyperpyrexia, anhidrosis, and mental status changes. Classic heatstroke is the result of an exogenous heat load overwhelming the body's ability to cope with it. In exertional heatstroke, which affects laborers and athletes, the exogenous heat load combined with the endogenous heat load, overwhelms the body's ability to dissipate heat. The key difference between classic and exertional heatstroke is the lack of anhidrosis. In exertional heatstroke, the majority of people will continue to sweat.[2,3,18]

There are no data that endurance athletes afflicted with exertional heatstroke are more dehydrated than those athletes who complete a race with normal body temperature. Many athletes dehydrate during endurance competitions but do not collapse.[11,19] Because of the rarity of heatstroke in endurance and ultra-endurance events, it has been proposed that there could be an acquired, genetic condition triggered by intense exercise such as malignant hyperthermia, which predisposes individuals to heatstroke.[11,19] Clinical in vitro testing of people at risk of malignant hyperthermia is not practical secondary to cost and low specificity; making it difficult to confirm this theory. More study is required to confirm the genetic correlate between theses two disease processes.[20]

It is imperative that heatstroke be recognized and treated promptly, as morbidity is directly proportional to peak core temperature and length of time spent in the hyperthermic state.[2,17,18] With prompt and proper treatment, the survival rate has increased significantly.[2,3,18] Persistent hyperthermia can lead to cellular damage and end organ failure in the form of cardiac myocyte damage, hepatic necrosis, rhabdomyolysis, disseminated intravascular coagulation, adult respiratory distress syndrome, renal failure, and seizures.[18] Immediate cooling to 38°C should be instituted when an athlete with an elevated temperature and mental status changes is encountered. Rapid reduction in body temperature reverses peripheral vasodilatation and restores central circulation, with a decrease in heart rate and increases in central volume, stroke volume, and blood pressure, thereby improving the prognosis.[17,21] The most effective cooling method proven in endurance athletes with heatstroke consists of immersing the athlete in an ice bath for 5 to 10 minutes. This method induces cooling at a rate of 1°C/min (1.8°F/min). It is imperative to watch for hypothermia. Because rectal temperatures lag behind esophageal (core) temperature, cooling should be terminated before the rectal temperature reaches normal body temperature. Shivering is an indication that the core temperature has decreased to 37°C (98.6°F).[17,21] The sidelines of high school or collegiate sports are not always comparative to the medical tents at endurance events and ice baths are not always available. The medical provider should first evaluate the ABCs (airway, breathing, circulation) and immediately move the athlete to a cool environment. As much as possible, the athlete's clothing should be removed and ice packs placed in areas of high heat dissipation (neck, axilla, and groin). Emergency medical services should be contacted and the athlete sprayed with cool water, while fanning to promote evaporative heat loss.[3,18]

For a comprehensive management plan for dealing with the collapsed athlete, the reader is referred to the proposal of Holzthausen and Noakes[17] for dealing with the collapsed athlete based on years of experience in managing competitive ultra-endurance events in South Africa. Their approach applies an evidence-based, rapid, and comprehensive means of assessing and treating athletes for common conditions who collapse during and after endurance events. The approach highlights pitfalls, such as knee jerk administration of IV fluids, which could exacerbate symptomatic hyponatremia in these athletes. As discussed earlier, with the emergence of the new breed of endurance athlete, the clinician needs to be aware of his or her patient population. The concerns in high school or collegiate athletes may not be the same as in the endurance athlete. The younger and less acclimated athlete is more apt to suffer from dehydration and hyperthermia.

The best treatment for heat illness is prevention. Because high humidity reduces the rate of evaporation and heat dissipation, exercise in hot and humid environments should be avoided based on using available objective measures of heat stress, the Wet Bulb Globe Temperature Index and Heat Index Chart. The Heat Index Chart takes into account air temperature and relative humidity and is the most economical means for assessing heat stress. [1,3,18] A copy of this chart can easily be obtained through the National Weather Service (www.weather.noaa.gov/). Prevention may require practicing/competing in the early morning or later in the evening when heat and humidity have decreased. Athletes should be acclimated to a warm environment and wear attire appropriate for exercise in heat. Any pre-existing condition should be treated prior to beginning any exercise program in the heat. There should be liberal use of fluids during practice and competition at regular intervals and when the athlete is thirsty. [1,3,18] Fluid hydration begins prior to exercising by incorporating a balanced diet into a healthy lifestyle and adequately hydrating. [1,22] Ingested fluids should be cooler than ambient temperature (15° to 22°C [59° to 72°F]). Flavoring the fluid can enhance palatability. [22] For endurance events lasting longer than 1 hour, it may be appropriate to add carbohydrates (4% to 8%) and electrolytes to fluid-replacement solutions. [22]

There are few studies documenting strategies for an athlete to return to competition following an episode of heat illness. Our best information comes from military studies involving soldiers collapsing from exertional heat illness. One study advocates exercise tolerance testing in soldiers 6 to 8 weeks after an initial event. [20] Another study showed weak and inconsistent associations between initial episodes of exertional heat illness and future hospitalization or recurrence of heat illness. [23]

HYPOTHERMIA

The classic definition of hypothermia is a decrease in core body temperature to less than 35°C (95°F). This develops when the rate of heat loss in an individual exceeds the rate at which the body can produce heat[24] and when the ambient temperature is less than the body's core temperature. [8] Classification is based on both cause and clinical severity. Primary, or accidental, hypothermia is what occurs in an otherwise healthy individual and is simply due to environmental exposure. Secondary hypothermia occurs in the face of a specific systemic disease or condition that may predispose one to heat loss. [25–27] Other classifications include acute versus chronic and immersion versus nonimmersion.

It is difficult to determine the exact worldwide incidence of hypothermia since it can be both a symptom as well as a disease entity. Deaths from secondary hypothermia are often considered as a natural complication of the underlying disease and often underreported. From the epidemiologic data that are available, the average annual incidence of fatal hypothermia in the United States during a 16-year period following 1979 was less than 750, and over half of these occurrences were in people older than the age of 65 years. [26] Mortality depends on the severity of hypothermia. An average 1.8% increase in mortality rate for every 1°C (1.8°F) drop in temperature has been reported and overall mortality is around 17%. [25] In the world of sports, the athletes most at risk tend to participate in outdoor or aquatic activities, such as skiing, mountaineering, snowmobiling, river rafting, and swimming.

The same four mechanisms of heat dispersion are at work during activity in cold environment as were discussed in the section on heat exposure. When the body cannot maintain heat production to match these four mechanisms, an individual is at risk of hypothermia. [8]

Hypothermia has an effect on multiple body systems including the central nervous, cardiovascular, renal, endocrine, respiratory, gastrointestinal, hematologic, and muscular. [28] This is due to a progressive metabolic depression in each system. [27] The clin-

ical presentation and associated pathology therefore vary based on the severity of the core temperature reduction. Based on that fact, hypothermia can be further classified into mild, moderate, and severe.

Mild hypothermia is defined as core temperature between 32°C (90°F) and 35°C (95°F). Patients in this temperature range generally exhibit pale, cool skin due to maximal vasoconstriction of the peripheral vessels. Uncontrollable shivering and varying degrees of alterations of mental status, such as confusion, amnesia, apathy, and impaired judgment, are usually present. [25,27,29] Tachycardia and hypertension may be present, but generally the cardiovascular system is stable. [25,28] A "cold diuresis" usually occurs at this stage of hypothermia. It is due to several mechanisms, including a defect in distal tubular sodium and water reabsorption, an increase in catecholamines, cold-induced glucosuria, and increases in glomerular filtration rate from the increase in cardiac output. [27,28] Neuromuscular effects include hypertonicity, ataxia, dysarthria, and deterioration of fine motor skills. [25,27]

More serious and life threatening, moderate hypothermia occurs when the core body temperature of an individual falls between 28°C (82°F) and 32°C (90°F). Within this temperature range, the body loses its ability to generate heat, becoming poikilothermic. [25] Reflexive shivering ceases and muscles become rigid. The central nervous system function declines precipitously. Pupillary dilation, decline in the level of consciousness to stupor or coma, hyporeflexia, paradoxical undressing, and hallucinations may all be present. Vital signs are also profoundly affected. Cardiovascularly, the cardiac cycle slows with prolongation of PR, QRS, and QT intervals. [8,25,27] On electrocardiography, the pathognomonic Osborn or J wave may also be present. These are thought to be due to a disturbance in ion fluxes that results in a late depolarization or an early repolarization of the left ventricle. [26] The result of all these effects is bradycardia and hypotension from a decrease in cardiac output. [9,27] The myocardium also becomes sensitive to minor insults and, as a result, is more susceptible to atrial or ventricular arrhythmias. [27,29] The respiratory system slows its normal function. Hypoventilation leads to respiratory acidosis and hypoxemia. The ability to adequately protect the airway is also compromised, increasing the risk of aspiration. [27,28] Renal function is relatively stable at this stage. Blood flow remains high despite the decrease in cardiac output, predominantly due to central vasodilatation. [27] Hyperkalemia, hyperglycemia, and lactic acidosis can be seen with the increase in load metabolic by-products and cellular injury. [28]

Severe hypothermia occurs when the core body temperature falls below 28°C (82°F). At this point, victims may appear dead. Decline in cerebral perfusion leads to a profound coma. [27] Pupils become unresponsive and extremities are rigid and areflexic. [25,29] Blood pressure is generally unobtainable and cardiac rhythm ranges from various degrees of heart block to pulseless electrical activity. [25,28] Respirations become slow and shallow and may progress to apnea. Oxygen consumption decreases to approximately 75% of baseline. Renal blood flow and thus renal function decrease in conjunction with the decrease in cardiac output. [27] Because of the clinical presentation of these victims, no patient should be pronounced dead until the core temperature has been raised to 30°C (84.2°F). [25]

The obvious goal of treatment for hypothermia is to rewarm the victim to a normal physiologic temperature range. That goal can be achieved through passive external, active external, and active core rewarming. The choice of method depends on the degree of hypothermia and on the setting where the treatment is taking place. Passive external rewarming is the easiest and most readily available method. It involves moving the victim into a warm, sheltered environment, removing all wet clothing, and covering with dry blankets.[8,29] It works best for the otherwise healthy individual with mild hypothermia. The rate of rewarming using this technique is usually in the range of 0.5° to 2°C (0.9°F–3.6°F) per hour.[28]

The active methods of rewarming both involve the application of an exogenous source of heat.[29] Active external rewarming methods include the use of warmed blankets, hot packs, radiant heat lamps, and partial warm water (40°C; 104°F) immersion. Total warm water immersion is not advised because it makes monitoring difficult and is associated with more frequent complications, including "after drop" and rewarming shock.[28,29] The phenomenon of "after drop" occurs when the victim's core temperature actually decreases due to rapid vasodilation in the extremities and the circulation of cool blood to the core.[27,28] Rewarming shock is also a result of rapid peripheral dilation and leads to relative hypotension and hypovolemia.[29] This method is required for any individual with moderate to severe hypothermia and should not be initiated until in a controlled environment (e.g., a tertiary care center). The rate of rewarming varies with each method.[29]

Active internal or core rewarming can be further differentiated as simple or invasive. Simple techniques include administration of warmed, humidified oxygen via mask or endotracheal tube and warmed intravenous fluid.[8,29] Initiation can be immediate, and the rate of rewarming is usually 1° to 2°C (1.8°F–3.6°F) per hour.[28] Invasive techniques include peritoneal dialysis and hemodialysis, extracorporeal circulation, venovenous circulation, and pleural and peritoneal lavage. Lavage of hollow viscous is no longer advised due to the potential for major electrolyte imbalances that may ensue.[8,27,29] All the fluids used for core rewarming should be in the range of 40° to 45°C (104°–113°F).[25] The rate of invasive core rewarming varies based on technique but can be as high as 1° to 2°C (1.8°F–3.6°F) per 5 minutes.[28] Some experts suggest that this rate is too rapid, and in order to avoid potential cardiovascular instability, a goal for rewarming rate should be 1° to 2°C (1.8°F–3.6°F) per hour.[8] Core warming methods are reserved for the victim with moderate to severe hypothermia and should be performed only when the victim has been transported to the appropriate facility.[28,29]

Frostbite

Frostbite is a localized lesion of the skin, predominantly of the periphery, caused by the direct effects of cold exposure. Enough heat is lost from the area that ice crystals are allowed to form in the tissues.[29] Most commonly affected are the feet and lower extremities, accounting for 57% of injuries. Also common are injuries of the hands (46%) and exposed areas of the face such as the nose, ears, and cheeks (17%).[30] Historically, frostbite has had its highest prevalence during military campaigns. Today, those most at risk are mountain climbers and cold-weather endurance athletes.[29]

Frostbite occurs with exposure to an ambient temperature of 0°C (32°F) or less for a moderate to long length of time.[29,30] Other factors that play a role in determining the time required to develop the lesion and the extent of injury include the windchill index, the humidity, and the wetness of the environment. As the cold exposure causes the skin temperature to drop, vasoconstriction occurs through stimulation by the sympathetic adrenergic nerve fibers.[31] At a skin temperature of 10°C (50°F),

peripheral vessels are maximally vasoconstricted.[25] Every 5 to 10 minutes, a period of vasodilation replaces maximal vasoconstriction. This is known as cold induced vasodilation or the "hunting response." There is considerable variability based on acclimatization and genetic factors, explaining differences in susceptibility to frostbite injury based on race and ethnicity.[25,31] Also, any factor, endogenous or exogenous, that affects peripheral circulation can predispose individuals to frostbite injury.[30,31]

Pathophysiologically, frostbite has four distinct phases. The first is the prefreeze phase. This occurs when the tissue temperature is in the range of 3° to 10°C (37° to 50°F). Sensation is generally absent. No ice crystal formation is present, but vasospasticity and cellular membrane instability cause plasma leakage and clinically obvious edema.[29,31] Tissue enters the freeze-thaw phase when it cools to the range of −15° to −6°C (5° to 21°F). Actual ice crystals begin to form. When cooling takes place slowly, extracellular crystals form and cause a movement of free water into the extracellular space. As the cells dehydrate and shrink, a toxic concentration of electrolytes build up.[25,31] With rapid cooling, ice crystals can form intracellularly, which is more damaging. Tissues most susceptible to injury include endothelial, bone marrow, and nerve tissue. The vascular stasis phase is a result of continued plasma leakage and ice crystal formation.[29,31] The blood vessels begin to spasm and dilate leading to stasis coagulation and shunting.[29,31] The last phase is the late ischemic phase. Progression to thrombosis formation and continued shunting of blood lead to tissue ischemia, gangrene, and autonomic dysfunction.[29–31]

Clinically, frostbite can be classified either by degree or by depth of injury. First- and second-degree injuries are considered superficial, whereas third- and fourth-degree injuries are considered deep.[29] At initial presentation, it is difficult to determine the true extent of injury and an accurate clinical classification of the injury may not be completely clear until days after rewarming.[30] First-degree injury presents with a firm, pale yellow to white plaque over the injured area. There is associated edema, erythema, and initial numbness followed by significant pain during rewarming. Ultimately little to no tissue loss is involved.[29,31] Second-degree injury also involves initial numbness, erythema, and edema, but rather than a plaque, vesicles filled with a clear to milky fluid form over the area.[31] Third-degree injury develops vesicles as well, but they characteristically contain a darker, purple fluid indicating that the injury is deeper, involving the vascularity of the dermis.[25,31] Fourth-degree injury remains cold and mottled after rewarming and eschar and mummification of the tissue develops in the area with involvement of muscle and bone.[31]

Treatment

The basic principle, regardless of clinical class, is rapid rewarming of the injured area. Before any attempt is made at rewarming, it is important to have the victim in an environment where there is little to no possibility that the involved tissue will have a chance to refreeze. A thaw-refreeze cycle carries with it significantly higher morbidity than does a period of extended freezing.[29] The first step in treatment is removal of all wet and binding clothing, replacing them with dry, loose wraps. This can be performed while in transit to a local medical facility as there is little risk of thawing-refreezing. On arrival, treatment begins immediately. Core body temperature should be initially measured, and if the temperature is less than 34°C (93°F), therapy should first be directed at treating hypothermia.[29,31] When core body temperature has been corrected, treatment is directed at rapid tissue rewarming. The most generally accepted method used is immersion of the injured area into a water bath warmed to between 40° and 42°C (104° and 108°F) for 15 to 30 minutes or until the involved skin becomes pliable.[25,28,31] It is important the water remain in such a narrow range for two reasons. If allowed to fall to a lower temperature, there is less benefit to potential tissue survival. On the other hand, if the temperature is allowed to go above the range, there is risk of compounding the injury with a thermal burn. Also, the higher the temperature, the less comfortable it is for the victim.[31] Following the initial thawing phase, treatment is focused on preventing the progressive phase of the injury. A protocol designed by McCauley et al[31] has been shown to decrease tissue loss, lower amputation rate, and decrease the hospital stay of victims (Table 6-2). The focus of this protocol is to inhibit the action of prostaglandins and thromboxanes that act locally to potentiate tissue damage.[29,31]

Surgery has little role in the acute treatment of frostbite. Deep injuries often require surgical treatment to remove nonviable or gangrenous tissue, but this is delayed at least 3 weeks and preferably later to allow the tissue to demarcate. Technetium bone scanning has shown some promise as a way to detect the line of demarcation earlier, but most experts still advise delayed amputation. Early postoperative prosthetics are advocated for the best fit.[25,30,31]

Long-term sequelae relate to the severity of the initial injury. Common problems include hyperhidrosis, increased sensitivity to cold exposure, skin color change, decreased sensation, and joint pain and stiffness.[25,31] Skeletally immature victims may develop premature epiphyseal closure in the area of injury, resulting in bone shortening or angular deformity.[31]

Nonfreezing Injuries

Immersion or "trench" foot is a significant cause of morbidity, particularly during military operations. Its name was first coined during World War I, after troops who stood in water-filled trenches for days developed this injury. It occurs in ambient temperatures of 0° to 10°C (32° to 50°F) and is caused by a prolonged exposure to cold water.[29,32] The exact pathophysiology remains somewhat controversial, but it is widely believed that the prolonged vasoconstriction causes an ischemic injury leading to demyelination of nerve fibers, muscle atrophy, skin atrophy, and decreased compliance of the small vessels.[24,25,32] On presentation, the affected limb appears mottled, pale, and cool to the touch. Sensation is impaired, and the victim will often describe the feeling as "walking on cotton wool." After rewarming, the involved area becomes warm, dry, erythematous, and excruciatingly painful. This may last several weeks. Long-term sequelae include cold sensitivity, hyperhidrosis, paresthesias, and chronic neuropathic pain.[32] Treatment of choice is removing the victim from the environment, elevating the affected extremity, and allowing passive rewarming.[24,32]

Although less severe, chilblains and pernio are also caused by prolonged exposure to a cold and wet environment. The ambient temperature is usually between 0° and 15°C (32° and 60°F) for these injuries to occur.[25,32] Chilblains are subcutaneous vesicles that appear after 3 to 6 hours of exposure. They are usually painless and resolve with no long-term sequelae. As length of exposure reaches 12 hours or more, partial thickness eschars and deep pain can develop. The eschars slough without scarring; however, the pain may persist and is termed pernio.[32] The major

---

Table 6-2 Protocol for Rapid Rewarming
1. Admit frostbite patients to a specialized unit if possible.
2. Do not discharge or transfer to another facility victims of acute frostbite requiring hospitalization unless it is necessary for specialized care. Transfer arrangements must protect the victim from cold exposure.
3. On admission, rapidly rewarm the affected areas in warm water at 40° to 42°C (104° to 108°F), usually for 15 to 30 minutes or until thawing is complete.

4. On completion of rewarming, treat the affected parts as follows:
a. Débride white blisters and institute topical treatment with aloe vera (Dermaide aloe) every 6 hours.
b. Leave hemorrhagic blisters intact and administer topical aloe vera (Dermaide aloe) every 6 hours.
c. Elevate the affected part(s) with splinting as indicated.
d. Administer antitetanus prophylaxis.
e. For analgesia, administer morphine or meperidine (Demerol) intravenously or intramuscularly as indicated.
f. Administer ibuprofen 400 mg orally every 12 hours.
g. Administer penicillin G 500,000 U intravenously every 6 hours for 48 to 72 hours.
h. Perform hydrotherapy daily for 30 to 45 minutes at 40°C (104°F). The solution should meet the following specifications:
  1. Large tank capacity: 425 gallons
    Fill level estimate: 285 gallons
    Sodium chloride: 9.7 kg
    Calcium hypochlorite solution: 95 mL
  2. Medium tank capacity: 270 gallons
    Fill level estimate: 108 gallons
    Sodium chloride: 3.7 kg
    Calcium hypochlorite solution: 36 mL
  3. Small tank capacity: 95 gallons
    Fill level estimate: 72 gallons
    Sodium chloride: 2.5 kg
    Potassium chloride: 71 g
    Calcium hypochlorite solution: 24 mL

5. For documentation, obtain photographs on admission, at 24 hours, and serially every 2 to 3 days until discharge.
6. Discharge patients with specific instructions for protection of the injured areas to avoid reinjury and follow up weekly until wounds are stable. If the patient is being discharged with no open lesions, instruct him or her to use wool socks, wear a hat, and use mittens instead of gloves to decrease the loss of heat between the fingers. Explain to patients that they are more susceptible to refreezing, so they should avoid exposure to cold and should wear warm clothing and shoes or boots if going outside is necessary. Give similar instructions to patients who are discharged with open lesions. Also instruct these patients to keep the affected extremity elevated and to take ibuprofen 400 mg orally every 12 hours. Aloe vera should be applied to the involved areas or scarlet red ointment used if the open areas are small.

From McCauley RL, Smith DJ, Robson MC, Heggers JP: Frostbite. In Auerbach PS (ed): Wilderness Medicine, 4th ed. St. Louis, Mosby, 2001, p. 188.

long-term complication associated with pernio is increased cold sensitivity. The pathology of these conditions is thought to be just like that of trench foot. The treatment is supportive, allowing passive rewarming.[29,33]

In addition to directly causing injury, the cold environment can stimulate other conditions in susceptible individuals. Cold urticaria with or without angioedema is produced by the degranulation of mast cells that are stimulated by the cold. Symptoms are generally mild and self-limited and may be relieved with the use of antihistamines.[25,29] Bronchospasm may also be induced, particularly with hyperventilation of cold air. Cold-induced asthma is considered a variant of exercise-induced asthma. The cold air causes a drying of the mucosa due to evaporative loss and local irritation of the mucosa leading to a cascade of immune response and ultimately to smooth muscle contraction in the bronchial tree. Preactivity use of inhaled β_2-agonist is the mainstay of treatment.[25,29,34] Raynaud's disease is a condition caused by intermittent vasospasm of the digital vessels and is often exacerbated by cold. It may be associated with an underlying medical condition but is mainly idiopathic. With exposure, the digits become pale and numb. After rewarming, redness, swelling, and throbbing pain are seen. The primary treatment is avoidance of cold exposure.[25,29] Cold air exposure of the nasal mucosa can stimulate an increase in mucous production resulting in rhinitis or "skier's nose." It causes no long-term problems and can be treated with nasal atropine sulfate.[29]

High-Altitude Illness

High altitude has captivated athletes and adventure seekers for years. Athletes subject themselves to living high and training low in the hopes of achieving that small edge to push them past their competitors. Extreme athletes traverse harsh and dangerous terrain, pushing the limits of human physiology in search of excitement and adventure. In recent years, the adventure travel industry has boomed by providing quick and rapid excursions for individuals who may not be prepared emotionally or physically to tackle the potential medical complications encountered at such extremes of altitude.[33]

It is generally agreed that high altitude ranges from 1500 to 3500 m (4921 to 11,483 feet). At this altitude, there is minor impairment of oxygen saturation (SaO_2 >90%). Manifestations of mountain sickness are common with rapid ascent above 2500 m (8202 feet). Very high altitude ranges from 3500 to 5500 m (11,483 to 18,045 feet) with maximum arterial oxygen saturation falling below 90% with concomitant decrease in PaO_2 to below 20 mm Hg. Hypoxemia is normally mild at this range, but severe altitude illness may present during exercise and sleep. Extreme altitude is marked by elevations over 5500 m (18,045 feet).[35,36] At this altitude, the benefits of acclimatization are overwhelmed by marked hypoxemia and physiologic decline,[35] making permanent human habitation impossible.[35,36]

High-altitude illness is a spectrum of conditions caused by a body's physiologic response to the hypobaric hypoxia environment of elevated altitude.[36] Because the same general pathologic mechanisms are at work in all these conditions, there is considerable overlap with no clear delineation between the different forms of illness.[33,35] Also, individuals presenting with altitude illness often have more than one of these conditions. The spectrum of diseases includes acute mountain sickness, high-altitude cerebral edema, and high-altitude pulmonary edema.

Acute mountain sickness (AMS) is the most common and most benign of the high altitude–induced illnesses. Typically symptoms will develop in an unacclimatized individual within 6 to 10 hours of arrival at an area of high altitude, usually at or above 2500 m (8202 feet).[36,37] The diagnosis of AMS is a clinical one based on setting and symptoms and exclusion of other illnesses.[36] There are no reliable findings on physical examination or from other diagnostic modalities to confirm or rule out the diagnosis.[38] Therefore, in 1991 (with revision in 1993), a group called the Lake Louise Consensus Committee proposed a definition of AMS as headache with at least one of the following symptoms: gastrointestinal upset (anorexia, nausea, and/or

vomiting), fatigue or weakness, dizziness or lightheadedness, and difficulty sleeping associated with an ascent in altitude.[37,39] The headache of victims of AMS is usually described as bitemporal or occipital, throbbing, worse with bending over or Valsalva maneuvers, and worse at night or on awakening.[35,40] The severity of the symptoms is based primarily on the rate of ascent and the ultimate altitude achieved. If no further ascent is attempted, symptoms usually resolve completely in 24 to 72 hours as acclimatization is achieved.[37,40] With continued ascent or when a very high altitude is achieved initially, symptoms may progress rapidly to one of the more life-threatening forms of high-altitude illness. Treatment depends on severity of symptoms. Proceeding to higher altitudes is absolutely contraindicated until the victim is symptom free.[39] Small descents of 500 m (1640 feet) or more often yield dramatic improvement and is the initial treatment of choice.[35-37] Acetazolamide (125 to 250 mg twice daily), a potent carbonic anhydrase inhibitor, improves symptoms and speeds acclimatization by producing a bicarbonate diuresis.[36,37,41] It can also be used as a prophylactic measure if started 24 to 48 hours prior to ascent and continued for 2 days at maximum altitude.[36,37] Dexamethasone (4 mg every 6 hours), a potent synthetic glucocorticoid, has a mechanism of action in AMS that is not entirely clear. Its proposed mechanism is a decrease in the permeability of the intracranial capillaries.[37] Effects may be additive when used with acetazolamide.[35] Unlike acetazolamide, it has no effect on acclimatization and there is a significant risk of rebound effects when discontinued.[35,37] If descent is not possible or the condition is deteriorating, low flow oxygen (0.5 to 4 L/min) may be useful in preventing further decompensation.[36,37] Portable hyperbaric chambers are also an option and have been shown to be as effective as oxygen in controlling symptoms while facilitating descent or other definitive treatment.[42] AMS, as well as the other high-altitude illnesses, is preventable. Acetazolamide can be used but is generally reserved for individuals with a history of AMS or other illness. The mainstays of prevention are proper acclimatization and a slow, graded ascent limiting gains to 300 to 800 m per 24-hour period.[35,41]

High-altitude pulmonary edema (HAPE) is the second most common form of high-altitude illness and is the most common cause of altitude-related death.[35,36,43] Just as with AMS, it is rarely seen in individuals below an altitude of 2500 m (8202 feet). The overall incidence depends greatly on individual susceptibility and rate of ascent, but has been estimated to be from 0.1 to 15% in those who ascend rapidly.[8] About 5% to 10% of those diagnosed with AMS will develop HAPE, and 50% of those with HAPE will also have symptoms of AMS.[33,36] Overall, mortality is estimated to be around 11% but can be more than 40% without proper treatment.[33,40] HAPE is a noncardiogenic form of pulmonary edema that usually presents on the second night at altitude. Early symptoms are mild and include exertional dyspnea, cough, and decreased exercise performance.[44,45] The Lake Louise Consensus diagnostic criteria for HAPE are at least two of the following symptoms: dyspnea at rest, cough, chest tightness or congestion, or weakness/decreased exertional performance. Also, the victim must have two of the following signs: rales or wheezing, central cyanosis, tachycardia, or tachypnea[37,40] The rales start localized to the area over the right middle lobe and as symptoms progress become more diffuse.[36] Symptoms are generally worse at night and may progress to include irrational behavior, orthopnea, and temperature elevated generally not higher than 38.5°C (101.3°F).[33,36] When available, a chest radiograph will show a patchy, peripheral infiltrate with normal cardiac size.[43,44] Electrocardiography shows a pattern of right ventricular strain.[43] The first priority in treatment is descent. When this is not immediately available, or while this is being planned, efforts must concentrate on improving oxygenation. This can be achieved directly by oxygen administration or indirectly by use of a portable hyperbaric chamber. The goal of therapy is to maintain oxygen saturation of at least 90%.[35,37,44] The calcium channel blocker nifedipine, given at a dose of 10 mg initially and then 30 mg in extended-release form every 12 hours, is a vasodilator that reduces pulmonary vascular resistance without causing hypotension.[35–37] Because of potential side effects, other medications are of little use until descent is achieved.[36] Measures taken to prevent HAPE, such as graded ascent and proper acclimatization, are especially important to those with a history of the illness because the recurrence rate has been estimated to be as high as 66%.[8,33]

Because it shares both clinical and pathophysiologic features with AMS, high-altitude cerebral edema (HACE) is considered by most experts to be an extension of the illness.[46] Therefore, HACE generally presents several hours to days after the first symptoms of AMS.[33,37] It is seen at the same altitudes at which both AMS and HAPE are seen, but it is far less common. Often victims will suffer from both HAPE and HACE. Case reports show that 13% to 20% of individuals treated for HAPE also had signs and symptoms of HACE, and an even higher percentage of HACE patients also had HAPE.[46] The hallmark features are varying degrees of confusion, altered consciousness, and ataxia, in addition to the symptoms common to AMS.[36,37,46] Victims may initially exhibit irrational behavior that progresses to severe lassitude, lethargy, obtundation, and ultimately coma over a period of hours to days.[33,35,37] The ataxia is nearly always truncal and affects tandem gait testing (no effect on the finger-to-nose test).[37,40] Because HACE is a global encephalopathy, focal neurologic signs are rarely present. Imaging studies are not necessary for the diagnosis, but one would expect to see evidence of edema in the white matter, specifically the corpus callosum, with no gray matter edema.[46] Treatment is essentially the same as for AMS, with more emphasis on descent as quickly as possible with other modalities used before and during transport.[36,37] The overall mortality of HACE is 13%, and for those who progress to coma, it is closer to 60%.[8] Because it is such a life-threatening illness and can have similar signs and symptoms of other serious illnesses, all but those with very mild cases who have a rapid and complete recovery on descent should be hospitalized for a full workup and observation.[46] Prevention is the same as for all the other altitude illnesses, particularly AMS.[36,37,46]

The high-altitude environment can pose other potential medical concerns. High-altitude retinopathy is a generally benign, asymptomatic condition that is relatively common, especially above 5000 m (16,000 feet). Blindness or scotomas may be present when the macula is involved, but these usually resolve with descent and cause no permanent sequelae.[35,40] Peripheral edema in the absence of any of the acute altitude illness is also common, especially in women, and can be treated with low-dose diuretics. It too will resolve on descent.[35,36] High-altitude pharyngitis and bronchitis can cause significant morbidity due to persistent coughing spasms. It is thought to be more related to the inspiration of large volumes of cold, dry air leading to a drying of the mucosa and is treated by staying well hydrated, using lozenges, and breathing through a scarf or cloth.[37,38] Susceptibility to bacterial infection is increased because of a mild reduction in T-lymphocyte function.[36] Dehydration, relative inactivity, polycythemia, and constrictive clothing increase the risk of thrombotic events.[35,36] Low temperatures increase the risk of hypothermia and frostbite.[35] Ultraviolet radiation is increased at altitude and usually enhanced when reflected off snow that is usually present. This increases the risk of ultraviolet keratitis (snow blindness) and significant sunburn.[35]

In order for an individual to reduce and/or avoid the symptoms associated with mountain sickness, a period of acclimatization to the environment at high altitude must be accomplished. The slow and gradual exposure to hypoxia through staged ascent maximizes oxygen delivery for a given altitude, thereby enhancing survival and performance.[8,36] This process involves a complex series of physiologic adjustments including hyperventilation and hypoxic ventilatory drive, circulation, and most importantly increased erythropoiesis resulting in increased hematocrit.[33,35,36] Acclimatization is an individual process. Study of populations who live at high altitudes suggest a possible genetic component. The severity of the hypoxic stress, rate of onset, and individual physiology determine whether the body successfully acclimatizes or is overwhelmed.[36] The role of staged ascent cannot be overemphasized. Guidelines for staging ascent are well published. A plan for acclimatization should be discussed with a trained medical professional knowledgeable in high-altitude medicine, taking into account altitude profile, the type of ascent, the performance capacity, the history of previous high-altitude illness, and the medical support available on the climb.[47] Pharmacologic prophylaxis with medication such as acetazolamide is a consideration for individuals who cannot stage their ascent or are at risk of high-altitude illness.[8] The most important method for avoiding high-altitude illness is careful preparation and education concerning proper climbing etiquette, signs and symptoms of AMS, and reaction if acute mountain illness is encountered by yourself or a fellow climber.[8,47]

Athletes and coaches alike have strived to achieve a performance edge by trying to harness the beneficial effects of intermittent hypoxic training as it affects the physiology of human adaptation to high altitude. The strategies of intermittent hypoxic training revolve around providing hypoxia at rest (living high/training low) or providing hypoxia during exercise (living low/training high).[48] Living high/training low has been shown to increase performance at sea level.[36,48,49] The benefit arises from increases in erythropoietin leading to increased red cell mass,[36,48,49] submaximal exercise efficiency,[36,50] and running performance.[36,48–50] Adequate iron stores are needed secondary to increased red cell mass production.[36] There have been no data supporting the benefit of training at altitudes above 2400 m (7874 feet). Training between 1500 to 2000 m (4921 to 6562 feet) maximizes the benefits of training in a hypoxic environment without substantial detriment.[36] These benefits can be quickly obtained (within 10 days of initiation of training)[36] and quickly diminish (within 3 weeks) with cessation of intermittent hypoxic training.[50] Athletes competing at high altitude will require a period of acclimatization. The duration and extent of acclimatization depend on the altitude of residence, the altitude of the athletic event, and the duration of the event.

REFERENCES

1. Martin TD: Special issues and concerns for the high school and college aged athletes. Pediatric Clin North Am 2002;49:533–552.
2. Vigil DV: Heat illness. In Puffer JC (ed): 20 Common Problems Sports Medicine. New York, McGraw Hill, 2002, pp 303–322.
3. Wexler R: Evaluation and treatment of heat-related illnesses. Am Fam Physician 2002;65:2307–2314.
4. Blows WT: Crowd physiology: The 'penguin effect.' Accid Emerg Nurs 1998;6:126–129.
5. Coyle EF: Thermoregulation. In Andenson SJ, Sullivan JA (eds): Care of the Young Athlete. Chicago, American Academy of Pediatrics and The American Academy of Orthopaedic Surgeons, 2001, pp 65–80.
6. Bar-Or O: Children's responses to exercise in hot climates: Implications for performance and health. Gatorade Sports Science Exchange 1994;7: No. 2.
7. Bar-Or O: Effects of age and gender on sweating pattern during exercise. Int J Sports Med 1998;19:S106–S107.
8. Tom PA, Garmel GM, Auerbach PS, et al: Environment dependent sports emergencies. Med Clin North Am 1994;78:305–325.
9. Noakes TD: Dehydration during exercise: What are the real dangers? Clin J Sport Med 1995;5:123–128.
10. Wyndham CH, Strydom NB: The danger of an inadequate water intake during marathon running. S Afr Med J 1969;43:893–896.
11. Noakes TD: Fluid and electrolyte disturbances in heat illness. Int J Sports Med 1998;19:S146–S149.
12. Walsh RM, Noakes TD, Hawley JA, Dennis SC: Impaired high-intensity cycling performance time at low levels of dehydration. Int J Sports Med 1994;15:392–398.
13. Eichner ER: Treatment of suspected heat illness. Int J Sports Med 1998;19:S150–S153.
14. Roberts WO: A 12 year profile of medical injury and illness for the Twin Cities Marathon. Med Sci Sports Exer 2000;32:1549–1555.
15. Holtzhausen LM, Noakes TD, Kronig B, et al: Clinical and biochemical characteristics of collapsed ultramarathon runners. Med Sci Sports Exerc 1994;26:1095–1101.
16. Roberts WO: Exercise-associated collapse in endurance events: A classification system. Phys Sport Med 1989;17:49–55.
17. Holtzhausen LM, Noakes TD: Collapsed ultraendurance athlete: Proposed mechanism and an approach to management. Clin J Sport Med 1997;7:292–301.
18. Sandor RP: Heat illness. On site diagnosis and cooling. Phys Sport Med 1997;25:35–41.
19. Bowden L, Canini F: On the nature of the link between malignant hyperthermia and exertional heat stroke. Med Hypoth 1995;45:268–270.
20. Porter AMW: Collapse from exertional heat illness: Implications and subsequent decisions. Mil Med 2003;168:76–81.
21. Armstrong CE, Crago AF, Adams R, et al: Whole-body cooling of hyperthermic runner: Comparison of two field therapies. Am J Emerg Med 1996;14:355–358.
22. American College of Sports Medicine: Position stand on exercise and fluid replacement. Med Sci Sports Exerc 1996;28:i–vii.
23. Phinney LT, Gardner JW, Kark JA, Wenger CB: Long-term follow-up after exertional heat illness during recruit training. Med Sci Sports Exerc 2001;33:1443–1448.
24. Lloyd EL: ABC of sports medicine: Temperature and performance I: Cold. BMJ 1994;309:531–534.
25. Hixson EG: Cold injury. In DeLee JC, Drez D (eds): Orthopaedic Sports Medicine Principles and Practice. Philadelphia, Elsevier Science, 2003, pp 305–325.
26. Danzl DF: Accidental hypothermia. In Auerbach PS (ed): Wilderness Medicine. St. Louis, Mosby, 2001, pp 135–177.
27. Danzl DF, Pozos RS: Accidental hypothermia. N Engl J Med 1994;331:1756–1760.
28. Bien J, Koehncke N, Dosman J: Out of the cold: Management of hypothermia and frostbite. CMAJ 2003;168:305–311.
29. Sallis R, Chassay CM: Recognizing and treating common cold-induced injury in outdoor sports. Med Sci Sports Exerc 1999;31:1367–1373.
30. Foray J: Mountain frostbite. Int J Sports Med 1992;13:S193–S196.
31. McCauley RL, Smith DJ, Robson MC, Heggers JP: Frostbite. In Auerbach PS (ed): Wilderness Medicine. St. Louis, Mosby, 2001, pp 178–196.
32. Hamlet MP: Nonfreezing cold injuries. In Auerbach PS (ed): Wilderness Medicine. St. Louis, Mosby, 2001, pp 129–134.
33. Bezruchka S: High altitude medicine. Med Clin North Am 1992;76:1481–1497.
34. Regnard J: Cold and the airways. Int J Sports Med 1992;13:S191–S193.
35. Zafren K, Honigman B: High-altitude medicine. Emerg Med Clin North Am 1997;15:191–222.
36. Hacket PH, Roach RC: High-altitude medicine. In Auerbach PS (ed): Wilderness Medicine. St. Louis, Mosby, 2001, pp 2–32.
37. Gallagher SA, Hacket PH: High-altitude illness. Emerg Med Clin North Am 2004;22:329–355.
38. Hacket PH, Roach RC: High-altitude illness. N Engl J Med 2001;345:107–114.
39. Bärtsch P, Bailey DM, Berger MM, et al: Acute mountain sickness: Controversies and advances. High Alt Med Biol 2004;5:110–124.
40. Harris MD, Terrio J, Miser WF, Yetter JF: High-altitude medicine. Am Fam Physician 1998;57:1907–1914.
41. Coote JH: Medicine and mechanism in altitude sickness. Sports Med 1995;20:148–159.
42. Bärtsch P, Merki B, Hofstetter D, et al: Treatment of acute mountain sickness by simulated descent: A randomized controlled trial. BMJ 1993;306:1098–1101.
43. Adelman DC, Spector SL: Acute respiratory emergencies in emergency treatment of the injured athlete. Clin Sports Med 1989;8:71–79.
44. Bärtsch P: High altitude pulmonary edema. Med Sci Sports Exerc 1999;31:S23–S27.
45. Bärtsch P: High altitude pulmonary edema. Respiration 1997;64:435–443.
46. Hackett PH, Roach RC: High altitude cerebral edema. High Alt Med Biol 2004;5:136–145.
47. Bärtsch P, Grunig E, Hoenhaus E, Dehnart C: Assessment of high altitude tolerance in healthy individuals. High Alt Med Biol 2001;2:287–296.
48. Levine BD: Intermittent hypoxic training: Fact and fancy. High Alt Med Biol 2002;3:177–193.
49. Levine BD, Stray-Gundersen J: A practical approach to altitude training: Where to live and train for optimal performance enhancement. Int J Sports Med 1992;13:S209–S212.
50. Katayama K, Matsuo H, Ishida K, et al: Intermittent hypoxia improves endurance performance and submaximal exercise efficiency. High Alt Med Biol 2003;4:291–304.

Psychological Aspects of Healing the Injured Athlete

J. Richard Steadman

In This Chapter

INTRODUCTION

- It is well-known that the psychological impact of serious injury on both the professional and amateur athlete must be dealt with if the patient is to achieve optimal healing and a timely return to sports.

- There are three types of rehabilitation: psychological, physiologic (aerobic conditioning, overall strength, and flexibility), and rehabilitation specific to the injured area.

- The athlete should be given a complete and honest explanation of the injury and rehabilitation process, allowing him or her to feel like a part of the team guiding the recovery.

- An understanding of the seven stages of injury and recovery is crucial in guiding the athlete toward a return to sport.

- The establishment of realistic, yet demanding goals helps the athlete to focus on each stage.

- The appropriate application of psychological precepts is critical to the successful treatment of the injured athlete. In fact, ignoring this facet of the rehabilitation process makes it less likely that the patient will make a full recovery.

In modern society, the pursuit of fitness, good health, and longevity is important to people of all ages who participate in many types of physical activity to reach these goals. Their identities are strongly tied to the sports they enjoy, and they are just as serious about them as professional athletes are about their careers. The dedicated amateur's eagerness to achieve full recovery and his or her previous activity level parallels that of the elite professional whose very livelihood depends on performance. Although there are greater psychological pressures on the pro who can lose his job if he or she returns to the game with diminished speed and skill, the injured amateur takes his or her performance level no less seriously. Thus, successful outcomes after sports injuries to professionals or amateurs require the same degree of dedication to the correct use of three types of postinjury rehabilitation.

ESTABLISHING REASONABLE GOALS

Being goal oriented, both types of athletes are highly motivated to improve the skills and speeds that lead to better scores. This focus on goal achievement can be harnessed in rehabilitation if the physician, sports medicine therapist, and athlete work together and are creative in their approach to the healing process. Goals give the athlete something concrete to work toward and require his or her active engagement in the rehabilitation process.

It is important that these goals be achievable. For example, in the early postoperative period, a goal of full motion may be unrealistic, yet the athlete may be able to achieve at least partial motion. Setting a goal that the athlete can reach helps to reestablish self-esteem and allows the patient to begin charting a course toward recovery. In general, early rehabilitation stages should focus on short-term goals, although long-term goals can be helpful in mental training techniques, such as visualization. As recovery progresses toward the specificity period, goals related to return to competition and athletic performance can be brought into progressively sharper focus.

STAGES OF INJURY AND RECOVERY

When planning a rehabilitation program, the rehabilitation team will find it helpful to identify and observe the relationship between specific time periods beginning with preinjury and ending with the athlete's return to sport. The stages of this process are shown in Figure 7-1.

During each of these periods, there is intense psychological pressure on the patient. A treatment approach that addresses the key psychological issues of each stage will optimize the outcomes of surgery and rehabilitation.

The treatment approach for injuries requiring surgery is similar to that employed for severe injuries that do not require surgery. With relatively minor injuries, rehabilitation moves more directly from treatment design and implementation toward the specificity period and return to play.

PREINJURY STAGE

Several studies have indicated that injury is often not purely accidental but is caused by a combination of factors, including loss of concentration, the pressures of performance, and fatigue. It is helpful for the practitioner to examine factors in the envi-

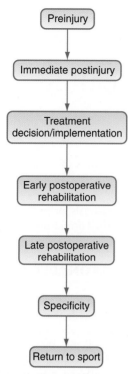

Figure 7-1 Stages of rehabilitation for the injured athlete.

ronment that may have affected the occurrence of the injury. If identified, preinjury factors may be addressed through psychological counseling during the course of treatment and rehabilitation.

IMMEDIATE POSTINJURY STAGE

This stage is characterized by fear and denial, which accompanies the immediate pain and disability caused by the injury. At this point, the patient will need an accurate diagnosis that is thoroughly explained to him or her, a proposed course of treatment, and an estimate of the duration of treatment. This estimate will be approximate, but it will give the athlete an idea of what to expect. Most athletes, particularly successful ones, realize that injury is often a part of athletics. It is a mistake, however, for clinicians to assume that athletes know much about injury, treatment, and rehabilitation. A patient's denial and fear can deter healing, though this can be countered by a plan that explains the severity of the injury, the duration of disability, and the expected recovery level. Such a plan gives the patient a measure of control and encourages active participation as an important part of the recovery team.

TREATMENT DECISION AND IMPLEMENTATION

Choosing treatment options is easier if the first two stages are managed satisfactorily, that is, if the patient has accepted the reality of the injury and is psychologically prepared to assume an analytical role in helping to choose the appropriate treatment. Treatment may be easily decided on in some cases, but when many issues are involved, the decision can be difficult to make. For instance, treatments may affect a patient's career or a team's performance and the physician should be aware of such

factors, which necessarily affect the final decision on a treatment course.

In some cases, injury at a critical point in a career may force an athlete to make a decision that may endanger his or her future physical well-being. This seemingly irresponsible decision may nonetheless be a good one for the athlete, especially one who feels strongly that an additional year's salary or other benefits may provide irresistible financial stability. Also, some athletes may view the psychological gratification gained from playing one more game or one more year as worth any risk. In cases like these, it is necessary for the athlete, agent, team management, and family to understand the hazards involved before a treatment course is chosen or rejected. The patient's input can only be truly effective if he or she has been fully apprised of the choices available and understands the risks involved with any course of action.

EARLY POSTOPERATIVE REHABILITATION STAGE

In the immediate postoperative phase, the rehabilitation team must consider more than the surgical event and its sequelae. The patient is affected in varying degrees by important psychological factors that can influence the final outcome of treatment.

If surgery is performed, the athlete is transformed from an athletic person (with the healthy self-image associated with physical activity) to a bedridden, disabled patient. To counteract the negative aspects of this stage (from both a physical and psychological standpoint), it is necessary to initiate a program of rehabilitation goals. Providing an athlete with well-leg aerobic workouts following knee surgery encourages a goal-seeking attitude and helps the athlete maintain aerobic conditioning. In addition, setting appropriate goals for the injured area, for example, achieving a certain range of motion or level of exer-cise intensity, permits the patient to take an active part in treatment and assume a level of control over the postoperative environment.

LATE POSTOPERATIVE REHABILITATION STAGE

During this phase, the drudgery of rehabilitation takes its toll. The physician must help the patient and the sports medicine therapist continue on a direct course to recovery. Continued goal orientation, provided by steadily increasing levels of activity, allows sustained patient input, and helps the patient to feel in control throughout rehabilitation. This emphasis on setting and achieving goals parallels the patient's preinjury mind set. For example, the athlete's preinjury goal may have been to run 5 miles in 30 minutes, and if he or she achieved this, confidence was increased. During rehabilitation, it is necessary to focus on different goals; for example, the completion of three sets of one-third knee bends becomes the mark of achievement. If goals are met, the patient feels empowered and enjoys a definite sense of accomplishment.

Achieving rehabilitation goals requires several elements. First, the milestones should be challenging but realistic and should be designed by the physician, sports medicine therapist, and patient working together. Second, goals should stretch the limits of what the injured area can tolerate (without causing deformation or further injury) but should not extend beyond these limits. This requires a thorough understanding of the physiology and biomechanics of the injured area. Third, the patient should strengthen uninjured parts of the body in aerobic training, which helps prevent reinjury while providing more goal orientation. In the case of a leg injury, this training can include well-leg biking or swimming with or without a float. The positive psychological effects of aerobic training are an important aspect of treatment during this period.

SPECIFICITY STAGE

This period is less challenging psychologically because, at this point, recovery is in sight. Exercise should become more specific for the sport, which entails a greater emphasis on patterns and muscle recruitment mimicking those used in the sport.

During this period, the athlete needs reassurance that he or she will return to sport and once again achieve success. The patient may fear that success will not occur and thus may need psychological reinforcement, which can be readily supplied by continued emphasis on reaching achievable goals. Psychological counseling may be required if the athlete's subconscious fears of failure are severe and seem obsessive.

RETURN TO SPORT STAGE

This period may require psychological counseling for several reasons. First, the athlete's lengthy absence from sport can produce fears, especially if success has not been reinforced in the earlier stages of rehabilitation. Second, the athlete may feel that peers have passed him or her by. Third, even though the rehabilitation program has been designed to return the athlete to a preinjury level, the absence of regular participation in a sport can create other realistic concerns.

If the road to recovery has been successfully navigated and the team (athlete, sports medicine therapist, physician, and psychologist) has provided appropriate standards for achievement at each level of rehabilitation, the experience will have served a useful psychological purpose. The athlete's ability to overcome the obstacles of injury and to gain a level of performance equal to or higher than preinjury levels can raise confidence that will enhance performance. It is unlikely that this success can be achieved, however, unless each stage of the rehabilitation program has been effectively followed.

CONCLUSIONS

This approach represents a physician's clinical perspective on the psychology of injury rehabilitation. The opportunities I have had to observe numerous world-class and dedicated recreational athletes have reinforced my appreciation for the role of psychological factors in active rehabilitation. In some cases, patients intuitively apply the principles mentioned here. This ability to structure their rehabilitation effectively is probably a reflection of the way in which they achieved their preinjury success.

In treating many athletes, I have observed quite a number who have returned to their sports at higher levels than they had achieved at the time of injury. This can be partially explained by the possibility that they were in an ascending curve of performance at the time of the accident, but this cannot be the entire explanation. Nor can good surgery and rehabilitation account for such successful recoveries. A multifaceted approach to rehabilitation provides a learning opportunity and helps create the psychological momentum that accompanies the athlete beyond rehabilitation and back to competition.

The psychological rehabilitation program is summarized in Box 7-1. Although this program seems simple, it requires careful judgment calls by the rehabilitation team at each treatment stage. This approach to treatment is based on over 25 years of clinical experience with most of the major world-class competitive sports as well as work with many recreational athletes. The careful use of standardized treatment methods along with personal attention to the athlete's needs during his or her different rehabilitation stages have proven effective. Our treatment team has contributed to some outstanding postinjury success stories. The return of several of our patients to top world-class performance levels after career threatening accidents is eloquent testimony to the validity of this approach as well as to the intensity of the athletes' motivation.

Box 7-1 Rehabilitation Program Summary

The patient's psychological rehabilitation includes the following steps:
1. Complete understanding of the injury, the treatment, and the stages of treatment. This allows the patient to feel like a real part of the team guiding the recovery process.
2. Establishment of attainable goals at each stage in rehabilitation. These are realistic but demanding goals that provide an immediate focus but do not look too far ahead.
3. Prompt initiation of an aerobic program to help avoid the depression associated with the immediate postinjury period. In addition, the aerobic program counters other stress-related psychological changes that occur due to the abrupt transition from intense physical activity to no activity at all.
4. Psychological counseling, when necessary, to help the patient deal with his or her altered status as an athlete, especially during extended periods of inactivity.

SUGGESTED READINGS

Hardy CJ, Crace RK: Dealing with injury. Sport Psychol Train Bull 1990;1:1–8.

Heil J (ed): Psychology of Sports Injury. Champaign, IL, Human Kinetics Publishers, 1993.

McGowan RW, Pierce EF, Williams M, et al: Athletic injury and self diminution. J Sports Med Phys Fitness 1994;34:299–304.

Pearson L, Jones G: Emotional effects of sports injuries: Implications for physiotherapists. Physiotherapy 1992;78:762–770.

Smith AM: Psychological impact of injuries in athletes. Sports Med 1996;22:391–405.

Smith AM, Scott SG, Wiese DM: The psychological effects of sports injuries. Coping. Sports Med 1990;9:352–369.

The Female Athlete

Letha Y. Griffin, James Kercher, and Fred Reifsteck

In This Chapter

INTRODUCTION

- With the recent explosion of participation in women's sports has come an understanding of musculoskeletal problems seen more commonly in the female athlete.

- The rate of noncontact ACL injuries has been found to be higher for women in numerous sports, and strategies for injury prevention have gained popularity.

- The medical issue of greatest concern in women has been termed the female athlete triad: disordered eating, amenorrhea, and osteoporosis.

The past 30 years has witnessed a tremendous growth in the participation of women in sports at all levels of play (middle school, high school, collegiate, professional, and recreational levels). According to U.S. government statistics, women's sport participation increased by 700% during the 1980s. In the 2003 to 2004 academic year, 2,865,299 girls participated in high school sports (National Federation of State High School Associations NFHS 2003 to 2004 High School Athletics Participation Survey, unpublished data, 2004). At the 2000 Olympic Games, 38% of the approximately 10,000 athletes were women, a far cry from the two dozen who competed in the 1928 games. Not only has the number of female athletes increased, but the level and intensity of play have also increased for most women's sports.

Although many of the musculoskeletal problems seen in women are similar to those seen in men, a few injuries and conditions appear to occur with greater frequency. These include scoliosis, shoulder laxity issues, patellofemoral problems (acute patellar instability and chronic overuse injuries), ACL injuries, and overuse problems of the forefoot.

Medical issues of note include anemia, disordered eating, and poor nutrition, the latter of which can result in osteopenia or even osteoporosis and can predispose the athlete to stress frac-

tures. Psychological stresses that can arise when young girls "grow out of their sport" is another area of concern that merits discussion as does sport burnout and overtraining syndrome. These topics are the focus of this chapter.

MUSCULOSKELETAL CONCERNS

Scoliosis

Knowledge of common spinal deformities and the effects strenuous sporting activities have on the developing spine is especially pertinent to diagnosis, outcomes, and level of participation in the female.

Scoliosis is defined as the lateral and rotational curvature of the spine. Idiopathic scoliosis refers to the presence of curvature in the absence of congenital or neurologic abnormalities. Idiopathic scoliosis is the most prevalent form of scoliosis, accounting for approximately 70% of all cases. The adolescent form of this disease is most common and is of particular concern for the female athlete due to the female-to-male ratio approaching 6:1. This is further compounded by the more aggressive progression pattern within the female gender.

The prevalence of adolescent idiopathic scoliosis is reported as 2% to 3% in the general population.[1] However, in certain female dominated sports such as gymnastics, ballet, and swimming, the prevalence has been found to be much higher.

In a study involving Junior Olympic swimmers, Becker[2] reported a 6.9% incidence of idiopathic scoliosis and a 16% incidence of mild functional curves. It was of particular importance that these curves were toward the swimmers' dominant hand side. This implicates muscle imbalance as a possible contributor to scoliosis. It has been postulated that the inequity of forces in these specific training regimens produces asymmetrical development of paraspinal musculature, thus creating a potential risk of the progression of spinal deformity.

Many athletes begin vigorous training in early childhood. It is thought that rapid growth makes immature bone more susceptible to intense training. Hellstrom et al[3] reviewed radiographs of competitive athletes and found abnormalities in the vertebral ring apophyses in gymnasts. In a study by Wojtys et al,[4] the authors correlated the amount of exposure to intense athletic training and the development of spinal curvatures in the immature spine. They found that increased spinal curvature was associated to cumulative hours spent in training; hence, biomechanical stresses may play a role in the progression.

In previous studies on ballet dancers, Warren et al[5] found the incidence of idiopathic scoliosis to be 24%. This was correlated to small body habitus and delayed menarche. It was found that dancers with scoliosis had a slightly higher prevalence of secondary amenorrhea. This suggests hypoestrogenism from delayed menarche and prolonged intervals of amenorrhea may predispose ballet dancers to scoliosis. Tanchev et al[6] found a 10-fold higher incidence of scoliosis in rhythmic gymnastic trainees, which they related to asymmetrical loading, delayed menarche, and ligamentous laxity.

Similar to the male athlete, the diagnosis of adolescent idiopathic scoliosis is made only after a thorough history, physical examination, and appropriate radiographs. The spine should be examined with particular attention given to the neurologic examination. Secondary sex characteristics should be assessed and the skin should be examined for café-au-lait spots, suggesting neurofibromatosis.

The Adams forward bend test is one of the most common screening tests used (Fig. 8-1). The patient bends forward as if to touch the toes. This enhances the spinal curve and demonstrates imbalances in the rib cage. This test is most sensitive to curves in the thoracic region.

Concern that significant deformity is present during screening justifies radiographic evaluation, typically a long anteroposterior and lateral radiograph of the torso that includes the thoracic and lumbar spines on one film and also includes the iliac crest. In addition to curve evaluation, radiographs are also useful for determining skeletal maturity. Additional tests such as a magnetic resonance imaging are indicated in patients with idiopathic scoliosis in the presence of neurologic abnormalities[7] or if the presenting complaint is back pain that does not respond to several weeks of conservative care (rest from activity, back exercises, and anti-inflammatory drugs). It is generally accepted that scoliosis is normally a painless condition.[1] The presence of pain may indicate an underlying condition such as fracture, tumor, spondylolysis, or disk herniation and therefore warrants investigation. Routine magnetic resonance imaging evaluation of all patients with adolescent idiopathic scoliosis is not recommended.

In the past, athletes identified with scoliosis were largely restricted from athletic participation. This philosophy was grandfathered from traditional teachings and based on studies demonstrating exercise was of no benefit in preventing progression. Experience and increasing understanding of scoliosis have begun to reverse this trend. Becker[2] believed that exercise and cross-training might help counteract overloading forces secondary to sport-specific training. Mooney et al[8] discuss this in a report on the effect of measured strength training in adolescent idiopathic scoliosis. These authors found measured strength differences between sides ranging from 12% to 47% and describe a benefit to rotary torso strengthening. Encouraging adolescents with scoliosis to participate in sports is now generally accepted as it is now thought that activity can help maintain endurance and flexibility, minimizing the asymmetrical forces on the spine.

The use of bracing has been shown in several studies to halt progression. Bracing is generally recommended in those whose curve is greater than 20 to 25 degrees. With the development of newer materials and evidence of the efficacy of nighttime brace wear, athletes now can participate both in and out of brace, depending on their unique situation (e.g., degree of curve, sport).

Discussion of specific indications and therapeutic options for athletes with progressive or severe curves is beyond the scope of this chapter. In deciding treatment, the type of sport and level of performance should be considered in combination with the severity of the deformity.[9] Much controversy exists over athletic participation after surgical intervention. Rubery and Bradford[10] polled members of the Scoliosis Research Society on athletic activity following spine surgery and presented the opinions of 261 surgeons active in treating spinal deformities. They discovered that the most common time to resume low-impact, noncontact sports was 6 months and that contact sports were generally allowed after 12 months. However, athletes were encouraged not to participate in collision sports.

In summary, increasing numbers of female athletes with idiopathic scoliosis are participating in sports. It is prudent for the treating physician to identify sport-specific risks associated with spinal deformity. Care for these athletes should be individualized. Increased knowledge and improvements in bracing protocols and surgical techniques have enhanced the quality of life for female athletes with scoliosis by allowing continued involvement in their athletic endeavors.

Shoulder Instability

Shoulder laxity has been traditionally associated with the female athlete. Hormonal factors such as progesterone, estrogen, and relaxin[11] as well as decreased upper extremity muscle mass[12] have all been implicated. Yet there has been much debate as to whether these gender-specific differences contribute to injury patterns. The shoulder is a complex, highly mobile structure. In order to accommodate for extremes in motion, there is a delicate dynamic between normal and pathologic. The glenohumeral joint is inherently unstable. Relative to the glenoid, the humeral head is very large, providing only a small contact surface area for bony support. Thus, the joint relies heavily on balanced contraction of rotator cuff musculature, coordinated scapulothoracic motion, and the integrity of the soft tissues. It has been proposed that the female athlete is predisposed to atraumatic or multidirectional shoulder instability due to laxity of capsuloligamentous constraints. McFarland et al[13] and Borsa et al[14] investigated these issues and found shoulders to be appreciably

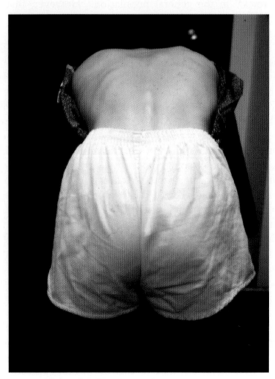

Figure 8-1 The Adams forward bend test.

more lax in females than males. However, it must be noted that the terms laxity and instability should not be interchanged.

While laxity describes the physiologic motions of the glenohumeral joint, it is not itself pathologic.[15] The term instability should be reserved for painful motion resulting in subluxation or dislocation.[11] In 1980, Neer and Foster[12] recognized multidirectional instability as a specific entity. While the essential lesion was initially thought to be capsular redundancy, operative findings of capsular tears and labral avulsions (Bankart lesions) have shown that the etiology is multifactorial.[11,16-18] It is thought that direct trauma or repetitive microtrauma, such as that found in overhead-throwing athletes, superimposed on a lax shoulder might result in instability.[18]

The physical examination is important in differentiating these two entities. The patient may present with vague complaints of pain, apprehension, and shoulder fatigue with or without voluntary subluxation. The shoulder should be assessed for range-of-motion deficits, rotator cuff weakness, and asymmetry of scapular motion. Excessive anterior and posterior motion of the humeral head and inferior translation with downward traction on the humerus (sulcus sign) can help identify laxity (Fig. 8-2). Many provocative tests such as the load and shift test, the apprehension relocation test, and the release test, described in the shoulder section of this book, can be used to elicit instability. In general, pain or apprehension while placing the shoulder in the abduction external rotation position is suggestive of instability.

Initial treatment for multidirectional instability should be conservative. With the assistance of a physical therapist, a program of mobilization, flexibility, and strengthening should be initiated. Graduated resistance training using elastic bands or weights through internal and external rotation motions are useful for strengthening the rotator cuff, thereby improving dynamic stability of the joint (Fig. 8-3). Scapular stabilizing muscles (trapezius, serratus anterior, rhomboids, and levator scapulae) must also be strengthened. Scapulothoracic motion is vital to overhead activity; in order to abduct the arm, the scapula must tilt and elevate. Failure of this motion can result in impingement on the underlying structures. To address this, activities such as pull backs, shoulder shrugs, and knee and wall push-ups, which emphasize protraction of the scapula as well as the correction of poor posture, are typically prescribed (Fig. 8-4). In addition, athletes should be enrolled in sport-specific training to enhance muscular control and proprioception.

Surgical treatment should be offered if the patient has not responded within 6 to 9 months of rehabilitation. The original surgical procedure was the open inferior capsular shift, aimed to reduce capsular redundancy.[12] Many authors report improvements in stability and return to preinjury activity level with this procedure or variations of open stabilization techniques.[17,19,20] Arthroscopic stabilization has been introduced as an alternative to established open procedures. The advantages include better identification of underlying intra-articular pathology,[16] less morbidity, and improved cosmesis. With the development of improved arthroscopic techniques, several clinical trials have reported excellent results for the treatment of multidirectional instability. Arthroscopic repair has also been shown to withstand the stress of sports activities.[21,22] Mazzocca et al[22] examined the results of arthroscopic anterior shoulder stabilization in collision and contact athletes. They reported 100% return to organized sports and believe that participation in collision and contact athletics was not a contraindication for arthroscopic repair. No gender-specific trials on the fate of patients treated operatively or nonoperatively are available.

Arthroscopic thermal capsulorrhaphy, which uses heat to shrink capsular volume, has been introduced in recent years. However, several authors have reported high failure rates and increased incidences of postoperative complications,[23,24] making this a less favored procedure.

Anterior Knee Pain

Difficulties with patellofemoral tracking can result in acute injuries (patellar subluxation or dislocation) or overuse problems (patellofemoral stress syndrome or anterior knee pain). Patellar subluxation and dislocation are discussed in detail in Chapter 57 and are not covered in this section.

Patellofemoral stress syndrome is a name given to the syndrome of anterior knee pain or patellofemoral pain associated with diffuse anterior knee pain that increases with such activities as squatting, kneeling, running, walking down steps, or walking downhill and is common in women athletes, especially young women. The diagnosis of patellofemoral stress is based on history and clinical examination (Table 8-1). Squats and lunges (i.e., those activities that increase patellofemoral forces) frequently enhance symptoms. Swelling is rarely present. Other symptoms of this syndrome include popping, catching, and snapping. Athletes may experience acute episodes of the knee giving out or giving way. Occasionally, crepitus may be present, although in general, this symptom more typically occurs in those with true softening and fraying of the retropatellar surfaces (chondromalacia) rather than the overuse problem of patellofemoral irritability, anterior knee pain, or patellofemoral stress syndrome.

Athletes will frequently report that they have a change in their exercise activity prior to the onset of symptoms with either

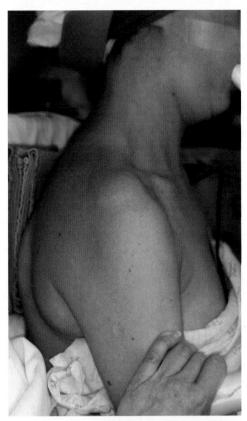

Figure 8-2 Sulcus sign. Note displacement of the humeral head inferiorly when traction is applied to the extremity.

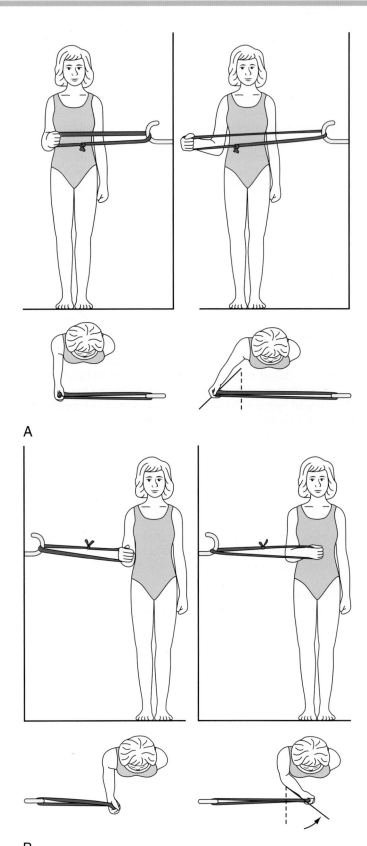

A

B

Figure 8-3 Exercises to strengthen the rotator cuff. **A,** External rotation: Stand with elbow at side and gently rotate arm out as illustrated. **B,** Internal rotation: Rotate arm across front of body as illustrated.

Table 8-1 Diagnosis of Patellofemoral Stress Syndrome
Frequent Symptoms
Locking
Catching
Giving out
Increased pain with flexion-extension movements (e.g., kicking, running)
Pain while squatting, kneeling, prolonged sitting, sitting cross-legged style, and climbing stairs
Physical Examination Features
Increased hip varus
Increased knee valgus
Vastus laterals > vastus medials
Foot pronation
Increased lumbar lordosis
Weak core strength
Increased tightness (apparent or real) of the hamstrings, iliotibial band and/or quadriceps

an increase in running-type activities or an increase in squats and lunges or knee extension exercises. They may report completing the same number of knee extensions but with a higher weight than what they would normally lift. Occasionally, and particularly in recreational athletes, the inciting factor may be related to job or home activities, for example, using a clutch car, moving to an upstairs apartment, or sitting more at work, even though the pain is elicited with sport.

The onset of pain in women is often during the mid-to-late teenage years at the time of transition from the narrower pelvis of adolescence into the wider pelvis of womanhood. College may bring a dramatic change in lifestyle to young women resulting in more seated study time and less active sport play or exercise, resulting in persistent patellofemoral forces from the bent knee position of studying and less vastus medialis obliquus strength.

The patella is guided in the trochlear groove by the bony anatomy of both the patella and the trochlear groove, by the surrounding quadriceps muscle and by the complex ligamentous structures that surround the patella, including the lateral patellofemoral ligament. If, during adolescence, the four heads of the quadriceps do not all develop symmetrically, the asymmetrical pull of the quadriceps can create abnormal patellofemoral forces or at least uneven patellofemoral forces.[25-27]

On physical examination, alignment and flexibility of the extremity should be carefully assessed. Hip varus, knee valgus, and foot pronation are frequently, but not always, present. The athlete may stand with her knees "locked" in hyperextension, a posture that is thought to be associated with increased patellofemoral forces. Tightness of the hamstring and quadriceps muscle groups can add to the abnormal mechanics about the knee and the increase or unequally distributed patellofemoral forces.[28] The normal progression of patellofemoral contact areas during knee flexion is illustrated in Figure 8-5.[29] As the knee

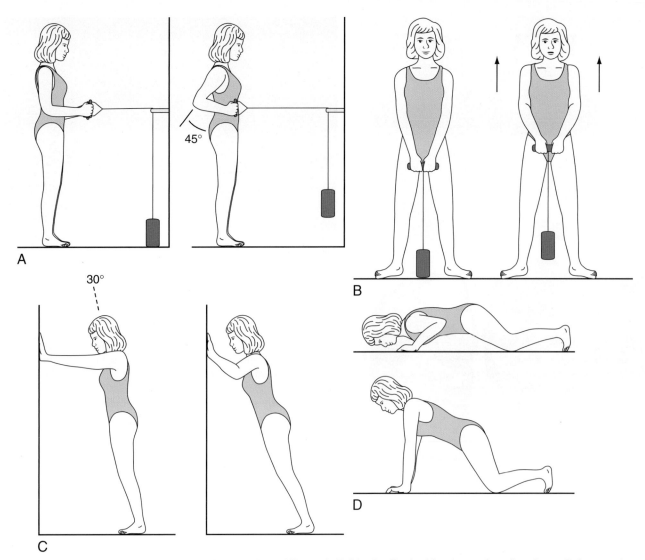

Figure 8-4 Exercises to strengthen the scapular stabilizers. **A,** Pull backs; **B,** shoulder shrugs; **C,** wall push-ups; **D,** knee push-ups.

flexes, the contact area on the patella moves proximally as the contact area on the femur moves inferiorly. At no time is the entire surface of the patella in contact with the trochlear groove of the femur.

Symptomatic athletes will generally have pain to palpation around and behind the patella. Infrequently they have apprehension with lateral deviation of the patella (i.e., a positive apprehension test). They do, however, have pain with slight downward pressure of the patella in the femoral groove. This sign can be enhanced by asking the patient to actively contract the quadriceps muscle while the examiner places an inferiorly directed force on the patella (Fig. 8-6). Typically, no effusion is present. The range of motion of the knee is full.

One theory of the cause of patellofemoral pain is based on the premise that abnormal patellofemoral mechanics can cause increased retropatellar forces that overwhelm the articular surface's ability to absorb the increased stress, resulting in increased pressure on the bone beneath. Dye,[30] who has done a great deal of research in this area, stresses the need to stay within one's "envelope of function." The envelope is determined not only by one's own personal anatomy but also can be influenced by exercise, braces, and orthotics, that is, by altering patellofemoral forces favorably, one can increase the envelope of function.

Radiographs can also be helpful as they may demonstrate an asymmetrical position of the patella in the trochlear groove (Fig. 8-7). Many different radiographic views have been used to describe the relationship of the patella to the trochlear groove. However, the degree of quadriceps contraction at the time the radiograph is taken can markedly change the patella's position in the trochlear groove.[31] Therefore, care must be taken in interpreting these views.

Skyline views of the patella are helpful, however, to provide indirect evidence of the thickness of the patellofemoral articular cartilage. With chondromalacia of the patella, this space may be diminished, but in the overuse syndrome of anterior knee pain or patellofemoral stress, the thickness of the patellofemoral articular cartilage should be normal, indicating a reversible situation (Fig. 8-8). The progression of patellofemoral stress syndrome to chondromalacia is not well known. Most young people

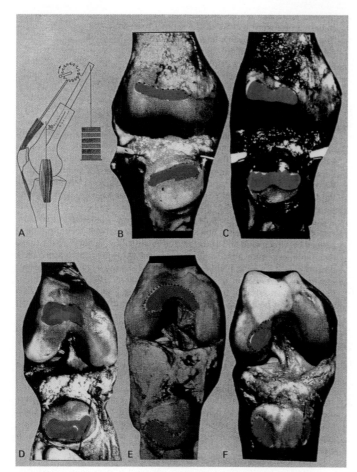

Figure 8-5 Normal progression of patellofemoral contact forces. **A,** Method of applying force to patellofemoral joint; **B,** 20 degrees of flexion; **C,** 60 degrees of flexion; **D,** 90 degrees of flexion; **E,** 120 degrees of flexion; **F,** 135 degrees of flexion. (Adapted from Ficat and Hungerford.[29])

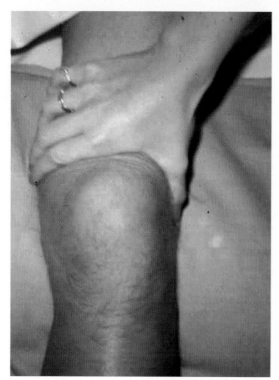

Figure 8-6 Patients with patellofemoral stress syndrome generally will have pain with downward pressure of the patella in the femoral groove.

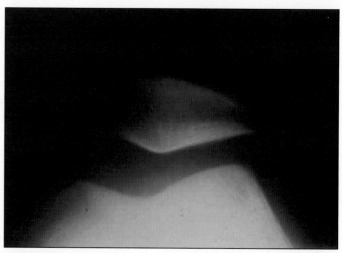

Figure 8-7 Note asymmetrical position of the patella in the trochlear groove.

with the overuse problem of anterior knee pain do not develop pathologic softening of the retropatellar surface (chondromalacia). More studies on the natural history of anterior knee pain are needed.

The treatment of athletes with patellofemoral pain centers on altering patellofemoral forces by altering the patella's position in the femoral groove (Table 8-2). Quadriceps strengthening, typically focused on the vastus medialis muscle, is combined with exercises to strengthen muscles of the hip and trunk. Exercise routines can employ machines, rubber tubing, or free weights.

Athletes should incorporate flexibility exercises for all muscles of the lower extremity and trunk into their program. A hyperextended lumbar spine (i.e., increased lumbar lordosis) can result in apparent shortening of hip external rotators including the iliotibial band and hamstrings and hence influence patellofemoral mechanics. A strong core (i.e., trunk muscles) to absorb impact force on landing may minimize increased stresses to the knee and foot. A good example to use for athletes is to explain that they need to land as "light as a feather" like the ballerina does when she lands en pointe.

Braces or tape are used to shift the patella's position to a more favorable one in the femoral groove.[32,33] Some patients prefer braces with a lateral pad; other patients prefer braces that have a pad about the entire patella. Others prefer an open patellar brace; some like merely an infrapatellar strap that lifts the patella superiorly in the groove or at least attempts to decrease pressure on the patellofemoral surface by elevating the patella (Fig. 8-9). A trial-and-error method in selecting a brace is often used as it may be difficult to predict which type of brace will be most helpful to the athlete. Orthotics to decrease foot pronation may be used to better align the patella as foot pronation can result in an increase in apparent knee valgus and hence lateral displacement of the patella in the groove.[34]

Oral nonsteroidal anti-inflammatory drugs can be used at a time of marked increased symptoms, but athletes must understand that these drugs do not alter the course of the overuse syndrome, but merely temporarily decrease symptoms caused by the inflammatory reaction. Therefore, it is essential to participate in an exercise program and incorporate other conservative measures into their routine. Activity modification, even if

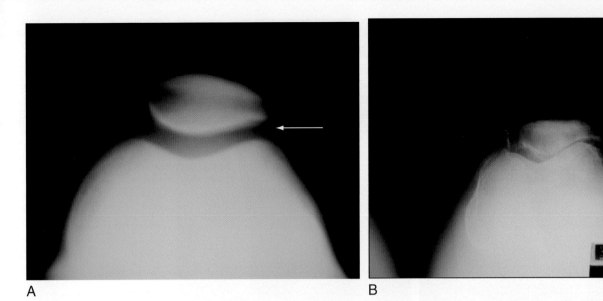

Figure 8-8 Skyline view of the patellofemoral joint. **A,** Note the width of the cartilage space *(arrow)* in a young knee with patellofemoral stress syndrome and no loss of articular cartilage space. **B,** Note the reduced width of the cartilage space *(arrow)* in the knee of a patient with significant chondromalacia.

only temporary, may be needed to decrease irritability until patellofemoral forces can be altered advantageously.

Anterior Cruciate Ligament Injuries

The rate of noncontact ACL injuries in high-risk sports such as soccer and basketball is greater in female than in male athletes.[35-37] The young appear to be most at risk, with the vast majority of ACL injuries occurring in those 15 to 45 years of age.[38] In one study, the average age of those who sustained an ACL injury was 26 years.[39] Neither risk factors nor the mechanism of injury is well defined for ACL noncontact injuries. Proposed risk factors include shoe-surface interactions and other environmental concerns; anatomic factors such as hip varus, knee valgus, foot pronation, femoral notch size, and size of the ACL; hormonal factors (levels of estrogen, progesterone, relaxin, and others); and neuromuscular factors such as upright posture, landing a jump and cutting on a straight knee, leg dominance, and poor hamstring strength relative to quadriceps strength (quadriceps dominance).[40,41]

Landing a jump, cutting, pivoting, or changing directions accounts for 80% to 85% of all noncontact ACL injuries. Often the athlete recalls that just prior to making a planned move, someone cut in front of her, bumped her, or in some similar way made her accommodate quickly to the change in direction of movement or landing.[42]

Men have less hip varus and knee valgus than women, and they appear to land a jump with their hips and knees more flexed than women.[43] Unlike women, men's strength is relatively equal in both lower extremities, and they fire their hamstrings more rapidly and prior to their quadriceps with an anteriorly directed tibial force, both appropriate responses to protect the ACL.[40,44] The diagnosis and management of ACL injuries in women are similar to those in men, as discussed in Chapter 51. Although at one time it was theorized that women would fare less well than men following ACL reconstruction, studies have not found this to be true. ACL reconstruction using autologous bone-patellar tendon-bone is as functionally stable in females as in males, and Tegner and Lysholm's scores after reconstruction are similar.[45,46] Although Barrett et al[47] reported increased laxity scores in women following ACL reconstruction with autologous quadruple hamstring tendon, others have reported equivalent results in males and females.[48-50]

During rehabilitation following ACL reconstruction, the therapist should emphasize avoidance of abnormal mechanics leading to ACL injury, substituting instead proper landing and cutting skills and agility skills minimizing dominant leg characteristics if such exist. Moreover, these same principles should be highlighted as a part of preseason conditioning programs. Drills to enhance balance and agility, incorporating plyometrics with an emphasis on proper landing techniques (i.e., landing light as a feather by contracting core muscles and with more hip and knee flexion and with the body balanced over the lower extremity) should be practiced.

In fact, a six-part preseason and in-season prevention program has been proposed by some and includes recognition of injury mechanics, flexibility and strengthening exercises, aerobic conditioning, plyometrics, and agility drills (Table 8-3).[51] These exercises should be incorporated into normal sport conditioning programs. Programs using these strategies or even those merely

Table 8-2 Overview of Treatment for Patellofemoral Stress Syndrome	
Strengthen	Quadriceps, particularly vastus medialis obliques and core
Increase flexibility	Trunk and lower extremities
Braces	To support, lift, or move the patella medially
Shoe orthotics	To decrease foot pronation
Activity modification	Decreased flexion/extension activities until acute symptoms subside
Nonsteroidal anti-inflammatory drugs	If no stomach irritability and no history of allergies to these medications

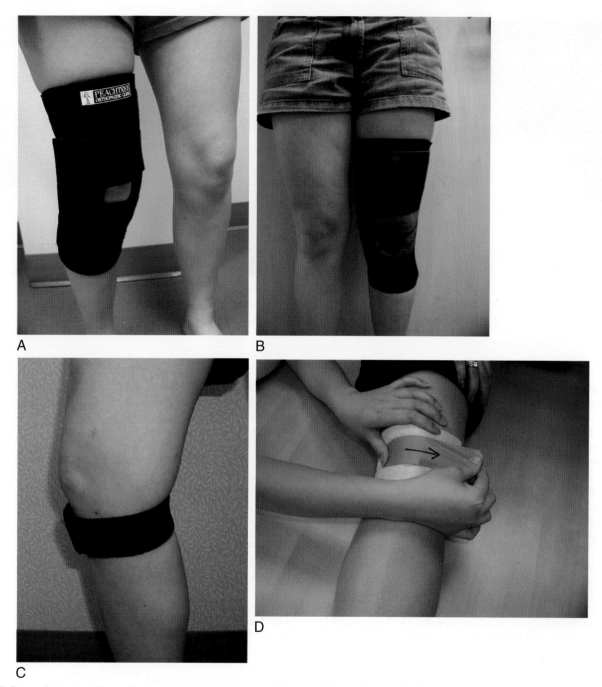

Figure 8-9 Braces/taping are frequently used as part of the treatment for patellofemoral stress. **A,** Brace with lateral pad; **B,** brace with a doughnut pad around patella; **C,** infrapatellar strap; **D,** patellar taping. The tape "pulls" the patella medially.

Table 8-3 Six-Part Alternative Warm-up Program for Anterior Cruciate Ligament Injury Prevention
Enhance recognition of injury mechanics
Increase flexibility of core and lower extremity muscles
Increase strength of core and lower extremity muscles
Aerobic conditioning
Incorporate plyometrics
Perform agility drills

incorporating simple balance drills into preseason and in-season condition routines have been reported to decrease the incidence of ACL noncontact injuries (Table 8-4).[41,52]

Some investigators have also proposed that those girls found to have poor landing skills and significant deficits in hamstring strength may benefit from participating in an intense therapy program prior to the beginning of the season or even during the season, in addition to performing an alternative in the field conditioning program.[53] More data from randomized, controlled trials with numbers sufficient to have adequate power from which to draw reliable conclusions are needed. However, early reports from trials of existing programs are very encouraging.

Forefoot Pain

It has been reported that 8% of all females wear shoes smaller than their feet and that this trend starts with adolescence. Girls also engage in more "foot abusive" sports than men. Although women spend more than men on athletic shoewear ($5.4 billion versus $5.3 billion), many shoe manufacturers do not make a last sized to a female's foot but merely scale down their male last. This results in a shoe with an inappropriate forefoot width-to-length ratio, predisposing female athletes to develop corns, calluses, bunions, bunionettes, and hammertoes.

Treatment of these forefoot abnormalities is generally symptomatic conservative care with pads, creams, moleskin, exercises, and shoe modification. Surgery should be approached with great caution as secondary biomechanical problems can result. Figure 8-10 is a radiograph of a young cross-country runner who had bunion surgery and then developed stress fractures in the second and thirds metatarsals from altered mechanical forces resulting from a shorter first metatarsal.

Stress fractures of the metatarsals are also frequent in dancers as well as runners and gymnasts. Bone is a dynamic tissue constantly repairing damage to its structure caused by activity. Stress fractures or microfractures of the bone occur when the rate of bone repair falls behind the rate of bone formation. This can occur if the athlete does too much too fast without proper conditioning or the repair processes are slowed secondary to one of several factors including inadequate sleep, a poor diet, or lack of adequate estrogen (as discussed in the section on the female athlete triad).

Clinically, the athlete with a forefoot stress fracture will complain of pain and swelling in the midfoot just behind the metatarsal heads. The swelling and pain increase with activity and improve with rest. They are better in the morning after a night's sleep. Initial radiographs may not demonstrate the early stress reaction, but if the athlete continues to participate in her sport despite pain, the increased insult to the bone results in a fracture line, which can be seen radiographically. If rest is instituted early when pain first begins, radiographs may never show a fracture line but instead may reveal an area of increased bone density indicative of healing. Because foot mobility is needed for performance by many female athletes (e.g., the gymnast, runner, and dancer), these athletes cannot perform in a hard-soled shoe, as might a football lineman, and will lose from 4 to 10 weeks from sport until their fracture heals. Preventing stress fractures by proper conditioning, adequate sleep, and appropriate diet and footwear is essential.

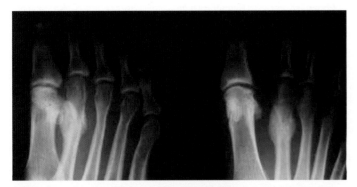

Figure 8-10 Runner who sustained a stress fracture of the second metatarsal after bunionectomy. Note shortening of the first metatarsal increasing stress to the second.

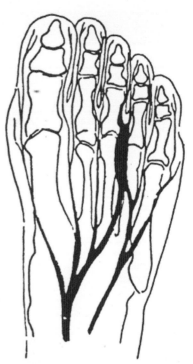

Figure 8-11 Schematic diagram of the compression of the interdigital nerve by adjacent metatarsal heads.

Interdigital neuroma or Morton's neuroma is a painful condition of the forefoot resulting from entrapment and perineural fibrosis of the interdigital nerve as it traverses the web space between the metatarsal heads (Fig. 8-11). This condition, which is eight times more prevalent in women than men, occurs most commonly between the second and third metatarsal heads but can also occur between the third and fourth metatarsal heads. The term neuroma, which is often used to describe this condition, is incorrect. The condition arises from entrapment and perineural fibrosis rather than a proliferation of neuronal tissue.

Patients will report paresthesias in the adjacent two toes as well as a vague pain relieved by removing the shoe and massaging the foot. On physical examination, swelling may be present between the metatarsal heads at the involved interspace, and pain can be reproduced by transverse pressure on the metatarsal heads while simultaneously placing upward pressure on the plantar surface of the foot at the site of discomfort (Fig. 8-12). Radiographs are normal but may show close proximity of the metatarsal heads at the involved site.

Conservative treatment includes the use of a wide toe box shoe, metatarsal pads, foot and toe exercises, and consideration of a steroid injection. If these measures fail to relieve symptoms, the most common surgical procedure is resection of the nerve in the intermetatarsal area, which can achieve satisfactory results.[54,55] Once again, caution should be exerted before surgery is undertaken as scar secondary to surgical intervention may alter performance in a female athlete who depends on mobility of the foot for her sport.

MEDICAL CONCERNS

The Female Athlete Triad

The term the female athlete triad was selected by a 1992 consensus conference called by the Task Force on Women's Issues

Table 8-4 Prevention Programs

No.	Author	Sport	No.	Duration	Sex	Random	Equipment	Strength	Flexibility	Agility	Plyometrics
1	Griffis et al (1989) S	Basketball	Not reported 2 teams	8 yr	F	No	Jump box, balance	No	No	Yes	No, landing technique
2	Ettinger et al (1995)	Alpine skiing	T: 4000 C: ?	1 yr with 2 yr of historic controls	M/F	No	Video clips of skiers sustaining ACL injuries and those who avoided injury in very similar falls	No	No	No	No
3	Caraffa et al (1996)	Soccer	T: 300 C: 300	3 seasons	M	No, prospective	Balance boards	PNF facilitation exercises	Yes	No	No
4	Hewett et al (1999) A	Basketball, volleyball, soccer	1263	1 yr	M/F	Yes	Jump box, balance	Yes	No	No	Yes
5	Heidt et al (2000) A, S	Soccer	300	1 yr intervention (7-wk period)	F	No	Sports cord, box jump	Yes	No	Yes	Yes
6	Söderman et al (2000) S	Soccer	T: 121 C: 100	1 season (Apr–Oct)	F	Yes	Balance board in addition to regular training	No	No	No	No
7	Myklebust et al (2003)	Team handball	900	3 yr	F	No	Wobble board, balance foam mats	No	Yes	Planting NM control	No, landing technique
8	Wedderkopp et al (2003) A, S	Team handball	236	10 mo	F	Yes, cluster RCT	Balance board (proprioceptive) in 4 levels	No	No	Yes	Yes
9	Gilchrist et al (2004)	Soccer	561	1 yr	F	Yes	Cones, soccer ball	Yes, glut med. abd, ext, hamstring, core	Yes	Deceleration, sport specific	No, landing technique, multiplanar
10	Pfeiffer et al (2004)	Soccer	1439	9 wk	F	No	No	No	Yes	Cut, NM control	No, landing technique
11	Mandelbaum et al (2005)	Soccer	T: 1041 C: 844	2 yr	F	No, voluntary enrollment	Cones, soccer ball	Hamstring, core	Yes	Soccer specific with dec tech	No, landing technique, multiplanar
12	Olsen et al (2005) A	Team handball	1837	1 yr	M/F	Yes, cluster RCT	Wobble board, balance foam mats	Yes	Yes	Cut, NM control	No, landing technique

A, Anterior cruciate ligament (ACL) injuries not specifically assessed; M, male; F, female; RCT, randomized controlled trial; S, sample size relatively small (power inadequate?).
From Griffin LY, Albohm MJ, Arendt EA, et al.[41]

Proprioception	Program/Study Strengths	Program/Study Weaknesses	Outcome
Yes, deceleration pattern (3-step shuffle)	Changing deceleration and landing technique (encouraged knee and hip flexion)	Not randomized, unpublished	89% decrease in noncontact ACL injury
No	Nonrandomized, controlled interventional study. Large number of injuries	Not randomized. Not all potential participants trained. Historic controls. Exact diagnosis of knee sprain not always available. Exact exposure to risk not precisely determined	Severe knee sprains were reduced by 62% among trained skiers (patrollers and instructors) compared to unperturbed group who had no improvement during the study period
Yes, balance board activities, multilevel	Mechanoreceptor/ proprioception training	Additional equipment; not cost-effective on large-scale basis	87% decrease in noncontact ACL injury, 1.15 rate reduced to 0.15/1000 AE
Yes	Decrease peak landing forces and valgus/varus perturbations, increase vertical leap, increase hamstring strength and decrease time to contraction	1-on-1 program in sports facility, not feasible to implement across large cohort	Female injury rates 0.43–0.12 (male = 0.9) over 6-wk program. Untrained group 3.6–4.8 higher rates of ACL injury
Yes	Increased strength, lower overall injury rates	Not statistically significant, 7 wk insufficient for NM education to occur at mechanoreceptor level	61.2% injuries in knee/ankle, 2.4% injury rate in intervention vs 3.1 in control
Yes, balance	Randomized	Small number, low overall injury incidence. 37% dropout rate, not all subjects received same amount of training. Unknown whether additional training was controlled	Intervention did not reduce risk of primary traumatic injuries to lower extremities; 4 of 5 ACL injuries in total sample occurred in intervention group
Balance activities on mats and boards	Compliance to program monitored; instructional video	Not randomized	In elite team division, risk of injury was reduced among those who completed program (odds ratio: 0.06 [0.01–0.54]) compared with control, overall reduction of ACL injury
Balance training with ankle disks	RCT	Injury types not specified. Description of ankle disk training not provided. Intervention group also did warm-up exercises but not specified. Compliance not assessed	Ankle injuries were significantly greater in control group (2.4 vs 0.2). Unspecified knee injuries were not significantly less in trained group (0.9 vs 0.6). Five knee sprains and 1 knee subluxation in control group vs 1 knee sprain in trained group
Strength on field perturbation on grass	Instructional video, Web site, compliance monitored (random site visits)	1 yr intervention, began at day 1 of season	Overall 72% reduction in ACL injury, 100% reduction in practice contact and noncontact ACL injury, 100% reduction in contact and noncontact ACL injury in last 6 wk of season
No	Compliance monitored; significant reduction in F & RFD in intervention	No decrease in injury, intervention performed at end of training, possible fatigue phenomenon	6 noncontact ACL injuries: 3 in treatment and 3 in control = no direct effect
Strength on field perturbation on grass	Instructional video, Web site, compliance monitored	Not randomized, inherent selection bias	Injury rates: yr 1: 88% reduction in noncontact ACL injury; yr 2: 74% reduction in noncontact ACL injury
Balance activity on mats and boards	Randomized, compliance monitored, reduction of injury	Efficacious component(s) of intervention not known	129 acute knee & ankle injuries overall, 81 in control (0.9 overall, 0.3 train, 5.3 match) vs 48 injuries in intervention (0.5 overall, 0.2 train, 2.5 match)

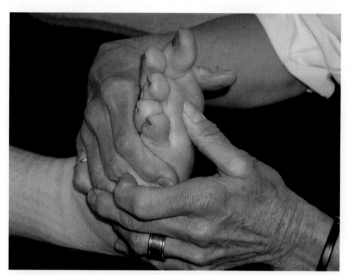

Figure 8-12 The pain from a Morton's neuroma can be elicited with upward pressure on the plantar aspect of the foot between the metatarsal heads simultaneously with transverse compression across the metatarsal heads.

of the American College of Sports Medicine to refer to the association of disordered eating, amenorrhea (lack of normal periods for three consecutive months), and osteoporosis (low bone mineral density), three conditions seen with increasing prevalence over the past several decades in female athletes, which individually, and certainly together, can result in impaired health and athletic performance.

Disordered eating can result in inadequate nutrition or energy, which can lead to abnormal menstrual function; abnormal menstrual function can result in low estrogen amenorrhea, which can result in osteopenia (minimally decrease bone mineral density) or even osteoporosis (more severe loss of bone mineral density). Stress fractures may be the consequence of the latter. Bone mass is influenced by estrogen, calcium, and exercise. Peak bone mineral density is achieved by age 25 after which premenopausal women lose 0.3% of their skeleton per year and postmenopausal women or those without periods (e.g., amenorrheic athletes) lose 2% of their bone mass per year. Therefore, concern has been raised that either inadequate calcium intake and/or inadequate estrogen from amenorrhea during the years of maximal bone mineral storage (young teens through 25) may lead to significant osteoporosis during the postmenopausal years. More recently, amenorrhea has been linked to cardiovascular disease and disordered eating to poor function of the immune system.

Athletes most at risk of developing the triad are young women involved in sports in which the lean look is thought to be advantageous (e.g., gymnastics, figure skating, dance, diving, and cheerleading), sports in which weight categories exists (e.g., rowing), and endurance sports (e.g., swimming and cross-country running).[56]

Disordered eating refers to a continuum of abnormal eating behaviors of which three categories have been recognized: anorexia nervosa, bulimia nervosa, and eating disorders not otherwise specified (Tables 8-5 through 8-8). The athlete with disordered eating has abnormal eating behaviors that may involve the quantity of food ingested; abnormal eating patterns (e.g., eating excessively and vomiting following eating); or inappropriate use of laxatives, diuretics, or other medical substances.

Table 8-5 Types of Eating Disorders
Anorexia nervosa 　Restricting type 　Binge eating/purging type
Bulimia nervosa 　Purging type 　Nonpurging type
Eating disorder not otherwise specified

The prevalence of disordered eating is higher for athletes than nonathletes; female athletes are more affected than male athletes. Studies have reported a 62% occurrence rate in female collegiate gymnasts, a 47% occurrence in long-distance female runners, and a 15.4% occurrence rate in elite female swimmers.[57,58] Overall, 32% to 64% of all female athletes have been reported to display some type of disordered eating.[59]

Recognition of the athlete with disordered eating is frequently difficult. Coaches may report a decrease in performance. Abnormal behavior during meals or a preoccupation with food may provide clues to the diagnosis. Once the diagnosis is made, treatment is provided through a team approach with a sports medicine physician, sports nutritionist, and mental health provider, preferably an eating disorder specialist.

Amenorrhea is defined as 3 or more months of missed menstrual cycles and has been associated with heavy physical training. Primary amenorrhea has been redefined by the American Society of Reproductive Medicine as the absence of menstrual cycles in a girl who has not menstruated by age 15. Secondary amenorrhea is cessation of menses after the first menstrual cycle.[60] Prevalence of amenorrhea has been documented as high as 65% in long-distance runners and 44% in dancers compared to 2% to 5% in nonathletic collegiate women.[60] Amenorrhea was

Table 8-6 Diagnostic Criteria for Anorexia Nervosa
Refusal to maintain body weight at or above a minimally normal weight for age and height (e.g., weight loss leading to maintenance of body weight less than 85% of that expected or failure to make expected weight gain during period of growth, leading to body weight less than 85% of that expected).
Intense fear of gaining weight or becoming fat, even though underweight.
Disturbance in the way in which one's body weight or shape is experienced, undue influence of body weight or shape on self-evaluation, or denial of the seriousness of the current low body weight.
In postmenarcheal females, amenorrhea, i.e., the absence of at least three consecutive menstrual cycles. (A woman is considered to have amenorrhea if her periods occur only following hormone, e.g., estrogen, administration.) 　Restricting type: During the current episode of anorexia nervosa, the person has not regularly engaged in binge eating or purging behavior (i.e., self-induced vomiting or the misuse of laxatives, diuretics, or enemas) 　Binge eating/purging type: During the current episode of anorexia nervosa, the person has regularly engaged in binge eating or purging behavior (i.e., self-induced vomiting or the misuse of laxatives, diuretics, or enemas)

American Psychiatric Association.[70]

Table 8-7 Diagnostic Criteria for Bulimia Nervosa

Recurrent episodes of binge eating. An episode of binge eating is characterized by both of the following:
  Eating, in a discrete period of time (e.g., within any 2-hour period), an amount of food that is definitely larger than most people would eat during a similar period of time and under similar circumstances.
  A sense of lack of control over eating during the episode (e.g., a feeling that one cannot stop eating or control what or how much one is eating).

Recurrent inappropriate compensatory behavior to prevent weight gain, such as self-induced vomiting; misuse of laxative, diuretics, enemas, or other medications; fasting; or excessive exercise.

The binge eating and inappropriate compensatory behaviors both occur, on average, at least twice a week for 3 months.

Self-evaluation is unduly influenced by body shape and weight.

The disturbance does not occur exclusively during episodes of anorexia nervosa.
  Purging type: During the current episode of bulimia nervosa, the person has regularly engaged in self-induced vomiting or the misuse of laxatives, diuretics, or enemas.
  Nonpurging type: During the current episode of bulimia nervosa, the person has used other inappropriate compensatory behaviors, such as fasting or excessive exercise, but has not regularly engaged in self-induced vomiting or the misuse of laxatives, diuretics, or enemas.

American Psychiatric Association.[70]

initially thought to result from low body weight and low body fat. More recently, its onset is thought to be more related to energy deficit. The energy deficit may be caused by inadequate energy intake (disordered eating).

Once thought to be a benign, reversible condition that many athletes considered a benefit for athletic participation, pro-

Table 8-8 Eating Disorder Not Otherwise Specified

This category is for those eating disorders that do not meet the criteria for any specific eating disorder. Examples include the following:
  For females, all the criteria for anorexia nervosa are met except that the individual has regular menses.
  All the criteria for anorexia nervosa are met except that, despite significant weight loss, the individual's current weight is in the normal range.
  All the criteria for bulimia nervosa are met except that the binge eating and inappropriate compensatory mechanisms occur at a frequency of less than twice a week or for a duration of less than 3 months.
  The regular use of inappropriate compensatory behavior by an individual of normal body weight after eating small amounts of food (e.g., self-induced vomiting after the consumption of two cookies).
  Repeatedly chewing and spitting out, but not swallowing, a large amount of food.
  Binge eating disorder: Recurrent episodes of binge eating in the absence of the regular use of inappropriate compensatory behaviors characteristic of bulimia nervosa.

American Psychiatric Association.[70]

longed amenorrhea is now thought to be a serious medical problem linked to diminished estrogen and a resultant loss of normal bone mineral density as well as to cardiovascular disease as occurs in postmenopausal women. Therefore, recognition and treatment are essential. Treatment consists of correcting the disordered eating and energy deficit, a major challenge in most of the athletes with this disorder.

Osteoporosis, the third component of the female athlete triad, is defined as decreased bone mass with disruption of the normal microarchitecture of bone. Bone is a living tissue and is continually undergoing remodeling and repair. Discrepancies that occur when the rate of bone resorption exceeds the rate of formation lead to the onset of diminished bone mineral density. The degree of loss of bone mass has been defined by the World Health Organization based on the amount of bone mineral density detected by bone densitometry. Bone densitometry measurements are most commonly done by dual-energy x-ray absorptiometry. In this technique, an aerial section of the spine or hip is analyzed for mineralized tissue. The results are compared with peers and against a young healthy adult population known to have peak bone mass, resulting in a value termed a *T* score (Fig. 8-13). Individuals found to be between 1 and 2.4 standard deviations below peak bone mass are considered to have osteopenia or low bone mineral density, and those with values greater than 2.5 standard deviations below peak bone mass are thought to have osteoporosis or severe loss of bone mineral density (Table 8-9). Recently, Khan et al[61] have suggested replacing the term osteoporosis in the triad with osteopenia, a far more common entity than osteoporosis among athletes and one that lends itself to early recognition and lifestyle changes to avoid further bone loss.

The International Society for Clinical Densitometry has recommended that the bone density of young women (adolescents and premenopausal women) be compared to that of women of their own age group. This is known as the *Z* score.[60] Values are interpreted according to the same scale as the *T* scores. A loss of 1 standard deviation of bone mineral density results in a 1.9 increased risk of spine fracture or a 2.4 increased risk of hip fracture in the elderly.[62] Such data are not available for young athletes, but inferences can be drawn.

As in the discussions on disordered eating and amenorrhea, detection of athletes with the female athlete triad is difficult. Screening athletes for menstrual, diet, and exercise history may be helpful (Table 8-10); however, frequently athletes with this disorder do not wish to be detected and will supply inaccurate answers. The sports medicine specialist must be alert to indirect signs of this disorder such as alteration in performance and secretive eating behaviors. A stress fracture in a lean female athlete should prompt further investigation into menstrual and dietary habits. Consideration of bone mineral density studies should be given to those following an initial stress fracture and indeed for those who have recurrent stress fractures.

Treatment intervention in the athlete diagnosed with the triad is frequently difficult and requires a multidisciplinary approach typically involving the physician, athletic trainer, physical therapist, coach, nutritionist, and sport psychologist. Improving the energy deficit through increasing caloric intake will help to establish regular periods and hence increase estrogen to improve bone health. A reasonable goal should be smaller amounts of food throughout the day to avoid the sensation of "overeating" or "being too full." Women athletes are not unique compared to men in needing to maintain a good nutritional state, but they are unique in regard to many medical conditions linked

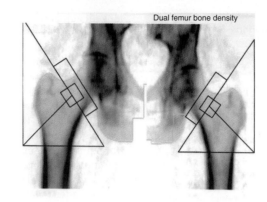

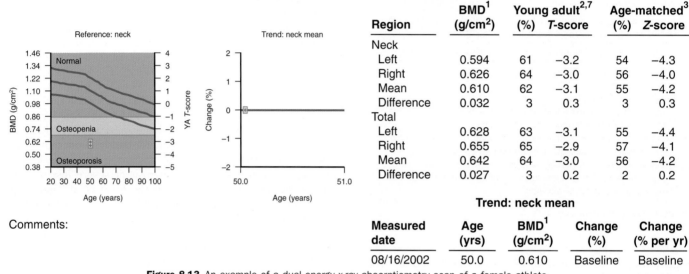

Region	BMD[1] (g/cm²)	Young adult[2,7] (%)	Young adult[2,7] T-score	Age-matched[3] (%)	Age-matched[3] Z-score
Neck					
Left	0.594	61	−3.2	54	−4.3
Right	0.626	64	−3.0	56	−4.0
Mean	0.610	62	−3.1	55	−4.2
Difference	0.032	3	0.3	3	0.3
Total					
Left	0.628	63	−3.1	55	−4.4
Right	0.655	65	−2.9	57	−4.1
Mean	0.642	64	−3.0	56	−4.2
Difference	0.027	3	0.2	2	0.2

Trend: neck mean

Comments:

Measured date	Age (yrs)	BMD[1] (g/cm²)	Change (%)	Change (% per yr)
08/16/2002	50.0	0.610	Baseline	Baseline

Figure 8-13 An example of a dual energy x-ray absorptiometry scan of a female athlete.

to poor nutritional or energy states. Athletes are frequently resistant to increasing calories for health reasons but frequently understand the need to improve energy for improved performance. (The analogy of a car being unable to go far without adequate fuel is often used.) Along with an increase in calories, athletes must also look at the quality of food ingested. A balance of protein, fats, and carbohydrates is needed, and adequate calcium is required, 1200 to 1500 mg daily (Tables 8-11 and 8-12), along with 400 to 800 IU of vitamin D.

Controversy surrounds the use of oral contraceptives in the treatment of athletes with the triad. One study reported an increase in the lumbar spine and total bone mineral density following their use,[60] while other studies have not shown an

Table 8-9 Definition of Normal Bone Mineral Density, Osteopenia, and Osteoporosis

Normal	BMD ≤1 SD below the mean peak bone mass in normal women
Osteopenia	BMD >1 but <2.5 SD below the mean peak bone mass
Osteoporosis	BMD ≥2.5 SD below the mean peak bone mass

BMD, bone mineral density; SD, standard deviation.

Table 8-10 Screening History for the Female Triad

Menstrual History

Age at menarche
Frequency and duration of menstrual cycles
Longest period of time without menstruation
Last menstrual period
Physical signs of ovulation, such as cervical mucus change or menstrual cramps
Hormone replacement therapy taken previously or currently

Diet History

What was eaten in the past 24 hours?
List of forbidden foods
Highest/lowest weight since menarche
Satisfaction with current weight
Ideal weight according to the patient
Disordered eating practices (binging and purging)
Use of laxatives, diuretics, or pills

Exercise History

Exercise patterns and training intensity for the sport (hours per day and days per week)
Additional exercise outside if required training
History of fractures
History of overuse injuries

Adapted from Hobart and Smucker.[71]

Table 8-11 Calcium-Rich Foods (Milligrams of Calcium per Serving)	
Milk	290 mg/cup
Yogurt	270 mg/cup
Cottage cheese	200 mg/cup
American cheese	170 mg/cup
Swiss cheese	270 mg/cup
Ice cream	200 mg/cup
Sardines (with bones)	370 mg/3 oz
Salmon (canned with bones)	170 mg/3 oz
Tofu	280 mg/cup
Oysters (raw)	110 mg/7–9 oz
Shrimp (canned)	100 mg/3 oz
Beans (dried, cooked)	90 mg/cup
Dark green leafy vegetables	200 mg/cup
Broccoli	150 mg/large stalk
Waffle	180 mg/waffle
Macaroni and cheese	360 mg/cup
Bread	25 mg/slice
Orange	50 mg/medium-sized orange

increase in bone mass.[63] Regardless of the controversy, many physicians use oral contraceptives as a part of their treatment programs for this disorder. Two treatments available to treat diminished bone mineral density in postmenopausal women, bisphosphonates and selective estrogen receptor modulators, are contraindicated for premenopausal female athletes. The female athlete triad remains a challenging diagnostic and therapeutic problem of female athletes.

Table 8-12 Guidelines for Calcium Requirements	
Group	*Daily Elemental Calcium Requirements (mg)**
Children	500–700
Growth spurt to young adult (10–25 yr of age)	1300
Adult male (25–65 yr of age) Adult female (25–65 yr of age)	750
Postmenopausal	1500
Elderly	1200
Pregnant	1500
Lactating	2000
Healing long bone fracture (women and men)	1500

*One daily equivalent of calcium is equal to 250 mg of elemental calcium; one equivalent is equal to an 8-oz glass of milk.
Adapted from Broström et al.[72]

Anemia

Anemia can negatively affect the female athlete's performance. Controversy surrounds whom to screen and when to screen. Four types of anemia that often affect female athletes are athletic pseudoanemia, sports anemia, iron deficiency anemia, and anemia from blood loss (Table 8-13).

Athletic pseudoanemia is a result of heavy aerobic training causing an increase in red blood cell mass and plasma volume. This dilutional effect is a physiologic adaptation to training and is not true anemia. No treatment is necessary, and the abnormalities should correct with elimination of the aerobic training.

Sports anemia is a condition of low ferritin and normal hemoglobin. Ferritin is a protein that binds iron and is a marker of stored iron. There has not been a consensus on the appropriate level of ferritin for the female athlete. It is generally believed that ferritin levels above 20 will improve performance. It is also not clear whether an increase in hemoglobin, in addition to an increase in ferritin, is needed to improve performance. It has been reported that an increase in ferritin concentration without an increase in hemoglobin concentration has not been shown to improve endurance performance.[64] At present, treatment is oral iron supplement to increase the ferritin.

Women especially are at risk of iron deficiency anemia. In most cases, this is an easily treatable condition. Iron deficiency anemia is the most common cause of true anemia in the female athlete, usually resulting from menstrual blood loss. If the female athlete has long-standing heavy menses, the anemia can be significant. The athlete does not have enough iron in the diet to keep up with the loss. Laboratory studies would show low hemoglobin, hematocrit, ferritin, and red blood cell levels. Treatment involves increasing dietary intake of iron and oral iron replacement (Table 8-14). It may take 6 to 12 months to normalize, depending on the severity of the deficit.

Anemia can also result from blood loss seen in other diseases. Gastrointestinal blood loss can come from peptic ulcer disease, diverticulitis, and inflammatory bowel disease, to name a few, or more acutely from diarrhea after prolonged endurance events such as marathons. Foot strike hemolysis is seen primarily in runners, but can be seen as a result of other sports without repetitive foot strike. The leading theory as to its cause is intravascular destruction of red blood cells. Other theories that have been proposed include intravascular turbulence, acidosis, and elevated temperature in muscle tissue.[65] Treatment consists of correcting or treating the underlying gastrointestinal condition if this is the cause. No treatment other than rest is necessary for foot strike hemolysis.

Table 8-13 Characteristics of Anemia Types			
Type	*Hemoglobin/ Hematocrit*	*Ferritin*	*Red Blood Cell Indices*
Pseudoanemia	Slightly decreased	Normal	Normal
Iron deficiency	Decreased	Decreased	Decreased
Sport anemia	Normal	Decreased	Normal
Blood loss Early	Normal	Normal	Normal
Late	Decreased	Decreased	MCV increased

Table 8-14 Iron Content of Foods	
Food	*Milligrams of Iron*
Liver (3 oz)	7
Turkey, pork, beef (3 oz)	4–5
Shrimp (3 oz)	3
Chicken breast (3 oz)	1
Fish (3 oz)	1
Egg (1)	1
Dried fruit (4 oz)	3–4
Kidney beans (½ cup)	3
Cream of Wheat (½ cup)	9
Fortified cereal (½ to ¾ cup)	18

PSYCHOLOGICAL ISSUES

"Growing Out" of One's Sport

Research studies have shown that girls play sports primarily to have fun, to exercise to get in shape, and to socialize with their peers. Boys reported that they play sports to have fun but also to gain improvement in sport skills and for the excitement of competition. When high school students were asked how they wished to be remembered, boys most frequently reported "for being an athlete"; girls answered "for being a leader in activities."[66] During puberty, boys generally get taller and stronger; however, girls may increase in size and weight, but frequently do not gain proportionally in strength. Moreover, for some sports such as ballet, dance, and ice skating, the change from adolescence to the more curvaceous figure of womanhood, especially if the change is not accompanied by a proportional increase in muscle mass and strength, may result in a loss of sports fitness and abilities. The female athlete may become frustrated as she tries to cope with her new body and she may not wish to continue in the sport in which she excelled as a youth.

Frequently, these young women have a difficult time with confronting the reality that their bodies no longer fit their sport. As noted previously in the female athlete triad discussion, eating disorders are common in this age group. Some girls, feeling no longer comfortable in their sport, will present to their physician complaining of various aches and pains that limit sport participation. Often one must see the deeper problem beneath these superficial complaints and help the young athlete and her family face the reality of this young girl not wishing or not being able to continue in her sport.

Sport Burnout

Since female athletes have less of their identity tied to sport, young female athletes, even those very good at their sport, may decide to stop sport participation to have more time to spend with friends, on academics, or in other extracurricular activities. This sport burnout or change of activity focus can be difficult for coaches and parents to accept. The young athlete may find

it more "socially acceptable" to have an "injury" that sidelines her. Once again, recognizing that the injury is merely a superficial expression of the deeper issue and helping the young athlete to recognize this as well are an important responsibility of the sports physician.

Overtraining Syndrome

Overtraining syndrome has been documented in elite athletes, especially endurance athletes such as runners or swimmers, or power athletes. This condition can have an impact on both the athlete's health and mental state. The athlete with this syndrome is training at such a high level of intensity that she is unable to adequately recover between sessions. The syndrome is a continuum from training fatigue to overload to full overtraining syndrome. The female athlete experiences worsening fatigue and inability to recover from the physical strain of workouts. Mental symptoms include fatigue, depression, anxiety, irritability, and difficulty concentrating.[67] Physical symptoms include increased resting blood pressure, increased heart rate, weight loss, muscle soreness, and frequent illnesses and injuries. Numerous theories have been proposed as to the cause of overtraining syndrome including hypothalamic dysfunction, amino acid imbalance, changes in the hypothalamic-pituitary axis, autonomic nervous system dysfunction, immune dysfunction, and others.[68,69]

The syndrome is difficult to diagnose because it has no diagnostic test. A careful patient history is needed. The diagnosis is one of exclusion and is made following exclusion of biochemical abnormalities with simple laboratory tests such as electrolytes, blood count, thyroid, iron studies, cortisol, and testosterone. Treatment in principle is simple, but sometimes difficult to accomplish. Although rest is the most important treatment, many female athletes do not want to follow this treatment suggestion. In some cases, it is only after the athlete's performance has significantly declined that she will rest. Therapeutic rest, which may be more acceptable to the athlete, is not total rest, but training at a much reduced level with more complete recovery periods. Treatment also includes ensuring that there is adequate nutrition, addressing depression, and improving sleep quality. Overtraining syndrome remains a well-recognized but difficult to understand problem (Table 8-15).

Table 8-15 Stages of Overtraining Syndrome
Fatigue
Overload Training volume/intensity Beyond normal levels
Overreaching Develops after intense training and overload
Overtraining syndrome "Staleness," not able to recover

REFERENCES

1. Lowe TG, Edgar ME, Marguiles JY, et al: Etiology of idiopathic scoliosis: Current trends in research. J Bone Joint Surg Am 2000;82:1157–1168.
2. Becker TJ: Scoliosis in swimmers. Clin Sports Med 1986;5:149–158.
3. Hellstrom M, Jacobsson B, Sward L: Radiologic abnormalities of the thoraco-lumbar spine in athletes. Acta Radiol 1990;31:127–132.
4. Wojtys EM, Ashton-Miller JA, Huston LJ, et al: The association between athletic training time and the sagittal curvature of the immature spine. Am J Sports Med 2000;28:490–498.
5. Warren MP, Brooks-Gunn J, Hamilton LH, et al: Scoliosis and fractures in young ballet dancers. Relation to delayed menarche and secondary amenorrhea. N Engl J Med 1986;314:1348–1353.
6. Tanchev PI, Dzherov AD, Parushev AD, et al: Scoliosis in rhythmic gymnasts. Spine 2000;25:1367–1372.
7. Davids JR, Chamberlin E, Blackhurst DW: Indications for magnetic resonance imaging in presumed adolescent idiopathic scoliosis. J Bone Joint Surg Am 2004;86:2187–2195.
8. Mooney V, Gulick J, Pozos R: A preliminary report on the effect of measured strength training in adolescent idiopathic scoliosis. J Spinal Disord 2000;3:102–107.
9. Omey ML, Micheli LJ, Gerbino PG 2nd: Idiopathic scoliosis and spondylolysis in the female athlete: Tips for treatment. Clin Orthop 2000;372:74–84.
10. Rubery PT, Bradford DS: Athletic activity after spine surgery in children and adolescents: Results of a survey. Spine 2002;27:423–427.
11. Flatow EL, Warner JJP: Instability of the shoulder: Complex problems and failed repairs. J Bone Joint Surg Am 1998;80:122–140.
12. Neer CS 2nd, Foster CR: Inferior capsular shift for involuntary inferior and multidirectional instability of the shoulder: A preliminary report. J Bone Joint Surg Am 1980;62:897–908.
13. McFarland EG, Kim TK, Park HB, et al: The effect of variation in definition on the diagnosis of multidirectional instability of the shoulder. J Bone Joint Surg Am 2003;85:2138–2144.
14. Borsa PA, Sauers EL, Herling DE: Patterns of glenohumeral joint laxity and stiffness in healthy men and women. Med Sci Sports Exerc 2000;32:1685–1690.
15. Brown GA, Tan JL, Kirkley A: The lax shoulder in females: Issues, answers, but many more questions. Clin Orthop 2000;372:110–122.
16. Kim SH, Kim HK, Sun JI, et al: Arthroscopic capsulolabroplasty for posteroinferior multidirectional instability of the shoulder. Am J Sports Med 2004;32:594–607.
17. Levine W, Flatow EL: The pathophysiology of shoulder instability. Am J Sports Med 2000;28:910–917.
18. Neer CS 2nd: Involuntary inferior and multidirectional instability of the shoulder: Etiology, recognition, and treatment. Instr Course Lect 1985;34:232–238.
19. Bak K, Spring BJ, Henderson JP: Inferior capsular shift procedure in athletes with multidirectional instability based on isolated capsular and ligamentous redundancy. Am J Sports Med 2000;28:466–471.
20. Choi CH, Ogilvie-Harris DJ: Inferior capsular shift operation for multidirectional instability of the shoulder in players of contact sports. Br J Sports Med 2002;36:290–294.
21. Ide J, Maeda S, Takagi K: Sports activity after arthroscopic superior labral repair using suture anchors in overhead-throwing athletes. Am J Sports Med 2005;33:507–514.
22. Mazzocca AD, Brown FM Jr, Carreira DS, et al: Arthroscopic anterior shoulder stabilization of collision and contact athletes. Am J Sports Med 2005;33:52–60.
23. D'Alessandro DF, Bradley JP, Fleischli JE, et al: Prospective evaluation of thermal capsulorrhaphy for shoulder instability: Indications and results, two- to five-year follow-up. Am J Sports Med 2004;32:21–33.
24. Miniaci A, McBirnie J: Thermal capsular shrinkage for treatment of multidirectional instability of the shoulder. J Bone Joint Surg Am 2003;85:2283–2287.
25. Bennett WF, Doherty N, Hallisey MJ, et al: Insertion orientation of terminal vastus lateralis oblique and vastus medialis oblique muscle fibers in human knee. Clin Anat 1993;6:129–134.
26. Powers CM: Patellar kinematics, part I: The influence of vastus muscle activity in subjects with and without patellofemoral pain. Phys Ther 2000;80:956–964.
27. Sakai N, Luo ZP, Rand JA, et al: The influence of weakness in the vastus medialis oblique muscle on the patellofemoral joint: An in vitro biomechanical study. Clin Biomech (Bristol, Avon) 2000;15:335–339.
28. Fulkerson JP, Arendt EA: Anterior knee pain in females. Clin Orthop 2000;372:69–73.
29. Ficat RP, Hungerford DS: Disorders of the Patellofemoral Joint. Baltimore, William & Wilkins, 1977, pp 22–35.
30. Dye SF: The knee as a biologic transmission with an envelope of function: A theory. Clin Orthop 1996;325:10–18.
31. Farahmand F, Senavongse W, Amis AA: Quantitative study of the quadriceps muscles and trochlear groove geometry related to instability of the patellofemoral joint. J Orthop Res 1998;16:136–143.
32. Crossley K, Cowan SM, Bennell KL, et al: Patellar taping: Is clinical success supported by scientific evidence? Man Ther 2000;5:142–150.
33. Salsich GB, Brechter JH, Farwell D, et al: The effects of patellar taping on knee kinetics, kinematics, and vastus lateralis muscle activity during stair ambulation in individuals with patellofemoral pain. J Orthop Sports Phys Ther 2002;32:3–10.
34. Saxena A, Haddad J: The effect of foot orthoses on patellofemoral pain syndrome. J Am Podiatr Med Assoc 2003;93:264–271.
35. Arendt E, Dick R: Knee injury patterns among men and women in collegiate basketball and soccer. NCAA data and review of literature. Am J Sports Med 1995;23:694–701.
36. DeHaven KE, Lintner DM: Athletic injuries: Comparison by age, sport, and gender. Am J Sports Med 1986;14:218–224.
37. Gomez E, DeLee JC, Farney WC: Incidence of injury in Texas girls' high school basketball. Am J Sports Med 1996;24:684–687.
38. Garrick JG, Lewis SL: Career hazards for the dancer. Occup Med 2001;16:609–618.
39. Daniel DM, Stone ML, Dobson BE, et al: Fate of the ACL-injured patient: A prospective outcome study. Am J Sports Med 1994;22:632–644.
40. Griffin LY, Agel J, Albohm MJ, et al: Noncontact anterior cruciate ligament injuries: Risk factors and prevention strategies. J Am Acad Orthop Surg 2000;8:141–150.
41. Griffin LY, Albohm MJ, Arendt EA, et al: Understanding and preventing non-contact ACL injuries: A review of the Hunt Valley II meeting, January 2005. Am J Sports Med (in press).
42. Garrett WE Jr: Non-contact ACL injuries in female athletes: Risk factors and biomechanical considerations. Instructional Course Lecture Series, 78th Annual American Academy of Orthopaedic Surgeons Meeting, New Orleans, LA, February 9, 2003.
43. Malinzak RA, Colby SM, Kirkendall DT, et al: A comparison of knee joint motion patterns between men and women in selected athletic tasks. Clin Biomech (Bristol, Avon) 2001;16:438–445.
44. Ireland M: The female ACL: Why is it more prone to injury? Orthop Clin North Am 2002;33:637–651.
45. Barber-Westin SD, Noyes FR, Andrews M: A rigorous comparison between the sexes of results and complications after anterior cruciate ligament reconstruction. Am J Sports Med 1997;25:514–526.
46. Ferrari JD, Bach BR, Bush-Joseph CA, et al: Anterior cruciate ligament reconstruction in men and women: An outcome analysis comparing gender. Arthroscopy 2001;17:588–596.
47. Barrett GR, Noojin FK, Hartzog CW, et al: Reconstruction of the anterior cruciate ligament in females: A comparison of hamstring versus patellar tendon autograft. Arthroscopy 2002;18:46–54.
48. Colombet P, Allard M, Bousquet V, et al: Anterior cruciate ligament reconstruction using four-strand semintendinosus and gracilis tendon grafts and metal interference screw fixation. Arthroscopy 2000;18:232–237.
49. Pinczewski LA, Deehan DJ, Salmon LJ, et al: A 5-year comparison of patellar tendon versus four-strand hamstring tendon autograft for arthroscopic reconstruction of the anterior cruciate ligament. Am J Sports Med 2002;30:523–536.

50. Siegel MG, Barber-Westin SD: Arthroscopic-assisted outpatient anterior cruciate ligament reconstruction using the semitendinosus and gracilis tendons. Arthroscopy 1998;14:268–277.

51. Mandelbaum BR, Silvers HJ, Watanabe DS, et al: Effectiveness of a neuromuscular and proprioceptive training program in preventing anterior cruciate ligament injuries in female athletes: 2-year follow-up. Am J Sports Med 2005;33:1003–1010.

52. Hewett TE, Myer GD, Ford KR: Current concepts: prevention programs; a meta-analysis of neuromuscular interventions aimed at the prevention of ACL injuries. Am J Sports Med (in press).

53. Hewett T, Myer G, Ford K: Prevention of anterior cruciate ligament injuries. Curr Womens Health Rep 2001;1:218–224.

54. Coughlin MJ, Pinsonneault T: Operative treatment of interdigital neuroma. A long-term follow-up study. J Bone Joint Surg Am 2001;83:1321–1328.

55. Stamatis ED, Karabalis C: Interdigital neuromas: Current state of the art-surgical. Foot Ankle Clin 2004;9:287–296.

56. Sundgot-Borgen J, Torstveit MK: Prevalence of eating disorders in elite athletes is higher than in the general population. Clin J Sport Med 2004;14:25–32.

57. Henriksson BG, Schnell C, Hirschberg AL: Women endurance runners with menstrual dysfunction have prolonged interruption of training due to injury. Gynecol Obstet Invest 2000;49:41–46.

58. Skolnick AA: 'Female athlete triad' risk for women. JAMA 1993;270:921–923.

59. Thomas DB, Taylor DC: The female athlete triad. In Garrick JG (ed): Orthopaedic Knowledge Update. Rosemont, IL, American Academy of Orthopaedic Surgems, 2004, pp 345–352.

60. Sangenis P, Drinkwater BL, Loucks A, et al: IOC Position Stand on The Female Athlete Triad. 2005. http://www.olympic.org/uk/organisation/commissions/medical/index_uk.asp.

61. Khan KM, Liu-Ambrose T, Sran MM, et al: New criteria for female athlete triad syndrome? As osteoporosis is rare, should osteopenia be among the criteria for defining the female athlete triad syndrome? Br J Sports Med 2002;36:10–13.

62. Lane JM, Russell L, Khan SN: Osteoporosis. Clin Orthop 2000;372:13–50.

63. Nolte RM, Fieseler CM: The female athlete. In O'Connor FG, Sallis RE, Wilder RP, et al (eds): Sports Medicine: Just the Facts. New York, McGraw-Hill, 2005, pp 573–581.

64. Garza D, Shrier I, Kohl HW III, et al: The clinical value of serum ferritin tests in endurance athletes. Clin J Sport Med 1997;7:46–53.

65. Adams WB: Hematology in the athlete. In O'Connor FG, Sallis RE, Wilder RP, et al (eds): Sports Medicine: Just the Facts. New York, McGraw-Hill, 2005, pp 193–199.

66. Kane, MJ: The female athletic role as a status determinant with the social system of high school adolescents. Adolescence 1998;23:253–264.

67. Hawley CJ, Schoene RB: Overtraining syndrome, a guide to diagnosis, treatment, and prevention. Phys Sports Med 2003;31:25–31.

68. Howard TM: Overtraining syndrome/chronic fatigue. In O'Connor FG, Sallis RE, Wilder RP, et al (eds): Sports Medicine: Just the Facts. New York, McGraw-Hill, 2005, pp 228–232.

69. Ketner JB: Overtraining. In Mellion MB, Walsh WM, Madden C, et al (eds): Team Physician Handbook, 3rd ed. Philadelphia, Hanley & Belfus, 2002, pp 215–218.

70. American Psychiatric Association: Diagnostic and Statistical Manual for Mental Disorders, 4th edition. Washington, DC, American Psychiatric Association, 1994.

71. Hobart JA, Smucker DS: The female athlete triad. Am Fam Physicians 2000;61:3357–3367.

72. Broström MPG, Boskey A, Kaufman J, Einhorn TA: Form and function of bone. In Buckwalter J, Einhorn T, Simon S (eds): Orthopaedic Basic Science: Biology and Biomechanics of the Musculoskeletal System. Rosemont, IL, American Academy of Orthopaedic Surgeons, 2000, p 356.

The Pediatric Athlete

Mininder Kocher, Rachael Tucker, and Patrick Siparsky

In This Chapter

Epidemiology
Exercise physiology
Psychosocial aspects of sports participation
Nutrition
Performance enhancing substances
Arthroscopy

INTRODUCTION

- Serious injuries are being seen with increased frequency in the pediatric athlete.

- The pediatric athlete differs from the adult athlete biologically, physiologically, and psychologically.

- Injury patterns in the pediatric athlete are age dependent and sport specific.

- Injury types include acute traumatic injuries and chronic overuse injuries.

- This chapter provides overviews of general issues of pediatric sports injury epidemiology, endurance training, flexibility, strength training, thermoregulation, psychology, nutrition, and performance-enhancing agents. In addition, common pediatric sports injuries are addressed by anatomic region.

EPIDEMIOLOGY

Epidemiology of Pediatric Sports Participation

Over the past 30 years, there has been a significant increase in the number of children and adolescents participating in physical activity and team sports, with the largest increase among adolescent females.[1] The overall trend has seen a shift from the largely unstructured, unsupervised "free play" of the early 20th century to the evolution of organized and highly structured youth sports activities.[2] It is estimated that at present as many as 30 million children and adolescents participate in organized sport in the United States. In 1995, reports indicated that 15 million 5- to 14-year-olds played baseball in the United States.[3]

The Youth Risk Behavior Survey (YRBS) was a large population-based study performed throughout the 1990s enabling accurate assessment of the emerging trends in youth sports participation. Results from the 1997 survey reported that 62% of U.S. high school students participated in one or more sports teams, with the majority playing in a combination of both school and nonschool teams.[4]

The YRBS study highlighted a number of significant demographic differences when results were compared for age, gender, and ethnicity. Although the number of women participating in sports teams has increased fivefold over the past 30 years, a disparity continues to exist between genders according to the 1997 YRBS study.[1] While almost 70% of male high school students participate in sports, only 53% of similarly aged females exhibit the same level of sporting interest.[1,4] This gender disparity was even more dramatic among ethnic minorities, with only 40% of Hispanic and African-American females participating compared to 62% and 71% of males, respectively.[4]

Furthermore, progression into adolescence was also associated with a reduction in the involvement of both males and females in vigorous sporting activities.[1,4] For males, there was a reduction in vigorous exercise participation from 81% in grade 9 to only 67% by grade 12.[1] Vigorous exercise was defined as activity causing shortness of breath, lasting at least 20 minutes, 3 days per week.[1] As expected, this trend was even greater in females with 61% of female ninth graders participating in vigorous exercise compared to only 41% by 12th grade.[1]

The growth and increasing popularity of school and community youth sports programs has become an integral part of American youth culture that has the potential to benefit the long-term physical and psychosocial health of those children and adolescents who participate.[4]

Epidemiology of Pediatric Sports Injury

Increased youth participation in sports and physical activities has resulted in an increase in sports-related injuries secondary to trauma and overuse.[2] The annual rate of sports injuries within the United States is estimated at approximately three million, with as many as 70% of those resulting from youth sports activities.[3] The financial costs of managing these injuries in 1996 was well in excess of $1 billion.[3]

Pediatric sports injuries are often unique not only in terms of the underlying pathology but also the challenges in managing these injuries. Many patients participate in multiple teams during a given season; the rest periods between seasons are short, if not nonexistent, and there is increasing demand for sporting success from parents, schools, and sporting establishments.[5]

Pediatric sports injuries can be classified according to the age of the athlete, the type of injury, and the sport/activity responsible for an injury.[6] From an epidemiology standpoint, these classifications assist in the identification of potential risk factors for injury and the implementation of prevention strategies and rehabilitation plans that are appropriate for the age of the patient and the sport they play.

Several studies have identified a correlation between increased risk of sports-related injury and increased age of the pediatric athlete.[6] A number of explanations to explain these findings have been postulated. These include greater opportunity for injury in the adolescent athlete due to longer game times and more frequent and intense practices.[6] The provision of medical assistance at many high school and college games allows for greater reporting of injuries.[6] It appears that anatomic factors such as the increased size of the athletes and the resultant increased force and speed of collisions play an insignificant role, as the same trend was noted for both contact and noncontact sports.[6]

Sports injuries can be broadly divided into acute traumatic and overuse type injuries according to their pathophysiology.[6] Whereas many acute traumatic injuries are the result of random events, overuse injuries are often the result of entrenched training errors and therefore have greater potential for prevention.[6] The difficulty lies in identifying these overuse injuries as initially they are only subtly disabling when compared to an immediate fall to the ground after a sprain.

It is important that an injury be viewed in context of the sport in which it occurred as an injury that may be functionally disabling for one sport may have no relevance in another sport.[6] Furthermore, it is important that physicians recognize that time lost from sports participation is often more of a concern to athletes and their coaches than the nature of the injury itself.[6] These perceived differences in injury severity will inevitably impact management programs.

Among school athletes, football has the highest rate of injury, with wrestling not far behind.[3] The rate of injury in both males and females at high school and college level are comparable with the exception of knee injuries, which are slightly greater in females at a college level.[7] Fortunately, fatal sports injuries are rare. A study conducted by Mueller et al[8] reported 160 nontraumatic deaths in high school and college athletes in the United States between 1983 and 1993, with the primary cause being cardiac death and only a small number of heat-related injuries. They also reported 53 traumatic deaths from 1982 to 1992 in football resulting primarily from head and neck trauma.[8]

EXERCISE PHYSIOLOGY

Endurance Training

The increased popularity of endurance sports such as swimming, running, rowing, and cycling among children and adolescents has heightened awareness of aerobic training as a means of maximizing performance.[9,10] The beneficial effect of aerobic training in adults is now well established, with increases in maximal oxygen uptake (VO_{2max}) of up to 15% to 20% reported in the literature.[10] The ability to enhance the aerobic capacity of children and adolescents through endurance training remains controversial, however, as many of the studies to date have been methodically flawed and largely neglected adolescents.[9–11]

While there are several physiologic parameters by which to measure aerobic fitness, maximal oxygen uptake (VO_{2max}) is the most commonly used in studies involving adult endurance.[9,10] The usefulness of this parameter in children was questioned as the majority of children fail to ever reach the plateau consistent with maximal oxygen uptake.[9,10] As a result, VO_{2max} has been replaced with peak VO_2 in pediatric endurance studies, which instead measure the highest VO_2 level achieved before the point of voluntary exhaustion.[9,10]

Despite the traditional view that prepubescent children are incapable of improving their aerobic capacity through endurance training, evidence is now emerging in the literature to the contrary.[9,10] A review of the 22 studies by Baquet et al[9] demonstrated that a 5% to 6% increase in peak VO_2 among both

children and adolescents is possible with appropriate aerobic training.[9] The ability to achieve these increases is influenced by several factors including baseline peak VO_2 levels, program design, maturity level, and genetics.[9,10]

The role of pubertal status on a child's ability to enhance aerobic capacity through endurance training remains unclear due to a lack of quality longitudinal data.[9,10] Early research indicated that for the same relative training intensity, greater gains in peak VO_2 were demonstrated for circumpubertal relative to prepubertal subjects.[9,10] Two theories have been used to explain this. First, a so-called maturational threshold below which training-induced adaptations in aerobic fitness were physiologically limited and, second, the greater level of habitual activity among children maintained their VO_2 closer of its maximum potential making additional increases in peak VO_2 more difficult to achieve.[9,10] Though limited, evidence is slowly emerging to contradict these theories as we gain a better understanding of the role of genetic, environmental, and endocrine influences.[9–11] High-quality longitudinal studies that document not only chronologic age but also maturity status are essential.[10]

Designing a program that incorporates appropriate levels of training duration, frequency, and intensity is essential to achieving the desired increase in aerobic capacity.[9–11] The literature review of Baquet et al[9] found that three to four sessions per week, lasting 30 to 60 minutes were optimal. Interestingly, no clear relationship was found between the length of training program and peak VO_2 improvement.[9] Training intensity is generally defined in terms of the percentage of maximal heart rate (% HR_{max}).[9,10] Several studies have confirmed that a heart rate that exceeds 80% of maximum is required to obtain significant increases in peak VO_2.[9]

Comparison between continuous and interval training and their effect on peak VO_2 is limited to prepubertal children.[9,11] Nine of the 16 studies reviewed by Baquet et al[9] demonstrated a significant increase in peak VO_2 after continuous training. However, only 3 of the 16 studies showed improvement when the heart rate was less than or equal to 80% of the maximum.[9] The implementation of continuous training among children poses difficulties with regards to compliance and motivation.[11] Interval training is not only easier to put into practice but has more consistently positive results. Programs that combine continuous and intermittent exercises make results difficult to interpret.[9]

The increasingly competitive nature of sports has resulted in a reluctance by athletes to take adequate breaks from training and performing.[12] The damaging effects of prolonged endurance training on skeletal muscle and function are well documented in the literature as is the huge capacity that human skeletal muscle has for repair and adaptation, given adequate recovery time.[12] A study by Grobler et al[12] demonstrated that although minor exercise-induced muscle damage is a precursor for adaptation, the reparative capacity of skeletal muscle is limited and the cumulative effects of repetitive trauma and injury to skeletal muscle may lead to reduced performance, especially in long distance runners. Further research is needed to investigate the limits of skeletal muscle regenerative capacity after chronic injury.[12]

Flexibility

Extremes of joint and ligament laxity have important implications for the pediatric athlete due to the increased risk of both acute traumatic and overuse type sporting injuries in addition to a number of degenerative orthopedic conditions, many of which have long-term implications for sports participation and performance.[13]

Childhood is associated with a gradual reduction in flexibility with the greatest loss occurring around puberty as a result of a growth-induced muscle-tendon imbalance.[14] This loss of flexibility is less pronounced in females.[14] Excessive tightness during this time of rapid growth is thought to play a major role in both acute and overuse type injuries affecting, in particular, the lower back, pelvis, and knee.[13] Slight improvements in flexibility are observed after the pubertal growth spurt in both males and females through early adulthood at which point it plateaus and then starts to decline once again.[14]

While only 4% to 7% of the general population meet all criteria for generalized ligament laxity, evaluation of flexibility still remains an essential component of the clinical assessment of a young athlete as it enables identification of those individuals at increased risk in addition to providing invaluable information for injury prevention and rehabilitation programs.[13,15] Studies performed by Marshall and his colleagues in 1980 demonstrated that increased flexibility was associated with a greater risk of sports-related injuries, particularly in those requiring rapid change of direction or acceleration.[13]

Although several instrumented tests are available to test the flexibility of individual joints, it is the use of simple screening tests such as the modified Marshall test devised in 1978 that are more commonly used as a routine part of the clinical assessment of the young athlete.[13] By measuring thumb to forearm apposition, the modified Marshall test can quickly identify extremes of flexibility that warrant further, more in-depth investigation and assessment relevant to their given sporting interest.[13]

Strength Training

Traditionally, strength training was discouraged among the pediatric population due to the perceived risk of growth disturbances and other injuries.[16] Research over the past 20 years, however, has demonstrated that not only can strength training be a safe and effective component of any comprehensive fitness program, but it can also provide clear health benefits to the pediatric age group.[16,17] These benefits include improved athletic performance as a result of increased coordination, muscle strength, and power in addition to enhancement of long-term health due to increased cardiorespiratory fitness, reduced risk of injury, improved bone mineral density, and blood lipid profile.[16-18]

Research shows that expertly tailored strength training programs in children and adolescents are associated with increased muscle strength and performance advantages in sports such as football and weight lifting.[18] Increases in strength of 50% to 65% above baseline have been reported in the prepubescent athlete over a 2- to 3-month training period.[19] Interestingly, in the preadolescent child, however, this increased strength occurs in the absence of muscle hypertrophy, highlighting the role of neurogenic adaptation as the likely cause. Neurogenic adaptation refers to the recruitment of increased motor neurons that can fire with each muscle contraction.[18] Moreover, the loss of benefits after the program is discontinued for 6 weeks provides further evidence in support of this hypothesis.[16] In contrast, strength training during and after puberty is further enhanced by the hormonally induced increase in muscle growth that occurs in both males and females.[18]

Although the risk of injury associated with strength training is real, research shows that it is no greater than in any other sport when adult supervision is available to ensure that proper technique and safety precautions are taken.[16,18] Data obtained by the National Electronic Injury Surveillance System between 1991 and 1996 estimated that strength training was responsible for more than 20,000 injuries annually in the under 21-year-old age group.[20] The usefulness of these results is limited, however, by the lack of distinction between competitive and recreational injuries or comment regarding the quality of the equipment being used or the presence of adult supervision.[18] Of note, 40% to 70% of those injuries were attributable to muscle strains, primarily within the lumbar area.[18] Case reports indicate that children and adolescents participating in strength training are at increased risk of specific lumbar injuries including herniated intervertebral disks, paraspinous muscle sprains, spondylolisthesis, and pars interarticularis stress fractures.[16]

Thermoregulation and Heat-Related Injuries

Heat-related illnesses are preventable.[21] However, heat stroke remains the third most common cause of exercise-related death among high school athletes in the United States, after head injuries and cardiac disorders.[22]

There are several physiologic characteristics unique to the pediatric population that contribute to the thermoregulatory disadvantage that they face in extreme climatic conditions including increased surface area–to–body mass ratio, reduced sweating capacity, greater generation of metabolic heat per mass unit, and a slower rate of heat acclimatization.[21,23] A large surface area–to–mass ratio is advantageous in mild to moderate climates due to the increased convective surface that it provides.[22] In hot humid weather, however, this provides a larger area for heat influx, thereby raising the core temperature and increasing the risk of heat-induced illnesses.[22] Conversely, in cold climates, enhanced metabolic heat production and cutaneous vasoconstriction are often insufficient to overcome the heat lost from their vast surface area, particularly in cold water.[24]

Sweat glands play a central role in the pediatric athlete's ability to thermoregulate. By 3 years of age, the number of sweat glands that a person will have is fixed.[22] Despite having a greater density of sweat glands per skin area than adults, the sweating capacity in children is restricted due to a lower sweating rate and a higher sweating threshold.[25] As a result, their ability to dissipate body heat by evaporation is reduced until the transition is made to an adult sweating pattern in late puberty.[21,23]

The reluctance of children to drink during prolonged exercise further exacerbates this thermoregulatory disadvantage.[26] The American Academy of Pediatrics recommends prehydration in addition to enforced periodic drinking during the course of prolonged exercise.[21] Although water is readily available, flavored drinks are often easier for children to tolerate.[21] Moreover, as the risk of dehydration is even greater in children with certain diseases or conditions such as cystic fibrosis, diabetes, and anorexia, the need for optimal fluid intake during exercise is essential.[21]

PSYCHOSOCIAL ASPECTS OF SPORTS PARTICIPATION

Psychosocial Development

Participation in sports activity is associated with a large number of health benefits that can influence both physical and psychosocial well-being. The social interaction associated with sports participation is instrumental in a child's psychosocial development including character development, self-discipline, emotion control, cooperation, empathy of others, and leadership skills.[25] The acquisition of new skills aids in building confidence and self-esteem.[25] It also allows children to experiment with success and failure in a low-risk environment.[27]

The YRBS study mentioned earlier in this chapter was a nationally representative study conducted throughout the 1990s by the Centers for Disease Control and Prevention. It evaluated the new trends in sports participation with particular focus on its effect on health behaviors.[4] It found a strong positive trend between sports participation and several types of positive health behaviors in both white males and females, including consumption of fruit and vegetables as part of a healthy diet as well as reduced levels of smoking or illegal drug use and a reduced risk of suicide.[4] This trend was not found among ethnic minorities, and, in fact, among Hispanics and African Americans, the risk of negative health behaviors actually increased with sports participation.[4]

Readiness for Sport

Knowledge of cognitive and motor developmental milestones as well as the factors that motivate children and adolescents to participate in sports is essential when designing sports activities that are both rewarding and beneficial.[24,27] Motor development is a sequential process like any other developmental milestone, and the rate of progression varies between children.[28] Participation in most sports require fundamental motor skills including kicking, throwing, running, jumping, and catching.[28] Most children will acquire these skills through informal play, but mastery often requires more formal instruction and repetition.[28] Although this process of acquisition and mastery can potentially be accelerated through intensive instruction and practice, research shows that it rarely speeds up motor development or leads to enhanced athletic performance.[28]

The principle motivating factors for young children to participate in sports activities are fun and enjoyment.[25] For an activity to be viewed as enjoyable, there must be a certain level of excitement but ultimately a sense of personal achievement associated with the improvement or mastery of specific skills.[25] We must acknowledge that although virtually all children have the ability to acquire new motor skills, the ease of acquisition and degree of mastery may vary among children.[27] Research has shown that children who feel less competent with one particular skill will be less likely to continue with that sport in the long term.[27] Therefore, it is important that young children are exposed to a range of sports that challenge and enable them to acquire a variety of fundamental motor skills.[27]

Progression into adolescence is not only associated with a number of physical changes resulting from the pubertal growth spurt but also a shift in the motivational factors influencing sports participation.[25,27,29] Cognitive and motor development is now sufficient to allow the incorporation of strategy into sports such as football or basketball.[28] The need for fun and excitement is overtaken by social factors such as interaction with friends and physical appearance, although mastery of skills still remains important.[25,28] Differing rates of progression through puberty can result in inequality within and between genders.[28] Those who experience earlier growth spurts may be temporarily taller, heavier, and stronger, which often leads to unrealistic expectations due to the erroneous conclusion that they are destined to become better athletes than their less mature peers.[28]

Adult Involvement

The level of adult involvement has increased significantly with the evolution of organized sports. Although the traditional role of supervisor still exists, the nature of adult involvement in youth sports has also evolved. An increased level of sophistication has developed due to the advent of specialized coaches, sports psychologists, nutritionists, and so on, all of which undoubtedly have an impact on the psychosocial development of the young athlete.

Adults are vital for the enforcement of rules and the creation of a safe, controlled environment in which to impart their knowledge and assist children and adolescents in the acquisition of new skills and development of appropriate attitudes toward sports.[27,28] Their involvement in sports activities can also have a detrimental impact on psychosocial development through the expression of negative and unsportsman-like behavior, negative reinforcement, and the enforcement of demands and expectations that exceed the child's abilities.[25,27]

In the early years of life, parental influence is instrumental in the development of lifelong core values and attitudes.[25] By 12 years of age, a child's attitudes toward winning are already well established and often directly reflect the values held by their parents.[25] These values and attitudes are often acquired through observation of parental behavior, and although extreme parental behavior is rare, the use of negative comments or reinforcements were negative, of which the majority were corrective in nature.[25] Variation was found between sporting codes with the greatest incidence among soccer and rugby players.[25] Children of relaxed and supportive parents who positively reinforce their child's performance are not only more self-confident but are more likely to be successful athletes.[25,27]

As the child progresses to adolescence, the role of parents starts to diminish as the role of the coach increases.[25] Coaches, through their provision of feedback and reinforcement, have a great impact on the confidence and self-perception of the young athlete.[25]

The increasingly competitive nature of sports has led to a shift in goals that are largely adult oriented and focused on winning at any cost.[3] Competitive behaviors start to emerge at 3 to 4 years of age, and the potential exists to either enhance or exploit this trait through the use of sports.[25] The danger arises when the demands and expectations placed on young athletes by their parents or coaches exceed their abilities.[25] This can result in the development of unhealthy competitive behavior with serious antisocial interpersonal consequences or even problems such as burnout and chronic stress.[25]

NUTRITION

The nutritional concerns of the pediatric athlete are complex and unique from those of their adult counterparts as it involves the interaction between normal growth and development and the optimization of athletic performance.[30,31]

During the 1980s, there was an erroneous belief that leanness correlated with enhanced athletic performance as a result of studies that demonstrated a positive correlation between running performance and percentage of body fat.[32] Not only is there a lack of scientific evidence to prove that reducing weight alone will improve athletic performance, but, in fact, deliberate caloric restriction in children and adolescents is likely to have detrimental implications, not only for their athletic performance but also their growth and development and general health.[32] Unfortunately, these erroneous beliefs are perpetuated today by coaches with little or usually no training in athlete nutrition.[32] In the case of school-based coaches, their employment is often dependent on the success of their teams and controlling an athlete's weight is often the easiest parameter by which a coach can try and ensure athletic success.[32] In fact, by reducing the dietary fat contribution, it is possible that essential sources of protein, as well as minerals and vitamins such as calcium, magnesium iron, zinc, and B_{12} and other fat-soluble vitamins, which are critical for growth, may be also eliminated from the diet.[31]

Diet should play an integral role in any comprehensive training program with specific attention to energy requirement including appropriate combinations of protein, carbohydrates, fat, vitamins, and minerals.[31] These requirements are often subject to large interindividual variation, not only between sporting codes but often within a given sport.[31]

Results from the YRBS study in the 1990s confirmed that children and adolescents involved in regular sporting activities not only maintain healthier diets consisting of greater amounts of fruit and vegetables but are often less concerned with caloric intake and energy balance.[33] For young athletes, the energy requirements must be sufficient to ensure normal growth and development but must also provide the additional calories to account for physical training.[31] The recommendations for estimated energy requirements in young athletes set by the Food and Nutrition Board are based on age, height, weight, and physical activity classification.[31]

Protein is an essential part of a young athlete's diet as it is required to build amino acids necessary for the growth and development of lean body mass and healthy bones but also as a alternative source of energy to carbohydrates.[31] There is a lack of research regarding the recommended daily protein intake for young athletes.[31] For adults, 12% to 15% of their dietary energy should come from protein; however, in children, the demands are greater, especially when involved in competitive, intensive training during periods of rapid growth.[31]

Research shows that children and adolescents up to the age of 13 to 15 years have restricted glycolytic capacity, which questions the role of high carbohydrate diets.[31] Regardless, nutritionists recommend that at least 50% of a young athlete's diet consist of carbohydrate due to the importance of this energy source during high-intensity training.[32] There remains a significant amount of research needed with regards to optimal nutrition of the pediatric athlete for enhancing performance and maximizing recovery.

PERFORMANCE-ENHANCING SUBSTANCES

The use of performance-enhancing substances among children and adolescents is increasing as a result of media exposure, the availability of so-called natural supplements, the absence of formal drug testing in schools, and the increasingly competitive nature of youth sports.[30,34] Pediatric athletes are at high risk due to increased susceptibility to societal pressures at a time when they are often dealing with complex developmental and psychosocial changes.

The term *ergogenic* is derived from the Greek "to make work" and refers to the inherent ability of many substances to enhance athletic power and/or endurance.[34] In many cases, the ergogenic effects of a substance are actually secondary to their intended use.[34] It is therefore essential that physicians dealing with athletes, especially those competing in high-level sports, have a working knowledge of substances that contain ergogenic properties, as inappropriate prescribing/counseling may result in an athlete's disqualification from a competition.[35]

Anabolic-Androgenic Steroids

Although a wide range of performance-enhancing substances are available in the United States, anabolic-androgenic steroids are by far the most publicized and intensely studied. Anabolic-androgenic steroids are synthetic analogues of the male hormone testosterone, and their use in the pediatric athlete for both performance and physique enhancement has been documented in the medical literature for well over 20 years.[34] The use of androgenic steroids is widespread, with an estimated 4% to 12% of male adolescents and 0.5% to 2% of female adolescents using anabolic-androgenic steroids in the 1990s despite being banned by almost every major athletic governing body.[35]

As the name suggests, anabolic-androgenic steroids have both masculinizing and tissue-building effects, such that when used in conjunction with adequate strength training and proper diet, they have the ability to increase muscle size and strength, enabling high-intensity workouts and possibly even a reduced recovery time after workouts.[34] As a result, it tends to be strength athletes (e.g., weight lifters, throwers, and football players) and those participating in sports such as swimming and running that require frequent, high-intensity workouts, who are attracted to the substance.[35]

Research demonstrated a significant correlation between the use of anabolic-androgenic steroids in adolescents and the abuse of other common drugs such as alcohol, tobacco, cannabis, and opioids.[35]

Although the perceived performance-enhancing benefits appear high, the side effects of using anabolic-androgenic steroids are extensive and often irreversible.[34] In addition to personality changes and psychological problems that are associated with steroid use, premature closure of epiphyseal plates with subsequent linear growth arrest, irreversible alopecia, gynaecomastia, acne, and irreversible masculinization of secondary sexual characteristics in females are just a few of the more dramatic and often psychologically devastating side effects of anabolic-androgenic steroids.[34]

Regulation of Performance-Enhancing Substances

Drug testing is both time-consuming and expensive, making the widespread testing of young athletes virtually impossible.[26] Despite this, many schools and youth organizations have implemented voluntary drug testing, which has a dual benefit of identifying and providing assistance for athletes with abuse problems as well as reducing the peer pressure to use drugs.[24]

With the introduction of the Dietary Supplement Health and Education Act in 1994, the role of the U.S. Food and Drug Administration in regulating "natural supplements" was eliminated.[12] Since that time, "natural agents" such as creatinine, androstenedione, and DHEA have been widely accessible via health stores and the Internet.[12] This accessibility results in an erroneous perception that these substances are "safe" even though the absence of regulatory control eliminates any legal requirement of manufacturers to declare all active ingredients and potential interactions and fully test their products for short- and long-term effects.[24]

The use of performance-enhancing drugs among athletes of any age is unethical, unhealthy, and potentially life threatening.[26] As physicians, we have a responsibility to acquire and impart factual knowledge to young athletes contemplating the use of these substances. Although the effectiveness of using scare tactics that emphasize the negative effects of substance use has been questioned, there is a clear role for positive counseling with regards to healthy alternatives such as strength training and conditioning, nutrition, and skill acquisition through coaching and camps.[26]

ARTHROSCOPY IN CHILDREN

The use of arthroscopy in the pediatric and adolescent population has dramatically expanded over the past decade as a result of increased youth participation in sports and the subsequent rise in sports-related injuries.[5] With the advent of smaller, more sophisticated arthroscopic instruments over the past decade, the major obstacle to its application in children was overcome.[5] In fact, Gross[36] noted that, after extensive experience, despite the difference in joint size, basic techniques of arthroscopy are largely the same in both children and adults. At present, arthroscopy is indicated in the management of severe shoulder, elbow, wrist, hip, knee, and ankle injuries in the pediatric population.[5] Advantages to arthroscopy in this population include reduced postoperative morbidity, smaller incisions, more rapid return to activities, decreased inflammatory response, and improved visualization of joint structures.[5]

Shoulder injuries in the pediatric athlete include acute fractures, overuse injuries such as little league shoulder (Fig. 9-1), and shoulder instability (Fig. 9-2). Most major shoulder injuries requiring arthroscopy are related to instability and can be divided into two descriptive groups: traumatic anterior instability and multidirectional instability.[5,29–42]

The incidence of elbow injuries continues to increase as a result of the growing popularity of youth sports. Many of the elbow injuries are repetitive, overuse type injuries, such as osteochondritis dissecans, which is prevalent in baseball, racket sports, and gymnastics.[43] In fact, the little league elbow is now an accepted term for a common overuse injury in young throwing athletes, with etiologies including fragmented medial epicondyle (Fig. 9-3), osteochondritis dissecans (Figs. 9-4 and 9-5), ulnar hypertrophy, and medial epicondylitis.[42–45]

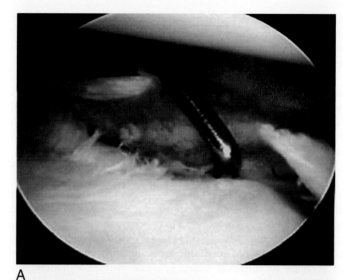

A

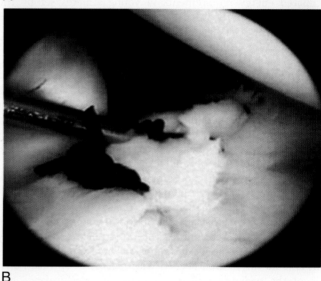

B

Figure 9-2 Traumatic anterior shoulder instability. **A,** Bankart lesion. **B,** Repair of Bankart lesion.

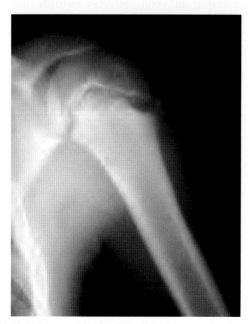

Figure 9-1 Little league shoulder. Widening of the proximal humeral physis associated with repetitive overuse.

Wrist arthroscopy is not a commonly practiced treatment modality among pediatric and adolescent patients because many injuries achieve successful healing nonoperatively and also because of the restricted size of the joint space.[45] Kocher et al[46] note an increasing incidence of repetitive use type injuries such as triangular fibrocartilage injuries (Fig. 9-6) and believe arthroscopy is indicated for débridement or determination of the extent of ligamentous injury in those patients failing nonoperative therapies.[47]

Although hip arthroscopy is a commonly used diagnostic and treatment modality for hip pathologies in the adult population, its application in the pediatric population is only beginning to increase. Indications in the pediatric population include isolated labral tears (Fig. 9-7), loose bodies, chondral injuries, and internal derangement associated with Perthes disease and epiphyseal dysplasias.[48–52] The risk of complications, although small, does exist; they include pudendal nerve irritation and recurrent injury.[5]

Currently, the largest application of arthroscopy in the pediatric and adolescent population is in the treatment of knee

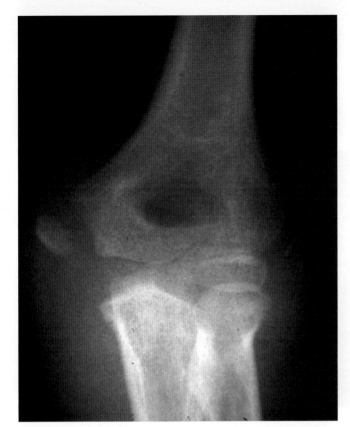

Figure 9-3 Medial epicondyle widening associated with little league elbow.

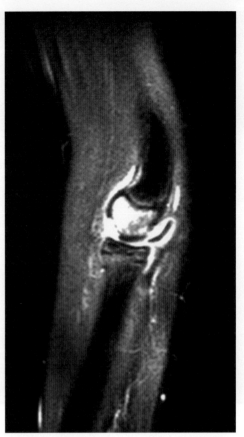

Figure 9-4 Sagittal magnetic resonance imaging of the elbow demonstrating chondral defect of the capitellum associated with osteochondritis dissecans.

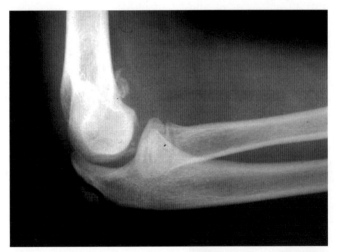

Figure 9-5 Lateral radiograph of the elbow demonstrating a loose body in the anterior elbow.

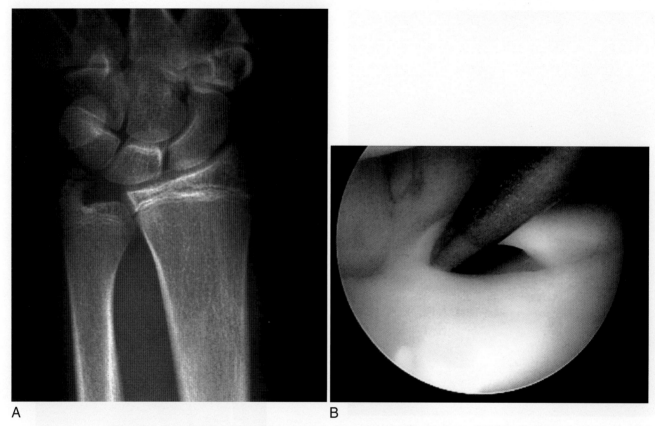

Figure 9-6 Ulnar styloid fracture **(A)** associated with a triangular fibrocartilage complex tear **(B)**.

pathology and is directly attributable to increased athletic activity.[37] Key indications for knee arthroscopy include osteochondritis dissecans (Figs. 9-8 and 9-9) discoid meniscus, tibial spine fractures (Figs. 9-10 and 9-11) and partial and complete anterior cruciate ligament tears.[53-62]

At present, the use of ankle arthroscopy in the pediatric population is restricted to a small number of conditions including osteochondritis dissecans, loose body removal, and triplane fracture repair due to technical challenges resulting from the size of the joint and the risk of neurovascular damage.[36,63-66]

CONCLUSIONS

Pediatric sports injuries are being seen with increased frequency. Just as the child is not a "little adult," the pediatric athlete is not a "little adult athlete." An understanding of the unique considerations of the pediatric athlete with respect to epidemiology, endurance, flexibility, strength, thermoregulation, psychology, and nutrition is important background knowledge. Recognition of common injury patterns of the shoulder, elbow, wrist, hip, knee, and ankle is essential to effective management.

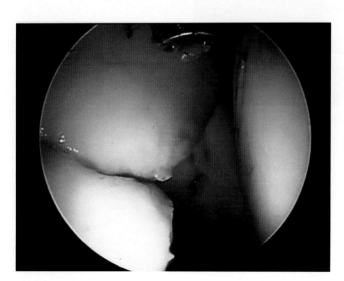

Figure 9-7 Radial labral tear of the hip.

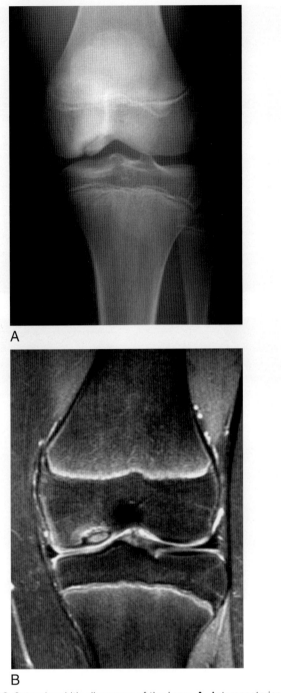

Figure 9-8 Osteochondritis dissecans of the knee. **A,** Anteroposterior radiograph. **B,** Corresponding coronal magnetic resonance imaging.

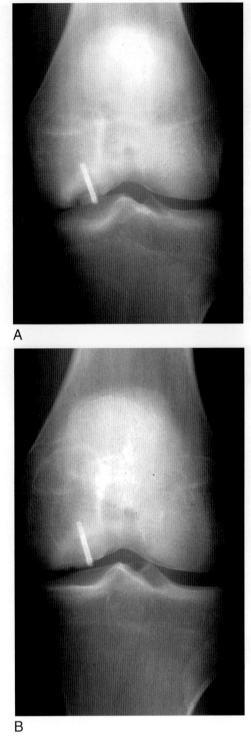

Figure 9-9 Fixation of unstable osteochondritis dissecans lesion of the knee. Immediate postoperative anteroposterior radiograph **(A)** and 3-month postoperative radiograph **(B)** demonstrating lesion healing.

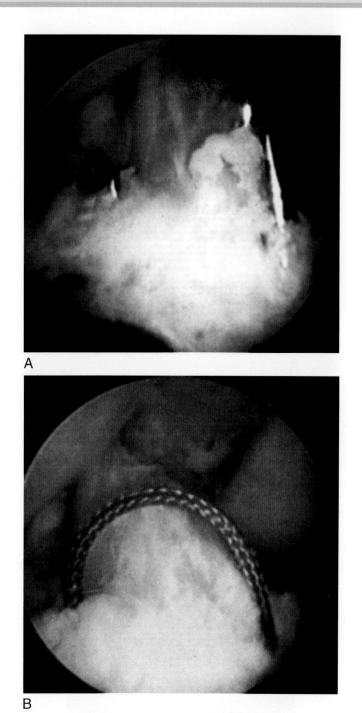

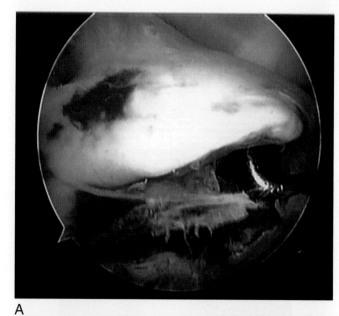

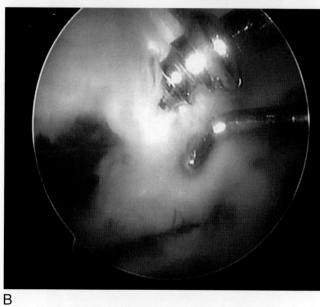

Figure 9-11 Epiphyseal cannulated screw fixation of tibial spine fracture. **A,** Displaced fracture. **B,** Screw fixation.

Figure 9-10 Suture fixation of tibial spine fracture. **A,** Guidewires brought through the tibial spine fragment. **B,** Suture fixation.

REFERENCES

1. Long B: Promoting physical activity. In Sullivan J, Anderson S (eds): Care of the Young Athlete. Chicago, American Academy of Pediatrics and the American Academy of Orthopaedic Surgeons, 2000, pp 33–34.
2. Washington RL, Bernhardt DT, Gomez J, et al: Organized sports for children and preadolescents. Pediatrics 2001;107:1459–1462.
3. Hergenroeder AC: Prevention of sports injuries. Pediatrics 1998;101:1057–1063.
4. Pate RR, Trost SG, Leven S, et al: Sports participation & health-related behaviors among U.S. youth. Arch Pediatr Adolesc Med 2000;154:904–911.
5. Kocher MS, Siparsky PN, Waters PM: Current concepts in pediatric arthroscopy. Arthroscopy 2006 (in press).
6. Garrick J: Epidemiology of sports injuries in the pediatric athlete. In Sullivan J, Grana W (eds): American Academy of Orthopaedic Surgeons Seminars: The Pediatric Athlete. Chicago, American Academy of Orthopaedic Surgeons, 1990, pp 123–132.
7. McClain LG, Reynolds S: Sports injuries in a high school. Pediatrics 1989;84:446–450.
8. Mueller FO, Cantu RC, Van Camp SP: Catastrophic injuries in high school and college sports. Philadelphia, Human Kinetics Sports Science Monograph Series, 1996, p 8.
9. Baquet G, Praagh EV, Berthoin S: Endurance training and aerobic fitness in young people. Sports Med 2003;33:1127–1143.
10. Baxter-Jones AD, Maffulli N: Endurance in young athletes: It can be trained. Br J Sports Med 2003;37:96–97.
11. Rowland TW, Boyajian A: Aerobic response to endurance exercise training in children. Pediatrics 1995;96:654–658.
12. Grobler LA, Collins M, Lambert MI, et al: Skeletal muscle pathology in endurance athletes with acquired training intolerance. Br J Sports Med 2004;38:697–703.
13. Micheli LJ, Greene HS, Cassella M, et al: Assessment of flexibility in young female skaters with the modified Marshall Test. J Pediatr Orthop 1999;19:665–668.
14. Kulling FA: Special considerations in the pediatric and adolescent athlete: Flexibility. In DeLee JC, Drez DD (eds): Orthopaedic Sports Medicine: Principles and Practices, vol 1, 2nd ed. Philadelphia, WB Saunders, 2003, pp 730–736.
15. Warner JJ, Micheli LJ, Arslanian LE, et al: Patterns of flexibility, laxity and strength in normal shoulders with instability and impingement. Am J Sports Med 1990;18:366–375.
16. Gyr BM: Strength training in children & adolescents. In DeLee JC, Drez DD (eds): Orthopaedic Sports Medicine: Principles & Practice, vol. 1, 2nd ed. Philadelphia, WB Saunders, 2003, pp 730–736.
17. Faigenbaum AD: Strength training for children & adolescents. Clin Sports Med 2000;19:593–619.
18. Washington RC, Bernhardt DT: Strength training by children & adolescents. Pediatrics 2001;107:1470–1472.
19. Metzel J: Age-specific concerns: Exercises in young and elderly athletes. In Arendt (ed): Orthopaedic Knowledge Update. Chicago, American Association of Orthopaedic Surgeons, 1999, pp 50–51.
20. Falk B, Tenenbaum G: The effectiveness of resistance training in children. A meta-analysis. Sports Med 1996;3:176–186.
21. Anderson SJ, Griesemer BA, Johnson MD, et al: Climatic heat stress & the exercising child and adolescent. Pediatrics 2000;106:158–159.
22. Coyle JF: Thermoregulation. In Sullivan J, Anderson S (eds): Care of the Young Athlete. Chicago, American Academy of Pediatrics and the American Academy of Orthopaedic Surgeons, 2000, pp 65–80.
23. Bar-Or O: Children's responses to exercise in hot climates: Implications for performance and health. Sports Science Exchange 7:86–87.
24. Bar-Or O: Children's responses to exercise in cold climates: Implications for performance and health. Sports Science Exchange 1999;7:90–92.
25. Elsass W, Wingler I: Psychological aspects of sports in children and adolescents. In DeLee J, Drez D (eds): Orthopaedic Sports Medicine: Principles & Practice. Philadelphia, WB Saunders, 1994, pp 687–702.
26. Bar-Or O, Dotan R, Inbar O: Voluntary hypohydration in 10- to 12-year-old boys. J Appl Physiol 1980;48:104–108.
27. Landry GL: Benefits of sports participation. In Sullivan J, Anderson S (eds): Care of the Young Athlete. Chicago, American Academy of Pediatrics and the American Academy of Orthopaedic Surgeons, 2000, pp 1–9.
28. Harris S: Readiness to participate in sports. In Sullivan J, Anderson S (eds): Care of the Young Athlete. Chicago, American Academy of Pediatrics and the American Academy of Orthopaedic Surgeons, 2000, pp 19–24.
29. Pease DG, Anderson DF: Longitudinal analysis of children's attitudes towards sports team involvement. J Sports Behav 1986;9:3–10.
30. Lombardo J: Drugs and ergogenic aids. In Sullivan J, Grana W (eds): American Academy of Orthopaedic Surgeons Seminars: The Pediatric Athlete. Chicago, American Academy of Orthopaedic Surgeons, 1990, pp 45–52.
31. Petrie HJ, Stover EA, Horswill CA: Nutritional concerns for the child and adolescent competitor. Nutrition 2004;20:620–631.
32. Gomez JE: ATHENA (Athletes Targetting Healthy Exercise and Nutritional Alternatives): A preliminary program up against stiff competition. Arch Pediatr Adolesc Med 2004;158:1084–1086.
33. Pate RR, Trost SG, Leven S, et al: Sports participation and health-related behaviours amongst US youth. Arch Pediatr Adolesc Med 2000;154:904–911.
34. Griesemer B: Performance enhancing substances. In Sullivan J, Anderson S (eds): Care of the Young Athlete. Chicago, American Academy of Pediatrics and the American Academy of Orthopaedic Surgeons, 2000, pp 95–104.
35. Tokish JM, Kocher MS, Hawkins RJ: Ergogenic aids: A review of basic science, performance, side effects, and status in sports. Am J Sports Med 2004;32:543–553.
36. Gross RL: Arthroscopy in children. In McGinty JB, Caspari RB, Jackson RW, Poehling GG (eds): Operative Arthroscopy. Philadelphia, Lippincott–Raven, 1996, pp 83–91.
37. Favorito PJ, Langenderfer MA, Colosimo AJ, et al: Arthroscopic laser-assisted capsular shift in the treatment of patients with multidirectional shoulder instability. Am J Sports Med 2002;30:322–328.
38. Hewitt M, Getelman MH, Snyder SJ: Arthroscopic management of multidirectional instability: Pancapsular plication. Orthop Clin North Am 2003;34:549–557.
39. DeBerardino TM, Arciero RA, Taylor DC, et al: Prospective evaluation of arthroscopic stabilization of acute, initial anterior shoulder dislocations in young athletes. Two- to five-year follow-up. Am J Sports Med 2001;29:586–592.
40. Deitch J, Mehlman CT, Foad SL, et al: Traumatic anterior shoulder dislocations in adolescents. Am J Sports Med 2003;31:758–763.
41. Larrain MV, Botto GJ, Montenegro HJ, et al: Arthroscopic repair of acute traumatic anterior shoulder dislocation in young athletes. Arthroscopy 2001;17:373–377.
42. Lawton RL, Choudhury S, Mansat P, et al: Pediatric shoulder instability: Presentation, findings, treatment and outcomes. J Pediatr Orthop 2002;22:52–61.
43. Hogan KA, Gross RH: Overuse injuries in pediatric athletes. Orthop Clin North Am 2003;34:405–415.
44. Klingele KE, Kocher MS: Little league elbow: Valgus overload injury in the pediatric athlete. Sports Med 2002;32:1005–1015.
45. Micheli LJ, Luke AC, Mintzer CM, et al: Elbow arthroscopy in the pediatric and adolescent population. Arthroscopy 2001;17:649–659.
46. Kocher MS, Waters PM, Micheli LJ: Upper extremity injuries in the pediatric athlete. Sports Med 2000;30:117–135.
47. Terry Cl, Waters PM: Triangular fibrocartilage injuries in pediatric and adolescent patients. J Hand Surg [Am] 1998;23:626–634.
48. DeAngelis NA, Busconi BD: Hip arthroscopy in the pediatric population. Clin Orthop 2003;406:60–63.
49. Schindler A, Lechevallier JJ, Raos NS, et al: Diagnostic and therapeutic arthroscopy of the hip in children and adolescents: Evaluation of results. J Pediatr Orthop 1995;15:317–321.
50. O'Leary JA, Berend K, Vail TP: The relationship between diagnosis and outcome in arthroscopy of the hip. Arthroscopy 2001;17:181–188.

51. Ikeda T, Awaya G, Suzuki S, et al: Torn acetabular labrum in young patients. Arthroscopic diagnosis and treatment. J Bone Joint Surg Br 1988;70:13–16.

52. Byrd JW, Jones KS: Hip arthroscopy in the presence of dysplasia. Arthroscopy 2003;19:1055–1060.

53. Aglietti P, Ciardullo A, Giron F, et al: Results of arthroscopic excision of the fragment in the treatment of osteochondritis dissecans of the knee. Arthroscopy 2001;17:741–746.

54. Flynn JM, Kocher MS, Ganley TJ: Osteochondritis of the knee. J Pediatr Orthop 2004;24:434–443.

55. Kocher MS, Micheli LJ, Yaniv M, et al. Functional and radiographic outcome of juvenile osteochondritis dissecans of the knee treated with transarticular arthroscopic drilling. Am J Sports Med 2001;29:562–566.

56. Aglietti P, Ciardullo A, Giron F, et al: Results of the arthroscopic excision of the fragment in the treatment of osteochondritis dissecans of the knee. Arthroscopy 2001;17:741–746.

57. Meyers MH: Fracture of the intercondylar eminence of the tibia. J Bone Joint Surg Am 1959;41:209–220.

58. Meyers MH, McKeever FM: Fracture of the intercondylar eminence of the tibia. J Bone Joint Surg Am 1970;52:1677–1684.

59. Kocher MS, Foreman ES, Micheli LJ: Laxity and functional outcome after arthroscopic reduction and internal fixation of displaced tibial spine fractures in children. Arthroscopy 2003;19:1085–1090.

60. Reynders P, Reynders K, Broos P: Pediatric and adolescent tibial eminence fractures: Arthroscopic cannulated screw fixation. J Trauma 2002;53:49–54.

61. Millet PJ, Willis AA, Warren RF: Associated injuries in pediatric and adolescent anterior cruciate ligament tears: Does a delay in treatment increase the risk of meniscal tear? Arthroscopy 2002;18:955–959.

62. Kocher MS, Micheli LJ, Zurakowski D, et al. Partial tears of the anterior cruciate ligament in children and adolescents. Am J Sports Med 2002;30:697–703.

63. Higuera J, Laguna R, Peral M, et al: Osteochondritis dissecans of the talus during childhood and adolescence. J Pediatr Orthop 1998;18:328–332.

64. Letts M, Davidson D, Ahmer A: Osteochondritis dissecans of the talus in children. J Pediatr Orthop 2003;23:617–625.

65. Whipple TL, Martin DR, McIntyre LF, et al: Arthroscopic treatment of triplane fractures of the ankle. Arthroscopy 1993;9:456–463.

66. Chambers HG: Ankle and foot disorders in skeletally immature athletes. Orthop Clin North Am 2003;34:445–459.

The Older Athlete

Greg Sassmannshausen

In This Chapter

Physiologic effects of aging
Athletic activity after total joint arthroplasty
    Hip replacement
    Knee replacement
    Shoulder replacement

INTRODUCTION

- The number of older individuals remaining active in sports is increasing.

- Muscles, tendons, and ligaments all have been found to show a decline in biomechanical properties with aging.

- Appropriate exercise can slow or prevent some age-related changes.

- Injuries in the older patient may require different treatment than similar injuries in the younger patient.

- Joint replacement surgery presents unique considerations with regard to athletics, as overly aggressive activities may result in early loosening or failure of the prosthesis.

- Education of the older athlete is important in allowing exercise while decreasing the risk of injury or adverse effects to replaced joints.

Over the past 20 years, the number of middle-aged individuals active in sports has undergone unprecedented growth. This has led to chronologically older patients subjecting their bodies to stresses seen previously only by their younger counterparts. A resultant increase in injuries previously reserved for younger athletes or injuries unique to the older athlete has occurred. While these patients continue to remain active, the physician must be aware of the physiologic changes that occur with aging that may predispose to more frequent injury, altered healing responses, and potential delay in recovery. This may require alternative treatment techniques and rehabilitation for soft-tissue injuries affecting the musculotendinous junction and ligaments.

As the average life expectancy of the population increases, the prevalence of symptomatic arthritis also increases. Joint replacement surgery has provided very predictable results in providing pain relief and increased function.[1,2] With this improvement in quality of life, patients continue to desire to remain physically active after arthroplasty. As joint replacement evolves with improvements in surgical technique, component

design, and component materials, the indications for arthroplasty have been expanded to younger, more active patients. Therefore, the demands on joint replacements continue to increase.

The purpose of this chapter is to make the physician aware of the physiologic changes of the musculoskeletal system with aging and the basic science of the aging soft-tissue response to injury and review common concerns with athletic activity after joint arthroplasty along with current recommendations for these activities. With better understanding of these processes, the physician should be able to make more timely diagnoses with appropriate and cost-effective treatment and rehabilitation in an attempt to return the mature athlete to the premorbid activity levels or activities that will not be detrimental to joint replacements.

EFFECTS OF AGING ON THE MUSCULOTENDINOUS UNIT, LIGAMENTS, AND BONE

Recently, a significant amount of basic science research has focused on the effects of aging on muscles, ligaments, and tendons. What was considered to be the physiology of "aging" is now being reevaluated as that of "disuse," with a very subtle distinction between the two.[3] While the changes of disuse may be reversed, it appears that age-related losses cannot be recovered. At some point, irrespective of activity level, muscle function will decline, making the muscle susceptible to injury (Table 10-1).[3] This is evident around the knee. The quadriceps of individuals older than 60 years are 25% to 30% smaller than those of 20-year-olds.[4,5] Along with a decrease in size comes a concomitant decrease in muscle strength and endurance. Total muscle mass appears to decrease gradually from age 20 to 50 and then drop more markedly from age 50 to 90.[6] Knee extensor muscles during jumping show gradually declining strength beyond age 30 and decline in endurance after age 20.[7,8] This loss of muscle mass, strength, and endurance is likely secondary to a decrease in the number of muscle fibers associated with aging. In a cadaveric study of physically active, apparently healthy men who suffered sudden death, Lexell et al[9] reported the vastus lateralis muscles of the older group of men had a 25% reduction in total number of muscle fibers compared to the younger group. The exact cause of this decrease in the number of muscle fibers remains unclear. However, with aging, there is a decrease in the number of motor units, which may explain the decrease in fiber number.[10] This "functional denervation" appears to result in decreased synaptic contact with aging muscle and subsequent loss of myofiber function, resulting in loss of strength and endurance.[10,11] The end result places the aging muscle at risk of

Table 10-1 Effects of Aging on Muscle
Decreased muscle size and mass
Decreased muscle strength
Decreased muscle endurance
Decreased number of muscle fibers

injury while participating in sports activities. However, data suggest exercise and strength training by older people may reverse some of the alterations normally associated with aging muscle, providing a protective effect.[12]

Muscles commonly become injured during eccentric contraction in which higher forces are generated using fewer motor units.[13] Typically, muscle failure occurs at the musculotendinous junction regardless of the rate of strain or architecture of the muscle.[14] These susceptible muscle groups tend to cross two joints. Conditions that predispose to muscle strain include muscle fatigue, weakness, prior injury, or systemic diseases that cause muscular or tendinous degeneration.[14-16] Therefore, the aging patient may be predestined to muscle strains if activities are performed that require significant eccentric contractions, including sprinting and cutting.

Age has a significant influence on tendons, with a resultant increased potential for injury (Table 10-2). Starting from the third decade of life, aging results in multiple changes in the collagen within the tendons, including decreased cross-link maturation, an increased amount of insoluble collagen, and decreased collagen turnover.[17,18] Proteoglycan and water content decrease along with a reduction in vascularity.[19] Systemic illnesses or medications may also contribute to tendon calcification, mucoid degeneration, and tendinosis. These age-related changes affect the biomechanical behavior, resulting in stiffer, less compliant, and weaker tendons susceptible to injury. Similar to muscle, exercise may actually slow the decline in biomechanical properties associated with aging.[19]

Aging also has significant effects on the biomechanical properties of ligaments. The stiffness and ultimate tensile load for the anterior cruciate ligament from donors aged 22 to 35 were nearly three times as high as those from older specimens aged 50 to 60.[20] This change in mechanical properties is thought to be secondary to a decrease in collagen fibril size and changes in collagen cross-linking that occur after skeletal maturity.[21]

The effects of aging on bone are well understood, with progressive loss in bone mineral density after the third decade of life. This provides unique challenges when surgical procedures require stabilization of soft tissues to bone. Significant osteopenia often requires surgeons to alter fixation methods, allowing for adequate repair stability in order to tolerate the rigors of postoperative rehabilitation.

Once injury has occurred, aging affects the healing potential for both muscle and tendon. While muscle can regenerate after injury in older patients, the morphology and function of the reparative tissue differ from those of younger people.[22] Aging results in reduced capillary density, decreased availability of reparative cells, altered responses of cells to cytokines and growth factors, and systemic endocrine changes leading to decreased efficiency of muscle or tendon repair.[23-25] These factors may delay healing and alter biomechanical properties of the healed tissue, leading the treating physician to adjust rehabilitation and potential return to sporting activities.

ATHLETIC ACTIVITY AFTER TOTAL JOINT ARTHROPLASTY

As the life expectancy in the United States continues to increase, the number of patients with symptomatic arthritis requiring arthroplasty is also on the rise. The main goals of joint arthroplasty are pain relief and increasing function. With this increase in function, patients often become more active after arthroplasty. Joint arthroplasty leads to significant improvements in exercise duration, maximum workload, and peak oxygen consumption.[26] Data show that activity, rather than age or body weight, is the main factor in predicting implant survival.[27,28]

Specific concerns following joint arthroplasty dictate recommendations for postoperative athletic activities. Early implants faced failure with catastrophic wear. However, improvements in conformity, appropriate polyethylene sterilization and thickness, and component design have improved wear characteristics. With repetitive cycles and increased joint reaction forces, the generation of wear debris and secondary osteolysis remains a concern with increased sporting activities after arthroplasty.[27] Traumatic complications, such as dislocation or fracture, may be increased with athletic activity. Often this may be secondary to a postoperative patient attempting new athletic activities as preoperative pain has resolved and function has increased. Therefore, it is recommended that patients not attempt new high-level athletic activities postoperatively unless they were facile at them preoperatively.[29]

TOTAL HIP ARTHROPLASTY

Total hip arthroplasty has become a successful, reproducible treatment for symptomatic arthritis with 90% good to excellent results for 10 to 20 years after surgery.[2,30] These results are consistent for cemented and ingrowth femoral components.[2,30]

With such success, patients continue to expect more after surgery, including resumption of physical activity. However, with increased physical activities come increased joint contact forces, ranging from two to three times body weight during walking, with a further increase of 43% with easy running.[31,32] This increase in activity has been demonstrated to cause increased polyethylene wear and earlier deterioration of functional results.[27,33] Because of this, new alternative bearing surfaces have been developed to help combat the potential of component wear and osteolysis (Fig. 10-1). However, the potential complications of the alternative bearing surfaces may be catastrophic in some cases and in other situations remain unknown.

Table 10-2 Effects of Aging on Tendons and Ligaments
Decreased collagen cross-linking
Increased amount of insoluble collagen
Decreased proteoglycan and water content
Decreased collagen turnover
Decreased stiffness
Decreased ultimate tensile load

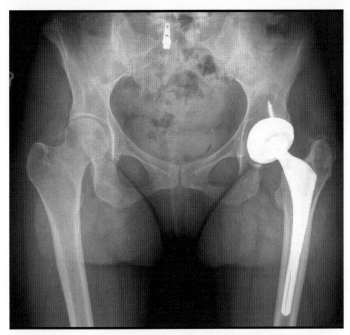

Figure 10-1 Total hip arthroplasty performed with a ceramic femoral head and acetabular liner. Ceramic components provide improved wear characteristics, as compared to traditional metals, with the potential for improved longevity in athletic individuals. However, these implants are more expensive, and fracture of the femoral head component has been reported.

There is limited literature evaluating athletic activity after hip arthroplasty. In one study, 70% of patients returned to participate in sports after hip replacement.[34] Low-impact sports after hip arthroplasty have not been shown to have a negative impact, with no difference in revision rates, and may provide potentially better outcomes as compared to patients not involved in sporting activities.[34,35] However, for active patients with cemented hips participating in higher impact sports, the risk of revision surgery is more than two times higher compared to less active patients.[36]

Current recommendations for activities after total hip arthroplasty discourage high-impact activities, while recommending low-impact activities. Surgeons must educate patients regarding risks of wear, loosening, and instability and must recommend athletic activities accordingly. A survey of 54 members of the Hip Society provides general guidelines for sport activities after hip arthroplasty (Table 10-3).[29]

TOTAL KNEE ARTHROPLASTY

Total knee arthroplasty has proven to be a consistent treatment providing improved function and pain relief for end-stage knee arthritis.[1] Knee arthroplasty has been shown to be effective in patients younger than 55 years old, with the primary concern being loosening and wear leading to revision surgery.[37] Both posterior cruciate ligament–sparing and –sacrificing designs have shown good long-term results in these younger patients.[1,38] However, with the potential of revision surgery, the choice of a posterior cruciate ligament–retaining knee does result in less loss of bone stock during femoral resurfacing.

Surgical technique geared to appropriate limb alignment and soft-tissue balancing is a prerequisite for ensuring long-term implant survival. Patients with tibiofemoral joint lines restored to normal and appropriate implant composite thickness have better function and better implant survival.[38]

The return to sports after knee arthroplasty has been evaluated, noting 91% of patients returning to low-impact activities such as bowling and 21% returning to high-impact activities such as tennis.[39] General recommendations after total knee arthroplasty discourage high-impact activities while recommending

Table 10-3 Activity after Total Hip Arthroplasty: 1999 Hip Society Survey			
Recommended/Allowed	*Allowed with Experience*	*Not Recommended*	*No Conclusion*
Stationary bicycling	Low-impact aerobics	High-impact aerobics	Jazz dancing
Croquet	Road bicycling	Baseball/softball	Square dancing
Ballroom dancing	Bowling	Basketball	Fencing
Golf	Canoeing	Football	Ice skating
Horseshoes	Hiking	Gymnastics	Roller/in-line skating
Shooting	Horseback riding	Handball	Rowing
Shuffleboard	Cross-country skiing	Hockey	Speed walking
Swimming		Jogging	Downhill skiing
Doubles tennis		Lacrosse	Stationary skiing*
Walking		Racquetball	Weight lifting
		Squash	Weight machines
		Rock climbing	
		Soccer	
		Singles tennis	
		Volleyball	

*NordicTrack, Logan, UT.
From Healy WL, Iorio R, Lemons MJ: Athletic activity after joint replacement. Am J Sports Med 2001;29:377–388.

Table 10-4 Activity after Total Knee Arthroplasty: 1999 Knee Society Survey			
Recommended/Allowed	*Allowed with Experience*	*Not Recommended*	*No Conclusion*
Low-impact aerobics	Road bicycling	Racquetball	Fencing
Stationary bicycling	Canoeing	Squash	Rollerblade/in-line skating
Bowling	Hiking	Rock climbing	Downhill skiing
Golf	Rowing	Soccer	Weight lifting
Dancing	Cross-country skiing	Singles tennis	
Horseback riding	Stationary skiing*	Volleyball	
Croquet	Speed walking	Football	
Walking	Tennis	Gymnastics	
Swimming	Weight machines	Lacrosse	
Shooting	Ice skating	Hockey	
Shuffleboard		Basketball	
Horseshoes		Jogging	
		Handball	

*NordicTrack, Logan, UT.
From Healy WL, Iorio R, Lemons MJ: Athletic activity after joint replacement. Am J Sports Med 2001;29:377–388.

no- or low-impact activities. A survey of 58 members of the Knee Society provides general guidelines for sport activities after knee arthroplasty (Table 10-4).[29]

TOTAL SHOULDER ARTHROPLASTY

Total shoulder arthroplasty presents a different dilemma for athletically active patients. While the shoulder does not generally bear weight, some sports create significant stresses on the joint nonetheless.[29] Recreating appropriate glenohumeral anatomy is important, as changes in the retroversion of the humeral component may cause up to a 300% increase in shoulder joint reaction forces (Fig. 10-2).[40]

Few data exist regarding shoulder replacement in athletically active patients. A review of 24 patients after shoulder arthroplasty showed that 96% of patients were able to return to playing golf.[41] These authors also noted no evidence of increase in radiographic lucencies between patients who did or did not play golf.

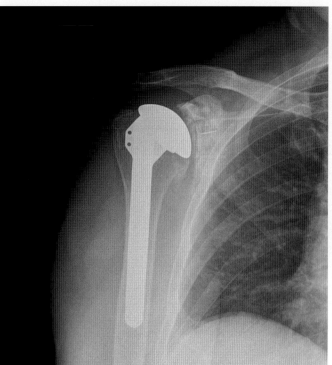

A

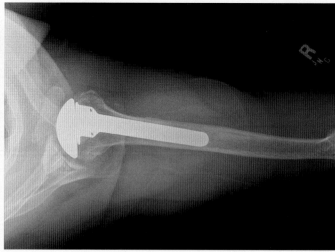

B

Figure 10-2 Total shoulder arthroplasty in a 62-year-old avid golfer. **A**, Anteroposterior radiograph. **B**, Axillary lateral radiograph.

Table 10-5 Activity after Total Shoulder Arthroplasty: 1999 American Shoulder and Elbow Surgeons Survey

Recommended/Allowed	Allowed with Experience	Not Recommended	No Conclusion
Cross-country skiing*	Golf	Football	High-impact aerobics
Stationary skiing	Ice skating	Gymnastics	Baseball/softball
Speed walking and jogging	Shooting	Hockey	Fencing
Swimming	Downhill skiing	Rock climbing	Handball
Doubles tennis			Horseback riding
Low-impact aerobics			Lacrosse
Bicycling, road and stationary			Racquetball, squash
Bowling			Skating, roller/in-line
Canoeing			Rowing
Croquet			Soccer
Shuffleboard			Tennis, singles
Horseshoes			Volleyball
Dancing: ballroom, square, and jazz			Weight training

*NordicTrack, Logan, UT.
From Healy WL, Iorio R, Lemons MJ: Athletic activity after joint replacement. Am J Sports Med 2001;29:377–388.

Current recommendations for young, active patients with symptomatic shoulder arthritis recalcitrant to nonoperative treatment is a modular uncemented humeral component with head sizes to allow adequate offset to achieve adequate tension on the soft tissues. Glenoid replacement is recommended with significant eccentric glenoid wear when there is adequate bone stock and an intact rotator cuff.

General recommendations for activity after shoulder arthroplasty are to avoid contact sports and high-impact loading sports affecting the shoulder. A survey of 35 members of the American Shoulder and Elbow Surgeons Society provides general guidelines for sport activities after shoulder arthroplasty (Table 10-5).[29]

CONCLUSIONS

The increasing activities of the middle-aged and older athlete, along with the age-related changes of the muscles, tendons, and ligaments, provide the potential for significant injury. The physician may see injuries typically found in younger patients, with the possibility of decreased healing ability or abnormally healed tissue. Therefore, the treating physician must be aware of the differences associated with aging tissues and their healing response and apply them to treatment and rehabilitative choices.

Most important to the treatment of injuries in the older athlete is prevention. Patient education and identification of medical conditions or medications predisposing to injury will assist the patient in choosing appropriate activities. If injury does occur, an honest discussion between the patient and physician regarding treatment options, published outcomes, and patient desires to return to premorbid activities will allow a timely and cost-effective treatment decision. On some occasions, this may include activity modifications or a lower demand sport.

As joint arthroplasty continues to improve and provide increased function, expectations of the athletic patient include returning to more demanding activities. These patient expectations must be addressed preoperatively and postoperatively with honest discussions regarding the potential for wear, loosening, or trauma about the replaced joint. With patient education about the risks associated with athletic activity, the ability of the patient to make a wise and appropriate choice of postoperative activities is improved.

REFERENCES

1. Colizza WA, Insall JN, Scuderi GR: The posterior stabilized total knee prosthesis: Assessment of polyethylene damage and osteolysis after a ten-year-minimum follow-up. J Bone Joint Surg Am 1995; 77:1713–1720.
2. Engh CA Jr, Culpepper WJ II, Engh CA: Long-term results of use of the anatomic medullary locking prosthesis in total hip arthroplasty. J Bone Joint Surg Am 1997;79:177–184.
3. Wilmore JH: The aging of bone and muscle. Clin Sport Med 1991;10:231–244.
4. Young A, Stokes M, Crowe M: The size and strength of the quadriceps muscles of old and young men. Clin Physiol 1985;5:145–154.
5. Rice CL, Cunningham DA, Paterson DH: Arm and leg composition determined by computed tomography in young and elderly. Clin Physiol 1989;9:207–220.
6. Tzankoff SP, Norris AH: Effect of muscle mass decrease on age-related BMR changes. J Appl Physiol 1977;43:1001–1006.
7. Bosco C, Komi PV: Influence of aging on the mechanical behavior of leg extensor muscles. Eur J Appl Physiol 1980;45:209–219.
8. Nakao M, Inoue Y, Murakami H: Aging process of leg muscle endurance in males and females. Eur J Appl Physiol 1989;59:209–214.
9. Lexell J, Henriksson-Larson K, Winblad B: Distribution of different fiber types in human skeletal muscles: Effects of aging studies in whole muscle cross sections. Muscle Nerve 1983;6:588–595.
10. Fitts RH: Aging and skeletal muscle. In Smith EL, Serfass RC (eds): Exercise and Aging: The Scientific Basis. Hillside, NJ, Enslow, 1981, pp 123–134.
11. Carlson BM: Factors influencing the repair and adaption of muscles in aged individuals: Satellite cells and innervation. J Gerontol 1995;50:96–100.

12. Frontera WR, Meredith CN, O'Reilly KP: Strength conditioning in older men: Skeletal muscle hypertrophy and improved function. J Appl Physiol 1988;64:1038–1044.

13. Stauber WT: Eccentric action of muscles: Physiology, injury, and adaptation. Exerc Sports Sci Rev 1989;17:157–185.

14. Garrett WE Jr: Muscle strain injuries. Am J Sports Med 1996;24:S2–S8.

15. Mair SD, Seaber AV, Glisson RR, et al: The role of fatigue in susceptibility to acute muscle strain injury. Am J Sports Med 1996;24:137–143.

16. Taylor DC, Dalton JD, Seaber AV, et al: Experimental muscle strain injury. Early functional and structural deficits and increased risk of reinjury. Am J Sports Med 1993;21:190–194.

17. Hamlin CR, Kohn RR, Luschin JH: Apparent accelerated aging of human collagen fibers. Diabetes 1975;24:902–904.

18. Shadwick RE: Elastic energy storage in tendons: Mechanical differences related to function and age. J Appl Physiol 1990;68:1033–1040.

19. Valias AC, Perrini VA, Pedrini-Mille A: Patellar tendon matrix changes associated with aging and voluntary exercise. J Appl Physiol 1985;58:1572–1576.

20. Woo SL-Y, Hollis JM, Adams DJ, et al: Tensile properties of the human femur-anterior cruciate ligament-tibia complex: The effects of specimen age and orientation. Am J Sports Med 1991;19:217–225.

21. Haut RC: Age-dependent influence of strain rate on the tensile failure of rat-tail tendon. J Biomech Eng 1983;105:296–299.

22. Sedah M: Effects of aging on skeletal muscle regeneration. J Neurol Sci 1988;87:67–74.

23. McCully KK, Posner JE: The application of blood flow measurements to the study of aging muscle. J Gerontol A Biol Sci Med Sci 1995;50:130–136.

24. Grounds MD: Age-associated changes in the response of skeletal muscle cells to exercise and regeneration. Ann N Y Acad Sci 1998;854:78–91.

25. Mezzogiorno A: Paracrine stimulation of senescent satellite cell proliferation by factors released by muscle of myotubes from young mice. Mech Ageing Dev 1993;70:35–44.

26. Ries MD, Philbin EF, Groff GD, et al: Effect of total hip arthroplasty on cardiovascular fitness. J Arthroplasty 1997;12:84–90.

27. Schmalzried TP, Shepherd EF, Dorey FJ, et al: Wear is a function of use, not time. Clin Orthop 2000;381:36–46.

28. Harris WH: Wear and periprosthetic osteolysis: The problem. Clin Orthop 2001;393:66–70.

29. Healy WL, Iorio R, Lemons MJ: Athletic activity after joint replacement. Am J Sports Med 2001;29:377–388.

30. Mulroy WF, Estok DM, Harris WH: Total hip arthroplasty with use of so-called second-generation cementing techniques. A fifteen-year-average follow-up study. J Bone Joint Surg Am 1995;77:1845–1852.

31. Brand RA, Pederson DR, Davy DT, et al: Comparison of hip force calculations and measurements in the same patient. J Arthroplasty 1994;9:45–51.

32. Rydell N: Biomechanics of the hip-joint. Clin Orthop 1973;92:6–15.

33. Dorr LD: Arthritis and athletics. Clin Sports Med 1991;10:343–357.

34. Dubs L, Gschwend N, Munzinger U: Sports after total hip arthroplasty. Arch Orthop Trauma Surg 1983;101:161–169.

35. Ritter MA, Meding JB: Total hip arthroplasty. Can the patient play sports again? Orthopaedics 1987;10:1447–1452.

36. Kilgus DJ, Dorey FJ, Fineman GA, et al: Patient activity, sports participation, and impact loading on the durability of cemented total hip arthroplasty. Clin Orthop 1991;269:25–31.

37. Duffy GP, Trousdale RT, Stuart MJ: Total knee arthroplasty in patients 55 years old and younger: 10- to 17-year results. Clin Orthop 1998;356:22–27.

38. Rand JA, Iistrup DM: Survivorship analysis of total knee arthroplasty. Cumulative rates of survival of 9200 total knee arthroplasties. J Bone Joint Surg Am 1991;73:397–409.

39. Bradbury N, Borton D, Spoo G, et al: Participation in sports after total knee replacement. Am J Sports Med 1998;26:530–535.

40. De Leest O, Rozing PM, Rozendaal LA, et al: Influence of glenohumeral prosthesis geometry and placement on shoulder muscle forces. Clin Orthop 1996;330:222–233.

41. Jensen KL, Rockwood CA Jr: Shoulder arthroplasty in recreational golfers. J Shoulder Elbow Surg 1998;7:362–367.

CHAPTER

11 Principles of Rehabilitation

Kevin E. Wilk, Michael M. Reinold, and Adam C. Olsen

In This Chapter

Creating a healing environment
Decreasing pain and effusion
Preventing deleterious effects of immobilization
Retarding muscle atrophy
Muscle strength and endurance
Soft tissue flexibility and mobility
Neuromuscular control
Entire kinetic chain
Return to functional activities

INTRODUCTION

- Rehabilitation is a multifaceted and ever-evolving process based on the basic science and general principles of tissue healing.

- The rehabilitation specialist must integrate the clinical diagnosis from the medical team with a full functional examination of the musculoskeletal system.

- The goal of rehabilitation is to enhance the recovery of injured tissues while avoiding stresses that may prove deleterious to the healing process. This is accomplished through a thorough understanding of the normal function, pathomechanics, and healing process of the specific tissue involved.

- The rehabilitation specialist must use current research and scientific evidence to establish guidelines to facilitate this process.

- In this chapter, we overview the most current evidence-based principles of rehabilitation with emphasis on clinical implication for sports medicine patients. The primary goal of this chapter is to discuss current concepts in rehabilitation.

PRINCIPLES OF REHABILITATION

Overview

Successful rehabilitation begins with communication among the sports medicine team and the establishment of an accurate and differential diagnosis. The key to successful rehabilitation is communication; to facilitate this interaction, the physician and rehabilitation specialist must communicate, providing information regarding the type of injury or surgical procedure performed, method of surgical fixation, the results of any diagnostic tests, the integrity and quality of the patient's tissue, and the

expectations of the physician for that specific patient. This information is invaluable to the rehabilitation specialist in designing and implementing a rehabilitation program.

The rehabilitation specialist must also perform a thorough and systematic physical examination to determine specific functional impairments, such as loss of motion or decreased strength of involved joints or muscles. Furthermore, the rehabilitation specialist must identify all involved structures that may be contributing to the patient's loss of motion, such as a tight joint capsule or muscular tightness. To obtain a successful outcome, the rehabilitation specialist must identify and treat the causes of the dysfunction. Then a thorough rehabilitation program can be outlined to address the individual diagnosis and functional needs of the athlete. It is imperative that the rehabilitation program be individualized based on each patient's unique response to injury.

For a patient to progress from one rehabilitation phase to the next, he or she must fulfill specific criteria. This progression allows the program to be individualized, based on the patient's unique healing rate and constraints. Programs are oftentimes broken up into phases such as acute postoperative phase or advanced strengthening phase, designed to emphasize goals that are specific to the proper time frame of tissue healing at that particular point in rehabilitation. Each phase has its unique goals that must be met in order to progress to the next phase, such as restoring full range of motion (ROM) or normalizing arthrokinematics. Each patient may reach these milestones at different times, which promotes a criteria-based rather than a time-based progression. The progression also helps to assist in locating areas in which the patient may be improving slowly and may need additional attention.

A fundamental concept that we use in developing a rehabilitation program at our center is to establish a differential diagnosis from the involved structures and causes contributing to the lesion. An example could be subacromial impingement. The cause of subacromial impingement is multifaceted.[1] Some possible causes are capsular tightness, capsular hypermobility, scapular position, and rotator cuff imbalances. To successfully treat this specific diagnosis, the rehabilitation specialist must treat the causes of the problem, thus normalizing joint function.

CREATING A HEALING ENVIRONMENT

The basis for all rehabilitation programs is to facilitate healing. It is imperative that the clinician promote healing but must be careful not to overstress the healing tissue. This first principle involves not just the facilitation of healing but also avoidance of excessive stresses that may be disadvantageous for tissue healing throughout the rehabilitation process. This may be illustrated in the rehabilitation of articular cartilage lesions. Controlled motion and gradual weight bearing progression is necessary to stimulate the healing process but must be progressed cautiously so that disadvantageous forces are not applied that will overload the tissue and inhibit healing. Thus, the program must be progressive and sequential, with each phase building from the previous one. Attempting to have a patient progress too quickly may result in inflammation, soreness, and potentially tissue failure, whereas the controlled application of specific stresses can benefit healing tissues. Another example of this is the rehabilitation of the anterior cruciate ligament (ACL) reconstruction patient. The graft must undergo revascularization as well as tissue remodeling before strenuous activities are allowed.

DECREASING PAIN AND EFFUSION

The first specific goal in most rehabilitation plans is to decrease the patient's pain and effusion resulting from the injury or pathology. Swelling at the injury site can stimulate sensory nerves leading to a further increase in the athlete's perception of pain. Pain and inflammation also work as muscle inhibitors, causing disuse atrophy the longer the effusion is present.

Numerous authors have studied the effect of joint effusion on muscle inhibition. DeAndrade et al[2] report that joint distention resulted in quadriceps muscle inhibition. A progressive decrease in quadriceps activity was noted as the knee exhibited increased distention. Spencer et al[3] found a similar decrease in quadriceps activation with joint effusion. The authors reported the threshold for inhibition of the vastus medialis to be approximately 20 to 30 mL of joint effusion and 50 to 60 mL for the rectus femoris and vastus lateralis. Similar results have been reported within the literature.[4-7]

Mangine et al (unpublished data, 1985) measured the peak torque and electromyographic activity of the quadriceps musculature while progressively effusing the knee joint. The authors noted that with the addition of 30 to 40 mL to the knee joint, quadriceps peak torque dramatically decreased by approximately 50% and continued to decrease with added effusion. Also, while the rectus femoris and vastus lateralis demonstrated mild decreases in muscle activity with the addition of joint effusion, the vastus medialis muscle activity decreased dramatically in proportion to the amount of joint effusion added. Vastus medialis oblique activity began to decrease with the addition of 20 mL while the rectus femoris and vastus lateralis required approximately 60 mL before a reduction in muscle activity was noted.

Thus, the reduction in knee joint swelling is crucial to restore normal voluntary quadriceps activity. Treatment options for swelling reduction include elevation, cryotherapy, high-voltage electrical stimulation, and joint compression through the use of a knee sleeve or compression wrap (Fig. 11-1). In patients who have undergone certain procedures for the knee, such as a lateral retinacular release, a foam wedge shaped to form around the lateral patella can be used in conjunction with a wrap to provide increased compression around the lateral genicular artery. Patients presenting with chronic joint effusion may also benefit from a knee sleeve or compression wrap to apply constant pressure while performing everyday activities in an attempt to minimize joint effusion. Conversely, patients with acute inflammation can benefit from ice and elevation.

Pain may also play a role in the inhibition of muscle activity observed with joint effusion. Young et al[8] examined the electromyographic activity of the quadriceps in the acutely swollen

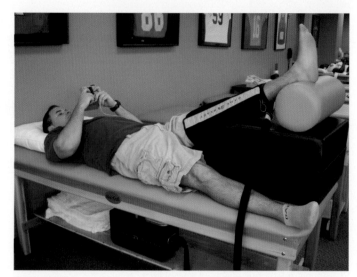

Figure 11-1 The application of cryotherapy and compression through a Game Ready commercial ice machine (Game Ready Inc., Berkeley, CA) with high-voltage electrical stimulation (300 PV; Empi Inc., St. Paul, MN) and elevation to minimize effusion.

and painful knee. An afferent block by local anesthesia was produced intraoperatively during medial meniscectomy. Patients in the control group reported significant pain postoperatively and pronounced inhibition of the quadriceps (30% to 76%). In contrast, patients with local anesthesia reported minimal pain and only mild quadriceps inhibition (5% to 31%). Thus, it appears that muscle inhibition may be attributed to a combination of joint pain and effusion.

Pain can be reduced passively through the use of cryotherapy and analgesic medication. Immediately following injury or surgery, the use of a commercial cold wrap can be extremely beneficial. Passive ROM may also provide neuromodulation of pain during acute or exacerbated conditions. Numerous studies have documented that passive ROM exercises reduce the need for pain medication.[9,10] Lastayo et al[11] report favorable results when continuous passive motion or manual passive ROM exercises are emphasized following repair of small, medium, or large tears of the rotator cuff. Therapeutic modalities such as ultrasound and electrical stimulation may also be used to control pain via the gate control theory.

The speed of progression of rehabilitation, particularly weight-bearing status and ROM, may also effect pain and swelling. Therefore, any increase in pain or effusion in the involved joint is monitored as the patient progresses through rehabilitation and begins new exercises. This is monitored to ensure that the pace of rehabilitation is appropriate and the tissue is not being overstressed. Persistent pain, inflammation, and swelling may result in long-term complications involving ROM, voluntary quadriceps control, and a delaying of the rehabilitation process; therefore, it is imperative that these symptoms be minimized.

BIOLOGY OF REHABILITATION

When progressing a patient through rehabilitation, thought must be given to the healing tissue itself. If a patient is progressing ahead of schedule and has no complaints, can he or she continue at an accelerated rate without compromising the long-term health of the tissues? Does an athlete returning to sport at 4 months mean a better outcome than returning at 6 months? Several characteristics must be considered when deciding the appropriate speed of rehabilitation. The patient's age, genetics, nutrition, concomitant injuries, and unique healing characteristics can all affect the rehabilitation time line.[12] Injuries to the meniscus or collateral ligaments may require a slower rehabilitation process following ACL reconstruction. Not all concomitant injuries are visible. Several authors[13,14] have reported that more than 80% of patients who sustain an acute ACL injury exhibit a bone bruise on magnetic resonance imaging. Johnson et al[13] have reported that patients with a bone bruise who underwent ACL reconstruction required a longer period to reduce effusion and pain and to return muscle function. Additional effects may not be seen for years after the initial injury such as articular cartilage lesions and the development of early knee osteoarthritis. Some authors believe that bone bruises resolve in several months,[15] whereas others believe the homeostasis of the bone may be altered for much longer[16] (Wojtys, unpublished data, 2004). The decisions made during rehabilitation may have significant effects on the metabolic activity of the injury site and the return to normal joint homeostasis.[16] Risks of an accelerated rehabilitation must be evaluated for each patient with careful consideration of the possible consequences. The rehabilitation specialist must be very careful when treating bone bruises. We recommend treating them with partial weight bearing, ice, compression, and control of aggressive loading for several months.

PREVENTING THE DELETERIOUS EFFECTS OF IMMOBILIZATION

In the acute stages of healing, it is often necessary to restrict motion of the injured tissues to promote healing (Fig. 11-2). While restricted, strength and muscular girth are quickly lost,

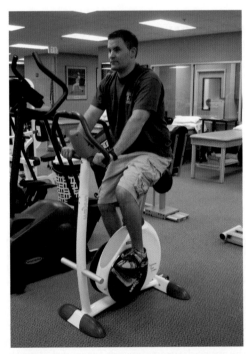

Figure 11-2 Range of motion performed on a Uni-Cam bicycle (Uni-Cam Inc., Ramsey, NJ). The axis of the pedals may be adjusted to allow for different range of motion for each extremity during the exercise. This can be used to protect specific areas within the joint range of motion.

and joint contracture and loss of ROM may occur. Furthermore, recent studies have documented that the combination of unloading and immobilization results in significant proteoglycan loss and weakening of the articular cartilage.[17,18] The deleterious effects of immobilization must therefore be minimized, and immobilization should be avoided in most cases.

Current research indicates immediate controlled motion is critical to a successful outcome.[19–23] Rehabilitation following ACL injury changed dramatically when it was found that patients who were taken through an accelerated program experienced a better outcome, including a decreased incidence of arthrofibrosis and quicker return to activity.[23] Immobilization is avoided in rehabilitation, with a greater emphasis on controlled ROM in a protected range. It is the authors' belief that the controlled application of ROM during the early phases of ROM is beneficial to avoid long-term loss of motion and to stimulate the synthesis, organization, and alignment of collagen tissue. Other benefits of early passive ROM include the reduction of pain and swelling, facilitation of a more normal gait pattern, and stimulation of collagen and cartilage repair. Beynnon et al[24] have documented with ACL subjects during passive ROM that there is no strain on the ACL with 0 to 125 degrees of motion.

Passive motion is most often performed by a skilled clinician but can also be performed by a continuous passive motion or by an isokinetic device set in the passive ROM setting. The use of continuous passive motion following surgery has several benefits including the avoidance of arthrofibrosis. In a study by Rodrigo et al,[25] patients undergoing a microfracture procedure of the knee who performed continuous passive motion for the first 8 weeks demonstrated 85% good to excellent results compared to a group of patients without continuous passive motion, who only had 55% good to excellent results. In the case of patients who underwent rotator cuff repair, restoring passive ROM is critical to the successful outcome of these patients.

RETARDING MUSCULAR ATROPHY

Rehabilitation should also emphasize the retardation of muscular atrophy and the facilitation of volitional muscle activity following an injury or surgical procedure. As previously mentioned, a small increase in pain and/or joint effusion can decrease the voluntary control of surrounding musculature. This can significantly affect the patient's ability to control the limb and ambulate with a normal gait pattern.

Exercises designed to enhance muscular volition begin with basic isometric contractions of the involved muscles. This isometric contraction allows firing of the muscle fibers without joint motion. This is a safe and effective method of exercise during the early phases of rehabilitation. Isometric contractions are performed for each muscle at multiple static angles throughout the available ROM. Isometric contraction has also been shown to be one of the most efficient forms of exercise for increasing muscular tension and improving strength.

Muscle re-education with electrical muscle stimulation (EMS) may assist in restoring the patient's voluntary control of inhibited musculature. EMS is often applied concomitantly during isometric and isotonic exercises to increase the recruitment of muscle fibers during the contraction.

Snyder-Mackler et al[26] studied the effects of electrical stimulation on quadriceps muscle strength following ACL reconstruction. Following a comparable 4-week training period, patients exercising with the adjunct of a high-intensity EMS unit exhibited quadriceps strength greater than 70% of the uninvolved lower extremity. Patients not using EMS presented with quadriceps strength of only 57% of the opposite knee in the same time period following surgery. The authors noted that the addition of neuromuscular electrical stimulation to postoperative exercises resulted in stronger quadriceps and more normal gait patterns than patients exercising without electrical stimulation. Several authors have also reported similar gains while integrating EMS into postoperative rehabilitation programs.[26–29]

Reinold et al (unpublished data, 2005) recently evaluated the use of EMS of the external rotators in the first 2 weeks following mini-open and arthroscopic rotator cuff repair surgery. The authors measured the amount of voluntary force generation by the patient during an isometric external rotation contraction with and without the application of EMS. Results revealed that patients were able to generate approximately 60% greater force production while using the EMS. This was a significant increase in force with the use of EMS superimposed on the muscular contraction.

Biofeedback may also be used to enhance the voluntary control of the injured musculature. Biofeedback is used to allow the patient to monitor the amount of force production throughout the exercise. Draper and Ballard[30] compared the use of EMS to biofeedback in the recovery of quadriceps strength following ACL reconstruction. Rehabilitation began immediately after surgery and continued for the first 6 weeks postoperatively. Both groups produced a significant increase in quadriceps peak torque. The group of patients using biofeedback showed slightly greater peak torque output of the quadriceps than did the group using EMS.

Clinically, we use EMS immediately following injury or surgery while performing isometric and isotonic upper and lower extremity exercises (Fig. 11-3A and B). EMS is used prior to biofeedback when the patient presents acutely with the inability to activate the musculature. Once independent muscle activation is present, biofeedback may be used to facilitate further neuromuscular activation. However, EMS may still be used to recruit more motor units, thus resulting in greater strength gains. Therefore, we use EMS for several weeks (4 to 8 weeks) following ACL surgery or selected shoulder surgeries. Conversely, biofeedback is used for patellofemoral rehabilitation patients when they are unable to actively recruit the vastus medialis (Fig. 11-3C). The patient must concentrate on neuromuscular control to independently activate the muscle during rehabilitation.

GRADUAL RESTORATION OF MUSCULAR STRENGTH AND ENDURANCE

After volitional control of muscle activity is achieved, emphasis is placed on gradually restoring muscular strength. A baseline level of muscular strength is needed before the athlete can progress to the later stages of rehabilitation that include advanced neuromuscular control drills. Strengthening can be performed through a variety of different methods of isotonic exercise. Weight is gradually applied and increased as the athlete progressively improves in strength to ensure that the exercise is constantly challenging. Isotonic exercises are generally performed as either isolated joint movements, such as knee extension, or multijoint movements, such as a squat. Furthermore, exercises can be performed in either an open or closed kinetic chain environment. An open kinetic chain exercise can be defined as a movement where the distal extremity is not fixed, such as knee extension. Conversely, a closed kinetic chain exer-

cise can be defined as a movement where the distal extremity is fixed, such as the leg press. Each of these modes of exercise have a place in rehabilitation, although all have a different effect on not only muscular activity, but also on the biomechanics of the joint. Wilk and Escamilla[31,32] have studied the EMG activity and biomechanical stresses during open and closed kinetic chain exercises for the lower extremities during various conditions. These authors noted that how the exercise is performed can significantly affect the exercise result. For example, during the vertical squat, by increasing the subject's hip flexion, the electromyographic activity of the hamstrings is increased and that of the quadriceps is slightly decreased. By performing a wall squat, the electromyographic activity of the quadriceps is extremely high and that of the hamstrings is lower and significantly different from the vertical squat.

Witvrouw et al[33] prospectively studied the efficacy of open and closed kinetic chain exercises during nonoperative patellofemoral rehabilitation. Sixty patients participated in a 5-week exercise program consisting of either open or closed kinetic chain exercises. Subjective pain scores, functional ability, quadriceps and hamstring peak torque, and hamstring, quadriceps, and gastrocnemius flexibility were all recorded prior to and following rehabilitation as well as at 3 months later. Both treatment groups reported a significant decrease in pain, increase in muscle strength, and increase in functional performance at 3 months following intervention.

Muscular endurance is also an important factor to emphasize in rehabilitation programs. Many of the activities that athletes participate in involve repetitive and microtraumatic events. Training the musculature to endure these events is necessary to prevent injuries. Fatigue has been shown to result in decreased proprioception and altered biomechanics of the joints, which may result in further pathology.[34–38] Murray et al[39] have reported significant changes in throwing mechanics, joint stresses, and velocity during overhead pitching once the thrower has fatigued.

NORMALIZATION OF SOFT-TISSUE MOBILITY AND FLEXIBILITY

Often times in rehabilitation, soft-tissue balance is emphasized. This applies to both the soft tissue around joints, such as the retinacular tissue surrounding the patella, and the muscular flexibility around each joint. Any deviations in the balance of soft-tissue forces will promote altered arthrokinematics and excessive forces to the joints. This can easily be illustrated in the patient with patellofemoral pain who presents with excessive lateral pressure syndrome and clinical signs of patellar tilting and lateral displacement due to tightness of the lateral retinacular tissue.

Another example of balancing the soft tissue about a joint is at the glenohumeral joint. Wilk et al[40] have referred to this concept as "asymmetrical capsular tightness." This means that if one side of the joint capsule is tight, then the arthrokinematics of the joint will be significantly affected. Thus, if the inferior capsule is tight, then the humeral head will translate superiorly during active arm motions. Harryman et al[41] have documented this concept with tightness of the posterior glenohumeral joint.

Muscular flexibility is also vital to normal joint function by allowing the musculature to absorb force and align the joint in a neutral position. For example, soft-tissue tightness of the quadriceps musculature is a common occurrence in patients with patellar tendonitis and patellofemoral pain.

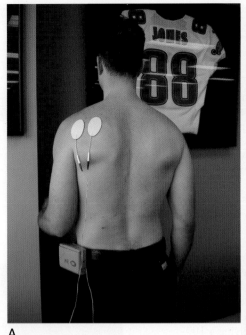

A

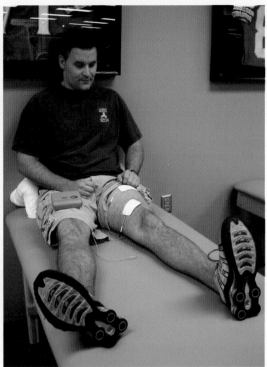

B

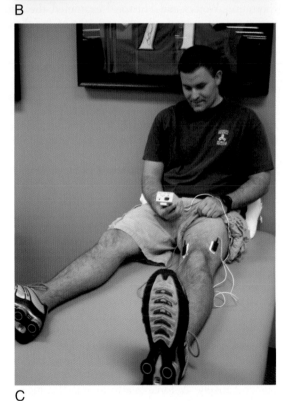

C

Figure 11-3 A, Neuromuscular electrical stimulation (300PV; Empi Inc., St. Paul, MN) of the infraspinatus during external rotation isometric exercise. **B,** Neuromuscular electrical stimulation (300PV, Empi Inc.) of the quadriceps during isometric quadriceps setting exercise. **C,** Biofeedback (Pathway MR-20, Prometheus Group, Dover, NH) on the vastus medialis obliquus and vastus lateralis during isometric quadriceps setting exercise to allow the patient to monitor the amount of muscle activity.

Witvrouw et al[42] prospectively studied the risk factors for the development of anterior knee pain in the athletic population over a 2-year period. A significant difference was noted in the flexibility of the quadriceps and gastrocnemius muscles between the group of subjects who developed patellofemoral pain and the control group, suggesting that athletes exhibiting tightness of specific muscles may be at risk of the development of patellofemoral disorders.

In the upper extremity, it is common to see patients who present with tightness in the anterior structures, such as the pectoralis musculature, and consequently exhibiting a protracted, forward head posture. This can lead to several shoulder pathologies, such as impingement due to the protracted and anteriorly tilted scapular position.[43] Furthermore, the authors believe that loss of internal rotation (IR) in most throwers is due to posterior rotator cuff tightness and osseous adaptation[44] and not from tightness of the posterior gleno-humeral joint.

RESTORATION OF NEUROMUSCULAR CONTROL

Early proprioception and kinesthesia exercises are important for patients returning to sporting activities. Basic exercises designed to enhance the athlete's ability to detect the joint position and movement in space are performed to establish a baseline of motor learning for further neuromuscular control exercises that will be integrated during the later phases of rehabilitation. Dynamic stability refers to the ability to stabilize a joint during functional activities to avoid injuries. This involves neuromuscular control and the efferent (motor) output to afferent (sensory) stimulation from the mechanoreceptors.

The emphasis of rehabilitation programs has shifted over the past several years to focus on restoring proprioception, dynamic stability, and neuromuscular control in patients. The neuromuscular control system may have a critical effect on the prevention of serious knee injuries.[45] Numerous authors have shown a decrease in proprioceptive and kinesthetic abilities following injury.[46-50] Beard et al[51] examined the effects of applying a 100-N anterior shear force on ACL-deficient knees and noted a deficit in reflexive activation of the hamstring musculature. Furthermore, Wojtys and Huston[52] examined the neuromuscular deficits in 40 normal subjects and 100 ACL-deficient subjects. In response to an anteriorly directed tibial force, the ACL-deficient group showed deficits in muscle timing and recruitment order. Proprioceptive deficits following shoulder dislocation have also been noted.[53]

We routinely begin basic proprioceptive training during the early phases of rehabilitation, such as the second postoperative week following ACL reconstruction, pending adequate normalization of pain, swelling, and quadriceps control. Proprioceptive training initially begins with basic exercises such as joint repositioning and closed kinetic chain weight shifting. Furthermore, Chmielewski et al[54] noted gait and weight-bearing drills are altered for several months following ACL injury.

Joint repositioning drills begin with the athlete's eyes closed. The rehabilitation specialist passively moves the extremity in various planes of motion, pauses, and then returns the extremity to the starting position. The patient is then instructed to actively reposition the extremity to the previous location. The rehabilitation specialist may perform these joint repositioning activities in variable degrees throughout the available ROM and notes the accuracy of the patient. Altering the patient's external stimulus such as vision and hearing may also provide increased challenge to the patient's proprioceptive system.

Weight shifts may be performed in the mediolateral direction and in diagonal patterns. Mini-squats are also performed early postoperatively. A force platform may be incorporated with weight shifts and mini-squats to measure the amount of weight distribution between the involved and uninvolved extremity (Fig. 11-4). Several authors have reported that an elastic bandage worn postoperatively has a positive impact on proprioception and joint position sense, and therefore our patients are encouraged to wear an elastic support wrap underneath their brace.[55,56]

As the patient advances, mini-squats are progressed onto an unstable surface such as foam or a tilt board. The patient is instructed to squat down to approximately 25 to 30 degrees and hold the position for 2 to 3 seconds while stabilizing the tilt

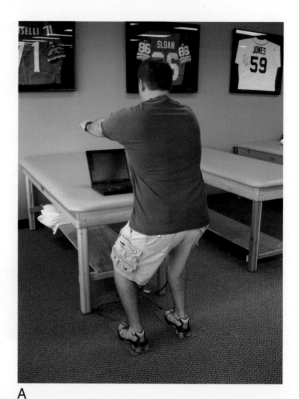

A

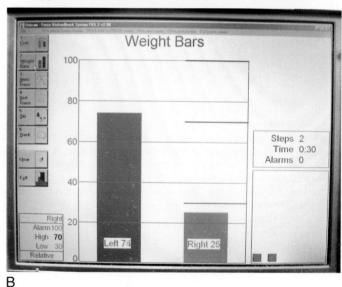

B

Figure 11-4 Mini-squats on a force platform **(A)** that can provide objective feedback of the amount of weight distributed between lower extremities **(B)** (Balance Trainer, Uni-Cam Inc., Ramsey, NJ).

board. Wilk et al[32] have shown the greatest amount of hamstring and quadriceps cocontraction occurred at approximately 30 degrees of knee flexion during the squat. Squats may be performed with the tilt board positioned in the mediolateral and anteroposterior directions. Wojtys et al[57] have shown that muscular contraction can decrease the anterior and posterior laxity in the knee joint by 275% to 450%. Also, Baratta et al[58] have shown an increased risk of ligamentous injury in knees with quadriceps to hamstring muscle strength imbalances. Thus, we believe by improving neuromuscular coactivation, stability is enhanced.

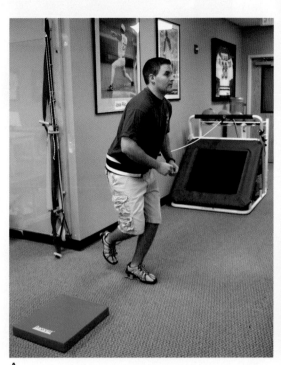 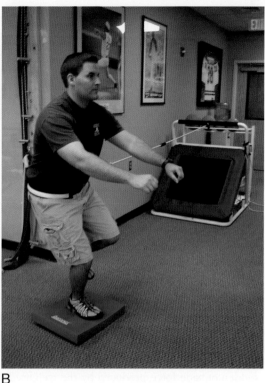

A   B

Figure 11-5 A and **B**, Lateral lunges using a sport cord onto an unstable surface.

As proprioception is advanced, drills to encourage preparatory agonist-antagonist coactivation during functional activities are incorporated. These dynamic stabilization drills for the lower extremity begin with single-leg stance on flat ground and unstable surfaces, cone stepping, and lateral lunge drills. The patient may perform forward, backward, and lateral cone stepover drills to facilitate gait training, enhance dynamic stability, and train the hip to help control forces at the knee joint. The patient is instructed to raise the knee up to the level of the hip and step over a series of cones, landing with a slightly flexed knee. These cone drills may also be performed at various speeds to train the lower extremity to dynamically stabilize with different amounts of momentum.

Lateral lunges are also performed with the patient instructed to lunge to the side, landing on a slightly flexed knee and holding that position for 1 to 2 seconds before returning to the start position. We use a functional progression for the lateral lunges: straight-plane lateral lunges are performed first, progressing to multiple-plane/diagonal lunges, lateral lunges with rotation, and finally lateral lunges onto foam (Fig. 11-5). As the patient progresses, concentration may be distracted by including a ball toss with any of these exercises to challenge the preparatory stabilization of the lower extremity with minimal conscious awareness.

Single-leg balance exercises are progressed by altering the patient's center of gravity and incorporating movement of the upper extremity and the uninvolved lower extremity. The patient stands on a piece of foam with the knee slightly flexed and performs random flexion, extension, abduction, adduction, and diagonal movement patterns of the upper extremity while holding weighted balls and maintaining control of the knee joint (Fig. 11-6). The uninvolved lower extremity may also be moved

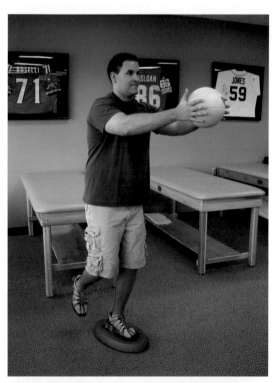

Figure 11-6 Single-leg balance on an unstable surface while incorporating alternating upper extremity movements with a weighted ball to alter the patient's center of gravity.

in the anteroposterior or mediolateral directions while maintaining control of the joint. Finally, both upper extremity and lower extremity movements may be combined. The patient again stabilizes the flexed knee on a piece of foam as the upper extremity moves forward with simultaneous extension of the lower extremity. This movement is followed by the upper extremity extending while the lower extremity moves forward. These single-leg balance drills are used with extremity movement to provide mild variations of the patient's center of gravity, thus altering the amount of dynamic stabilization needed as well as recruiting various muscle groups to provide the majority of neuromuscular control. Medicine balls of progressive weight may be incorporated to provide further challenge to the neuromuscular control system.

Perturbation training may also be incorporated. Fitzgerald et al[28] examined the efficacy of perturbation training in the rehabilitation program of ACL-deficient knees. The authors reported that perturbation training resulted in more satisfactory outcomes and lessened the frequency of subsequent giving way episodes in ACL-deficient knees. We incorporate perturbations while the patient performs double- or single-leg balance on a tilt board. While flexing the knee to approximately 30 degrees, the patient stabilizes the tilt board with an isometric hold at 30 degrees of flexion and throws and catches a lightweight medicine ball. The patient is instructed to stabilize the tilt board in reaction to the sudden outside force produced by the weighted ball. The rehabilitation specialist may also provide manual perturbations by striking the tilt board with his or her foot to create a sudden disturbance in the static support of the lower extremity, requiring the patient to stabilize the tilt board with dynamic muscular contractions (Fig. 11-7). Perturbations may also be performed during this drill by tapping the patient at the hips to provide proximal and distal perturbation forces.

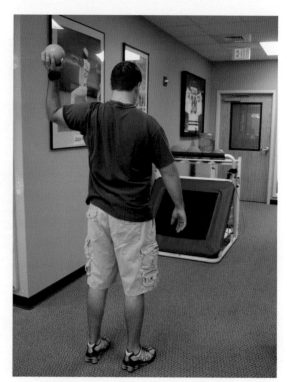

Figure 11-8 Upper extremity plyometrics.

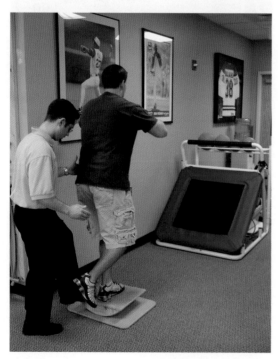

Figure 11-7 Single-leg balance on a tilt board while the patient tosses a ball against a rebound device. The rehabilitation specialist can create a perturbation by striking the board.

Exercises such as balance beam walking, lunges onto an unstable surface, and step-up exercises while standing on an unstable surface are also used to strengthen the knee musculature while requiring the muscles located proximally and distally within the kinetic chain to stabilize and allow coordinated functional movement patterns. For a complete description and progression to neuromuscular control drills for the ACL patient, Wilk et al[59-61] have published several articles.

Plyometric jumping drills may also be performed to facilitate dynamic stabilization and neuromuscular control of the knee joint. Plyometric exercises use the muscle's stretch-shortening properties to produce maximal concentric contraction following a rapid eccentric loading of the muscle tissues.[61,62] Plyometric training is used to train the extremities to produce and dissipate forces to avoid injury (Fig. 11-8).

Hewett et al[63] examined the effects of a 6-week plyometric training program on the landing mechanics and strength of female athletes. The authors reported a 22% decrease in peak ground reaction forces and a 50% decrease in the abduction/adduction moments at the knee during landing. Also, significant increases in hamstring isokinetic strength, hamstring-to-quadriceps ratio, and vertical jump height were reported.

Using the same plyometric program, Hewett et al[64] prospectively analyzed the effect of neuromuscular training on serious knee injuries in female athletes. The authors reported a statistically significant decrease in the amount of knee injuries in the trained group compared to the control group.

The final aspect of rehabilitation regarding neuromuscular control involves enhancing muscular endurance. Proprioceptive and neuromuscular control has been shown to diminish once muscular fatigue occurs.[65-67] Exercises such as bicycling, stair climbing, and elliptical machines may be used for long durations to increase endurance as well as high repetition, low weight

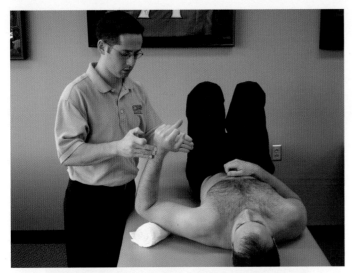

Figure 11-9 Rhythmic stabilization to promote cocontraction of the rotator cuff.

Dynamic stabilization exercises for the upper extremity also begin with baseline proprioception and kinesthesia drills to maximize the athlete's awareness of joint position and movement in space. In addition to joint repositioning and closed kinetic chain drills, rhythmic stabilizations are incorporated to facilitate cocontraction of the rotator cuff and dynamic stability of the glenohumeral joint. This exercise involves alternating isometric contractions designed to promote cocontraction and basic reactive neuromuscular control (Fig. 11-9). These dynamic stabilization techniques may be applied as the athlete progresses to provide advancing challenge to the neuromuscular control system. As the athlete progresses, it is necessary to train the upper extremity to provide adequate dynamic stabilization in response to sudden forces, particularly at end ROM (Fig. 11-10). We refer to this as reactive neuromuscular control.

EMPHASIS ON THE ENTIRE KINETIC CHAIN

Rehabilitation must be focused on not only regaining strength and neuromuscular control of the affected joint, but also include attention to the surrounding areas. For example, neuromuscular control of the shoulder involves stability of not only the glenohumeral joint but also the scapulothoracic joint. The scapula serves to provide a stable base of support for muscular attachment and dynamically positions the glenohumeral joint during upper extremity movement. Scapular strength and stability are essential to proper function of the glenohumeral joint. Therefore, isotonic strengthening and dynamic stabilization of the scapular musculature should also be included in rehabilitation programs for the athlete's shoulder to ensure proximal stability. Furthermore, the core of the body should be emphasized to enhance scapular control.

Additionally, altered forces at the knee joint may be the result of several biomechanical faults, both distal and proximal in the kinetic chain. These include rearfoot and tibial rotation distally and femoral rotation, hip control, and core stability proximally.

resistance strengthening. Additionally, we frequently recommend performing neuromuscular control drills toward the end of a treatment session, after cardiovascular training. This type of training is performed to challenge the neuromuscular control of the knee joint when the dynamic stabilizers have been adequately fatigued.

The enhancement of neuromuscular control is equally important in the upper extremity, and many of the previously mentioned techniques can also be applied to the upper extremity. The excessive mobility and compromised static stability observed within the glenohumeral joint often result in numerous injuries to the capsulolabral and musculotendinous structures of the shoulder. Efficient dynamic stabilization and neuromuscular control of the glenohumeral joint is necessary for athletes to avoid injuries during competition.[19]

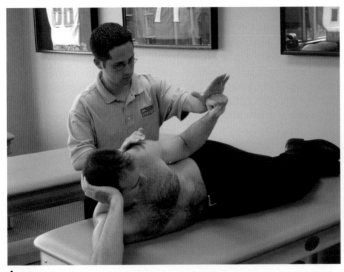

A

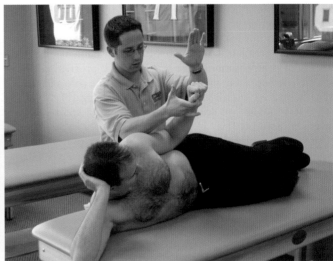

B

Figure 11-10 A, Manual resistance during side-lying external resistance; the rehabilitation specialist resisted both external rotation and retraction of the scapula. **B**, Rhythmic stabilizations may also be performed at end range.

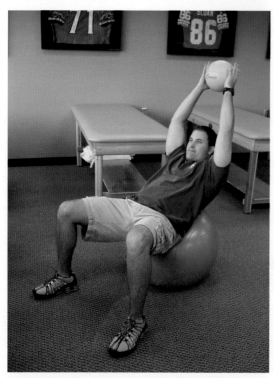

Figure 11-11 Abdominal exercises on a Swiss ball while holding a weighted ball.

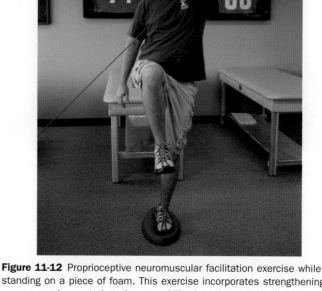

Figure 11-12 Proprioceptive neuromuscular facilitation exercise while standing on a piece of foam. This exercise incorporates strengthening, neuromuscular control, and core stabilization while simulating the stance position of baseball pitching.

The senior author of this chapter (K.W.) believes that the way to control varus and valgus at the tibiofemoral joint is either proximally (through pelvic and hip control) and/or distally with foot mechanics (e.g., controlling hyperpronation). Thus, we emphasize hip rotation strengthening exercises and foot biomechanical correction.

Core stabilization drills are used to further enhance proximal stability with distal mobility of the extremities. Core stabilization is used based on the kinetic chain concept where imbalance within any point of the kinetic chain may result in pathology throughout. Movement patterns, such as throwing, require a precise interaction of the entire body kinetic chain to perform efficiently. An imbalance of strength, flexibility, endurance, or stability may result in fatigue, abnormal arthrokinematics, and subsequent compensation. Core stabilization is progressed using a multiphase approach, progressing from baseline core and trunk strengthening to intermediate core strengthening (Fig. 11-11) with distal mobility to advanced stabilization in sport-specific movement patterns (Fig. 11-12).

Also, during rehabilitation, it is important not to neglect the uninjured extremity. Studies have pointed to a crossover effect when the contralateral extremity is exercised, which may result in improvements in proprioception and strength.[68–71] Preliminary studies at our center have shown a decrease in proprioception of the uninvolved extremity following ACL injury. This has also been reported with unilateral ankle sprains. It appears that the neuromuscular control system may have a certain amount of central mediating function that may be receptive to bilateral training techniques. Thus, when rehabilitating a patient with a joint injury, the rehabilitation specialist must consider the

patient performing either bilateral exercises or unilateral reciprocal exercises (Fig. 11-13).

GRADUAL RECONDITIONING THROUGH APPLIED LOADS AND STRESSES

Rehabilitation must be performed in a gradual manner. Tissues are best reconditioned through progressive loading and stressing. The rehabilitation process involves a progressive application of therapeutic exercises designed to gradually increase function in the athlete. As previously discussed, an overaggressive approach early within the rehabilitation program may result in increased pain, inflammation, and effusion. This simple concept may also be applied to the progression of strengthening exercises, proprioception training, neuromuscular control drills, functional drills, and sport-specific training. For example, exercises such as weight shifts and lunges are progressed from straight plane anteroposterior or mediolateral directions to involve multiplane and rotational movements. Two-legged exercises, such as leg press, knee extension, balance activities, and plyometric jumps, are progressed to single-leg exercises. Thus, the progression through the postoperative rehabilitation program involves a gradual progression of applied and functional stresses. This progression is used to provide a healthy stimulus for healing tissues while ensuring that forces are gradually applied without causing damage. This ensures that the patient has ample time to develop the neuromuscular control and dynamic stabilization needed to perform these drills.

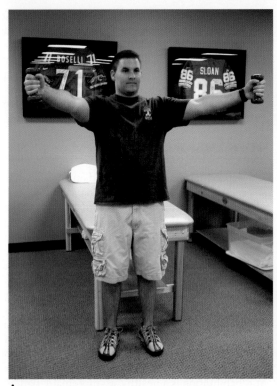
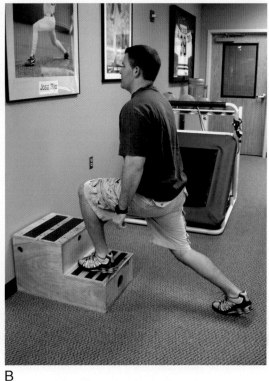

A   B

Figure 11-13 Examples of exercises performed bilaterally, the standing "full can" exercise (**A**) and forward lunging onto a box (**B**).

GRADUAL RETURN TO FUNCTIONAL ACTIVITIES

Following the successful completion of a rehabilitation program, the athlete must begin a gradual return to sport activities. Interval sport programs (ISPs) are designed to gradually return motion, function, and confidence to the athlete after injury or surgery by slowly progressing through graduated sport-specific activities.[72] The goal of this phase is to gradually and progressively increase the functional demands on the athlete to return the patient to full, unrestricted sport or daily activities. The criteria established before a patient's return to sport activities are (1) full functional ROM, (2) adequate static stability, (3) satisfactory muscular strength and endurance (Fig. 11-14), (4) adequate dynamic stability, and (5) a satisfactory clinical examination. Once these criteria are successfully met, the patient may initiate a gradual return to sport activity in a controlled manner. Healing constraints based on surgical technique and fixation, as well as the patient's tissue status, should be considered before a functional program can be initiated.

The interval sport program is set up to minimize the chance of reinjury and emphasize precompetition warm-up and stretching. Because there is an individual variability in all athletes, there is no set timetable for completion of the program. Variability will exist based on the skill level, goals, and injury of each athlete. ISPs may be developed based on the specific sport and stresses observed during these athletic activities. For example, overhead athletes perform an interval throwing program that begins with a limited amount of throws using a flat-ground long-toss program. As the distance of throws is progressed from 45, 60, 90, and 120 feet, the athlete may progress to begin throwing from a mound.

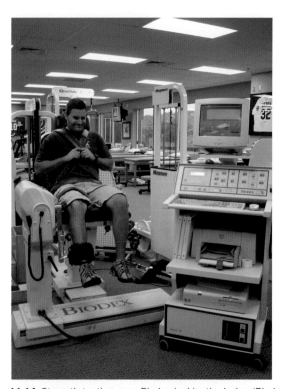

Figure 11-14 Strength testing on a Biodex isokinetic device (Biodex Corp., Shirley, NY).

Again, a gradual approach is applied by limiting the amount of throws and the intensity of throws is progressed.

Other goals of this phase are to maintain the patient's muscular strength, dynamic stability, and functional motion established in the previous phase. A stretching and strengthening program should be performed on an ongoing basis to maintain and continue to improve on these goals. The rate of progression with functional activities is dictated by the patient's unique tolerance to the activities. Exercise must be performed at a tolerable level without overstressing the healing tissues; this is referred to as the patient's envelope of function.

The athlete's return to sport-specific drills progresses through a series of transitional drills designed to progressively challenge the neuromuscular control system. Pool running is performed prior to flat-ground running, backward and lateral running is performed prior to forward running, plyometrics are performed prior to running and cutting drills, and finally sport-specific agility drills are performed. The integration of functional activities is necessary to train the injured patient to perform specific movement patterns necessary for everyday activities. The intention of sport-specific training is to simulate the functional activities associated with sports while incorporating peripheral afferent stimulation with reflexive and preprogrammed muscle control and coactivation. Many of the drills, such as cone drills, lunges with sport cord, plyometrics drills, and the running and agility progression may be modified based on the specific functional movement patterns associated with the patient's unique

sport. Some of the sport-specific running and agility drills incorporated include side shuffle, cariocas, sudden starts and stops, 45-degree cutting, 90-degree cutting, and various combinations of the previous drills. The specific movement patterns learned throughout the rehabilitation program are integrated to provide challenge in a controlled setting. These drills are performed to train the neuromuscular control system to perform during competition in a reflexive pattern to prevent injuries.

CONCLUSIONS

The rehabilitation process is based on our knowledge of the basic science of injury and tissue healing as well as an understanding of the general principles discussed in this chapter. Team communication and the gradual application of these principles in a well-designed rehabilitation program based on the individual needs of each patient are essential to ensure successful results. The goal of this chapter was to discuss current concepts in the rehabilitation process.

The ultimate goal of the rehabilitation process is not getting the patient or athlete back to work or sport as fast as possible, but rather returning the patient to function when it is safe and appropriate. For example, returning someone to running or jumping while the patient exhibits a femoral bone bruise can lead to long-term articular cartilage problems. The ultimate goal of rehabilitation is a healthy, asymptomatic patient 5 to 10 years after surgery, not just at 6 months.

REFERENCES

1. Wilk KE, Andrews JR: Rehabilitation following arthroscopic subacromial decompression. Orthopedics 1993;16:49–58.
2. DeAndrade JR, Grant C, Dixon A: Joint distension and reflex muscle inhibition in the knee. J Bone Joint Surg Am 1965;47:313–320.
3. Spencer JD, Hayes KC, Alexander IJ: Knee joint effusion and quadriceps reflex inhibition in man. Arch Phys Med Rehabil 1984;65:171–177.
4. Fahrer H, Rentsch HU, Gerber NJ, et al: Knee effusion and reflex inhibition of the quadriceps: A bar to effective retraining. J Bone Joint Surg Br 1988;70:635–638.
5. Hopkins JT, Ingersoll CD, Krause BA, et al: Effect of knee joint effusion on quadriceps and soleus motoneuron pool excitability. Med Sci Sports Exerc 2001;33:123–126.
6. Jensen K, Graf BK: The effects of knee effusion on quadriceps strength and knee intraarticular pressure. Arthroscopy 1993;9:52–56.
7. Torry MR, Decker MY, Viola RW, et al: Intra-articular knee joint effusion induces quadriceps avoidance gait patterns. Clin Biomech 2000;15:147–159.
8. Young A, Stokes M, Shakespeare DT, Sherman KP: The effect of intra-articular bupivacaine on quadriceps inhibition after meniscectomy. Med Sci Sports Exerc 1983;15:154.
9. Colwell CW, Morris BA: The influence of continuous passive motion on the results of total knee arthroplasty. Clin Orthop 1992;276:225–228.
10. McCarthy MR, Yates CK, Anderson MA, et al: The effects of immediate continuous passive motion on pain during the inflammatory phase of soft tissue healing following anterior cruciate ligament reconstruction. J Orthop Sports Phys Ther 1993;17:96–101.
11. Lastayo PC, Wright T, Jaffe R, et al: Continuous passive motion after repair of the rotator cuff. J Bone Joint Surg Am 1998;80:1002–1011.
12. Wilk KE: Are there speed limits in rehabilitation? J Orthop Sports Phys Ther 2005;35:50–51.
13. Johnson DL, Bealle DP, Brand JC Jr, et al: The effect of a geographic lateral bone bruise on knee inflammation after acute anterior cruciate ligament rupture. Am J Sports Med 2000;28:152–155.
14. Spindler KP, Schils JP, Bergfeld JA, et al: Prospective study of osseous, articular, and meniscal lesions in recent anterior cruciate ligament tears by magnetic resonance imaging and arthroscopy. Am J Sports Med 1993;21:551–557.
15. Davies NH, Niall D, King LJ, et al: Magnetic resonance imaging of bone bruising in the acutely injured knee-short-term outcome. Clin Radiol 2004;59:439–445.
16. Dye SF, Wojtys EM, Fu FH, et al: Factors contributing to function of the knee joint after injury or reconstruction of the anterior cruciate ligament. Instr Course Lect 1999;48:185–198.
17. Buckwalter JA, Stanish WD, Rosier RN, et al: The increasing need for nonoperative treatment of patients with osteoarthritis. Clin Orthop 2001;385:36–45.
18. Buckwalter JA: Articular cartilage: Injuries and potential for healing. J Orthop Sports Phys Ther 1998;28:192–202.
19. Cosgarea AJ, Sebastianelli WJ, DeHaven KE: Prevention of arthrofibrosis after anterior cruciate ligament reconstruction using the central third patellar tendon autograft. Am J Sports Med 1995;23:87–92.
20. Millett PJ, Wickiewicz TL, Warren RF: Motion loss after ligament injuries to the knee. Part I: Causes. Am J Sports Med 2001;29:664–675.
21. Millett PJ, Wickiewicz TL, Warren RF: Motion loss after ligament injuries to the knee. Part II: Prevention and treatment. Am J Sports Med 2001;29:822–828.
22. Shelbourne KD, Gray T: Anterior cruciate ligament reconstruction with autogenous patellar tendon graft followed by accelerated rehabilitation. A two- to nine-year followup. Am J Sports Med 1997;25:786–795.
23. Shelbourne KD, Wickens JH, Mollabashy A, et al: Arthrofibrosis in acute anterior cruciate ligament reconstruction. The effect of timing of reconstruction and rehabilitation. Am J Sports Med 1991;19:332–336.
24. Beynnon BD, Johnson RJ, Stankewich CJ, et al: The strain behavior of the anterior cruciate ligament during squatting and active flexion-extension. A comparison of an open and a closed kinetic chain exercise. Am J Sports Med 1997;25:823–829.

25. Rodrigo JJ, Steadman JR, Sillman JF, et al: Improvement of full-thickness chondral defect healing in the human knee after debridement and microfracture using continuous passive motion. Am J Knee Surg 1994;7:109–116.

26. Snyder-Mackler L, Delitto A, Bailey SL, Stralka SW: Strength of the quadriceps femoris muscle and functional recovery after reconstruction of the anterior cruciate ligament. A prospective, randomized clinical trial of electrical stimulation. J Bone Joint Surg Am 1995;77:166–173.

27. Delitto A, Rose SJ, McKowen LM, et al: Electrical stimulation versus voluntary exercise in strengthening thigh musculature after anterior cruciate ligament surgery. Phys Ther 1988;68:660–663.

28. Fitzgerald GK, Axe MJ, Snyder-Mackler L: The efficacy of perturbation training in nonoperative anterior cruciate ligament rehabilitation programs for physical active individuals. Phys Ther 2000;80:128–140.

29. Snyder-Mackler L, Ladin Z, Schepsis AA, Young JC: Electrical stimulation of the thigh muscles after reconstructing the anterior cruciate ligament. Effects of electrically elicited contraction of the quadriceps femoris and hamstring muscles on gait and on strength of the thigh muscles. J Bone Joint Surg Am 1991;73:1025–1036.

30. Draper V, Ballard L: Electrical stimulation versus electromyographic biofeedback in the recovery of quadriceps femoris muscle function following anterior cruciate ligament surgery. Phys Ther 1991;71:455–461.

31. Escamilla RF, Fleisig GS, Zheng N, et al: Biomechanics of the knee during closed kinetic chain and open kinetic chain exercises. Med Sci Sports Exerc 1998;30:556–569.

32. Wilk KE, Escamilla RF, Fleisig GS, et al: A comparison of tibiofemoral joint forces and electromyographic activity during open and closed kinetic chain exercises. Am J Sports Med 1996;24:518–527.

33. Witvrouw E, Lysens R, Bellemans J, et al: Open versus closed kinetic chain exercises for patellofemoral pain. Am J Sports Med 2000;28:687–694.

34. Carpenter JE, Blasier RB, Pellizzon GG: The effects of muscle fatigue on shoulder joint position sense. Am J Sports Med 1998;26:262–265.

35. Cools AM, Witvrouw EE, De Clercq GA, et al: Scapular muscle recruitment pattern: Electromyographic response of the trapezius muscle to sudden shoulder movement before and after a fatiguing exercise. J Orthop Sports Phys Ther 2002;32:221–229.

36. Hiemstra LA, Lo IK, Fowler PJ: Effect of fatigue on knee proprioception implications for dynamic stabilization. J Orthop Sports Phys Ther 2001;31:598–605.

37. Sterner RL, Pincivero DM, Lephart SM: The effects of muscular fatigue on shoulder proprioception. Clin J Sport Med 1998;8:96–101.

38. Voight ML, Hardin JA, Blackburn TA, et al: The effects of muscle fatigue on and the relationship of arm dominance to shoulder proprioception. J Orthop Sports Phys Ther 1996;23:348–352.

39. Murray TA, Cook TD, Werner SL, et al: The effects of extended play on professional baseball pitchers. Am J Sports Med 2001;29:137–142.

40. Wilk KE, Andrews JR, Arrigo CA: The physical examination of the glenohumeral joint: Emphasis on the stabilizing structures. J Orthop Sports Phys Ther 1997;25:380–389.

41. Harryman DT 2nd, Sidles JA, Clark JM, et al: Translation of the humeral head on the glenoid with passive glenohumeral motion. J Bone Joint Surg Am 1990;72:1334–1343.

42. Witvrouw EE, Lysens R, Bellemans J, et al: Intrinsic risk factors for the development of anterior knee pain in an athletic population. Am J Sports Med 2000;28:480–489.

43. Lukasiewicz AC, McClure P, Michener L, et al: Comparison of 3-dimensional scapular position and orientation between subjects with and without shoulder impingement. J Orthop Sports Phys Ther 1999;29:574–583.

44. Crockett HC, Gross LB, Wilk KE, et al: Osseous adaptation and range of motion at the glenohumeral joint in professional baseball pitchers. Am J Sports Med 2002;30:20–26.

45. Lephart SM, Pincivero DM, Giraldo JL, et al: The role of proprioception in the management and rehabilitation of athletic injuries. Am J Sports Med 1997;25:130–137.

46. Barrack RL, Skinner HB, Buckly SL: Proprioception in the anterior cruciate deficient knee. Am J Sports Med 1989;17:1–6.

47. Barrett DS, Cobb AG, Bentley G: Joint proprioception in normal, osteoarthritic and replaced knees. J Bone Joint Surg Br 1991;73:53–56.

48. Beard DJ, Dodd CA, Trundle HR, et al: Proprioception enhancement for anterior cruciate ligament deficiency. A prospective randomized trial of two physiotherapy regimes. J Bone Joint Surg Br 1994;76:654–659.

49. Beard DJ, Kyberd PJ, Dodd CA, et al: Proprioception in the knee. J Bone Joint Surg Br 1994;76:992–993.

50. Beard DJ, Kyberd PJ, Fergusson CM: Proprioception after rupture of the anterior cruciate ligament. An objective indication of the need for surgery? J Bone Joint Surg Br 1993;75:311–315.

51. Beard DJ, Kyberd PJ, O'Connor JJ, et al: Reflex hamstring contraction latency in anterior cruciate ligament deficiency. J Orthop Res 1994;12:219–228.

52. Wojtys EM, Huston LJ: Neuromuscular performance in normal and anterior cruciate ligament-deficient lower extremities. Am J Sports Med 1994;22:89–104.

53. Myers JB, Lephart SM: The role of the sensorimotor system in the athletic shoulder. J Athl Train 2000;35:351.

54. Chmielewski TL, Wilk KE, Snyder-Mackler L: Changes in weight-bearing following injury or surgical reconstruction of the ACL: Relationship to quadriceps strength and function. Gait Posture 2002;16:87–95.

55. Beynnon BD, Good L, Risberg MA: The effect of bracing on proprioception of knees with anterior cruciate ligament injury. J Orthop Sports Phys Ther 2002;32:11–15.

56. Kuster MS, Grob K, Kuster M, et al: The benefits of wearing a compression sleeve after ACL reconstruction. Med Sci Sports Exerc 1999;31:368–371.

57. Wojtys EM, Ashton-Miller JA, Huston LJ: A gender-related difference in the contribution of the knee musculature to sagittal-plane shear stiffness in subjects with similar knee laxity. J Bone Joint Surg Am 2002;84:10–16.

58. Baratta R, Solomonow M, Zhou BH, et al: Muscular coactivation. The role of the antagonist musculature in maintaining knee stability. Am J Sports Med 1988;16:113–122.

59. Wilk KE, Arrigo C, Andrews JR, et al: Rehabilitation after anterior cruciate ligament reconstruction in the female athlete. J Athl Train 1999;34:177–193.

60. Wilk KE, Reinold MM, Hooks TR: Recent advances in the rehabilitation of isolated and combined anterior cruciate ligament injuries. Orthop Clin North Am 2003;34:107–137.

61. Wilk KE, Reinold MM: Plyometric and closed kinetic chain exercise. In Brandy WD (ed): Therapeutic Exercises: Techniques for Intervention. Philadelphia, Lippincott Williams & Wilkins, 2001.

62. Wilk KE, Voight ML, Keirns MA, et al: Stretch-shortening drills for the upper extremities: Theory and clinical application. J Orthop Sports Phys Ther 1993;17:225–239.

63. Hewett TE, Stroupe AL, Nance TA, et al: Plyometric training in female athletes. Decreased impact forces and increased hamstring torques. Am J Sports Med 1996;24:765–775.

64. Hewett TE, Lindenfeld TN, Riccobene JV, et al: The effect of neuromuscular training on the incidence of knee injury in female athletes. A prospective study. Am J Sports Med 1999;27:699–706.

65. Lattanzio PJ, Petrella RJ, Sproule JR, et al: Effects of fatigue on knee proprioception. Clin J Sports Med 1997;7:22–27.

66. Lattanzio PJ, Petrella RJ: Knee proprioception: A review of mechanisms, measurements, and implications of muscular fatigue. Orthopedics 1998;21:463–470.

67. Skinner HB, Wyatt MP, Hodgdon JA, et al: Effect of fatigue on joint position sense of the knee. J Orthop Res 1986;4:112–118.

68. Kannus P, Alosa D, Cook L, et al: Effect of one-legged exercise on the strength, power and endurance of the contralateral leg. A randomized, controlled study using isometric and concentric isokinetic training. Eur J Appl Physiol Occup Physiol 1992;6:117–126.

69. Nagel MJ, Rice MS: Cross-transfer effects in the upper extremity during an occupationally embedded exercise. Am J Occup Ther 2001;55:317–323.

70. Stromberg BV: Contralateral therapy in upper extremity rehabilitation. Am J Phys Med 1986;65:135–143.

71. Stromberg BV: Influence of cross-education training in postoperative hand therapy. South Med J 1988;81:989–991.

72. Reinold MM, Wilk KE, Reed J, et al: Interval sport programs: Guidelines for baseball, tennis, and golf. J Orthop Sports Phys Ther 2002;32:293–298.

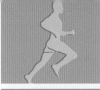

12

Safety Issues for Musculoskeletal Allografts

Craig S. Mauro, Jeffrey A. Rihn, and Christopher D. Harner

In This Chapter

Bacterial infection
Viral infection
Immunologic concerns
Tissue bank regulation
Tissue procurement
Aseptic tissue processing
Secondary tissue sterilization
Tissue storage

INTRODUCTION

- Musculoskeletal allograft tissue has become increasingly popular, with approximately 350,000 allografts distributed in 1990 and 875,000 in 2001.[1]

- The advantages of allograft tissue include decreased operating time, no donor-site morbidity, and increased availability of tissue in complex multiligament or revision surgery.

- Clinical studies have demonstrated results comparable with those of autograft tissue.[2-4]

- Allograft tissue is associated with the risk of disease transmission and the potential for immune reaction.

- We describe the reported cases of infection and the risk for immune reaction from allograft tissue transplantation before outlining the current state of tissue bank regulation and tissue procurement, processing, sterilization, and storage.

BACTERIAL INFECTION

In the December 7, 2001, *Morbidity and Mortality Weekly Report*, the Centers for Disease Control and Prevention (CDC) described four cases of septic arthritis following anterior cruciate ligament (ACL) reconstruction using allograft tissue, bringing this issue to national attention.[5] Each of the patients in this series underwent ACL reconstruction using a bone-patellar tendon-bone (BPTB) allograft. The allografts used in two of the patients were supplied from one Texas tissue bank and had been harvested from a common donor. The grafts had been irradiated and processed according to standard procedures. The cultures from the surgical site infections of these patients grew *Pseudomonas aeruginosa* that had indistinguishable genotypic patterns. The grafts used in the other two patients in this series also were supplied from another common donor and processed through one Florida tissue bank. These allografts had not received terminal sterilization with gamma irradiation.

Subsequently, in March 2002, the CDC reported having identified 26 patients who had developed allograft-associated infections.[6] This investigation was prompted by the death of a 23-year-old man who received a femoral condyle bone-cartilage allograft and died on postoperative day 4 with blood cultures growing *Clostridium sordellii*.[7,8] The allograft implanted into this patient was from a donor whose tissues were transplanted into eight other patients. Of these patients, only one other patient, who had received a femoral condyle allograft and a meniscus allograft, developed an infection. His cultures also grew *C. sordellii*, but he was treated with ampicillin-sulbactam and recovered. Of these 26 cases identified by the CDC, 13 were infections with *Clostridium* spp. and 14 were associated with a single tissue processor. Eleven of the 13 allografts associated with the *Clostridium* spp. infections were processed by a single tissue bank. Eight of the 13 allografts associated with the *Clostridium* spp. infections were tendons used for ACL reconstructions. The allografts in remaining five patients with *Clostridium* spp. infections were from femoral condyles (two), bone (two), and meniscus (one).

Following the report by the CDC describing the allograft associated *Clostridium* spp. infections, Kainer et al[9] further traced these infected tissues to tissue banks and reported their findings in 2004. They identified 14 patients who developed culture-proven *Clostridium* spp. infection of a surgical site within 1 year of allograft implantation between 1998 and 2002. These 14 allografts were from nine donors and were processed by a single tissue bank. The authors estimated the rates of *Clostridium* spp. infection in patients receiving an allograft from the implicated tissue bank in 2001 to be 0.12% for all sports-medicine tissues. Barbour and King[10] had previously described four of these cases in detail, demonstrating the morbidity caused by such an infection.

The CDC again reported on a case of infection following ACL reconstruction with allograft tissue in December 2003.[11] In this case, the affected individual's cultures grew *Streptococcus pyogenes* (group A streptococcus). This bacterium had been identified in the preprocessing cultures of the tissues recovered from the donor. Since all postprocessing tissue cultures were negative, the tissues were distributed. Tendon allografts from the donor had also been implanted in five other patients, but there have been no reports of infection in these patients.

VIRAL INFECTION

Transmission of viral infections through musculoskeletal allograft tissue has been occasionally reported in the literature. There have been several cases of transmission of hepatitis C virus (HCV) and one unidentified case of hepatitis in 1954.[12-16] In 2003, the CDC reported on the most recent case of HCV transmission, which occurred through a patellar tendon allograft from a donor in the window period between infection and detectable HCV-antibody response.[15] The other tissues from this donor included 44 organs and tissues that had been transplanted into 40 recipients. Thirty-two patients received tissues and five probable cases of HCV infection developed: in all three recipients of tendon with bone, in one of three recipients of tendon, and in one of three recipients of saphenous vein.

Two cases of human immunodeficiency virus (HIV),[17–19] and one case of human T-lymphotrophic virus (HTLV)[20] transmission through allograft tissue have been reported to date. The first case of HIV transmission reported involved a patient who received bone from a femoral head of an unscreened donor for a spinal fusion in 1984.[17] The second case is one of a young male donor who was screened and found to be seronegative by enzyme-linked immunosorbent assay HIV antibody testing after being shot to death in 1985.[18,19] Fifty-two of his tissues were transplanted into recipients, and three patients who received tissue from a femoral head or a BPTB ultimately tested positive for the HIV antibody. The case of HTLV transmission was through a femoral head allograft in 1991.[20] Except for the most recent case of hepatitis C transmission, the viral transmissions occurred before current serologic tests were available and before the implementation of guidelines for donor screening for viruses and bacteria.

IMMUNOLOGIC CONCERNS

Animal and clinical studies of menisci, tendons, cartilage, and bone have demonstrated a localized immune response associated with allograft transplantation.[21–23] Rodeo et al[23] demonstrated the presence of histocompatibility antigens on the donor meniscal surface at the time of transplantation and immunoreactive lymphocytes in the meniscus or synovial tissue of the recipient at follow-up. This response did not, however, affect the clinical outcome of these patients. Friedlaender et al[22] confirmed the immunogenicity of bone allografts, and Vasseur et al[21] identified the presence of antibodies to donor leukocyte antigens in the synovial fluid of dogs following allograft ACL transplantation. Although a histologically evident immune response seems to be elicited by all allograft material, this immune response does not appear to affect clinical outcome.

TISSUE BANK REGULATION

A tissue bank is an organization that provides donor screening, recovery, processing, storage, and/or distribution of allograft tissue. The first tissue bank, a dedicated bone bank, was described by Inclan[24] in 1942. A 2001 report by the Department of Health and Human Services (HHS) Office of Inspector General identified 154 tissue banks.[25] Regulation of tissue banks has developed concurrently with their increasing number.

Currently, there are three levels of tissue bank regulation: the U.S. Food and Drug Administration (FDA), the American Association of Tissue Banks (AATB), and the state governments. The FDA seeks to prevent communicable diseases by requiring donor screening and testing. Further, the FDA began inspecting tissue banks in 1993 and has the power to halt operations at a bank, recall tissue, and punish owners/operators. The 2001 HHS report identified that the FDA had never inspected at least 36 of the 154 identified tissue banks. Further, of the 118 banks that had been inspected, 68 had been inspected only once. The

limitations of the FDA oversight identified in the report were identification of banks, because banks were not required to register with the FDA, and insufficient funds to expand the inspection program.[25]

In January 2004, the FDA Good Tissue Practices broadened the scope of tissue establishments, as regulations became effective requiring tissue bank registration with the agency and disclosure of each cell or tissue produced.[26] The FDA's new comprehensive framework also proposed establishment of donor suitability criteria for donors of human cellular and tissue-based products and requirement of manufacturers to follow current good tissue practices.

In May 2004, the donor suitability regulations requiring human cell, tissue, and cellular and tissue-based product establishments to screen and test cell and tissue donors for risk factors for, and clinical evidence of, relevant communicable disease agents and diseases became effective.[27] Further, in May 2005, the FDA began requiring human cell, tissue, and cellular and tissue-based product establishments to follow current good tissue practices.[28] This requirement governs the methods used in, and the facilities and controls used for, the manufacture of human cell, tissue, and cellular and tissue-based products; record keeping; and the establishment of a quality program. With this regulation the FDA also issued new regulations pertaining to labeling, reporting, inspections, and enforcement that apply to manufacturers of certain human cell, tissue, and cellular and tissue-based products.

The AATB is a not-for-profit organization that was founded in 1976 to facilitate the provision of transplantable cells and tissues of uniform high quality in quantities sufficient to meet national needs. The AATB began offering inspection and accreditation of tissue banks in 1986. Following an application process, banks may undergo an on-site inspection of facilities and operations, including record keeping, quality control, quality assurance, donor and tissue suitability determination, and safety. Tissue banks may receive accreditation for their operations including retrieval, processing, storage, and/or distribution of tissue. Currently, the AATB also offers a program of certification of tissue bank personnel through an examination that tests candidates on their knowledge in all areas of tissue banking. The AATB currently has 85 members on its accredited bank list. Tissue banks are not required to apply for accreditation by the AATB, and nonaccredited tissue banks are under no obligation to meet the policies or standards of the AATB.

New York and Florida are the only two states that require licensure and inspection of tissue banks. They address issues such as tissue procurement process, tracking practices, emergency procedures, equipment standards, conflict of interest, laboratory testing, and disposition of unused tissue. In addition, these states require banks to report adverse incidents. Less stringent requirements exist in California, Georgia, and Maryland, where tissue banks must be licensed by the state. There is no licensure or inspection of tissue banks at the state level in the other 45 states.

TISSUE PROCUREMENT

Tissue procurement is coordinated through the nationwide Organ Procurement and Transplantation Network, to which organ procurement organizations belong. Organ procurement organizations are responsible for first evaluating potential donors and discussing donation with family members, and, ultimately, arranging for the surgical removal of donated organs. These

Box 12-1 Window Periods for Detection of Antibodies

	Standard	With Nucleic Acid Amplification
Human immunodeficiency virus	22 days	7–12 days
Hepatitis B	56 days	41–50 days
Hepatitis C	70 days	10–29 days

organizations are also important for the procurement of musculoskeletal tissue because they refer potential donors to tissue banks. The tissue bank is then responsible for the procurement process.

The FDA requires that tissue donors must be screened for HIV, hepatitis B virus (HBV), HCV, *Treponema pallidum* (syphilis), HTLV I and II, and human transmissible spongiform encephalopathy, including Creutzfeldt-Jakob disease. This screening is accomplished through a medical history and physical examination. The FDA also requires serologic testing for HIV, HBV, HCV, and *Treponema pallidum*, and, in viable, leukocyte-rich tissues, cytomegalovirus and HTLV I and II. One limitation with the screening process is the window period, the time period between which an individual is infected with a virus and the virus becomes detectable by screening tests. Traditionally, the detection of antibodies to a virus marked the end of the window period. This period is about 22 days for HIV, 56 days for HBV, and 70 days for HCV.[29] The window period may be shortened by using nucleic acid amplification testing, but it still remains 7 to 12 days for HIV, 41 to 50 days for HBV, and 10 to 29 days for HCV (Box 12-1).[29]

Once the donor is deemed free of risk factors, tissue processing begins. Despite this screening, contamination inherent to the graft may be the result of occult infection in the donor or postmortem invasion by organisms from the donor's gastrointestinal or respiratory tract. The latter risk increases with time postmortem, so most banks have a 24-hour postmortem limit during which tissue may be procured.[30] However, this regulation is variable and difficult to monitor. Following recovery, the tissues are transported under conditions designed to maintain tissue integrity.

ASEPTIC TISSUE PROCESSING

Aseptic tissue processing is the most common method of preparation employed by tissue banks to minimize contamination of tissue. The technique does not remove contaminants; rather, the process seeks to prepare the tissue without adding further contaminants to it. The CDC stressed this fact in the December 2001 *Morbidity and Mortality Weekly Report*, stating, "Although aseptic processing avoids contamination of tissue at the tissue bank, it does not eliminate contamination originating from the donor that might be inherent to the graft."[5] The technique removes only surface lipids and blood and does not penetrate the tissue.

Following aseptic processing but before the application of antibiotics, disinfectants, or sterilizing agents, swab culturing for bacteria and fungi is performed. The results are maintained in the donor's records and are reviewed before the tissue is released. However, the sensitivity of swab cultures of allograft tissue has been reported to be as low as 10%, suggesting inadequacy of this instrument of allograft contamination identification.[31] Following culturing, some tissue processors apply antiseptic and/or antibiotic solutions. These solutions may kill some surface microbes, but they do not kill viruses and do not fully penetrate the tissue.

SECONDARY TISSUE STERILIZATION

Sterilization is a process that results in the killing or inactivation of all life forms. The American National Standard Institute and the Association for the Advancement of Medical Instrumentation define sterility in terms of a sterility assurance level. They have established the industry standard sterility assurance level for medical devices as 10^{-6}, which means that the probability of a single viable organism being present on an item is one in one million after the item has undergone a terminal sterilization process validated to that level.[32]

Secondary tissue sterilization is used because of the limitations described in donor screening, graft harvesting, and microbial testing. Ideally, this terminal sterilization would eliminate all pathogens without affecting the biologic and biomechanical properties of the tissues. However, such ideal sterilization, as conventionally performed on medical devices, may not truly exist for tissues. With tissue sterilization, this balance between tissue sterility and tissue properties must always be considered. Further, most sterilization techniques are validated by a log-reduction assay that uses spiked tissue samples. These samples are immersed into known concentrations of bacterial and/or viral cultures before being treated and then recultured for the presence of the organisms. Systemically infected tissue is not routinely tested for validation, possibly compromising the validity of this assay for testing allograft tissue sterilization techniques.

Traditionally, ethylene oxide and gamma irradiation have been used in the tissue sterilization process. Recently, low-temperature chemical sterilization methods have also been developed.

Ethlyene Oxide

Ethylene oxide has historically been the most common method of tissue sterilization. It causes DNA and RNA dysfunction through alkylation of purine and pyrimidine moieties. The solution kills bacteria, fungi, and spores and preserves the tissue strength and biocompatibility, although biocompatibility may be dose dependent. However, it does not kill viruses and has a limited ability to fully penetrate tissue. Further, reports have noted that ethylene oxide and its byproducts (ethylene glycol and ethylene chlorohydrin) may be toxic, which prompted the FDA to regulate residual levels of ethylene oxide and its byproducts.[33] Since ethylene oxide has been shown to incite a chronic synovitis, it has largely been abandoned as a sterilizing agent for tissue used for reconstruction of intra-articular ligaments.[33] Consequently, most tissue banks use other methods of tissue sterilization.

Gamma Irradiation

Gamma irradiation is typically delivered to tissue at levels of 1.0 to 3.5 mrad.[30] It fully penetrates tissue, preserves biocompatibility, and kills bacteria, fungi, and spores at relatively low doses (1.5 to 2.0 mrad). Further, gamma irradiation kills viruses in a dose-dependent manner. Studies suggest that doses greater than 2.5 mrad are required to inactivate HIV in allograft tissue.[34,35]

Gamma irradiation also decreases tissue strength in a dose-dependent manner.[36–38] Doses as low as 2.0 mrad have been shown to reduce the structural properties of BPTB allograft.[37,38]

In 1995, Fideler et al[37] demonstrated a dose-dependent effect of irradiation on both the structural and mechanical properties of a human BPTB allograft. A dose of 2.0 mrad resulted in a statistically significant reduction in four of seven biomechanical parameters tested, including modulus and maximum stress to failure of the tissue. All seven parameters were reduced in a dose-dependent fashion after 3.0 and 4.0 mrad of irradiation. More recently, Curran et al[38] studied the effect of 2.0 mrad on the cyclic and failure properties of human BPTB allograft. This low dose of irradiation resulted in a 27% increase in elongation after cyclic loading and a 20% decrease in strength compared to nonirradiated grafts. The authors believed that these effects may be detrimental to graft function and could lead to graft failure when used to reconstruct the ACL. They suggested the use of nonirradiated rather than irradiated allograft to avoid such problems.

It is unknown whether this alteration in biomechanical properties has an effect on clinical outcome. Rihn et al[39] recently presented a study comparing the clinical outcome of patients who underwent ACL reconstruction with irradiated allograft BPTB with those who underwent ACL reconstruction with autograft BPTB. The allograft BPTB grafts used had been irradiated with 2.5 mrad prior to distribution from the tissue bank. They found both the patient-reported and objective outcomes of irradiated BPTB allograft ACL reconstruction were statistically and clinically similar to those obtained using autograft BPTB. They concluded that irradiation may be used as a means of sterilization of allograft BPTB without compromising the clinical outcome of ACL surgery, but the optimal dose of irradiation necessary for true sterilization remains unclear. Therefore, the dose of gamma irradiation must be considered when using this method of tissue sterilization.

Low Temperature Chemical Sterilization

The newest methods developed for tissue sterilization use low temperature chemical sterilization. These techniques are designed to kill spores but preserve the biomechanical integrity of the tissue. Allowash XG (Lifenet, Virginia Beach, VA), BioCleanse (Regeneration Technologies Incorporated, Alachua, FL), Tutoplast (Tutogen Medical, Inc., West Paterson, NJ), and NovaSterilis (NovaSterilis, Lansing, NY) are examples of these processes. The Allowash formula combines biologic detergents, alcohol, and hydrogen peroxide with ultrasonics, centrifugation, and negative pressure. The BioCleanse tissue sterilization process relies on the low-temperature chemicals to completely penetrate the tissue. The Tutoplast process uses solvent dehydration with acetone baths and low-dose gamma irradiation. The NovaSterilis process uses supercritical CO_2 to kill microorganisms through transient acidification by carbonic acid formation. Initial reports suggest that these chemical sterilization techniques are effective in sterilizing tissue and have no effect on the biomechanical properties of tissue. However, further evaluation of these techniques is warranted to confirm their effectiveness and identify any risks.

Other techniques currently being used for tissue sterilization include the Clearant Process (Clearant, Inc., Los Angeles, CA) and peracetic acid–ethanol. The Clearant Process uses a process of high-dose irradiation under conditions optimized to minimize damage to the tissue. Free radicals and reactive oxygen species are secondary products of standard gamma irradiation techniques that are thought to cause the deleterious biomechanical effects. The Clearant Process seeks to minimize this secondary chemistry. The tissues are incubated in a solution containing

---

Box 12-2 Tissue Storage Options

- Deep-freezing: tissue frozen to –80°C, most common method, grafts stored 3–5 years
- Freeze-drying: moisture removed, vacuum packaged, can be stored 3–5 years (room temperature)
- Cryopreservation: controlled-rate freezing, preserves cells, grafts stored 10 years

---

radioprotectants, including propylene glycol and dimethyl sulfoxide. They are then dehydrated to 8% residual moisture before being irradiated with 5.0 mrad at –65°C. The process has been shown to have no effects on the mechanical properties of tendon and bone.[40] Peracetic acid–ethanol has been used for more than 20 years in Europe to sterilize bone allografts. Recently, it has been applied to BPTB grafts without any apparent effect on the biomechanical properties of the tissue.

TISSUE STORAGE

The current methods of allograft tissue storage include deep-freezing, freeze-drying, and cryopreservation. Each of these techniques may be used for storage of ligament and meniscal allografts. Deep-freezing is the most widely used storage method for ligament and meniscal allografts, entailing simply freezing the tissue to –80°C. The grafts typically can be stored for 3 to 5 years. In the freeze-drying process, moisture is removed from the tissue and the graft is vacuum packaged. It may be stored at room temperature for 3 to 5 years but requires rehydration before implantation. Deep-freezing and freeze-drying allograft tissue decreases immunogenicity by killing antigen-bearing cells. Cryopreservation is a process of controlled-rate freezing with extraction of cellular water by means of dimethyl sulfoxide and

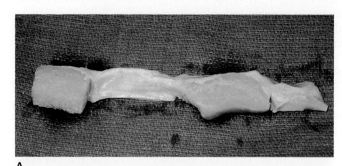
A

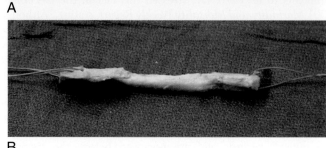
B

Figure 12-1 A, Bone-patellar tendon-bone allograft prior to preparation. **B,** Allograft prepared at time of surgery, ready for implantation in anterior cruciate ligament reconstruction.

glycerol. This process preserves some cells and offers a 10-year storage life.

Fresh transplantation is popular for osteochondral allografts because it better preserves cartilage cells and matrix. However, fresh allograft tissue, particularly osteochondral allografts, contains viable blood-borne cells, known to be highly immunogenic. Further, fresh allografts have a questionable shelf life, necessitating use within days of harvesting. It is often difficult to complete required serologic screening tests and adequately prepare, size match, and distribute fresh tissue within this short period of time (Box 12-2).

CONCLUSIONS

Allograft use has been increasing worldwide because of such advantages as decreased operating time, no donor-site morbidity, and availability for complex cases (Fig. 12-1). Although infection is rare, it has occurred several times recently, as reported by the CDC and other authors. Donor screening and serologic testing continue to expand, and sterilization techniques continue to develop. The role of the FDA has increased, as with the 2004 Good Tissue Practices, and most likely will continue to expand in this arena in years to come.

REFERENCES

1. Organ transplants and grafts, 1990 to 2000. No. 161. Statistical Abstracts of the United States: 2003. Washington, DC, Census Bureau, 2002, p 113.
2. Harner CD, Olson E, Irrgang JJ, et al: Allograft versus autograft anterior cruciate ligament reconstruction: 3- to 5-year outcome. Clin Orthop 1996;134–144.
3. Shelton WR, Papendick L, Dukes AD: Autograft versus allograft anterior cruciate ligament reconstruction. Arthroscopy 1997;13:446–449.
4. Peterson RK, Shelton WR, Bomboy AL: Allograft versus autograft patellar tendon anterior cruciate ligament reconstruction: A 5-year follow-up. Arthroscopy 2001;17:9–13.
5. Septic arthritis following anterior cruciate ligament reconstruction using tendon allografts—Florida and Louisiana, 2000. Morb Mortal Wkly Rep 2001;50:1081–1083.
6. Update: Allograft-associated bacterial infections—United States, 2002. Morb Mortal Wkly Rep 2002;51:207–210.
7. Unexplained deaths following knee surgery—Minnesota, November 2001. Morb Mortal Wkly Rep 2001;50:1035–1036.
8. Update: Unexplained deaths following knee surgery—Minnesota, 2001, Morb Mortal Wkly Rep. 2001;50:1080.
9. Kainer MA, Linden JV, Whaley DN, et al: *Clostridium* infections associated with musculoskeletal-tissue allografts. N Engl J Med 2004;350:2564–2571.
10. Barbour SA, King W: The safe and effective use of allograft tissue—An update. Am J Sports Med 2003;31:791–797.
11. Invasive *Streptococcus pyogenes* after allograft implantation—Colorado, 2003. Morb Mortal Wkly Rep 2003;52:1174–1176.
12. Conrad EU, Gretch DR, Obermeyer KR, et al: Transmission of the hepatitis-C virus by tissue transplantation. J Bone Joint Surg Am 1995;77:214–224.
13. Pereira BJ, Milford EL, Kirkman RL, et al: Low risk of liver disease after tissue transplantation from donors with HCV. Lancet 1993;341:903–904.
14. Eggen BM, Nordbo SA: Transmission of HCV by organ transplantation. N Engl J Med 1992;326:411–413.
15. Hepatitis C virus transmission from an antibody-negative organ and tissue donor—United States, 2000–2002. Morb Mortal Wkly Rep 2003;52:273–276.
16. Shutkin NM: Homologous-serum hepatitis following the use of refrigerated bone-bank bone. J Bone Joint Surg Am 1954;36:160–162.
17. Transmission of HIV through bone transplantation: Case report and public health recommendations. Morb Mortal Wkly Rep 1988;37:597–599.
18. Simonds RJ, Holmberg SD, Hurwitz RL, et al: Transmission of human immunodeficiency virus type 1 from a seronegative organ and tissue donor. N Engl J Med 1992;326:726–732.
19. Asselmeier MA, Caspari RB, Bottenfield S: A review of allograft processing and sterilization techniques and their role in transmission of the human immunodeficiency virus. Am J Sports Med 1993;21:170–175.
20. Sanzen L, Carlsson A: Transmission of human T-cell lymphotrophic virus type 1 by a deep-frozen bone allograft. Acta Orthop Scand 1997;68:72–74.
21. Vasseur PB, Rodrigo JJ, Stevenson S, et al: Replacement of the anterior cruciate ligament with a bone-ligament-bone anterior cruciate ligament allograft in dogs. Clin Orthop 1987;268–277.
22. Friedlaender GE, Strong DM, Tomford WW, Mankin HJ: Long-term follow-up of patients with osteochondral allografts. A correlation between immunologic responses and clinical outcome. Orthop Clin North Am 1999;30:583–588.
23. Rodeo SA, Seneviratne A, Suzuki K, et al: Histological analysis of human meniscal allografts. A preliminary report. J Bone Joint Surg Am 2000;82A:1071–1082.
24. Inclan A: The use of preserved bone grafts in orthopaedic surgery. J Bone Joint Surg Am 1942;24:81–96.
25. Department of Health and Human Services Office of Inspector General: Oversight of Tissue Banking, vol. OEI-01-00-00441. 2001, p 17.
26. U.S. Food and Drug Administration: Human cells, tissues, and cellular and tissue-based products; establishment registration and listing; final rule. Fed Register 2001;66:5447–5469.
27. U.S. Food and Drug Administration: Eligibility determination for donors of human cells, tissues, and cellular and tissue-based products; final rule and notice. Fed Register 2004;69:29785–29834.
28. U.S. Food and Drug Administration: Current good tissue practice for human cell, tissue, and cellular and tissue-based product establishments; inspection and enforcement; final rule. Fed Register 2004;69:68611–68688.
29. Busch MP, Kleinman SH, Jackson B, et al: Committee report. Nucleic acid amplification testing of blood donors for transfusion-transmitted infectious diseases: Report of the Interorganizational Task Force on Nucleic Acid Amplification Testing of Blood Donors. Transfusion 2000;40:143–159.
30. Vangsness CT Jr, Triffon MJ, Joyce MJ, Moore TM: Soft tissue for allograft reconstruction of the human knee: A survey of the American Association of Tissue Banks. Am J Sports Med 1996;24:230–234.
31. Veen MR, Bloem RM, Petit PL: Sensitivity and negative predictive value of swab cultures in musculoskeletal allograft procurement. Clin Orthop 1994;(300):259–263.
32. Association for the Advancement of Medical Instrumentation: Sterilization of Health Care Products—Requirements for Products Labeled 'Sterile.' ANSI/AAMI ST67:2003. Arlington, VA, Association for the Advancement of Medical Instrumentation, 2003, p 10.
33. Jackson DW, Windler GE, Simon TM: Intraarticular reaction associated with the use of freeze-dried, ethylene oxide-sterilized bone-patella tendon-bone allografts in the reconstruction of the anterior cruciate ligament. Am J Sports Med 1990;18:1–11.
34. Fideler BM, Vangsness CT Jr, Moore T, et al: Effects of gamma irradiation on the human immunodeficiency virus. A study in frozen human bone-patellar ligament-bone grafts obtained from infected cadavers. J Bone Joint Surg Am 1994;76:1032–1035.
35. Smith RA, Ingels J, Lochemes JJ, et al: Gamma irradiation of HIV-1. J Orthop Res 2001;19:815–819.
36. Salehpour A, Butler DL, Proch FS, et al: Dose-dependent response of gamma irradiation on mechanical properties and related biochemical

composition of goat bone-patellar tendon-bone allografts. J Orthop Res 1995;13:898–906.

37. Fideler BM, Vangsness CT Jr, Lu B, et al: Gamma irradiation: Effects on biomechanical properties of human bone-patellar tendon-bone allografts. Am J Sports Med 1995;23:643–646.

38. Curran AR, Adams DJ, Gill JL, et al: The biomechanical effects of low-dose irradiation on bone-patellar tendon-bone allografts. Am J Sports Med 2004;32:1131–1135.

39. Rihn JA, Chabra A, Fu FH, et al: Does irradiation affect the clinical outcome of patellar tendon allograft ACL reconstruction? Program and abstracts of the American Orthopaedic Society of Sports Medicine Annual Meeting, Keystone, CO, July 14–17, 2005.

40. Grieb TA, Forng RY, Stafford RE, et al: Effective use of optimized, high-dose (50 kGy) gamma irradiation for pathogen inactivation of human bone allografts. Biomaterials 2005;26:2033–2042.

13 Muscle Injuries

Steven J. Svoboda and Dean C. Taylor

In This Chapter

INTRODUCTION

- Muscle composes 40% to 45% of total body weight and represents the single largest tissue mass in the body.[1]

- Common types of muscle injuries can be broken down into several categories (Table 13-1).

- The purpose of this chapter is to discuss the most common forms of muscle injury presenting within a sports medicine practice.

- Indirect injuries include delayed-onset muscle soreness and muscle strain injuries.

- Direct injuries include contusions and myositis ossificans.

MUSCLE STRUCTURE AND FUNCTION, INJURY AND REPAIR

Muscle-tendon units originate from bone and usually insert onto another bone through a second tendon. Muscle contraction serves to produce torque about a joint leading to limb motion. Muscle consists of both contractile proteins including myosin, actin, troponin, and tropomyosin and a connective tissue matrix.[2] A muscle fiber is a syncytium of fused, multinucleated muscle cells and is the basic structural element of skeletal muscle. The muscle fibers can be arranged in parallel to a muscle's direction (unipennate) or oblique to the muscle's direction (bipennate; Fig. 13-1). The surrounding connective tissue includes the endomysium, which invests the individual fibers, the perimysium, which surrounds fascicles of muscle fibers, and the epimysium, which surrounds the entire muscle.[2]

The sarcolemma is a plasma membrane surrounding the muscle fiber whose nuclei are eccentrically located immediately beneath the sarcolemma. Also along the periphery of the fiber are satellite cells whose predominant function is to provide stem cells during times of muscle proliferation and regeneration. There are two major fiber types of skeletal muscle. Type I fibers are considered slow twitch and fatigue resistant due to their high mitochondrial and myoglobin content; however, they have the slowest contraction time and the lowest concentration of glycogen and glycolytic enzymes. Type II fibers are considered fast twitch with type IIA consisting of fast-twitch oxidative glycolytic fibers and type IIB consisting of fast-twitch glycolytic fibers. Type II fibers contract with the highest velocity and are most at risk of fatigue. Fiber composition, among other properties, has been implicated as a critical factor in susceptibility to certain muscle injuries.[3]

Regardless of which mechanism of injury to muscle one considers, there is a common response. The initial injury to muscle fibers stimulates mononucleated cells that typically reside within muscle to release chemotactic factors that initiate a three-stage inflammatory response. First, neutrophils invade the injury site, releasing cytokines that attract additional cells to the area. In addition to promoting inflammation, these neutrophils release oxygen free radicals that cause further damage to the cell membrane. The second stage is represented by an increase in macrophage migration to the injury site to phagocytose cellular debris. The third phase of inflammation begins when a subpopulation of macrophages increases in number. These macrophages are associated with muscle regeneration. Substances released by the injured muscle and attracted inflammatory cells have been likened to "wound hormones."[4] Muscle regeneration occurs within this milieu, with satellite cells providing the necessary stem cells. In a mouse model, this process appears to be limited to muscles weighing less than 1.5 g and, therefore, does not play a significant role in human muscle healing. In the case of human muscle healing, repair by connective tissue fibrosis or scar often predominates, beginning at 2 days after injury and increasing over the next 2 weeks with fibroblasts the important cell type. Satellite cell proliferation that accounts for muscle regeneration peaks at 2 to 4 days after injury, implying that there is a fine balance between the two processes.[2] The remainder of the chapter analyzes specific subtypes of muscle injuries to highlight their similarities and differences as they apply to the clinical situation.

INDIRECT MUSCLE INJURY

Indirect muscle injuries occur in response to too much strain or force within the muscle without direct contact. These injuries occur near the muscle-tendon junction despite distant application of force, whereas injury occurs at the site of force application in direct injuries.[5]

Delayed-onset Muscle Soreness

Pain localized to a muscle that occurs 24 to 48 hours after a bout of unaccustomed exercise and resolves over 5 to 7 days without

Table 13-1 Common Types of Muscle Injury
Indirect
Delayed-onset muscle soreness
Muscle strain
Direct
Contusion
Laceration
Vascular
Traumatic
Tourniquet
Exercise-induced compartment syndrome
Infectious
Neurologic
Denervation
Central or peripheral
Viral or traumatic
Neuropathic
Metabolic
Viral
Genetic
Myopathies

From Beiner JM, Jokl P: Muscle contusion injuries: Current treatment options. J Am Acad Orthop Surg 2001;9:227–237.

intervention is the hallmark of delayed-onset muscle soreness (DOMS).[6] DOMS occurs more frequently with eccentric exercise, meaning that the involved muscle is lengthening while it is being activated.[5] After DOMS develops, passive stretching and resumption of activity aggravate the pain. Palpation of the muscle is painful and is associated with a reduced range of motion and prolonged strength loss. Laboratory testing reveals an elevated level of creatine kinase. This increase is thought to

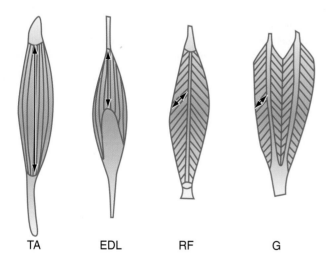

Figure 13-1 Muscle architecture varies from fusiform (TA, tibialis anterior) and unipennate (EDL, extensor digitorum longus) with muscle fiber direction and pull in line with the muscle-tendon unit to bipennate (RF, rectus femoris) and multipennate (G, gastrocnemius) with muscle fiber direction and pull oblique to the muscle-tendon unit. Arrows indicate fiber length and orientation. (From Garrett WE Jr, Nikolaou PK, Ribbeck BM, et al: The effect of muscle architecture on the biomechanical failure properties of skeletal muscle under passive extension. Am J Sports Med 1988;16:7–12.)

be due to increased permeability or breakdown of the sarcolemma due to the excessive eccentric loads that disrupt the z lines within the fibril.[7] Calcium ions accumulate within the muscle due to the disrupted sarcolemma and this results in activation of calcium-dependent proteolytic enzymes that allow release of the creatine kinase. The creatine kinase attracts monocytes that convert to macrophages, contributing to local inflammation.[7] The inflammatory mediators contribute to pain perception, as they are noxious to nociceptors within muscle. Further, the acute clinical finding of generalized swelling of the affected muscle is significant and thought to be due to this inflammatory process. Interestingly, a recent study has described a persistent loss of muscle volume of 7% to 10% between 2 and 8 weeks after exercise. A small population of "susceptible" muscle fibers is thought to be injured initially and necrose, leading to fewer muscle fibers within the muscle. This loss of volume persisted after recovery and after a second bout of eccentric exercise at 8 weeks.[8]

Individuals who are in excellent general aerobic condition are susceptible to DOMS if they engage in novel, eccentric exercise just the same as generally untrained individuals. However, training of a muscle group eccentrically confers a highly specific protective effect on that muscle for a prolonged period of time. This protective effect manifests itself as decreased pain reporting, decreased muscle swelling, and decreased serum creatine kinase levels up to at least 8 weeks after the initial bout.[8] Muscle fiber type is also a factor in DOMS with type II muscle implicated as more susceptible to such injuries.

Treatment

No single therapy has been shown to unequivocally resolve DOMS faster than the currently understood natural history of the condition. Nonsteroidal anti-inflammatory drugs (NSAIDs) have shown early subjective benefit that is minimized by prolonged administration that tends to inhibit the healing process. Exercise is thought to be the single intervention with the most promise of ameliorating the symptoms of DOMS. The mechanism by which exercise reduces symptoms is unclear but is thought to be due to breaking up adhesions within the muscle, increasing noxious waste removal from the area by improved local blood flow, or endorphin release, which decreases the perception of pain.[7]

Muscle-Tendon Strains

Muscle-tendon strain injuries are stretch-induced injuries that are noncontact in nature. While understanding of this class of injuries is incomplete, much basic science as well as clinical research has been completed to assist in their management.

Mechanism

A muscle-tendon unit can be injured when it is either passively stretched or is stretched while activated. Further, a strain injury frequently occurs in light of eccentric contraction. It is known that forces generated within eccentrically activated muscle are higher than in a concentrically activated muscle.[5] Maximal nerve stimulation, which generates concentric loading within a muscle, does not generate enough muscle activation to cause disruption of muscle.[5] In order to cause either partial or complete muscle injury, some type of stretch must be added. Pulling passive muscles until failure generates loads several times greater than the maximal isometric force that an activated muscle can generate. This suggests that the passive forces within muscle in addition to the active forces generated by the muscle are important in muscle strain injury.[9] Passive stretching of muscle results in ruptures near to, but not exactly at, the muscle-tendon junction. This location of failure is constant regardless of strain rate or type of muscle being stretched.[10] Active muscles, when stretched to failure, generate failure loads only moderately above those generated within stretched resting muscle; however, activated muscle absorbs significantly more energy prior to failure than resting muscle.[11] The relevance of this to clinical practice lies in the consideration of muscle as a shock absorber and implies that larger and stronger muscles resist injury better. In addition to these features of muscle undergoing complete disruption, muscle undergoing nondisruptive injury also has unique features. First, muscle strained to 80% of failure load exhibits a change in the linearity of the force-displacement curve that indicates the muscle has undergone plastic deformation and a subsequent change in material structure.[12,13] In animal models, muscle-tendon units stretched into plastic deformation are able to generate only 70% of the load of uninjured muscle immediately after injury. At 24 hours after stretch injury, it can generate only 50% of normal load and then begins to improve over the ensuing days and at 7 days following injury can generate loads equal to 90% of controls. Stretching unstimulated muscle to failure 7 days after nondisruptive injury requires only 77% of the force required to rupture uninjured muscle.[12] This suggests that healing muscle is at risk of reinjury, which is discussed in more detail later.

Predisposing Factors

There are several factors that have been implicated as predisposing a muscle to injury. These factors can be considered both as intrinsic characteristics of a muscle and extrinsic factors acting on the muscle. Intrinsic characteristics of muscles that predispose them to injury include gross anatomic characteristics, basic functional characteristics, and muscle architecture. Extrinsic factors include a history of injury and the presence of fatigue.

Several muscles by nature of their anatomic origins and insertions are frequently implicated as being at risk of muscle strain injury. Notable among them are the hamstrings (most frequently the biceps femoris), the rectus femoris, the gastrocnemius, the adductor longus, the pectoralis major, and the triceps brachii muscles.[14] The former three are the muscles that are most commonly affected by strain injuries. One theory as to why these three muscles are selectively involved is their common characteristics of muscle-tendon units that span two joints from origin to insertion and their more superficial location.[2,15] It has been suggested that the adductor longus owes its increased risk of muscle strain injury to its complex architecture.[10]

With respect to basic muscle function, it must be understood that these two-joint muscles act predominantly as limiters of joint range of motion. For example, the hamstring muscles during sprinting, rather than acting to actively flex the knee, work more to decelerate knee extension.[14] Another example is the quadriceps muscle group during running that acts to limit knee flexion after heel strike rather than powering knee extension.[5,14] Referring back to the basic science of muscle injury, we see that this role as a limiter of joint motion forces the muscle to activate eccentrically and as a result puts it at increased risk of muscle strain injury.

Muscle architecture also has been found to be a factor implicated in muscle strain injury. Injured muscle, regardless of architectural type (i.e., fusiform, unipennate, bipennate, and multipennate) fails at the musculotendinous junction.[9] Typically, the affected muscle-tendon junction is the distal one except in the case of the gastrocnemius, which fails variably at the distal or proximal junction or even at the musculotendinous junction between the medial and lateral heads. This variability is thought to be due to the complex multipennate architecture of the gastrocnemius.[9] More pennate muscles (such as the tibialis anterior, extensor digitorum longus, and rectus femoris) were found to have a greater percentage of elongation prior to failure than less pennate muscles. In one specific case of muscle strain injury, rectus femoris injuries occurring at its proximal end were investigated as they represented a different pattern of injury than that of the typical distal rectus femoris injury.[16] Anatomic dissections confirmed that the classic description of the proximal rectus femoris anatomy was imprecise and that, indeed, these proximal injuries were adjacent to the musculotendinous junction, like other muscle strain injuries.[17] The fiber type composition of a muscle also affects a muscle's susceptibility to strain injury. Muscles with a high percentage of type II (fast-twitch) fibers are more commonly injured, which may be due to the fact that type II fibers are preferentially recruited during high-speed activities.[3,18]

When muscle has been injured, it is susceptible to further injury if it is placed under high-level stresses too soon. As mentioned earlier, muscle's ability to resist stretch equates to its ability to absorb energy. This resistance derives from its passive connective tissue elements and its active contraction against the lengthening force. Most physiologic activity in eccentrically contracting muscle occurs at small deformations, and this is when the active component of muscle absorbs the most energy. Thus, a weakened muscle from previous injury will be more susceptible to further injury.[3] Fatigued muscle has also been found to be at risk of muscle strain injury. While control muscle and fatigued muscle fail at the same length, fatigued muscle has been found to absorb less energy prior to reaching the degree of stretch that causes injuries.[19] Further, a fatigued muscle is not as efficient in its function, and this may interfere with the storage and retrieval of elastic energy by muscle, resulting in loss of athletic function.[19]

Preventive Measures

Various prevention methods exist to minimize the risk of acute strain injuries. While it has been commonly thought that there was a neuromuscular response resulting from stretching, more recent literature has shown that muscle is viscoelastic in nature. This means that if a constant load is applied to muscle passively, the muscle will slowly elongate; similarly, if muscle is repeatedly stretched to a specified length, it will require less load to achieve this length as the number of cycles increases. This effect has been noted to achieve approximately 80% of its maximum level after four cycles in experimental animals and accounts for approximately a 4% increase in length.[20] The persistence of this effect has not been well established. It appears that stretching may afford muscle some protective effects due to this phenomenon, although there is no clear consensus in the literature to support this. In fact, preinjury stretching in a mouse extensor digitorum longus muscle model was not effective in preventing muscle injury.[21] While there are some distinctions between animal species tested and strain rate applied, static stretching does not appear to be harmful in any study. A warm-up period has also been recommended prior to exercise or competition, with research showing that an increase of 1 degree within muscle increases the peak load at failure compared to muscle that has not been warmed up.[22] This study used muscle preconditioning in the form of repeated isometric contractions to raise temperature, and this may also influence the muscle's resistance to injury. Another study used warm (40°C) and cold (25°C) muscle to show that warm muscle has less stiffness and as a result generates lower loads as it is deformed.[23] This is protective against muscle strain injury as it is thought that there is a critical load threshold above which muscle will be injured.[23] Thus, a prudent strategy prior to exercise would be to include a period of warm-up consisting of moderate activity followed by a period of static stretching prior to initiating intense sport or exercise. Muscle strength also exists as a relative preventive measure owing to the fact that this is typically accompanied by increased muscle bulk, which allows increased energy absorption by the muscle.

Clinical Features and Evaluation
History
Muscle strain injuries typically occur to athletes engaged in explosive activities such as sprinting or sports such as football, rugby, or soccer. A complete tear of the muscle can be quite remarkable to witness, and the athlete usually has no difficulty identifying the specific moment that he or she was injured. The athlete will complain of a sudden, intense pain in the affected muscle and occasionally will be able to describe a "pop" with ensuing tightness in that muscle.[2] These are typically noncontact injuries causing the injured athlete to complain of pain localized to the region of the muscle-tendon junction of the affected muscle. The most commonly affected muscle is the hamstring muscle, specifically the biceps femoris. Hamstring strains occur most commonly during sprinting and during football and rugby. Other muscles commonly affected include the rectus femoris and the adductor longus. This is often associated with kicking a soccer ball. A complete rupture of the hamstrings from their proximal insertion on the ischial tuberosity has been described in water skiers when transitioning from being in the water to being up on skis. It typically occurs in novice skiers and is a result of excessive hip flexion with extended knees.[24]

Physical Examination
Athletes sustaining a muscle strain injury can have variable presentation, from requiring assistance off the field to nearly being able to return to immediate play. Pain will be localized to a specific region, typically near the muscle-tendon junction. There may be a palpable defect, as in the case of a complete rupture, or there may be no palpable defect, just localized pain. Passive extension of the muscle is painful as is active contraction of the same muscle. After 24 hours, significant ecchymosis may be evident over the muscle within the subcutaneous space as a result of the intermuscular hemorrhage. This ecchymosis can propagate distally along the subcutaneous plane. In the case of a hamstring strain, this ecchymosis may extend to the foot over time.

Imaging
Imaging studies have shown that in the vast majority of muscle strain injuries, only a single muscle is affected.[15] Plain radiographic imaging may show soft-tissue swelling and in the case of a complete rupture may suggest a defect. Computed tomography imaging can also show soft-tissue swelling and define the extent of a complete tear, but magnetic resonance imaging (MRI) is the preferred method of imaging a muscle strain injury.[15] Most muscle strains will not require imaging. Such

imaging is rarely indicated in an acute muscle strain unless there is a need for greater information in situations in which time to return to sports is critical as in professional or high-level college athletics.[25] MRI performed immediately after injury may also be difficult to interpret as the acute hemorrhage may not have the increased T2 signal typically noted after 24 hours following injury.[15] MRI may be most helpful in those muscle strain injuries that do not initially respond to usual therapy in order to rule out concomitant injuries and to most objectively define the location and extent.[15]

Classification
There is no classification scheme that is predictive of outcome and no evidence-based research has been performed to assist in treating these injuries. The most easily communicated classification was established by the American Medical Association and consists of three grades: I, mild interstitial strain; II, moderate partial muscle disruption; and III, severe complete disruption.[26]

Treatment Options
The vast majority of muscle strain injuries will require nonoperative management with operative management being reserved for selected complete ruptures. The basic scheme for nonoperative treatment includes the RICE mnemonic, which stands for rest, ice, compression, and elevation, and, additionally, a short course of NSAIDs[2,3,5,18,27,28] (Table 13-2).

While relative rest is paramount in the treatment of muscle strain injuries, the degree of rest should not be taken to the extreme as this may hasten atrophy and loss of strength. Taylor et al[29] determined that, immediately after a severe strain injury, muscle had 63% of the peak tensile load and 79% of the elongation to failure of control muscle. This relative preservation of muscle integrity supports the notion of functional rehabilitation to preserve range of motion and muscle tone in the affected muscle.

The use of NSAIDs can be advocated over the first 48 to 72 hours after injury; however, their long-term effects would suggest that they delay healing of the injured tissue and result in lower peak failure loads. Their use should be closely monitored and discontinued as early as appropriate. The use of judicious physical therapy cannot be overemphasized. Early active assisted range of motion exercises should be instituted, but forced passive range of motion beyond the pain-free extremes of motion should be avoided.

Criteria for Return to Sports
Return to sports should not be attempted until the following three criteria are met: full, pain-free range of motion; return of strength; and ability to perform the sporting activity without pain. An acceptable rule of thumb for the degree of strength required to return to activity is at least 80% of the contralateral side, although for some athletes, it may be more appropriate to delay activity return until nearly 100% strength is attained.

Complications
The most common complication after a muscle strain injury is reinjury and the most significant predictor of reinjury is premature return to competitive activity before full pain-free motion, strength, and pain-free activity are attained. Adequate rest and supervised physical therapy with frequent reevaluation can ensure that return to activity is not done too early.

Table 13-2 Treatment Protocol for Hamstring Strains*			
Phase		Goals	Treatment
I (acute)	3–5 days 1–5 days After 1–5 days Up to 1 wk	Control pain and edema Limit hemorrhage and inflammation Prevent muscle fiber adhesions Normal gait	Rest, ice, compression, elevation Immobilization in extension, NSAIDs Pain-free PROM (gentle stretching), AAROM (Crutches)
II (subacute)	Day 3 to >3 wk	Control pain and edema Full AROM Alignment of collagen Increase collagen strength Maintain cardiovascular conditioning	Ice, compression, and electrical stimulation Pain-free pool activities Pain-free PROM, AAROM Pain-free submaximal isometrics, stationary bike Well-leg stationary bike, swimming with pull buoys, upper body exercise
III (remodeling)	1–6 wk	Achieve phase II goals Control pain and edema Increase collagen strength Increase hamstring flexibility Increase eccentric loading	Ice and compression Ice and electrical stimulation Prone concentric isotonic exercises, isokinetic exercise Moist heat or exercise prior to pelvic-tilt hamstring stretching Prone eccentric exercises, jump rope
IV (functional)	2 wk to 6 mo	Return to sport without reinjury Increase hamstring flexibility Increase hamstring strength Control pain	Walk/jog, jog/sprint, sport-specific skills and drills Pelvic-tilt hamstring stretching Prone concentric and eccentric exercises Heat, ice, and modalities; NSAIDs as needed
V (return to competition)	3 wk to 6 mo	Avoid reinjury	Maintenance stretching and strengthening

AAROM, active-assisted range of motion; AROM, active range of motion; NSAIDs, nonsteroidal anti-inflammatory drugs; PROM, passive range of motion.
*Concentric high speeds at first, proceeding to eccentric low speeds.
From Clanton TO, Coupe KJ: Hamstring strains in athletes: Diagnosis and treatment. J Am Acad Orthop Surg 1998;6:237–248.

SURGICAL TREATMENT OF INDIRECT MUSCLE INJURIES

It is beyond the scope of a chapter such as this to discuss all aspects of complete muscle injury as it pertains to each anatomic region and the specifics of diagnosis and management of each. Direct surgical repair of indirect muscle-tendon unit injuries is not commonly advocated; however, bony avulsions of muscle-tendon units are an exception. Distal biceps brachii and proximal hamstring injuries are two examples of injuries that should be considered for surgical repair. Other regions where surgical treatment is an option include the pectoralis major tendon, patellar tendon, quadriceps tendon, and the Achilles tendon.

Repair of Proximal Hamstring Avulsion
The proximal hamstring avulsion injury also represents an uncommon muscle injury that is associated with significant disability. It is included in this chapter as it represents the extreme result of muscle overload injury.

Clinical Features and Evaluation
While most hamstring strains occur at the muscle-tendon junction as discussed previously, the avulsion of the proximal hamstring occurs from the ischial tuberosity involving a fairly predictable mechanism. Forced hip flexion with maintained knee extension is described most commonly.[24] When combined with eccentric contraction of the hamstring muscles, avulsion of the common hamstring origin can occur. The largest series of proximal hamstring avulsions described injuries to water skiers. While the aforementioned mechanism was most common among inexperienced water skiers and typically occurred while the skier was attempting takeoff (five of six injuries), experienced water skiers were placed into the position of injury when they caught their ski tip in the water while skiing at high speed and their foot was not released from the binding.[24] The role of muscle fatigue in these injuries among the experienced skiers was implicated as all their injuries occurred at the end of a day of skiing. Other activities resulting in rupture of the common hamstring origin include motor vehicle crashes,[30] sprinting, falls from heights, horseback riding, volleyball, martial arts, jet skiing, and tennis.[24]

Patients typically present in a delayed fashion to the orthopedic surgeon. When seen acutely, the surgeon must have a high index of suspicion for these injuries when the patient describes an injury mechanism similar to that described previously. There is often ecchymosis over the posterior gluteal region, and a defect is palpable distal to the ischial tuberosity and proximal to the distally retracted muscle belly. Asking the patient to flex the knee results in retraction of the hamstring muscle belly and tendons of origin distally, with an increase in the length of the defect distal to the ischial tuberosity (Fig. 13-2).

Plain radiographs may reveal a shell of cortical bone avulsed from the ischial tuberosity (Fig. 13-3). MRI should confirm a complete rupture of the origin and in one series was able to identify both proximal hamstring tendon rupture and myotendinous junction injury within the same muscle.[24]

When seen chronically, patients complain of awkwardness or a sense of poor leg control during walking and running. This may be due to the loss of the hamstring's ability to decelerate the extending knee during the terminal swing phase of gait and the float phase of running.[24] These patients often report inability to return to high demand physical activities or athletics despite referral for physical therapy.

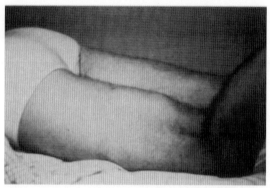

Figure 13-2 Clinical photograph of a patient with a chronic complete hamstring tendon avulsion. Note the retracted muscle belly distally and the depression distal to the buttocks accentuated by active knee flexion. (From Sallay PI, Friedman RL, Coogan PG, Garrett WE: Hamstring muscle injuries among water skiers. Functional outcome and prevention. Am J Sports Med 1996;24:130–136.)

Relevant Anatomy

The semitendinosus and biceps femoris muscles share a common insertion on the posterolateral aspect of the ischial tuberosity. The semimembranosus muscle may form a portion of this common tendon or may be independent, inserting anteriorly and medially to the common tendon. This common origin may be a factor in the hamstring failing in certain scenarios from its tendon-bone interface and not at its myotendinous junction (Fig. 13-4).

Treatment Options

Few comprehensive studies exist to guide decision making with this injury. In a retrospective study of a series of water skiing–related proximal hamstring ruptures,[24] 12 patients were studied, and it was found that only seven patients (58%) were able to return to most of their preinjury sports at a reduced level. Six of these seven had partial ruptures, and the one complete rupture that returned to preinjury sports did not participate in

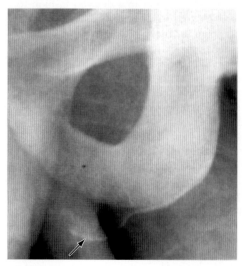

Figure 13-3 Radiographic appearance of a complete avulsion injury (arrow) of the common hamstring origin. (From Clanton TO, Coupe KJ: Hamstring strains in athletes: Diagnosis and treatment. J Am Acad Orthop Surg 1998;6:237–248.)

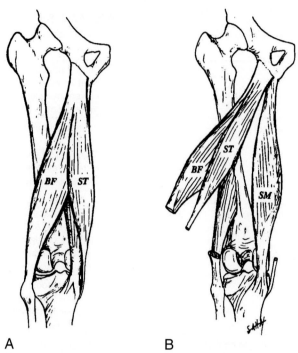

A   B

Figure 13-4 A, Origin of the proximal hamstring tendons on the ischial tuberosity with the biceps femoris (BF) and semitendinosus (ST) in place. **B,** BF and ST reflected to reveal the origin of the semimembranosus (SM) tendon deeper and more medial. Note that the BF and ST share a common tendon. (From Sallay PI, Friedman RL, Coogan PG, Garrett WE: Hamstring muscle injuries among water skiers. Functional outcome and prevention. Am J Sports Med 1996;24: 130–136.)

high demand, acceleration sports. Only three of these seven returned to regular water skiing. Five of 12 patients (42%) were significantly limited and unable to run or perform agility sports. They had pain, cramping, and poor leg control with attempts to run. All five of these patients had complete ruptures. Notably, only two patients in this series had surgical repair. Both of these were performed chronically, and one patient continued to have pain and weakness with sporting activities, while the second reported no limitation in sporting participation.

While there is no outcome measure commonly accepted to compare methods of treatment, the preceding series highlights the fact that nonoperative management should only be associated with limited goals following treatment. For athletes with complete ruptures desiring return to high-demand sporting activity, injuries can be divided into acute (less than 4 weeks from injury) and chronic (more than 4 weeks from injury). This distinction has been suggested based on the increased scar formation seen within the muscle and degree of scar surrounding the sciatic nerve seen more than 4 weeks after injury.[31] For individuals seen acutely, surgery may be recommended for those individuals who are physically fit and desire to return to high-demand activities, especially running activities. For chronic injuries, surgery is indicated if the patient is unable to return to desired activity due to pain or weakness despite physical therapy.

Surgery

After obtaining informed consent and after identifying the surgical site by signing it, the patient is brought to the operating

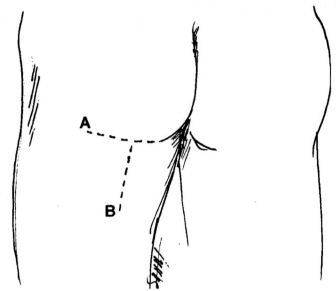

Figure 13-5 Common skin incisions for repair of proximal hamstring avulsion injuries. Incision A is transverse within the gluteal crease and is most appropriate for acute repairs and incision B is a vertical incision over the posterior thigh and is most appropriate for chronic hamstring avulsions requiring sciatic neurolysis. (From Klingele KE, Sallay PI: Surgical repair of complete proximal hamstring tendon rupture. Am J Sports Med 2002;30:742–747.)

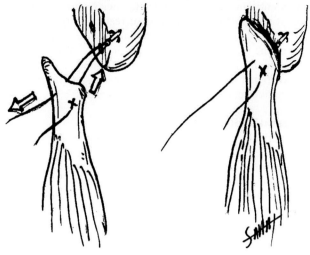

Figure 13-7 Use of simple and locking stitches through suture anchors to repair the tendon to the ischium. Tension placed on the simple suture reduces the tendon to the insertion site. (From Klingele KE, Sallay PI: Surgical repair of complete proximal hamstring tendon rupture. Am J Sports Med 2002;30:742–747.)

room and placed prone. For acute injuries, a transverse incision may be made in the gluteal crease as it is more cosmetic; however, for chronic tears or tears with concern for sciatic nerve involvement, an extensile incision made over the posterior thigh should be employed (Fig. 13-5). The inferior border of the gluteus maximus muscle is mobilized superiorly by dividing the posterior fascia. The combined tendon is avulsed from the lateral aspect of the ischium and usually does not contain a bony fragment.[31] The tendon can be anatomically reattached using any common method of tendon fixation to bone such as two or three large suture anchors loaded with heavy nonabsorbable sutures[31] (Figs. 13-6 and 13-7) or with two or three heavy nonabsorbable sutures via bone tunnels.[30] A locking stitch should be used with each suture. In the case of suture anchors, one limb of the suture can be passed through the tendon using a Mason-Allen stitch

while the other limb is passed in a simple fashion. This suture is then tensioned, reducing the proximal tendon end to its insertion site and finally tied to the suture limb that was passed as a Mason-Allen stitch.[31]

In the event of a chronic avulsion, using an extensile incision, the scarred hamstring tendons are identified from distal to proximal. The sciatic nerve is typically encased in dense scar tissue adherent to the scarred hamstring muscles (Fig. 13-8). In these

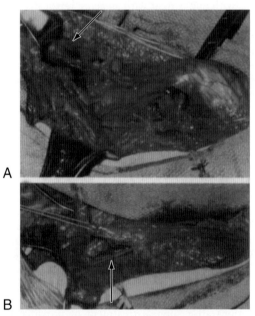

Figure 13-8 A, Intraoperative view of a chronic proximal hamstring rupture with the clamp beneath the retracted tendon. Arrow points to the insertion site. **B,** Suture in tendon reduced to the common hamstring origin. Arrow points to the sciatic nerve. (From Sallay PI, Friedman RL, Coogan PG, Garrett WE: Hamstring muscle injuries among water skiers. Functional outcome and prevention. Am J Sports Med 1996;24:130–136.)

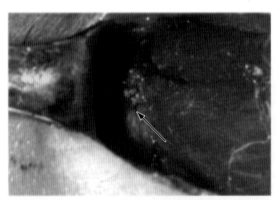

Figure 13-6 Appearance of the repaired proximal hamstring origin using two suture anchors. Arrow points to the repaired tendon. (From Klingele KE, Sallay PI: Surgical repair of complete proximal hamstring tendon rupture. Am J Sports Med 2002;30:742–747.)

cases, identifying the normal sciatic nerve distally and then tracing it proximally through the scar region are recommended. A nerve stimulator has been recommended as an adjunct to neurolysis of the sciatic nerve from the scar bed.[31] With the sciatic nerve isolated, the tendon can then be repaired as for the acute case. Fractional lengthening of these muscles at the myotendinous junction may be required in chronic cases.

Postoperative Rehabilitation

Postoperatively, the repair should be braced for 4 to 6 weeks. Harness suspension devices that maintain the knee in flexion during crutch ambulation[31] and braces that prevent simultaneous hip flexion and knee extension[30] have been advocated during this period. Passive range of motion exercises can be initiated as well as gait training with the goal of full weight bearing and normal gait being attained by 6 to 12 weeks. Strength training may then be initiated as tolerated by the patient.

Criteria for Return to Sports

There are no validated measures to determine absolute criteria for return to sport. Given return of normal motion, gait, and subjective strength, patients have returned to sport and high-demand activities by 3 months.[31] In a report of an airman injured in a motor vehicle crash, full military duties were resumed 6 months postoperatively.[30] Johnson et al[30] advocate that return to activity be limited until the hamstring-to-quadriceps strength ratio is 50% to 60% on the repaired side and when the isokinetic strength of the injured side is at least 90% of the uninjured side.

Results and Outcomes

In the largest series reported to date, seven of nine athletically active patients were able to return to full sport in 6 months (range, 3 to 10 months).[31] Ten of 11 patients were satisfied with the result, with one patient with an acute repair dissatisfied due to sciatic nerve paresthesia. These results suggest that both early and late proximal hamstring repairs can expect to have satisfactory results, contrary to previous reports that found uniformly poor results in cases treated more than 12 weeks after injury.[30] Klingele and Sallay[31] reported the isokinetic testing results at 1 year postoperatively to be 85.3% (range, 50% to 98%) of the nonoperative side. For acute repairs, isokinetic strength was 83% (range, 50% to 100%) of the unaffected side and for chronic repairs, it was 89% (range, 72% to 98%). This difference was not statistically significant due to the small sample size. While side-to-side strength has been advocated to be greater than 90% before return to sport,[30] it is interesting to compare this value to the mean values determined in the series of Klingele and Sallay at 1 year, when patients had been released from activity restriction. The utility of isokinetic strength testing as a predictor of appropriate time to return to sport may be limited, but certainly should be considered the most conservative and risk-free decision point.

Complications

Complications after surgical treatment of proximal hamstring ruptures include stiffness (either occurring when awakening or after strenuous exercise), incisional paresthesia, and residual deformity.[24] One case of an acute repair complicated with distal paresthesia has been treated with a sciatic nerve exploration and neurolysis. This patient had subsequent improvement of symptoms but was still dissatisfied overall.

DIRECT MUSCLE INJURY

The aforementioned disorders share an indirect mechanism of injury, primarily eccentric loading. The final portion of this chapter deals with direct muscle injuries, which primarily present as lacerations and contusions. It is beyond the scope of this chapter to discuss lacerations, and readers are referred to general trauma texts. In cases of closed transactions of the biceps brachii muscle, surgical repair has been described with good results.[32] This injury is uncommon and affects the unique population of static line parachute jumpers such as those found in airborne infantry units. While this particular injury may be unique to a military setting, the poor outcomes seen in those managed nonoperatively stimulated the interest in developing a surgical technique to improve function, and this, in turn, has stimulated further interest in basic science research of surgical muscle repair.[33,34] Research efforts such as this can be expanded on and their findings applied to the treatment of muscle disruptions. Contusions resulting from sports participation are extremely common and deserve specific attention in a sports text.

Contusion Injury
Clinical Features and Evaluation

Muscle contusions represent the second most common form of muscle injury after strain injuries.[35,36] This injury typically involves the anterior, posterior, and lateral thigh, as well as the anterior arm.[35] In animal models of contusion, crush mechanisms result in muscle fiber rupture leading to an intramuscular hematoma, edema, and inflammation.[37] Due to the hematoma formation, contusion injury is often complicated by the development of myositis ossificans. Myositis ossificans is discussed in more detail later. Muscle healing after contusion is similar to that seen after strain injuries but is associated with less scar formation.

Contusion injuries have been reported to occur in virtually all contact sports. They are clinically diagnosed almost universally by localized pain, swelling, limited range of motion of the joints involving the affected muscle, and, often, a palpable mass.[38] There should be a high degree of suspicion for a contusion in contact athletes sustaining any injury, even if that athlete does not relate a specific injury. In a series of 117 quadriceps contusions in military academy cadets, the most common mechanism of injury was a knee to the thigh (48 of 117) followed by helmet (31 of 117), shoulder (12 of 117), direct blow (8 of 117), object (6 of 117), ground contact (5 of 117), kicking (2 of 117), and other (5 of 117).[38] The highest injury rate was among rugby players (4.7%), but the greatest number of injuries in this patient population occurred during contact football.[38]

While clinical diagnosis of contusion injury is straightforward, assessing the extent of injury is not as easily established and imaging studies may be of utility in this regard.[35] Ultrasonography can distinguish a focal hematoma from diffuse swelling and edema, and MRI can assist in resolving a diagnosis given limited medical history, determining the extent of initial injury, and in following resolution of injury over time periods.[35,39] It should be stressed that findings on MRI persist beyond the period of clinical symptoms and that there are reports of athletes performing at the professional level without limitations despite persistent MRI findings.[39] This study also demonstrated that contusions may involve only one muscle group, despite diffuse swelling in an entire compartment.

Treatment Options

The goal of treatment of muscle contusions is to limit swelling and hemorrhage, minimize the amount of scar formation, and preserve bioelasticity, contractility, and strength of the injured and uninjured muscle tissue. The balanced use of early, short-term immobilization followed by accelerated motion is critical (Fig. 13-9). An early report in cadets described short periods of quadriceps immobilization with the knee in extension[38]; however, this protocol was changed to 24 to 48 hours of immobilization with the hip and knee flexed as far as comfortable to maintain the quadriceps under tension.[38] This change was driven by the clinical observation after immobilization in extension that flexion was the slowest motion to return. Flexion is thought to minimize the bleeding into the muscle.

Management of muscle contusions is driven by the classification of the initial injury. Common to all treatment algorithms is the liberal use of cryotherapy to reduce microvascular perfusion and subsequent edema formation,[35] compression, elevation, and relative rest. The classification scheme of Ryan et al[38] for quadriceps contusions is most widely used and applied to other areas of the body as well. Mild contusions are defined as active knee motion greater than 90 degrees, moderate contusions 45 to 90 degrees, and severe contusions less than 45 degrees. Table 13-3 contains the management protocol for quadriceps contusions. This is a progressive protocol consisting of three phases: phase I, limitation of hemorrhage; phase II, restoration of pain-free motion; and phase III, functional rehabilitation of strength and endurance. Severe contusions require bed rest with hip and knee flexion to tolerance. In military cadets, this is accomplished with admission to the hospital; outside the military, this may be achieved with bed rest at home with excuse from classes or work. Mild and moderate contusions are managed similarly; however, the strict call for bed rest is not indicated. This initial period of treatment progresses to the second phase when thigh girth is stable and the patient is pain free at rest. Phase I typically is 24 to 48 hours in length. Phase II initiates motion and for severe contusions begins with continuous passive motion until painless passive range of motion is achieved from 0 to 90 degrees, and then continues phase II exercises for the outpatient condition using supine and prone active flexion and well-leg gravity-assisted motion with a stationary bike. All injuries progress to phase III when 120 degrees of pain-free active knee flexion and equal thigh girths are obtained. Phase III involves graded return to activities with the underlying requirement that they are always performed pain free. These activities include increasing resistance on the stationary bike, isokinetic exercise, swimming, walking, jogging (pool then surface), and running. During any phase, should the patient experience pain or loss of motion, they are moved back to the previous level.

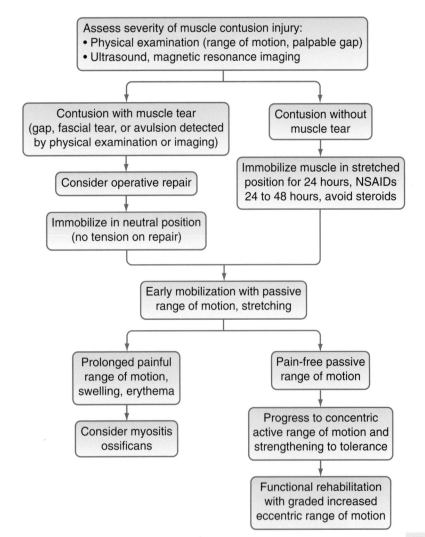

Figure 13-9 Algorithm for the evaluation and management of muscle contusion injuries. (From Beiner JM, Jokl P: Muscle contusion injuries: Current treatment options. J Am Acad Orthop Surg 2001;9:227–237.)

Table 13-3 Treatment Protocols for Management of Quadriceps Contusions

	Phase I	Phase II
Inpatient Quadriceps Contusion Therapy		
Purpose	Limit hemorrhage	Restoration of pain-free motion
Modalities	Rest; bed rest; ice: ice pack applied to injured area; compression: thigh-length support hose and Ace wrap entire thigh; elevation: hip and knee flexed to tolerance	Continuous passive motion; well-leg gravity-assisted motion; supine and prone active knee flexion; isometric quadriceps contraction; ice, crutch ambulation; Ace wrap
Advance to next phase when	Comfortable; pain free at rest; stabilized thigh girth	Pain-free passive range of motion 0 to 90 degrees; good quadriceps control; crutch ambulation with patient weight bearing to tolerance and negotiating steps Continue Phase II as outpatient

	Phase I	Phase II	Phase III
Outpatient Quadriceps Contusion Therapy			
Purpose	Limit hemorrhage	Restoration of pain-free motion	Functional rehabilitation: strength and endurance
Modalities	Rest; weight bearing to tolerance, crutch ambulation if limp present; ice: ice massage for 10 min; cold pack/cool whirlpool for 20 min; compression: Ace wrap entire thigh (occasional use: long-leg support hose, confirm taping); elevation: in class and in barracks, hip and knee flexed to tolerance; isometric quadriceps contracture <10 reps	Ice or cool whirlpool, 15–20 min; isometric quadriceps exercises, 15–20 min; supine and prone active flexion; well-leg gravity-assisted motion; static cycle: minimum resistance; discard: (1) crutches when range of motion >90 degrees, no limp, good quadriceps control, and pain free, with flexed weight-bearing gait; (2) Ace, when thigh girth reduced to equivalent of uninjured thigh	Always pain free: static cycle with increasing resistance; Cybex; swim; walk; jog (pool and surface); run
Advance to next phase when	Comfortable; pain free at rest; stabilized thigh girth	>120 degrees pain-free active knee motion; equal thigh girth bilaterally	Full active range of motion; full squat; pain free in all activities; wear thigh girdle with thick pad 3–6 mo for all contact sports

Mild and moderate, treat daily; severe, treat twice daily.
From Ryan JB, Wheeler JH, Hopkinson WJ, et al: Quadriceps contusions. West Point update. Am J Sports Med 1991;19:299–304.

As in the treatment of muscle strain injury, the use of NSAIDs is controversial. The West Point series used no medications in the treatment of quadriceps contusions and experienced no loss to activity return.[38] There are no other large clinical series from which to draw inferences about NSAID use, although there is some animal research in this area. NSAIDs have been found to decrease the catabolic loss of protein in the early postinjury period as well as the degree of inflammatory response, but this has also led to a decrease in tensile muscle strength in the long term.[35] Thus, the beneficial effect in the short term may be overshadowed by the longer term inhibition of the normal muscle regeneration cascade.[36] While no firm evidence supports this application, at our institution, we currently begin a course of NSAIDs 2 days after injury to limit formation of myositis ossificans.

Surgery   The operative treatment of contusions is controversial. Anecdotal descriptions exist of large hematomas being evacuated after contusions,[35] and in the face of large spatial defect within a contused muscle, direct suturing of muscle may be indicated, but more work is needed to make a generalization about

surgery for this problem. The incidence of compartment syndrome in the thigh after contusion is not well described, but in rare instances may occur and must then be treated with fasciotomy. Most authors advocate a high clinical suspicion for compartment syndrome in limbs where thigh girth fails to stabilize after contusion and recommend compartment pressure monitoring; however, no report of anterior thigh compartment release for contusion related compartment syndrome has demonstrated muscle injury at the time of surgery.[39] None of the major series describing treatment of quadriceps contusions report any cases of compartment syndrome or the completion of thigh fasciotomies.[38–40] In cases in which arterial injury is suspected, fasciotomy should still be considered as a treatment option. Arteriography is a useful study in this unlikely scenario.

Criteria for Return to Sports
Noncontact sports participation may be resumed once the patient advances to the functional rehabilitation portion of his or her treatment. Once full strength, motion, and endurance are achieved, contact sports may be resumed. For individuals playing

contact sports, a football thigh girdle is worn for 3 to 6 months during contact sports.

Results and Outcomes

In the series of 117 quadriceps contusions treated in West Point cadets, all returned to full activity to include performing as well or better on their Army Physical Fitness Test (2-mile run, 2 minutes of sit-ups, 2 minutes of push-ups) and Indoor Obstacle Course Test. For the 71 mild contusions, average disability time was 13 days. For the 38 moderate contusions, the average disability time was 19 days, and for the eight severe contusions, it was 21 days. The disability time was defined as the amount of time a cadet was unable to participate fully in the cadet activity schedule due to injury. The disability times for the moderate and severe contusions seen in this later study are much shorter than those noted in the first series (56 and 72 days, respectively). This has been attributed to the change in the initial position of immobilization from unstretched (knee extended) to stretched (knee flexed). Subjectively, two cadets had subjective weakness, two complained of endurance issues, and one complained of numbness in the area of the contusion after 5 miles of jogging.

Complications

The most significant, yet uncommon, complication associated with muscle contusion is myositis ossificans, also referred to as myositis ossificans traumatica or post-traumatic ectopic calcification.[41]

Myositis Ossificans

Risk Factors   Five factors have been described for the development of myositis ossificans after contusion by Ryan et al.[38] These authors determined that range of motion less than 120 degrees at classification, participation in football, history of a contusion injury to the same site, sympathetic knee effusion, and delayed treatment for 3 or more days were associated with the occurrence of myositis ossificans. By themselves, each risk factor was not significant; however, cadets with myositis ossificans averaged 3.3 risk factors, while cadets in whom myositis ossificans did not develop averaged only 1.6. The application of aggressive, passive stretching past the pain-free region of motion should be strictly avoided as this also has been linked to the onset of myositis ossificans.

Incidence   Myositis ossificans developed in 11 of 117 (9%) of the cadets sustaining quadriceps contusions in the most recent West Point study.[38] This occurred in 18% of moderate contusions and 13% of severe contusions, but only 4% of mild contusions. Myositis ossificans developed in none of the cadets with more than 120 degrees of knee range of motion at presentation, and it should be noted that the 4% of cadets with mild contusions in whom myositis ossificans developed had knee range of motion between 90 and 120 degrees. The primary location of myositis ossificans correlates with the most common sites of contusion, namely, the anterior thigh followed by the brachialis.[38,40,41]

Etiology   Intramuscular hematoma, most commonly occurring with muscle contusion injury, is the major etiology of myositis ossificans.[41] The pathway for this at the molecular level is unknown.[42] Enchondral bone formation is the predominant mechanism of osteoid production and, in its early stages, may be mistaken for extraosseous osteosarcoma. A key distinguishing factor between osteosarcoma and myositis ossificans is the pattern of ossification seen both radiographically and histopathologically; it is characterized by maturation from the outside to inside in myositis ossificans and maturation from inside to outside in osteosarcoma.[18]

Clinical Features and Evaluation   The most common presentation is after a severe contusion and, while it is developing, persistent swelling is the norm with the thigh becoming increasingly tender and warm.[40] Radiographic evidence of myositis ossificans can be noted between 2 and 4 weeks after injury. Radiographs reveal three forms of myositis ossificans: a stalk type, a periosteal type in which all ectopic bone is in continuity with underlying bone, and a broad-based type transitional between the first two types.[18,40] It has been suggested that the stalk type and broad-based type may present symptomatically due to the increased risk of a mechanical block to gliding within the affected muscle.[41] The utility of bone scan in the evaluation of myositis ossificans is equivocal, but MRI can be useful to localize the affected muscle in the acute phase. It has also been suggested that the erythrocyte sedimentation rate and serum alkaline phosphatase activity are increased in the early process of myositis ossificans.[18]

Treatment Options   Early treatment of injuries suspicious for myositis ossificans is similar to the initial treatment of contusions including rest, ice, compression, and elevation. Use of indomethacin has been advocated to reduce heterotopic calcification after total hip replacement and acetabular fracture open reduction and internal fixation. It may be effective in preventing myositis ossificans after contusion injuries. It is unclear whether indomethacin's increased efficacy over other drugs in its class is due to increased potency or having a different specific action.[41]

Surgery   Surgery is indicated only for lesions associated with significant activity limiting pain and loss of function due to muscle tethering. It should never be done in the acute phase because, postoperatively, the lesion is likely to recur. A bone scan should be performed to determine whether the lesion is mature. Resection of mature lesions should be performed with meticulous hemostasis and suction drainage with the goal of limiting the amount of postoperative hematoma formation. No clear objective guidance, other than the application of bone scan, has been published to facilitate the evaluation of this ectopic bone in order to characterize it as mature.

Criteria for Return to Sports   The criteria for return to sport are the same as for muscle contusion. Return of full motion and activity does not depend on reabsorption or excision of the ectopic bone.[18]

Results and Outcomes   Resection of the symptomatic, mature myositis ossificans lesion should result in adequate return of function, assuming no postoperative recurrence of the lesion. No series documenting outcomes after resection of myositis ossificans have been published.

REFERENCES

1. Garrett WE, Best TM: Anatomy, physiology, and mechanics of skeletal muscle. In Buckwalter JA, Einhorn TA, Simon SR (eds): Orthopaedic Basic Science, 2nd ed. Chicago, American Academy of Orthopaedic Surgeons, 2000, p 683.

2. Best TM: Soft-tissue injuries and muscle tears. Clin Sports Med 1997;16:419–434.

3. Noonan TJ, Garrett WE Jr: Muscle strain injury: Diagnosis and treatment. J Am Acad Orthop Surg 1999;7:262–269.

4. Tidball JG: Inflammatory cell response to acute muscle injury. Med Sci Sports Exerc 1995;27:1022–1032.

5. Noonan TJ, Garrett WE Jr: Injuries at the myotendinous junction. Clin Sports Med 1992;11:783–806.

6. Lieber RL, Friden J: Morphologic and mechanical basis of delayed-onset muscle soreness. J Am Acad Orthop Surg 2002;10:67–73.

7. Cheung K, Hume P, Maxwell L: Delayed onset muscle soreness: Treatment strategies and performance factors. Sports Med 2003;33: 145–164.

8. Foley JM, Jayaraman RC, Prior BM, et al: MR measurements of muscle damage and adaptation after eccentric exercise. J Appl Physiol 1999;87:2311–2318.

9. Garrett WE Jr, Nikolaou PK, Ribbeck BM, et al: The effect of muscle architecture on the biomechanical failure properties of skeletal muscle under passive extension. Am J Sports Med 1988;16:7–12.

10. Garrett WE Jr: Muscle strain injuries. Am J Sports Med 1996;24: S2–S8.

11. Garrett WE Jr, Safran MR, Seaber AV, et al: Biomechanical comparison of stimulated and nonstimulated skeletal muscle pulled to failure. Am J Sports Med 1987;15:448–454.

12. Nikolaou PK, Macdonald BL, Glisson RR, et al: Biomechanical and histological evaluation of muscle after controlled strain injury. Am J Sports Med 1987;15:9–14.

13. Obremsky WT, Seaber AV, Ribbeck BM, et al: Biomechanical and histologic assessment of a controlled muscle strain injury treated with piroxicam. Am J Sports Med 1994;22:558–561.

14. Garrett WE Jr: Muscle strain injuries: Clinical and basic aspects. Med Sci Sports Exerc 1990;22:436–443.

15. Speer KP, Lohnes J, Garrett WE Jr: Radiographic imaging of muscle strain injury. Am J Sports Med 1993;21:89–95.

16. Hughes CT, Hasselman CT, Best TM, et al: Incomplete, intrasubstance strain injuries of the rectus femoris muscle. Am J Sports Med 1995;23:500–506.

17. Hasselman CT, Best TM, Hughes CT, et al: An explanation for various rectus femoris strain injuries using previously undescribed muscle architecture. Am J Sports Med 1995;23:493–499.

18. Arrington ED, Miller MD: Skeletal muscle injuries. Orthop Clin North Am 1995;26:411–419.

19. Mair SD, Seaber AV, Glisson RR, et al: The role of fatigue in susceptibility to acute muscle strain injury. Am J Sports Med 1996;24:137–143.

20. Taylor DC, Dalton JD Jr, Seaber AV, et al: Viscoelastic properties of muscle-tendon units. The biomechanical effects of stretching. Am J Sports Med 1990;18:300–309.

21. Black JD, Stevens ED: Passive stretching does not protect against acute contraction-induced injury in mouse EDL muscle. J Muscle Res Cell Motil 2001;22:301–310.

22. Safran MR, Garrett WE Jr, Seaber AV, et al: The role of warmup in muscular injury prevention. Am J Sports Med 1988;16:123–129.

23. Noonan TJ, Best TM, Seaber AV, et al: Thermal effects on skeletal muscle tensile behavior. Am J Sports Med 1993;21:517–522.

24. Sallay PI, Friedman RL, Coogan PG, et al: Hamstring muscle injuries among water skiers. Functional outcome and prevention. Am J Sports Med 1996;24:130–136.

25. Cross TM, Gibbs N, Houang MT, et al: Acute quadriceps muscle strains: Magnetic resonance imaging features and prognosis. Am J Sports Med 2004;32:710–719.

26. Standard Nomenclature of Athletic Injuries. Chicago, American Medical Association, 1968.

27. Clanton TO, Coupe KJ: Hamstring strains in athletes: Diagnosis and treatment. J Am Acad Orthop Surg 1998;6:237–248.

28. Kujala UM, Orava S, Jarvinen M: Hamstring injuries. Current trends in treatment and prevention. Sports Med 1997;23:397–404.

29. Taylor DC, Dalton JD Jr, Seaber AV, et al: Experimental muscle strain injury. Early functional and structural deficits and the increased risk for reinjury. Am J Sports Med 1993;21:190–194.

30. Johnson AE, Granville RR, DeBerardino TM: Avulsion of the common hamstring tendon origin in an active duty airman. Mil Med 2003;168: 40–42.

31. Klingele KE, Sallay PI: Surgical repair of complete proximal hamstring tendon rupture. Am J Sports Med 2002;30:742–747.

32. Kragh JF Jr, Basamania CJ: Surgical repair of acute traumatic closed transection of the biceps brachii. J Bone Joint Surg Am 2002;84:992–998.

33. Kragh JF Jr, Svoboda SJ, Wenke JC, et al: The role of epimysium in suturing skeletal muscle lacerations. J Am Coll Surg 2005;200:38–44.

34. Kragh JF Jr, Svoboda SJ, Wenke JC, et al: Passive biomechanical properties of sutured mammalian muscle lacerations. J Invest Surg 2005;18:19–23.

35. Beiner JM, Jokl P: Muscle contusion injuries: Current treatment options. J Am Acad Orthop Surg 2001;9:227–237.

36. Beiner JM, Jokl P: Muscle contusion injury and myositis ossificans traumatica. Clin Orthop 2002;S110–S119.

37. Walton M, Rothwell AG: Reactions of thigh tissues of sheep to blunt trauma. Clin Orthop 1983;(176):273–278.

38. Ryan JB, Wheeler JH, Hopkinson WJ, et al: Quadriceps contusions. West Point update. Am J Sports Med 1991;19:299–304.

39. Diaz JA, Fischer DA, Rettig AC, et al: Severe quadriceps muscle contusions in athletes. A report of three cases. Am J Sports Med 2003;31:289–293.

40. Jackson DW, Feagin JA: Quadriceps contusions in young athletes. Relation of severity of injury to treatment and prognosis. J Bone Joint Surg Am 1973;55:95–105.

41. King JB: Post-traumatic ectopic calcification in the muscles of athletes: A review. Br J Sports Med 1998;32:287–290.

42. Kaplan FS, Glaser DL, Hebela N, et al: Heterotopic ossification. J Am Acad Orthop Surg 2004;12:116–125.

14 Head Injuries

Kevin M. Guskiewicz

In This Chapter

INTRODUCTION

- Signs and symptoms of significant head injury include loss of consciousness (LOC), cranial nerve deficit, mental status deterioration, and worsening symptoms.

- The most common head injury is a cerebral concussion.

- Serial assessment is critical in classification and management of concussion.

- Grading of head injury is done only after symptoms have resolved.

- No athlete should return to participation while still experiencing symptoms of a head injury.

- Decisions about return to play follow established guidelines but are made on an individual basis.

The immediate management of the head-injured athlete depends on the nature and severity of the injury. It is therefore important for the sports medicine clinician to be skilled in the early detection and follow-up evaluation procedures of these injuries.[1] Several terms are used to describe the injury, the most global being traumatic brain injury, which can be classified into two types: focal and diffuse. Focal or post-traumatic intracranial mass lesions include subdural hematomas, epidural hematomas, cerebral contusions, and intracerebral hemorrhages and hematomas. These are considered uncommon in sport but are serious injuries; the sports medicine clinician must be able to detect signs of clinical deterioration or worsening symptoms during serial assessments in order to classify the injury and manage it appropriately. Signs and symptoms of these focal vascular emergencies can include LOC, cranial nerve deficits, mental status deterioration, and worsening symptoms. Concern for a significant focal injury should also be raised if the signs or symptoms occur after an initial lucid period in which the athlete seemed normal.[1]

Diffuse brain injuries can result in widespread or global disruption of neurologic function and are not usually associated with macroscopically visible brain lesions except in the most severe cases. Most diffuse injuries involve an acceleration/deceleration motion, in a linear plane, a rotational direction, or both. In these cases, lesions are caused by the brain being shaken within the skull.[2,3] The brain is suspended within the skull in cerebrospinal fluid (CSF) and has several dural attachments to bony ridges that make up the inner contours of the skull. With a linear acceleration/deceleration mechanism (side to side or front to back), the brain experiences a sudden momentum change that can result in tissue damage. The key elements of injury mechanism are the velocity of the head before impact, the time over which the force is applied, and the magnitude of the force.[2,3] Rotational acceleration/deceleration injuries are believed to be the primary injury mechanism for the most severe diffuse brain injuries. Structural diffuse brain injury (diffuse axonal injury) is the most severe type of diffuse injury because axonal disruption occurs, typically resulting in disturbance of cognitive functions, such as concentration and memory. In its most severe form, diffuse axonal injury can disrupt the brain stem centers responsible for breathing, heart rate, and wakefulness.[2,3]

CEREBRAL CONCUSSION

The most common type of head injury sustained by athletes is a cerebral concussion. Cerebral concussion can best be classified as a mild diffuse injury and is often referred to as mild traumatic brain injury. The injury involves an acceleration/deceleration mechanism in which a blow to the head or the head striking an object results in one or more of the following conditions: headache, nausea, vomiting, dizziness, balance problems, feeling "slowed down," fatigue, trouble sleeping, drowsiness, sensitivity to light or noise, LOC, blurred vision, difficulty remembering, or difficulty concentrating.[4] It is often reported that there is no universal agreement on the standard definition or nature of concussion; however, agreement does exist on several features that incorporate clinical, pathologic, and biomechanical injury constructs associated with head injury:

1. Concussion may be caused by a direct blow to the head or elsewhere on the body from an "impulsive" force transmitted to the head.

2. Concussion may cause an immediate and short-lived impairment of neurologic function.

3. Concussion may cause neuropathologic changes; however, the acute clinical symptoms largely reflect a functional disturbance rather than a structural injury.

4. Concussion may cause a gradient of clinical syndromes that may or may not involve LOC. Resolution of the clinical and cognitive symptoms typically follows a sequential course.

5. Concussion is most often associated with normal results on conventional neuroimaging studies.[5]

Classification of Cerebral Concussion

Occasionally, players sustain a blow to the head resulting in a stunned confusional state that resolves within minutes. The colloquial term "ding" is often used to describe this initial state. However, the use of this term is not recommended because this stunned confusional state is still considered a concussion resulting in symptoms, although only very short in duration, which should not be dismissed in a cavalier fashion.[1] It is essential that this injury be reevaluated frequently to determine whether a more serious injury has occurred because often the evolving signs and symptoms of a concussion are not evident until several minutes to hours later.

Although it is important for the sports medicine clinician to recognize and eventually classify the concussive injury, it is equally important for the athlete to understand the signs and symptoms of a concussion, as well as the potential negative consequences (e.g., second-impact syndrome, predisposition to future concussions) of not reporting a concussive injury. Once the athlete has a better understanding of the injury, he or she can provide a more accurate report of the concussion history.[1]

Several grading scales have been proposed for classifying and managing cerebral concussions.[4,6–14] None of the scales have been universally accepted or followed with any consistency by the sports medicine community. Some of the scales are more conservative than others; however, most of them are believed to be useful in the management of concussion. It is recommended that athletic trainers and team physicians working together choose one scale, while ensuring consistent use of that scale. Although most scales are based primarily on level of consciousness and amnesia, it is very important to consider other signs and symptoms associated with concussion because the majority of concussions will not involve LOC or observable amnesia. It is reported that only 8.9% involve LOC and only 27.7% involve amnesia.[15] Regardless of the grade of injury, clinicians should focus on the duration of any and all symptoms associated with the injury. Table 14-1 contains a list of signs and symptoms associated with cerebral concussion, which can be checked off or graded for severity on an hourly or daily basis following an injury. The graded symptom checklist is best used in conjunction with the Cantu evidence-based grading system for concussion[6] (Table 14-2), which very appropriately emphasizes signs and symptoms other than LOC and amnesia in the grading of the injury. It is also important to grade the concussion only *after* the athlete's symptoms have resolved, as the duration of symptoms are believed to be a good indicator of overall outcome.[6,16]

Table 14-1 Graded Symptom Checklist for Concussion					
Symptom	Time of Injury	2–3 Hr Postinjury	24 Hr Postinjury	48 Hr Postinjury	72 Hr Postinjury
Blurred vision					
Dizziness					
Drowsiness					
Fatigue					
Feel "in a fog"					
Feel "slowed down"					
Headache					
Irritability					
Loss of consciousness					
Memory problems					
Nausea					
Poor balance/coordination					
Poor concentration					
Ringing in ears					
Sadness					
Sensitivity to light					
Sensitivity to noise					
Sleep disturbance					
Vomiting					

A postconcussion signs and symptoms checklist is used not only for the initial evaluation but for each subsequent follow-up assessment, which is periodically repeated until all postconcussion signs and symptoms have returned to baseline or cleared at rest and during physical exertion.

Table 14-2 Cantu Evidence-based Grading System for Concussion[6]	
Grade 1 (mild)	No LOC, PTA <30 min, PCSS <24 hr
Grade 2 (moderate)	LOC <1 min **or** PTA ≥30 min <24 hr **or** PCSS ≥24 hr <7 days
Grade 3 (severe)	LOC ≥1 min **or** PTA ≥24 hr **or** PCSS ≥7 days

LOC, loss of consciousness; PTA, post-traumatic amnesia (anterograde/ retrograde); PCSS, postconcussion signs/symptoms other than amnesia.

Mild Concussion

The mild concussion, which is the most frequently occurring (approximately 85%), is the most difficult head injury to recognize and diagnose.[15-17] The force of impact causes a transient aberration in the electrophysiology of the brain substance, creating an alteration in mental status. Although mild concussion involves no LOC, the athlete may experience impaired cognitive function, especially in remembering recent events (post-traumatic amnesia) and in assimilating and interpreting new information.[6,17-19] Dizziness and tinnitus (ringing in the ears) may also occur, but there is rarely a gross loss of coordination that can be detected with a Romberg test. The clinician should never underestimate the presence of a headache, which presents to some degree with nearly all concussions.[15] The intensity and duration of the headache can be an indication of whether the injury is improving or worsening with time.

Moderate Concussion

The moderate concussion is often associated with transient mental confusion, tinnitus, moderate dizziness, unsteadiness, and prolonged post-traumatic amnesia (>30 minutes). A momentary LOC often results, lasting from several seconds up to 1 minute. Blurred vision, dizziness, balance disturbances, and nausea may also be present. Moderate concussions demand careful clinical observation and skillful judgment, especially regarding return to play at a later date.

Severe Concussion

It is not difficult to recognize a severe concussion, as these injuries present with signs and symptoms lasting significantly longer than mild and moderate concussions. The athlete will often experience more signs and symptoms than described in the previous two levels, and blurred vision, nausea, and tinnitus are more likely to be present. Most experts agree that a concussion resulting in prolonged LOC should be classified as a severe concussion. Some authors[1,9] classify *brief* LOC (including momentary blackout) as a severe concussion instead of the more widely accepted moderate classification. The severe concussion may also involve post-traumatic amnesia lasting longer than 24 hours, as well as some retrograde amnesia (memory loss of events occurring prior to injury). In addition, neuromuscular coordination is markedly compromised, with severe mental confusion, tinnitus, and dizziness. Again, despite the emphasis often placed on LOC and amnesia, it is important to consider the duration of all signs and symptoms when classifying the injury. Serial observations (repeated assessments) for signs and symptoms should be conducted in an attempt to identify progressive underlying brain damage.

Management of the three types of concussive injuries is not all that different, as rest and serial evaluations are the standard of care. In the event of prolonged LOC (severe concussion), the athlete should be evaluated by a physician, with consideration given to neuroimaging of the brain. No athlete should return to participation while still experiencing symptoms. More specific assessment guidelines are presented in the section on management in this chapter.

CEREBRAL CONTUSION

The brain substance may suffer a cerebral contusion (bruising) when an object hits the skull or vice versa. The impact causes injured vessels to bleed internally, and there is a concomitant LOC. A cerebral contusion may be associated with partial paralysis or hemiplegia (paralysis of one side of the body), one-sided pupil dilation, or altered vital signs and may last for a prolonged period of time. Progressive swelling (edema) may further compromise brain tissue not injured in the original trauma. Even with severe contusions, however, eventual recovery without intercranial surgery is typical. The prognosis is often determined by the supportive care delivered from the moment of injury, including adequate ventilation and cardiopulmonary resuscitation if necessary.

CEREBRAL HEMATOMA

The skull fits the brain like a custom-made helmet, leaving little room for space-occupying lesions like blood clots. Blood clots, or hematomas, are of two types, epidural and subdural, depending on whether they are outside or inside the dura mater. Each of these can cause an increase in intracranial pressure and shifting of the cerebral hemispheres away from the hematoma. The development of the hematoma may lead to deteriorating neurologic signs and symptoms typically related to the intracranial pressure.

Epidural Hematoma

An epidural hematoma in the athlete most commonly results from a severe blow to the head that typically produces a skull fracture in the temporoparietal region. These are usually isolated injuries involving acceleration/deceleration of the head, with the skull sustaining the major impact forces and absorbing the resultant kinetic energy. The epidural hematoma involves an accumulation of blood between the dura mater and the inner surface of the skull as a result of an arterial bleed, most often from the middle meningeal artery. The hemorrhage results in the classic computed tomography appearance of a biconvex or lenticular shape of the hematoma[20] (Fig. 14-1). These are typically fast developing hematomas leading to a deteriorating neurologic status within 10 minutes to 2 hours. The athlete may or may not lose consciousness during this time but will most likely have a lucid interval or altered state of consciousness. The athlete may subsequently appear asymptomatic and have a normal neurologic examination.[20] The problem arises when the injury leads to a slow accumulation of blood in the epidural space, causing the athlete to appear asymptomatic until the hematoma reaches a critically large size and begins to compress the underlying

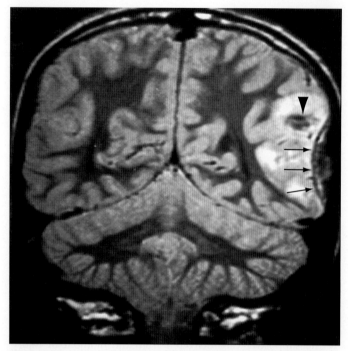

Figure 14-1 Epidural hematoma compressing the underlying brain tissue.

brain.[21] Immediate surgery may be required to decompress the hematoma and to control the hemorrhage. The clinical manifestations of epidural hematoma depend on the type and amount of energy transferred, the time course of the hematoma formation, and the presence of simultaneous brain injuries. Often the size of the hematoma determines the clinical effects.[22,23]

Subdural Hematoma
The mechanism of the subdural hematoma is more complex. The force of a blow to the skull thrusts the brain against the point of impact. As a result, the subdural vessels stretch and tear, leading to a hematoma developing in the subdural space. The injury has been divided into acute subdural hematoma, which presents in 48 to 72 hours after injury, and chronic subdural hematoma, which occurs in a later time frame with more variable clinical manifestations.[20] As bleeding produces low pressure with slow clot formation, symptoms may not become evident until hours or days (acute), or even weeks later (chronic), when the clot may absorb fluid and expand. The clinical presentation of an athlete with acute subdural hematoma can vary and includes those who are awake and alert with no focal neurologic deficits, but typically individuals with any sizable acute subdural hematoma have a significant neurologic deficit. This may consist of alteration of consciousness, often to a state of coma or major focal neurologic deficit.[20] Treatment for any athlete who has suffered LOC or altered mental status should include prolonged (several days) observation and monitoring because slow bleeding will cause subsequent deterioration of mental status. In such a case, surgical intervention may be necessary to evacuate (drain) the hematoma and decompress the brain.

Intracerebral Hemorrhage
A cerebral contusion is a heterogeneous zone of brain damage that consists of hemorrhage, cerebral infarction, necrosis, and edema. Cerebral contusion is a frequent sequela of head injury and is often considered the most common traumatic lesion of the brain visualized on radiographic evaluation.[20,24] Typically, these are a result of an inward deformation of the skull at the impact site. Contusions can vary from small, localized areas of injury to large, extensive areas of involvement. Intracerebral hematomas are similar in pathophysiology and radiographic appearance to a cerebral contusion. The intracerebral hematoma, which is a localized collection of blood within the brain tissue itself, is usually caused by a torn artery from a depressed skull fracture, penetrating wound, or acceleration/deceleration. These injuries are not usually associated with a lucid interval and are often rapidly progressive; however, there can be a delayed traumatic intracerebral hematoma. Intracerebral hematomas have been, along with subdural hematoma, the most common cause of sport-related lethal brain injuries.[20]

SECOND IMPACT SYNDROME

A special condition involves that of second impact syndrome (SIS). There has been much discussion and debate over the past two decades about SIS in sport.[4,12,14,17,19,25-27] SIS occurs when an athlete who has sustained an initial head trauma, most often a concussion, sustains a second injury before symptoms associated with the first have totally resolved. Often times the first injury was unreported or unrecognized. SIS usually occurs within 1 week of the initial injury and involves rapid brain swelling and herniation due to the brain losing autoregulation of its blood supply. Brain stem failure develops in a matter of 2 to 5 minutes, causing rapidly dilating pupils, loss of eye movement, respiratory failure, and eventually coma. On-field management of SIS should include removal of any helmet or pads so the athlete can be rapidly intubated. Unfortunately, the mortality rate of SIS is 50%, and the morbidity rate is 100%. While the number of reported cases is relatively low, the potential for SIS to occur in mildly head-injured athletes should be a major consideration when making return-to-play decisions.[8]

While the involved structures of these nonconcussive head injuries may vary depending on the impact acceleration/deceleration and the mechanism, the presentation of signs and symptoms and recommended care are rather standard (Table 14-3).

PATHOMECHANICS OF TRAUMATIC BRAIN INJURY

A forceful blow to the resting movable head usually produces maximal brain injury beneath the point of cranial impact (coup injury). A moving head hitting against an unyielding object usually produces maximal brain injury opposite the site of cranial impact (contrecoup injury) as the brain bounces within the cranium. When the head is accelerated prior to impact, the brain lags toward the trailing surface, thus squeezing away the CSF and allowing for the shearing forces to be maximal at this site. This brain lag actually thickens the layer of CSF under the point of impact, which explains the lack of coup injury in the moving head injury. On the other hand, when the head is stationary prior to impact, there is neither brain lag nor disproportionate distribution of CSF, accounting for the absence of contrecoup injury and the presence of coup injury. Many sport-related concussions involve a combined coup-contrecoup mechanism but are not considered to be necessarily more serious than an isolated coup or contrecoup injury.[28] If a skull fracture is

Table 14-3 Traumatic Intracranial Lesions			
Type	Mechanism	Injured Structures	Signs and Symptoms
Cerebral contusion	Object hits skull Skull hits object	Injured vessels bleed internally Progressive swelling may injure brain tissue not originally harmed	Loss of consciousness, partial paralysis, hemiplegia, unilateral pupil dilation, altered vital signs
Cerebral hematoma Epidural	Severe blow to head; skull fracture	Middle meningeal artery	Neurologic status deteriorates in 10 min–2 hr
Subdural	Force of blow thrusts brain against point of impact	Subdural vessels tear and result in venous bleeding	Neurologic status deteriorates in hours, days, or weeks
Intracerebral	Depressed skull fracture, penetrating wound, acceleration-deceleraton injury	Torn artery bleeds within brain substance	Rapid deterioration of neurologic status
Second impact syndrome	Sustains second injury before symptoms from first injury resolve	Brain loses autoregulation of blood supply; rapidly swells and herniates	Typically occurs within 1 wk of first injury; pupils rapidly dilate, loss of eye movement, respiratory failure, eventual coma

Table 14-4 Types of Skull Fractures	
Type	Description
Depressed	Portion of the skull is indented toward the brain
Linear	Minimal indentation of skull toward the brain
Nondepressed	Minimal indentation of skull toward the brain
Comminuted	Multiple fracture fragments
Basal/basilar	Involves base of skull

present, the first two scenarios do not pertain because the bone itself, either transiently (linear skull fracture) or permanently (depressed skull fracture) displaced at the moment of impact, may absorb much of the trauma energy or may directly injure the brain tissue (Table 14-4). Focal lesions are most common at the anterior tips and the inferior surfaces of the frontal and temporal lobes because the associated cranial bones have irregular surfaces.[19,20]

There are three types of stresses that can be generated by an applied force when considering injury to the brain: compressive, tensile, and shearing. *Compression* involves a crushing force whereby the tissue cannot absorb any additional force or load. *Tension* involves pulling or stretching of tissue, and *shearing* involves a force that moves across the parallel organization of the tissue. Uniform compressive stresses are fairly well tolerated by neural tissue, but shearing stresses are very poorly tolerated.[17,19,20]

IMMEDIATE MANAGEMENT OF SPORT-RELATED CONCUSSION

Recognition of a concussion is straightforward if the athlete has an LOC; however, 90% of all cerebral concussions involve no LOC but rather only a transient loss of alertness or the presence of mental confusion. The athlete will likely appear dazed, dizzy, and disoriented. These injuries are more difficult to recognize and even more challenging to classify, given the numerous grading scales available and inability to quantify most of the signs and symptoms.

There are three primary objectives for the clinician dealing with a head injured athlete: (1) assessing the injury and its severity, (2) determining whether the athlete requires additional attention and/or assessment, and (3) deciding when the athlete may return to sports activity. The first of these objectives can be met by performing a thorough initial evaluation. A well-prepared protocol is the key to the successful initial evaluation of an athlete who has suffered a head injury or any other type of trauma. During the secondary survey, a seven-step protocol (history, observation, palpation, special tests, active/passive range of motion, strength tests, and functional tests) should be strictly followed to ensure that nothing has been overlooked.

INITIAL ON-SITE ASSESSMENT

Your approach to the initial assessment may differ depending whether you are dealing with an athlete-down or ambulatory condition. Athlete-down conditions are signified by the athletic trainer and/or team physician responding to the athlete on the field or court. Ambulatory conditions involve the athlete being seen by the clinician at some point following the injury. Head trauma in an athletic situation requires immediate assessment for appropriate emergency action, and if at all possible, the athletic trainer or team physician should perform the initial evaluation of the athlete at the site of injury.

A primary survey involving basic life support should be performed first. This is easily performed and usually takes only a matter of 10 to 15 seconds, as respiration and cardiac status are assessed to rule out a life-threatening condition. Once this has been ruled out, the secondary survey can begin.

The secondary survey begins with the clinician performing a thorough history. The history is thought to be the most important step of the evaluation because it can narrow down the assessment very quickly. The clinician should attempt to gain as much information as possible about any mental confusion, LOC, or amnesia. Confusion can be determined rather quickly by noting facial expression (dazed, stunned, "glassy-eyed") and any inappropriate behavior such as running the wrong play or returning to the wrong huddle. Some physicians monitor level of consciousness through the use of a neural watch chart (Table 14-5).

If the athlete is unconscious or is regaining consciousness but still disoriented and confused, the injury should be managed similar to that of a cervical spine injury because the clinician may not be able to rule out an associated cervical spine injury. Therefore, the unconscious athlete should be transported from the field or court on a spine board with the head and neck immobilized. Vital signs should be monitored at regular intervals (1 to 2 minutes), as the clinician talks to the athlete in an attempt to help bring about full consciousness. If the athlete is in a state of lethargy or stupor and appears to be unconscious, the athlete should not be shaken in an attempt to arouse him or her. Shaking the athlete is contraindicated when a cervical spine injury is suspected. If LOC is brief, lasting less than 1 minute, and the remainder of the examination is normal, the athlete may be observed on the sideline and referred to a physician at a later time. Prolonged unconsciousness, lasting 1 minute or longer, requires immobilization and transfer to an emergency facility so the athlete can undergo a thorough neurologic examination.

Table 14-6 On-site Assessment

Primary Survey	Secondary Survey
Rule out life-threatening condition Check respirations (breathing) Check cardiac status	History Mental confusion Loss of consciousness Amnesia
	Observation Monitor eyes Graded symptom checklist Deformities, abnormal facial expressions, speech patterns, respirations, extremity movement
	Palpation Skull and cervical spine abnormalities Pulse and blood pressure (if deteriorating)

The clinician can perform amnesia testing by first asking the athlete simple questions directed toward recent memory and progressing to more involved questions. Asking the athlete what the first thing he or she remembered after the injury will test for length of post-traumatic amnesia. Asking what the play was before the injury or who the opponent was last week will test for retrograde amnesia. Retrograde amnesia is generally associated with a more serious head injury. Questions of orientation (name, date, time, and place) may be asked; however, research suggests that orientation questions are not good discriminators between injured and noninjured athletes.[29] Facing the athlete away from the field and asking the name of the team being played may be helpful. The athlete should also be asked whether he or she is experiencing any tinnitus, blurred vision, or nausea. The clinician should use a concussion symptom checklist similar to that found in Table 14-1 to facilitate the follow-up assessment of signs and symptoms.

Portions of the observation and palpation plan should take place during the initial on-site evaluation. The clinician should look for any deformities and check for abnormal facial expressions (cranial nerve VII), speech patterns, respirations, and movement of the extremities, which can be done while asking the athlete questions. Additionally, gentle palpation of the skull and cervical spine should be performed to rule out an associated fracture. The athlete who is conscious or who was momentarily unconscious should be transported to the sidelines or locker room for further evaluation after the initial on-site evaluation. If the athlete is unconscious, moving and positioning should be done carefully, assuming possible associated cervical injury. A helmet does not have to be removed at this time unless in some way it compromises maintenance of adequate ventilation. Often an adequate airway can be maintained just by removing the face mask or strap. Any unconscious player must be moved with care, avoiding motion of the neck by gentle, firm support, and transported on a spine board. Table 14-6 highlights the primary and secondary survey.

Table 14-5 Neural Watch Chart

Unit	Time
1. Vital signs	
Blood pressure	_____
Pulse	_____
Respiration	_____
Temperature	_____
2. Conscious and	_____
Oriented	_____
Disoriented	_____
Restless	_____
Combative	_____
3. Speech	_____
Clear	_____
Rambling	_____
Garbled	_____
None	_____
4. Will awaken to	_____
Name	_____
Shaking	_____
Light pain	_____
Strong pain	_____
5. Nonverbal reaction to	_____
Appropriate	_____
Inappropriate	_____
Decerebrate	_____
None	_____
6. Pupils	_____
Size on right	_____
Size on left	_____
Reacts on right	_____
Reacts on left	_____
7. Ability to move	_____
Right arm	_____
Left arm	_____
Right leg	_____
Left leg	_____

SIDELINE ASSESSMENT

A more detailed examination can be conducted on the sideline or in the training room once the helmet has been removed. At this time, the clinician can proceed with the remainder of the observation and palpation. A quick cranial nerve assessment should first be conducted. Visual acuity (cranial nerve II: optic) can be checked by asking the athlete to read or identify selected objects (at near range and far range). Eye movement (cranial nerves III and IV: oculomotor and trochlear) should be checked for coordination and a purposeful appearance by asking the athlete to track a moving object. The pupils also should be observed to determine whether they are equal in size and equally reactive to light; the pupils should constrict when light is shined into the eyes. Observation of the pupils also assesses the oculomotor nerve. Abnormal movement of the eyes, changes in pupil size, or reaction to light often indicate increased intracranial pressure. The clinician should also look for any signs indicating a potential basilar skull fracture, including battle's sign (posterior auricular hematoma), otorrhea (CSF draining from the ear canal), CSF rhinorrhea (CSF draining from the nose), and "raccoon eyes" (periorbital ecchymosis secondary to blood leaking from the anterior fossa of the skull). If the athlete's condition appears to be worsening, the pulse and blood pressure should be taken. The development of an unusually slow heart rate or an increased pulse pressure (increased systolic and decreased diastolic) after the athlete has calmed down may be signs of increasing intracranial involvement. The overwhelming majority of cerebral concussions will not reveal positive results for these tests; however, they are important considerations for detecting a more serious injury such as an epidural or subdural hematoma.

SPECIAL TESTS FOR THE ASSESSMENT OF COORDINATION

The inclusion of objective balance testing in the assessment of concussion is recommended. The Balance Error Scoring System is recommended over the standard Romberg test, which for years has been used as a subjective tool for the assessment of balance. The Balance Error Scoring System was developed to provide clinicians with a rapid, cost-effective method of objectively assessing postural stability in athletes on the sports sideline or training room after a concussion. Three different stances (double, single, and tandem) are completed twice, once while on a firm surface and once while on a 10-cm thick piece of medium density foam (Airex, Inc.) for a total of six trials (Fig. 14-2). The total test time is approximately 6 minutes; the athlete is asked to assume the required stance by placing his or her hands on the iliac crests and on eye closure, the 20-second test begins. During the single-leg stances, the subject is asked to maintain the contralateral limb in 20 to 30 degrees of hip flexion and 40 and 50 degrees of knee flexion. Additionally, the athlete is asked to stand quietly and as motionless as possible in the stance position, keeping his or her hands on the iliac crests and eyes closed. The single-limb stance tests are performed on the nondominant foot. This same foot is placed toward the rear on the tandem stances. The subject is told that on losing his or her balance, they are to make any necessary adjustments and return to the testing position as quickly as possible. Performance is scored by adding one error point for each error committed (Table 14-7). Trials are considered to be incomplete if the athlete is unable to sustain the stance position for longer than 5 seconds during the entire 20-second testing period. These trials are assigned a standard maximum error score of 10. Balance test results during injury recovery are best used when compared to baseline measurements, and clinicians working with athletes or patients on a regular basis should attempt to obtain baseline

Table 14-7 Balance Error Scoring System
Errors
Hands lifted off iliac crests
Opening eyes
Step, stumble, or fall
Moving hip into >30 degrees of flexion or abduction
Lifting forefoot or heel
Remaining out of testing position for move than 5 sec

The Balance Error Scoring System score is calculated by adding one error point for each error or any combination of errors occurring during a movement.

measurements whenever possible. Research findings have found this to be a reliable and valid assessment tool for the management of sport-related concussion.[30-32]

More sophisticated balance assessment using computerized force plate systems and sensory organization testing has identified balance deficits in athletes up to 3 days following a mild concussion.[30,33,34] These tests are recommended for making return-to-play decisions, especially when preseason baseline measurements are available for comparison. The finger-to-nose test is also considered to be a good test for combining cognitive processing and balance. The clinician asks the athlete to stand with his or her eyes closed and arms out to the side. The athlete is then asked to touch the index finger of one hand to the nose and then to touch the index finger of the other hand to the nose. The athlete is then asked to open his or her eyes and touch the index finger of the evaluator (placed at varying ranges in the peripheral view) to test acuity and depth perception. Inability to perform any of these tasks may be an indication of physical disorientation secondary to intracranial involvement.

SPECIAL TESTS FOR ASSESSMENT OF COGNITION

The cognitive evaluation should begin by giving the athlete three words (e.g., pig, blue, hat) to remember because he or she will be asked to recall the words at the conclusion of the assessment. A brief mental status examination should be conducted using the Standardized Assessment of Concussion (SAC). The SAC is a brief screening instrument designed for the neurocognitive assessment of concussion by a medical professional with no prior expertise in neuropsychological testing.[35,36] Studies have demonstrated the psychometric properties and clinical sensitivity of the SAC in assessing concussion and tracking postinjury recovery.[37-40] The SAC requires approximately 5 minutes to administer and assesses four domains: cognition including orientation, immediate memory, concentration, and delayed recall. A composite total score of 30 possible points is summed to provide an overall index of cognitive impairment and injury severity. The SAC also contains a brief neurologic screening and documentation of injury-related factors (e.g., LOC, post-traumatic amnesia, retrograde amnesia; Table 14-8). Equivalent alternate forms of the SAC are available and should be used to minimize practice effects from serial testing after an injury. The authors identified significant differences between concussed athletes and nonconcussed controls as well as between preseason baselines and postinjury scores.[38,40] In lieu of using the SAC, the clinician can consider using a series of questions for concentration (Table 14-9) and recent memory (Table 14-10).

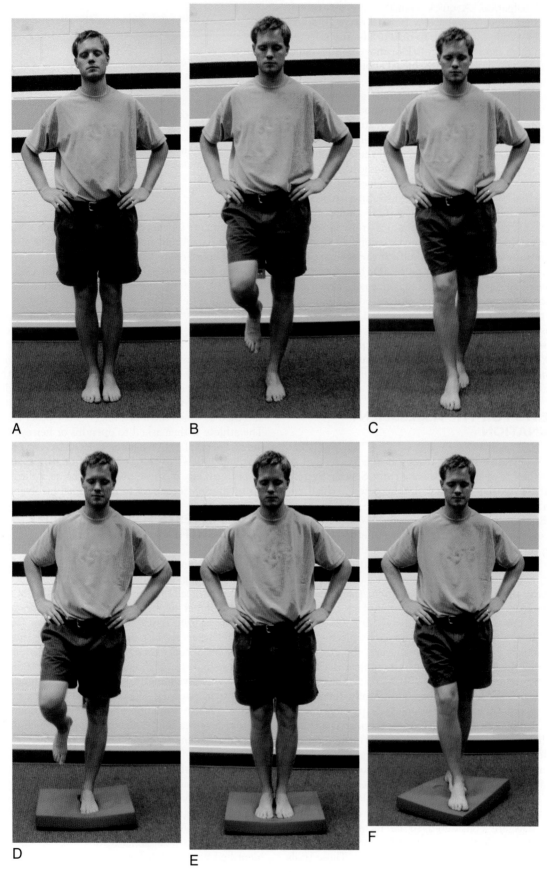

Figure 14-2 A–F, Six testing conditions for the Balance Error Scoring System.

Table 14-8 Standardized Assessment of Concussion

1. Orientation

Month:		0	1
Date:		0	1
Day of week:		0	1
Year:		0	1
Time (within 1 hr.):		0	1
Orientation Total Score	/	5	

2. Immediate memory (all 3 trials are completed regardless of score on trials 1 and 2; total score equals sum across all 3 trials)

List	Trial 1		Trial 2		Trial 3	
Word 1	0	1	0	1	0	1
Word 2	0	1	0	1	0	1
Word 3	0	1	0	1	0	1
Word 4	0	1	0	1	0	1
Word 5	0	1	0	1	0	1
Total						
Immediate Memory Total Score ____ / 15						

(Note: Subject is not informed of delayed recall testing of memory)

Neurologic screening

Loss of consciousness (occurrence, duration)
Pre- and post-traumatic amnesia (recollection of events pre- and postinjury)
Strength:
Sensation:
Coordination:

3. Concentration

Digits backward (If correct, go to next string length; if incorrect, read trial 2. Stop if incorrect on both trials)

4-9-3	6-2-9	0	1
3-8-1-4	3-2-7-9	0	1
6-2-9-7-1	1-5-2-8-6	0	1
7-1-8-4-6-2	5-3-9-1-4-8	0	1

Months in reverse order (entire sequence correct for 1 point)
Dec-Nov-Oct-Sep-Aug-Jul
Jun-May-Apr-Mar-Feb-Jan _____ 0 1

Concentration total score _____ / 5

Exertional maneuvers

(when appropriate)

5 jumping jacks	5 push-ups
5 sit-ups	5 knee-bends

4. Delayed recall

Word 1	0	1
Word 2	0	1
Word 3	0	1
Word 4	0	1
Word 5	0	1
Delayed recall total score	/	5

Summary of total scores

Orientation	/	5
Immediate Memory	/	15
Concentration	/	5
Delayed Recall	/	5
Total score	/	30

Data from McCrea, Kelly, Randolph, 1997.[35]

Computerized Neuropsychological Tests

Recently, a number of computerized neuropsychological testing programs have been designed for the assessment of athletes after concussion. The Automated Neuropsychological Assessment Metrics, CogState, Concussion Resolution Index, and Immediate Postconcussion Assessment and Cognitive Testing are all currently available and have shown promise for reliable and valid concussion assessment (Table 14-11).[41-54] The primary advantages to computerized testing are the ease of administration, ability to baseline test a large number of athletes in a short period of time, and multiple forms used within the testing paradigm to reduce the practice effects. Collie et al[48] summarized

the advantage and disadvantages of computerized versus traditional paper-and-pencil testing.

As outlined previously, in the case of conventional neuropsychological testing, several of the same challenges must be addressed before computerized testing becomes a widely used method of sport concussion assessment. Issues requiring further consideration include demonstrated test reliability; validity, sensitivity, and specificity in the peer-reviewed literature; required user training and qualifications; the necessary role of the licensed psychologist for clinical interpretation of postinjury test results; hardware and software issues inherent to computerized testing; and user costs.[1] Progress is being made on many of these issues,

Table 14-9 Tests of Concentration

Questions	Correct Response?
1. Recite the days of the week backward beginning with today.	
2. Recite the months of the year backward beginning with this month.	
3. Serial 3s—count backward from 100 by 3s until you get to single digits.	
4. Serial 7s—count backward from 100 by 7s until you get to single digits.	

Table 14-10 Test of Recent Memory

Questions	Correct Response?
1. Where are we playing (name of field or site)?	
2. Which quarter (period, inning, etc.) is it?	
3. Who scored last?	
4. Who did we play last week?	
5. Who won last week?	
6. Recite the three words given at the start of the examination.	

Table 14-11 Computerized Neuropsychological Tests		
Neuropsychologic Test	*Developer (Contact Information)*	*Cognitive Tests*
Automated Neuropsychological Assessment Metrics (ANAM)	National Rehabilitation Hospital Assistive Technology and Neuroscience Center, Washington, DC (jsb2@mhg.edu)	Simple reaction metrics Sternberg memory Math processing Continuous performance Matching to sample Spatial processing Code substitution
CogSport	CogState Ltd., Victoria, Australia (www.cogsport.com)	Simple reaction time Complex reaction time One-back Continuous learning
Concussion Resolution Index	HeadMinder Inc., New York, NY (www.headminder.com)	Reaction time Cued reaction time Visual recognition 1 Visual recognition 2 Animal decoding Symbol scanning
ImPACT	University of Pittsburgh Medical Center, Pittsburgh, PA (www.impacttest.com)	Verbal memory Visual memory Information processing speed Reaction time Impulse control

but further clinical research is required to provide clinicians with the most effective neuropsychological assessment tools and maintain the testing standards of neuropsychology.

OTHER TESTS

If the athlete successfully completes the special tests and return to participation on the same day is anticipated, sensory (dermatome) testing and range of motion (ROM) testing should be performed followed by strength testing. These tests are performed to ensure that the athlete has normal sensory/motor function, which could have been compromised due to an associated brachial plexus injury. These tests can be performed in a systematic order, as described for upper and lower quarter screenings.

If the athlete has been asymptomatic for at least 20 minutes and has been cleared on all tests to this point, functional tests may be performed to assess the athlete's readiness to return to participation.[1] Functional testing should include exertional tests on the sideline such as sit-ups, push-ups, short sprints, and sport-specific tasks. The objective of these tests is to seek evidence of early postconcussive symptoms. Often these exercises will increase intracranial pressure in the head-injured athlete and cause symptoms to increase.

It is essential that the clinician document and record the initial findings and subsequent monitoring of any athlete with head injury.

Medications

At this time, the clinician has no evidence-based pharmacologic treatment options for an athlete with a concussion.[55] Most pharmacologic studies have been performed in severely head-injured patients. It has been suggested that athletes with concussion avoid medications containing aspirin or nonsteroidal anti-inflammatories, which decrease platelet function and potentially increase intracranial bleeding, mask the severity and duration of symptoms, and possibly lead to a more severe injury. It is also recommended that acetaminophen (Tylenol) be used sparingly in the treatment of headache-like symptoms in the athlete with a concussion. Other medications to avoid during the acute post-concussion period include those that adversely affect central nervous function, in particular alcohol and narcotics.

Wake-ups and Rest

Once it has been determined that a concussion has been sustained, a decision must be made as to whether the athlete can return home or should be considered for overnight observation or admission to the hospital. For more severe injuries, the athlete should be evaluated by the team physician or emergency department physician if the team physician is not available. If the athlete is allowed to return home or to the dormitory room, the athletic trainer should counsel a friend, teammate, or parent to closely monitor the athlete. Traditionally, part of these instructions included a recommendation to wake up the athlete every 3 to 4 hours during the night to evaluate changes in symptoms and rule out the possibility of an intracranial bleed, such as a subdural hematoma. This recommendation has raised some debate about unnecessary wake-ups that disrupt the athlete's sleep pattern and may increase symptoms the next day due to the combined effects of the injury and sleep deprivation. It is further suggested that the concussed athlete have a teammate or friend stay during the night and that the athlete not be left alone. No documented evidence suggests what severity of injury requires this treatment. However, a good rule to use is if the athlete experienced LOC, had prolonged periods of amnesia, or is still experiencing significant symptoms, he or she should be awakened during the night.[1] Both oral and written instructions should be given to both the athlete and caregiver regarding waking.[1,56] The use of written and oral instructions increases the compliance to 55% for purposeful waking in the middle of the night. In the treatment of concussion, complete bed rest was ineffective in decreasing postconcussion signs and symptoms.[57] The athlete should avoid activities that may increase symptoms (e.g., staying up late studying, physical education class) and should resume normal activities of daily living, such as attending class or driving, once symptoms begin to resolve or decrease in severity. As previously discussed, a graded test of exertion should be used to determine the athlete's ability to safely return to full activity.[1]

RETURN TO COMPETITION AFTER SPORT-RELATED CONCUSSION

Over the past two decades, a number of grading scales for severity of concussion and return to play have been proposed.[4,6,8–14] The lack of consensus among experts lies in the fact that few of the scales or guidelines are derived from conclusive scientific data but rather developed from anecdotal literature and clinical experience. The Cantu evidence-based grading scale (see Table 14-2) is currently recommended because it emphasizes all signs and symptoms, without placing too much weight on LOC and amnesia. This scale should be used to grade the injury only after the athlete is declared symptom free, as duration of symptoms is important in grading the injury. No athlete should return to participation while still symptomatic.

The question of return to competition after a head injury is handled on an individual basis, although conservatism seems the wisest course in all cases. The athlete whose confusion resolves promptly (20 minutes) and has no associated symptoms at rest or during or following functional testing may be considered a candidate to return to play. Any LOC should eliminate a player from participation that day. Table 14-12 offers a guide to making restricted and unrestricted return-to-play decisions following concussion. The following factors should also be considered when making decisions regarding an athlete's readiness to return following head injury:

1. Athlete's history of concussion.
2. The sport of participation (contact versus noncontact).
3. Availability of experienced personnel to observe and monitor the athlete during recovery.
4. Early follow-up to determine when a disqualified athlete can return to participation.
5. Repeated assessment should be the rule. The athletic trainer and team physician must be assured that the athlete is asymptomatic before a return to participation is permitted. This can be done through the use of neuropsychological testing and postural stability assessment.
6. Any athlete who has experience LOC should not be permitted to return to play on that day.
7. Any athlete with a concussion that evolves downward should be sent for neurologic evaluation and/or hospital admission.

Athletes who are unconscious for a period of time or those who have headaches require evaluation and monitoring by a physician. Although the majority of people with head trauma recover without any permanent neurologic deficit or need for surgery, head trauma can be very serious and perhaps life threatening. Several guidelines have been proposed for return to play following multiple head injuries in the same season.[4,8,9] Most experts agree that athletes should be held from competition for extended periods of time (1 to 3 additional weeks) following a second concussion to ensure that all postconcussive symptoms

Table 14-12 Guidelines for Return to Play after Concussion*
Mild
Remove from contest. Examine immediately and at 5-min intervals for development of abnormal concussive symptoms at rest and with exertion. May return to contest if examination is normal and no symptoms develop for at least 20 minutes.
If any symptoms develop within the initial 20 minutes, return on that day should not be permitted.
If the athlete is removed from participation as a result of developing symptoms, follow-up evaluations should be conducted daily. May return to *restricted* participation when the athletic trainer and team physician are assured that the athlete has been asymptomatic† at rest and with exertion for at least 2 days, followed by return to *unrestricted* participation if asymptomatic for 1 additional day. Neuropsychological assessment and balance/coordination testing are valuable criteria, especially if preseason baseline measures are available.
Moderate
Remove from contest and prohibit return on that day. Examine immediately and at 5-min intervals for signs of evolving intracranial pathology. Re-examine daily. May return to *restricted* participation when the athletic trainer and team physician are assured that the athlete has been asymptomatic at rest and with exertion for at least 4 days, followed by return to *unrestricted* participation if asymptomatic for an additional 2 days. The performance during restricted participation should be used as a guide for making the decision for unrestricted participation. Neuropsychological assessment and balance/coordination testing are valuable criteria, especially if preseason baseline measures are available.
Severe
Treat on field/court as if there has been a cervical spine injury. Examine immediately and at 5-min intervals for signs of evolving intracranial pathology. Re-examine daily. Return to play is based on how quickly the athlete's initial symptoms resolve:
1. If symptoms totally resolve within the first week, athlete may return to *restricted* participation when the athletic trainer and team physician are assured that the athlete has been asymptomatic at rest and with exertion for at least 10 days, followed by return to *unrestricted* participation if asymptomatic for an additional 3 days.
2. If symptoms fail to totally resolve within the first week, athlete may return to *restricted* participation when the athletic trainer and team physician are assured that the athlete has been asymptomatic at rest and with exertion for at least 17 days, followed by return to *unrestricted* participation if asymptomatic for an additional 3 days.
The performance during restricted participation should be used as a guide for making the decision for unrestricted participation. Neuropsychological assessment and balance/coordination testing are valuable criteria, especially if preseason baseline measures are available.

*Refer to Table 14-2 for grade/level.
†*Asymptomatic means that the athlete has returned to baseline scores on the Graded Symptom Checklist. Any second concussion sustained within a 3-month period of the first concussion requires that the athlete rest for twice the maximum number of days recommended for the respective severity level.*

have resolved and that participation in contact sports should be terminated for the season after three concussions.

IMPORTANT CONCEPTS

1. Cerebral concussions are basic injuries to the brain itself and are classified by severity, as mild, moderate, or severe. These injuries should be graded only after the athlete is asymptomatic.
2. Cerebral hematomas are blood clots that form when the middle meningeal artery severs (epidural hematoma) or when subdural vessels tear and cause a clot to form several hours, days, or even weeks later (subdural hematoma).
3. Decisions about when and if a concussed athlete can return to competition have to be made on an individual basis, depending on the athlete's concussion history, the severity of the injury, duration of signs and symptoms, time between injuries, and availability of experienced personnel to conduct repeated assessments and monitor recovery. It is important to combine tests of cognitive function, postural stability, and symptomatology to determine the athlete's status.
4. The injury should be graded or classified only after the athlete has been rendered asymptomatic, whether it is 5 minutes, 5 hours, 5 days, or 5 weeks following the injury. Your goal should always be to try to prevent a recurrent injury, and research suggests that all the aforementioned factors can influence the outcome.
5. Athletic trainers, team physicians, neurosurgeons, and neuropsychologists should work together as a team to determine the athlete's readiness to return safely to competition following a head injury.

REFERENCES

1. Guskiewicz KM, Bruce SL, Cantu RC, et al: National Athletic Trainers' Association position statement: Management of sport-related concussion. J Athl Train 2004;39:280–297.
2. Gennarelli T: Mechanisms of brain injury. J Emerg Med 1993;11(Suppl 1):5–11.
3. Schneider RC: Head and Neck Injuries in Football: Mechanisms, Treatment and Prevention. Baltimore, Williams & Wilkins, 1973.
4. American Academy of Neurology: Practice parameter: The management of concussion in sports (summary statement). Neurology 1997;48:581–585.
5. Aubry M, Cantu R, Dvorak J, et al: Summary and agreement statement of the First International Conference on Concussion in Sport, Vienna 2001: Recommendations for the improvement of safety and health of athletes who may suffer concussive injuries. Br J Sports Med 2002;36:6–10.
6. Cantu R: Post-traumatic retrograde and anterograde amnesia: Pathophysiology and implications in grading and safe return to play. J Athl Train 2001;36:244–248.
7. Ommaya A: Biomechanical aspects of head injuries in Sports. In Jordan B, Tsairis P, Warren R (eds): Sports Neurology. Rockville, MD, Aspen Publishers, 1990.
8. Cantu R: Guidelines for return to contact sports after a cerebral concussion. Physician Sportsmed 1986;14:75–83.
9. Colorado Medical Society: Report of the Sports Medicine Committee: Guidelines for the management of concussion in sports (revised). Paper presented at the Colorado Medical Society, 1991, Denver.
10. Jordan B: Head injuries in sports. In Jordan B, Tsairis P, Warren R (eds): Sports Neurology. Rockville, MD, Aspen Publishers, 1989.
11. Nelson W, Jane J, Gieck J: Minor head injuries in sports: A new system of classification and management. Physician Sportsmed 1984;12:103–107.
12. Roberts W: Who plays? Who sits? Managing concussion on the sidelines. Physician Sportsmed 1992;20:66–72.
13. Torg J (ed): Athletic Injuries to the Head, Neck & Face. St. Louis, Mosby-Year Book, 1991.
14. Wilberger JJ, Maroon J: Head injuries in athletes. Clin Sports Med 1989;8:1–9.
15. Guskiewicz KM, Weaver N, Padua DA, Garrett WE: Epidemiology of concussion in collegiate and high school football players. Am J Sports Med 2000;28:643–650.
16. Guskiewicz KM, McCrea M, Marshall SW, et al: Cumulative consequences of recurrent concussion in collegiate football players: The NCAA Concussion Study. JAMA 2003;290:2549–2555.
17. Cantu R: Athletic head injuries. Clin Sports Med 1997;16:531–542.
18. Lovell M, Maroon JC: Does loss of consciousness predict neuropsychological decrements of concussion. Clin J Sports Med 1999;9:193–198.
19. Cantu R: Reflections on head injuries in sport and the concussion controversy. Clin J Sports Med 1997;7:83–84.
20. Bailes JE, Hudson V: Classification of sport-related head trauma: A spectrum of mild to severe injury. J Athl Train 2001;36:236–243.
21. Jamieson KG, Yelland JDN: Extradural hematoma: Report of 167 cases. J Neurosurg 1968;29:13–23.
22. Bricolo A, Pasut LM: Extradural hematoma: Toward zero mortality, a prospective study. Neurosurgery 1984;14:8–12.
23. Servadei F: Prognostic factors in severely head injured adult patients with epidural hematomas. Acta Neurochir (Wien) 1997;139:273–278.
24. Schonauer M, Schisano G, Cimino R, Viola L: Space occupying contusions of cerebral lobes after closed head brain injury: Considerations about 51 cases. J Neurosurg Sci 1979;23:279–288.
25. Mueller FO: Catastrophic head injuries in high school and collegiate sports. J Athl Train 2001;36:312–315.
26. Kelly J, Nichols J, Filley C, et al: Concussion in sports: Guidelines for the prevention of catastrophic outcome. JAMA 1991;226:2867–2869.
27. Saunders R, Harbaugh R: The second impact in catastrophic contact-sports head injuries. JAMA 1984;252:538–539.
28. Barr WB, McCrea M: Sensitivity and specificity of standardized neurocognitive testing immediately following sports concussion. J Int Neuropsychol Soc 2001;7:693–702.
29. Maddocks D, Saling M: Neuropsychological sequelae following concussion in Australian rules footballers. J Clin Exp Neuropsychol. 1991;13:439–442.
30. Guskiewicz KM, Ross SE, Marshall SW: Postural stability and neuropsychological deficits after concussion in collegiate athletes. J Athl Train 2001;36:263–273.
31. Riemann BL, Guskiewicz KM, Shields EW: Relationship between clinical and forceplate measures of postural stability. J Sport Rehabil 1998;8:71–82.
32. Riemann BL, Guskiewicz KM: Objective assessment of mild head injury using a clinical battery of postural stability tests. J Athl Train 2000;35:19–25.
33. Guskiewicz K, Perrin D, Gansneder B: Effect of mild head injury on postural sway. J Athl Train 1996;31:300–306.
34. Guskiewicz K, Riemann V, Perrin D, Nashner L: Alternative approaches to the assessment of mild head injuries in athletes. Med Sci Sports Exerc 1997;29:S213–S221.
35. McCrea M, Kelly JP, Randolph C, et al: Standardized Assessment of Concussion (SAC): On-site mental status evaluation of the athlete. J Head Trauma Rehabil 1998;13:27–35.
36. McCrea M, Randolph C, Kelly JP: The Standardized Assessment of Concussion (SAC): Manual for Administration, Scoring and Interpretation. 1997.
37. McCrea M: Standardized mental status assessment of sports concussion. Clin J Sport Med 2001;11:176–181.
38. McCrea M: Standardized mental status testing on the sideline after sport-related concussion. J Athl Train 2001;36:274–279.

39. McCrea M, Kelly JP, Randolph C, et al: Immediate neurocognitive effects of concussion. Neurosurgery 2002;50:1032–1042.

40. McCrea M, Kelly JP, Kluge J, et al: Standardized assessment of concussion in football players. Neurology 1997;48:586–588.

41. Bleiberg J, Halpern E, Reeves D, Daniel JC: Future directions for neuropsychological assessment of sports concussion. J Head Trauma Rehabil 1998;13:36–44.

42. Erlanger D, Saliba E, Barth J, et al: Monitoring resolution of postconcussion symptoms in athletes: Preliminary results of a web-based neuropsychological test protocol. J Athl Train 2001;36:280–287.

43. Lovell MR, Collins MW, Iverson GL, et al: Recovery from mild concussion in high school athletes. J Neurosurg 2003;98:296–301.

44. Bleiberg J, Garmoe W, Halpern E, et al: Consistency of within-day and across-day performance after mild brain injury. Neuropsychiatry Neuropsychol Behav Neurol 1997;10:247–253.

45. Erlanger D, Kaushik T, Cantu R, et al: Symptom-based assessment of the severity of a concussion. J Neurosurg 2003;98:477–484.

46. Collins MW, Field M, Lovell MR et al: Relationship between postconcussion headache and neuropsychological test performance in high school athletes. Am J Sports Med 2003;31:168–173.

47. Bleiberg J, Cernich AN, Cameron K, et al: Duration of cognitive impairment after sports concussion. Neurosurgery 2004;54:5073–1080.

48. Collie A, Darby D, Maruff P: Computerised cognitive assessment of athletes with sports related head injury. Br J Sports Med 2001;35:297–302.

49. Collie A, Maruff P, Makdissi M, et al: CogSport: Reliability and correlation with conventional cognitive tests used in postconcussion medical evaluations. Clin J Sport Med 2003;13:28–32.

50. Makdissi M, Collie A, Maruff P, et al: Computerised cognitive assessment of concussed Australian rules footballers. Br J Sports Med 2001;35:354–360.

51. Bleiberg J, Kane RL, Reeves DL, et al: Factor analysis of computerized and traditional tests used in mild brain injury research. Clin Neuropsychol 2000;14:287–294.

52. Collie A, Maruff P, Darby DG, McStephen M: The effects of practice on the cognitive test performance of neurologically normal individuals assessed at brief test-retest intervals. J Int Neuropsychol Soc 2003;9:419–428.

53. Daniel JC, Olesniewicz MH, Reeves DL, et al: Repeated measures of cognitive processing efficiency in adolescent athletes: Implications for monitoring recovery from concussion. Neuropsychiatry Neuropsychol Behav Neurol 1999;12:167–169.

54. Reeves D, Thorne R, Winter S, Hegge F: Cognitive Performance Assessment Battery (UTC-PAB). Report 89-1. San Diego, CA: Naval Aerospace Medical Research Laboratory and Walter Reed Army Institute of Research, 1989.

55. McCrory P: New treatments for concussion: The next millennium beckons. Clin J Sport Med 2001;11:190–193.

56. de Louw A, Twijnstra A, Leffers P: Lack of uniformity and low compliance concerning wake-up advice following head trauma. Ned Tijdschr Geneeskd 1994;138:2197–2199.

57. de Kruijk JR, Leffers P, Meerhoff S, et al: Effectiveness of bed rest after mild traumatic brain injury: A randomised trial of no versus six days of bed rest. J Neurol Neurosurg Psychiatry 2002;73:167–172.

15 Cervical Spine

Adam C. Crowl and James D. Kang

In This Chapter

INTRODUCTION

- Cervical spine injuries are common in athletes.

- The anatomy of the cervical spine is unique and predominantly based on ligamentous restraints with little inherent bony stability.

- Cervical sprains and strains are best managed conservatively.

- The majority of simple fractures can be managed with cervical collar immobilization for 6 weeks.

- The incidence of catastrophic neurologic injury is low.

- Degenerative changes are more frequent in athletes of high-impact sports.

- Return to play criteria continue to be controversial.

EPIDEMIOLOGY

In modern society, the term *athlete* continues to evolve. In decades past, the descriptor athlete was applied only to those individuals currently or previously engaged in an organized sport. Today, due to the widespread increase in physical fitness activities, athletes now encompass a much larger population of people with vastly different interests, levels of participation, and conditioning. As musculoskeletal specialists, we are called on to apply our knowledge of the literature across this spectrum, from a National Football League athlete to a "weekend warrior." Fortunately, although cervical spine injuries are relatively common in athletes, the majority are self-limited strains and sprains; however, catastrophic injuries can and do occur.

The true incidence of cervical spine injuries in athletes is difficult to determine because of underreporting secondary to fears of restriction from play. Kuhlman and McKeag[1] demonstrated that although 65% of college football players had at least one episode of neurologic symptoms during their career, only 30% reported the injury. Symptomatic cervical spine injuries are reported at the rate of 7% to 18%, with a threefold increase in the risk of recurrent injury.[2] Albright et al[3] examined high

school and college freshman football players and found 32% had radiographic evidence of previous neck injury. Catastrophic (quadriparesis) spinal injuries have been most recently estimated at a rate of one in 200,000.[3] The incidence however, is proportional to the level of play.

During the late 1960s and early 1970s, much attention was given to improving helmet design to prevent closed head injuries. Although successful in decreasing the rate of intracranial hemorrhage and head injury–related deaths, the incidence of serious cervical spine injury increased from 1.36 per 100,000 athletes to 4.14 per 100,000 from 1971 to 1975.[4] It appeared that athletes were using the helmet as a battering ram. In 1976, rules were changed to eliminate dangerous tackling techniques such as spearing. Over the next decade, the rate of cervical spine injuries decreased 70% and the rate of quadriplegia decreased 82%.[5] Although American football commonly comes to mind when discussing cervical injuries, ice hockey, gymnastics, equestrian sports, recreational diving, bicycling, rugby, wrestling, and skiing/snowboarding all have reported cases of catastrophic spinal cord injury.[6]

RELEVANT ANATOMY

The cervical spine is composed of seven specialized vertebrae that provide a wide range of possible motions. Approximately 50% of cervical flexion-extension and rotation occurs in the upper cervical spine (occiput-C2), with the remainder distributed among the subaxial segments. Ligamentous structures provide the main support to the cervical spine as there is little inherent bony stability. This is especially true in the upper cervical spine where the transverse ligament prevents atlantoaxial subluxation. The subaxial cervical spine relies on static stabilizers such as the anterior longitudinal ligament, intervertebral disk, posterior longitudinal ligament, facet joint capsules, and interspinous and supraspinous ligaments to maintain stability while providing maximum flexibility. Important dynamic stabilizers include the sternocleidomastoid, paraspinal, strap, and trapezius muscles. These dynamic stabilizers are important in the acute evaluation as spasm in these muscles can mask ligamentous injury.[7] Accordingly, rehabilitation and strengthening of these muscles can decrease the risk of future injury. An assessment of both the osseous and ligamentous structures before determining the treatment plan is critical as unrecognized ligamentous injury can lead to late instability and neurologic compromise.[8]

CLINICAL FEATURES AND EVALUATION

The on-the-field examination of suspected head and spinal cord injury has been addressed previously in this text. As mentioned,

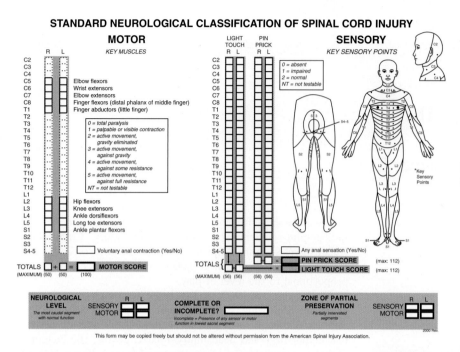

Figure 15-1 American Spinal Cord Injury Association classification of spinal cord injury.

maintaining in-line cervical immobilization with log rolling, leaving the shoulder pads and helmet in place with face mask removal is important in the prehospital care of athletes suspected of a head or spinal injury. Several studies have demonstrated that trying to remove the helmet with the shoulder pads left in place causes unacceptable degrees of motion of the cervical spine that may compromise the injured cervical spine.[9-11] A well-rehearsed action plan for suspected head or cervical spine injury cannot be overemphasized. Athletes with altered mental status, neck pain, tenderness or limited motion, or neurologic deficits should be transported to a medical facility while maintaining cervical spine immobilization with continued evaluation of airway, breathing, and circulation.

A complete neurologic examination including cranial nerve and orientation testing is mandatory. Active range of cervical motion should be evaluated within the levels of comfort. The examiner should palpate the athlete's neck both in the midline and paraspinal regions to assess for tenderness, step-off, hematoma, and muscular spasm. Upper and lower extremity strength testing should be graded and recorded. Sensory testing to light touch, temperature, and pinprick is also performed. An evaluation for abnormal reflexes such as a Hoffman's sign, Babinski's response, and spasticity should be performed. Spurling's maneuver may be performed and may indicate nerve root irritation secondary to spondylosis or acute disk herniation. If deficits are present, they are usually radicular. More profound deficits such as an incomplete spinal cord injury should be further characterized as central cord, Brown-Sequard, anterior, or posterior spinal cord syndromes as these categories have different prognoses for recovery. All findings should be recorded according to the American Spinal Cord Injury Association scoring system[12] (Fig. 15-1).

IMAGING OF THE CERVICAL SPINE

Imaging of the cervical spine has been a topic of considerable debate in the athlete. The favorable natural history of neck pain and the high incidence of false-positive findings should temper the use of advanced imaging. Gore et al[13] demonstrated that

95% of asymptomatic male and 75% of asymptomatic female subjects had evidence of degenerative changes on plain films by the age of 65. Friedenberg and Miller[14] showed that 25% of men and women have degenerative changes of the cervical spine by the fifth decade of life increasing to 75% by the seventh decade. Healy et al[15] demonstrated that 15 of 19 asymptomatic lifelong noncontact sport athletes had abnormalities on cervical magnetic resonance imaging (MRI). Berge et al[16] demonstrated a higher incidence of degenerative changes of the cervical spine by MRI in high-level front-line rugby players than in age-matched controls.

The radiographic evaluation of neck pain should begin with plain radiographs including anteroposterior, lateral, and oblique views. Evaluation should include a check of overall alignment (lordosis 21 ± 13 degrees) as well as for instability (>3 mm translation, >11-degree kyphosis), fracture, spondylosis, congenital malformations, or ankylosed segments. Radiographic clues to potential stenosis include canal diameter less than 17 mm, Pavlov ratio greater than 0.85 (sagittal canal diameter to sagittal vertebral body width), and encroachment of the facet joints on the spinolaminar line (Fig. 15-2). If plain films demonstrate fracture, computed tomography is recommended to improve detail of the extent of bony injury.[17]

MRI is indicated if the patient has a neurologic deficit, disabling weakness, persistent radiculopathy, or long tract signs.[18] MRI may demonstrate acute soft disk herniations, edema, central or foraminal stenosis, syringomyelia, hematoma, or spinal cord edema. However, one must interpret findings in light of the clinical picture. Boden et al[19] demonstrated that 14% of asymptomatic subjects younger than 40 years old had abnormalities as well as 28% of those older than 40 years of age.

CERVICAL STENOSIS

The diagnosis, management, interpretation, and implications of cervical stenosis have caused significant debate and controversy over the past several decades. The concept of cervical stenosis is simple; the spinal canal is narrow. However, the answer to the question of how narrow is too narrow is quite complex.

body. A Pavlov ratio of less than 0.85 qualified as stenosis and a ratio of more than 0.8 was reported to place athletes at risk of catastrophic neurologic injury. Herzog et al[24] recognized that football players generally have larger vertebral bodies and that even if these athletes had normal canal measurements, the Pavlov ratio could be less than 0.8, a false-positive result that may prevent an asymptomatic athlete from participating in contact sports. Computed tomography and MRI have been subsequently used to determine ranges of "normal" canal diameter. The average spinal cord diameter ranges from 5.0 to 11.5 mm (mean, 10 mm).[20] The average canal diameter from C3–C7 is 15 to 25 mm (mean, 17 mm).[25,26] A canal diameter less than 13 mm is considered stenotic and absolute stenosis considered to be less than 10 mm.[27,28] Blackley et al[29] showed a poor correlation between Pavlov's ratio and computed tomography scan measurements of canal diameter. Prasad et al[30] demonstrated that Pavlov's ratio correlated poorly with MRI measurements of the space available for the cord. Matsuura et al[31] demonstrated that the anteroposterior diameter of the spinal canal on computed tomography was less in patients with spinal cord injury than in controls. Of importance in this topic is that the overall space available for the cord is dependent on the sagittal and transverse diameters of the canal. Cantu,[32] expounding Burrows'[33] ideas, proposed the concept of "functional stenosis." This concept takes into account the variability in anatomy of the canal and cord among athletes and states that the more important factor is whether there is enough spinal fluid surrounding the cord to protect it from injury. Functional stenosis must be determined on a case-by-case basis, as the predictability of absolute measurements and ratios is moderate at best.

Stenosis may be either acquired, congenital, or a combination of both. Acquired causes include disk pathology, osteophytes, degenerative subluxation, hypertrophic ligamentum flavum, fracture, or ossification of the posterior longitudinal ligament. Congenital causes may vary from shortened pedicles, Klippel-Feil syndrome, or other congenital anomalies.

Previously, stenosis alone was thought to be a contraindication to contact sports, but more recent literature has suggested a revision of that doctrine.[4,34] Currently, the use of Pavlov's ratio should not be used as a screen for prediction of spinal cord injury given its low positive predictive value (0.2%). A ratio of less than 0.8 has, however, been demonstrated to have reasonable predictive value for a recurrent episode of either transient neurapraxia or burner syndrome but not catastrophic injury.[35,36] Kang et al[37] demonstrated that the canal diameter at the time of injury was positively correlated to the severity of the neurologic injury sustained. Higher energy injuries were associated with smaller canal diameters and more severe neurologic injuries. This study raises concern for athletes with severe stenosis who wish to participate in collision sports.[37] Some authors continue to recommend that asymptomatic athletes with stenosis not participate in contact sports.[38] A proven screening tool for prediction of catastrophic injury remains elusive. In the existing literature, quadriplegia has been more closely associated with axial loading from poor tackling techniques, such as spearing, that lead to catastrophic vertebral body fracture than to stenosis.[39]

TRANSIENT QUADRIPARESIS

Temporary paralysis after a collision in sports with rapid and *complete* resolution of symptoms within 10 to 48 hours after injury has been termed transient quadriparesis or cervical cord

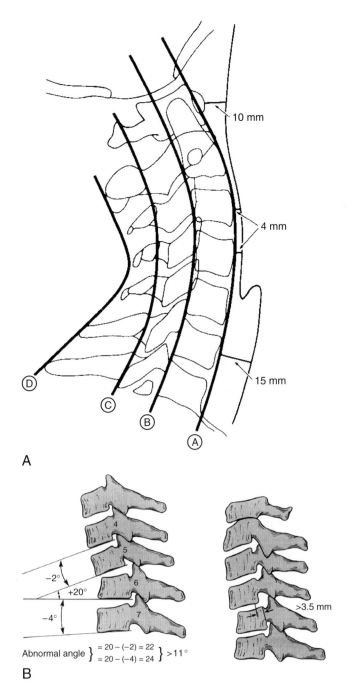

Figure 15-2 Radiographic assessment of cervical spine alignment. **A,** The anterior vertebral line, posterior vertebral line, spinolaminar line, and spinous process line should be smooth and continuous without step-off. **B,** Sagittal displacement greater than 3.5 mm or angular deformity greater than 11 degrees indicates an unstable injury of the cervical spine.

The definition of stenosis has generated considerable debate. Originally, stenosis was diagnosed from measurements of the transverse spinal canal diameter on plain radiographs.[20] Wolfe et al[21] and Penning[22] recognized the relations between radiographic measurements and myelopathy as early as 1956 and 1962, respectively. Gore et al[13] understood that technique factors in obtaining plain radiographs could cause significant discrepancies in absolute measurements obtained from them. Torg and Pavlov in 1987 put forth the Pavlov ratio as a method to avoid problems of magnification when evaluating for possible stenosis.[23] This is the ratio of the spinal canal to the vertebral neurapraxia.[23] The incidence in collegiate football players has been estimated to be 7.3 in 10,000 athletes. The mechanism of injury is usually axially loading of the cervical spine in flexion or extension. Penning[22] described the pathoanatomy of the "pincer mechanism" of hyperextension on the cervical cord. Taylor reported that infolding of the ligamentum flavum can reduce canal diameter up to 30%. The cervical spinal cord gets pinched between the inferior aspect of the superior vertebral body and the anterosuperior aspect of the spinolaminar line of the inferior adjacent vertebra. Similarly, with hyperflexion the cervical cord gets pinched between the anterosuperior aspect of the spinolaminar line of the superior vertebrae and the posterior superior aspect of the vertebral body of the inferior vertebrae.[22,40]

Although the precise etiology of transient quadriparesis remains elusive, Torg has postulated that cord function is disrupted because of local cord anoxia and the increased concentration of intracellular calcium.[41] Zwimpfer and Bernstein[42] described a "postconcussive state" of the spinal cord after brief conduction block causing axon dysfunction.

Transient quadriparesis encompasses a spectrum of neurologic dysfunction. Motor dysfunction ranges from bilateral upper and lower extremity weakness to complete paralysis. Sensory dysfunction ranges from dysesthesias to complete absence of sensation. Deficits may resolve in as little as 10 minutes but may persist for up to 48 hours. Deficits lasting longer than 48 hours are not due to transient quadriparesis.[43]

Radiographic evaluation of patients with transient quadriparesis or an abnormal neurologic examination includes plain radiographs and MRI. Imaging is negative for fractures but may reveal congenital anomalies (Klippel-Feil), congenital stenosis (canal diameter <13 mm), acquired stenosis, a herniated disk, or cervical instability. As previously stated, considerable controversy currently exists regarding the use of spinal canal measurements to predict risk of catastrophic neurologic injury. Torg et al[43] reported that 56% of players of contact sports with transient quadriparesis experienced a recurrence; however, none suffered a permanent neurologic injury. Risk factors for recurrence included a small Torg ratio (<0.8) as well as acquired stenosis from spondylotic changes.[43] For a first-time occurrence, if the athlete's symptoms resolve quickly and he or she is asymptomatic and imaging studies do not demonstrate contraindications, the athlete should be allowed to return to play. Prolonged quadriparesis of 24 to 48 hours, two or more previous episodes of transient neuropraxia, or an increase in baseline neck discomfort are relative contraindications to return to play. Absolute contraindications include persistent pain, abnormal neurologic examination, spear tackler's spine, instability, acute fracture, or malalignment.[44]

CERVICAL SPRAINS

The majority of athletes with cervical sprains will complain of neck stiffness, "kinking," or a "jammed" feeling in the neck. Most cervical sprains occur from collisions in contact sports but can also occur from acute twisting injuries in noncollision sports. Athletes will demonstrate diminished cervical range of motion, but the neurologic examination should not demonstrate abnormality. Significant midline or paraspinal muscle tenderness should alert the physician to the possibility of ligamentous injury. Collar immobilization followed by radiographic examination including anteroposterior, lateral, oblique, and open mouth odontoid views should be obtained. Nonsteroidal anti-inflammatory medication and immobilization should be continued

until the acute symptoms subside. Dynamic flexion and extension radiographs should then be obtained. Anteroposterior translation of more than 3 mm or angulation of more than 10 degrees indicates instability and the need for MRI. On ruling out ligamentous injury, treatment then becomes supportive. Conservative measures including palliative, rehabilitative, and maintenance protocols are used until painless range of motion is achieved.[45]

SPEAR TACKLER'S SPINE

Torg et al[46] in 1993, after reviewing the National Football Head and Neck Injury Registry, identified a subset of athletes with an increased risk of permanent neurologic injury. These athletes had a spectrum of radiographic findings including congenital and acquired stenosis, loss of cervical lordosis, spondylosis, healed compression fractures, and instability (Fig. 15-3). In and of themselves, these abnormalities are not always associated with neurologic injury; however, in combination with poor tackling technique such as "spearing" in which the top of the head is used as a battering ram can result in spinal cord injury. When repetitive axial loads are applied to the straightened cervical spine, catastrophic injury can occur. Torg et al[46] have recommended that these athletes should be withheld from contact sports and return to play considered only if the loss of lordosis was reversible and the athlete could demonstrate proper and safe tackling techniques.

CERVICAL DISK HERNIATIONS

Cervical disk injuries occur with higher frequency in high-performance athletes playing football or wrestling than the general population.[3] Cervical disk disease is generally categorized into soft versus hard disk disease. Acute disk herniations in sports are thought to occur from uncontrolled lateral bending[3] (Fig. 15-4). Hard disk disease (disco-osteophytic disease) can become symptomatic through various mechanisms (Fig. 15-5). Both entities can cause varying amounts of neck and arm pain. Athletes with radicular symptoms or long tract signs should undergo MRI examination.[17] It can be difficult to differentiate

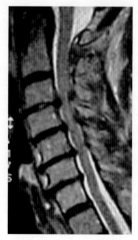

Figure 15-3 Spear tackler's spine. The sagittal magnetic resonance imaging demonstrates loss of the normal cervical lordosis, multilevel spondylosis leading to cervical stenosis. Torg et al[46] showed that athletes with radiographic findings of stenosis, spondylosis, and loss of cervical lordosis were at increased risk of permanent neurologic injury when combined with poor tackling techniques such as "spearing."

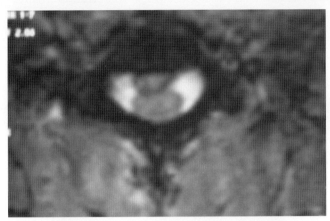

Figure 15-4 Axial magnetic resonance image of a large extruded soft disk herniation at C6–C7.

between an acute herniation and symptomatic hard disk disease in patients with significant spondylosis. Regardless, initial treatment is generally nonoperative with few exceptions. Treatment includes rest, short-term immobilization, activity modifications, anti-inflammatory medications, cervical traction, and possibly selective nerve root injections and is successful in the majority of patients.[17] Once initial symptoms improve, a three-phase rehabilitation program of stretching, range of motion, and isometric strengthening is performed. The athlete should be allowed to return to play once symptoms have resolved, the neurologic examination is normal, and painless full range of motion has been restored.[44]

Surgical indications include progressive neurologic deficits, disabling motor deficits at presentation, acute myelopathy, or persistent or recurrent radicular symptoms despite 6 weeks of nonoperative treatment.[47] The two most common surgical procedures performed for cervical herniated disk are anterior cervical diskectomy and fusion and posterior lamino-

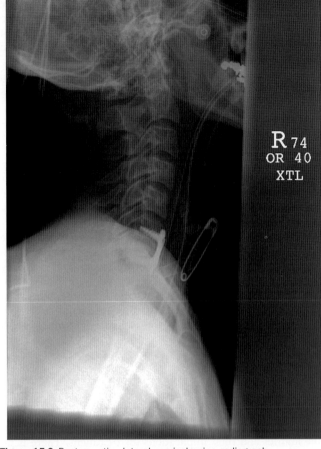

Figure 15-6 Postoperative lateral cervical spine radiograph demonstrating anterior cervical diskectomy and fusion. The patient's iliac crest was used as the interbody bone graft and a small anterior cervical plate applied to prevent extrusion and enhance healing.

foraminotomy[17] (Fig. 15-6). After a healed single-level anterior diskectomy and fusion or posterior laminoforaminotomy, an athlete should be able to return to play after appropriate rehabilitation.[44] Relative contraindications to return to play after cervical surgery include two-level anterior cervical procedures or single-level posterior fusion procedures. Absolute contraindications include single-level fusions with surrounding congenital stenosis, multilevel posterior fusion procedures, and circumferential fusions.[44]

MINOR FRACTURES

Compression fractures, spinous process fractures (clayshoveler's), and lamina fractures can occur during athletic participation. Hyperflexion can lead to both compression or spinous process fractures, and axial loading is associated with lamina fracture.[48,49] Cervical immobilization should be maintained throughout the evaluation. Plain radiographs and computed tomography scanning should be performed and scrutinized for evidence of instability or associated ligamentous injuries. Nondisplaced compression and lamina and spinous process fractures can be successfully treated with cervical collar immobilization for 6 weeks followed by flexion and extension views.[45,50] If no instability is present, the athlete should begin rehabilita-

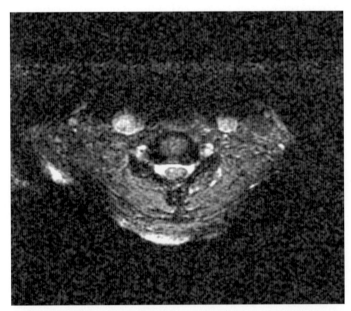

Figure 15-5 Axial magnetic resonance image of the cervical spine demonstrating hypertrophy of the uncovertebral joints causing narrowing of the neuroforamen and radiculopathy.

tion. Once asymptomatic and painless range of motion and protective strength have been restored, the athlete should be able to return to competition. Healed, nondisplaced compression fractures and lamina and spinous process fractures should not be a contraindication to return to play.[44] Fractures with mild height loss, mild malalignment, and facet fractures are relative contraindications. Absolute contraindications include sagittal malalignment, canal encroachment from healed fractures, radiographic instability, and upper cervical spine fractures.[44]

MAJOR FRACTURES

Major fractures and fracture dislocations do occur in sports. Although discussion of these injuries is beyond the scope of this text, most major fractures are the result of flexion and axial loading. Rotational forces also may cause major fracture dislocations. These fractures include compression and burst fractures, facet fractures, and dislocations as well as extension-type injuries. The majority of these injuries ultimately require surgical intervention for decompression of the spinal cord and bony stabilization (Fig. 15-7). Maintenance of in-line cervical immobilization and support of the airway, breathing, and circulation is critical. Emergency transport to a medical facility with specialists in spine care maximizes the athlete's opportunity for a successful outcome.

SUMMARY

Cervical spine injuries are relatively common in athletes today. Fortunately, the vast majority are minor without long-term morbidity. It is critical to understand the pathoanatomy of cervical spine injuries and their implications for treatment. There is no universal agreement on return to play criteria. The decision to

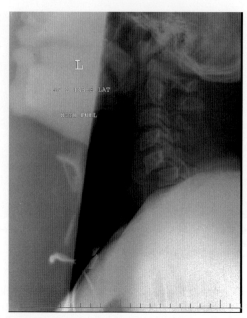

Figure 15-7 Lateral cervical spine radiograph demonstrating bilateral facet dislocation. Note greater than 50% anterolisthesis of the C5 vertebral body on the C6 vertebral body. This patient suffered a C6 complete permanent spinal cord injury.

return to play after a cervical spine injury is dependent on several factors: severity of injury, treatment response, congenital anatomy, and the athlete's career aspirations and expectations. These decisions should not be made in a vacuum. Emphasis should be placed on truthful, realistic, and candid discussions with the athlete, the athlete's family, and coach.

REFERENCES

1. Kuhlman GS, McKeag DB: The "burner": A common nerve injury in contact sports. Am Fam Physician 1999;60:2035–2042.
2. Castro FP: Stingers, cervical cord neurapraxia, and stenosis. Clin Sports Med 2003;22:483–492.
3. Albright JP, Moses JM, Feldick HG, et al: Nonfatal cervical spine injuries in interscholastic football. JAMA 1976;236:1243–1245.
4. Torg JS, Guille JT, Jaffe S: Injuries to the cervical spine in American football players. J Bone Joint Surg Am 2002;84:112–122.
5. Torg JS, Vegso JJ, O'Neill MJ, et al: The epidemiologic, pathologic, biomechanical, and cinematographic analysis of football-induced cervical spine trauma. Am J Sports Med 1990;18:50–57.
6. Cooper MT, McGee KM, Anderson DG: Epidemiology of athletic head and neck injuries. Clin Sports Med 2003;22:427–443.
7. Wang JC, Hatch JD, Sandhu HS, et al: Cervical flexion and extension radiographs in acutely injured patients. Clin Orthop 1999;365:111–116.
8. Gerrelts BD, Petersen EU, Mabry J, et al: Delayed diagnosis of cervical spine injuries. J Trauma 1991;31:1622–1626.
9. Swenson TM, Lauerman WC, Blanc RO, et al: Cervical spine alignment in the immobilized football player. Radiographic analysis before and after helmet removal. Am J Sports Med 1997;25:226–230.
10. Donaldson WF 3rd, Lauerman WC, Heil B, et al: Helmet and shoulder pad removal from a player with suspected cervical spine injury. A cadaveric model. Spine 1998;23:1729–1732.
11. Peris MD, Donaldson WF 3rd, Towers J, et al: Helmet and shoulder pad removal in suspected cervical spine injury: Human control model. Spine 2002;27:995–998.
12. American Spinal Injury Association, International Medical Society of Paraplegia: International Standards for Neurological and Functional Classification of Spinal Cord Injury, Revised 1996. Chicago, American Spinal Injury Association, 1996.
13. Gore DR, Sepic SB, Gardner GM: Radiographic findings of the cervical spine in asymptomatic people. Spine 1986;11:521–524.
14. Friedenberg ZB, Miller WT: Degenerative disk disease of the cervical spine: A comparative study of asymptomatic and symptomatic patients. J Bone Joint Surg Am 1963;45:1171–1178.
15. Healy JF, Healy B, Wong WH, et al: Cervical and lumbar MRI in asymptomatic older male lifelong athletes: Frequency of degenerative findings. J Comp Assist Tomogr 1996;20:107–112.
16. Berge J, Marque B, Vital JM, et al: Age related changes in the cervical spine of front-line rugby players. Am J Sport Med 1999;27:422–429.
17. Wang JC, Boyce RH: Evaluation of neck pain, radiculopathy, and myelopathy: Imaging, conservative treatment, and surgical indications. In An H (ed): Instructional Course Lectures: Spine. Chicago, American Academy of Orthopaedic Surgeons, 2003, pp 15–21.
18. Levine MJ, Albert TJ, Smith MD: Cervical radiculopathy: Diagnosis and nonoperative management. J Am Acad Orthop Surg 1996;4:305–316.
19. Boden SD, McCowin PR, Davis DO, et al: Abnormal magnetic resonance scans of the cervical spine in asymptomatic subjects: A prospective investigation. J Bone Joint Surg Am 1990;72:1178–1184.
20. Mintz DN: Magnetic resonance imaging of sports injuries of the cervical spine. Semin Musculoskelet Radiol 2004;8:99–110.
21. Wolf BS, Khilnani M, Malis L: The sagittal diameter of the bony cervical spinal canal and its significance in cervical spondylosis. J Mt Sinai Hosp NY 1956;23:283–292.
22. Penning L: Some aspects of plain radiography of the cervical spine in chronic myelopathy. Neurology 1962;12:513–519.

23. Torg JS, Pavlov HK, Genuario SE, et al: Neurapraxia of the cervical spinal cord with transient quadriplegia. J Bone Joint Surg Am 1986;68:1354–1370.

24. Herzog RJ, Wiens JJ, Dillingham MF, et al: Normal cervical spine morphometry and cervical spinal stenosis in asymptomatic professional football players. Plain film radiography, multiplanar, computed tomography, and magnetic resonance imaging. Spine 1991:16(Suppl):S178–S186.

25. Payne E, Spillane J: The cervical spine and anatomico-pathological study of 70 specimens with particular reference to the problem of cervical spondylolysis. Brain 1957;80:571–596.

26. Moiel R, Raso E, Waltz T: Central cord syndrome resulting from congenital narrowness of the cervical spinal canal. J Trauma 1970;10:502–510.

27. Dee R, Hurst LC, Bruber MA, et al: Principles of Orthopaedic Practice, 2nd ed. New York, McGraw-Hill, 1997, p 1352.

28. Murone I: The importance of the sagittal diameters of the cervical canal in relation to spondylosis and myelopathy. J Bone Joint Surg Br 1974;56:30–36.

29. Blackley HR, Plank LD, Robertson PA. Determining the sagittal dimensions of the cervical spine. J Bone Joint Surg Br 1999;81:110–112.

30. Prasad SS, O'Malley M, Caplan M, et al: MRI measurements of the cervical spine and their relation to Pavlov's ration. Spine 2003;28:1263–1268.

31. Matsuura P, Waters RL, Adkins RH, et al: Comparison of computerized tomography parameters of the cervical spine in normal control subjects and spinal cord injured patients. J Bone Joint Surg Am 1989;71:183–188.

32. Cantu RC: Functional cervical spinal stenosis: A contraindication to participation in contact sports. Med Sci Sports Exerc 1993;25:316–317.

33. Burrows EH: The sagittal diameter of the spinal canal in cervical spondylosis. Clin Radiol 1963;14:77–86.

34. Cantu RC: The cervical spinal stenosis controversy. Clin Sports Med 1998;17:121–126.

35. Torg JS, Naranja RJ, Pavlov H, et al: The relationship of developmental narrowing of the cervical spinal canal to reversible and irreversible injury of the cervical spinal cord in football players. An epidemiological study. J Bone Joint Surg Am 1996;78:1308–1314.

36. Torg JS, Ramsey-Emrhein JA: Cervical spine and brachial plexus injuries: Return to play recommendations. Phys Sport Med 1997;25:61–88.

37. Kang JD, Figgie MP, Bohlman HH: Sagittal measurements of the cervical spine in subaxial fractures and dislocations. An analysis of two hundred and eighty-eight patients with and without neurological deficits. J Bone Joint Surg Am 1994;76:1617–1628.

38. Cantu RC, Mueller FO: Catastrophic football injuries 1977–1988. Neurosurgery 2000;47:673–677.

39. Curl LA: Side line decisions and close encounters. Presented at the 2003 Annual Meeting of the American Academy of Orthopaedic Surgeons, New Orleans, LA.

40. Taylor AR: The mechanism of injury to the spinal cord in the neck without damage to the vertebral column. J Bone Joint Surg Br 1951;33B:543–547.

41. Torg JS, Thibault L, Sennett B, et al: The pathomechanics and pathophysiology of cervical spinal cord injury. Clin Orthop 1995;321:259–269.

42. Zwimpfer TJ, Bernstein M: Spinal cord concussion. J Neurosurg 1990;72:894–900.

43. Torg JS, Corcoran TA, Thibault LE, et al: Cervical cord neurapraxia: Classification, pathomechanics, morbidity and management guidelines. J Neurosurg 1997;87:843–850.

44. Vaccaro AR, Watkins B, Albert TJ, et al: Cervical spine injuries in athletes: Current return to play criteria. Orthopedics 2001;24:699–703.

45. Zmurko MG, Tannoury TY, Tannoury CA, et al: Cervical sprains, disc herniations, minor fractures, and other cervical injuries in the athlete. Clin Sports Med 2003;22:513–523.

46. Torg JS, Sennett B, Pavlov H, et al: Spear tackler's spine: An entity precluding participation in tackle football and collision activities that expose the cervical spine to axial energy inputs. Am J Sports Med 1993;21:640–649.

47. Albert TJ, Murrell SE: Surgical management of cervical radiculopathy. J Am Acad Orthop Surg 1999;7:368–376.

48. Marks MR, Bell GR, Boumphrey FR: Cervical spine injuries and their neurologic implications. Clin Sports Med 1990;9:263–278.

49. Mazur JM, Stauffer ES: Unrecognized spinal instability associated with seemingly "simple" cervical compression fractures. Spine 1983;8:687–692.

50. Laporte C, Laville C, Lazennee JY, et al: Severe hyperflexion sprains of the lower cervical spine in adults. Clin Orthop 1999;363:126–134.

Shoulder

II Shoulder

CHAPTER

16 Physical Examination and Evaluation

Sumant G. Krishnan, John M. Tokish, and Richard J. Hawkins

In This Chapter

INTRODUCTION

- This chapter on the physical examination of the athlete's shoulder is different from the more traditional "textbook" approach. Although we remain committed to a comprehensive, organized approach to the shoulder, the direction here is driven by the chief complaint, such that a differential diagnosis is deduced at the beginning of the interview rather than at the end.

- This "differential-directed" approach allows the examiner to test the premise of the initial diagnosis throughout the history and physical and allows a more focused approach to the shoulder as it pertains to the athlete (and, specifically, the overhead athlete).

- Although this differs in style from established texts that describe the history and physical followed by formation of the differential diagnosis, we hope that this approach leads to the same destination: an accurate diagnosis for an athlete with shoulder dysfunction.

- For an organized, comprehensive, and traditional approach to examination of the shoulder, we refer readers to "Clinical Evaluation of Shoulder Problems" (Krishnan SG, Hawkins RJ, Bokor DJ: In Rockwood CA, Matsen FA [eds]: The Shoulder, 3rd ed. Philadelphia, Elsevier, 2004).

Physical examination of the injured shoulder for some has unfortunately become somewhat of a lost art because of the difficulty of the examination itself, the subtleties of the normal athletic shoulder that often make comparison to the opposite side unreliable, and the ever-increasing reliance on magnetic resonance imaging (MRI) for definitive diagnosis. As helpful a tool as the MRI is, it is of concern that completely asymptomatic shoulders demonstrate pathology that might be erroneously attributed to an athlete with symptoms. Sher et al[1] demonstrated a 34% rate of tears of the rotator cuff in painless volunteers. Miniaci et al[2] showed that 79% of asymptomatic professional baseball pitch-

ers had abnormalities of the glenoid labrum. Furthermore, partial-thickness rotator cuff tears, a diagnosis common to the throwing and overhead shoulder, may be missed by MRI as much as 44% of the time.[3] Hence, even with the technologic advances available, we remain convinced that the diagnosis of a shoulder problem in the athlete is made by a proper history and physical examination and not in the scanner.

Although a classic tenet of physical examination is to compare the symptomatic side to the opposite normal side, this is not always reliable in the overhead athlete. There are a number of physiologic adaptations that occur in throwers and other overhead athletes that, although asymmetrical, are not pathologic. These include hypertrophy of the dominant arm, elbow flexion contracture, increased external rotation, and decreased internal rotation.[4] Striving to create symmetry in these athletes may "correct" physiologic adaptations that protect the overhead arm and might lead to further problems and dysfunction.

One theme that is emphasized in this chapter is the importance of communication with the athlete to arrive at a correct understanding of the athlete's problem. Many athletes present with shoulders that contain multiple pathologies such as labral tears, impingement, and instability. Communication with the athlete is critical to understand which of these may be the most important in their disability. Communication is also critical in differentiating between objective signs on physical examination and clinical symptoms. For example, laxity (a physical examination sign) is present in many overhead athletes. It can often be demonstrated on physical examination as a positive sulcus sign or increased translation of the humeral head on the glenoid. Although often more pronounced than in the nonathlete, this finding may be totally asymptomatic, and attempts to "correct" it may do more harm than good. This is in contrast to symptomatic laxity, which is instability (a clinical *symptom*). The key difference is obviously symptomatology. An athlete who can be shifted over the glenoid rim with a posterior translation maneuver demonstrates laxity. This patient must demonstrate reproduction of symptoms with such a maneuver to raise the level of suspicion to diagnose instability.[5] It is only with communication during such maneuvers that these subtle differences can be reliably interpreted (Box 16-1).

Another important area of communication exists between physicians and the athlete's team trainers and/or physical therapists. A treating physician might be unimpressed with a pitcher's signs or symptoms in the office only to find out that, once the player throws at more than half speed, he becomes ineffective. Trainers/therapists can often provide key feedback on the mechanism of injury, the degree of disability, and the athlete's progression with conservative treatment. They are helpful with decisions concerning return to play or in determining when rehabilitation is not working and other options should be considered. Such benefits only happen with open lines of communication.

This chapter begins with a throwing athlete who cannot throw well. From this initial presentation, we hope to describe an organized yet focused differential-directed approach to understanding the cause of the dysfunction, which forms the basis for how to resolve the problem. Although much of this chapter is focused on the overhead shoulder, it is important to keep in mind that these principles apply both to the examination of shoulders involved in any repetitive overhead activity (such as tennis, volleyball, handball, and swimming) and also to athletes of all ages and levels of participation with shoulder problems.

RATIONALE FOR THE DIFFERENTIAL-DIRECTED APPROACH

One of the early skills taught to medical students is how to perform a history and physical examination. It forms the structure and base of the clinical encounter in which a diagnosis is formulated and treatment subsequently planned. Students are taught to be organized and thorough, and although much of the necessary knowledge base will come later, the structure must be stressed early and often to have a framework in which to fill in new knowledge. Traditionally, this framework follows a fairly strict order of history, physical examination, review of imaging, and the creation of a differential diagnosis. This differential is the end result of the sum total of information gained throughout the encounter. One common directive in teaching students is to not let them see any of the past notes or diagnostic conclusions during their evaluation, as such information might "tip them off" as to what to look for during the encounter, leading the student to focus on the expected findings of the examination and be too quickly directed toward the diagnosis. This is helpful for the young clinician, as it teaches completeness and avoids the pitfall of jumping to conclusions or making assumptions that the diagnosis purported by another clinician is correct. While we agree that this process is valuable to the young development of any promising diagnostician, once the framework is ingrained, the clinician will learn which findings in each specific clinical encounter are pertinent and which are superfluous. To perform every aspect of the physical examination on every patient is unrealistic, and often results in a great amount of data with no comprehension of what the data mean. It is far easier "to find what you are looking for when you know what you seek." This premise is the basis for the differential-directed approach. If one can be taught to develop a suspicion of what may be the problem(s) in the athletic shoulder at the beginning of the clinical encounter, one will stay directed, efficient, and accurate. We *do not* sacrifice thoroughness and completeness because other pathologic diagnoses often may not have been suspected at the beginning of the examination and may only be elucidated with appropriate physical examination maneuvers. However, we use this differential-directed approach to allow for

patient-appropriate specific versus "screening" examination techniques, and we believe that the development of these initial suspicions is not only possible but is the natural history of becoming more "focused" as a diagnostician. This focus comes with experience but can be accelerated by modifying the approach to both the history and physical examination. It will become readily obvious that the success of the evaluation is directly related to the initial differential. The quality of the differential is dependent on the clinician's understanding of shoulder pathology and the various tests that are available for each. The better one's understanding is of the shoulder pathologies presented in this book, the higher the quality of the initial differential and the better the clinician becomes. This creates a dynamic relationship between knowledge and skill that can continue to improve throughout one's career. The experienced clinician learns to "go for the money" and yet not miss more subtle diagnoses.

The initial pathologic differential in the athlete's shoulder is formed from two important pieces of information: (1) the athlete's age and (2) the athlete's chief complaint. One simple example of this is the 60-year-old male tennis player with shoulder pain. Certainly the diagnosis is not guaranteed with such limited information, but the astute clinician has a working differential from the very start. Throughout the examination, the clinician has certain findings that he or she is expecting may be positive. In this example, impingement signs with associated weakness with supraspinatus testing would strongly suggest a rotator cuff tear. At the same time, features of the examination that focus on subtle glenohumeral instability might be less emphasized. This format emphasizes attention to a set of expected findings and makes the diagnosis that much more specific.

The first step in the differential-directed approach is to understand how pathologies present as chief complaints, so that the initial differential is complete but focused. It should be noted that this is rarely as easy as the example given. This is clearly illustrated if we substitute a 20-year-old baseball pitcher with pain into the example. Rather than suspecting just a rotator cuff tear, the initial diagnosis might include instability, labral pathology, impingement, internal impingement, or a combination of these. Thus, a deeper understanding of the chief complaint and how it relates to the history is necessary to come to an accurate differential. Even in difficult presentations, we still formulate an initial differential that may "tip us off" to what we are looking for while keeping us directed toward the appropriate diagnosis.

Once this differential is formulated, the remainder of the history proceeds in an organized fashion with expectations already in mind. If the differential is correct, answers to queries within the history will serve to validate the initial diagnosis. If, however, the answers given by the athlete are not what were expected, the clinician will be alerted very early to suspect another diagnosis and thus take the examination in a different direction. By the completion of the history, the clinician should have clear expectations of what to look for and emphasize in the physical examination.

It would be ideal if we could exactly reproduce an athlete's symptoms during the physical examination, but this is only occasionally possible. Many tests for pain are not specific enough to be reliable, and patients with instability are often too guarded to allow provocative testing. In the throwing and overhead athletic population, many pathologies coexist and make presentations confusing. It is therefore important that the physical

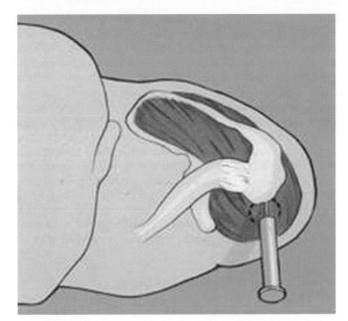

Figure 16-1 Neer impingement test: Instillation of local anesthetic into the subacromial space alleviates the previous pain that was demonstrated with the Neer impingement sign, indicating the pathology of subacromial impingement.

examination remain organized and systematic. One of the dangers of having a short list of differential diagnoses in mind is that the clinician's attempts to be focused could result in an examination that is incomplete. Although we recommend reorganizing the examination according to the differential, the essential tenets of "inspect, palpate, and move" the shoulder remain.[5,6]

Diagnostic injections can be very helpful in determining the source of symptoms. The goal is to eliminate the athlete's clinical signs and physical symptoms with the use of a short-acting local anesthetic placed in the specific anatomic area that seems to be responsible for the symptoms. This maneuver is the equivalent of the Neer subacromial "impingement test" (Fig. 16-1) and can be applied to a variety of other conditions in the differential diagnoses. There are limitations to this, as differential injections are time-consuming and often are not applicable for diagnoses such as instability. When pain is the presenting complaint, a diagnostic injection in a specific location that quickly (within 5 to 10 minutes) takes away nearly 100% of the athlete's pain often leads to the area of pathology and the correct diagnosis.

The organization of this chapter is according to chief complaint, followed by the specific historical questions and physical examination maneuvers that are applicable to each entity. This is an alternative approach from traditional texts where it is more common to separate the history from the physical examination and from diagnostic injections. Nevertheless, we believe that this organization more closely resembles how we approach the evaluation of the athlete's shoulder.

PRINCIPLES OF THE HISTORY

Regardless of how one approaches the history, it is crucial that this approach is organized and systematic so that the clinician is thorough yet efficient. The general categories of chief complaint,

history of present illness, medical history, and review of systems (followed by the physical examination) remain the backbone of the clinical evaluation. We organize this evaluation according to the chief complaint for several reasons:

1. It is the impetus behind the athlete's request for help, so organization by chief complaint keeps the interview patient directed.
2. Organization by chief complaint keeps the clinician focused and efficient.
3. Knowing the age and the chief complaint provides a high index of suspicion for the diagnostic probabilities.[1,3,5,6] Such an understanding provides an immediate differential diagnosis that can be tested throughout the history and physical examination to arrive at the correct diagnosis. It allows each step in the examination to help confirm or refute the diagnosis, providing dynamic confirmation when the initial diagnosis is right and a series of red flags throughout the examination when the initial diagnosis is erroneous.

Chief Complaint

A complete understanding of the chief complaint is critical to arriving at the correct diagnosis. This cannot be overemphasized due to the multiple pathologies in the shoulder of the throwing and overhead athlete. An operative "shotgun" approach to the wrong problems can end such an athlete's career, as more surgery that is undertaken in these patients lowers the chances of returning to high levels of participation. These overlapping pathologies present the so-called athlete's dilemma, emphasizing why the athlete's shoulder is so challenging. It is therefore critical to sort out which pathologies are dominant and might be corrected surgically and which should be left for rehabilitation.

These are difficult decisions that can be successfully made only with a thorough understanding of the athlete's chief complaint and how it relates to the rest of his or her history. For example, a chief complaint of pain in the shoulder may intimidate a novice examiner because there are so many possibilities. This assumption would be compounded if the examiner went from the chief complaint of pain directly to an MRI that showed AC degenerative changes, a partial-thickness undersurface tear of the rotator cuff, and a patulous capsule. However, if that same examiner seeks to gain a thorough understanding of the chief complaint, he or she might ask where exactly is the pain, when does it hurt, and how is the pain produced. These simple questions might reveal an athlete who has pain on the top of the shoulder with a bench press and is tender to palpation of the AC joint, leading to an initial suspicion of AC pathology. In contrast, the patient might say the shoulder hurts at the back when he or she starts to come forward with a fastball pitch, in which case the initial suspicion might be one of internal impingement. Thus, understanding the chief complaint should give the examiner a reliable early differential of the problem.

Once this is established, this differential can guide the examiner through the physical examination, providing clues to which findings should be positive on provocative testing and which should be negative. The first patient described suggested symptoms of AC joint pathology. The examiner notes this by the chief complaint of pain on top of the AC joint and reproduction with the bench press. He or she then expects that during the physical examination the patient is likely to have tenderness to palpation of the AC joint and reproduction with crossed-arm adduction and an "augmented" AC joint maneuver. It does not mean that the clinician neglects to examine for symptoms of instability or impingement; it just highlights and sharpens the focus for the upcoming remainder of the history and physical examination. If the examiner notes that these findings on examination are indeed positive, especially in the absence of other findings, his or her suspicion is strengthened and he or she is closer to arriving at a correct diagnosis. If, however, the physical examination does not show these findings, the clinician must reconsider the diagnosis and perhaps move to one of the other ones in the differential. Perhaps the chief complaint was not fully understood, and one should revisit this first step before proceeding with the workup.

History of Present Illness and Injury

After the chief complaint, the next step of the history should be the history of the present illness. The purpose of the history of the present illness is to reconstruct the story of the chief complaint (from onset to present) so that the examiner has a clear understanding of how things started, what has been previously done, and the current state of the problem. The athlete may be unclear as to how or why symptoms started and may describe an insidious onset. When a single traumatic event is responsible for the injury, appropriate time spent on the mechanism, degree, and events surrounding the event provides reliable information. For example, in the patient whose chief complaint is that his shoulder "came out," appropriate questions might include those shown in Box 16-2.

The answers to these questions not only may establish the diagnosis but also may determine different courses of treatment. For example, an athlete who presents with a shoulder that came "partly" out of joint 1 week ago in a posterior direction, then spontaneously reduced, would be approached differently from the same athlete who complains of the shoulder coming "all the way" out of joint on the field. This short illustration demonstrates how similar chief complaints could result in entirely different management plans based on an appropriate history of present illness.

Clinical Course and Progression of the Problem

Once the circumstances surrounding the onset are established, the clinical course of the complaint is determined from its inception to the present. During this period, the effects and timing of various treatments are carefully considered. Any response to treatment, even if temporary, is important. For example, if a lidocaine and steroid injection was administered to the subacromial space for shoulder pain, it is important to note whether this was effective, even if only temporarily, as this will yield diagnostic as well as therapeutic information. One should evaluate other interventions such as the effect of anti-inflammatories, modalities, and physical therapy. This information should lead the examiner to an understanding of what has already been done, and the progression of the treatment instituted. A patient who is improving after 6 weeks of physical therapy prescribed for impingement is a much different case from a patient who is getting worse with 6 months of the same therapy. It is important to realize that, while some athletes have the luxury of having highly trained therapists and athletic trainers who supervise their rehabilitation on a daily basis, others are often left on an independent, poorly guided therapy regimen that is often incomplete or even misdirected. It is not enough to ask whether "physical therapy" has been done. One must delve into the specifics of that therapy to make an accurate assessment of whether it was an adequate regimen that was correctly followed.

Current Status of the Problem and Degree of Disability

Finally, before leaving the clinical course section of the history, it is important to note the current status of the complaint. This current status should be understood in light of the athlete's current level of activity, where he or she is in relation to the season, and how long he or she has until the shoulder has to be in "playing condition." A college football quarterback who dislocates his shoulder for the first time early in his senior year might pursue a different treatment course from that of the same player who dislocates in the first week of the off-season after his junior year. Such an understanding requires thorough communication with the athlete and an understanding of his or her goals and guides the patient and the physician to the best choice for their desired outcome.

The final aspect to the current status of the problem is the *degree of disability* incurred by the athlete from his or her injury. Athletes, and patients in general, present with complaints on the spectrum from minimal annoyance with high-level sports to complete disability with activities of daily living. Understanding where the patient is on this spectrum greatly aids in guiding how aggressive the diagnostic workup and how invasive the treatment plan should be. It is important to note that an accurate assessment of the degree of disability may require communication with the athletic trainer and/or physical therapist, as some athletes may attempt to "play through" injuries that render them ineffective and put themselves in danger of further injury. These are sometimes difficult decisions for an athlete to make, and often a trainer's input is very valuable in defining the degree of disability.

Medical History and Review of Systems

Although we should be confident with a solid differential diagnosis at this point, and although athletes are among the healthiest patients in our population, questions about medical history should not be neglected. These include questions about medications, allergies, and congenital or other medical problems. Finding out that a swimmer with shoulder pain has Ehlers-Danlos syndrome might not only point to multidirectional instability (MDI) as a diagnosis but might also influence the treatment of such a shoulder. Although often negative, a review of systems and queries regarding medical history can avoid missing key aspects affecting the diagnosis and eventual treatment of the athlete.

Box 16-2

- Did the shoulder "come out" because of a significant injury?
- What position was the arm in when it "came out?"
- Could you move the shoulder after the injury?
- Did it "slide out of joint" or did it "pop?"
- Did the shoulder feel like it came all the way out of joint?
- Did you feel any numbness or tingling in the arm or hand?
- Did you have to go to the hospital or have something else done to have it "put back in?"
- Did you have radiographs?
- Has this ever happened to your shoulder before?

PRINCIPLES OF THE PHYSICAL EXAMINATION

Once the examiner completes an organized history, there should be a clear idea of the differential, and this should direct which aspects of the physical examination should be emphasized. Just as in the history, there are certain expected responses (both positive and negative) for the differential-directed physical examination. During the examination, one should note whether the physical examination expectations are met (in which case the suspicion of the correct diagnosis is strengthened) or whether the expectations are not met (in which case, one must reconsider the appropriate diagnosis). Although we organize our approach based on complaint, there are certain aspects to the physical examination that should be ingrained in any competent examiner. Depending on the differential, some of these areas are emphasized more than others. Nevertheless, especially in the overhead athlete in whom multiple pathologies often exist and there is considerable overlap for many chief complaints, we repeatedly emphasize that the following tenets should be remembered:

1. *Introduction to the patient and cursory assessment of general aspects.* This allows the examiner to see the "big picture," to remember the whole patient, and to avoid making the mistake of focusing too narrowly on the shoulder.
2. *Features of inspection such as muscle wasting, deformity, and previous surgical scars.* This is especially important when the chief complaint is weakness related, which can lead to a number of other chief complaints such as pain and instability.
3. *Palpation of known anatomic sites.* This is crucial in the patient who complains of pain, but also can be used for other pathologies (e.g., to diagnose rotator cuff tears in patients complaining of weakness).
4. *Range of motion (active and passive) with careful documentation.* This is an often overlooked area of the examination but is often the key finding in overhead athletes with tight posterior capsules leading to pain and other complaints.
5. *Strength testing and neurologic examination.* These should be a part of every shoulder examination in the athlete.
6. *Stability assessment and laxity measurements.* Because laxity and "microinstability" are the "great imitators" in the athlete's shoulder, this is critical to every examination. Instability can underlie many chief complaints in the overhead athlete.
7. *Special tests.* These tests may be the decisive blow in ruling a diagnosis in or out; familiarity with the special tests for each diagnosis separates the beginner from the advanced diagnostician.
8. *Lower extremities and trunk.* Although outside the scope of this chapter, it is emphasized that the kinetic chain begins in the legs and proceeds through the trunk before it ever gets to the shoulder. The examiner is reminded that problems in the shoulder may only be a manifestation of more proximal pathology in the chain that must be corrected to allow the athlete to return to proper performance.

The patient should be prepared by removing the outer garment for a view of the bare shoulders. For women, a sports bra or designed halter top type gown will preserve modesty while allowing the examiner to pick up on often subtle aspects of the examination like atrophy or winging (Fig. 16-2). Attention to the asymptomatic side remains important to note, but the examiner must remember those physiologic adaptations that often are present in overhead athletes. With this in mind, the examiner should attempt to reproduce the conditions that bring on the chief complaint. This may involve more emphasis on range of motion when instability is suspected or palpation and special tests when pain is the chief complaint. This does not mean that we ignore range of motion in the patient with pain or palpation in the patient with instability; it is just that a dif-

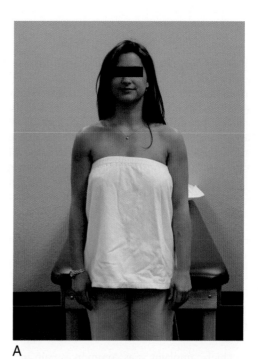

A

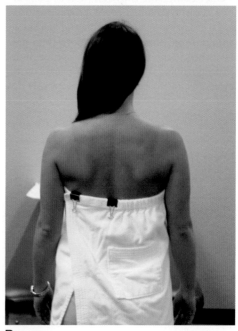

B

Figure 16-2 A and **B,** Direct inspection of shoulder.

Table 16-1 Common Descriptions of Shoulder-Area Pain	
Patient Description	*Likely Source of Pain*
Whole hand over deltoid in rubbing motion	Impingement/rotator cuff
Greater tuberosity	Impingement/rotator cuff
One finger on top of distal clavicle	Acromioclavicular joint
In the back when the arm is in the throwing position (points to posterior capsule with arm abduction/external rotation)	Internal impingement/superior labrum anterior to posterior tear
Down the neck and scapula medial border	Neck pathology
In front within deltopectoral groove	Biceps tendon, subscapularis pathology
"Deep inside"	Labral or articular cartilage pathology
Vague and diffuse down arm	Brachial neuritis/thoracic outlet syndrome (neurologic)

ferent set of red flags and expectations arise for each patient with this approach.

We now define the various chief complaints common to the athletic shoulder (and, specifically, the overhead shoulder) and discuss which initial differential corresponds to each chief complaint. Next, we describe the specific historical questions that should narrow the focus and sharpen the differential. Finally, we demonstrate the various physical examination techniques that may rule a specific diagnosis in or rule out in the athlete. We hope that this differential-directed approach provides an organized template for the correct diagnosis right from the initial history, tips off the examiner on what to expect and what not to expect throughout the physical examination, reinforces each step of the workup, and creates solid evidence for the diagnosis by the completion of the encounter.

CHIEF COMPLAINT: PAIN

Perhaps no chief complaint is as common as pain in the shoulder and none with a broader list of possible causes. Many of these causes overlap or play a role in the pathology of other processes. In addition, there is often more than one source of pain in the overhead athlete, making the approach not nearly as clear as one would like.[2] We begin with pain, describe the differential, and endeavor to describe how to narrow down the list

to a few diagnoses to test on physical examination. A list of common causes for pain as chief complaint follows:

- *Impingement*: classic outlet impingement, internal impingement, subcoracoid impingement
- *Rotator cuff*: tendinosis, partial-thickness tearing, full-thickness tearing
- *Instability*: anterior, posterior, MDI
- *AC joint pathology*
- *Biceps and labral pathology*
- *Chondral defects*
- *Neurologic*: cervical spine nerve root compression, brachial neuritis, thoracic outlet syndrome, suprascapular nerve entrapment

Such a list can be quite daunting unless the examiner stays organized. With a few early questions, the differential can be established and narrowed down. One question to begin with is, simply, "Where is the pain?" Although a seemingly basic question, it is often difficult to get the patient to be specific. We often ask patients to point with one finger to the area. Most patients will respond in any of the ways described in Table 16-1.

Palpation to Reproduce Pain

Once the patient has identified the area of the pain, the next step may be to find the point of maximal tenderness by palpating each of the following areas. Keep in mind that some areas of the shoulder are naturally tender, so comparison to the asymptomatic side might be helpful (Table 16-2; Fig. 16-3).

Table 16-2 Common Sites of Tenderness and Locations/Pearls	
Point of Maximal Tenderness	*Location/Pearl*
Greater tuberosity (Codman's point) (see Fig. 16-3)	Just anterior to anterolateral corner of acromion with dorsum of hand on buttock. Codman's point is the insertion of supraspinatus tendon on greater tuberosity.
Lesser tuberosity	Subscapularis pathology, biceps
AC joint	Follow posterior part of clavicle to acromion. AC joint just anterior to this; push the clavicle down hard enough to move it
Acromion	Do not forget about symptomatic os acromiale
Posterior capsule	Internal impingement lesions are tender posteriorly; SLAP tears may also be tender here
Biceps tendon/bicipital groove	Directly anterior when arm internally rotated 10 degrees
Coracoid	Subcoracoid impingement
Erb's point	Medial to coracoid, inferior to clavicle

AC, acromioclavicular; SLAP, superior labrum anterior to posterior.

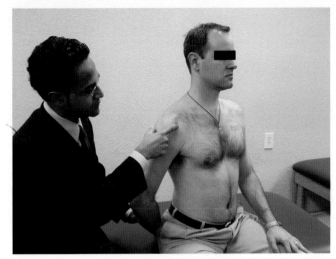

Figure 16-3 Codman's point.

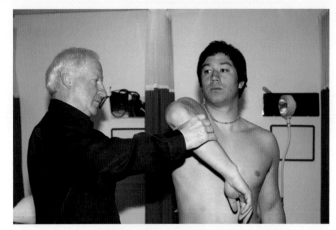

Figure 16-5 Hawkins sign.

Remember that the patient may say that their pain is "deep" and not really palpable (think intra-articular superior labrum anterior to posterior [SLAP], labral tear, articular cartilage injury). In addition to finding (or not finding) the point of maximal tenderness, there are a number of additional maneuvers that should be performed to further narrow the differential.

Provocative Tests to Reproduce Pain
Subacromial Impingement-Producing Maneuvers
When an athlete presents with tenderness over the greater tuberosity (especially with vague complaints involving the whole deltoid with overhead activity), one should already strongly suspect impingement. The following are provocative maneuvers that should lead one toward the diagnosis of subacromial impingement.

Neer Sign   This test is performed by placing the symptomatic arm in maximum passive forward flexion while stabilizing the scapula (Fig. 16-4). A positive test is signified by production of pain. The Neer sign has been shown to be 88.7% sensitive for

subacromial impingement and 85% sensitive for rotator cuff tearing but has poor specificity.[7,8]

Hawkins Sign   This test is performed by placing the arm in 90 degrees of forward flexion, with the elbow flexed 90 degrees. The examiner then internally rotates the arm maximally (Fig. 16-5). A positive test is signified by production of pain. This test has been shown to reflect contact between rotator cuff and the coracoacromial ligament.[5] It has been shown to have a sensitivity of 92% for subacromial impingement and 88% for rotator cuff tearing.[8] Like the Neer sign, however, this test is not very specific for these conditions.

Painful Abduction Arc Sign   This test is performed by having the patient perform resisted abduction in or just posterior to the coronal plane (Fig. 16-6). Reproduction of the patient's symptoms of pain constitutes a positive sign.[5,9] Unlike the Neer and Hawkins signs, this test is more specific than it is sensitive.[7]

If these signs are positive, subacromial impingement may be strongly suspected. Suspicion can be strengthened further with a Neer impingement test (see Fig. 16-1), especially if the test becomes negative after injection.

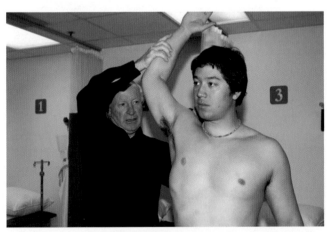

Figure 16-4 Neer sign.

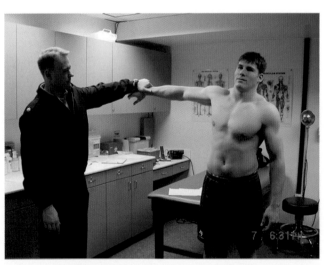

Figure 16-6 Painful abduction arc sign.

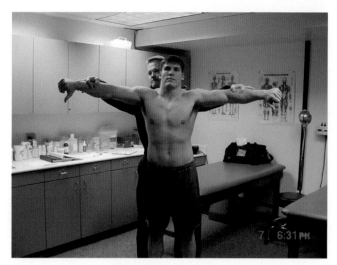

Figure 16-7 Jobe's test.

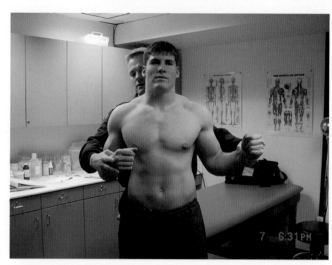

Figure 16-9 Resisted external rotation. Right side is abnormal.

One should be mindful that subacromial impingement syndrome may be associated with a tear of the rotator cuff. Because rotator cuffs are often painful, any workup for impingement should include testing for a tear of the cuff. Although these tests are usually looking for weakness, any impingement examination should include an evaluation of the cuff.

Tests for Weakness

Jobe's Test

This test is performed by placing the patient in 90 degrees of elevation in the scapular plane, classically with the thumbs pointed down (Fig. 16-7). This position is held against downward resistance. This test isolates the supraspinatus to a degree[10] and is positive when there is asymmetrical weakness. Caution should be used in the patient with pain, as it can simulate weakness in patients with painful subacromial impingement.

Full Can Test

Because Jobe's test can be painful in patients with impingement, the full can test has been proposed as an alternative (Fig. 16-8). This test is performed exactly like Jobe's test, except that the

thumbs are pointed up. This test has been shown to isolate the supraspinatus as well as Jobe's test, while producing less pain.[11]

Resisted External Rotation

This test is performed with the patient's elbows at his or her side, flexed 90 degrees (Fig. 16-9). A positive test is signified by asymmetrical weakness and indicates weakness of the infraspinatus and posterior cuff.

Lift-off Test

This test is performed by having the patient place his or her arm behind the back, resting on the small of the lumbar spine. The patient's hand is lifted off the back, without extending the elbow, and the patient attempts to hold the arm off of the back once the examiner lets go (Fig. 16-10). Gerber et al[12] found that this test reliably diagnosed or ruled out clinically significant subscapularis ruptures. This test is of limited value in patients with painful internal rotation or with stiffness that does not allow the patient to achieve the starting position. Careful attention should be paid to the technique, as it is possible to "lift off" the hand by extending the elbow, which can be misleading.

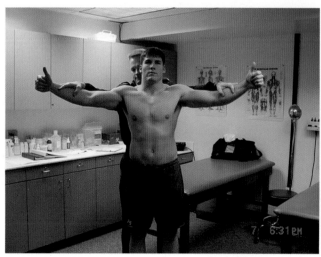

Figure 16-8 Full can test.

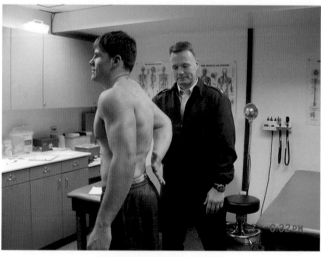

Figure 16-10 Lift-off test.

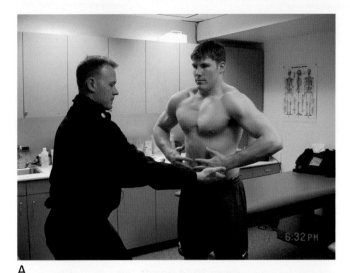

A

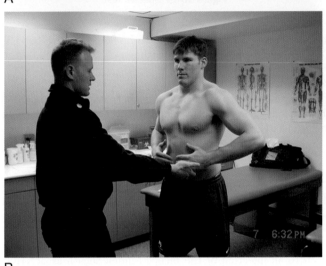

B

Figure 16-11 Belly press test. **A,** Normal; **B,** abnormal right side.

Belly Press Test

This test has been proposed as an alternative to the lift-off test in patients with either too much pain or stiffness to attempt the lift-off maneuver (Fig. 16-11). It is performed by having the patient place both hands on the belly with flat wrists. The elbows should remain anterior to the trunk while the patient pushes posteriorly against the belly. Patients with subscapularis weakness will demonstrate a dropped elbow because they use shoulder extension to compensate for weak internal rotation.

The belly press and lift-off tests tests have both been validated as tests for the subscapularis. The lift-off test is more specific for the lower subscapularis, and the belly press test is superior for the upper subscapularis.[13]

Lag Signs

These are three signs that have been shown to be reliable and efficient alternatives to more traditional rotator cuff testing.[14] The external rotation lag sign is performed by placing a patient in 20 degrees of elevation, 90 degrees of elbow flexion and near maximal external rotation. A patient who cannot maintain this position (even with a 5-degree lag) has a positive test suggesting a supraspinatus or infraspinatus tear.[14] The drop sign (or hornblower's sign) is evaluated much the same way, except that

the patient holds the affected arm in 90 degrees of elevation, 90 degrees of elbow flexion, and near full external rotation. If a drop occurs when the examiner releases the wrist, the sign is considered positive for infraspinatus and posterior cuff (infraspinatus/teres minor) weakness. Finally, the internal rotation lag sign is very similar to the description of the lift-off test, noting a 5-degree drop toward the back. Hertel et al[14] noted that the external rotation lag sign and drop sign had a positive predictive value of 100% and a negative predictive value of 56% and 32%, respectively. They also noted that the internal rotation lag sign had a positive predictive value of 97% and a negative predictive value of 69%.

Rent Test

This test, described by Codman,[5,15] attempts to palpate a "rent" through the deltoid in a patient with a supraspinatus tear. Palpation is accomplished in a relaxed patient at Codman's point, just anterior to the anterolateral border of the acromion with the dorsum of the hand on the buttock. Wolf et al[16] have reported on the diagnostic accuracy of this test, noting a sensitivity of 95.7%, a specificity of 96.8%, and a diagnostic accuracy of 96.3% for a rotator cuff tear.

It should be noted that patients may demonstrate pseudo-weakness on examination because many of these tests are subacromial impingement producing. It can be difficult to distinguish true weakness due to a rotator cuff tear from pseudo-weakness due to impingement-type pain. In those cases, use of the Neer impingement test, as described later, can be very helpful, as it may eliminate the pain, differentiating true weakness from that produced by pain.

Acromioclavicular Joint Testing

If the patient has complaints of pain on the top of the shoulder, which is reproduced with pressing down on the clavicle, one should consider AC joint pathology. Palpation tenderness is quite a reliable sign for this condition because a clinically significant AC joint problem is rarely nontender.[17] Three additional tests are good stressors of the AC joint.

Compression Test

This is a cross-body adduction maneuver that compresses the AC joint (Fig. 16-12). A positive test produces pain on top of the shoulder. An "augmented" AC compression test can be per-

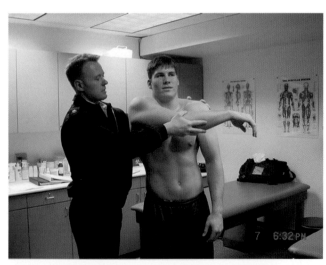

Figure 16-12 Acromioclavicular joint compression.

formed with palpation of the AC joint during forced cross-body adduction.

Distraction Test ("Bad Cop" Test)

This is accomplished by placing the arm in maximal internal rotation and applying slight pressure upward. Again, a positive test is signified by pain on top of the shoulder.

Active Compression Test (O'Brien's Test)

This test is performed by having the patient place his or her arm forward flexed to 90 degrees with 10 degrees of horizontal adduction and internal rotation (thumb down; Fig. 16-13). A positive test is signified by pain on top of the shoulder when the arm is pushed in a downward direction, which is lessened when the test is repeated with the arm in external rotation (thumb up). This test has been shown to be positive in 89% of patients successfully treated for AC joint pathology.[18]

When performing these tests, it is very important that the examiner specifically look for pain at the top of the shoulder at the AC joint because the first two tests will often produce pain in the shoulder with impingement, whereas O'Brien's test will often produce "deep" pain in the presence of a SLAP tear (see "Superior Labral Pathology Tears"). When the previously described tests are positive, strong consideration should be given to injecting the AC joint with 1 to 3 mL lidocaine (as described later) to help confirm the diagnosis.

Biceps Tendon Pathology (Nonanchor Related)

If the presenting complaint is pain at the front of the shoulder, especially if the point of maximal tenderness is reproduced with palpation in the area of the biceps tendon as described previously, a biceps tendon problem should be considered. Although the biceps tendon is normally difficult to palpate, there are a number of provocative maneuvers that can be considered to help confirm or rule out biceps tendon pathology. It should be remembered that many of these signs coexist with subacromial impingement.

Speed's Test

This is accomplished by having the patient hold the supinated arm in 90 degrees of forward flexion (Fig. 16-14). A positive test is marked by reproduction of pain with resisted forward

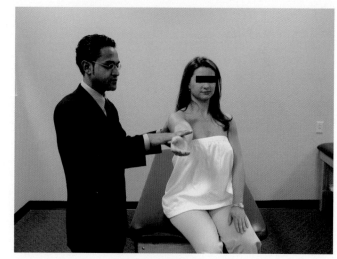

Figure 16-14 Speed's test.

flexion. This test has been shown to be 90% sensitive but only 14% specific for biceps tendon pathology.[19]

Yergason's Test

This test is performed by grasping the patient's hand as if to shake hands. The patient is asked to supinate while the examiner resists (Fig. 16-15). A positive test is reproduction of the pain at the front of the shoulder.

Ludington's Test

This is an observational test to look for a ruptured long head of the biceps. The patient is asked to place both palms of the hands on his or her head and flex the biceps. A positive test is marked by an asymmetrical biceps contour.

If these tests are positive, strong consideration should be given to an injection of the biceps tendon sheath as described later. If such an injection provides nearly complete relief in the office, especially with the subsequent normalization of the previously mentioned tests, one can be confident that the diagnosis of biceps tendon pathology is correct. This does not always address intra-articular biceps pathology (see SLAP Tears), and this differentiation can be confusing.

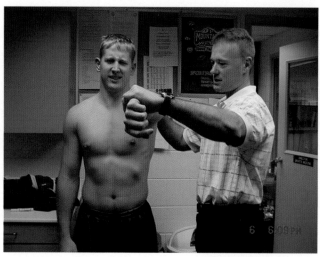

Figure 16-13 Active compression test (O'Brien's test).

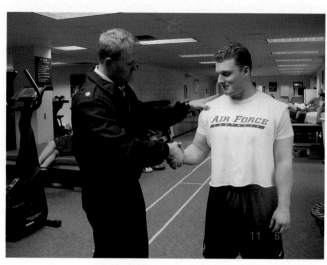

Figure 16-15 Yergason's test.

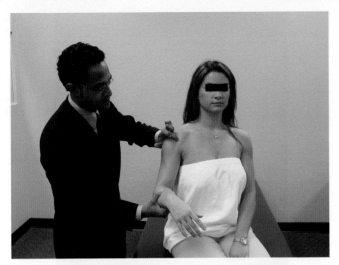

Figure 16-16 Palpation of bicipital groove.

It is difficult to exactly palpate the biceps tendon in its groove, and, thus, an injection can be difficult to place in the right anatomic location. The location of the biceps tendon and bicipital groove is commonly found with direct anterior palpation approximately 2 cm distal to the anterolateral corner of the acromion when the arm is in 10 degrees of internal rotation[5,20] (Fig. 16-16). As this is very close to the insertions of the subscapularis and pectoralis major, care must be taken to rule out strains of these two muscles before assuming a diagnosis of biceps tendonitis.

Superior Labral Pathology Tears

When a patient presents with a complaint of "deep" pain in the shoulder, especially in the absence of impingement signs or specific palpable points of tenderness, consideration should be given to the possibility of a SLAP tear. Since its description in 1990,[21] there has been an aggressive search by authors to find an accurate physical examination technique for superior labral tears. Some of the more commonly used are described in the following.

When these tests are strongly positive, especially in the relative absence of impingement signs, consideration should be given to performing an intra-articular injection, as described later. Complete relief suggests an intra-articular source and points strongly to a diagnosis of a SLAP tear or internal impingement.

Active Compression Test (O'Brien's Test)

Described previously as an AC joint provocative test, this test will often produce dramatic pain "deep inside" in the presence of a SLAP tear (see Fig. 16-13). This test has been shown to be positive in 95% of patients who demonstrate superior labral pathology at arthroscopy.[18] We find this test to be sensitive for labral tears, but not very specific, as it is often positive in patients with impingement.

"SLAP"-prehension Test

This test is similar to the active compression test, but the arm is placed in 45 degrees of adduction and 90 degrees of shoulder flexion, with the elbow extended and forearm pronated, and a downward force on the arm is resisted by the patient. A positive test produces apprehension, pain referable to the bicipital groove, and/or an audible or palpable click. The test is repeated

with the forearm supinated, which must cause diminution of the pain. The creators of this test found it to be 87.5% sensitive for unstable SLAP lesions.[5,22]

Biceps Load Test

This test is performed by placing the supine patient's arm in 120 degrees of elevation and maximal external rotation with the elbow flexed 90 degrees and the forearm supinated. The patient is asked to flex the elbow against resistance, and the test is considered positive if this reproduces or accentuates the patient's pain. In one prospective study, this test was shown to be 90% sensitive and 97% specific for a type II SLAP lesion.[5,23] We have not been able to reproduce the accuracy of this test for SLAP lesions in our practice.

Anterior Slide Test

This test is performed by having the patient place both hands on the hips with the thumbs facing forward. The examiner directs an axial force at the elbow in an anterior and superior direction. A positive test is marked by pain with this maneuver. The anterior slide test has been shown to be 78% sensitive and 92% specific[24] for lesions of the superior labrum in throwing athletes.

O'Driscoll's Superior Labral Pathology Test

This test is similar to the test for valgus instability of the elbow. The patient is supine or upright, and the shoulder is placed in the extreme abducted, externally rotated position. From this position, a moving valgus stress is applied, and a positive response is signified by pain in the shoulder. We have found this test to be quite sensitive but not very specific for SLAP lesions.[5]

Pain at the Coracoid (Subcoracoid Impingement)

Although a rare cause of pathology, subcoracoid impingement has been recognized as a source of anterior shoulder pain.[25] One test for this is the coracoid impingement sign, which is performed with the patient standing with the shoulder abducted 90 degrees with horizontal adduction in the coronal plane and maximally internally rotated (tennis follow-through position, similar to the Hawkins sign with less horizontal adduction). A positive test is marked by pain around the coracoid process.

Pain Secondary to Instability

As stated from the outset of this chapter, we believe that the best approach to problems with the evaluation of the shoulder is to begin with the patient's chief complaint, allowing it to immediately focus the clinical examination. It may seem odd, then, to describe a few tests for instability in a section on pain, but as pain is often the chief complaint in the athlete with instability, we remain consistent in our approach. Instability can coexist with conditions such as internal impingement or SLAP tears, which often present as posterior pain when the patient is in maximum abduction and external rotation. In addition, athletes are not immune from the diagnosis of MDI, which can present with pain. Thus, although we recommend tests that traditionally produce instability, pain in these positions may have instability as the underlying cause.

Relocation Test for Pain (Posterior Impingement Test)

This test is performed by placing the patient supine in maximum abduction and external rotation (Fig. 16-17). If this position pro-

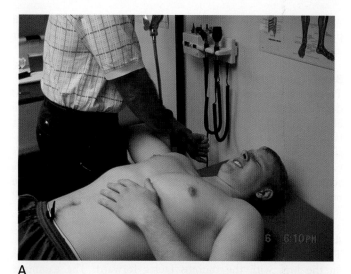

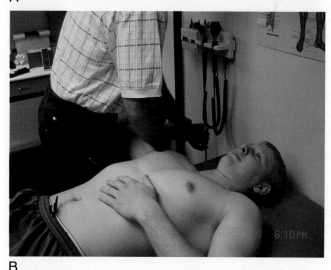

Figure 16-17 Relocation test for pain (posterior impingement test). **A,** With anterior translation; **B,** with posterior stabilization.

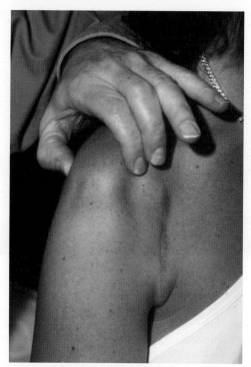

Figure 16-18 Sulcus sign.

duces posterior pain that is relieved by a posteriorly directed force on the humerus, and again recreated by removing the pressure and allowing the humerus to slide forward, then a diagnosis of internal impingement and/or posterosuperior labral pathology may be considered. Paley et al[26] demonstrated contact of the undersurface of the rotator cuff and the posterosuperior glenoid in the relocation position in 100% of patients undergoing arthroscopy for internal impingement. It should be noted that this test is differentiated from a standard apprehension test, which is a measure of instability and described later.

Inferior Sulcus Test for Pain
This test is performed by applying downward pressure on the humerus, at both 0 and 90 degrees of abduction. Patients with MDI will usually have reproduction of their symptoms with this maneuver with a positive sulcus sign (Fig. 16-18). It is critical to keep in mind that a positive sulcus sign or visible dimpling between the inferior acromion and superior humeral head in and of itself is not enough to establish the diagnosis of MDI. Patients with a combined SLAP and Bankart lesion will often show an increase in the sulcus sign, as do some asymptomatic patients.

It is therefore important to differentiate between shoulder laxity, which is a sign, and instability, which is a symptom. As MDI requires inferior instability plus at least one other direction of instability, the reproduction of the patient's pain with a sulcus test suggests the diagnosis.

The inferior sulcus test can also be used to diagnose pain secondary to rotator interval laxity and pathology. A sulcus sign (with the shoulder in the standard position of adduction and neutral rotation) that does not disappear when the sulcus is again tested in adduction and 25 to 30 degrees of external rotation indicates a deficient or lax rotator interval.

Pain Secondary to Cervical Spine Pathology
One potentially confusing cause of pain in the shoulder is that which is referred from the cervical spine. Herniated disks can cause pressure on the C5-T1 nerve roots, which can cause vague symptoms in the anterior and posterior shoulder girdle. Patients may interpret this as shoulder pain, and thus it is incumbent on the examiner to determine exactly where the pain comes from. In such cases, the patient will not often localize the pain. The various tests that are good indicators of cervical pathology are described.

Provocative Tests
In patients in whom the examiner suspects cervical pathology, testing should begin with gently stressing the limits of range of motion, especially in extension, where patients with cervical pathology will often have pain. In addition, posterior cervical tenderness is often present in these patients. Finally, there are some specific maneuvers (discussed following) that can help to define cervical pathology as the source of the pain.

The Neer Relief Test In patients with cervical spine pathology, symptoms will often be relieved when the patient places his or

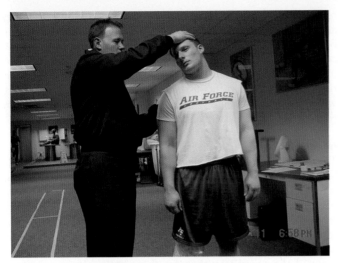

Figure 16-19 Spurling's test.

her arm above the head. This maneuver may relieve tension on an inflamed nerve and would be expected to exacerbate pain in the shoulder with impingement. This test may help differentiate between pain from a cervical spine source and pain from shoulder pathology and can be elicited by history as well as on physical examination.

Spurling's Test   This test is performed by stressing the neck in lateral flexion, rotation to the side tested, and compression (Fig. 16-19). A positive test is heralded by reproduction of the patient's specific symptoms with special attention to radiation of pain or numbness into the dermatome of a specific nerve root or into the shoulder. In one evaluation of Spurling's test,[27] it was shown to have a sensitivity of only 30% but showed a specificity of 93%. The authors therefore concluded that the test is not useful as a screening test but may be helpful in confirming the diagnosis of cervical radiculopathy. We find this test, when positive, to be the most helpful to us in determining the presence of cervical spine disease.

Valsalva Maneuver   This maneuver is performed by asking the patient to bear down, thereby increasing intrathecal pressure. Such an increase would be more likely to exacerbate pain from a cervical spine source than a shoulder cause.

Compression and Distraction Tests   In the patient with cervical pain, compression of the top of the spine in extension would be expected to exacerbate the patient's symptoms, while distraction in flexion might provide relief.

Pain Secondary to Other Neurologic Conditions

It will be noted by the reader that the organization of this chapter by chief complaint requires some redundancy, as some underlying conditions may lead to several chief complaints. One such area is neurologic pathology of the shoulder. Some neurologic conditions present primarily as pain, although they may also present as weakness and paresthesias.[28]

In addition to nerve compression at the level of the cervical spine, athletes can present with neurologic pain that is from a more distal source. The initial differential diagnosis might include compression of the suprascapular nerve, burners or stingers, thoracic outlet syndrome, and brachial neuritis.

Compression of the Suprascapular Nerve

This condition more commonly presents as weakness and atrophy in the supraspinatus, infraspinatus, or both and is therefore covered more extensively in the section on weakness. However, when an athlete presents with posterior shoulder pain, especially in the presence of weakness of the spinatii, consideration of compression of this nerve should be considered.[29-31] There are no provocative maneuvers that exacerbate the specific pain associated with compression of the suprascapular nerve, but, with a high index of suspicion, an injection of lidocaine into the area of the suprascapular notch may alleviate shoulder pain and be diagnostic. There are two common sites of compression for this nerve. The proximal site, at the suprascapular notch, both the nerve to the supraspinatus and infraspinatus can be compressed, leading to pain and weakness of both muscles. More distal compression can occur at the spinoglenoid notch, most commonly from a spinoglenoid notch cyst (usually associated with a posterosuperior labral tear), and can lead to isolated infraspinatus weakness.

Burners (Stingers)

Burners or stingers are common causes of pain and burning dysesthesias in the upper extremity. These injuries are most commonly the result of a violent stretch[31] of the brachial plexus. These injuries are usually transient, lasting only a few seconds. As these often occur in game situations, especially in football, the athlete should be kept out of competition until symptoms resolve. The diagnosis of this condition is made almost on history alone, although a player might run off the field with a characteristic "dead arm" at his or her side. Symptoms should be unilateral, extremely painful with burning and paresthesias down the extremity, and transient. They may also be accompanied by weakness of the deltoid, biceps, spinatii, and brachioradialis. It is very important to distinguish a burner from cervical radiculopathy caused by compression of a nerve root. The former is usually self-limiting, while the latter is of more concern. Most patients with findings attributable to cervical radiculopathy, such as tenderness in the cervical spine, pain with motion, a positive Spurling's test, or pain with compression, should be considered for early workup with cervical spine radiographs, MRI, and electromyography.

Thoracic Outlet Syndrome

This condition should be suspected in a patient who complains of diffuse shoulder pain, especially accompanied by radiating paresthesias in the ulnar nerve distribution below the elbow. As paresthesias are more frequently the chief complaint with this condition, it is covered in detail in that section.

Brachial Neuritis

Occasionally, athletes will present with an acute onset of severe pain with no apparent traumatic history. This pain can be severe and will follow a variable distribution throughout the brachial plexus. In such a patient, a brachial neuritis can be the source. It has no known etiology and usually resolves over several weeks. In addition, it can often present with accompanying weakness, especially of the proximal musculature. This is generally a diagnosis of exclusion, and the examiner often makes this diagnosis only after obtaining imaging studies of the neck and elec-

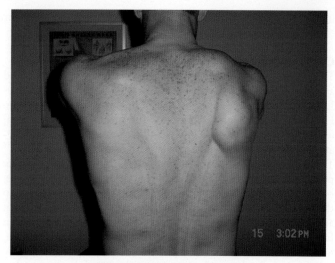

Figure 16-20 Scapular winging.

tromyographic studies to rule out a specific source of compression.

Pain in the Presence of Scapular Dyskinesia

Most overhead athletes with shoulder problems have some degree of scapular dysfunction. Given this, it is important to examine all athletes and any patient with shoulder pain for scapular winging. Although it is discussed more thoroughly in the section on weakness, winging can be either the cause or the effect of shoulder pain. Thus, it is incumbent on the examiner to determine whether scapular winging, when present, contributes to a patient's symptomatology. This is done by examining the patient from the back and asking the patient to elevate the arms at about half speed. Winging can be maximally demonstrated with resisted forward flexion at approximately 30 degrees of forward flexion (Fig. 16-20). It can also be observed with a push-up or wall push or when patients use their arms to rise from a seated position.

Scapular Stabilization Test

This test is performed by asking the patient to elevate the painful shoulder both before and after the examiner stabilizes the scapula against the thorax (Fig. 16-21). If the patient's pain is relieved by this maneuver, then it is likely that the source of the pain is the dysfunctional scapular platform.

Pain of Uncertain Origin

There are some pain evaluations that remain difficult even when armed with all the techniques described. Some patients simply cannot specifically describe their pain, and in others, the shoulder is so inflamed that everything seems to produce positive signs. It is in these patients that the injection tests may have their greatest utility. Before discussing these, however, there is an additional test that is reported to accurately delineate between intra- and extra-articular sources of pain. This test is called the internal rotation resisted strength test.[32] It is performed by asking the patient to place his or her shoulder in a position of 90 degrees abduction and 80 to 85 degrees of external rotation, with the elbow at 90 degrees flexion. A manual isometric muscle test is performed for external rotation and then compared to one for internal rotation in the same position. Apparent weakness in internal rotation compared to external

rotation signals a positive internal rotation resisted strength test, and intra-articular pathology is then suspected. This test has been reported to be 88% sensitive, 96% specific, and 94.5% accurate in differentiating between intra-articular and subacromial sources for shoulder pain.[32] We occasionally use this test in the presence of a difficult examination, often to help direct which injection to begin with, although we rely more heavily on the subsequent injection test to delineate the source of pain.

Injection Tests

The injection of a short-acting local anesthetic provides an excellent litmus test of one's clinical examination. The presumption is that if a local anesthetic is specifically placed in an area causing pain, that pain will be temporarily and nearly completely relieved. As important, the converse is true, making injection tests sensitive and specific. Performing a successful injection test has several important principles including the accurate placement of the anesthetic, time for this to take effect, re-examination for the elimination of the various provocative maneuvers, and subjective assessment of the patient's relief.

Accurate placement of the anesthetic takes time and experience to achieve consistency. One study has shown that attempts

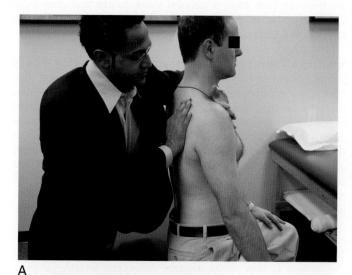

A

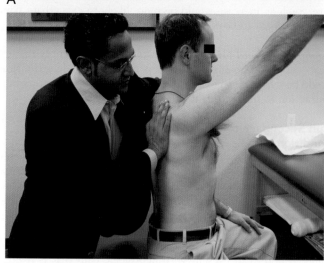

B

Figure 16-21 **A** and **B**, Scapular stabilization test.

at subacromial injection can be unsuccessful in 17% of shoulders, and attempts at AC injections can be unsuccessful 33% of the time.[33] Therefore, meticulous attention must be paid to technique. A second pitfall to the successful employment of the injection test is a failure to give the anesthetic time to take effect. With today's emphasis on the 10-minute office visit, the importance of providing this time is often put aside, and the outcome of the injection test is postponed for a future visit. Asking the patient to recall the immediate response to the injection several weeks after the fact may be inaccurate and misleading. Finally, accuracy of interpretation of the injection test demands that the patient be re-examined during the same office visit. Particular diagnostic maneuvers that were specific to the patient's symptoms are repeated. The patient is asked what percentage of the symptoms were relieved by the injection, and the agreed-on level is recorded in the note. In our experience, 80% to 100% relief should be obtained by the injection test. If significantly less relief is gained, the examiner should reconsider the diagnosis and consider an additional injection.

Subacromial Injection

We normally perform this injection from the back using the posterior lateral angle of the acromion as a landmark, although an anterior approach was originally described by Neer (Fig. 16-22). The area is prepped sterilely, and 5 mL of 1% lidocaine and 5 mL of 0.25% Marcaine are placed in the subacromial space by advancing the needle directly under the acromion anteriorly and slightly medially. Care must be taken in the exceptionally large individual that the needle be long enough to reach the anterior one third of the subacromial area since the pathology exists anteriorly. Alternatively, lateral and anterior injections can be placed in the subacromial space. Once an adequate amount of time has passed (usually 5 minutes), re-examination of the patient is performed. We inquire about any resting relief that the patient experiences with the injection. Next, we ask the patient to move the arm into positions that caused pain before the injection to see whether he or she obtained relief. This generally includes reassessment of Neer and Hawkins signs and painful abduction arc tests, as well as palpation over the greater tuberosity (Codman's point). The patient is asked to grade the relief as less than 25%, 25% to 75%, or greater than 75% relief. Rotator cuff strength testing is also repeated. Weakness in these tests when there is no pain is highly suggestive of rotator cuff tear and is often met with a more aggressive treatment plan.

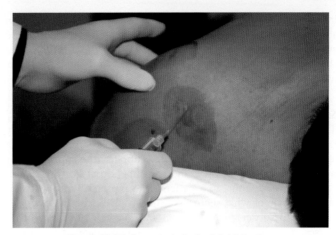

Figure 16-23 Acromioclavicular joint injection.

Acromioclavicular Joint Injection

Injection of the AC joint is performed by palpating the end of the clavicle, prepping the area sterilely, and attempting to inject 3 mL lidocaine into the joint (Fig. 16-23). This can be a tricky joint to inject because there may be considerable degenerative spurring or an abnormal angle of entry. Plain radiographs of the area will help direct the angle of injection. In addition, if in the joint, one should be able to perform a "refill test." This is done by allowing the increased intra-articular pressure created by the injection to refill the syringe when pressure is taken away from the piston. This test is positive whenever a closed space is entered and distended and is a routine part of any closed-space injection that we perform. The AC joint is variable in its volume, and enough local anesthetic should be used to meet firm resistance with a 20-gauge needle. This injection test is among the most dramatic in the office when positive and, when steroid is added, often provides dramatic lasting relief.

Biceps Tendon Sheath Injection

As previously mentioned, the biceps tendon is very difficult to feel in all but the thinnest individuals. However, the position of the tendon and its groove have been shown to be reproducibly located directly anterior on the shoulder, 2 cm distal to the anterolateral corner of the acromion, when the arm is held in 10 degrees of internal rotation.[20] Injection is accomplished by sterilely prepping the area, and placing a 20-gauge needle down to bone, then drawing back until resistance is released (Fig. 16-24). This step is important as it is not desirable to inject directly

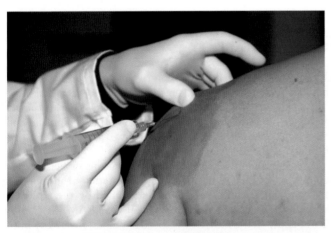

Figure 16-22 Subacromial injection.

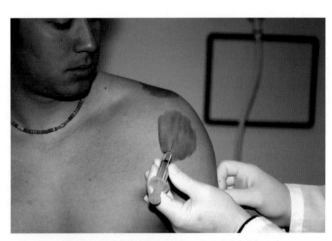

Figure 16-24 Biceps tendon sheath injection.

into the tendon, and the release of tension during injection should signify the needle moving out of the tendon and into the surrounding area. We have seen several tendons rupture after this injection, and although this is of concern if the patient has not given consent properly, it often provides lasting relief.

Suprascapular Nerve Injection

This is a rarely used injection because it serves to diagnose a very rare condition—a suprascapular nerve compression that presents as pain. Although primarily a motor supplier, the suprascapular nerve does contain sensory and pain fibers that go to the subacromial bursa. Thus, in a patient who presents with posterior shoulder pain or what seems like subacromial pain that does not respond to subacromial injection and one has ruled out other causes, consideration may be given to compression of the suprascapular nerve as the source of the pain.[29] The diagnostic injection to confirm this is performed by palpation of the AC joint and injecting 5 mL of 1% lidocaine beginning at a point just posterior to this joint with the needle directed 2 cm medially and 2 cm inferiorly. Weakness of the spinatii confirms infiltration of the nerve, and temporary resolution of symptoms confirms the diagnosis of entrapment.

Intra-articular Glenohumeral Joint Injection

This injection can be very effective in isolating the source of pain to an intra-articular location. Internal impingement, SLAP and other labral tears, and chondral lesions will all show relief with an intra-articular injection. This injection can be difficult for the inexperienced clinician because the joint is deep and the injection is uncomfortable for the patient. We stress the importance of intra-articular placement of the local anesthetic by injecting 10 to 20 mL of fluid into the joint and allowing the refill test to confirm this placement.

We approach this injection anteriorly. The coracoid process and the anterolateral corner of the acromion are identified and sterilely prepped. With the forearm in neutral rotation, a point halfway between the coracoid and the acromion is identified and infiltrated with 5 mL lidocaine in the skin along the path of the needle. An 18-gauge needle is then introduced and directed posteriorly perpendicular to the plane of the body. If a bony stop is encountered, it is likely the humeral head and the arm is internally rotated allowing the needle to "fall" into the glenohumeral joint. This technique is the same as that used to establish an anterior portal for shoulder arthroscopy and has been demonstrated to be the most accurate method for entering the glenohumeral joint without fluoroscopic assistance.

The glenohumeral joint may also be injected from a posterior approach, although this has demonstrated far less accuracy when compared to an anterior approach. The posterolateral corner of the acromion is identified and sterilely prepped. Next, a point 2 cm inferior and 1 cm medial to this point is identified and infiltrated with 5 mL lidocaine in the skin and along the path of the needle. An 18-gauge spinal needle is then introduced and directed anteriorly, aiming for the coracoid process. Often, the needle will hit a bony stop, and it must be determined whether this is the humerus or the glenoid. This can be determined by rotating the arm slightly internally and externally. If the needle moves with this rotation, the path must be redirected more medially to avoid the humerus. If it does not, it signifies that the needle is in the glenoid and must be directed more laterally. This is the same technique that we use to establish a posterior portal for shoulder arthroscopy.

Our choice of an 18-gauge needle is important for several reasons. First, a smaller gauge needle may not be stout enough to maintain its shape as it traverses through the posterior muscle mass and can be bent along its course. Second, an 18-gauge needle is large enough that once in the joint, intra-articular distention will provide enough pressure to refill the syringe, where a smaller gauge needle often will provide too much resistance to do this. Because the intra-articular placement of the needle is so critical, its position must be confirmed by this maneuver. Again it is critical to allow time for the local anesthetic to set up in the shoulder and then to re-examine the patient, especially those maneuvers that reproduced the patient's symptoms prior to the injection. If those provocative tests have been eliminated by the injection, one can be quite confident that the source of the pain is intra-articular. Given the high incidence of so-called pathologic findings on MRI of asymptomatic individuals, such injections can differentiate between variations of anatomy and symptomatic pathology. Such differentiation is the key to the clinical evaluation.

It must be remembered that if an abnormal connection exists between two distinct anatomic spaces, an injection in one may relieve pain in another, leading to confusion in the interpretation of the injection test. An example of this is in the patient with a full-thickness rotator cuff tear who receives a subacromial injection. The tear will allow infiltration not only in the subacromial space, but also in the shoulder joint proper. Thus, it is incumbent on the examiner to interpret the result of an injection in light of these possibilities.

Subscapular Injection

In patients who present with posterior scapular pain with or without an associated "snapping scapula" (see "Chief Complaint: Noise"), subscapular bursitis may be considered. This condition may produce impressive popping and may have associated pain. Five milliliters of 1% lidocaine can be directed into the more common superomedial or less common inferior angle bursa. This is done by palpating the medial border of the scapula and inserting the needle 1 cm medial to this. The goal is to hit the most anterior portion of the scapula and slide just anterior to this for medication infiltration. Care should be taken not to direct the needle too anteriorly, as penetration of the thoracic cavity is an undesired consequence. The patient should wait several minutes and attempt to reproduce the pain and noise from the shoulder. Relief of pain helps to confirm a subscapular source.

CHIEF COMPLAINT: SLIPPING, LOOSENESS, AND/OR COMING OUT OF JOINT—INSTABILITY

One of the most challenging culprits in the athletic overhead shoulder seeking treatment is instability. Note that instability is a diagnosis and not generally a chief complaint. As it is the goal of this chapter to begin always with the chief complaint, one must understand the multitude of ways that the athlete can communicate underlying instability.

Although the athlete may complain that his or her shoulder "comes out of joint," most often a presentation of instability is far more subtle and often is not understood by the patient as instability. The classic patterns of TUBS and AMBRI[5,34] often do not apply to the athletic overhead shoulder. Instability in the overhead athlete is usually more subtle than complete dislocation and may present as pain, slipping, sliding, or even as numbness or loss of control or velocity. Conditions such as the dead arm syndrome are also indicative of instability. With such a varied complaint set, the astute examiner must remain adherent to the principles of understanding the chief complaint and attempting to reproduce symptoms on physical examination. Instability may be the great imitator of the athletic shoulder because it can lead to so many different chief complaints. Because it underlies so many pathologies, it is important to look for it in most situations. For example, a patient with internal impingement will complain of pain, but the pain may be associated with underlying instability. Some surgeons address this assumption surgically by doing thermal capsulorrhaphy or capsular plication to stabilize all patients with internal impingement, while others do so only in the presence of internal impingement and increased laxity compared to the opposite side. While it is not yet clear how aggressive one should be with subtle instability that underlies other pathologies, it is important that the examiner be aware of its many forms and become skilled in laxity testing and the findings of instability on examination.

Finally, when an athlete complains that the shoulder "comes out," one should also consider a large labral tear or chondral defect because these pathologies can sometimes masquerade as feelings of instability.

Pertinent Questions Regarding Instability

When the chief complaint leads to the suspicion of instability, the examiner often does not have the luxury of being able to palpate for symptom reproduction, as is the case with other causes of pain. As instability is a dynamic process, our approach begins with asking the patient to reproduce the sensation. Particular attention is paid to the position that the patient assumes when attempting to reproduce the symptoms, and in throwers, the phase of throwing when problems arise. Often patients will know that their shoulder slides, and they are usually right. Determining which direction their shoulder slides can be more difficult to discern.

In the majority of cases in which anterior instability is the underlying problem, symptoms will be maximally reproduced in the abducted externally rotated position—the apprehension position. Patients may place their arm in the cocking position of throwing or state that symptoms occur when they move into the acceleration of the throw. Follow-up questions should include whether the symptoms happen at the beginning of activity in this position or whether the symptoms get worse as activity continues. The former is consistent with static sources and more severe instability, while the latter may represent instability that is masked by dynamic stabilizers like the rotator cuff until they become fatigued.

Although anterior instability is far more common than other directions, posterior instability and MDI may occur in the athlete. Throwers with posterior instability may describe the sensation occurring during the follow-through phase of a throwing motion, and other athletes may describe their symptoms as taking place during punching maneuvers or when the arm is forward flexed, adducted, and internally rotated. An additional curious complaint is of sliding or a "hitch" in the lead arm at the top of an aggressive golf swing.[35] Although atypical, these patients can be greatly helped if a correct diagnosis is made. Patients with MDI often have problems in all extremes of range of motion and can be some of the more difficult patients to evaluate and treat.

Examination of the Shoulder for Laxity and Instability

With laxity testing, it is important that the patient be as relaxed as possible. We use a consistent grading system (described later) and ask the patient whether he or she can appreciate the translation.[5] We then ask whether the translation reproduces the symptoms. It is important to note that although we use these tests primarily for laxity, grinding, clicking, or pain may represent labral tears or chondral defects.

Anterior Tests

Apprehension Test   This test is performed with the patient either supine (fulcrum) or sitting (crank) by stressing the symptomatic shoulder in maximum abduction and external rotation (Fig. 16-25). The patient may exhibit guarding or other actions that may make the patient or the examiner apprehensive, resulting in a positive test. We believe that this is the best clinical test for anterior instability because it is easy to perform and is very sensitive for producing symptoms in the anteriorly unstable patient. We believe that it is also quite specific, with the exception that the apprehension position is a possible impingement position, and thus one must be specific in asking the patient the nature of his or her symptomatology. It should be remembered that pain in this position is different from the feeling that the shoulder is going to come out of the joint.

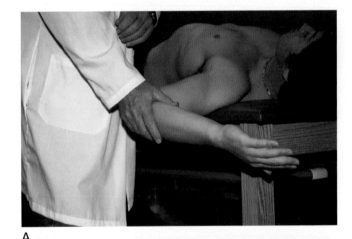

A

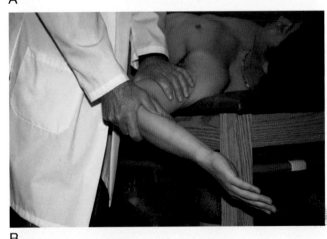

B

Figure 16-25 A, Apprehension test. **B,** Relocation test for instability.

Relocation Test for Instability This test is performed just as was described previously for pain, except that a positive sign here is signified by apprehension or a feeling that the shoulder will come out if further external rotation is applied (see Fig. 16-25). Such apprehension should disappear with a posteriorly directed force while holding the arm in the same degree of external rotation; with this posteriorly directed force, the arm can be moved into further external rotation without discomfort. We will often increase the external rotation slightly while holding the humerus back, then release this posterior pressure. This often reproduces the patient's symptoms exactly. We have found this test to be highly suggestive of anterior instability and place a great deal of emphasis on it during our examination.

Load and Shift Test The load and shift test is a test for laxity or translation of the shoulder. It is performed with the patient in the supine and seated positions at various levels of glenohumeral abduction. In the seated position, the examiner stands behind the affected shoulder (Fig. 16-26). One hand is used to stabilize the scapula by grasping the anterior and posterior acromion between the fingers. The other hand grasps the humeral head and by applying compression along with anterior and posterior force, the translational movement of the humerus on the glenoid can be appreciated. Grading of this passive translation includes motion up the face (normal or grade 0), up the face to the glenoid rim (grade 1), over the rim but spontaneously reducible (grade 2), and over the rim into a position of fixed dislocation that will not spontaneously reduce (grade 3).[5] This test can be repeated posteriorly, with a similar grading system. It is important to compare the translational grades to the asymptomatic side, as gross differences may suggest abnormal laxity.

The load and shift test may be repeated supine (our preference). In this position, the examiner holds the patient's wrist with one hand while the other hand grasps the humerus and again provides some load with translational force. The test is done with the arm at the side, at 45 degrees, and at 90 degrees. We will occasionally "dial in" the laxity by progressively abducting and also rotating the arm while performing the load and shift test. Patients who continue to translate at increased glenohumeral abduction angles compared to the opposite side may indicate laxity of the inferior glenohumeral ligament. We always ask the patient whether he or she can appreciate the translation, and if the patient responds "yes," we ask whether this sensation reproduces the symptoms.

There are several aspects to this test that may limit its clinical utility. First, any patient who is at all guarded can make the

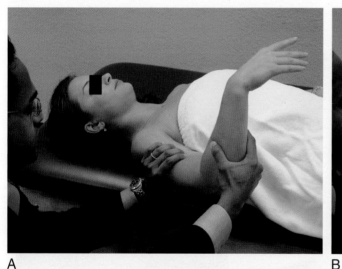

A

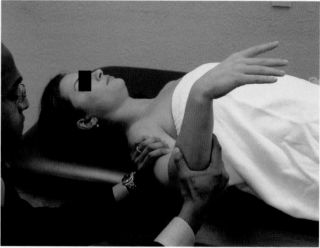

B

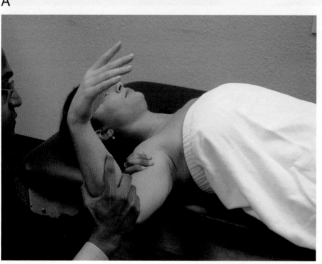

C

Figure 16-26 Load and shift test. **A,** Abduction supine. **B,** 45 degrees supine. **C,** 90 degrees supine.

test unreliable. Second, as anterior instability is normally a problem with the inferior glenohumeral ligament, it would make sense that the most useful portion of the test would be done at 90 degrees of abduction. Unfortunately, achieving this position requires that one of the examiner's hands hold the patient's arm there, which then prevents it from being used to stabilize the scapula. Thus, the mobility of the scapula on the thorax decreases the sensitivity of the test. Finally, although the load and shift test can be learned to detect subtle differences in side-to-side laxity, we do not treat laxity. As stated before, laxity is a clinical *sign* and instability is a *symptom*.

Posterior Tests

The workhorse test for posterior instability is the push-pull test (Fig. 16-27). This is performed in the supine patient by holding the patient's arm at the wrist at 90 degrees abduction and neutral rotation.[5,9] The examiner places the other hand on the proximal humerus and, while pulling with the arm holding the patient's wrist, pushes with the arm on the proximal humerus. This is often enough to maximally translate the patient's humeral head posteriorly. Again, the test is positive only when the maneuver reproduces the patient's symptoms, and in our experience, the patient's response to this test is not subtle. The only caution here is to be sure to differentiate between pain and instability because we have found the former to be consistently present with posterosuperior labral tears.

Jahnke or "Jerk" Test   This test is performed in the seated or supine patient by placing the affected arm in maximal horizontal adduction with internal rotation.[5,9] A posterior force is then applied (Fig. 16-28). In the patient with posterior instability, this starting position will sublux or dislocate the shoulder posteriorly, and care is taken to ask the patient whether this maneuver reproduces specific symptoms. Next, the shoulder is brought back from horizontal adduction while maintaining the posterior force on the humerus at the elbow. As the shoulder approaches normal, a clunk may herald the reduction of the subluxed shoulder, which is a positive test. In our experience, this test has few false-positive results and therefore has a good positive predictive value.

Tests for Multidirectional Instability

As patients with MDI often present with a chief complaint of pain, we believe that such tests are more appropriately discussed

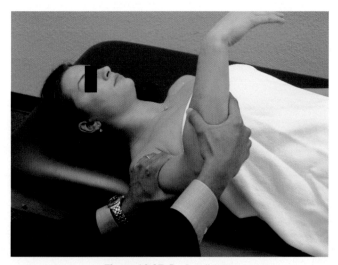

Figure 16-27 Push-pull test.

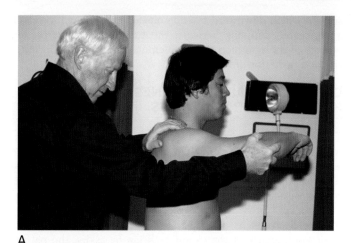

A

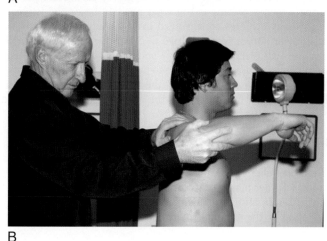

B

Figure 16-28 A and **B,** Jahnke (jerk) test.

in the preceding section. However, there are complementary data that should be included in the evaluation of the patient with MDI. The classic finding associated with MDI is a positive sulcus sign (see Fig. 16-18). This is a visible dimpling between the bottom of the acromion and the top of the humeral head when an inferior traction force is placed on the arm. This is quantified by measuring this acromiohumeral distance in millimeters. It should be remembered that the normal shoulder sits approximately 7 to 8 mm below the acromion, so that an acromiohumeral distance of 1.5 cm is really only 7 to 8 mm of excursion. It is again emphasized that instability implies symptoms and that a positive sulcus sign is not enough to make the diagnosis. Nevertheless, it is an important adjunctive clue for the diagnosis, and when positive, attempts should be made to correlate it with symptoms. When instability is the underlying diagnosis in MDI, patients often will complain that their shoulder comes "out the bottom," and we therefore ask patients this specific question if we are concerned that MDI is the underlying diagnosis.

There are other clues and complexes to note when entertaining the diagnosis of MDI. Many of these patients have generalized ligamentous laxity, which can be measured with such tests as an ability to touch the thumb to the forearm[5,9,23] and hyperextension of the elbow or knee. These patients often will have reproduction of their symptoms in all directions of translational testing and can be difficult to manage conservatively or operatively. Often patients with MDI will demonstrate a sulcus sign, in which downward traction on the humerus will produce a noticeable dimpling between the top of the humerus and bottom of the acromion and will demonstrate laxity in the anterior and posterior directions.

CHIEF COMPLAINT: WEAKNESS, HEAVINESS, OR TIREDNESS

These chief complaints can have several sources. With such complaints, we formulate an initial differential diagnosis of a muscle problem such as scapular dyskinesia, a neurologic problem like suprascapular nerve palsy, or in rare cases (especially with tiredness) a vascular problem, and our workup proceeds from here.

Muscle Sources

We recommend that the examiner begin by asking the patient during which activities and in what position he or she is weak. As so many athletes are involved in year-round strength training, they are often very sensitive to changes in their lifting abilities and will often present early and with subtle findings. The examiner must use enough force to overcome the tested muscle. We use a standard approach to the muscular examination[36] as shown in Table 16-3 (as well as the rotator cuff tests employed as previously described).

Scapular Dyskinesia

The function of the upper extremity is dependent on a number of factors. One of the most important of these is a stable and strong scapular platform to support the motions of the shoulder joint. Abnormalities of this platform may be as subtle as early activation of the scapular rotators to assist in glenohumeral ele-

vation or as pronounced as severe and fixed scapular winging. Such dyskinesia can lead to a variety of chief complaints including pain, weakness, loss of control, and crepitance, among others. Given such a wide variety of chief complaints that can be attributed to this problem, it is rare for any patient *not* to warrant a careful look at the scapular platform.

Scapular dyskinesia is best tested by examining the disrobed patient from behind. The patient is asked to repeatedly elevate and lower the arms at a moderate pace, while the examiner notes the scapula for signs of dyskinesia or winging. Static winging will often signify either a long thoracic or spinal accessory nerve palsy, while dynamic winging or early substitution will often point to compensation for a glenohumeral joint abnormality. Winging can be maximized by performing resisted shoulder flexion at about 30 degrees of elevation (see Fig. 16-20), by asking the patient to perform a wall push-up, or by having the patient use his or her arms to rise from a chair.

When winging is noted on examination, it is helpful to guess whether it is primary, as in a nerve palsy, or secondary, in compensating for a diseased glenohumeral joint. Findings associated with a primary cause include a static or fixed scapular wing that is often painless, while a compensatory dyskinesia is often more subtle, presenting as early substitution during elevation with associated glenohumeral abnormalities. In either case, it is important for the examiner to note these findings to suggest correction of both the dyskinesia and the underlying shoulder abnormality.

Neurologic Sources of Weakness

Any athlete who presents with weakness about the shoulder should also be suspected of having a neurologic cause. The most common sources of this in the athlete are compression at the level of the cervical spine and neuropathy of the suprascapular nerve.[4,37]

A thorough understanding of the cervical spine neurologic examination is a baseline requirement for any shoulder examiner. Since cervical spine pathology can present as pain, paresthesias, or weakness about the shoulder, it is therefore a part of the shoulder workup. Although provocative maneuvers for reproduction of radiculopathy were presented in the section on pain, the specific neuroanatomy pertinent to the sensory and motor examination of the cervical spine is listed in Table 16-4.

It is uncommon that a radiculopathy will result in weakness without pain, and the examiner is referred to the cervical spine sources for shoulder pain in the previous section. Any findings of weakness should be cross-checked for pain with the various cervical spine provocative tests to strengthen or discredit the suspicion of a cervical source for the shoulder symptoms.

Table 16-3 Muscle Tests around the Shoulder Area	
Muscle	*Test*
Trapezius	Shoulder shrug
Deltoid	Resisted abduction
Biceps	Resisted forearm supination
Triceps	Resisted elbow flexion
Brachialis	Resisted elbow extension
Wrist flexors	Resisted wrist flexion
Wrist extensors	Resisted wrist extension
Interossei	Resisted finger abduction

Table 16-4 Neurologic Levels in the Upper Extremity			
Nerve Root	*Sensory*	*Motor*	*Reflex*
C5	Lateral deltoid	Deltoid abduction	Biceps
C6	Thumb	Biceps/wrist extension	Brachioradialis/biceps
C7	Middle finger	Triceps/wrist flexors/finger extension	Triceps
C8	Ulnar border of middle finger	Finger flexors	—
T1	Medial side proximal arm	Finger abduction	—

Suprascapular Nerve

This is a common cause of weakness in the athlete and should be considered high on the list when an athlete presents with a complaint of weakness in external rotation or elevation, especially with an intact rotator cuff. The examiner should be mindful of the anatomy of the nerve and recall that it has two chief sites of entrapment. The first is at the suprascapular notch, where such compression would result in both supraspinatus and infraspinatus weakness and possibly atrophy, while the second site of entrapment, the spinoglenoid notch, will usually spare the supraspinatus. Thus, if one notes weakness in Jobe's position and in external rotation, the differential might include either a large tear of the rotator cuff or a suprascapular nerve entrapment. Such a large tear would normally require a history of significant trauma in the young athlete, and therefore the two diagnoses are often easily differentiated. Compression of this nerve has been reported in volleyball players,[38] baseball players,[39] and gymnasts.[40] Sometimes a patient will present with isolated infraspinatus atrophy and weakness. In such patients, consideration should be given to an isolated compression of the suprascapular nerve at the spinoglenoid notch. A common cause of this in athletes is a ganglion cyst in conjunction with a posterior or posterosuperior labral tear.[38] These tears usually cause pain and often can demonstrate tenderness, atrophy, and weakness on examination.[41]

Brachial Neuritis

Although not a true compressive neuropathy, the acute onset of brachial neuritis has been documented in athletes[42] and may manifest as weakness in a patchy distribution of C5 to T1 neurologic levels. A more complete discussion of this condition is presented in the section on pain, as that is the far more common presentation of this condition.

Finally, chief complaints of weakness, heaviness, or tiredness should lead the examiner to think of a vascular source. One such source is "effort thrombosis,"[43] which is venous thrombosis of the axillary or subclavian veins in close proximity to the intersection of the clavicle and first rib. Specific findings in this diagnosis include venous engorgement of the arm, upper extremity swelling of several centimeters, discoloration, and palpable cords.

CHIEF COMPLAINT: NUMBNESS OR TINGLING—PARESTHESIAS

There are a number of conditions that may lead the athlete to seek treatment for numbness or tingling. If one rules out the possible cervical pathologies discussed previously, then the initial differential should concentrate on sources of peripheral nerve compression. The pertinent sources include thoracic outlet syndrome, burners, and brachial neuritis. If distal in the arm, compression of the median and ulnar nerves may also be considered.

Thoracic outlet syndrome is an uncommon, but important source of paresthesias in the athlete. It is associated with neurologic symptoms in over 90% of patients and presents with primary vascular symptoms in only 3% to 5% of cases.[43] This syndrome often presents in throwers and racquet sports athletes, is often insidious, and can present as pain or heaviness. Neurologic findings can vary, but usually involve the lower brachial plexus and affect the forearm and hand.[44] However, thoracic outlet syndrome has also been reported to manifest as a high radial nerve palsy with triceps weakness in tennis players.[45,46]

Provocative Maneuvers for Thoracic Outlet Syndrome

Perhaps the best test for thoracic outlet syndrome is with overhead exercises consisting of slow, repetitive opening and closing of the hand in the elevated position looking for reproduction of symptoms.[9] In addition, several maneuvers have been described to detect the neurovascular symptoms that result from compression of the thoracic outlet.

Adson's Maneuver

This is accomplished by palpating the patient's radial pulse in a seated position with the arm at the side (Fig. 16-29). The patient is instructed to hold his or her breath while the arm is extended and the head rotated toward the side being examined. The examiner documents a diminution in the radial pulse, which is recorded as a positive finding for vascular compression (Fielding's modification). We modify this test by turning the patient's head away from the side being examined[5,9] and deem a positive test not only by a decrease in pulse, but by reproduction of symptoms.

Hyperabduction Syndrome Test

In this test, the radial pulses are again monitored for change with the arms brought from resting to a hyperabducted position. It should be noted that 20% of individuals will demonstrate a diminution of the radial pulse in this position, so attention should be paid to asymmetry.[5]

Wright's Test

This test is performed by abducting, extending, and externally rotating the arm.[47] It is traditionally a test to monitor decrease in radial pulse, but we again modify this for reproduction of the patient's specific symptoms to call the test positive.

In addition to these findings, thoracic outlet syndrome can rarely present with vascular symptoms like engorgement and increased arm circumference, raising suspicion of thrombosis as described previously.

It is important to note that although burners and brachial neuritis more commonly present as pain and dysesthesias, some patients have a difficult time describing their symptoms, so that such complaints should illicit some suspicion of these diagnoses.

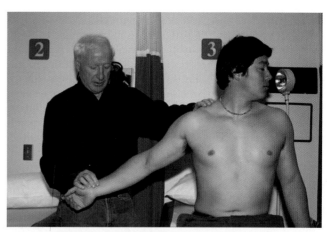

Figure 16-29 Modified Adson's maneuver.

CHIEF COMPLAINT: CATCHING OR CLUNKING

When a patient presents with catching or clunking, the differential should include a SLAP tear or other labral lesions, a loose body, an osteochondral defect, or instability. Note that these mechanical symptoms are different from the "popping" or "crackling" that is such a common finding with subacromial crepitance. It is usually not difficult to differentiate between the two, as usually the noise from the subacromial space is not accompanied by much disability, while true mechanical symptoms generally are immediately, though often temporarily, disabling. The patient should be asked to attempt to reproduce the symptoms. This is an important step, as the active shoulder motions that can get the shoulder to catch are often not demonstrated on passive movement of the joint. If the symptoms can be reproduced by the patient, we attempt to temporarily provide relief with an injection. As most causes of mechanical symptoms of the shoulder are intra-articular, we generally begin with an intra-articular injection. The injection should relieve any painful or disabling symptoms with the provocative maneuvers and also may temporarily relieve the mechanical symptom itself because the increase in intra-articular fluid often cushions the inside of the joint. If the injection is effective, an imaging modality will sometimes provide the specific cause of the mechanical symptom.

CHIEF COMPLAINT: NOISE

One very common chief complaint, or at least a common concern, for athletes is "popping," "crunching," or "grinding" in the shoulder. This can run the spectrum from completely asymptomatic, inaudible noise to painful cracks that concern the patient and the examiner alike. Crepitus in the shoulder girdle should suggest an initial differential of subacromial (impingement), glenohumeral (degenerative arthritis, chondral defect, loose body), or scapulothoracic (subscapular bursitis) source. The goal of the examiner with these patients is to find out whether the noise is associated with an additional chief complaint such as pain. By having the patient or examiner reproduce the noise, it can usually be localized to its origin. The examiner should ask the patient whether the popping is associated with the pain or simply occurs but is not painful in and of itself. One might ask if the popping is taken away, would the shoulder be perfect, that is, is the patient there regarding the noise or some other reason like pain? The most common source of crepitus in the shoulder is subacromial associated with impingement. It is important to note that although the patient may associate the noise with symptoms, the patient with impingement will often demonstrate the crepitus for the examiner to hear and will not be nearly as painful demonstrating the crepitus as during maneuvers like the Neer sign. This is in contrast with the patient who is reluctant to demonstrate his or her crepitus because each and every time they do, it hurts. This is often less like grinding and more like a series of larger "cracks" that will be obviously painful with each iteration. This second type may be associated with an intra-articular source, and one should think of a loose body or a cartilage defect. It is rare to treat such noise in the absence of pain or disability.

Once the examiner has a good sense of the degree of disability of the popping as an isolated entity, he or she should move on to trying to reproduce the popping. This may be done by placing a hand on the top of the shoulder and asking the patient to reproduce the noise. A patient who moves his or her glenohumeral joint through a range of motion to demonstrate the noise is likely to have a subacromial source. This is a softer crepitus than the patient who has the painful bone-on-bone grind of arthritis. The examiner should pay particular attention to a patient who, when asked to reproduce the noise, moves only slightly from the glenohumeral joint, but reproduces the crepitus by moving the scapula or shrugging the shoulders. This is a classic finding in a patient with subscapular crepitus.

Once demonstrated, the examiner should specifically ask whether the crepitus is the chief complaint. Patients with subacromial symptoms will often be able to differentiate the two, but patients with intra-articular sources often will not. If pain is the true chief complaint, with the crepitus coexistent, the examiner should attempt to use the previously illustrated techniques to narrow the source of the pain and to use various injection tests to eliminate the pain and arrive at a diagnosis. It should be noted that crepitus may or may not be silenced by the injection, and attention should again be directed to alleviation of the patient's symptoms, not the associated noise.

CHIEF COMPLAINT: LOSS OF CONTROL AND/OR VELOCITY

When a patient presents with this complaint, the initial differential should include dynamic instability often associated with SLAP tears and internal impingement as well as muscle weakness and scapular dyskinesia. Throwing is an extremely complex athletic maneuver and relies on the specific coordination of the entire kinetic chain. This chief complaint is often among the most difficult to discern because, by its nature, it implies that the athlete is able to throw, and thus the impediment is usually a subtle one. In addition, as this often is a dynamic complaint (i.e., only demonstrated when the patient is throwing), reproducing the patient's symptoms may not be possible in the office. It is sometimes necessary to go to the field or the weight room to illicit signs or reproduce the patient's symptoms. In spite of the difficulty of symptom reproduction, there are some techniques that will help in the approach to this chief complaint.

Does the loss of control/decreased speed happen in initial or in later innings? In the thrower who complains of decreased velocity or loss of control that is present at the outset of throwing, the initial differential should point more toward a static condition affecting the kinetic chain. It is important to remember that the chain starts in the core with the legs and trunk, and although here we emphasize the shoulder, it is important to appreciate that such problems often originate lower in the chain. The astute examiner will do well to inquire and examine the lower extremities and trunk for causes of shoulder pathology. If the core is functioning properly, then the shoulder differential should include causes of weakness, subtle instability, SLAP tears, and cuff problems. We refer the reader to those sections for the focused examinations for those pathologies.

If a pitcher starts out normally but loses command later, the problem is more likely dynamic. This makes the evaluation more challenging because findings may be minimal in an office evaluation. The importance of "revving up" the shoulder is emphasized. The initial differential includes dynamic fatigue or instability. As a pitcher continues to throw, he may become fatigued in any segment of his kinetic chain, leading to compensatory maneuvers like "dropping the elbow," a straighter lead leg, or less external rotation at the shoulder.[48] Although it is beyond the scope of this chapter to specifically address these

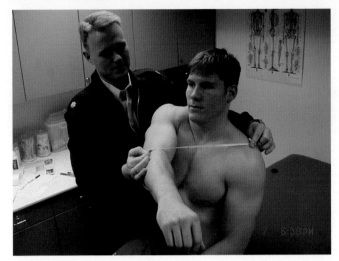

Figure 16-30 Coracoantecubital distance for measurement of posterior capsular tightness.

compensations, they have been noted by pitching coaches for years and lead to increasing strains in the shoulder should the athlete continue to pitch. This may lead to new shoulder problems that will be difficult to completely eliminate until the more proximal elements of the chain are evaluated and rehabilitated.

CHIEF COMPLAINT: STIFFNESS

True stiffness, defined as a mechanical block to passive motion, can present with or without pain and can be global or in selected motions. In most athletes, stiffness occurs in the presence of a painful shoulder. When stiffness does coincide with pain, the reader is directed to the pain as chief complaint section, as diagnosis and treatment of the pain source will often lead to resolution of the stiffness. Occasionally, stiffness can contribute to pain, especially in the throwing athlete. One example of this is the development of posterior capsular tightness in pitchers. This is likely an adaptive change from the powerful forces created in repetitive pitching. This stiffness can be measured as the distance between the coracoid and the antecubital fossa when the athlete is in a position of maximal horizontal adduction with a straight elbow (Fig. 16-30). Other causes of stiffness in the shoulder include adhesive capsulitis, osteoarthritis, or synovitis. In addition, patients who have had previous anterior stabiliza-

tions should be closely examined for overtightening, especially limiting external rotation, as these patients can present with such selective stiffness.

CONCLUSIONS

Over the course of this chapter, we have attempted to present a focused approach to the evaluation of the athlete's shoulder that begins with an understanding of the patient's chief complaint and, based on this, immediately forms a differential diagnosis. The accuracy of this differential is enhanced by asking the right questions in the history such as onset, character, duration, clinical course, degree of disability, and response to clinical intervention. This differential-directed approach then guides the remainder of the encounter.

The physical examination of the overhead and throwing athlete remains an even more challenging art. However, with knowledge of various tests and techniques, the examiner can often narrow its focus. The examination should be organized and comprehensive, but with expectations for findings directed by the differential ("going for the money"). Finally, when possible, and especially when pain is a chief complaint, we are liberal in our use of local anesthetic to temporarily and completely relieve the patient's chief complaint as an aid to narrowing the diagnosis.

The advantage of the differential-directed approach is that it establishes a suspected diagnosis at the beginning of the encounter and guides the examiner as to what to look for during the examination. When one elicits expected positive findings, one's suspicions of the diagnosis are strengthened. However, even when the examiner is surprised by unexpected findings, it will redirect him or her toward another diagnosis that is also in the differential.

Formulating a differential at the beginning of the encounter, however, does have its risks. One must be careful not to be convinced too quickly, as overconfidence will lead to a biased interpretation of the physical examination findings and can result in a misdiagnosis. In addition, the quality of the differential and the skill of validating it depend largely on the examiner's knowledge of shoulder pathology and the various forms in which it presents. We have attempted to describe the process of this focused approach and hope that by formulating a short list of diagnoses early in the encounter, the examiner will be more directed, efficient, and accurate in the approach to the athlete's shoulder.

REFERENCES

1. Sher JS, Uribe JW, Posada A, et al: Abnormal findings on magnetic resonance images of asymptomatic shoulders. J Bone Joint Surg Am 1995;77:10–15.
2. Miniaci A, Mascia AT, Salonen DC, Becker EJ: Magnetic resonance imaging of the shoulder in asymptomatic professional baseball pitchers. Am J Sports Med 2002;30:66–73.
3. Traughber PD, Goodwin TE: Shoulder MRI: Arthroscopic correlation with emphasis on partial tears. J Comput Assist Tomogr 1992;16:129–133.
4. King JW, Brelsford HJ, Tullos HS: Analysis of the pitching arm of the professional baseball pitcher. Clin Orthop 1969;67:116–123.
5. Krishnan SG, Hawkins RJ, Bokor DJ: Clinical evaluation of shoulder problems. In Rockwood CA, Matsen FA (eds): The Shoulder, 3rd ed. Philadelphia, Elsevier, 2004.
6. Hawkins RJ: Musculoskeletal Examination: An Organized Approach to Musculoskeletal Examination and History Taking. Boston, Mosby-Year Book, 1995.
7. Calis M, Akgun K, Birtane M, et al: Diagnostic values of clinical diagnostic tests in subacromial impingement syndrome. Ann Rheum Dis 2000;59:44–47.
8. MacDonald PB, Clark P, Sutherland K: An analysis of the diagnostic accuracy of the Hawkins and Neer subacromial impingement signs. J Shoulder Elbow Surg 2000;9:299–301.
9. Boublik M, Silliman JF: History and physical examination. In Hawkins RJ, Misamore GW (eds): Shoulder Injuries in the Athlete. New York, Churchill Livingstone, 1996, pp 9–22.
10. Yocum LA: Assessing the shoulder. History, physical examination, differential diagnosis, and special tests used. Clin Sports Med 1983;2:281–289.
11. Itoi E, Kido T, Sano A, et al: Which is more useful, the "full can test" or the "empty can test," in detecting the torn supraspinatus tendon? Am J Sports Med 1999;27:65–68.
12. Gerber C, Krushell RJ: Isolated rupture of the tendon of the sub-

scapularis muscle. Clinical features in 16 cases. J Bone Joint Surg (Am) 1991;73:389–394.

13. Tokish JM, Decker M, Ellis H, et al: The belly press test for the physical examination of the subscapularis muscle: Electromyographic validation and comparison to the lift-off test. Paper presented at the American Shoulder and Elbow Surgeons 3rd Biennial Open Meeting, 2002, Orlando, FL.

14. Hertel R, Ballmer FT, Lombert SM, Gerber C: Lag signs in the diagnosis of rotator cuff rupture. J Shoulder Elbow Surg 1996;5:307–313.

15. Codman EA: The Shoulder: Rupture of the Supraspinatus Tendon and Other Lesions in or about the Subacromial Bursa. Boston, Thomas Todd, 1934.

16. Wolf EM, Agrawal V: Transdeltoid palpation (the rent test) in the diagnosis of rotator cuff tears. J Shoulder Elbow Surg 2001;10:470–473.

17. Petersson CJ: The acromioclavicular joint in rheumatoid arthritis. Clin Orthop 1987;223:86–93.

18. O'Brien SJ, Pagnani MJ, Fealy S, et al: The active compression test: A new and effective test for diagnosing labral tears and acromioclavicular joint abnormality. Am J Sports Med 1998;26:610–613.

19. Bennett WF: Specificity of the Speed's test: Arthroscopic technique for evaluation the biceps tendon at the level of the bicipital groove. Arthroscopy 1998;14:789–796.

20. Matsen FA, Kirby R: Office evaluation and management of shoulder pain. Orthop Clin North Am 1982;13:453–475.

21. Snyder SJ, Karzel RP, Del Pizzo W, et al: SLAP lesions of the shoulder. Arthroscopy 1990;6:274–279.

22. Berg EE, Ciullo JV: A clinical test for superior glenoid labral or 'SLAP' lesions. Clin J Sport Med 1998;8:121–123.

23. Kim SH, Ha KI, Ahn JH, et al: Biceps load test II: A clinical test for SLAP lesions of the shoulder. Arthroscopy 2001;17:160–164.

24. Kibler WB: Specificity and sensitivity of the anterior slide test in throwing athletes with superior glenoid labral tears. Arthroscopy 1995;11:296–300.

25. Dines DM, Warren RF, Inglis AE, et al: The coracoid impingement syndrome. J Bone Joint Surg Br 1990;72:314–316.

26. Paley KJ, Jobe FW, Pink MM, et al: Arthroscopic findings in the overhand throwing athlete: Evidence for posterior internal impingement of the rotator cuff. Arthroscopy 2000;16:35–40.

27. Tong HC, Haig AJ, Yamakawa K: The Spurling test and cervical radiculopathy. Spine 2002;15:156–159.

28. Porter P, Fernandez GN: Stretch-induced spinal accessory nerve palsy: A case report. J Shoulder Elbow Surg 2001;10:92–93.

29. Post M, Mayer J: Suprascapular nerve entrapment: Diagnosis and treatment. Clin Orthop 1987;223:125–136.

30. Ringel SP, Treihaft M, Carry M, et al: Suprascapular neuropathy in pitchers. Am J Sports Med 1990;18:80–86.

31. Rowe CR (ed): The Shoulder. New York, Churchill Livingstone, 1988, p 419.

32. Zaslav KR: Internal rotation resistance strength test: A new diagnostic test to differentiate intra-articular pathology from outlet (Neer) impingement syndrome in the shoulder. J Shoulder Elbow Surg 2001;10:23–27.

33. Partington PF, Broome GH: Diagnostic injection around the shoulder: Hit and miss? A cadaveric study of injection accuracy. J Shoulder Elbow Surg 1998;7:147–150.

34. Matsen FA, Thomas SC, Rockwood CA, Wirth MA: Glenohumeral instability. In Rockwood CA, Matsen FA (eds): The Shoulder, 2nd ed. Philadelphia, WB Saunders, 1998, pp 611–754.

35. Hovis WD, Dean MT, Mallon WJ, Hawkins RJ: Posterior instability of the shoulder with secondary impingement in elite golfers. Am J Sports Med 2002;30:886–890.

36. Netter FH: The CIBA Collection of Medical Illustrations: Musculoskeletal System Part I: Anatomy, Physiology and Metabolic Disorders. Ciba-Geigy Corporation, 1991, p 29.

37. Fielding JW, Francis WR, Hensinger RN: The cervical and thoracic spine. In Cruess RJ, Rennie WRJ (eds): Adult Orthopaedics, vol 2. New York, Churchill Livingstone, 1984, pp 747–841.

38. Feretti A, Cerullo G, Russo G: Suprascapular neuropathy in volleyball players. J Bone Joint Surg Am 1987;69:260–263.

39. Bryan WJ, Wild JJ: Isolated infraspinatus atrophy: A common cause of posterior shoulder pain and weakness in the throwing athlete. Am J Sports Med 1989;17:130–131.

40. Lauland T, Fedders O, Sgaard I, Kornum M: Suprascapular nerve compression syndrome. Surg Neurol 1984;22:308–310.

41. Piatt BE, Hawkins RJ, Fritz RC, et al: Clinical evaluation and treatment of spinoglenoid notch ganglion cysts. J Shoulder Elbow Surg 2002;11:600–604.

42. Hershman EB, Wilbourn AJ, Bergfeld JA: Acute brachial neuropathy in athletes. Am J Sports Med 1989;17:655–659.

43. DiFelice GS, Paletta GA, Phillips BB, Wright RW: Effort thrombosis in the elite throwing athlete. Am J Sports Med 2002;30:708–712.

44. Duralde XA, Bigliani LU: Neurologic disorders. In Hawkins RJ, Misamore GW (eds): Shoulder Injuries in the Athlete. New York, Churchill Livingstone, 1996, pp 243–265.

45. Mitsunga MM, Nakano K: High radial nerve palsy following strenuous muscular activity. Clin Orthop 1982;98:39–42.

46. Priest JD: The shoulder of the tennis player. Clin Sports Med 1988;7:387–402.

47. Wright IS: The neurovascular syndrome produced by hyperabduction of the arm. Am Heart J 1945;29:1–4.

48. Murray TA, Cook TD, Werner SL, et al: The effects of extended play on professional pitchers. Am J Sports Med 2001;29:137–142.

In This Chapter

INTRODUCTION

- A reproducible, consistent setup facilitates successful shoulder arthroscopy.

- Adherence to several simple principles and techniques optimizes visualization and access to shoulder pathology.

- Familiarity with a variety of hardware, knot-tying principles, and suture management gives the surgeon the flexibility to complete most arthroscopic shoulder procedures efficiently and successfully.

PREOPERATIVE PREPARATION

Positioning

Positioning the patient may seem trivial, but if done inappropriately, it may aggravate cervical spine, lumbar spine, or other patient pathology. In addition, poor positioning adds to the difficulty of the procedure.

Patients may be positioned in either the lateral decubitus or beach chair position. Other positions have been described including hybrids of the beach chair and lateral decubitus positions.[1] We perform all shoulder arthroscopy in the beach chair position.

A Schloein positioner (Orthopedic Systems, Union City, CA) is used to support the patient in a seated position (Fig. 17-1). The design of the Schloein allows easy access to the posterior aspect of the shoulder. Once the patient is asleep, the back of the Schloein is lifted to place the patient in a seated position. The bed controls are adjusted to flex the torso at the waist and lower the legs slightly. A pillow is placed beneath the knees to minimize strain on the lower back. The headrest is adjusted and foam is placed behind the head if necessary to keep the neck in a neutral position in the sagittal plane. A forehead strap and chin strap with Velcro control the head and a chest strap, waist strap, and leg strap control the torso. These steps are essential to allow for ease of arthroscopy while minimizing stress on the patient's cervical or lumbar spine during the procedure. If the patient is not secure or is leaning to one side, the procedure becomes significantly more difficult and a successful shoulder procedure may be tainted by complaints of neck and back pain (Box 17-1).

Special Equipment

Once the patient is in position, accessory equipment is arranged appropriately. We use a McConnell arm holder (McConnell Orthopedics, Greenville, TX; see Fig. 17-1C) or a Spider Limb Positioner (Smith-Nephew Endoscopy, Andover, MA) to optimize the use of the first assistant. A standard arthroscopic tower is positioned toward the patient's feet on the contralateral side to allow a good view for the surgeon. An arthroscopy pump is used to allow the surgeon to control pressure and flow to optimize visualization.

Interscalene Block

An interscalene block is beneficial prior to all arthroscopic shoulder procedures. This decreases pain, which may elevate blood pressure during the procedure. By helping to control the blood pressure, the interscalene block improves visualization.

Preparing and Draping the Patient

The most important principle of sterilely cleaning and draping the patient is to ensure that the surgeon has easy access to all potential portal sites. The Schloein positioner allows for ample posterior access. We use split sheets to drape the patient, but any drape that allows ample access is sufficient. An arthroscopy pouch is also useful to keep the floor dry. Care should also be taken to cover the patient toward the head to minimize the possibility of contamination during the procedure from the anesthesia poles and other equipment.

Personnel

The essential elements of the operative team include the surgeon, the scrub nurse, the circulator, the first assistant, and the anesthesiologist.[2] Each must be in tune with the operative procedure to minimize surgeon anxiety and optimize the surgical results. Both the circulator and the scrub nurse must be familiar not only with the equipment, but also with the steps of the given procedure to ensure that the surgeon receives the appropriate equipment in a timely fashion. The first assistant must be capable, at a minimum, of holding the arthroscopic camera appropriately during knot tying and retrieving suture during suture passage. In addition, simple maneuvers such as providing counterpressure for instrument passage or holding a cannula steady as an instrument is passed in or out of the joint can greatly facilitate the procedure.

The anesthesiologist plays the essential role of maintaining a systolic blood pressure as close to 90 to 100 mm Hg as possible

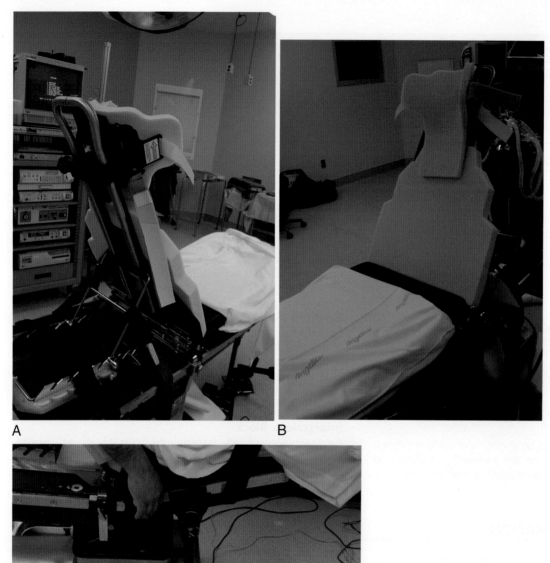

A

B

C

Figure 17-1 **A,** Posterior view of Schloein positioner. **B,** Anterior view. **C,** McConnell arm holder.

if not contraindicated for the patient. As mentioned previously, the interscalene block is one measure that helps to achieve this goal. By keeping the blood pressure low, intra-articular bleeding is minimized, which allows the surgeon to adequately visualize the joint with an intra-articular pump pressure between 40 and 60 mm Hg.[3]

Examination under Anesthesia

The procedure actually begins prior to making an incision. The shoulder should always be examined. The contralateral shoulder is also examined to allow comparison of shoulder translation and range of motion. The examination under anesthesia may iden-

tify stiffness not recognized previously due to pain. A simple manipulation at the beginning of the procedure may be of great benefit. For instability procedures, it defines the degree of instability and the existing range of motion, which dictate the goals of the procedure.

OPERATIVE PEARLS

Portals

Poor portal position can easily convert a relatively simple procedure to a very difficult one. Beginner arthroscopists may

Box 17-1 Preparation

- Proper positioning is critical.
- Lateral decubitus or beach chair position is ideal.
- Interscalene block allows for better blood pressure control and helps with visualization.

Box 17-2 Primary Portals

- Posterior, in the "soft spot," superior and lateral for primarily subacromial procedures
- Anteroinferior, just about subscapularis
- Anterosuperior, high in the rotator interval
- Lateral, parallel to the undersurface of the acromion

benefit from marking the skin. Landmarks include the clavicle, acromioclavicular joint, acromion, and coracoid (Fig. 17-2A). Most procedures can be done using three portals, but these portals differ based on the procedure. We use posterior, anteroinferior, anterosuperior, and lateral portals (Box 17-2). A variety of other portals have been described including the Neviaser portal and the port of Wilmington.[4]

The standard posterior portal is generally placed in the soft spot in the posterior aspect of the shoulder. A reasonable landmark is 1.5 to 2 cm inferior and 1.5 to 2 cm medial to the posterolateral acromion. The arthroscope is inserted, aiming slightly medially on an imaginary line directed toward the coracoid. This portal works well for glenohumeral procedures, but we have found that it is a little inferior and medial for subacromial procedures. Consequently, if the anticipated procedure will require more work to be done in the subacromial space, the portal is best placed only 1 cm medial and inferior to the posterolateral corner of the acromion[5] (see Fig. 17-2B).

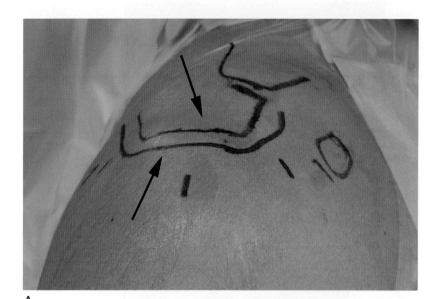

A

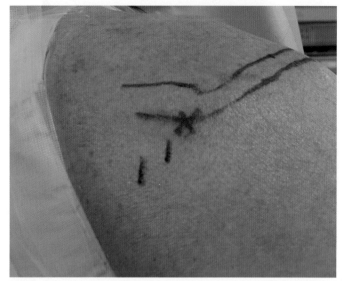

B

Figure 17-2 A, Preoperative marking of a right shoulder. The anterior circle is the coracoid. *Arrows* indicate the superior and inferior edges of the acromion. The portal sites are marked. **B,** Standard and modified posterior portal. The inferomedial portal works best for glenohumeral arthroscopy. The superolateral portal works best for subacromial arthroscopy. (From Gartsman G: Shoulder Arthroscopy. Philadelphia, WB Saunders, 2003.)

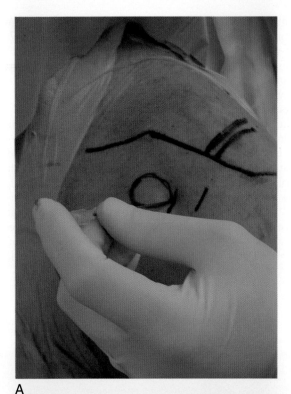

A

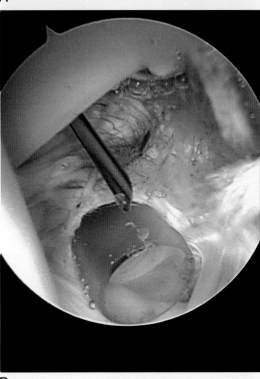

B

Figure 17-3 A, Surface view demonstrating outside-in technique to establish anteroinferior portal. **B,** Articular view through the posterior portal of a left shoulder demonstrating anterosuperior portal relationship to anteroinferior portal. (From Gartsman G: Shoulder Arthroscopy. Philadelphia, WB Saunders, 2003.)

The remaining portals are placed in an outside-in fashion. An inside-out technique may be used, but this may limit the angle of approach for the given pathology. A spinal needle is placed through the skin to ensure not only the correct entry site but also to ensure that the instruments are directed appropriately to address the pathology. The location of the portal is determined by the procedure. For glenohumeral procedures, an anteroinferior portal is established first (Fig. 17-3A). This portal is just above the intra-articular subscapularis and is slightly lateral to the glenoid face. The anterosuperior portal is placed in the rotator interval just anterior to the biceps tendon and more lateral to the inferior portal (see Fig. 17-3B). This allows an appropriate angle to place anchors in the superior and inferior glenoid without injury to the articular surface of the glenoid. Generally, at least a 2-cm skin bridge is maintained between portals to minimize difficulty with instrument manipulation (Fig. 17-4).

A lateral portal is generally used for subacromial pathology. It is established under direct visualization once the arthroscope is placed in the subacromial space. Optimal position is determined with a spinal needle (Fig. 17-5). This portal will be used to perform a bursectomy and place anchors in the greater tuberosity; therefore, it should be high, but it should also be parallel to the undersurface of the acromion. Once each portal is established, we place a cannula to prevent soft-tissue swelling, which may complicate the procedure.[3] The cannulas also facilitate suture management and instrument access to the joint (Fig. 17-6).

Visualization

Visualization is critical to simplifying shoulder arthroscopy. Several maneuvers discussed previously help facilitate good visualization. These include positioning the patient, portal placement, and the use of the outside-in technique, interscalene block, use of a pump to control the pressure, controlled hypotension by the anesthesiologist, and the use of cannulas to control tissue swelling. If these maneuvers fail, other techniques may be implemented. For example, the fluid temperature may be kept lower to prevent bleeding.[3] Additionally, epinephrine may be added to selected bags of fluid. A typical concentration is 1 mg epinephrine in one 3-L bag of saline (0.33 mg/L).[6]

Knot Tying

New instruments and implants are constantly being introduced to facilitate shoulder arthroscopy. However, there is no good substitute for the ability to tie an arthroscopic knot (Box 17-3). This skill adds flexibility to the surgeon's ability to address most shoulder pathology.

Knots can generally be divided into two broad types. These are sliding and nonsliding knots. Nonsliding knots can be referred to as locking knots. A third type of knot is the sliding locking knot. A surgeon should be able to tie at least one slid-

Box 17-3 Knot Tying

- Surgeon should know one sliding knot and one nonsliding knot.
- Sliding knots require a suture to slide through tissue and the suture anchor.
- After the initial locking knot, three half hitches with alternate posts back it up.

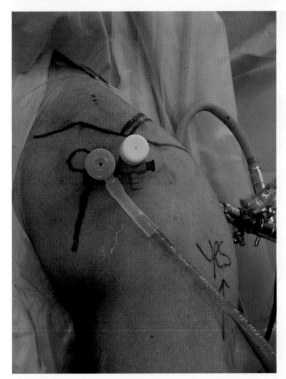

Figure 17-4 A skin bridge is maintained between the two anterior portals. (From Gartsman G: Shoulder Arthroscopy. Philadelphia, WB Saunders, 2003.)

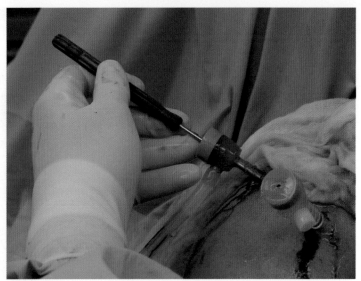

Figure 17-6 Cannulas facilitate passage of instruments into the joint. (From Gartsman G: Shoulder Arthroscopy. Philadelphia, WB Saunders, 2003.)

ing and one nonsliding knot to successfully complete most procedures.

A sliding knot may only be thrown if the suture can slide through the tissue and anchor. This knot is used first to bring the repaired tissue in close apposition with the suture anchor or with other tissue. Locking knots prevent the sliding knot from sliding away from the tissue and losing tension of

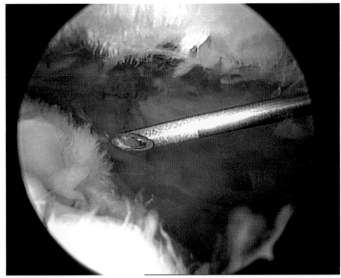

Figure 17-5 Spinal needle used to localize the position of the lateral portal. (From Gartsman G: Shoulder Arthroscopy. Philadelphia, WB Saunders, 2003.)

the repair. We generally use a half hitch followed by square knots for most procedures.[5] The sliding knots are reserved for occasions when we may be tying a knot blindly such as in a closure of a portal.

The first important premise in tying knots is understanding the concept of post and nonpost strands. When a half hitch is created, the two strands of suture may have one of three relationships. In the first two relationships, one suture is wrapped around the second suture (Fig. 17-7A). This is the most common event. The third relationship occurs when each suture is under the same tension and neither suture is wrapped around the other (see Fig. 17-7B). The first two events result in a half-hitch knot (see Fig. 17-7C). The last relationship results in a flat throw designated as half of a square knot (see Fig. 17-7D). If the two sutures are under unequal tension, the suture wrapped around the second suture is designated as the nonpost strand and the other suture is the post strand. The post strand is under more tension than the nonpost strand. The post strand may change at any point in passing the suture by simply altering the tension on each suture. The tension may be manipulated either by pulling on one strand with a hand or using the knot pusher. The post strand is not defined by which strand is manipulated by the knot pusher.

This concept is important because certain configurations of knots have been shown to be biomechanically superior and resist unraveling. Generally, it has been shown that once the tissue is apposed with an initial locking knot, three half hitches with alternate posts and directions of the throw are sufficient to prevent the knot from unraveling and maintaining tissue apposition.[7,8]

We prefer to place the knot pusher on the strand that comes directly from an anchor and does not pass through any tissue (Fig. 17-8A). The initial post strand is the second suture. Two half hitches are thrown sequentially in the same direction while maintaining tension on the post strand (see Fig. 17-8B). As tension is placed on the post strand, the two half hitches will

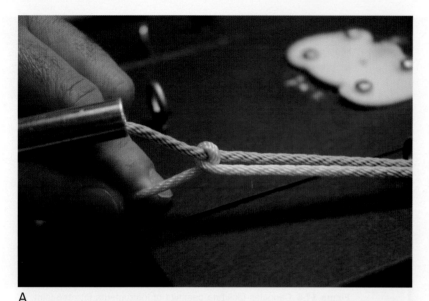

A

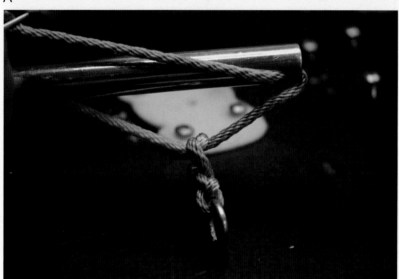

B

Figure 17-7 Rope and a practice board used to demonstrate knot tying concepts. **A,** Two strands under unequal tension. The knot pusher is on the post strand. **B,** Both strands under equal tension. **C,** Two half hitches in same direction posted on the white strand. This can slide down the post before it is locked.

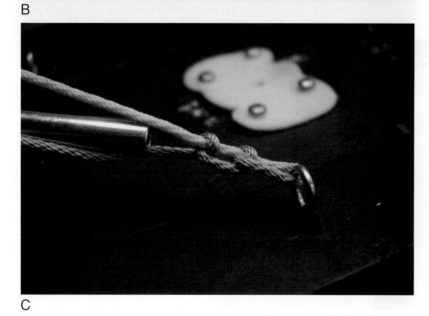

C

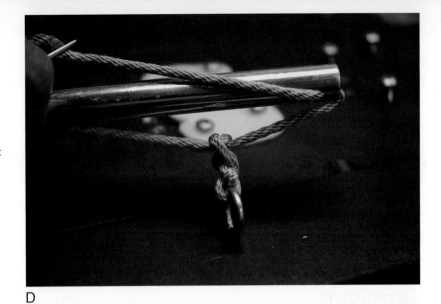

D

Figure 17-7—Cont'd D, Strands under equal tension result in a square throw.

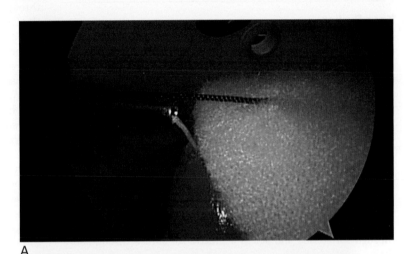

A

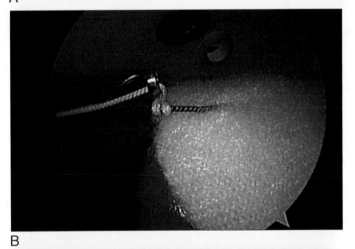

B

Figure 17-8 Arthroscopic model demonstrating knot tying. **A,** Knot pusher is placed on suture coming directly from anchor in tuberosity. **B,** Knot pusher on the nonpost strand slides two half hitches down the post strand. **C,** Arthroscopic square knot.

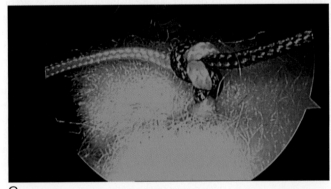

C

not lock. However, if tension is lost on the post strand, the half hitches will prematurely lock, resulting in poor tissue apposition. Once the tissue is apposed, the knot pusher is pushed past the knot to equalize tension and lock the knot in place. Alternatively, a sliding or sliding locking knot may be used on the initial throw. Several of these knots have been published in the literature.[8] This initial knot should be backed up with three more knots. These knots are thrown in alternate directions. Once thrown, the tension should be manipulated to either change post strands on each throw or to equalize the tension. Changing the tension results in a pattern of knots with alternating directions and posts. This is biomechanically sound. However, we prefer to alternate directions and equalize the tension to create sequential square knots (see Fig. 17-8C).

INSTRUMENTS

Knot Pusher

This device is simply used to push the knot through the cannula and into the joint. Several variations have been manufactured. We prefer a simple closed ring. The knot pusher can be used as more than simply an instrument to tie knots. It may also be used to deliver suture to a grasper or even to redirect a suture through fragile soft tissue such as the labrum.[9]

Suture Graspers

These are generally instruments with either an open loop or a closed loop that can be opened. Suture is grasped atraumatically with these instruments. The three types that we use are the crochet hook, the suture grasper, and the Arthropierce device (Smith and Nephew Endoscopy, Andover, MA; Fig. 17-9). The Arthropierce device has a sharp tip that allows it to pass through soft tissue and act as a shuttle for suture through soft tissue.

Suture Cutters

Suture may be cut with a standard arthroscopic scissors. Additionally, an end-cutting device should be available to cut suture blindly such as in a portal closure. Additionally, with the development of new, stronger suture types, specialized cutters may be needed (Arthrex, Naples, FL; Fig. 17-10).

Suture-Passing Instruments

Several instruments have been devised to pass suture through tissue for arthroscopic shoulder surgery. We highlight a few of the devices that we use. Several other companies create devices with a similar concept.

Spectrum (Linvatec, Largo, FL)

The Spectrum set is a cannulated set of curved or straight trocars used to pierce tissue and deliver suture using a manual wheeling mechanism (Fig. 17-11). It is most useful for labral repairs or capsular plications. It may also be useful in side-to-side rotator cuff repairs.

Cuff Stitch (Smith and Nephew Endoscopy)

The cuff stitch is a device with a sharp trocar tip and a needle eye used to pass suture (Fig. 17-12). It has a concave side and convex side. This instrument allows the user to pass a stitch through soft tissue and retrieve it with a grasper. Applications include soft tissue-to-soft tissue repair such as in a side-to-side rotator cuff repair or the passage of suture from suture anchors

through soft tissue such as in a labral or rotator cuff repair. The one technical obstacle is to understand how to load and unload the instrument. The instrument is loaded and unloaded on the same side. For example, if it is loaded through the convex side, it should be unloaded with a grasper from the convex side. Otherwise, the suture traps the instrument in the joint and the suture must be repassed.[10]

Caspari Suture Punch (Linvatec)

The Caspari punch has a manual wheel mechanism similar to the Spectrum devices (Fig. 17-13). It has a jaw that opens and uses a cannulated needle tip to pierce soft tissue.

Elite Pass (Smith and Nephew Endoscopy) and ExpresSew Suture Passer (Surgical Solutions, Valencia, CA)

These devices have a disposable needle that delivers the repair through tissue (Fig. 17-14). They confer a few advantages over the Caspari punch. No suture shuttling is necessary. The needle on each device is longer and, with a triggering device, capable of penetrating thicker tissue. Additionally, the jaws of the ExpresSew and Elite Pass are longer, allowing more substantial inclusion of soft tissue in the repair. The disadvantage of the ExpresSew and Elite Pass when compared with the Caspari punch is the cost of using a disposable needle for each procedure.

When the suture is passed using the ExpresSew or the Elite Pass, it can be retrieved with a hook on the upper jaw of the instrument. However, it may also be retrieved with a tissue grasper and taken out another portal to simplify suture management.

IMPLANTS

These refer to materials left in situ to maintain the repair. For arthroscopic shoulder surgery, these include suture and suture anchors. Most suture that we use is nonabsorbable, braided multifilament suture. Generally, no. 2 suture is used for rotator cuff repairs and 2-0 suture is used for labral repairs. Some new suture types such as FiberWire (Arthrex, Naples, FL) confer greater failure strength. Capsular plications may also be done with no. 1 or 0 polydiaxone suture.

Anchors are either bioabsorbable or metal. Either type may be used, although we prefer metal for rotator cuff repairs. Larger 5.0-mm anchors are used to repair the rotator cuff and smaller 2.8- mm to 3.5-mm anchors are used for glenohumeral repairs.

PRACTICAL CONCEPTS

Organization and consistency are the key to successful shoulder arthroscopy. Certainly, the surgeon must be flexible to deal with a variety of pathologies; however, certain concepts pervade arthroscopic procedures. These include arm positioning (particularly for beach chair), suture management, and shuttling techniques.

Arm position plays an important role in rotator cuff and labral repairs. For rotator cuff repairs, the arm position is varied with some abduction and internal/external rotation to place the greater tuberosity beneath the lateral portal to allow a 90-degree angle of entry into the tuberosity (Fig. 17-15). For labral repairs, the arm is positioned in mild external rotation prior to tying knots to avoid constraining the joint.

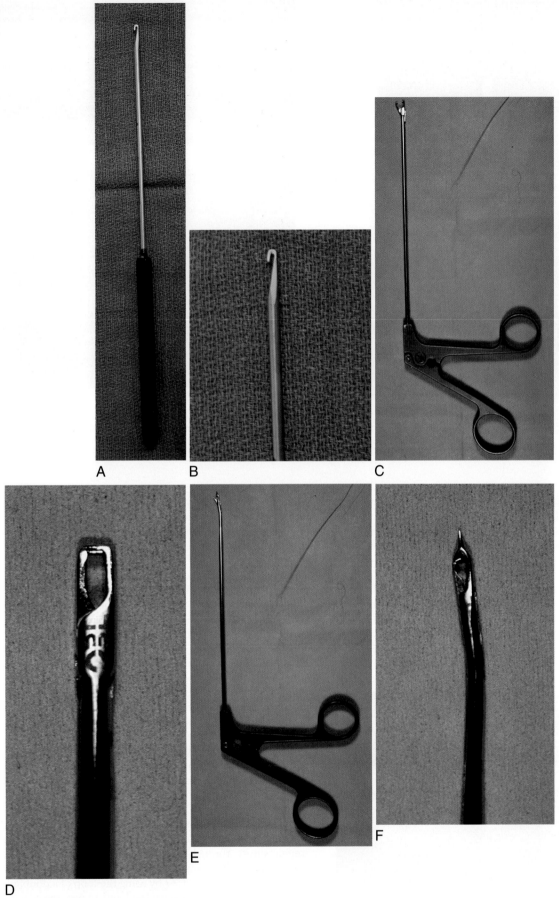

Figure 17-9 A, Crochet hook. **B,** Close-up of crochet hook tip. **C,** Suture grasper. **D,** Close-up of suture grasper tip. **E,** Arthropierce. **F,** Close-up of Arthropierce tip. (**C–F,** From Gartsman G: Shoulder Arthroscopy. Philadelphia, WB Saunders, 2003.)

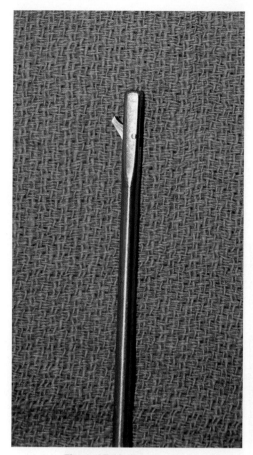

Figure 17-10 Suture cutter.

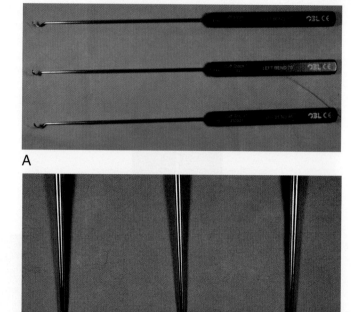

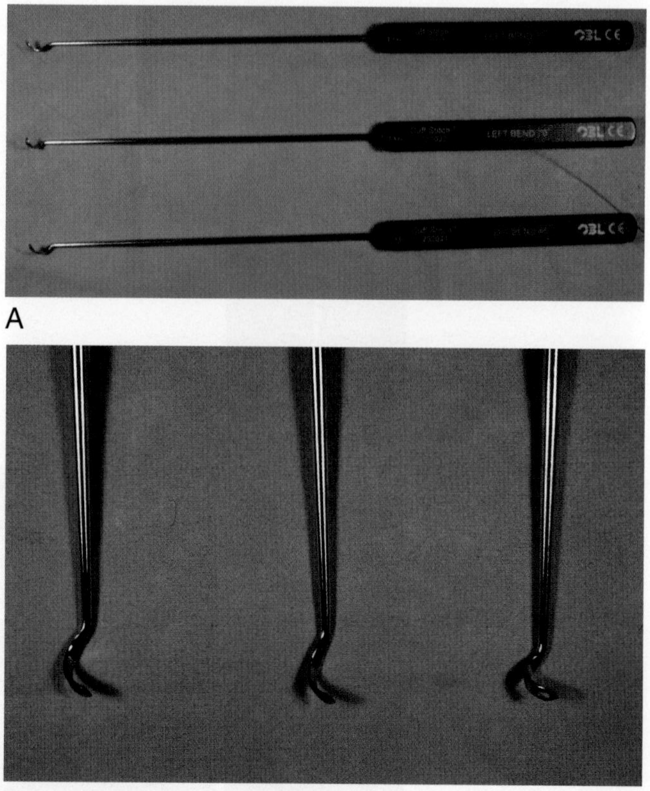

Figure 17-12 A, Cuff stitches. **B,** Close-up view of cuff stitch tips. (From Gartsman G: Shoulder Arthroscopy. Philadelphia, WB Saunders, 2003.)

Suture management is perhaps the most complex and difficult concept to successfully achieve. Anchors need to be placed in a logical progression, and the sutures need to be tied at specific intervals to avoid tangling suture. Judicious use of accessory and working portals helps to minimize tangles. For example, in a rotator cuff repair, we place all the anchors first and group all the sutures in separate clamps in the anterior portal. Sutures are sequentially passed through the rotator cuff from anterior to posterior. Once all sutures are passed, they are sequentially tied down from posterior to anterior. When tying the suture, two important principles should be kept in mind. First, never tie

suture when another suture is in the cannula. This may result in a tangled mess. Second, a suture grasper or knot pusher should be passed into the joint first to remove any twists that may be present between the two sutures to be tied.

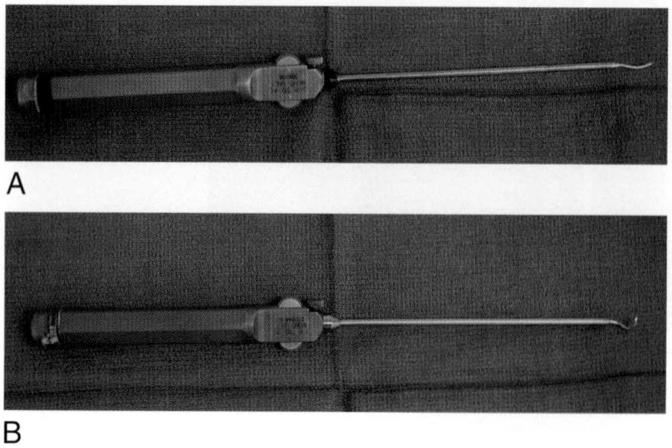

Unlike rotator cuff repairs, all the anchors for a labral repair are not placed prior to passing the suture. This would result in tangled suture. For this reason, generally, the suture from the first anchor is passed through the labral tissue prior to placing the second anchor. Once the suture is passed, the second anchor is placed. The first suture is tied down prior to passing the suture of the second anchor. The same procedure is done with a third anchor. Generally, it is easiest to place the most inferior anchor first and progress superiorly for an anterior labral repair. It is easiest to place the posterior anchor first for a superior labrum anterior to posterior (SLAP) repair if two anchors are to be used.

Suture can be passed through tissue directly or shuttled through tissue indirectly. The ExpresSew, Elite Pass, Cuff Stitch, and several other devices allow direct passage of suture through the rotator cuff, for example. In addition, graspers such as the Arthropierce may pass suture directly through labral, capsular, or rotator cuff tissue. However, suture may also be shuttled through tissue. Devices such as the Caspari or Spectrum may be used to pierce tissue and pass a firm suture such as a single or doubled nylon. This suture can be used to pass the repair suture through the tissue either by tying it directly to the repair suture, using the loop of a doubled suture to lasso the repair suture and pass it, or by using the loop of a doubled suture to pass a second loop (reverse the loop) to pass the repair suture. The final technique is done to facilitate the use of the passing

Figure 17-11 A, Straight spectrum. **B,** Curved spectrum.

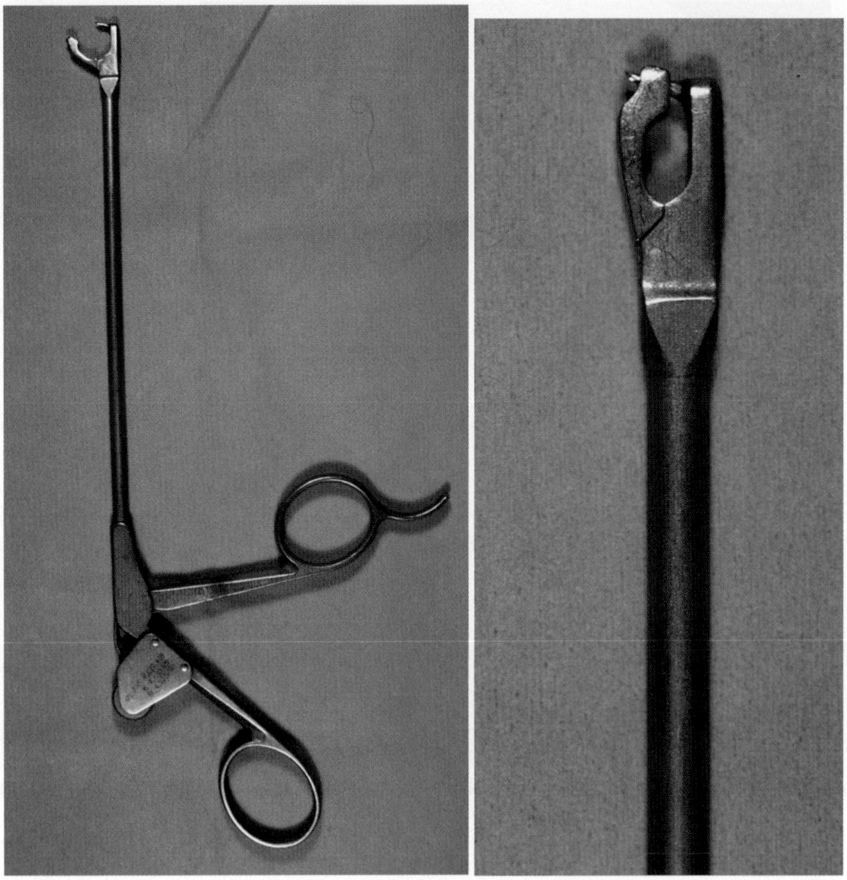

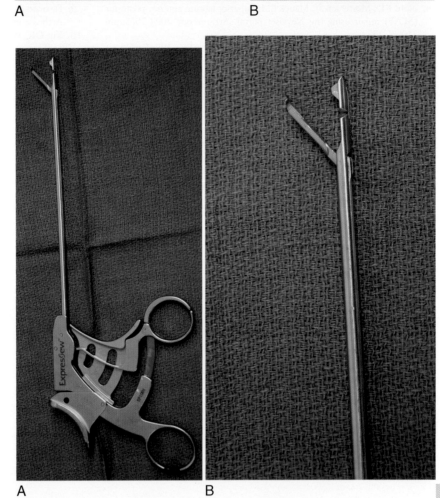

Figure 17-13 A, Caspari suture punch. **B,** Close-up view of Caspari suture punch tip. (From Gartsman G: Shoulder Arthroscopy. Philadelphia, WB Saunders, 2003.)

Figure 17-14 A, ExpresSew. **B,** Close-up view of ExpresSew tip.

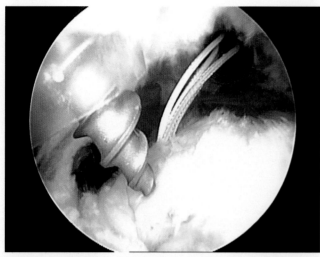

Figure 17-15 Anchor placed 90 degrees to tuberosity. (From Gartsman G: Shoulder Arthroscopy. Philadelphia, WB Saunders, 2003.)

device. For example, it is often easier to pierce labral tissue from the capsular surface. When this is done, the two free ends of a nylon suture are passed from the capsular surface of the labrum to the articular surface. To shuttle a suture from the anchor from the articular surface, a second loop of nylon must be passed first using the initial nylon. This places the loop of the shuttle suture on the articular side. This is termed reversing the loop. This concept may be used for many applications.

CONCLUSIONS

Many factors contribute to the success or failure of shoulder arthroscopy. The surgeon can help him- or herself by ensuring that the patient is appropriately positioned, communicating with the surgical team, being able to use a variety of equipment, and, most importantly, understanding and adhering to a few basic principles. The simple principles outlined in this chapter should provide a foundation for more advanced surgical techniques.

REFERENCES

1. Hoenecke HR, Fronek J, Hardwick M: The modified beach chair position for arthroscopic shoulder surgery: The La Jolla beach chair. Arthroscopy 2004;20(Suppl 2):113–115.
2. Hasan S, Gartsman G: Pearls and pitfalls of arthroscopic rotator cuff repair. Oper Tech Orthop 2002;12:176–185.
3. Boszotta H, Prunner K: Arthroscopically assisted rotator cuff repair. Arthroscopy 2004;20:620–626.
4. Nord KD, Masterson JP, Mauck BM: Superior labrum anterior posterior (SLAP) repair using the Neviaser portal. Arthroscopy 2004;20(Suppl 2):129–133.
5. Gartsman GM: Shoulder Arthroscopy. Philadelphia, WB Saunders, 2003, p 286.
6. Jensen KH, Werther K, Stryger V, et al: Arthroscopic shoulder surgery with epinephrine saline irrigation. Arthroscopy 2001;17:578–581.
7. Loutzenheiser TD, Harryman DT 2nd, Yung SW, et al: Optimizing arthroscopic knots. Arthroscopy 1995;11:199–206.
8. Elkousy H, Sekiya J, Stabile K, et al: A biomechanical comparison of arthroscopic sliding and sliding-locking knots. Arthroscopy 2005;21: 204–210.
9. Favorito PJ: Simplifying arthroscopic suture retrieval with a knot pusher. Arthroscopy 2004;20(Suppl 2):208–209.
10. Yip DK, Wong JW, Kong JK: How to use cuff suture instruments: The concept of "concave in and concave out." Arthroscopy 2004;20(Suppl 2):100–102.

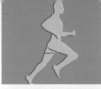

18 Anterior Instability

Craig R. Bottoni

In This Chapter

INTRODUCTION

- Anterior shoulder instability is defined as symptomatic anterior translation of the humerus, most commonly reproduced with the arm in an abducted, externally rotated position.

- Anterior instability is often the sequela of a traumatic glenohumeral dislocation or subluxation episode.

- Patients present with a history of one or several dislocation episodes. On examination, patients may have a limited range of motion, especially external rotation with humeral abduction due to apprehension or a feeling that their shoulder is "coming out of joint."

- Age is the primary determinant of instability. The younger the athlete is at the time of his or her first dislocation episode, the greater is the risk of developing recurrent instability.

- In some cases, surgery after a single dislocation is selected by the athlete in order to decrease the risk of recurrent dislocation and subsequent time lost from sport.

- Surgical options to address recurrent anterior instability include traditional open and newer arthroscopic techniques. Higher recurrence rates have been reported with arthroscopic repairs, but more recent reports have demonstrated comparable results between open and arthroscopic techniques for anterior instability.

HISTORICAL PERSPECTIVE

In 1938, Bankart[1] suggested that the result of a traumatic anterior dislocation of the shoulder joint in most cases was recurrent instability. He stated that a rent in the capsule healed readily and that dislocation never recurred unless a tear in the glenoid labrum was present. Recurrence seems, however, to be significantly influenced by the age at which the first dislocation occurs. There are numerous reports in the literature supporting arthro-scopic repair following a first-time traumatic shoulder dislocation in a young athlete. Regardless of the controversy concerning the treatment of an initial dislocation and the subsequent recurrence rate, several conclusions can be made. First, age of the patient at the first dislocation is the primary prognostic factor for recurrent instability. Second, nonoperative treatment has little predictable effect on recurrence. Finally, the patient's activity level and type of sport may also play a role in determining risk of recurrent instability.

The ideal patient for surgical stabilization is a young athlete who has sustained a limited number of documented dislocations, has clear unidirectional instability, and has failed nonoperative treatment. Additionally, the ideal shoulder for an anterior stabilization procedure has a Bankart lesion (detachment of the anterior-inferior labrum) with robust labral tissue for repair and no concomitant intra-articular pathology. Given this scenario, the procedure to repair the capsulolabral injury and decrease the capsular volume, whether done open or arthroscopically, should produce comparable clinical outcomes. Irrespective of the technique chosen, the surgeon needs to be prepared to address all pathoanatomic findings in these shoulders. The broad spectrum of intra-articular injuries that will be encountered by a surgeon treating instability is well described in other chapters. This chapter focuses on arthroscopic and open capsulolabral repair in anterior unidirectional instability.

CLINICAL FEATURES AND EVALUATION

Acute Shoulder Dislocation

The presentation of an anterior glenohumeral dislocation is typically not subtle. A significant force is required to produce a dislocation. The patient presents with an internally rotated arm that is usually splinted by the contralateral hand. Any manipulation causes discomfort. In many cases, the athlete will know that the shoulder is dislocated.

There is a myriad of reduction techniques; however, a gentle reduction of the joint with traction-countertraction or by slow forward elevation and in-line traction is recommended. The reduction is facilitated by either intravenous sedation or intra-articular xylocaine.

The decision to reduce an on-field dislocation without prereduction radiographs can be problematic. A reduction is easier if done soon after the injury. However, an unusual concomitant injury such as greater tuberosity or proximal humeral fracture cannot be ruled out until radiographs are taken. Although it is unlikely that these injuries can result from a reduction attempt, a litigious patient or his lawyer can claim otherwise.

Anterior Instability

Traumatic anterior shoulder dislocations and subluxations are common injuries in young athletes. Contact sports provide frequent opportunities for these injuries to occur. The first or primary dislocation may involve a collision or a fall typically with the arm in an abducted and externally rotated position. Despite a period of immobilization and rehabilitation following a traumatic dislocation, recurrent instability often results and can lead to significant disability.

Evaluation of a shoulder in a patient with instability should follow the systematic approach as outlined in Chapter 16. A specific test used to diagnose anterior instability is the apprehension/relocation test of Jobe.[2] The patient is placed supine with his or her humerus abducted to 90 degrees. The arm is then slowly externally rotated to elicit a feeling of apprehension as the humerus begins to subluxate anteriorly. The relocation component of the test is positive if a posterior force applied to the proximal humerus alleviates the feelings of apprehension. This maneuver reduces the humerus in the glenoid and prevents anterior subluxation. The load and shift test is used to grade humeral translation, the results of which are usually compared to the contralateral shoulder. With the patient supine or sitting and his or her arm abducted at 70 to 90 degrees, the proximal humerus is translated anteriorly, posteriorly, and inferiorly. The amount of humeral translation is graded according to the system by Altchek and Dines.[3] A 1+ shift defines a shoulder that can be brought to the anterior glenoid rim. A 2+ shift is translation over the glenoid rim with spontaneous reduction. A 3+ shift designates glenohumeral dislocation without spontaneous reduction.

Another maneuver we have found useful in assessing anterior instability is the scapular protraction test. With the patient sitting up, the arm is slowly abducted and externally rotated. In an unstable joint, when the shoulder begins to subluxate anteriorly, the patient will involuntarily protract the scapula to maintain the reduced position of the glenohumeral joint. This can be identified from the back of the patient and more easily elicited in a thin patient.

Radiographic assessment should include at least three projections: scapular anteroposterior, scapular lateral, and axillary views (Fig. 18-1A–D). Additionally, a West Point axillary lateral view can be used to assess for a bony avulsion of the anteroinferior glenoid (see Fig. 18-1E). Conventional radiography, however, is not useful for evaluating labral or capsular pathology in the shoulder. Magnetic resonance imaging is the gold standard to evaluate the soft-tissue injuries associated with anterior instability, and specific imaging sequences have been developed that allow a more precise depiction of intra-articular pathology in the unstable shoulder.

Recently, the use of intra-articular gadolinium to further elucidate glenohumeral pathoanatomy has added an additional dimension to conventional magnetic resonance imaging. Magnetic resonance arthrography offers even greater accuracy in evaluating the anatomic structures of the shoulder in patients with anterior glenohumeral instability. Multiple studies have found magnetic resonance arthrography to be better than magnetic resonance imaging without gadolinium enhancement for diagnosing capsulolabral injury.[4–6] The distention of the joint with fluid outlines and separates the anatomic labroligamentous structures that otherwise lie closely opposed, especially if scarring or partial healing has already ensued. Furthermore, magnetic resonance arthrographic evaluation with the patient's shoulder in the abducted and externally rotated position has been shown to be of particular benefit in evaluating the glenoid labrum and the integrity of the attachment of the anterior capsulolabral complex (Fig. 18-2).[7]

RELEVANT ANATOMY

Turkel et al[8] demonstrated that the anterior band of the inferior glenohumeral ligament is the primary restraint to anterior glenohumeral translation, especially with the arm in an abducted position. Anterior dislocation usually results from an indirect force with the arm in the abducted, externally rotated position. In this position, the anterior band of the inferior glenohumeral ligament is tensioned across the front of the glenoid. This checkrein, in conjunction with the glenoid labrum, normally prevents further anterior translation of the humeral head. With sufficient force, however, the anterior band of the inferior glenohumeral ligament traumatically fails, and the humerus is levered over the anterior glenoid rim resulting in dislocation. This capsulolabral injury, the Bankart or Perthes lesion, is the salient pathoanatomic feature of anterior instability and is seen in a very high percentage of traumatic shoulder dislocations.[9–13]

In addition to the anteroinferior lesion, the injury may extend superiorly into the labral attachment of the biceps tendon producing a concomitant superior labrum anterior posterior (SLAP) lesion as described by Snyder et al.[14] Another injury variant is the detachment laterally of the inferior glenohumeral ligament from the humeral neck, a humeral avulsion of glenohumeral ligament lesion, as described by Bach et al[15] and subsequently by Wolf et al.[16]

A traumatic humeral dislocation typically results in posterolateral humeral head compression against the bony glenoid rim. This produces the classic Hill-Sachs lesion, a chondral or osteochondral compression fracture. Arthroscopically, this lesion can be differentiated from the normal, nonarticular "bare area" of the humeral head by the appearance of articular cartilage on both sides of the lesion. Arthroscopically, the acute Hill-Sachs lesion will have an irregular appearance with bleeding, exposed cancellous bone (Fig. 18-3). A large Hill-Sachs lesion may engage the anterior glenoid with humeral abduction and external rotation and produce a subjective clunk and a sensation of glenohumeral dislocation.

TREATMENT OPTIONS

Nonoperative Treatment
Acute Shoulder Dislocation

Initial management of an acute shoulder dislocation consists of a variable period of immobilization followed by rehabilitation focused on restoration of active motion and periscapular muscle strengthening. The duration of immobilization does not appear to alter the recurrence rate. A recent report by Itoi et al[17] suggests immobilization in a position of humeral external rotation may result in a lower rate of recurrence compared to traditional immobilization in internal rotation. Several studies are ongoing to compare immobilization in internal and external rotation. The most important factor associated with recurrence is the age at the time of the first dislocation. It has been well established that the younger the patient is at the time of the first dislocation, the greater is the recurrence rate.

After an acute anterior shoulder dislocation, we recommend immobilization in a sling for comfort for about 1 week, followed by range-of-motion exercises as tolerated and progression to strengthening exercises.

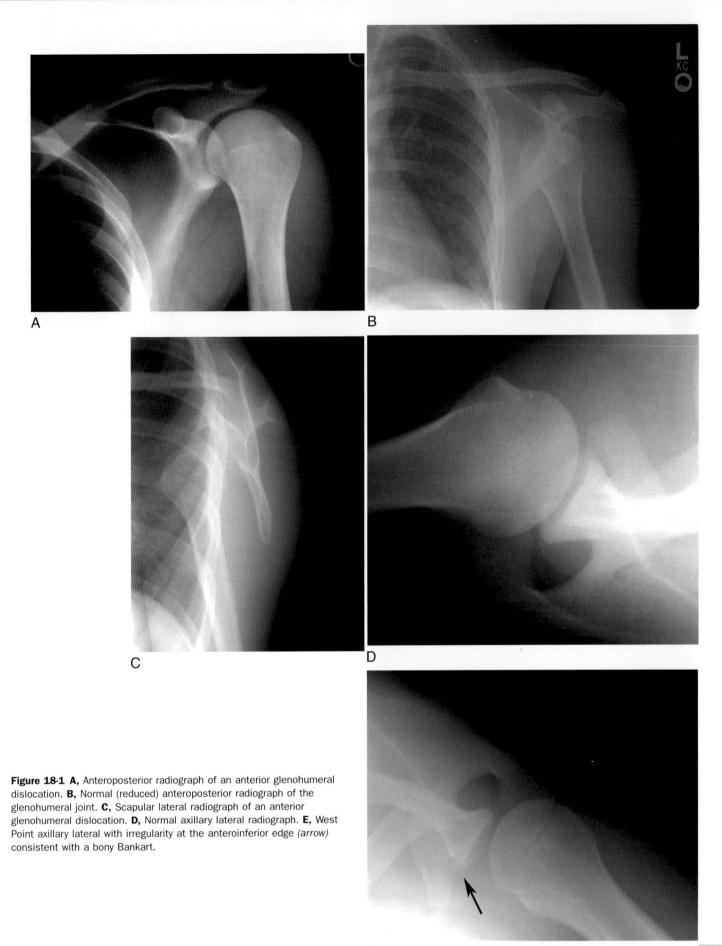

Figure 18-1 A, Anteroposterior radiograph of an anterior glenohumeral dislocation. **B,** Normal (reduced) anteroposterior radiograph of the glenohumeral joint. **C,** Scapular lateral radiograph of an anterior glenohumeral dislocation. **D,** Normal axillary lateral radiograph. **E,** West Point axillary lateral with irregularity at the anteroinferior edge *(arrow)* consistent with a bony Bankart.

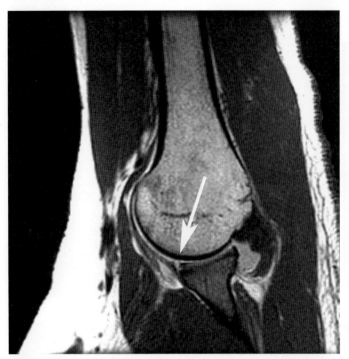

Figure 18-2 A magnetic resonance arthrogram with the shoulder in an abducted and externally rotated position demonstrating a Bankart lesion (arrow).

Anterior Instability

Rehabilitation with an emphasis on periscapular muscle strengthening is typically the first course of treatment prescribed for patients with anterior shoulder instability. The improvement in periscapular muscles and proprioception can allow a patient to function with the instability. With an increased awareness of the provocative position of humeral abduction and external rota-

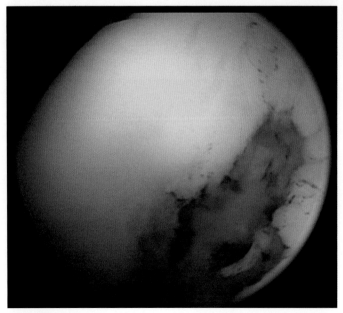

Figure 18-3 Arthroscopic image of a Hill-Sachs lesion following a traumatic dislocation. Note cartilage on both sides of the osteochondral injury.

tion, patients can, at times, return to sports. Orthotics that limit humeral abduction and/or external rotation can be used to allow an athlete to complete a season. However, many athletes have persistent symptoms that preclude return to their prior sports or activities despite a course of physical therapy. In these cases, a surgical repair is recommended. Indications for surgical stabilization include shoulder instability that has failed nonoperative treatment and precludes return to preinjury activities.

First-Time Shoulder Dislocations

Controversy exists as to whether athletes should be offered surgical stabilization after a single first-time anterior shoulder dislocation. Nonoperative treatment, which typically entails a brief period of immobilization, followed by a variable duration of rehabilitation, has resulted in recurrent instability rates ranging from 17% to 96% in patients younger than 30 years of age. Because of this high rate of recurrence in young patients, some authors have investigated the role of arthroscopic treatment of shoulders following dislocation. The Bankart lesion has been demonstrated to occur in over 95% of traumatic dislocations. In two prospective, randomized studies of young, first-time dislocators, Kirkley et al[18] and Bottoni et al[19] reported significantly lower recurrence rates following arthroscopic Bankart repair when compared to nonoperative treatment. Additionally, patients treated surgically demonstrated a superior outcome compared to the nonoperative group using a quality-of-life assessment.

The decision to surgically stabilize a shoulder that has recently dislocated is made with the expectation that the risks incurred by nonoperative treatment outweigh those incurred by surgery. The major risk of nonoperative treatment is recurrent instability and the additional glenohumeral injury sustained by repeated dislocation episodes. Although the rate of recurrence is high in young athletes, it is not 100%. Therefore, an unknown number of patients will be undertaking surgery unnecessarily, the chief argument for those advocating nonoperative management. However, given the high rate of recurrence and the disability following any subsequent episodes of instability, a patient may conclude that choosing the time of disability, i.e., postoperative rehabilitation, will most likely decrease the risk of subsequent instability episodes significantly. This is the argument presented for operative stabilization. In certain situations, such as the collegiate athlete with a limited number of seasons of competition available, the risk of recurrence in the following season is not acceptable to the athlete and early stabilization is often selected.

Operative Treatment and Preoperative Assessment

Traditionally, open Bankart repair with capsulorrhaphy has been the most reliable technique to restore stability. The goal, whether approached via open or arthroscopic means, is to anatomically repair the avulsion of the anteroinferior capsulolabral complex and to eliminate capsular redundancy that can contribute to increased anterior humeral translation. All shoulders undergoing stabilization should be examined under anesthesia to assess glenohumeral laxity. This allows an accurate assessment of humeral translation without the effect of muscular contractions in an apprehensive patient. The examination should be compared to the contralateral shoulder (assuming it is normal) to determine asymmetrical increased glenohumeral laxity.

An initial diagnostic glenohumeral arthroscopy should be performed to assess intra-articular pathoanatomy in all patients. This provides several benefits including the opportunity to assess the intra-articular anatomy, confirm the presence of a Bankart lesion, and contrast intraoperative findings with preoperative radiographic studies. Most importantly, the superior labrum is best evaluated and treated arthroscopically. The repair of an unstable SLAP lesion is nearly impossible from an open approach. Additionally, the rest of the intra-articular structures including the posterior labral attachment can be quickly and easily assessed from an initial arthroscopic glenohumeral evaluation.

Operative Techniques
Open Anterior Stabilization
The beach chair position for the initial glenohumeral arthroscopy will facilitate positioning for the open procedure. After arthroscopic evaluation and superior labral repair, if indicated, the back of the surgical table is lowered to a recumbent position. The operative extremity can be supported on a padded Mayo stand or a commercially available arm holder. Through a deltopectoral approach, the cephalic vein is identified and retracted laterally. A self-retraining retractor is used to maintain the conjoined tendon medially. The clavipectoral fascia is cleared to allow identification of the anterior humeral circumflex vessels (often referred to as the "three sisters"). These vessels can be safely cauterized without risk to the humeral head. For better exposure inferiorly, the superior portion of the pectoralis tendon as it inserts into the humerus can be incised.

With the arm in adduction and slight external rotation, the subscapularis tendon is tensioned and then longitudinally sectioned approximately 1 cm from its insertion on the lesser tuberosity. Typically, only the superior two thirds of the tendon is transected since the inferior third is mostly muscle. The subscapularis is then carefully separated from the underlying capsule. This is more easily performed from inferior to superior. The lateral end of the sectioned subscapularis tendon is secured with three no. 2 nonabsorbable sutures (FiberWire, Arthrex, Inc., Naples, FL). The tendon is retracted medially and secured beneath the self-retaining retractor. Superiorly, between the anterior edge of the supraspinatus and the superior edge of the subscapularis, the rotator interval, a variable area of capsular deficiency often exists. The rotator interval capsular defect, if present, is closed in a side-to-side manner with nonabsorbable sutures. Next, a longitudinal capsulotomy, 5 mm medial to the humeral capsular insertion, is made. Perpendicular to this capsulotomy, a horizontal capsular incision is made to the anteroinferior glenoid to allow adequate exposure of the Bankart lesion. This horizontal capsulotomy is made at the level of the inferior glenoid to facilitate exposure and repair of the Bankart lesion. A humeral head retractor locked on the posterior glenoid maintains this exposure (Fig. 18-4). Diligent hemostasis is maintained throughout the approach to ensure adequate visualization of the capsulolabral repair.

Anatomic labral repair is next performed using bone tunnels or, more commonly, suture anchors (Fig. 18-5). Typically three anchors are used to repair the Bankart lesion. We prefer bioabsorbable suture anchors (Bio-FASTak, Arthrex, Inc.) for all labral repairs. The anchors do not obstruct any future radiographic studies and allow strong fixation of soft tissue to bone. Following Bankart repair, a lateral-based capsular shift is used to eliminate redundancy while the humerus is maintained in at least 45 degrees of abduction and 45 degrees of external rotation. The

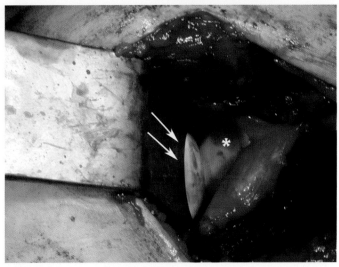

Figure 18-4 The humeral head retractor levers on the anterior edge of the glenoid and retracts the head *(arrows)* laterally. This maneuver facilitates the Bankart repair to the glenoid *(asterisk).*

axillary pouch is palpated with one finger while the sutures secured to the lateral edge of the capsule are pulled superiorly. The capsule is sharply released from its humeral insertion, and nonabsorbable sutures are placed along the lateral edge every centimeter. An adequate capsular shift is accomplished when the capsular redundancy is eliminated through superior advancement of the inferior capsular leaf. While releasing the inferior capsule, the axillary nerve, coursing just distal to the inferior glenoid, is identified and protected. Capsular imbrication is then performed in a "pants over vest" technique by advancing the inferior leaflet superiorly along the lateral capsular margin and then reinforcing the repair with the overlapping superior leaflet. If the lateral edge of the tendon is tenuous, a suture anchor can be inserted into the humerus at the 6 o'clock position. We prefer a double-loaded bioabsorbable anchor (Bio-Corkscrew, Arthrex, Inc.). This provides secure capsular fixation at the lateral capsular margin. Anatomic repair of the subscapularis is performed in an end-to-end fashion with the previously placed sutures.

Arthroscopic Technique
Arthroscopic labral repair can be performed in the beach chair or lateral decubitus position. The beach chair position facilitates conversion, if necessary, to an open procedure more easily. However, the lateral decubitus position with overhead traction allows for greater joint distraction and better visualization. Following an examination under anesthesia in the supine position, the patient is then placed in either the lateral decubitus or upright beach chair position. In the lateral position, the patient's operative extremity is maintained in 40 degrees of abduction and slight forward flexion with an overhead traction crane (Fig. 18-6; 3-Point Shoulder Distraction System, Arthrex, Inc.). A standard posterior arthroscopy portal is established first. Two anterior portals are then established from the outside in after proper localization with an 18-gauge spinal needle. A 6.5-mm clear cannula (Stryker Endoscopy, San Jose, CA) is inserted anterosuperiorly at the level of the long head of the biceps tendon. This is called the anterosuperior portal. An 8.4-mm clear cannula (Linvatec, Largo, FL) is inserted just above the subscapularis tendon (Fig. 18-7). This is called the anteroinferior portal. A systematic glenohumeral examination from both

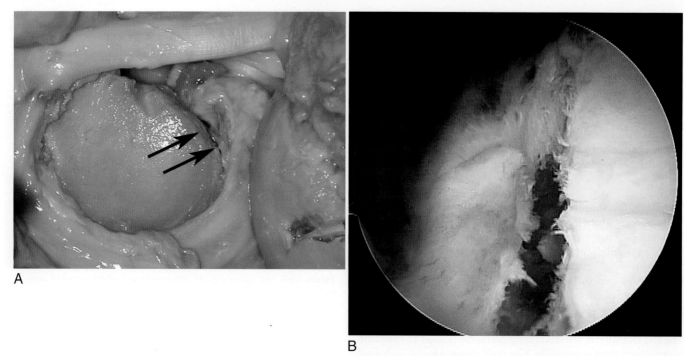

Figure 18-5 A, Cadaveric right shoulder with a Bankart lesion *(arrows).* **B,** An arthroscopic image from the anterosuperior portal of a right shoulder with a Bankart lesion.

the anterior and posterior portals is conducted. If an unstable superior labral lesion is found, it is repaired prior to the anterior stabilization. The technique for SLAP repairs is well described in Chapter 22.

The anteroinferior labral attachment often heals along the medial face of the glenoid following traumatic disruption from a dislocation. The anterior labral-periosteal sleeve avulsion (ALPSA) lesion needs to be completely released from the underlying glenoid (Fig. 18-8). The anteroinferior labrum is separated completely from the glenoid with an arthroscopic eleva-

tor (Fig. 18-9). The capsulolabral attachment, once completely free, should easily be brought up onto the glenoid with an arthroscopic grasper inserted through the anterosuperior portal. Following release of the capsular soft tissue, an aggressive shaver or bur is used to decorticate the anterior glenoid and stimulate a bleeding bed to which the capsulolabral tissue will be reattached (Fig. 18-10A). To better visualize the anterior glenoid

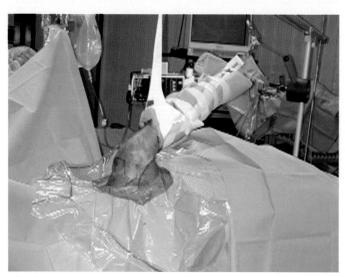

Figure 18-6 Intraoperative radiograph demonstrating lateral decubitus positioning of patient using the shoulder distraction crane. The bony landmarks have been identified to assist with portal placement. Additionally, the edges of the sterile drape have been sealed with loban strips to prevent leakage of arthroscopic fluid onto the patient.

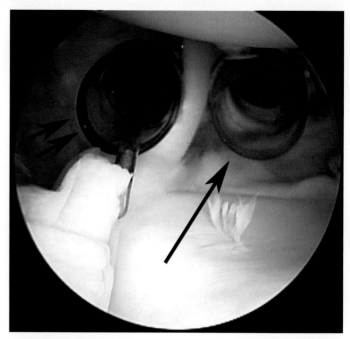

Figure 18-7 Arthroscopic image of the two anterior cannulas. The smaller cannula *(double arrows),* the anterosuperior portal, is positioned superior to the biceps tendon, and the larger of the two *(single arrow)* is the anteroinferior portal and is used for instrumentation.

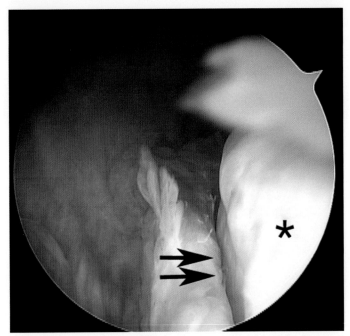

Figure 18-8 Arthroscopic image of a right shoulder from the anterosuperior portal with an anterior labral-periosteal sleeve avulsion (ALPSA) lesion *(arrows)*. The labral attachment was avulsed from the glenoid *(asterisk)* and subsequently healed in a nonanatomic, medial location.

during preparation, the 30-degree arthroscope can be inserted down the anterosuperior portal (see Fig. 18-10B); alternatively, a 70-degree arthroscope will allow excellent visualization from the posterior portal.

Serving as a temporary shuttle stitch, a no. 1 PDS II (Ethicon, Inc., Somerville, NJ) suture is passed through the capsule and

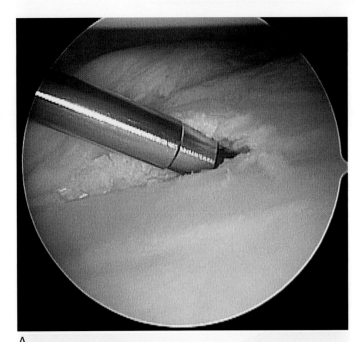

A

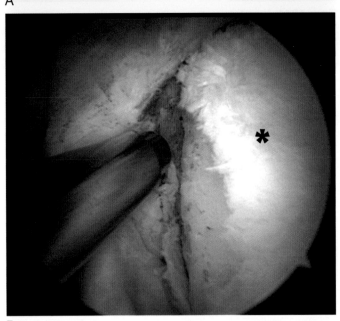

B

Figure 18-10 A, Arthroscopic image of the glenoid abrasion and release of the labrum viewed from the posterior portal. **B,** Arthroscopic image of the glenoid abrasion viewed from the anterosuperior portal. The labrum is completely released from the glenoid *(asterisk)*.

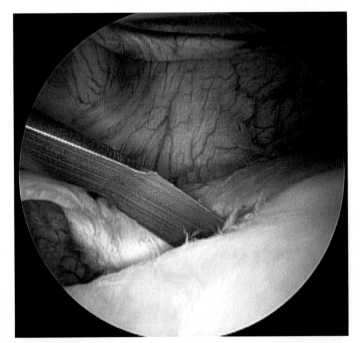

Figure 18-9 Arthroscopic image of a right shoulder demonstrating the use of an arthroscopic elevator (Liberator, Linvatec, Largo, FL) to release the labrum from the glenoid in preparation for the repair.

labrum in separate passes using a 45-degree Spectrum Shuttle (Linvatec, Largo, FL) inserted through the anteroinferior portal (Fig. 18-11). Through the anteroinferior portal, a bioabsorbable suture anchor (Bio-FASTak, Arthrex, Inc.) is then inserted at the articular margin of the glenoid (Fig. 18-12). The inferior limb of the permanent suture from the anchor is then retrieved out the anterosuperior portal with a ring grasper (Fig. 18-13). Outside the cannula, the PDS shuttle suture is tied to the

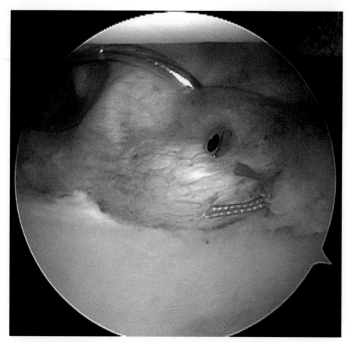

Figure 18-11 Arthroscopic image of the suture hook inserted through the anteroinferior portal and passed through the capsule. The second passage will be through the labrum. One suture has been already completed.

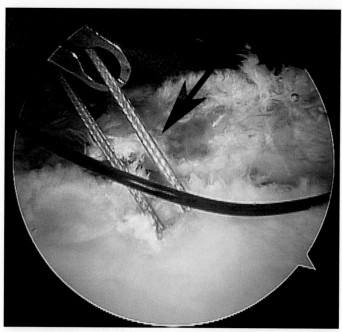

Figure 18-13 Through the anterosuperior portal, a ring grasper is used to retrieve one limb of the permanent suture and pull it out the anterosuperior portal. This limb is anterior or the one closer to the capsulolabral complex *(arrow)*.

suture limb from the anchor with a leading dilation knot that will facilitate passage of both sutures back through the tissue (Fig. 18-14). The shuttle suture is then pulled back through the anteroinferior portal, thus pulling the permanent anchor suture through the labrum and capsule. From the anteroinferior portal, an arthroscopic sliding knot with alternating half hitches secures

the tissue to the bone. This process is repeated to effect a capsular imbrication of the anteroinferior capsule and anatomic Bankart repair (Fig. 18-15).

Postoperative Treatment

Following anterior stabilization with either open or arthroscopic techniques, we immobilize the shoulder in a Cryo/Cuff sling (Aircast, Inc., Summit, NJ). The rehabilitation protocol consists of three stages, each lasting approximately 1 month. The first stage consists of immobilization in a sling where we encour-

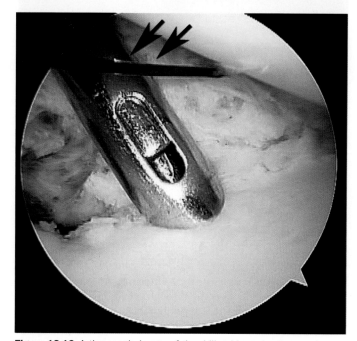

Figure 18-12 Arthroscopic image of the drill guide and suture anchor drill. Note placement several millimeters onto articular margin. The purple PDS II shuttle suture is passing across the guide into the anterosuperior portal.

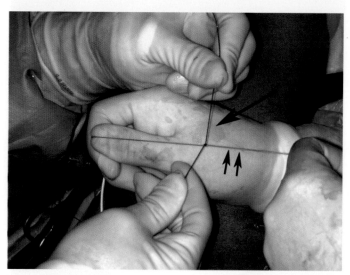

Figure 18-14 The PDS suture *(single arrow)* is tied to the permanent suture *(double arrows)* outside of the anterosuperior portal cannula. This allows the PDS II to pull the permanent suture back into the joint and through the capsulolabral tissue.

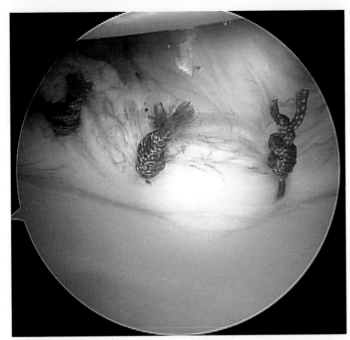

Figure 18-15 Arthroscopic image of completed Bankart repair with capsular plication.

age pendulum and elbow exercises. Immediate active motion in the forward plane is allowed, but abduction and external rotation are avoided. The second stage involves restoration of a full active range of motion while protecting the repair from aggressive abduction or external rotation. In the third stage, the focus is on periscapular muscular strengthening. Slight modifications by the therapists are allowed based on each individual's progress. Return to sport activities is permitted at 4 to 6 months depending on return of function and strength.

Revision Stabilization

The approach to revision surgery for recurrent anterior instability should begin with a careful assessment of why the instability recurred and whether another surgical procedure will improve the patient's function. The following questions need to be answered to determine the cause and to plan the treatment of the recurrent instability.

1. Did the patient return to normal function and shoulder stability following the previous surgery?
2. Did a subsequent glenohumeral dislocation or subluxation occur?
3. What is the direction of instability, i.e., anterior, posterior, or inferior?
4. Does the patient have generalized ligamentous laxity or a collagen disorder?
5. Are there any radiographic findings that intimate problems with the previous surgery?

Preoperative Assessment

Revision surgery, whether performed open or arthroscopically, is typically more challenging than primary stabilization. The direction of the instability is an important determination. Missed posterior labral injuries or anterior repairs made too tightly can result in postoperative posterior instability. Specific tests to evaluate for posterior glenohumeral pathology, as described in Chapter 19, are performed. The patient should be queried as

to the timing of the recurrent instability. For recurrent anterior instability due to subsequent trauma when normal function and stability were restored after the surgery, a recurrent capsulolabral injury is a likely cause. For recurrent instability that develops insidiously without a definitive traumatic event, a specific cause for the failed surgery needs to be ascertained. Generalized ligamentous laxity and multidirectional instability can be a difficult problem to tackle. More information and surgical tips to address multidirectional instability and capsular injuries are offered in Chapter 20.

Preoperative evaluation of recurrent anterior instability should follow that prescribed for primary instability. The operative report, if available, should be obtained to ascertain what type of approach and fixation were used in the previous surgery. Plain radiographs should be used to assess bony injuries or glenoid insufficiency as well as retained hardware. Placement of suture anchors can provide clues for failure of the previous surgery. Suture anchors placed too far medially (Fig. 18-16) instead of up on the articular margin or placed too superiorly to adequately address the anteroinferior capsulolabral laxity may contribute to recurrent instability. If metallic suture anchors are in the correct position, they may preclude placement of new suture anchors or necessitate alternative methods of fixation in the revision surgery. Although postoperative changes may make the interpretation more difficult, magnetic resonance imaging or preferably magnetic resonance arthrography should be obtained to assess for capsulolabral reinjury. Superior labral injuries, if not addressed at the time of the previous surgery, can also be a source of persistent pain and instability.

Either an open or arthroscopic approach for revision surgery can be used to address recurrent instability; however, scarring and disruption of normal tissue planes can complicate an open revision. If an open approach is chosen, an initial arthroscopy can be beneficial. The posterior and superior labral attachments should be evaluated. Although the surgical approach for open revision stabilization is the same as previously described, the separation of the capsule from the subscapularis is inherently more difficult. The Bankart lesion, if present, is repaired and a capsulorrhaphy to eliminate capsular redundancy is performed.

The ability to visualize and address all intra-articular structures makes the arthroscopic approach desirable for revision surgery. If a nonanatomic open technique such as a coracoid transfer (Bristow) had been used, the alteration in the normal anatomy makes the arthroscopic approach much safer than revision open surgery. The arthroscopic surgical technique is the same as previously described. If posterior or inferior capsular laxity is present, it is addressed prior to the anterior structures. The posterior labral repair is well described in Chapter 19. If a capsulolabral injury is present, it is repaired in the same fashion as the primary injury. The anteroinferior capsulolabral complex is completely separated from the glenoid. If hardware is exposed or if it obstructs appropriate placement of new anchors, an attempt can be made to remove it. In most cases, the new anchors can be adequately placed without undue difficulty. The anteroinferior capsule is incorporated into the labral repair as previously described to effect a reduction in the capsular volume.

Complications

Arthroscopic stabilization is a technically demanding procedure. The surgeon should be well versed in shoulder arthroscopy, be knowledgeable about the arthroscopic equipment, and ideally have a well-trained assistant prior to embarking on this proce-

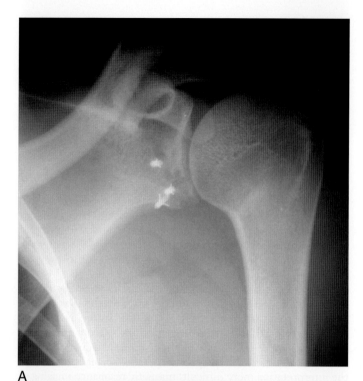

A

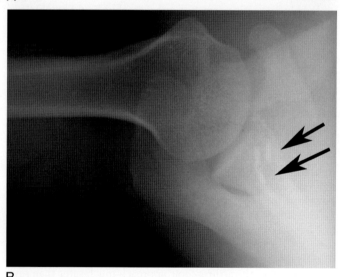

B

Figure 18-16 A and **B,** Anteroposterior and axillary lateral radiographs of a shoulder with metal suture anchors *(arrows)* placed too far medially. The patient developed recurrent instability and required revision stabilization.

Replacement parts should be readily available to allow continuation of the procedure.

Complications associated with either technique include inadequate tissue preparation leading to an inability to properly mobilize the capsulolabral complex. Inadequate tensioning of the capsulolabral complex can lead to suture breakage or recurrent laxity in the tissue. This may lead to an inadequate repair and surgery failure. Metallic anchors, if left protruding above the articular cartilage, can result in disastrous consequences for the humeral articular cartilage. Even slight prominence can result in a destruction of the humeral cartilage as the shoulder abrades on the metallic edge. Additionally, improperly placed metallic or bioabsorbable anchors can dislodge and become loose bodies that result in destruction of articular cartilage. Some bioabsorbable fixation devices have been associated with a reactive synovitis as they are hydrolyzed. This may be manifested clinically as an increase in shoulder pain at 4 to 6 weeks postoperatively and a loss of glenohumeral motion.

RESULTS AND OUTCOMES

Over the past decade, rates of recurrent instability with nonoperative treatment following a traumatic anterior dislocation in several studies have been reported to be between 50% and 92%. The difference in reported recurrence rates is often correlated with the age of the patients at the time of the first dislocation. In a study of young Swedish hockey players, Cvitanic et al[7] reported the recurrence rate with nonoperative treatment in players younger than the age of 20 to be greater than 90%. The level of activity a patient resumes after an initial shoulder dislocation may determine his or her risk for reinjury. Once recurrent instability fails nonoperative treatment and is symptomatic, an operative approach is recommended.

For recurrent instability, numerous open and arthroscopic techniques have been reported. Historically, the lowest recurrence rates have been reported with open techniques. However, most studies comparing open and arthroscopic results have included arthroscopic techniques that poorly mimicked the anatomic labral repair and capsulorrhaphy of the open procedure. The traditional open Bankart repair, however, is not an easy surgical procedure and can be complicated by neurovascular injury, postoperative stiffness, and long-term glenohumeral arthritis. Arthroscopic Bankart repairs have been reported to decrease operative time, blood loss, postoperative narcotic use, and time off from work.[20] The evolution of arthroscopic stabilization has progressed from glenoid abrasion to the use of various devices to repair the labral injury including arthroscopic staples[4] and transglenoid labral fixation where sutures are passed across the glenoid and then tied over the posterior fascia of the shoulder.[21] In 1991, Warner and Warren[22] introduced a bioabsorbable tack (Suretac, Acufex Microsurgical, Mansfield, MA) that can be inserted arthroscopically to repair Bankart lesions. The tacks eliminate the need to tie arthroscopic knots but have limited initial strength, degrade quickly, and do not effect a reduction in capsular volume. Although good results were reported in acute stabilization of first-time dislocations, the results for recurrent instability were much less promising.[19,23-26] None of these techniques paralleled that which was done via an open approach.

The use of suture anchors for shoulder stabilization was first reported by Weber et al[27] in 1991. Their use provides strong fixation of soft tissue to bone and allows tensioning of the anteroinferior capsulolabral complex. Metallic and bioabsorbable

dure. Because of the learning curve associated with arthroscopic stabilization, a surgeon should have a low threshold for converting to an open shoulder reconstruction if satisfactory repair is not achieved. Prerequisite arthroscopic skills include the following: (1) ability to visualize an instrument from anterior and posterior portals, (2) ability to shuttle and pass monofilament and permanent braided suture, and (3) arthroscopic knot tying.

The complications associated with arthroscopic stabilization include not only problems associated with the actual performance of the steps required to repair the injured tissue, but also include problems associated with the equipment required to maintain adequate visualization during the procedure. The camera, monitor, and arthroscopic equipment may malfunction.

anchors with either absorbable or nonabsorbable sutures are available. A myriad of surgical instruments are available to pass and retrieve sutures for shoulder repairs. Most devices require the ability to reliably tie arthroscopic knots. Stronger suture, color-coding of each suture limb, and double-loaded anchors have been some recent advances that facilitate arthroscopic stabilization.

Several recently published studies assessing results between open and arthroscopic repairs in patients with recurrent anterior instability demonstrated comparable outcomes with both techniques.[13,24,28]

CONCLUSIONS

Anterior shoulder instability is a common problem encountered by orthopedic surgeons. Although nonoperative treatment should be the initial course, when necessary, operative stabilization can provide a return to preinjury sporting activities in a high percentage of patients. Whether an open or arthroscopic technique is chosen, careful attention to operative principles is imperative. Arthroscopic repair techniques are now approaching the reliability of the traditional open procedure with advantages of a quicker procedure, better cosmetic results, and decreased morbidity. However, it is technically demanding and fraught with potential complications.

The approach to revision anterior stabilization parallels that done for the primary procedure. However, both a clear etiology for the surgical failure and a definitive surgical need to be ascertained before embarking on revision stabilization. Concomitant intra-articular pathology such as superior and posterior capsulolabral lesions need to be addressed at the time of the revision. Scarring and distortion of normal anatomy can make revision surgery much more difficult than primary procedures.

REFERENCES

1. Bankart ASB: The pathology and treatment of recurrent dislocation of the shoulder-joint. Br J Surg 1938;26:23–29.
2. Jobe FW, Kvitne RS, Giangarra CE: Shoulder pain in the overhand or throwing athlete. The relationship of anterior instability and rotator cuff impingement. Orthop Rev 1989;18:963–975.
3. Altchek DW, Dines DM: Shoulder injuries in the throwing athlete. J Am Acad Orthop Surg 1995;3:159–165.
4. Chandnani VP, Gagliardi JA, Murnane TG, et al: Glenohumeral ligaments and shoulder capsular mechanism: Evaluation with MR arthrography. Radiology 1995;196:27–32.
5. Chandnani VP, Yeager TD, DeBerardino T, et al: Glenoid labral tears: Prospective evaluation with MRI imaging, MR arthrography, and CT arthrography. Am J Roentgenol 1993;161:1229–1235.
6. Choi JA, Suh SI, Kim BH, et al: Comparison between conventional MR arthrography and abduction and external rotation MR arthrography in revealing tears of the antero-inferior glenoid labrum. Korean J Radiol 2001;2:216–221.
7. Cvitanic O, Tirman PF, Feller JF, et al: Using abduction and external rotation of the shoulder to increase the sensitivity of MR arthrography in revealing tears of the anterior glenoid labrum. Am J Roentgenol 1997;169:837–844.
8. Turkel SJ, Panio MW, Marshall JL, et al: Stabilizing mechanisms preventing anterior dislocation of the glenohumeral joint. J Bone Joint Surg Am 1981;63:1208–1217.
9. Arciero RA, St Pierre P: Acute shoulder dislocation. Indications and techniques for operative management. Clin Sports Med 1005;14:937–953.
10. Arciero RA, Taylor DC: Primary anterior dislocation of the shoulder in young patients. A ten-year prospective study. J Bone Joint Surg Am 1998;80:299–300.
11. Bottoni CR, Arciero RA: Arthroscopic repair of primary anterior dislocations of the shoulder. Tech Shoulder Elbow Surg 2001;2:2–16.
12. Cole BJ, Romeo AA: Arthroscopic shoulder stabilization with suture anchors: Technique, technology, and pitfalls. Clin Orthop 2001;390:17–30.
13. Fabbriciani C, Milano G, Demontis A, et al: Arthroscopic versus open treatment of Bankart lesion of the shoulder: A prospective randomized study. Arthroscopy 2004;20:456–462.
14. Snyder SJ, Karzel RP, Del Pizzo W, et al: SLAP lesions of the shoulder. Arthroscopy 1990;6:274–279.
15. Bach BR, Warren RF, Fronek J: Disruption of the lateral capsule of the shoulder. A cause of recurrent dislocation. J Bone Joint Surg Br 1988;70:274–276.
16. Wolf EM, Cheng JC, Dickson K: Humeral avulsion of glenohumeral ligaments as a cause of anterior shoulder instability. Arthroscopy 1995;11:600–607.
17. Itoi E, Hatakeyama Y, Kido T, et al: A new method of immobilization after traumatic anterior dislocation of the shoulder: A preliminary study. J Shoulder Elbow Surg 2003;12:413–415.
18. Kirkley A, Griffin S, Richards C, et al: Prospective randomized clinical trial comparing the effectiveness of immediate arthroscopic stabilization versus immobilization and rehabilitation in first traumatic anterior dislocations of the shoulder. Arthroscopy 1999;15:507–514.
19. Bottoni CR, Wilckens JH, DeBerardino TM, et al: A prospective, randomized evaluation of arthroscopic stabilization versus nonoperative treatment of acute, first-time shoulder dislocations. Paper presented at the 26th annual meeting of the American Orthopaedic Society for Sports Medicine, 2000, Sun Valley, ID.
20. Green MR, Christensen KP: Arthroscopic versus open Bankart procedures: A comparison of early morbidity and complications. Arthroscopy 1993;9:371–374.
21. Morgan CD, Bodenstab AB: Arthroscopic Bankart suture repair: Technique and early results. Arthroscopy 1987;3:111–122.
22. Warner JJ, Warren RF: Arthroscopic Bankart repair using a cannulated, absorbable fixation device. Op Tech Orthop 1991;1:192–198.
23. Arciero RA, Wheeler JH, Ryan JB, et al: Arthroscopic Bankart repair versus nonoperative treatment for acute, initial anterior shoulder dislocations. Am J Sports Med 1994;22:589–594.
24. Cole BJ, Romeo AA, Warner JJ: Arthroscopic Bankart repair with the Suretac device for traumatic anterior shoulder instability in athletes. Orthop Clin North Am 2001;32:411–421.
25. Fealy S, Drakos MC, Allen AA, et al: Arthroscopic Bankart repair: Experience with an absorbable, transfixing implant. Clin Orthop 2001;390:31–41.
26. Karlsson J, Magnusson L, Ejerhed L, et al: Comparison of open and arthroscopic stabilization for recurrent shoulder dislocation in patients with a Bankart lesion. Am J Sports Med 2001;29:538–542.
27. Weber EM, Wilk RM, Richmond JC: Arthroscopic Bankart repair using suture anchors. Op Tech Orthop 1991;1:194.
28. Tauro JC: Arthroscopic inferior capsular split and advancement for anterior and inferior shoulder instability: Technique and results at 2- to 5-year follow-up. Arthroscopy 2000;16:451–456.

In This Chapter

INTRODUCTION

- Posterior instability is defined as symptoms resulting from excessive posterior glenohumeral translation.[1]

- Posterior shoulder instability is less common than its anterior counterpart and is frequently difficult to diagnose.

- Patients with symptoms originating from excessive posterior translation of the shoulder rarely present with a history of dislocation requiring reduction.[2,3] Instead, the patient with posterior instability more commonly presents with symptoms related to recurrent subluxation events.

- Posterior instability is more common in athletes who frequently place a posteriorly directed force on their shoulders, such as football offensive linemen and weight lifters.

- Treatment generally starts with a rehabilitation program, unless significant trauma initiates the instability.

- When rehabilitation fails, both open and arthroscopic surgical techniques are available. Recent studies have reported improved results for surgical posterior stabilization.

CLINICAL FEATURES AND EVALUATION

Posterior Subluxation

The majority of patients do not recall an inciting event, but patients should be queried regarding a posteriorly directed force, which can occur with a fall on an outstretched arm or during athletic activity. The most common complaint at presentation is pain with activity. Symptoms are often vague and are generally not localized to the posterior aspect of the shoulder. Chronic subluxation episodes lead to pain secondary to inflammation of the capsule, rotator cuff, and/or biceps tendon.[4,5] Many patients do report a feeling that the shoulder is "slipping" posteriorly. In patients who describe a feeling of instability, the position of the arm when this occurs is an important clue as to diagnosis. A combination of flexion and internal rotation of the adducted arm is the classic position for allowing posterior translation of the

humeral head. Patients frequently report clicking or crepitus, which can be related to subluxation about the posterior glenoid rim or may occur with mechanical symptoms related to posterior labral pathology.

A complete physical examination, as described in Chapter 16, is necessary in evaluating for posterior instability. The examination components most important to this diagnosis involve tests for posterior translation. In general, patients with posterior instability are better able to relax their musculature than their anterior counterparts, likely owing to less apprehension about dislocation during the physical examination. Posterior apprehension or a reproduction of symptoms may occur with flexion and internal rotation of the adducted arm and a posteriorly directed force. Load and shift testing is evaluated for translation. Finally, the "jerk" test result is frequently positive. In patients in whom one shoulder is symptomatic, careful comparison to the opposite shoulder is essential in order to confirm that the physical examination findings are the source of symptoms.

Radiographs are usually normal in patients with posterior instability. Occasionally, posterior glenoid erosion or avulsion may be seen, more commonly in patients with a defined traumatic event. Magnetic resonance imaging is useful in evaluating for posterior labral detachment (reverse Bankart lesion; Fig. 19-1). In many cases, labral pathology is subtle and may be difficult to appreciate on magnetic resonance imaging.[6]

Posterior Dislocation

Acute shoulder pain after a history of a posteriorly directed force on an adducted arm or indirect muscle forces from seizure or electrical shock should raise suspicion for posterior dislocation. Patients generally present with the arm in a "sling" position, adducted and internally rotated. Classic examination findings include a limitation of external rotation short of neutral, painful limited elevation of the arm, an anterior void or prominence of the coracoid, and posterior fullness. Radiographic evaluation must include a lateral view to assess the relationship of the humeral head and glenoid. The anteroposterior view may show overlap of the humeral head on the glenoid rim (Fig. 19-2). Isolated fracture of the lesser tuberosity is nearly pathognomic for posterior dislocation, and a reverse Hill-Sachs lesion is frequently seen. In cases in which an acceptable lateral view cannot be obtained, a computed tomography scan is necessary. It has been reported that as many as 50% of posterior dislocations are missed on initial assessment, and this is a frequent source of litigation.[7]

RELEVANT ANATOMY

Anatomic lesions associated with posterior shoulder instability involve injury to the posterior labrum, inferior glenohumeral

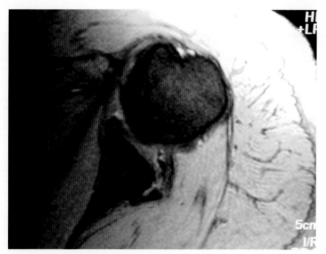

Figure 19-1 Magnetic resonance imaging shows detachment of the posterior labrum (reverse Bankart lesion) in a 20-year-old football lineman with posterior instability.

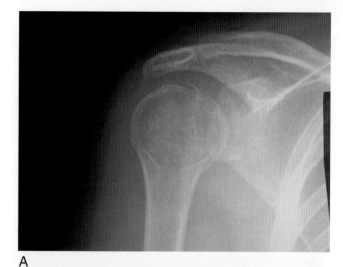

A

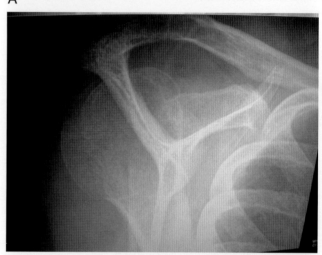

B

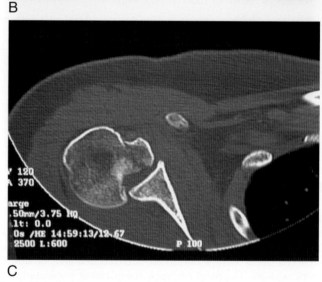

C

Figure 19-2 A, Anteroposterior view of the shoulder in a 29-year-old patient with shoulder pain after a seizure. **B,** In the same patient, adequate axillary lateral view could not be obtained. Transthoracic lateral view remains inconclusive. **C,** Computed tomography scan done 1 month after injury shows the posterior dislocation with a large reverse Hill-Sachs lesion.

ligament, and capsule. Posterior labral detachment (the reverse Bankart lesion) has been described in approximately 50% of patients. This lesion is commonly more subtle and less displaced than the standard anterior Bankart lesion. With the advent of arthroscopy, subtle irregularity of the posterior labrum is more easily appreciated. Posterior capsular laxity or plastic deformation has been implicated in many patients with posterior instability, and tightening of the posterior capsule is a component of the many surgical procedures described for posterior instability.

TREATMENT OPTIONS

The initial treatment of posterior subluxation is usually nonoperative.[8] Pain is treated with relative rest, avoidance of provocative activities and arm position, and anti-inflammatory medications. Physical therapy is initiated with an emphasis on strength and endurance of the parascapular musculature and rotator cuff. Improvement in the scapular muscles helps to create a stable platform for the humeral head. The rotator cuff is important in fine-tuning shoulder stability through a range of motion and also provides a compressive effect, helping to center the humeral head. In general, research has supported the belief that posterior subluxation responds better to rehabilitation than does its anterior counterpart. Clearly, patients with a history of a significant traumatic event are less likely to respond to nonoperative treatment.[9,10] In these patients, surgery is considered earlier if response to conservative treatment is unsuccessful.

The indications for surgical treatment of patients with posterior shoulder instability are subjective and must be individualized. Many patients choose to live with occasional episodes of subluxation, and there are few data to support operative intervention to prevent future complications such as arthritis or rotator cuff injury. The patient who has undergone an appropriate period of rehabilitation and is not satisfied with his or her shoulder function is a candidate for surgery. This includes those who have pain with use of the shoulder or those who are unable to participate in desired activities due to episodes of instability. Football players, particularly offensive linemen, and weight lifters generally tolerate posterior instability poorly. In patients in whom a defined traumatic event has led to posterior instability, early surgery without a course of nonoperative treatment is considered. This is particularly true if magnetic resonance imaging shows evidence of a posterior labral detachment.

There are several contraindications to surgical treatment of posterior glenohumeral instability. Patients who have not undergone an adequate course of rehabilitation are not surgical candidates, nor are those who are unable to complete an adequate postoperative rehabilitation program. Surgery is also contraindicated in the patient with a seizure disorder that has not been medically controlled because a seizure in the postoperative period will almost certainly result in failure of the repair. A documented period of 3 to 6 months without a seizure is required before elective surgical intervention.

As many as 50% of patients with posterior instability can voluntarily subluxate the shoulder.[9,10] This is not an absolute contraindication to surgery, as this finding can be present despite the best intentions of the patient, after an aggressive rehabilitation program, and may occur with a pathologic lesion (posterior labral detachment). However, patients who voluntarily or habitually subluxate or dislocate the shoulder often have psychological problems or do so for issues involving secondary gain, whether it be attention, narcotic medication, or issues of compensation. These patients are very poor surgical candidates.

Posterior Dislocation

Initial management of acute posterior dislocation is attempted closed reduction. Adequate anesthesia and relaxation are required. The humeral head is often perched on the glenoid rim, impacted in the area of the reverse Hill-Sachs lesion. For reduction, the arm is adducted and gently flexed to 90 degrees as lateral distraction is applied to disimpact the humeral head. Once this is accomplished, the humeral head is translated anteriorly and gradually externally rotated, and the arm is brought down to the side. The arm is generally held in a brace in neutral rotation for about a month before initiating physical therapy. In the presence of a lesser tuberosity fracture or a reverse Hill-Sachs lesion involving more than 30% to 40% of the humeral head, early surgery is indicated. In cases of chronic locked posterior dislocation, generally present for more than 1 to 2 weeks, surgical open reduction is necessary.

SURGERY

Open versus Arthroscopic Treatment

Surgical treatment of posterior glenohumeral instability has traditionally been performed through an open posterior approach to the shoulder. In general, this surgery is less predictable with regard to successful stabilization of the shoulder compared to surgery for anterior instability.[11] Posterior stabilization surgery generally involves posterior capsulorraphy, with concomitant repair of the reverse Bankart lesion when present. Some authors have advocated augmentation of the thin posterior capsule with an infraspinatus tenodesis, and others have transferred bone to form a "block" against posterior dislocation.[12]

There are two primary difficulties with open posterior stabilization. The first relates to the technically demanding nature of the approach, as it can be difficult to gain adequate exposure. Second, the posterior capsule is quite thin, making it difficult to perform the capsulorraphy. Given these difficulties, along with the advancement of arthroscopic suturing techniques, methods of arthroscopic posterior stabilization have gained popularity over the past several years. Arthroscopy allows improved visualization of the labrum and ligamentous structures and improves accuracy in diagnosing other intra-articular pathologic lesions.[11]

Other potential advantages include less postoperative pain and scar tissue formation. While few studies are available with which to make conclusions regarding the efficacy of posterior arthroscopic stabilization, early results have been quite favorable. As techniques continue to improve, it is likely that the majority of surgery for posterior instability will be performed arthroscopically.

TECHNIQUES

Open Posterior Stabilization

The posterior approach to the shoulder begins with a vertical incision extending from approximately 1 cm medial to the posterolateral corner of the acromion and extends down toward the posterior axillary fold. Dissection is carried down to the deltoid muscle, which is split in line with its fibers from the scapular spine extending inferiorly. Classically, the approach is then continued in the internervous plane between the infraspinatus and teres minor, dividing this interval transversely to expose the underlying posterior capsule (Fig. 19-3). Care must be taken not to stray inferiorly because the axillary nerve and posterior humeral circumflex artery exit the quadrilateral space below the teres minor.

An alternative approach involves splitting the infraspinatus in line with its fibers.[13] This allows for a more direct approach to the posterior capsule, but the split must not be carried more than 1.5 cm medial to the glenoid in order to avoid injury to the suprascapular nerve.

The capsule is opened and retractors placed to expose the posterior glenoid. If a reverse Bankart lesion is present, it is repaired. Suture anchors are placed at the glenoid margin. The sutures are passed around the labrum and knots tied sequentially. A posterior capsular shift is then performed to address capsular laxity. Because the posterior capsule is quite thin, this repair can appear to be somewhat tenuous. To combat this, some surgeons prefer to divide the infraspinatus tendon vertically, incorporating this tendon into the repair by repairing the lateral flap to the glenoid, then taking the medial flap and suturing it over the top of the lateral flap.[12]

Arthroscopic Posterior Stabilization

Arthroscopic posterior stabilization may be performed in the beach chair or lateral decubitus position. Use of the beach chair position prevents potential distortion of normal anatomy, allows the arm to be free to dynamically evaluate the glenohumeral ligaments throughout a range of motion, and provides easier conversion to an open procedure. The primary advantage of the lateral position is that distraction of the joint is obtained, allowing easier access to the inferior aspect of the posterior labrum, glenoid, glenohumeral ligaments, and capsule, the most important part of the repair.

A standard diagnostic arthroscopy, starting with visualization from the posterior portal, is performed first. An anterosuperior portal is placed within the rotator interval. A second anterior portal, placed just above the subscapularis tendon, is helpful in allowing the shuttling of sutures. After inspection of the entire joint, the arthroscope is then placed in the anterosuperior portal, allowing a view to the posterior aspect of the shoulder. The posterior glenoid, labrum, and capsule are carefully inspected. If a posterior labral detachment is present, surgical stabilization involves repair of the labrum back to the glenoid, with incorporation of the capsule into the repair in order to perform a capsulorraphy. The posterior glenoid rim is abraded with a shaver

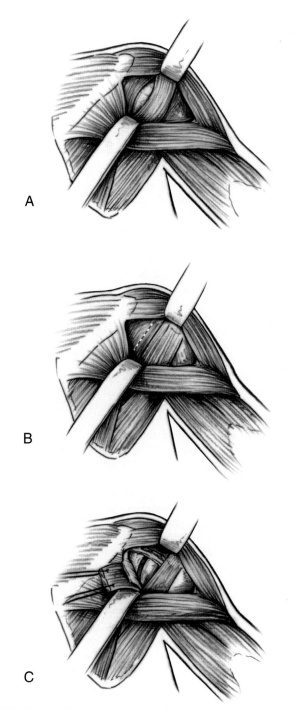

Figure 19-3 A, The capsule is approached between the infraspinatus and teres minor. **B,** Alternative approach, splitting the infraspinatus transversely. **C,** The infraspinatus and capsule are divided vertically as one layer. The lateral flap is then sutured to the glenoid to bolster the posterior capsular repair.

or rasp to expose bleeding bone. In order to place suture anchors posteriorly, an accessory posterior portal is made more laterally than the portal made for the diagnostic arthroscopy. It is remarkable how steep the angle must be with regard to the arm in order to place the anchors. A drill guide is placed, a hole drilled, and suture anchor positioned near the inferior aspect of the detachment, often as low as the 7 o'clock position (right shoulder). The suture from the anchor is passed through the labrum and a portion of the capsule (Fig. 19-4). Several variations of suture

passers are available. Often a suture is passed, then used to "shuttle" the suture from the anchor through the tissue. An arthroscopic knot is then tied. This process is repeated, moving superiorly, with three anchors commonly placed.

In cases in which no posterior labral detachment is present, capsulorrhaphy is performed without labral repair. Many surgeons still place anchors at the glenoid margin and perform the repair as described previously. Alternatively, the posterior capsule may be plicated, with sutures passed through the capsule and labrum and knots tied (Fig. 19-5). The capsule is simply folded over to reduce the size of the posterior recess. Suture capsulorrhaphy in the rotator interval, the area between the subscapularis and supraspinatus tendons, has also been advocated in addressing posterior instability. Rotator interval plication has been shown to decrease posterior translation of the glenohumeral joint.[14]

Some authors have advocated thermal treatment of the capsule to perform capsulorrhaphy. This technique is controversial, and its efficacy is undetermined, particularly relating to the posterior capsule. A cadaveric study found that posterior translation was not decreased with thermal treatment.[15] These authors postulated that the lack of substantial collagenous material in the thin posterior capsule may account for the ineffectiveness of thermal treatment posteriorly. Given these findings, along with concerns about the long-term effectiveness of thermal capsulorrhaphy in general, as well as the potential for complications, this technique is not recommended.

Open Reduction of Chronic Dislocation

When a posterior dislocation cannot be reduced through closed means, open reduction is generally performed through an anterior approach. A standard deltopectoral approached is used. If the lesser tuberosity is fractured, this fragment is identified and dissected free working on its lateral side to allow repair with the subscapularis tendon remaining attached. Releases are performed to regain length of the subscapularis. The glenohumeral joint is entered lateral to the fragment, and the humeral head is carefully levered laterally and externally rotated to allow it to be reduced to the glenoid. The lesser tuberosity is then sutured back to the defect from the fracture. When dislocation occurs without fracture of the lesser tuberosity, the subscapularis tendon may be divided off of the lesser tuberosity. After reduction of the humeral head back into the glenoid fossa, the subscapularis is mobilized, then transferred into the reverse Hill-Sachs lesion, which is lateral to the lesser tuberosity. Alternatively, the lesser tuberosity may be osteotomized and transferred into the defect, with the subscapularis remaining attached (Fig. 19-6).

POSTOPERATIVE REHABILITATION

Patients undergoing posterior stabilization are frequently placed into a "gunslinger" type of brace postoperatively to keep the arm in slight external rotation. The brace should be fitted to the patient before surgery. Patients are immobilized for 4 to 6 weeks. Passive and active-assisted ranges of motion are then initiated. Around 12 weeks, strengthening is begun, and stretches are performed if range of motion remains limited.

CRITERIA FOR RETURN TO SPORTS

Return to sports is not considered until shoulder range of motion and strength are regained. In general, a minimum of 4 months after surgery is required to reach these parameters, as well as to

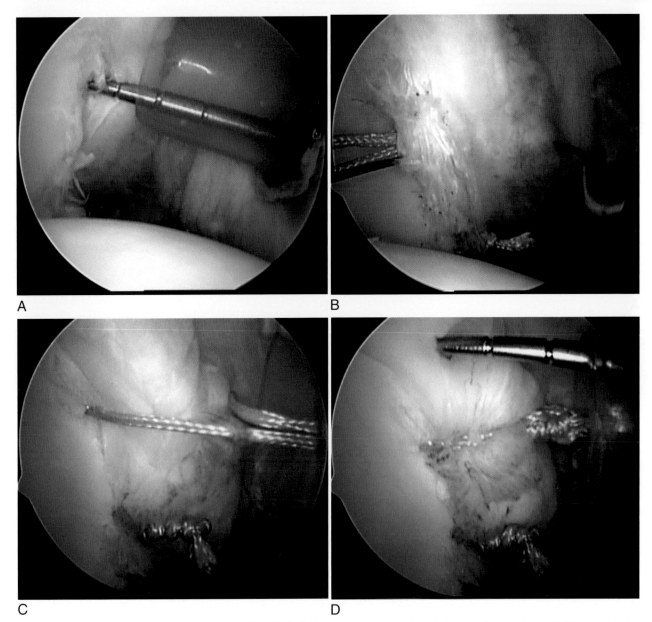

A

B

C

D

Figure 19-4 Shoulder of 20-year-old football player (from Fig. 19-1). **A,** Posterior labral detachment viewed arthroscopically. **B,** With two inferior sutures already placed and tied, final anchor has been placed and suture passed through labrum and capsule to be used as "shuttle" suture. **C,** Suture from anchor after being passed through labrum and capsule. **D,** Final posterior repair.

allow adequate healing of the repaired tissues. In many cases, return to sports is delayed for 6 months or longer.

RESULTS AND OUTCOMES

In general, posterior stabilization procedures have been reported to be less predictable than their anterior counterparts. However, many recent series have reported relatively good results. In three of the largest series of patients undergoing open stabilization, satisfactory results were obtained in 88% to 93% of patients.[9,12,16] Recent reports of arthroscopic techniques also show promise. Wolf and Eakin[17] reported on 14 patients treated with posterior suture anchor repair, 12 were graded as having

excellent results and two as having fair results. One patient required a second procedure to stabilize the shoulder. Williams et al[18] reported on 27 patients treated with arthroscopic tack stabilization of a posterior labral detachment with instability. Twenty-four patients had excellent results, and two required further surgery.

COMPLICATIONS

The most common complication of surgical posterior stabilization is recurrent instability. Postoperative stiffness is rare. With open surgery, neurologic injury can occur to the suprascapular

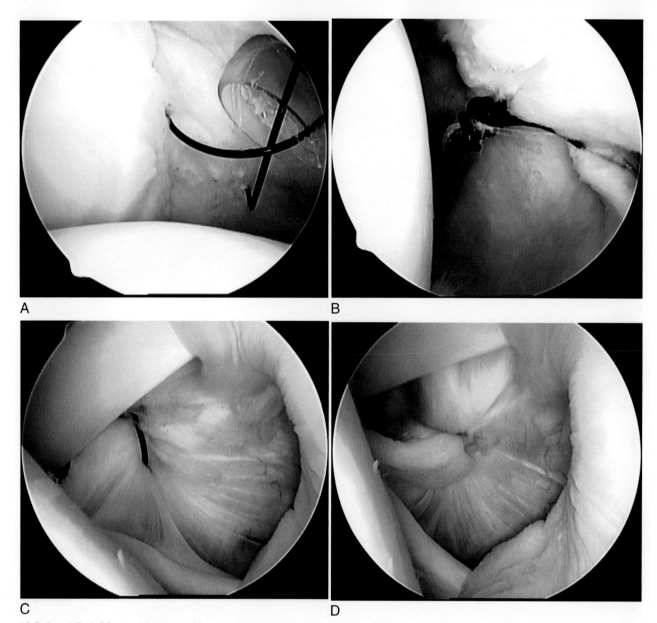

A

B

C

D

Figure 19-5 A and **B,** A 26-year-old laborer with posterior instability, no labral injury. Sutures are passed through the posterior capsule and tied (suture plication). **C** and **D,** Closure of the rotator interval in the same patient.

nerve with excessive medial dissection or the axillary nerve if care is not taken inferiorly.

CONCLUSIONS

Posterior shoulder instability is less common than its anterior counterpart. Unless it is preceded by significant trauma, a course of rehabilitation is often successful in restoring stability. When surgery is required, both open and arthroscopic stabilization procedures are available. Given the difficulties inherent in open posterior stabilization, along with promising results in recent studies of arthroscopic techniques, arthroscopic labral repair and capsular plication are likely to become more common in the future.

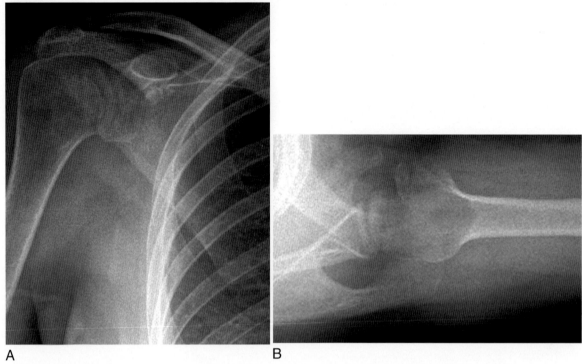

A   B

Figure 19-6 A and **B,** Postoperative radiographs of patient from Figure 19-2. Open reduction of dislocation performed, followed by transfer of lesser tuberosity and subscapularis into the defect.

REFERENCES

1. Ramsey M, Klimkiewicz J: Posterior instability: Diagnosis and management. In Iannotti J, Williams G (eds): Disorders of the Shoulder: Diagnosis and Management. Philadelphia, Lippincott Williams & Wilkins, 1999, pp 295–315.
2. Hawkins R, Koppert G, Johnston G: Recurrent posterior instability of the shoulder. J Bone Joint Surg Am 1984;66:169–174.
3. Rowe C, Pierce D, Clark J: Voluntary dislocation of the shoulder. A preliminary report on a clinical, electromyographic, and psychiatric study of twenty-six patients. J Bone Joint Surg Am 1973;55:445–460.
4. Hawkins R, McCormack R: Posterior shoulder instability. Orthopedics 1988;2:101–107.
5. Tibone J, Bradley J: The treatment of posterior subluxation in athletes. Clin Orthop 1993;291:124–137.
6. Mair S, Zarzour R, Speer K: Posterior labral injury in contact athletes. Am J Sports Med 1998;26:753–758.
7. Hawkins R, Neer C, Pianta R, Mendoza F: Locked posterior dislocation of the shoulder. J Bone Joint Surg Am 1987;69:9–18.
8. Noble J, Morin W: Surgery for posterior instability. In Hawkins R, Misamore G (eds): Shoulder Injuries in the Athlete. New York, Churchill Livingstone, 1996, pp 173–187.
9. Bowen M, Warren R: Recurrent posterior subluxation—Open surgical treatment. In Warren R, Craig E, Altchek D (eds): The Unstable Shoulder. Philadelphia, Lippincott–Raven, 1999, pp 237–247.
10. Fronek J, Warren R, Bowen M: Posterior subluxation of the glenohumeral joint. J Bone Joint Surg Am 1989;71:205–216.
11. Metcalf M, Savoie F, Field L: Arthroscopic stabilization in posterior or multidirectional instability of the shoulder. Instr Course Lect 2003;52:17–23.
12. Hawkins R, Janda D: Posterior instability of the glenohumeral joint. A technique of repair. Am J Sports Med 1996;24:275–278.
13. Shaffer B, Conway J, Jobe F, et al: Infraspinatus muscle-splitting incision in posterior shoulder surgery. Am J Sports Med 1994;22:113–120.
14. Harryman D, Sidles J, Harris S, Matsen F: The role of the rotator interval capsule in passive motion and stability of the shoulder. J Bone Joint Surg Am 1992;74:53–66.
15. Selecky M, Tibone J, Yang B, et al: Glenohumeral joint translation after arthroscopic thermal capsuloplasty of the posterior capsule. J Shoulder Elbow Surg 2003;12:242–246.
16. Bigliani L, Pollock R, McIlveen S, et al: Shift of the posteroinferior aspect of the capsule for recurrent posterior glenohumeral instability. J Bone Joint Surg Am 1995;77:1101–1120.
17. Wolf E, Eakin C: Arthroscopic capsular plication for posterior shoulder instability. Arthroscopy 1998;14:153–163.
18. Williams R, Strickland S, Cohen, M, et al: Arthroscopic repair for traumatic posterior shoulder instability. Am J Sports Med 2003; 31:203–209.

REFERENCES

Multidirectional Instability

Spero G. Karas and Jeffrey T. Spang

In This Chapter

Nonoperative management
Surgery
  Open capsular shift
  Arthroscopic stabilization

Introduction

- Multidirectional instability (MDI) of the shoulder has become an increasingly recognized source of shoulder disability.

- In general, patients are thought to have excessive generalized laxity of the glenohumeral joint capsule.

- If unrecognized MDI patients are treated as simple anterior dislocators, the underlying causes of shoulder pain and instability will not be correctly addressed.

- Common misdiagnoses for MDI include impingement, brachial plexitis, thoracic outlet syndrome, and unidirectional instability.[1] Thus, recognizing pathology unique to the MDI patient is critical to achieve successful management.

Neer and Foster[2] reported the first series of MDI patients in 1980 and coined the term that remains in use today. However, the exact definition of MDI is not clear. MDI may be defined as the ability to dislocate or subluxate the glenohumeral joint in three directions (anteriorly, inferiorly, and posteriorly) with reproduction of symptoms in one or more of these directions.[2] Some authors believe that MDI patients have a primary direction of symptomatic instability in conjunction with other areas of significant laxity. However, these patients rarely present with complete or global symptomatic laxity.[3] It is important to recognize the difference between laxity (joint mobility objectively described) and instability (an abnormal increase in glenohumeral translation that causes symptoms).[1,3,4] Although treated as a distinct entity, MDI may represent the extreme on a graduated spectrum of joint laxity.[5] The distinction between traditional anteroinferior shoulder instability and MDI can be subtle and spotlights the importance of the clinical examination in differentiating the two.

ETIOLOGY

Shoulder laxity can be congenital, acquired, or some combination of both.[1] Acquired laxity has been shown to occur in athletes with repetitive shoulder motions (gymnasts, swimmers, throwers) and manual laborers. It is possible that repetitive use patterns involving the extremes of glenohumeral motion lead to tissue laxity.[1]

Patients may also have joint laxity due to a collagen disorder (i.e., Ehlers-Danlos syndrome). These patients may also present with a history of recurrent ankle sprains and patellar dislocations.[6] Congenital collagen abnormalities are thought to represent a small fraction of MDI patients.[7]

An analysis of shoulder capsular tissue from patients with MDI reveals some collagen differences when compared to asymptomatic shoulders, thus supporting a biochemical etiology of MDI. Tsutsui[8] found no differences in the amount of collagen but did find significantly reduced collagen cross-links in the glenohumeral joint capsules of patients with MDI. Bell and Hawkins[9] also noted similar collagen types and quantities but described significantly decreased collagen formation in the MDI samples. Rodeo et al[10] found no major differences with regard to collagen types when comparing typical anterior dislocators with MDI patients, but skin analysis of MDI patients indicated a significantly smaller mean collagen fibril diameter, thus suggesting the possibility of an underlying connective tissue disorder. It is unclear from these biochemical studies whether the difference between MDI capsular tissue and normal shoulder tissue contributes to shoulder laxity or results from increased joint mobility.

Authors have noted that the definitive etiology of MDI is likely multifactorial.[11] The approach of Neer and Foster remains instructive. They concluded that MDI is based on two major factors in varying proportions: the inherent laxity of the shoulder tissue and the activity level of the individual patient.[2]

RELEVANT ANATOMY AND PATHOPHYSIOLOGY

Schenk et al[1] noted "the anatomic lesion found in MDI is a large, patulous inferior capsular pouch" that is often associated with a deficient rotator interval. These two pathologic findings contribute to an overall increase in capsular volume and glenohumeral laxity. The voluminous capsule and rotator interval lesion act to disrupt the complex components that serve to stabilize the glenohumeral joint.

In MDI, all components that contribute to stability are affected at some level. Glenohumeral stability is established by the static stabilizers (bony architecture, labral support, and ligamentous structures) and by dynamic muscular control. Static stabilizers such as the inferior labrum and the inferior and superior capsular structures resist inferior translation of the humeral head. The inferior labrum is an important extension of the glenoid, providing depth and a buttress to humeral head translation.[12] The superior capsular elements, including the superior

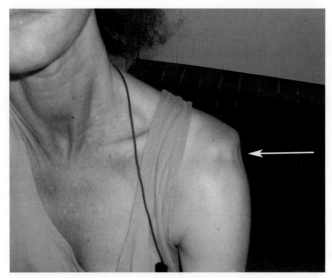

Figure 20-1 The sulcus sign. Traction on the adducted arm produces a conspicuous sulcus *(arrow)* between the acromion and humeral head. This is a classic physical examination finding in multidirectional instability.

glenohumeral ligament and the other structures of the rotator interval, prevent the humerus from translating inferiorly and posteriorly when the arm is in adduction. Failure of these superior elements leads to the classic "sulcus sign" on physical examination (Fig. 20-1).[13] The intact rotator interval also serves to maintain the normal negative pressure environment that exists in the glenohumeral joint, thus enhancing stability. As the arm is abducted, the rotator interval structures play a decreasing role in glenohumeral stability. In abduction, the anterior and posterior inferior glenohumeral ligaments become increasingly important in preventing inferior migration.[13] Other sectioning studies have also confirmed the importance of the rotator interval to overall shoulder stability.[14]

As Neer and Foster originally proposed, injury to the stabilizing structures likely occurs with repetitive microtrauma, thus rendering the superior and inferior capsular structures unable to provide adequate stability.[2] This may in turn lead to gradual failure of the posterior stabilizers of the shoulder. The combination of events may lead to symptomatic glenohumeral laxity.

The dynamic component of shoulder stabilization is the rotator cuff–deltoid coupling. The combined effect of the rotator cuff musculature is to create a glenohumeral joint compressive force.[15] It has been proposed that MDI patients have poor muscular control of shoulder function. Others have noted that patients with instability show decreased proprioception with shoulder movement.[3,16] Failure of the active stabilizers in the shoulder likely comprises a significant portion of the global laxity associated with MDI.

CLINICAL FEATURES AND EVALUATION

Patients with MDI may report recurrent subluxations with minimal trauma and a *sense* of instability rather than frank dislocations that require reduction. While occasionally caused by a single large traumatic event, most MDI patients do not present with a high-energy dislocation. When dislocations do occur, they usually require minimal force and frequently spontaneously reduce. Patients may not describe individual episodes of subluxation and may instead complain of a "dead arm" or pain after

episodes of physical activity.[17] Some authors report that patients typically are symptomatic in the midrange positions of glenohumeral motion and can be symptomatic during activities of daily living.[1] It is particularly important to obtain information about the activities and arm positions that are associated with symptoms. This may provide clues to the direction of instability. An important part of the initial patient evaluation involves recognizing the voluntary dislocating patient. This subgroup of patients frequently has secondary gain issues and will not be compliant with treatment regimens.[6]

The physical examination of the patient must elicit nonvolitional glenohumeral translation that reproduces the patient's symptoms.[6] Again, the key factor is to separate asymptomatic joint laxity from symptomatic instability. It is critical to examine the asymptomatic shoulder to establish a baseline understanding of the patient's natural laxity. However, it is not uncommon to note bilateral symptoms in patients with MDI.

Neer and Foster hypothesized that a patulous inferior capsule was the cardinal lesion in the MDI shoulder.[2] Inferior laxity must be assessed by applying inferior traction to the adducted arm in a bid to cause inferior humeral migration. If inferior translation of 1 to 2 cm occurs with the appearance of skin indentation under the acromion (sulcus sign), the patient is thought to have inferior capsular laxity, an important component of MDI (see Fig. 20-1).[2] Inferior laxity may also be evaluated by abducting the arm 90 degrees and directing an inferior force on the proximal humerus in an effort to promote excessive inferior translation.[13] A careful examination of anterior and posterior glenohumeral stability should also be performed. Multiple maneuvers exist that can help define anterior and posterior laxity, including the apprehension-relocation test, the load and shift test, and the push-pull test.

Plain radiographs are typically normal in patients with MDI. In patients with a documented traumatic dislocation superimposed on the clinical setting of MDI, a humeral head defect (Hill-Sachs lesion) or glenoid injury may be noted. Mag-

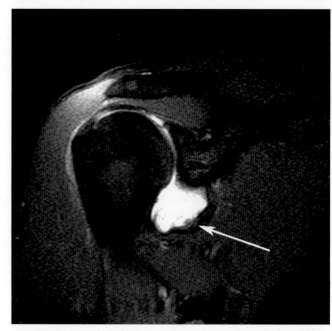

Figure 20-2 Contrast-enhanced magnetic resonance coronal image of a patient with symptomatic multidirectional instability. Contrast distends the voluminous capsule *(arrow)*. Frequently, this is the only pathologic radiographic finding in patients with multidirectional instability.

netic resonance imaging may also be noncontributory in the diagnosis of MDI. However, contrast-enhanced magnetic resonance imaging may reveal a voluminous capsule or labral injury (Fig. 20-2).

TREATMENT OPTIONS

Nonoperative Management

Nonoperative management with targeted physical therapy is the first step in treatment. Kronberg et al[18] and Burkhead and Rockwood[19] have concluded that the majority of patients with generalized instability will respond favorably to a physical therapy regimen. In particular, Burkhead and Rockwood[19] reported satisfactory results in 88% of their patients with MDI. Thus, a structured course of physical therapy is likely to provide relief in the majority of patients.

Any physical therapy protocol should combine rotator cuff strengthening with scapular stabilization to improve humeral-scapular coordination and glenohumeral stabilization.

Surgical Management

Historically, when compared with anterior instability, uniformly excellent results have been difficult to achieve in the surgical management of MDI. The reason for the relatively high failure rates seen in the surgical repair of MDI is multifactorial but likely stems from the complex array of pathophysiologic processes that contribute to the condition.[1,2,6,8–10,12,14,16,18]

Indications for the surgical management of MDI include those patients with symptomatic capsular laxity who have failed a 6-month course of formal, supervised physiotherapy. It is important to counsel surgical candidates that MDI, especially severe cases with large glenohumeral translational displacements, has a higher rate of failure than surgery for anterior instability.

Surgical contraindications for MDI include those patients who are unwilling or unable to perform a rigorous postoperative physiotherapy program. Similarly, patients who were noncompliant with a prescribed preoperative physiotherapy program may be deemed inappropriate surgical candidates. Patients with voluntary dislocation, especially those who use shoulder instability for secondary gain, are also typically poor candidates for surgical intervention.

SURGERY

Open Stabilization

The standard technique for open capsular shift has changed little since its original description in 1980.[2] An incision is made in the axillary fold, and the cephalic vein is located and protected during retraction. The deltopectoral interval is used to access the subscapularis, which is incised and retracted medially. The capsule is divided in a T fashion to form inferior and superior flaps. The inferior flap is then mobilized from the inferior humeral neck. Superior advancement of the mobilized inferior flap serves to decrease the volume of the axillary pouch. Once the inferior flap is advanced, it is secured to the humeral neck with strong nonabsorbable sutures. The superior flap is then placed over the top of the inferior flap to reinforce the repair. The subscapularis is reattached anatomically (Fig. 20-3).

An alternative technique approaches the capsule by splitting the subscapularis tendon in line with its fibers. This approach is theorized to provide less surgical trauma to the subscapularis tendon, which may be favorable in throwing athletes undergoing open inferior capsular shift.[20]

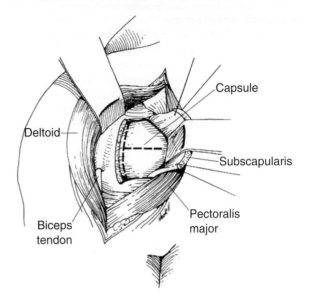

A

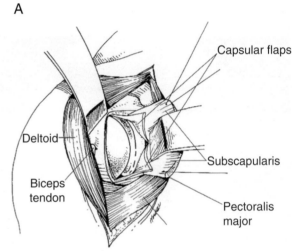

B

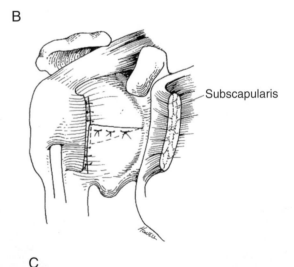

C

Figure 20-3 Open capsular shift. **A,** The subscapularis is incised to expose the anterior capsule. **B,** A laterally based T-capsulotomy produces superior and inferior capsular flaps. **C,** After the inferior flap is released from the humeral neck, it is advanced superior to reduce the volume of the axillary pouch and tighten the inferior and middle glenohumeral ligaments. (From Hawkins RJ, Bell RH, Lippitt SB: Instability. In Hawkins RJ, Bell RH, Lippitt SB [eds]: Atlas of Shoulder Surgery. Philadelphia, Mosby, 1996, pp 65–67.)

Arthroscopic Stabilization

Arthroscopic reconstruction for MDI typically involves *pancapsular plication* of the glenohumeral capsule. Due to global laxity in the MDI shoulder, the posterior, anterior, inferior, and superior (rotator interval) structures must be addressed. We prefer the lateral position for all intra-articular reconstructions due to the enhanced field of vision that joint distraction provides.

A standard posterior arthroscopic portal is used to inspect the articular surfaces, labral rim, rotator interval and biceps, rotator cuff articular side, and the axillary pouch. Placing the arthroscope into the anterior portal will also facilitate improved visualization of the posterior labrum, the posterior band of the inferior glenohumeral ligament, and the posterior capsule. In classic MDI, there are few anatomic lesions. The most commonly encountered finding is a voluminous axillary recess, the classically defined entity in MDI.

We prefer to address the voluminous pouch with a series of "pinch tucks" or capsular plications. A suture shuttle device is passed through a fold of capsular tissue that will be folded over itself toward the labrum. These 1- to 2-cm tissue advancements begin at the 6 o'clock position on the glenoid and proceed superoanteriorly and superoposteriorly until adequate ligamentous tensioning is achieved. For most moderate to severe cases of MDI, we also incorporate a previously described method of interval closure[21] (Fig. 20-4).

Thermal treatment of collagenous structures was originally met with great enthusiasm. The concept is straightforward; the glenohumeral ligaments are heated with an arthroscopic laser or radiofrequency device. This thermal energy causes the ligaments to contract and become tighter, thus rendering the shoulder more stable. The technique is simple and minimally invasive and does not require tying intra-articular knots. Unfortunately, with longer follow-up, few authors have noted uniformly good results. Others believe that there may still be a limited role for thermal energy in addressing subtle instability in throwing athletes.[22] However, a number of authors have recently reported on the relatively poor surgical results for MDI treated with thermal capsulorrhaphy.[23–25]

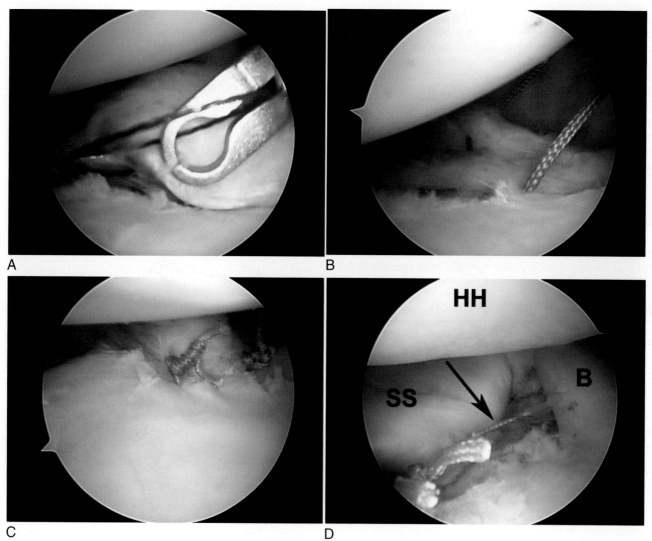

Figure 20-4 Arthroscopic capsular plication. **A,** A shuttle device is passed through the capsule and labrum. **B,** The shuttle device is used to pass a strong, braided polyester suture through the capsulolabral complex. **C,** Completed arthroscopic reconstruction. Multiple "pinch tucks" are performed to tighten the glenohumeral ligaments and reduce the volume of the glenohumeral joint. **D,** Arthroscopic sutures in the rotator interval *(arrow)* further reduce capsular volume and serve to eliminate pathologic translation of the glenohumeral joint. B, biceps; HH, humeral head; SS, intra-articular subscapularis tendon. (Courtesy of Dr. John W. Xerogeanes.)

POSTOPERATIVE REHABILITATION

The postoperative rehabilitation program is composed of four phases.

In phase I, the patient undergoes a period of immobilization with a sling or orthosis. Immobilization can last from 1 to 8 weeks, depending on the degree of instability and demands of the patient. During phase II, the patient begins range of motion exercise to achieve full, pain-free range of motion. In phase III, the patient begins resistance exercise with rubber tubing or weights. Full return of strength is the goal in phase III rehabilitation. Finally, in phase IV, athletes perform sport-specific therapy. Phase IV will restore proprioception and motor control as a means to return the athlete to his or her particular sport.

CRITERIA FOR RETURN TO SPORTS

Athletes undergoing open or arthroscopic reconstruction for MDI must complete the four-phase rehabilitation program. Full range of motion and strength should be achieved prior to athletic participation. In patients with low-grade MDI, this can take as little as 6 months. Throwing athletes or those participating in overhead sports (tennis, swimming, volleyball) should be counseled that return to play can take as long as 12 to 18 months.

RESULTS OF SURGICAL TREATMENT

Historically, the outcomes for surgical management have been difficult to characterize due to the wide spectrum of pathology inherent to MDI. Patients with underlying collagen disorders and high-grade laxity are among the most difficult to treat, and the results in this patient population have been variable.

However, patients with more subtle forms of MDI have been successfully managed with open and arthroscopic techniques. In the original description of Neer and Foster[2] of the open capsular shift, 32 shoulders were followed for a minimum of 1 year. Only one patient developed recurrent instability, but 23 of these patients were followed for less than 2 years. Altchek et al[7] described a T-plasty modification of the Bankart procedure for the management of MDI.[1] Of 42 shoulders in 40 patients, only four shoulders had recurrence of instability postoperatively. More recently, Treacey et al.[26] and McIntyre et al[27] have described arthroscopic techniques for the management of MDI. They noted low recurrence rates and high patient satisfaction, comparable with the results for open reconstruction.

COMPLICATIONS

The most common complication of surgical management is recurrence of instability. This is particularly the case in patients with collagen disorders or high-grade instability. While rare, infection, axillary nerve injury, and postoperative stiffness are also potential complications of instability surgery for MDI.

CONCLUSIONS

MDI is a complex form of shoulder instability that ranges from subtle increases in glenohumeral translation to severe instability of the glenohumeral joint. Multiple factors have been implicated in the etiology of MDI, which makes it a challenging diagnostic and therapeutic entity. Correctly diagnosed patients should initiate treatment with a formal physiotherapy program. Open and arthroscopic surgical reconstructive techniques may be necessary in those patients who fail nonoperative rehabilitation.

REFERENCES

1. Schenk TJ, Brems JJ: Multidirectional instability of the shoulder: Pathophysiology, diagnosis, and management. J Am Acad Orthop Surg 1998;6:65–72.
2. Neer CS 2nd, Foster CR: Inferior capsular shift for involuntary inferior and multidirectional instability of the shoulder. A preliminary report. J Bone Joint Surg Am 1980;62:897–908.
3. Mallon WJ, Speer KP: Multidirectional instability: Current concepts. J Shoulder Elbow Surg 1995;4:54–64.
4. Fu FH, Burkhead WZ, Flatow EL, et al: Controversies in reconstruction of the unstable shoulder: Mobility vs. instability. Contemp Orthop 1993;26:301–322.
5. Bigliani LU, Kurzweil PR, Schwartzbach CC, et al: Inferior capsular shift procedure for anterior-inferior shoulder instability in athletes. Am J Sports Med 1994;22:578–584.
6. Flatow EL, Warner JJ: Instability of the shoulder: Complex problems and failed repairs. Part I. Relevant biomechanics, multidirectional instability, and severe glenoid loss. Instr Course Lect 1998;47:97–112.
7. Altchek DW, Warren RF, Skyhar MJ, et al: T-plasty modification of the Bankart procedure for multidirectional instability of the anterior and inferior types. J Bone Joint Surg Am 1991;73:105–112.
8. Tsutsui H: Biochemical study on collagen from the loose shoulder joint capsule. In Morrey BF, Hawkins RJ (eds): Surgery of the Shoulder. Philadelphia, Mosby, 1991, pp 108–111.
9. Bell RM, Hawkins RJ: Collagen typing and production in multidirectional instability of the shoulder. Orthop Trans 1991;15:188.
10. Rodeo SA, Suzuki K, Yamauchi M, et al: Analysis of collagen and elastic fibers in shoulder capsule in patients with shoulder instability. Am J Sports Med 1998;26:634–643.
11. Paxinos A, Walton J, Tzannes A, et al: Advances in the management of traumatic anterior and atraumatic multidirectional shoulder instability. Sports Med 2001;31:819–828.
12. Cooper DE, Arnoczky SP, O'Brien SJ, et al: Anatomy, histology, and vascularity of the glenoid labrum. An anatomical study. J Bone Joint Surg Am 1992;74:46–52.
13. Warner JJ, Deng XH, Warren RF, et al: Static capsuloligamentous restraints to superior-inferior translation of the glenohumeral joint. Am J Sports Med 1992;20:675–685.
14. Harryman DT 2nd, Sidles JA, Harris SL, et al: The role of the rotator interval capsule in passive motion and stability of the shoulder. J Bone Joint Surg Am 1992;74:53–66.
15. Gibb TD, Sidles JA, Harryman DT 2nd, et al: The effect of capsular venting on glenohumeral laxity. Clin Orthop 1991;(268):120–127.
16. Warner JJ, Lephart S, Fu FH: Role of proprioception in pathoetiology of shoulder instability. Clin Orthop 1996;(330):35–39.
17. Hawkins RJ, Abrams JS, Schutte J: Multidirectional instability of the shoulder—An approach to diagnosis. Orthop Trans 1987;11:246.
18. Kronberg M, Brostrom LA, Nemeth G: Differences in shoulder muscle activity between patients with generalized joint laxity and normal controls. Clin Orthop 1991;269:181–192.
19. Burkhead WZ Jr, Rockwood CA Jr: Treatment of instability of the shoulder with an exercise program. J Bone Joint Surg Am 1992;74:890–896.
20. Kvitne RS, Jobe FW: Anterior capsulolabral reconstruction for instability in the throwing athlete. In Craig E (ed): The Shoulder. New York, Lippincott Williams & Wilkins, 1997, pp 89–108.
21. Karas SG: Arthroscopic rotator interval repair and anterior portal closure: An alternative technique. Arthroscopy 2002;18:436–439.

22. Reinhold MM, Wilk KE, Hooks TR, et al: Thermal-assisted capsular shrinkage of the glenohumeral joint in overhead athletes: A 15- to 47-month follow-up. J Orthop Sports Phys Ther 2003;33:455–467.

23. D'Alessandro DF, Bradley JP, Fleischli JE, et al: Prospective evaluation of thermal capsulorrhaphy for shoulder instability: Indications and results, two- to five-year follow-up. Am J Sports Med 2004;32:21–33.

24. Miniaci A, McBirnie J: Thermal capsular shrinkage for treatment of multidirectional instability of the shoulder. J Bone Joint Surg Am 2003;85:2283–2287.

25. Noonan TJ, Tokish JM, Briggs KK, Hawkins RJ: Laser-assisted thermal capsulorrhaphy. Arthroscopy 2003;19:815–819.

26. Treacy SH, Savoie FH 3rd, Field LD: Arthroscopic treatment of multi-directional instability. J Shoulder Elbow Surg 1999;8:345–350.

27. McIntyre LF, Caspari RB, Savoie FH 3rd: The arthroscopic treatment of multidirectional shoulder instability: Two-year results of a multiple suture technique. Arthroscopy 1997;13:418–425.

21 Overuse Injuries

Philip C. Forno and Jeffrey A. Guy

In This Chapter

INTRODUCTION

- The focus on proper training of the athlete has become increasingly important in recent years as the rapid growth of participatory sports has placed increasing demands on the mature and immature skeleton.

- The continued growth of organized sports is now clearly evident throughout the world. Given this growth, the future promises to see the majority of athletes in developed countries spending their physical activity and exercise time involved in organized sports.

- As the numbers of adult and pediatric athletes continue to rise, the patterns of their participation have changed as well. The concept of "free play" and the notion of participating in a variety of sporting activities have been replaced with "sports-pecificity" and concentration on excellence in a single sport. Compounding the problem is the development of summer sports camps, "showcase games," and "traveling All Star teams."

- The media-generated concept of the "elite athlete" encourages many to strive toward unrealistic goals. The intensity of competition and the pressure to perform seem to only increase with age and ability.

- With widespread interest and focus on excellence in sports, it becomes increasingly important that parents, coaches, trainers, and health professionals look to accept responsibility for the health and well-being of young athletes as they continue to physically and mentally mature.

- The following chapter outlines the musculoskeletal characteristics of overuse shoulder injuries in the athlete and provides a brief description of common injuries and disorders seen in this population. In addition, the general physical characteristics and therapeutic options are provided to promote the early identification and prompt institution of therapy necessary to return the injured athlete back to sport.

RISK FACTORS FOR OVERUSE INJURY

Over 25 million young athletes participate in school sponsored sports and an additional 20 million participate in extracurricular organized sports. The past decade has seen a continued increase in organized sports with more pressure to succeed, more organized and advanced leagues, more opportunities for structured play, and traveling teams. This increase in activity and participation has led to a corresponding increase in overuse injuries in this young population.

Until recently, sports medicine has been primarily focused on the treatment of acute injuries or those injuries that occur in a single episode or event. These injuries most often occur during full-contact sports like football, soccer, and hockey. However, the focus on acute injuries is not as relevant as it once was. The recreational athlete of today is typically involved in repetitive sports such as running, aerobics, swimming, and/or overhead sports. Athletes involved in these sports are less likely to experience an acute injury, yet are more susceptible to injury secondary to repetitive microtrauma. Younger athletes continue to involve themselves in organized year-round sports and are predisposed to similar overuse injuries.

Overuse injuries can be characterized as the accumulation of microtrauma in a setting that does not allow for adequate repair of normal musculoskeletal tissue. The overuse or perhaps "misuse" of musculotendinous units in the upper extremity can lead to chronic tendon, muscle, and ligament disease. Some overuse injuries are specific to children and adolescents, such as damage to the apophysis and physis.

The etiology of overuse is often multifactorial, including repetitive mechanical load, anatomic malalignment, training errors, and equipment problems (Table 21-1). A resulting muscle imbalance may lead to abnormal kinematics or repetitive tensile failure. Overuse injuries can be insidious and difficult to diagnose. Acute injuries often force an athlete out of play and demand immediate attention. Continued slow accumulation of microinjury may be easily overlooked by both athlete and physician. Early diagnosis and prevention remain paramount. When overuse injuries are caught early in their course, the athlete will most often respond favorably to conservative treatment with minimal time out of play. When diagnosed late, the injury complex may have progressed to the point of requiring significant time off for rest, rehabilitation, and possibly surgery. Recognition of poor technique or inadequate stretching, proper strength training, and reduction of excessive play are all key to preventing overuse injuries.

Table 21-1 Risk Factors for Overuse Injuries
Extrinsic
• Poor coaching
• Improper equipment/clothing
• Errors in training, frequency, duration, intensity
Intrinsic
• History of injury
• Poor technique
• Poor flexibility
• Muscle imbalance
• Anatomic abnormality
• Associated illness
• Poor conditioning

Table 21-3 Organized Baseball	
1970s	*1990s*
• Start at 9 years old	• Start at 5 years old
• Two leagues	• Multiple leagues
• Bimodal	• Year round
• Multisport involvement	• Sport specific

SHOULDER

The shoulder joint sits at the "center of action" for most sports involving the upper extremity. Baseball pitching, tennis, gymnastics, and competitive swimming are sports that share certain similarities (Table 21-2). These overhead endeavors, while all unique, rely heavily on individual accomplishment and intensive, repetitive training. Athletes in these sports may have lengthy careers beginning at a very young age. These sports all require coordinated unrestricted shoulder motion for full participation and success. The capacity for nearly global range of motion is impressive and unique to the shoulder joint. This range of motion allows an athlete to perform the specialized maneuvers necessary to throw a baseball, serve a tennis ball, or swim a race.

As a joint capable of extremes of motion, the shoulder is inherently unstable. Capsuloligamentous structures and muscular stabilizers outweigh bony contact, providing the majority of stability. Dysfunction of these soft-tissue structures, whether through attenuation or imbalance, can lead to instability, impingement, or injury. Healthy, coordinated activity of muscle, ligament, and tendon are all essential to maintain normal pain-free function in the shoulder.

BASEBALL

Perhaps the classic sports model for overuse is baseball pitching. During recent years, new understanding of the biomechanics and pathoanatomy of throwing injury have given us insight into the causes of shoulder pain in the athlete. A thorough understanding of these advances is essential to the successful approach to treating overuse injury in the baseball pitcher.

Of the capsuloligamentous structures in the shoulder, the anterior glenohumeral ligament seems to play a crucial role in overuse-related instability. During late cocking, this ligament sees high tensile forces as it prevents anterior translation of the abducted, externally rotated humerus. Posterior capsular contracture, common in the pitching shoulder, acts to further lever the humerus anteriorly. With time, repetitive stretching of this structure may lead to chronic laxity and plastic deformation. In an attempt to maintain stability, the dynamic stabilizers of the rotator cuff must compensate, rendering them vulnerable to fatigue and discoordination, eventually resulting in more damage to ligamentous restraints and recurrent instability.

Throwing sports continue to contribute significantly to the overall incidence of shoulder injury. In particular, the past 30 years has seen a significant growth in organized baseball. Children as young as 5 years old are involved and soon after may participate in multiple leagues. This is in contrast to 30 years ago when organized baseball was not available until the athletes reached the age of 9 (Table 21-3). In general, young athletes today tend to focus on single-sport specialization rather than the "free-play" concept of multisport involvement. Those athletes involved in "free play" tend to play multiple sports in a seasonal pattern, thereby resting one body part that may be emphasized during one sport and not during another. Those athletes who select one sport at an early age are at high risk of overuse injuries (Table 21-4). Compounding the problem, young athletes in their early teens are often faced with the option of playing on multiple teams at a time. While guidelines exist limiting the number of appearances or pitches during a season, there are no such rules limiting the number of teams that one may play on. The emphasis on year-round play and high-level training are a recipe for overuse injury in the throwing athlete. This vicious cycle needs to be recognized early and treated with appropriate active rest and rehabilitation.

Most cases of instability related overuse can be treated with a program of active rest and supervised rehabilitation focusing on strengthening of the rotator cuff musculature and scapular stabilizers. Posterior capsular stretching can aid in reduction of anterior translational forces. This cool down phase should be continued through the initial stages of pain and inflammation, with commencement of a staged throwing program only after restoring strength, normal kinematics, and painless motion. Reinstitution of pitching too quickly will inevitably only restart the cycle of capsular and tendon degeneration and pain. Rarely, overuse instability refractory to conservative measures may require surgical intervention.

Table 21-2 Overuse Sports	
• Gymnastics	• Volleyball
• Baseball	• Tennis
• Softball	• Swimming

Table 21-4 Overuse Factors	
• Age at start of sport	• Ovehead sport
• Frequency	• Duration
• Repetitive nature	• Year round play

Table 21-5 Organized Swimming		
U.S. Club: Practice Year Round		
• 7–10 years old	1.5 hr/day	3–5 x/wk
• 11–14 years old	2 hr/day	6–7 x/wk
• 15–18 years old	3–4 hr/day	8–10 x/wk
• College	4–5 hr/day	8–10 x/wk

SWIMMING

Shoulder pain among swimmers is a frequent cause of missed practice and time away from the sport. At least 50% of college swimmers have reported pain lasting 3 weeks or more. Among elite level swimmers, nearly 25% have reported pain interfering with practice. During a typical season, the college level swimmer can expect to cover a distance of 9000 meters per practice, participate in five to 10 practices per week, and train for 6 to 11 months per year. This amounts to nearly 1500 miles and over 1 million strokes per arm each year (Tables 21-5 and 21-6). The frequency and intensity of repetitive sport-specific training may predispose swimmers to several discrete pathologies about the shoulder. Fortunately, most overuse injuries of the shoulder in swimmers will respond favorably to an early and aggressive regimen of rest, physical therapy, retraining, and reintroduction to competition.

Endurance is a major goal of the swimmer. As such, training routines often focus on maximal power output for extended periods of time, throughout multiple contiguous sessions. The competition level athlete may expect to spend in excess of 30 hours per week in the pool. Such intense stress can rapidly overcome the intrinsic ability of musculoskeletal tissue for self-repair leading to cumulative microtrauma. Overtraining may not only exacerbate pre-existing injury, but also form an important secondary cause of shoulder pathology and pain—fatigue.

The rotator cuff musculature is responsible for retaining the highly mobile humeral head within the glenoid, while the periscapular stabilizers work to position the glenoid in space for maximal congruity of the glenohumeral joint. Weakness or fatigue of these dynamic stabilizers may result in subluxation and impingement, precipitating more pain and increased discoordination. Studies using real-time electromyography have shown altered muscle recruitment and increased impingement among painful shoulders. Continuing to swim through a period of pain or weakness may therefore lead to dyskinetic shoulder mechanics and additional injury and inflammation.

Table 21-6 Overuse Factors
Swimming
• Typical practice, 7000–9000 m
• 5–10 practices per week
• 6–11 months of training per year
• 1000–1500 miles per year
• Approximately 1,000,000 arm cycles per year

Several adaptations that allow for increased speed and strength may also predispose the swimmer to overuse injury. Unlike locomotion on land, swimmers propel themselves primarily with their upper body, essentially "pulling" themselves through a relatively viscous medium. The pectoralis major and latissimus dorsi are responsible for the strong adduction, internal rotation, and extension movement of the arm necessary for this forward motion. Studies have shown a direct correlation between strength of these muscles and swimming speed. A lax anterior and tight posterior capsule is frequently noted. The combination of laxity, posterior capsular tightness, and increased internal rotation power may predispose the swimmer to increased anterior glenohumeral translation and subsequent secondary coracoacromial impingement. In one cinematographic study, front-crawl swimmers were found to actively impinge 25% of their total stroke time.

Treatment of swimmer's shoulder begins with a mandatory period of "shut down" in which the athlete must be counseled to reduce or modify all activities to a level where no pain is experienced. This is combined with modalities and medication to reduce inflammation and break the cycle of overuse. Once the shoulder has "cooled down" from the acute episode of pain and inflammation, an aggressive schedule of stretching, strengthening, and proprioceptive exercise is begun. The swimmer's often tight posterior capsule must be stretched to reduce the anterior translation moment on the humerus. Muscle imbalance must be addressed with particular attention to strengthening the external rotators and scapular stabilizers, including the serratus anterior and teres minor, both of which have been implicated in early fatigue leading to impingement. Proprioceptive exercises and technique modification, including instruction on proper stroke mechanics and the use of body roll to properly position the scapula in space without excessive protraction, are emphasized. Ice and anti-inflammatories are useful to help break the cycle of inflammation and tendinosis. Surgery is normally reserved for severe demonstrable pathology refractory to continued conservative care.

PEDIATRIC OVERUSE INJURIES

Earlier age of participation in sports, increased number of leagues, year-round play, and sport specialization in the young athlete all cause increased demands on an immature athlete's shoulder and psyche. Pressure to succeed from role models, peers, parents, and coaches may force young athletes into unrealistic expectations of themselves and their performance. Overtraining, injury, and psychological burnout may be consequences of these pressures. In addition, skeletally immature athletes, by virtue of their evolving anatomy, are prone to certain overuse injuries not seen in more mature athletes.

A number of intrinsic factors in the growing athlete make them especially prone to injury. Growth spurts in children allow for rapid rates of bony growth, with a lag in soft-tissue adaptation of muscle and tendon. Increased stretch across the musculotendinous unit results in periods of relative inflexibility, predisposing the young athlete to muscle strains, avulsions, and strains. The rapidly growing child may feel uncoordinated during these times of intense growth leading to decreased proprioception, improper technique, and eventual overuse. The cartilaginous physis is relatively less resilient than osseous and soft-tissue structures to both mechanical and vascular stress and is thus easily injured.

There has been an increasing awareness of pediatric overuse injuries and their consequences in maturation over the past decade. This has led to increasing amounts of knowledge concerning the pathophysiology and predisposing factors to injury and pain in the adolescent athlete. Injuries sustained at the youth level may not be transient, but may affect the lifelong function of the athlete. Recent studies have postulated a relationship between humeral head remodeling in pitchers in response to lifelong throwing. A positive association has been found between risk of injury and increasing level of competition and age, possibly from the results of cumulative microtrauma. Several studies have shown a direct correlation between number and type of pitches thrown and risk of shoulder pain. These have led to recommendations limiting the number of pitches thrown per game and age recommendations for beginning certain high-risk pitches.

Probably the best known overuse injury in children is "Little Leaguer's shoulder," a repetitive strain of submaximal load to the proximal humeral physis, resulting in fatigue fracture and separation. Children typically have a long history of shoulder pain, but will sometimes report a specific throw that "set it off." There is tenderness to palpation at the physis, and radiographs reveal widening of the proximal physis. Treatment consists of active rest and avoidance of all throwing for a minimum of 6 weeks or until complete resolution of symptoms.

Proximal humeral osteochondrosis is a somewhat more rare entity, thought to result from repetitive mechanical stress across a young physis predisposed to vascular injury. Pain is the presenting complaint, localized to the epiphysis, and radiographs will reveal fragmentation of the head. The process may be similar to avascular necrosis and seems to have a poorer prognosis than Little Leaguer's shoulder.

Treatment of most pediatric overuse injuries is similar to that of the adult, and a good overall prognosis can be expected. Due to the growing athlete's high capacity for repair and regeneration, surgical intervention is very rare. Treatment begins with a period of active rest, in which all inciting activities are stopped while general strength and mobility conditioning are encouraged. Various modalities including ice, anti-inflammatories, ultrasound therapy, and massage are used to overcome the acute stages of inflammation. Progressive reintroduction of the inciting activity is then begun, with emphasis on body mechanics, proprioception, and strengthening of stabilizer muscles. Finally, gradual reintroduction to play is allowed.

The approach to overuse injuries of the pediatric shoulder must focus not only on the anatomic pathology, but on the factors predisposing the young athlete to injury. Parents and coaches must be counseled along with the child to the risk of lifelong consequences from overuse as a youth. Psychosocial pressures on the young athlete need to be recognized and addressed. Finally, a team approach using the parents, coaches, trainers, physical therapists, and athlete must be sought with the intention of returning the child to healthy, active play.

PREVENTION

Overuse injuries represent a continuum from muscle soreness and fatigue to mechanical failure of anatomic structures. Similarly, treatment and prevention span the spectrum from maintaining good sport-specific mechanics and strengthening exercises to complete rest from the sport. Central to all strategies is prevention of the initial injury cycle. While most athletes

Table 21-7 Periodization: Four Phases
• General preparation Sport unrelated fitness, general conditioning
• Specific preparation Moderate sport-specific conditioning, continue general fitness
• Early competition Gradually increasing specific exercises at below maximum level (preseason, exhibition games, etc.)
• Peak Competitive season; sport focused

train for sport-specific excellence, few concentrate on general conditioning and development of antagonistic and synergistic muscle groups. As the name implies, overuse injuries result from repetitive stress without sufficient time for reparative processes. Contributors to this problem are poor kinematics, inadequate preparation, and muscle imbalance.

Technique needs to be monitored carefully, with attention to potential motions or "habits" that place the athlete at risk. Proper mechanics, emphasizing balance and control, are taught. Beginning aggressive competition or training at high levels during early season without appropriate time for adaptation should be avoided. Similarly, within each game or training session, the athlete needs sufficient warm-up time. Attention to stabilizing and antagonist muscle groups is vital to guard against relative hypertrophy of sport-specific muscles with resulting atrophy of others. This may create dangerous imbalances, predisposing musculotendinous units to abnormal loading forces.

Recently, the concept of periodization has been proposed as a training regimen that allows for both sport-specific gains in fitness as well as prevention of overuse injury (Table 21-7). The concept classically involves four phases: general preparative, specific preparative, early competitive, and peak. The stages progress from general fitness exercises, which become increasingly sport specific, culminating in a final, very limited phase of peak power. By allowing for periods of relative rest between competition, this process allows time for muscle adaptation and repair. Continued high output without adequate time for rest is a set up for injury. In addition, by stressing general fitness, programs such as these address muscle imbalance in the single-sport athlete.

CONCLUSIONS

Overuse injuries are multifactorial and preventable. Proper attention to antagonist muscle groups, stretching, correct form, and avoidance of excessive play and training all lower the risk of developing overuse. A careful and coordinated team approach by the athlete, trainer, coach, and physician will ensure timely recognition, diagnosis, and recovery from such an injury. Proper treatment requires assessment of the athlete's entire training and playing regimen with elucidation of the etiologic factors of overuse. Only after recognition and modification of these factors can further injury be prevented.

SUGGESTED READINGS

Abrams J: Special shoulder problems in the throwing athlete: Pathology, diagnosis, and nonoperative management. Clin Sports Med 1991;10: 839–861.

Burkhart SS, Morgan CD, Kibler WB: The disabled throwing shoulder: Spectrum of pathology. Part 1: Pathoanatomy and biomechanics. Arthroscopy 2003;19:404–420.

Burkhart SS, Morgan CD, Kibler WB: The disabled throwing shoulder: Spectrum of pathology. Part 3: The SICK scapula, scapular dyskinesis, the kinetic chain, and rehabilitation. Arthroscopy 2003;19:641–661.

Crockett HC, Gross LB, Wilk KE, et al: Osseous adaptation and range of motion at the glenohumeral joint in professional baseball pitchers. Am J Sports Med 2002;30:20–26.

Hawley JA, Williams MM: Relationship between upper body anaerobic power and freestyle swimming. Int J Sports Med 1991;12:1–5.

Kibler WB, Chandler TJ: Sport-specific conditioning. Am J Sports Med 1994;22:424–432.

Lyman S, Fleisig GS, Andrews JR, et al: Effect of pitch type, pitch count, and pitching mechanics on risk of elbow and shoulder pain in youth baseball pitchers. Am J Sports Med 2002;30:463–468.

Mair SD, Uhl TL, Robbe RG, Brindle KA: Physeal changes and range-of-motion differences in the dominant shoulders of skeletally immature baseball players. J Shoulder Elbow Surg 2004;13:487–491.

Micheli LJ: The Sports Medicine Bible: Prevent, Detect, and Treat Your Sports Injuries through the Latest Medical Techniques. New York, Harper Collins, 1995.

Osbahr DC, Cannon DL, Speer KP: Retroversion of the humerus in the throwing shoulder of college baseball pitchers. Am J Sports Med 2002;30:347–353.

Reagan KM, Meister K, Horodyski MB, et al: Humeral retroversion and its relationship to glenohumeral rotation in the shoulder of college baseball players. Am J Sports Med 2002;30:354–360.

Richardson AB, Jobe FW, Collins HR: The shoulder in competitive swimming. Am J Sports Med 1980;8:159–163.

Ross JG, Gilbert GG: The National Children and Youth Fitness Study: A summary of findings. J Phys Ed, Recreation, and Dance 1985;56:45–50.

Scovazzo ML, Browne A, Pink M, et al: The painful shoulder during freestyle swimming. An electromyographic cinematographic analysis of twelve muscles. Am J Sports Med 1991;19:577–582.

Stanitski CL: Overuse injuries in the skeletally immature athlete. In DeLee JC, Drez D (eds): Orthopaedic Sports Medicine. Philadelphia, WB Saunders, 2003, pp 703–712.

Wadsworth DJ, Bullock-Saxton JE: Recruitment patterns of the scapular rotator muscles in freestyle swimmers with subacromial impingement. Int J Sports Med 1997;18:618–624.

Superior Labrum Anterior to Posterior Lesions

Walter R. Lowe and David R. Anderson

In This Chapter

Nonoperative management
Surgery—superior labrum anterior to posterior (SLAP) repair

INTRODUCTION

- A SLAP lesion is defined as a superior labrum tear that may or may not involve the long head of the biceps attachment.

- Overhead throwing athletes may develop SLAP tears from overuse and without specific injury. Traumatic shoulder injuries can cause superior labrum tears via compression or traction. Some patients develop SLAP lesions without a history of overuse or trauma.[1–3]

- Patients with SLAP tears frequently experience symptoms consistent with impingement and glenohumeral instability. As a result, the clinical diagnosis of a symptomatic SLAP tear can be difficult. Physical examination findings specific to superior labrum pathology have debatable accuracy and reliability.[3,4]

- Conservative treatment involves rest, anti-inflammatory medication, and a rehabilitation program.[3,4]

- Surgery is appropriate for patients that fail nonoperative management. Arthroscopic repair should be performed for patients with detachment of the superior labrum and biceps anchor (types II and IV). Arthroscopic débridement is appropriate for SLAP tears with an intact labrum and biceps attachment (types I and III).[3,4]

CLINICAL FEATURES AND EVALUATION

SLAP lesions have received significant attention from shoulder surgeons over the past 20 years. Andrews et al[1] initially described superior labrum tears at the insertion point of the long head of the biceps tendon in 1985. Snyder et al[3] subsequently defined the SLAP lesion in 1990, outlining four types. This chapter provides an overview of the diagnostic criteria, pertinent anatomy, treatment options including operative technique, and postsurgical rehabilitation program. Anterior and posterior labral tears and their association with glenohumeral instability are specifically addressed in Chapters 18 and 19, respectively.

Patients with superior labral tears will typically present with deep anterior shoulder pain, most pronounced with overhead activities. Clicking, catching, or popping may trouble the patient

as well. The patient may report a history of specific injury.[3,4] Overhead-throwing athletes may develop superior labral tears without specific injury. Andrews et al[1] suggest that the long head of the biceps tendon places traction on the superior labrum during the deceleration phase of throwing. Repetitive throwing may lead to superior labrum and biceps anchor detachment. Capsular tightness and poor throwing mechanics may contribute to the problem. Traumatic injuries may cause SLAP tears through traction or compression. The labrum may be pulled off the glenoid from an inferiorly directed traction force, such as catching a heavy falling object. A superiorly directed traction force could have the same effect, as in an attempt to prevent a fall by holding onto an overhead object. A fall onto an outstretched arm or a direct blow to the lateral shoulder may tear the superior labrum through a compressive load. Some patients develop SLAP tears with no history of overuse or trauma.[2,5]

A detailed shoulder physical examination, as described in Chapter 16, should be performed. Examination findings specific to superior labral pathology remain somewhat controversial. SLAP tears are commonly associated with other pathology, which complicates the interpretation of the examination.[6] The combination of history and physical examination findings should raise suspicion for SLAP injuries and direct further evaluation and treatment. Table 22-1 includes several signs and symptoms that are commonly seen with SLAP tears. Anterior tenderness in the bicipital groove, pain with resisted forward elevation (Speed's test), and pain with resisted forearm supination (Yergason's test) suggest biceps anchor pathology. Pain with resisted forward elevation in adduction and internal rotation, which is more intense than when repeated in external rotation (O'Brien's test), has been popularized as a specific test for SLAP tears.[7] Rotation and a compressive force applied to the humerus in abduction may elicit a painful click (compression rotation test). A positive apprehension/relocation test may be demonstrated in patients with SLAP tears and associated anterior instability. Physical examination findings consistent with subacromial impingement or internal impingement may be seen. An abnormal arc of motion with an internal rotation deficit may be identified in throwers.

Plain radiographs of the shoulder are typically normal in patients with SLAP lesions. Magnetic resonance imaging is the gold standard study for the radiographic diagnosis of a SLAP tear.[8] Intra-articular contrast may improve the ability to identify labral pathology. A positive study will demonstrate increased signal extending into the superior labral tissue. While the sagittal and axial images may demonstrate the tear, the coronal images are typically the most sensitive. Paralabral cysts visualized in the proximity of the superior labrum should raise suspicion of a SLAP tear.

Table 22-1 SLAP Lesions: Signs and Symptoms
History of overuse (overhead athlete) or trauma
Pain with activity
Popping, snapping, grinding
Positive Speed's, Yergason's, O'Brien's tests
Magnetic resonance imaging: Irregular appearance on coronal images
Associated pathology common (glenohumeral instability)

SLAP, superior labrum anterior to posterior.

Table 22-3 SLAP Lesions: Treatment Options
Conservative treatment: rest, nonsteroidal anti-inflammatory drugs, rehabilitation
Surgery appropriate for patients with persistent symptoms
Consider early surgery for high-demand patients
Contraindications: unclear diagnosis, inability to adhere to postoperative rehabilitation and restrictions

SLAP, superior labrum anterior to posterior.

RELEVANT ANATOMY

The glenoid labrum is a circumferential rim of fibrous tissue that surrounds the glenoid. The superior labrum is typically loosely attached to the glenoid with a triangular or wedge shape. In contrast, the inferior labrum is more securely attached to the glenoid and has a rounded appearance. The superior and anterior labra are less vascular compared to the inferior and posterior labra.[9-11]

The labrum serves as a point of attachment for several structures in the shoulder. The long head of the biceps tendon typically inserts near the 12 o'clock position. A recent study has shown that the biceps tendon originates from the supraglenoid tubercle alone in 30%, from both the supraglenoid tubercle and the superior labrum in 25%, and from the superior labrum alone in 45% of shoulders.[12] Moreover, another study has demonstrated variability in the anterior versus posterior labral contribution to the biceps tendon attachment.[13] The labrum also serves as an anchor for the superior, middle, and inferior glenohumeral ligaments. By increasing the depth of the glenoid fossa, and through its attachments to the capsuloligamentous complex, the labrum significantly contributes to glenohumeral stability.[11,14]

Snyder et al[15] classified superior labrum anterior to posterior (SLAP) tears into four types (Table 22-2). Type I lesions involve degenerative fraying of the superior labrum with an intact biceps anchor. Type II lesions involve detachment of the superior labrum and the biceps anchor from the glenoid rim. Type III lesions involve a bucket-handle superior labrum tear with an intact biceps anchor. Type IV lesions involve a bucket-handle superior labrum tear that extends into the biceps anchor.[3] Maffet et al[2] described other SLAP tear patterns that do no fit into this classification. Morgan et al[16] further divided type II SLAP tears into three subgroups based on the location of the labrum-glenoid detachment. For the purposes of this chapter, types I through IV are addressed.

Table 22-2 SLAP Lesions: Classification[15]	
Type I	Torn superior labrum, no detachment
Type II	Detached superior labrum ± biceps anchor
Type III	Bucket-handle tear superior labrum, no detachment
Type IV	Bucket-handle tear superior labrum, extension into biceps anchor

SLAP, superior labrum anterior to posterior.

TREATMENT OPTIONS

Initial conservative treatment should be considered for most patients. Nonsurgical treatment should consist of rest, anti-inflammatory medication, and a rehabilitation program emphasizing scapular stabilization, capsular stretching, rotator cuff strengthening, and modalities. Many patients, including overhead athletes, will respond well to these measures, with complete resolution of symptoms and full return to activities. Patients should be counseled that the rehabilitation program might take several weeks before results are evident. Maintenance of shoulder conditioning will minimize the chance of further pain and dysfunction. Treatment options are outlined in Table 22-3.

Patients with persistent symptoms unresponsive to conservative measures should be considered for surgical management.[4,9] Similar to other elective musculoskeletal procedures, the indications for surgery must be individualized. While some patients may be content to experience an occasional recurrence of symptoms to avoid surgery, others may prefer to optimize their outcome and minimize the risk of further symptoms by undergoing surgery. Patients who perform high-demand physical work or sports activities and those with a history of high-energy traumatic injury may be considered for early surgical treatment. This is especially true for those patients with associated glenohumeral instability and radiographic evidence of anterior/posterior labral detachment.[4,9]

As discussed previously, careful attention must be given to the evaluation of the symptoms, physical examination, and imaging. The true cause of a patient's shoulder pain can be elusive. Surgical repair of a SLAP lesion will not alleviate a patient's symptoms if the SLAP lesion is not the pain generator. Thus, surgical treatment of a SLAP tear is contraindicated if the diagnosis has not been appropriately made and other shoulder conditions have not been appropriately evaluated and treated. Operative management is contraindicated in patients with medical conditions that preclude elective surgery. Patients who are unable or unwilling to participate in postoperative rehabilitation and adhere to activity restrictions should not be treated surgically.

SURGERY

Arthroscopic Repair versus Débridement
Surgical treatment of SLAP lesions is performed arthroscopically. Characteristics of the tear pattern dictate the specific management. In general, SLAP tears that involve superior labrum and biceps tendon anchor detachment should be repaired. If the

Table 22-4 SLAP Lesions: Surgical Treatment Algorithm[15]	
Type I	Débridement
Type II	Suture anchor repair
Type III	Débridement
Type IV	Débridement (less than one third of biceps involved) Repair (more than one third of biceps involved)

SLAP, superior labrum anterior to posterior.

Table 22-5 SLAP Lesions: Surgical Equipment
Arthrex Bio-SutureTak anchors threaded with FiberWire suture
Arthrex Bio-SutureTak instrumentation
Arthrex 90-degree suture lasso
Arthroscopic cannulas (Accufex, 5 × 76 mm and 8 × 76 mm)
Arthroscopic elevators
Beach chair table attachment (Schlein)
Knot pusher
Mallet
McConnell arm holder set
Shaver (Stryker 3.5 Aggressive Plus)
Standard arthroscopy equipment
Suture retriever ×2
Two-lead arthroscopy tubing ×2

SLAP, superior labrum anterior to posterior.

superior labrum and biceps tendon anchor are firmly attached to the glenoid rim, the SLAP tear should be débrided.[3,4] Table 22-4 outlines appropriate surgical treatment for different types of SLAP lesions.

Type I SLAP lesions involve degenerative fraying of the superior labrum with no labral or biceps detachment from the glenoid rim. Therefore, type I lesions should be treated with débridement as opposed to repair. Similarly, type III SLAP lesions involve a bucket-handle tear of the superior labrum with no labral or biceps detachment from the glenoid rim. Consequently, type III lesions should also be débrided to a smooth stable border of healthy tissue. In contrast, type II SLAP lesions involve detachment of the superior labrum and biceps anchor from the glenoid rim. Thus, type II lesions should be repaired. Type IV SLAP lesions involve a bucket-handle tear of the superior labrum that extends into the biceps anchor, effectively detaching the biceps tendon attachment from the glenoid. In general, if one third or more of the biceps tendon is involved, repair should be considered. Tears involving less than one third of the tendon may be débrided.[3,4]

Technique: Arthroscopic Superior Labrum Anterior to Posterior Lesion Repair

Regardless of technique used for the repair of type II SLAP lesions, direct repair of the biceps anchor to the superior glenoid is paramount. A recent biomechanical cadaveric study emphasized the importance of biceps anchor reattachment. The study demonstrated biomechanical failure after SLAP repair at the point of biceps tendon attachment regardless of repair technique.[17]

It is essential that all required instruments and implants are available and ready to use. There are several available instrument and anchor systems that can be used to perform an arthroscopic SLAP repair. A list of the authors' preferred equipment is provided in Table 22-5.

The patient may receive a general or regional anesthetic. Our preference is for a combined general anesthetic augmented with a regional interscalene block. The patient may be positioned in the sitting beach chair or lateral decubitus position. Our preference is the sitting beach chair position. Place the arm in the McConnell arm holder under moderate longitudinal traction in line with the torso and with the shoulder in 30 degrees of abduction.

Establish a standard posterior glenohumeral portal. Insert the arthroscope into the glenohumeral joint and perform a complete intra-articular examination. Carefully inspect the articular surfaces, biceps tendon, superior labrum, subscapularis tendon, rotator cuff undersurface and insertion, axillary recess, anterior labrum, and posterior labrum. Establish an anterior portal using the outside-in technique with spinal needle localization. This portal should be positioned high in the rotator interval. Proper portal placement is critical to achieve the angles required for effective SLAP repair. Insert an arthroscopic cannula (Accufex, 5 × 76 mm). Attach a second two-lead arthroscopy tubing to this cannula for additional inflow and improved visualization. Insert an arthroscopic probe and repeat the arthroscopic examination paying close attention to injured structures. Probe the superior labrum and identify the size and location of the area of detachment (Fig. 22-1).

Establish a lateral (transrotator cuff) portal through the subacromial space and the myotendinous portion of the supraspinatus. Insert a spinal needle just lateral to the palpable acromial edge. Advance the needle through the supraspinatus directed toward the torn superior labrum. The needle angle should be very flat and perpendicular to the floor. Remove the needle and incise the skin longitudinally with a no. 11 blade scalpel. Advance the scalpel through the supraspinatus longitudinally at the same trajectory. Remove the scalpel and insert a switching stick into the joint through the incision and supraspinatus. Insert

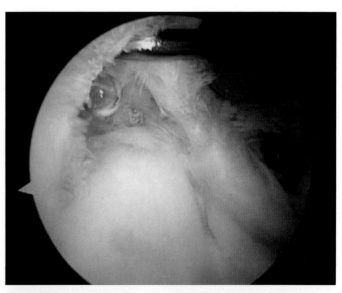

Figure 22-1 Arthroscopic view of a type II SLAP (superior labrum anterior to posterior) lesion.

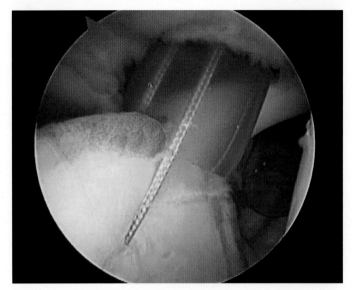

Figure 22-2 Suture anchor has been placed through the cannula and seated into the superior glenoid, and one limb of the suture passed through the labrum (simple suture repair).

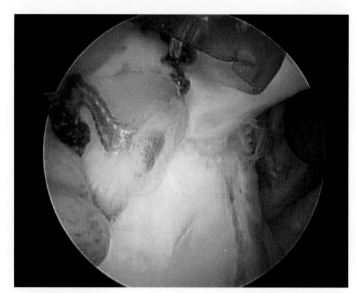

Figure 22-4 Final completed repair with two simple sutures.

an arthroscopic cannula (Accufex, 8 × 76 mm) over the switching stick.

Insert a shaver (Stryker 3.5 Aggressive Plus) through the anterior portal and gently débride the torn superior labrum. Use the shaver to prepare the repair site by exposing and decorticating the glenoid rim in the zone of detachment. An arthroscopic elevator may also be used. Evaluate the size of the tear and decide how many anchors will be necessary to achieve a stable repair. In general, two anchors are typically used for a tear that extends from the 11 o'clock to the 1 o'clock positions.

Insert the Arthrex Bio-SutureTak metal cannulated guide through the lateral cannula and position it on the glenoid rim at the location for the anterior-most anchor. Insert the punch through the guide to create a small pilot hole. Insert the 2.75-mm drill and advance until the chuck is flush with the guide. Remove the drill and insert a Bio-SutureTak anchor loaded with a single no. 2 FiberWire suture through the guide. Push the

anchor into the hole and advance with a mallet until the laser mark on the anchor inserter is flush with bone. Remove the anchor inserter. Shuttle the limbs of suture out the anterior cannula with a suture retriever.

Insert the Arthrex 90-degree suture lasso loaded with a looped no. 1 Prolene suture through the lateral cannula. Pierce the labrum superiorly with the suture lasso and advance the tip of the instrument under the detached labrum directed toward the anchor. Once the tip of the suture lasso is visible under the labrum, advance the Prolene suture loop into the joint. Grasp the loop with a suture retriever and shuttle the loop out of the anterior cannula. Select the posterior-most limb of FiberWire suture from the anchor and pass it through the prolene suture loop. Shuttle this limb of FiberWire suture through the labrum by removing the suture lasso and Prolene suture from the lateral cannula. Repeat the preceding steps to pass the second limb of FiberWire suture through the labrum. Shuttle the FiberWire suture limbs out the anterior cannula with a suture retriever. Superior labral lesions can be repaired with simple or mattress type sutures. Our preferred method is to use mattress for meniscoid type labrum anatomy and simple for smaller more atrophic labral anatomy (Fig. 22-2).

If additional anchors are required for stable repair, repeat the preceding steps for anchor insertion and suture placement. Once sufficient anchors and suture have been placed, secure the labrum down to the glenoid rim with standard arthroscopic knot-tying technique. Knots may be tied from either the anterior or lateral portal, depending on the location of the anchor and knot to be tied. The arthroscopic knot should be tied through the same portal that the anchor was placed (Fig. 22-3). When tying knots, start with the anterior-most anchor and work posteriorly. After tying each knot, cut the excess suture with the FiberWire arthroscopic suture cutter, leaving a short tail. Insert the arthroscopic probe and inspect the repair. The labrum should be firmly secured to the glenoid rim (Fig. 22-4).

POSTOPERATIVE REHABILITATION

Physical therapy is initiated within the first week after surgery. The program is divided into several phases. The patient is

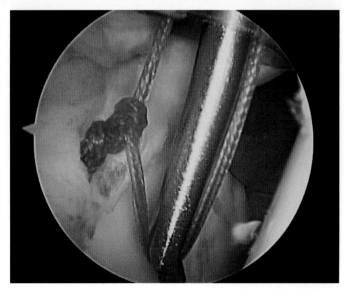

Figure 22-3 An arthroscopic knot is tied.

encouraged to perform exercises at home or at a gym between supervised physical therapy appointments. In general, the program is designed to optimize early passive and active-assisted range of motion while keeping stress off the repair during the first 6 weeks. The program is individualized to each patient, with respect to their speed of recovery and the integrity of the repair.

During the first 3 weeks after surgery (phase I), the patient wears the sling full-time except when participating in therapy. Passive range of motion, submaximal isometric, and scapular stabilization exercises are performed. Between weeks 3 and 6 (phase II), passive and active-assisted range of motion exercises are advanced, and specific strengthening exercises are initiated. Between weeks 6 and 12 (phase III), additional strengthening exercises are added and advanced. After week 12 (phase IV), gym exercises such as bench presses, lat pull-downs, and military presses are initiated. An interval-throwing program may be started at week 16. Rotator cuff strengthening and scapular stabilization exercises are continued throughout the program.

CRITERIA FOR RETURN TO SPORTS

Return of full range of motion and strength are required before return to athletic participation. Patients should be advised that 4 to 6 months are typically required before return to play. Throwing athletes must be encouraged to be patient, closely following the sequential steps of an interval-throwing program, and avoiding the tendency to throw too much too soon. An interval-throwing program can begin at 3 months postoperatively. Return to full throwing off a mound may take as long as 6 months.

RESULTS AND OUTCOMES

Several studies have documented successful surgical treatment of SLAP lesions.[15,18,19] The majority of publications address results following surgical repair of type II SLAP lesions. In general, approximately 90% of patients demonstrate good or excellent results at short to intermediate follow-up. Nevertheless, no long-term follow-up studies have been published to date. Recent publications are, however, providing additional insight into our understanding of surgical results. Kim et al[20] evaluated 34 patients at a mean of 33 months after surgical repair of type II SLAP lesions. While the overall results were good (94% satisfactory UCLA shoulder score, 91% return to preinjury shoul-

der function), significant differences were seen between patients who participated in different types of athletics. Specifically, throwing athletes had lower shoulder scores and a lower percentage of return to their preinjury level of shoulder function than patients who were not involved in overhead sports. Ide et al[21] evaluated 40 patients at a mean of 41 months after surgical repair of type II SLAP lesions. All subjects in this study were overhead athletes. Again, overall results were favorable (90% good or excellent modified Rowe score, 75% return to preinjury shoulder function). However, throwers without a specific traumatic injury had lower scores and a lower return to preinjury function rate than throwers with a history of specific traumatic injury. These publications suggest that surgical repair of type II SLAP tears in overhead athletes with an overuse-related cause may less successful than in other patients.

COMPLICATIONS

Failure to address associated pathology may result in persistent pain and dysfunction. Noncompliance with postoperative activity restrictions may lead to a recurrence of the SLAP tear. Poor participation with physical therapy or refusal to perform exercises can result in postoperative stiffness. The transrotator cuff portal has not been shown to compromise rotator cuff function or affect rehabilitation or outcomes after SLAP repair. If paralabral cyst decompression is performed, neurologic injury to the suprascapular nerve is a potential risk if an instrument is passed too far medially under the torn labrum.

CONCLUSIONS

SLAP tears may be caused by overuse such as in an overhead athlete. Conversely, SLAP tears may be the result of a traction or traumatic compression injury. Oftentimes, SLAP tears are identified in patients with no history of overuse or trauma. For many patients, initial conservative treatment consisting of rest, anti-inflammatory medication, and physical therapy is appropriate. Patients who do not respond to these conservative measures should be considered for surgery. Patients with high-demand work or athletic activities may be considered for early surgical treatment. SLAP tears with superior labrum and/or biceps anchor detachment from the glenoid rim should be arthroscopically repaired. SLAP lesions without labrum or biceps detachment may be treated with débridement.

REFERENCES

1. Andrews JR, Carson WG, McLeod WD: Glenoid labrum tears related to the long head of the biceps. Am J Sports Med 1985;13:337–340, 1985.
2. Maffet MW, Gartsman GM, Moseley B: Superior labrum-biceps tendon complex lesions of the shoulder. Am J Sports Med 1995;23:93–98.
3. Snyder SJ, Karzel RP, Del Pizzo W, et al: SLAP lesions of the shoulder. Arthroscopy 1990;6:274–279.
4. Peterson CA II, Altchek DW, Warren RF: Shoulder arthroscopy. In Rockwood CA, Matsen FA III (eds): The Shoulder, vol 2. Philadelphia, WB Saunders, 1998, pp 290–335.
5. Cheng JC, Karzel MD: Superior labrum anterior posterior lesions of the shoulder: Operative techniques and management. Oper Tech Sports Med 1997;5:249–256.
6. Kim TK, Queale WS, Cosgarea AJ, et al: Clinical features of the different types of SLAP lesions: An analysis of one hundred and thirty-nine cases. J Bone Joint Surg Am 2003;85:66–71.
7. O'Brien SJ, Pagnani MJ, Fealy S, et al: The active compression test: A new and effective test for diagnosing labral tears and acromioclavicular joint abnormality. Am J Sports Med 1998;26:610–613.
8. Connell DA, Potter HG, Wickiewicz TL, et al: Noncontrast magnetic resonance imaging of superior labral lesions: 102 cases confirmed at arthroscopic surgery. Am J Sports Med, 1999;27:208–213.
9. Burkhead WZ, Arcand MA, Zeman C, et al: The biceps tendon. In Rockwood CA, Matsen FA III (eds): The Shoulder, vol 2. Philadelphia, WB Saunders, 1998, pp 1009–1063.
10. Cooper DE, Arnoczky SP, O'Brien SJ, et al: Anatomy, histology, and vascularity of the glenoid labrum. J Bone Joint Surg Am 1992;74:46–52.
11. Pollock RG: Tissues of the shoulder and their structure. In Norris TR (ed): OKU Shoulder and Elbow, vol 2. Rosemont, IL, AAOS, 2002, pp 3–12.
12. Habermeyer P, Kaiser E, Knappe M, et al: Functional anatomy and biomechanics of the long biceps tendon. Unfallchirurg 1997;90:319–329.

13. Vangsness CT Jr, Jorgenson SS, Watson T, Johnson DL: The origin of the long head of the biceps from the scapula and glenoid labrum. J Bone Joint Surg Br 1994;76:951–954.

14. Gerber A, Apreleva M, Warner JP: Basic science of glenohumeral instability. In Norris TR (ed): OKU Shoulder and Elbow, vol 2. Rosemont, IL, AAOS, 2002, pp 13–22.

15. Snyder SJ, Banas MP, Karzel RP: An analysis of 140 injuries to the superior glenoid labrum. J Shoulder Elbow Surg 1995;4:243–248.

16. Morgan CD, Burkhart SS, Palmeri M, et al: Type II SLAP lesions: Three subtypes and their relationships to superior instability and rotator cuff tears. Arthroscopy 1998;14:553–565.

17. DiRaimondo CA, Alexander JW, Noble PC, et al: A biomechanical comparison of repair techniques for type II SLAP lesions. Am J Sports Med 2004;32:727–733.

18. O'Brien SJ, Allen AA, Coleman SH, et al: The trans-rotator cuff approach to SLAP lesions: Technical aspects for repair and a clinical follow-up or 31 patients at a minimum of 2 years. Arthroscopy 2002; 18:372–377.

19. Samani J, Marston S, Buss D: Arthroscopic stabilization of type II SLAP lesions using an absorbable tack. Arthroscopy 2001;17:19–24.

20. Kim SH, Ha KI, Kim SH, et al: Results of arthroscopic treatment of superior labrum lesions. J Bone Joint Surg Am 2002;84:981–985.

21. Ide J, Maeda S, Takagi K: Sports activity after arthroscopic superior labral repair using suture anchors in overhead-throwing athletes. Am J Sports Med 2005;33:507–514.

CHAPTER

23 Internal Impingement

E. Lyle Cain, Jr. and Ryan C. Meis

In This Chapter

Signs and symptoms
Anatomic lesions
Nonoperative management
Surgery—arthroscopic management

INTRODUCTION

- Internal impingement is defined as intra-articular contact between the posterosuperior rotator cuff and posterior glenoid labrum that occurs with the shoulder in the abducted externally rotated position (Fig. 23-1).

- Internal impingement is a common pathologic entity seen primarily in overhead athletes, especially baseball pitchers and tennis players.

- Patients with internal impingement often present with "dead arm syndrome" consisting of loss of ability to meet previous performance levels (velocity and control) with pain during the late cocking and acceleration phases of throwing.

- The pathophysiology of internal impingement often includes excessive rotational laxity with subclinical anterior capsular laxity and resultant hyperexternal rotation in the abducted position. Posterior capsular contracture and loss of internal rotation with posterosuperior translation of the humeral head has also been proposed as a potential etiology.

- The end-result is articular-sided pathology of the infraspinatus and supraspinatus in combination with posterior superior labral injury.

- Rehabilitation, focusing on gradually decreasing inflammation and normalizing shoulder motion, rotator cuff strength, scapular conditioning, and throwing biomechanics is often successful in allowing return to previous competitive levels.

- In cases of failed conservative treatment, arthroscopic shoulder surgery is the treatment of choice. Surgical treatment includes débridement or repair of the rotator cuff injury (most often partial articular-side tearing) and labral pathology (posterosuperior labral fraying or detachment).

- Thermal-assisted capsular shrinkage (TACS) or arthroscopic suture plication may be used as adjunctive treatments to reduce excessive capsular laxity in some patients.

- Surgery is effective in allowing the majority of athletes to return to previous levels of performance.

CLINICAL FEATURES AND EVALUATION

Internal impingement is a pathologic condition typically seen in overhead throwing athletes. Baseball pitchers are most commonly afflicted, although athletes participating in other sports requiring repetitive shoulder abduction and external rotation such as tennis, volleyball, javelin throwing, and swimming are at risk.[1–6] Patients typically present with complaints of posterior shoulder pain when the arm is abducted and maximally externally rotated (late cocking and acceleration phases of throwing). Symptoms may be vague and reported by the athlete only as a gradual onset of loss of velocity or control during competition, often known as dead arm syndrome (Box 23-1). Other common complaints are feeling tight and uncomfortable while throwing, along with difficulty warming up.[7] The majority of athletes do not recall a single acute event, but many report an acute exacerbation of previous lesser symptoms as the impetus for seeking medical attention. Concomitant labral injury is not uncommon and may be identified by mechanical catching or popping during the follow-through phase of throwing if an unstable lesion is present (superior labrum anterior and posterior, or SLAP). Tennis players often report pain with the overhead serve, but no difficulty with ground strokes. Athletes occasionally acknowledge a recent episode of overuse and should specifically be asked about changes in throwing habits, training, or mechanics prior to the onset of symptoms. Knowing the duration of symptoms, precise anatomic location of pain, and any previous treatment, including periods of rest, is beneficial.

Once the history is completed, a thorough physical examination is carried out as noted in Chapter 16. Specific physical examination testing for internal impingement involves eliciting pain attributed to the infraspinatus tendon and posterior superior labrum. Active range of motion of both shoulders should be carefully measured and documented, along with measures of passive internal rotation and external rotation with the shoulder in abduction and the scapula stabilized in order to mimic the position the arm reaches during the late cocking phase. Most throwers have significantly increased external rotation and concomitant decreased internal rotation in the dominant throwing shoulder due to skeletal and soft-tissue adaptations that develop over time.[6,8,9] It is not uncommon for external rotation with the shoulder abducted 90 degrees to reach 130 to 155 degrees, with limited internal rotation in the range of 40 to 55 degrees. However, the total arc of motion (external rotation + internal rotation) should be equal in both shoulders.[8,10] Asymmetrical total motion may be caused by pathologic decrease in internal rotation due to posterior capsular contracture, which Burkhart et al[11] believe is the primary underlying pathologic process driving this entity. In addition, posterior musculature contrac-

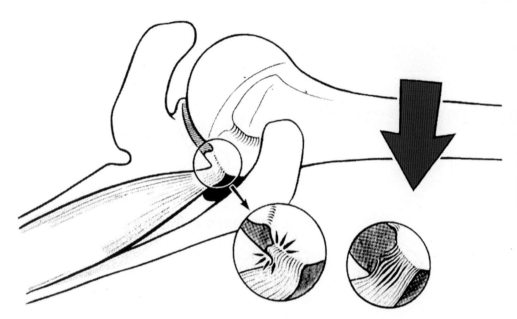

Figure 23-1 Schematic representation of posterosuperior glenoid impingement: The posterior edge of the glenoid and the deep surface of the supraspinatus and infraspinatus are directly in contact with one another. (From Walch G, Boileau P, Noel E, et al: Impingement of the deep surface of the supraspinatus tendon on the posterosuperior glenoid rim: An arthroscopic study. J Shoulder Elbow Surg 1992;1:238–245.)

ture due to the eccentric forces driving deceleration can contribute to the loss of motion.

If the patient experiences posterior pain with maximal external rotation at 90 to 110 degrees of abduction, the posterior impingement test is considered positive (Fig. 23-2).[3,12,13] Tenderness to palpation is usually located at the infraspinatus insertion on the humeral head, just inferior to the posterolateral acromial margin. This can best be elicited by having the patient lie prone with the arm hanging free over the edge of the examination table, and then palpating the posterior joint line.

Testing for labral pathology should be performed due to the strong association between internal impingement and SLAP lesions. A multitude of tests have been reported with varying degrees of sensitivity and specificity.[14] We use several including the active compression (O'Brien's), Meyer's, Mimori's, and Clunk tests, but caution the reader that no single test is adequately sensitive or specific to make the diagnosis with a high degree of certainty.[14,15] Resisted testing of the supraspinatus, infraspinatus, and subscapularis should be performed to document any side-to-side differences, although a strength deficit of at least 20% must be present to be appreciated by manual muscle testing.[16] Affected athletes often have weakness and pain with external rotation strength testing, particularly at 90 degrees

of abduction. Stability testing should be performed to assess not only the amount of translation in the glenohumeral joint, but also the endpoint of that translation. It is not uncommon for a thrower to have symmetrical, natural increases in posterior translation in both shoulders; however, most throwers do not have significant inferior translation (negative sulcus sign). Scapular motion should also be assessed by a sitting lift-off test or a wall push-up. Weakened scapular retractors and elevators can contribute to internal impingement by leading to increased compression between the posterior glenoid and humeral structures in the cocking phase.[17,18]

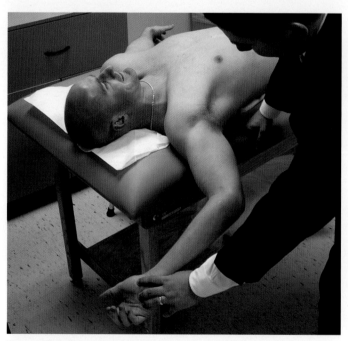

Figure 23-2 The posterior impingement test is performed with the shoulder abducted 90 to 110 degrees and in maximal external rotation. Posterosuperior shoulder pain in this position indicates a positive test.[19,23]

Box 23-1 Internal Impingement:
Signs and Symptoms

- Vague shoulder pain that later localizes posteriorly
- Stiffness and difficulty warming up to throw
- "Dead arm" or decreased throwing velocity, control, and effectiveness
- Pain in late cocking and early acceleration
- Positive posterior impingement sign
- Excessive external rotation
- Mild anterior instability and rotational instability
- Glenohumeral internal rotation deficit without corresponding increase in external rotation

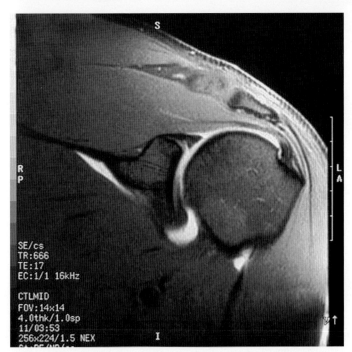

Figure 23-3 Arthrographic magnetic resonance image demonstrating a SLAP (superior labrum anterior to posterior) lesion. Less well visualized is an articular side partial-thickness rotator cuff tear.

Plain radiographs of the shoulder may show cystic changes at the insertion of the infraspinatus tendon on the humeral head, but are usually unremarkable. Our radiographic series includes four views: a Stryker notch view, an anteroposterior view in external rotation, a West Point view, and a glenoid view (Neer anteroposterior). Radiographs should be obtained to exclude other pathology, especially a posterior glenoid exostosis or Bennett's lesion, which can be a marker of internal impingement.[19] Arthrographic magnetic resonance imaging (MRI) is the best diagnostic test to evaluate potential changes associated with internal impingement. Findings on MRI most often include articular-side rotator cuff (infraspinatus) injury, posterior and superior labral injury or detachment, and cystic changes in the humeral head (Fig. 23-3).[20] Labral pathology is often subtle and difficult to diagnose accurately by nonarthrographic MRI evaluation. Special MRI sequences, especially in shoulder abduction-external rotation (ABER) views, may be useful to demonstrate common pathology. MRI results must be interpreted with caution and correlated with clinical findings because as many as 40% of asymptomatic throwers will have pathologic changes noted on MRI.[21]

RELEVANT ANATOMY

Walch et al[6] first described internal impingement as intra-articular contact between the posterosuperior rotator cuff (infraspinatus) and posterior glenoid labrum at maximal shoulder abduction and external rotation in tennis players. Anatomic lesions associated with internal impingement include injury to the articular surface of the rotator cuff (especially the infraspinatus tendon in throwers and the supraspinatus tendon in tennis players), posterior and superior labrum, and anterior capsular structures. Posterior capsular thickening and contracture have also been reported as common findings[11] (Box 23-2).

The biomechanical etiology for injury to these structures is controversial. Two possible causes have been reported, although neither is universally accepted. The most prevalent theory has been termed rotational instability, which describes the ability of the throwing shoulder to overrotate into a position of hyperexternal rotation during the late cocking and acceleration phases of the throwing motion. At maximal external rotation, the undersurface of the rotator cuff becomes entrapped between the humeral head and posterior superior glenoid labrum. This extreme position is resisted actively by the subscapularis and passively by the anterior band of the inferior glenohumeral ligament. Most shoulders, even those without symptoms, can achieve this position, and it is not considered pathologic.[2,22] However, this physiologic posture gradually creates pathology in overhead throwers because throwing imparts progressive microtrauma to the anterior capsular structures. Fatigue of the subscapularis or overload of the inferior glenohumeral ligament may lead to subtle anterior instability that can worsen the impingement by facilitating this rotational instability. If these restraints fail to keep the humeral head centered in the glenoid, then the amount of external rotation will be accentuated.[23] This, in turn, imparts even greater stress to the rotator cuff and labrum. Repetitive posterior impingement, particularly the aggressive act of throwing a baseball, may lead to fraying of either the labrum or rotator cuff and eventually pain. This cascade can result in altered mechanics, which will further irritate and fatigue the rotator cuff and scapular musculature, increase pain, and decrease effectiveness.

Another hypothesis to explain the injury cascade of internal impingement has focused on the presence of posterior capsular tightness and contracture as the predominant cause of injury.[11] Burkhart and Morgan theorized that repetitive distraction microtrauma in tension that occurs in the follow-through phase of the throwing motion in the posterior shoulder leads to scarring and capsular contracture posteroinferiorly. This has been demonstrated to cause obligate posterior and superior migration of the humeral head on the glenoid, allowing relaxation of the anterior capsule, and excessive external rotation, which may lead to injury of the posterior labrum and rotator cuff.[12,24] In addition to excessive external rotation, there is a disproportionate loss of internal rotation that they termed glenohumeral internal rotation deficit (GIRD). However, the authors of this chapter believe that overhand athletes, particularly baseball players, do not commonly present with clinical tightness of the posterior capsule.

TREATMENT OPTIONS

Nonoperative Treatment

Mild symptoms and early phases of the disorder are treated conservatively with "active rest," which includes a complete break

---

Box 23-3 Internal Impingement: Nonoperative Treatment Options

- Initially treated with anti-inflammatory modalities nonsteroidal anti-inflammatory drugs, ice, iontophoresis, and occasionally a corticosteroid injection)
- Throwing cessation
- Therapy emphasizing scapular and rotator cuff strengthening, posterior shoulder flexibility, and end-range dynamic stability
- Gradual return to throwing; interval throwing program

---

from throwing along with physical therapy. The length of time off of throwing varies. Axe[25] proposes 2 days off for every day that symptoms have been present (maximum 12 weeks), but in general 2 to 6 weeks is appropriate, based on the severity and chronicity of the symptoms (Box 23-3). Anti-inflammatory measures to "cool down" the irritated shoulder can be beneficial in accelerating the rehabilitative process. This includes nonsteroidal anti-inflammatory drugs, occasionally a corticosteroid injection, and physical therapy modalities like iontophoresis. Wilk et al[10] described a rehabilitation protocol for the conservative management of internal impingement that emphasizes dynamic stability, rotator cuff strengthening (targeting the posterior cuff), and a scapular stabilization program. Stretching to improve soft-tissue flexibility in internal rotation and horizontal adduction is also initiated with avoidance of aggressive mobilization of anterior and inferior glenohumeral structures. Drills using proprioceptive neuromuscular facilitation patterns and rhythmic stabilization are included. Perturbation and stabilization drills at end-range external rotation are essential to improve proprioception, neuromuscular control, and dynamic stability.

A formal throwing mechanics evaluation may be helpful, particularly in the younger athlete with less specialized training. The mature athlete with altered or poor throwing mechanics may also benefit from biomechanical and professional evaluation. Once an appropriate "rest" period has passed and symptoms are relieved, throwing is resumed with an interval throwing program; however, the shoulder should be completely pain free prior to resuming any throwing activities. Intensity is advanced based on symptoms, or the lack thereof, with the goal of returning to effective throwing.[26,27]

Surgical Treatment

One of the most challenging decisions facing clinicians who treat throwing athletes is whether surgical treatment is indicated and when the most appropriate time for surgery might be. Timing is based on a number of issues including injury pattern, degree of injury, potential for improvement without surgery, and temporal issues regarding the current and future seasons. Surgical intervention (Box 23-4) for internal impingement should be

---

Box 23-4 Internal Impingement: Surgical Indications

- Failure of a comprehensive nonoperative treatment program of at least 3 months' duration
- Mechanical symptoms with posterior labral signs
- Magnetic resonance imaging and examination findings consistent with internal impingement

---

undertaken only when 3 months of a solid nonoperative protocol have failed to allow a return to activity and the physical examination and radiographic studies are consistent with this particular diagnosis. The clinician must be aware that SLAP lesions often are present in this population and will typically present with mechanical symptoms and positive labral findings on examination, thus differentiating them from internal impingement alone. Experience has taught us that throwing athletes with SLAP lesions generally fare poorly without surgical repair and a more aggressive strategy should be employed.[28,29]

The goal of surgery is aimed at repairing or removing any abnormalities encountered in the shoulder and addressing the underlying pathologic process, which is often anterior and inferior laxity. The difficulty managing patients with internal impingement centers on what Wilk et al[10] have termed the thrower's paradox. This refers to the need for a thrower to have enough laxity so as to achieve the extreme external rotation necessary to maintain velocity, while at the same time avoiding pathologic laxity or instability. With that in mind, a detailed and closely supervised postoperative rehabilitation protocol is of paramount importance.

Our surgical approach begins with an examination under anesthesia, followed by arthroscopy in the lateral decubitus position (Box 23-5). A standard posterior portal in the soft spot is established, and a complete diagnostic arthroscopy is performed. The rotator cuff and labrum are carefully viewed from both anterior and posterior portals to gain a complete understanding of the pathology present. Rotator cuff tears are described by their location, depth, and quality of tissue. It is rare to have a partial tear in this younger population that is both less than 33% thickness and of sufficient quality to repair. Therefore, we commonly proceed with débridement of the tear back to healthy tissue. When the delaminated tissue from the torn fragment is retracted and of good quality or the tear exceeds 50% of the thickness of the cuff, then arthroscopic repair should be undertaken. This usually consists of a suture anchor at the articular margin, and horizontal mattress sutures securing the delaminated portion of the tendon back to the intact cuff.

Labral fraying can be débrided, but the labrum must be inspected carefully for any evidence of instability or a SLAP tear (Fig. 23-4). Failure to recognize and treat an unstable superior labrum will likely result in treatment failure.[28] Techniques for repair of SLAP lesions can be found in Chapter 22.

Again, it is essential to understand that the underlying pathology frequently revolves around mild anteroinferior instability.[12,30,31] Failure to address this problem, when present, will lead

---

Box 23-5 Internal Impingement: Operative Treatment

- Débride or fix the partial-thickness rotator cuff tear
- Débridement of labral fraying and stabilization of SLAP (superior labrum anterior to posterior) lesion, if present
- Arthroscopic capsular plication or thermal-assisted capsular shrinkage, when appropriate
- Strict postoperative adherence to the physical therapy protocol and close monitoring of progress is essential in obtaining a successful outcome
- Adjust therapy on an individual basis to avoid excessive laxity or stiffness

---

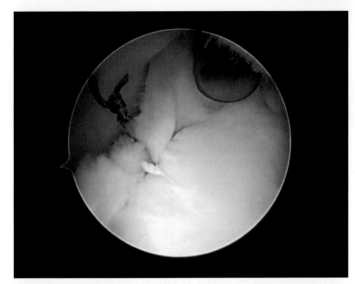

Figure 23-4 Arthroscopic image taken during the repair of a SLAP (superior labrum anterior to posterior) lesion in a patient with internal impingement. Undersurface fraying of the rotator cuff is also noted.

to compromised results.[32] Excess laxity can be treated with suture plication of the capsule, but we prefer to use limited TACS with a monopolar device (Oratec TAC-S, Menlo Park, CA). Perhaps the most difficult aspect of the decision-making process is determining who needs to have capsular laxity addressed and just how much of a shift to perform. In general, we try to have a good feel for the amount of laxity present in the shoulder based on examination in the clinic and the examination performed under anesthesia. Intraoperatively, assessing the capsular redundancy and getting a feel for the pathology present can help direct treatment. Our technique involves prebending the application probe 20 to 30 degrees a few centimeters from the tip; this allows adequate application of the tip of the probe to the capsule around the curvature of the humeral head. Although the probe may be used through a cannula, we prefer to place it directly through the portals without cannulas in order to improve maneuverability. Initially, we employed a "painting" technique of the anterior, inferior, and posterior capsule; however, we now believe that the majority of patients require only selective treatment of the anteroinferior capsule, and we use a "striping" or "cornrow" technique. The camera is placed in the posterior portal and the anterior and inferior portions of the capsule are treated with the probe set at 75°C. Thermal treatment must be tailored to each individual shoulder, and in those that display a more global laxity picture, a portion of the posterior capsule may also need to be treated.

Burkhart et al[11] have proposed that the essential lesion of internal impingement is posteroinferior capsular contracture that leads to decreased internal rotation in abduction and excessive external rotation. This, in turn, will produce a SLAP lesion and the resulting increase in shoulder laxity can be erroneously interpreted as anteroinferior instability.[11,24] Their data indicate that 90% of these patients can be successfully treated with a nonoperative program emphasizing posteroinferior capsular stretching to reduce glenohumeral internal rotation deficit to an acceptable level. They believe that the 10% that fail such treatment can undergo an arthroscopic posterior capsulotomy through the diseased, contracted tissue to improve internal rotation and alleviate the problem.[11]

POSTOPERATIVE REHABILITATION

Following surgery, patients are immediately placed into a shoulder immobilizer and begin a strict physical therapy regimen on the first postoperative day. The rehabilitation protocol is tailored to the exact nature of the surgery with alterations for other included procedures such as a SLAP repair. Again, the importance of closely supervised rehabilitation cannot be overemphasized in the presence of a thermally treated shoulder. Both surgeon and therapist must be familiar with the nuances involved in nurturing TACS patients because they represent one of the greatest therapy challenges in all of orthopedics—"loose enough to throw, but stable enough to prevent symptoms."[10,33] Essentially, we are seeking to reach a "normal" rotational laxity for throwers, which certainly differs from the nonthrowing population.

Complete details of the rehabilitation protocol following TACS are beyond the scope of this chapter, but some of the basic principles follow.[10,26,33,34] During the first 4 weeks, a simple sling is worn during the day, while a shoulder immobilizer is used for sleeping. Weeks 1 and 2 focus on gentle passive and active-assisted range-of-motion exercises, but not stretching, along with anti-inflammatory modalities. Excessive external rotation and abduction are avoided. Weeks 3 and 4 see a progression of motion to established goals, but not beyond. Light external/internal rotation tubing is begun with gradual progression of applied loads. Motion continues to advance during weeks 5 and 6 with progression to 75 degrees of external rotation (with the shoulder abducted 90 degrees) by the end of week 6. The Thrower's Ten program can be started in the sixth week. Full range of motion is expected by week 8, and full functional overhead thrower's range of motion by week 12. More aggressive strengthening can be undertaken by week 10. Weeks 12 to 22 are spent maintaining range of motion, improving dynamic stability, and increasing muscular strength. If satisfactory stability and strength have been achieved by 4 months following surgery and the patient is completely pain and GIRD free, an interval throwing program is initiated. The interval throwing program must be highly structured with advancement based on the individual's symptoms. Return to competition is rarely accomplished in less than 7 months, with pitchers and catchers expected to be closer to 11 months from their surgical date.

CRITERIA FOR RETURN TO SPORTS

Pain-free completion of the interval throwing program is required prior to providing medical clearance. In addition, sport-specific drills should be performed under supervision.[27]

RESULTS AND OUTCOMES

Shoulder pain in the throwing athlete was at one time attributed to subacromial impingement, even though we now know that this is a rare entity in the young population. Tibone et al[35] were the first to report the lack of success treating throwers with "chronic overuse disorders" by acromioplasty. Only 43% of the patients (including just 4 of 14 pitchers) returned to their preoperative level of competition following surgery. Acromioplasty alone was used with unflattering results by Kvitne et al.[4] Andrews et al[36] treated athletes with débridement of both rotator cuff and labral pathology, resulting in a 76% return to same level sport. Payne et al[22] reported on débridement of partial-thickness rotator cuff tears, noting decreased return to competition when instability was present in addition to a tear. The patients with a history of an insidious onset of symptoms were much less likely to return to their preinjury sports level (45%), and this probably represents the patients with true internal impingement. Glasgow et al[29] identified similar findings when studying débridement of labral tears; patients with increased glenohumeral laxity did not fare as well postoperatively when compared to throwers with stable shoulders.

It was becoming clear that the rotator cuff tears and labral pathology noted in throwers' shoulders were not the primary underlying problem, but instead the result of a cascade of events leading to mild anteroinferior instability. Failure to recognize and address this pathologic laxity has compromised surgical outcomes. Armed with that knowledge, Jobe et al[31] retrospectively reviewed the cases of 25 overhand-throwing athletes who failed conservative management and were then treated with an open capsulolabral reconstruction. Eighteen of the 25 athletes returned to their prior competitive level for at least 1 year. Altchek et al[37] proposed a less invasive method of addressing the anterior capsule through a horizontal capsular incision. The use of open stabilization was improving overall results, but continued to be somewhat unpredictable in returning athletes to the same level of play.

At our institution, James Andrews began using TACS to address the instability associated with internal impingement in overhead athletes in July 1997. The addition of thermal energy represented an evolution in the overall approach to athletes with this malady. This prompted us to undertake a two-phase retrospective study to investigate the effects of adding TACS to standard treatment for internal impingement in the thrower's shoulder.[32] In phase I, group A consisted of 51 baseball players treated surgically between January 1, 1995 and December 31, 1996. Forty-nine of the 51 patients demonstrated increased glenohumeral laxity on examination under anesthesia. Forty-four of the 51 demonstrated partial-thickness rotator cuff tears that were débrided, and 40 of 51 had evidence of labral pathology (13 treated with repair and 37 with débridement). Capsular laxity was not addressed in this subset of patients. The phase I, group B patients included 31 baseball players who underwent shoulder arthroscopy between July 1997 and December 1997. Treatment was the same as group A except for the addition of TACS to address capsular laxity. Both groups maintained at least 2-year follow-up.

In phase I, group A (no TACS), 80% (41/51) of players returned to play. The mean time to return to competition was 7.2 months. At 2 years postoperatively, 67% of individuals were still competing, with 61% at the presurgical level or higher. In group B (TACS), 97% (30/31) returned to competition at an average of 7.4 months, and 87% were still competing at the same level or higher 2 years after the procedure. Although patients treated without TACS fared relatively well initially, they began to lose their ability to compete at the same level over time much more so than the TACS subjects. Of the group A patients without a repairable SLAP lesion, 71% were still competing at 2 years versus 100% of similar patients in group B. If a SLAP repair was performed, the numbers worsened for both subsets of patients (group A, 50% and group B, 73% at 2 years). Average loss of external rotation measured 7 degrees.[34]

Phase II of the study addressed the association of SLAP lesions and anterior capsular laxity. This limb of the study dealt with elite throwers and found that adding TACS to a SLAP repair in throwers with internal impingement increased return to play from 42% (no TACS) to 91% (with TACS augmentation). This retrospective study provides strong evidence that addressing capsular laxity at the time of arthroscopy can significantly improve the most important outcome measure in this population—return to play at the preoperative level of competition.

Reinold et al[34] studied 130 overhead athletes at an average of 29.3 months following the use of TACS to augment treatment of internal impingement. Eighty-seven percent of subjects returned to competition at average of 8.4 months following the procedure, and at latest follow-up, 88% reported a good or excellent result. They concluded that TACS of the glenohumeral joint is a viable option for overhead athletes with pathologic instability.

COMPLICATIONS

Treatment of internal impingement carries the same inherent risks of all arthroscopic shoulder procedures, in addition to some hazards particular to the use of thermal energy.[38] The risk of partial-thickness rotator cuff tears progressing to full-thickness lesions over time certainly exists but is somewhat difficult to quantify. Complete tears are devastating, and often career-ending, injuries for elite throwers.[39] Carefully assessing the percentage of the partial tear and repairing it when appropriate will help to decrease the chance of progression. Discussing the operative findings and their meaning openly with the patient will provide realistic expectations of future performance in this population.

As noted in the study from our institution, SLAP repair has the potential to decrease the overall success rate even without intervening complications.[32] In addition, the anchors used to repair the lesion can become loose, break, or instigate a synovitic reaction, a problem that was specifically noted with the use of Suretac anchors.[40] Positioning anchors in the proper orientation can also be difficult, leading to implants that are directed out the front or back side of the glenoid.

The complications with the use of thermal energy in the shoulder are well documented and include axillary neuropathy, capsular ablation, recurrent instability, and stiffness.[17,21,41,42] Although these risks are pertinent to our discussion, much of the data collected in which the complications have occurred in the past involved the use of thermal energy to treat multidirectional instability. Transient neuritis rates have been documented as high as 8%.[22] We reviewed 140 consecutive patients treated with TACS as an augmentation procedure for internal impingement or for instability alone between January 1, 1995 and December 31, 1998. In this series, just one case of transient axillary nerve neuritis (complete resolution within 6 weeks) was encountered. In addition, there were no episodes of axillary nerve injury in the 130 patients with internal impingement studied by Reinold et al.[34] Postoperative stiffness and recurrent laxity are concerns that we attempt to address with our detailed and vigilant physical therapy. Complete capsular ablation has been reported[17] and is more likely to occur in the face of prior techniques such as "painting" the entire capsule rather than the selective "striping" or "cornrow" technique that is used today.

CONCLUSIONS

Internal impingement is pathologic contact of the posterosuperior rotator cuff against the posterior glenoid labrum in the maximal abducted externally rotated position. Overhead athletes often present with loss of ability to perform due to early fatigue and posterior shoulder pain, previously known as dead arm syndrome. Symptoms usually occur during the late cocking and acceleration phases of the throwing motion or tennis serve. Clinical examination and diagnostic studies most often demonstrate partial articular-side tearing of the infraspinatus tendon and posterosuperior labral fraying or detachment. Rehabilitation is focused on normalizing the static restraints and muscular coordination of the shoulder during the overhead throwing. Surgical treatment of rotator cuff and labral pathology with potential additional methods to decrease capsular laxity are effective in allowing the majority of athletes to return to previous levels of function.

REFERENCES

1. Andrews JR, Dugas JR: Diagnosis and treatment of shoulder injuries in the throwing athlete: The role of thermal-assisted capsular shrinkage. AAOS Instr Course Lect 2001;50:17–21.
2. Halbrecht JL, Tirman P, Atkin D: Internal impingement of the shoulder: Comparison of findings between the throwing and nonthrowing shoulders of college baseball players. Arthroscopy 1999;15:253–258.
3. Jazrawi LM, McCluskey GM III, Andrews JR: Superior labral anterior and posterior lesion and internal impingement in the overhead athlete. AAOS Instr Course Lect 2003;52:43–63.
4. Kvitne RS, Jobe FW, Jobe CM: Shoulder instability in the overhand or throwing athlete. Clin Sports Med 1995;14:917–935.
5. Paley KJ, Jobe FW, Pink MM, et al: Arthroscopic findings in the overhand throwing athlete: Evidence for posterior internal impingement of the rotator cuff. Arthroscopy 2000;16:35–40.
6. Walch G, Boileau P, Noel E, et al: Impingement of the deep surface of the supraspinatus tendon on the posterosuperior glenoid rim: An arthroscopic study. J Shoulder Elbow Surg 1992;1:238–245.
7. Meister K: Internal impingement in the shoulder of the overhand athlete: Pathophysiology, diagnosis, and treatment. Am J Orthop 2000; 29:433–439.
8. Crockett HC, Gross LB, Wilk KE, et al: Osseous adaptation and range of motion at the glenohumeral joint in professional baseball pitchers. Am J Sports Med 2002;30:20–26.
9. Jobe CM, Sidles J: Evidence for a superior glenoid impingement upon the rotator cuff: Anatomic, kinesiologic, MRI, and arthroscopic findings (abstract). Paper presented at the 5th International Conference on Surgery of the Shoulder, 1992, Paris, France.
10. Wilk KE, Meister K, Andrews JR: Current concepts in the rehabilitation of the overhead throwing athlete. Am J Orthop 2002;30:135–151.
11. Burkhart SS, Morgan CD, Kibler WB: The disabled throwing shoulder: Spectrum of pathology. Part I: Pathoanatomy and biomechanics. Arthroscopy 2003;19:404–420.
12. Jobe FW, Kivitne R, Giangarra C: Shoulder pain in the overhand or throwing athlete: The relationship of anterior instability and rotator cuff impingement. Orthop Rev 1989;18:963–975.
13. Meister K, Buckley B, Batts J: The posterior impingement sign: Diagnosis of rotator cuff and posterior labral tears secondary to internal impingement in overhead athletes. Am J Orthop 2004;33:412–415.
14. Guanche CA, Jones DC: Clinical testing for tears of the glenoid labrum. Arthroscopy 2003;19:517–523.
15. O'Brien SJ, Pagnani MJ, Fealy S, et al: The active compression test: A new and effective test for diagnosing labral tears and acromioclavicular joint abnormality. Am J Sports Med 1998;26:610–613.
16. Ellenbecker TS: Muscular strength relationship between normal grade manual muscle testing & isokinetic measurement of the shoulder internal & external rotators. Isokin Exerc Sci 1996;6:51–56.
17. Savoie FH: Failed thermal procedures: Absent capsule preliminary experience in 20 cases. Paper presented at Shoulder Surgery Controversies, 2000, Laguna Hills, CA.
18. Warner JJP, Micheli LJ, Arslenian LE, et al: Scapulothoracic motion in normal shoulders and shoulders with glenohumeral instability and impingement syndrome: A study using Moire topographic analysis. Clin Orthop 1992;285:191–199.
19. Meister K, Andrews JR, Batts J, et al: Symptomatic thrower's exostosis: Arthroscopic evaluation and treatment. Am J Sports Med 1999;27:133–137.
20. Kaplan LD, McMahon PJ, Towers J, et al: Internal impingement: Findings on magnetic resonance imaging and arthroscopic evaluation. Arthroscopy 2004;20:701–704.
21. D'Alessandro DF, Bradley JP, Fleischli JF, et al: Prospective evaluation of electrothermal arthroscopic capsulorrhaphy (ETAC) for shoulder instability: Indications, technique, and preliminary results. Paper presented at Annual Closed Meeting of American Shoulder and Elbow Surgeons, 1998, New York, NY.
22. Payne LZ, Altchek DW, Craig EV, et al: Arthroscopic treatment of partial rotator cuff tears in young athletes. Am J Sports Med 1997;25:299–305.
23. Mihata T, Lee Y, McGarry MH, et al: Excessive humeral external rotation results in increased shoulder laxity. Am J Sports Med 2004; 32:1278–1282.
24. Barber AF, Morgan CD, Burkhart SS, et al: Current controversies point counterpoint: Labrum/biceps/cuff dysfunction on the throwing athlete. Arthroscopy 1999;15:852–857.
25. Axe MJ: Throwing programs for Adolescents. Paper presented at 23rd Annual ASMI Injuries in Baseball Course, 2005, Scottsdale, AZ.
26. Reinold MM, Wilk KE, Hooks TR, et al: Interval sports programs: Guidelines for baseball, tennis, and golf. J Orthop Sports Phys Ther 2002;32:293–298.
27. Wilk KE (ed): Interval throwing program for baseball players. In Preventive and Rehabilitative Exercises for the Shoulder and Elbow. Birmingham, AL, American Sports Medicine Institute, 2001.
28. Cordasco FA, Steinmann S, Flatow EL, et al: Arthroscopic treatment of glenoid labrum tears. Am J Sports Med 1993;21:425–431.
29. Glasgow SG, Bruce RA, Yacobucci GN, et al: Arthroscopic resection of glenoid labral tears in the athlete: A review of 29 cases. Arthroscopy 1992;8:48–54.
30. Jobe CM: Posterior superior glenoid impingement: Expanded spectrum. Arthroscopy 1995;11:530–537.
31. Jobe FW, Giangarra CE, Kvitne RS, et al: Anterior capsulolabral reconstruction of the shoulder in athletes in overhead sports. Am J Sports Med 1991;19:428–434.
32. Levitz CL, Dugas JD, Andrews JR: The use of arthroscopic thermal capsulorrhaphy to treat internal impingement in baseball players. Arthroscopy 2001;17:573–577.
33. Wilk KE, Reinold MM, Dugas JR, et al: Rehabilitation following thermal-assisted capsular shrinkage of the glenohumeral joint: Current concepts. J Orthop Sports Phys Ther 2002;32:268–292.
34. Reinold MM, Wilk KE, Hooks TR, et al: Thermal-assisted capsular shrinkage of the glenohumeral joint in overhead athletes: A 15- to 47-month follow-up. J Orthop Sports Phys Ther 2003;33:455–467.
35. Tibone JE, Jobe FW, Kerlan RK, et al: Shoulder impingement syndrome in athletes treated by anterior acromioplasty. Clin Orthop 1985;198:134–140.
36. Andrews JR, Broussard TS, Carson WG: Arthroscopy of the shoulder in the management of partial tears of the rotator cuff: A preliminary report. Arthroscopy 1985;1:117–122.
37. Altchek DW, Warren RF, Wickiewicz TL, et al: T-plasty modification of the Bankart procedure for multidirectional instability of the anterior and inferior types. J Bone Joint Surg Am 1991;73:105–112.
38. Ruotolo C, Penna J, Namkoong S, et al: Shoulder pain and the overhead athlete. Am J Orthop 2003;32:248–258.

39. Mazoue CG, Andrews JR: Repair of full-thickness rotator cuff tears in professional baseball players. Paper presented at 23rd Annual ASMI Injuries in Baseball Course, 2005, Scottsdale, AZ.

40. Burkhart SS: The evolution of clinical applications of biodegradable implants in arthroscopic surgery. Biomaterials 2000;21:2631–2634.

41. McCarty EC, Warren RF, Deng XH, et al: Temperature along the axillary nerve during radiofrequency-induced thermal capsular shrinkage. Am J Sports Med 2004;32:909–1914.

42. Weber SC: Complications of thermal surgery. Paper presented at Fall Course of the Arthroscopy Association of North America, 2000, Palm Desert, CA.

24 Biceps Tendon Disorders

Daniel E. Weiland and Mark W. Rodosky

In This Chapter

The role of the biceps tendon
Proximal biceps tendon rupture
Partial tears/tendonopathy
Nonoperative management
Surgery—biceps tenodesis

INTRODUCTION

- Although the functional significance of the long head of the biceps has been a controversial topic in the orthopedic literature for some time, the anatomy and pathology are well described, and there is no debate that the biceps tendon can be a significant source of pain and disability in the shoulder.

- Athletes who participate in overhead activities repetitively place increased forces on their shoulders, which can lead to a vast array of pathologic changes.

- Injuries of the biceps tendon often occur concurrently with a complete spectrum of shoulder disorders, which at times makes diagnosis quite challenging.

- The treatment of biceps tendon injuries requires the ability to manage rotator cuff tears, subacromial impingement, instability, and lesions of the biceps anchor.

RELEVANT ANATOMY AND BIOMECHANICS

The biceps brachii muscle is composed of two origins. The short head of the biceps arises from the coracoid process along with the coracobrachialis to form the conjoined tendon. The long head of the biceps originates in the glenohumeral joint from the supraglenoid tubercle and posterior labrum and travels in the rotator interval obliquely from posteromedial to anterolateral over the humeral head. The tendon then exits the joint beneath the transverse humeral ligament, entering the bicipital groove (also known as intertubercular groove) between the greater and lesser tuberosities. The bicipital groove has an average depth of 4 mm and a medial wall angle of 56 degrees.[1] The tendons of both the long and short heads of the biceps travel distally to their respective muscle bellies that converge as they approach the elbow before inserting on the bicipital tuberosity of the radius and the fascia of the forearm via the bicipital aponeurosis. The biceps is innervated by the musculocutaneous nerve

(C5–C7), the first branch off the lateral cord of the brachial plexus. The proximal portion of the long head of the biceps receives its blood supply from the anterior circumflex humeral artery and distally from branches of the deep brachial artery.

Within the glenohumeral joint, the biceps tendon is surrounded by a synovial sheath that is continuous with the capsular lining.[2] The capsuloligamentous restraints in the rotator interval retain the biceps in its proper location as it courses toward the bicipital groove. The rotator interval itself is a triangular area of fibrous tissue that is positioned between the supraspinatus and the subscapularis. The interval is composed mainly of the biceps tendon and the superior glenohumeral ligament. This triangular area is bordered medially by the coracohumeral ligament and apexed laterally by the transverse humeral ligament.[3] The coracohumeral and the superior glenohumeral ligaments form a sling around the biceps tendon and are the most important structures in preventing medial subluxation.[3]

The biceps muscle takes origin from the scapula, spans two joints, and inserts in the forearm. At the elbow, it is well established that the biceps functions as both a forearm flexor and supinator. Its precise function about the shoulder remains controversial. It has been postulated that the long head of the biceps acts as both a humeral head depressor and stabilizer of the glenohumeral joint. The biceps has also been shown to have a primary role in the deceleration of the elbow during throwing, suggesting that this high-strain activity might be responsible for generating superior labrum anterior to posterior (SLAP) lesions.[4]

Using a cadaveric model, many authors have shown the stabilizing effect of the long head of the biceps on the glenohumeral joint. Creating simulated contractures in a cadaveric model, Rodosky et al[5] demonstrated that the biceps contributed to anterior stability of the glenohumeral joint by increasing resistance to torsional forces in the abducted and externally rotated position. They also showed that the detachment of the biceps anchor at the superior labrum was associated with an increased magnitude of strain in the inferior glenohumeral ligament.[5] Pagnani et al[6] used a cadaveric model to demonstrate simulated biceps contractions decreased the amount of humeral head translation. This stabilizing effect, however, was more pronounced when the humerus was placed at middle and lower elevation angles. In a selective cutting experiment using 13 cadaveric shoulders, Itoi et al[7] were able to show that the biceps becomes a more important glenohumeral stabilizer as the stability of anterior structures decreases. Cadaveric studies using simulated contractions can be difficult to interpret due to the inability to replicate in vivo resting tension and the complex force couple generated about the shoulder.

In an in vivo model, the long head of the biceps has been shown to be a static and dynamic restraint to superior migration of the humeral head. Warner and McMahon[8] evaluated seven patients with isolated loss of the proximal attachment of the long head of the biceps and noted significant superior migration of the humeral head when compared to the contralateral shoulder as a normal control. Andrews et al[4] showed compression of the humeral head by the long head of the biceps during electrical stimulation during arthroscopy. These interpretations of the role of biceps tendon are in contradiction to Yamaguchi et al, who showed no significant electromyographic activity in the biceps with shoulder activity when the elbow and forearm position was controlled.[9]

CLINICAL FEATURES

Shoulder pain secondary to biceps tendon pathology can be quite severe, causing significant disability. Often the exact etiology of the pain is not clear, as the pathogenesis of biceps tendonopathy is intimately related to existence of other shoulder disorders. Yamaguchi and Bendra[10] classified three major groups of pathologic processes in order to help describe and manage biceps disorders: inflammatory, instability, and traumatic. This classification system was designed to characterize the pathologic process present in the biceps tendon, taking into account that overlapping conditions may exist.

Primary bicipital tendonitis, where there is isolated inflammation of the long head of the biceps with no identifiable inciting cause, is rare. In younger athletes, biceps inflammation is usually caused by repeated microtrauma from overuse activities. The development of subacromial impingement is a more common scenario, which can be potentiated by weak periscapular musculature that fatigues with repetitive use. Rotator cuff muscle fatigue results in an elevation of the humeral head further potentiating the impingement. In older patients, degenerative changes of the biceps are frequently associated with impingement and rotator cuff disease. Many times the cause of biceps inflammation is multifactorial.

The long head of the biceps is surrounded by a synovial extension of the glenohumeral joint, and the development of an inflammatory process can be directly related to the structures in proximity. Inflammatory tenosynovitis almost always occurs with concomitant rotator cuff disease as the biceps is subject to the same mechanical wear from the undersurface of the acromion. Neer's[11] opinion was that biceps tendonitis was intimately associated with subacromial impingement, and he noted that biceps tendonopathy rarely occurs without a tear of the supraspinatus tendon. With associated tears of the supraspinatus tendon, the biceps can subluxate medially over the lesser tuberosity. In an autopsy study of 77 cadavers, Petersson[12] noted that medial displacement of the tendon was always found in connection with full-thickness supraspinatus tendon ruptures.

In the acute painful stage of biceps tendonitis, inflammation is usually found initially along the tendon in the bicipital groove. This can be easily visualized arthroscopically by using a probe to pull the tendon back into the glenohumeral joint (Fig. 24-1). The biceps tendon can appear swollen, partially frayed, or synovitic. Later on in the course of disease, the tendon can further degenerate and become adherent to the surrounding soft tissue. Microscopic changes include atrophy of collagen fibers, fibrinoid necrosis, and fibrocyte proliferation.[13] In the prerupture stage, the tendon can appear either hypertrophic or atrophic and have multiple fissures. In cases of spontaneous rupture, symptoms will often completely resolve.

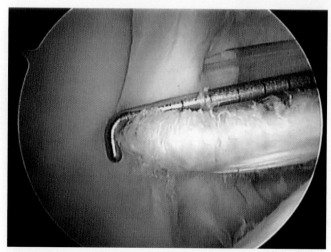

Figure 24-1 Arthroscopic photograph showing a diseased biceps tendon.

As the biceps travels from the supraglenoid tubercle to the intertubercular groove, it turns and angles 35 degrees anteriorly. Any damage to the soft-tissue restraints in the rotator interval can cause medial subluxation and even dislocation of the biceps tendon. Patients with this condition usually present with pain and tenderness over the bicipital groove, and a reproducible pop during rotation of the humeral head. When the shoulder is in abduction and external rotation, the biceps is forced medially. During internal rotation, the biceps is forced laterally in the bicipital groove.[14] Although this entity has been reported in younger athletes who participate in throwing sports, the cause is not well defined.[15] Fixed subluxation of the biceps tendon occurs with complete loss of soft-tissue constraints and is often seen in patients with a disrupted rotator interval or degenerative rotator cuff tears.[16] Frank dislocation is almost always associated with a complete tear of the subscapularis tendon or a complete rotator cuff tear involving the rotator interval. The position of the dislocated tendon will usually be evident on magnetic resonance imaging.

Traumatic rupture of the biceps tendon requires a high-energy force, and this is uncommon with no history of biceps tendonitis and degeneration. The mechanism can be a powerful deceleration of the forearm while throwing or in forced supination. Full-thickness tears can be less symptomatic than partial tears. As the biceps originates from the glenoid labrum and the supraglenoid tubercle, many biceps tears are intimately associated with SLAP lesions, as described by Snyder et al.[17] In 140 cases of injuries to the superior labrum, the most common cause was a fall or direct blow to the shoulder.[18]

CLINICAL EVALUATION

The evaluation of biceps disorders requires a detailed history and physical examination as symptoms can be vague. It is important to determine when the onset of pain occurred and how it has progressed. Was there a traumatic event? Are the symptoms activity related? The level of athletic participation can play an integral role in the diagnosis and treatment of biceps disorder. Some patients will describe a popping or clicking sensation, but this has to be differentiated from other shoulder disorders. It is difficult to differentiate bicipital groove pain from impingement and anterior cuff pain. With disorders specific to the biceps tendon, pain often radiates down to the muscle belly. Patients can also give a long history of anterior shoulder pain and popping that spontaneously resolved after a specific incident requiring elbow flexion. This is a classic story of a patient with chronic biceps tendonitis who ruptured his or her biceps tendon. Instability of the biceps tendon can sometimes be difficult to assess clinically. Often the patient will describe a history of painful snapping when moving from an abducted externally rotated position to internal rotation, a motion that is replicated frequently in overhead athletes.

On physical examination, the patient should be inspected for symmetry of both upper extremities. A ruptured long head of the biceps can result in the classic "Popeye" deformity in which the muscle of the long head of the biceps is retracted distally leaving a characteristic bulge in the distal arm (Fig. 24-2). Strength and range of motion of both shoulders should be documented. Changes in range of motion are variable and are often in conjunction with rotator cuff disease. Impingement as well as stability testing must be included in the examination. Direct palpation of the biceps tendon can sometimes be difficult. The bicipital groove faces anteriorly when the arm is in slight internal rotation. Pain consistent with biceps tendonopathy will move laterally as the arm is externally rotated. Biceps pain can sometimes be elicited with shoulder extension and internal rotation.

Due to the difficulty in isolating biceps tendonopathy, diagnostic tests designed specific to the biceps tendon have been described to help localize shoulder pain. The clinical effective-ness of these tests, however, is examiner dependent, and many clinicians find them nonspecific.[19] Speed's test is attempted elevation of the arm against resistance with the elbow extended and the forearm supinated. A positive test is elicited when there is pain in the anterior aspect of the shoulder, and this is suggestive of biceps tendonopathy. The Yergason test is resisted forearm supination with the elbow flexed at 90 degrees. The test is positive when there is pain in the biceps.

Differential injections may also be useful in diagnosing biceps disorders. An injection into the subacromial space should have no effect on biceps pain unless a full-thickness rotator cuff tear is present. Conversely, assuming no other intra-articular pathology, an intra-articular injection of local anesthetic should resolve any symptoms caused by the biceps tendon. A more accurate diagnosis can be obtained from an injection of local anesthetic directly into the sheath of the biceps tendon. It is important, however, to avoid an intertendinous injection. A helpful injection technique is to place the patient supine on the examining table with the elbow flexed 90 degrees and internally rotated 10 degrees. In this position, the bicipital groove can on occasion be palpated. When the local anesthetic is introduced, there should be no resistance to flow if the needle is correctly placed in the sheath. In large patients with excessive soft tissue overlying the anterior aspect of the shoulder, ultrasonography-guided injections are sometimes required.

Patients with biceps instability will usually present with a history of shoulder pain associated with popping and catching. One method for testing biceps stability is to position the arm in

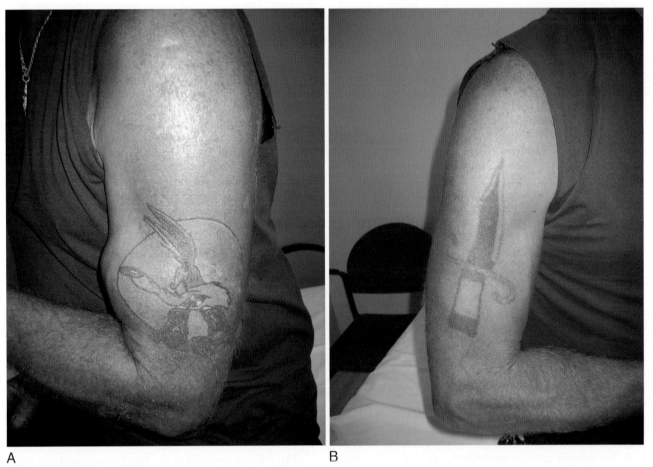

A   B

Figure 24-2 Patient demonstrating a characteristic Popeye deformity **(A)**. Compare to the contralateral normal side **(B)**.

abduction and external rotation while palpating the bicipital groove. In cases of instability, as the arm approaches 90 degrees of abduction and external rotation, a palpable clunk will be appreciated at the anterior edge of the acromion.[20] In the evaluation for biceps stability, an essential aspect of the physical examination is to assess the integrity of the subscapularis tendon with the Gerber lift-off test.[21] This test is performed by bringing the patient's arm into maximum internal rotation behind the back, with the hand away from the back. The patient's ability to maintain the position after the examiner releases the hand is indicative of an intact subscapularis tendon. The combination of a detailed history and complete physical examination is essential in the workup of biceps tendon disorders and should help narrow the differential diagnosis.

Plain film radiographs should always be the first set of images obtained in the evaluation of shoulder pathology. The standard three views of the shoulder: a true anteroposterior, scapular outlet, and axillary views are the minimum requirements to rule out any associated conditions. The plain films will help evaluate the glenohumeral joint for any degenerative changes, acromion morphology, and evidence of acromioclavicular (AC) joint arthrosis, but plain films will rarely be able to provide any information that is specific to the biceps tendon. Radiographs may offer hints about other osseous abnormalities such as a Hill-Sachs lesion or a bony Bankart lesion. In cases in which there is a suspected abnormality of the bicipital groove, a specific view has been developed by Cone et al.[1] This view is obtained by placing the radiographic cassette at the apex of the shoulder with the arm externally rotated. The beam is then aimed along the medial axis of the long axis of the humerus, allowing visualization of any osteophytes or narrowing of the bicipital groove. Ultrasonography has the benefit of being noninvasive and the ability to detect tendon size as well as the presence of fluid in the tendon sheath. Although it is user dependent, studies have shown ultrasonography to be effective in the evaluation of biceps tendonopathy as well as concurrent rotator cuff disease.[22]

Due to its rapidly advancing technology, magnetic resonance imaging has become the gold standard for visualizing the surrounding soft-tissue anatomy of the shoulder. Magnetic resonance imaging has the ability to evaluate for rotator cuff pathology, including intrasubstance signal changes that are consistent with tendonosis.[23] Biceps subluxations are best seen on oblique and sagittal views. Edema associated with tendonitis is visible on the T2-weighted images. Tendon ruptures are easy to visualize and are represented by a discontinuity of the tendon along its course.

TREATMENT OPTIONS

Nonoperative treatment of disorders of the long head of the biceps is usually directed by the treatment for concomitant rotator cuff disease. Initially ice, rest, and anti-inflammatory medications in conjunction with a well-supervised physical therapy program should be prescribed. Athletic activity that incites shoulder pain should be temporarily curtailed. Patients who fail a trial of rest and physical therapy may require a subacromial steroid injection to help control the inflammation. Injections can also be given in the glenohumeral joint or directly into the tendon sheath. During the acute phase of inflammation, physical therapy begins with range-of-motion exercises of the shoulder before moving on to strengthening of periscapular musculature. The serratus anterior and trapezius muscles help create a stable platform for the scapula. Strengthening exercises can

gradually progress to repetitive eccentric loading of the biceps to build endurance in preparation for strenuous activities. Overhead athletic activity is allowed once the strength is fully restored. In many cases, conservative management will be curative, but occasionally biceps tendonitis may persist or even worsen. Nonoperative management of biceps instability is usually unsuccessful as there is almost always an associated tear of the rotator cuff. Symptomatic biceps tendonopathy that is resistant to well-supervised nonoperative measures is an indication for surgical management.

Isolated spontaneous ruptures of the biceps can occur and the mode of treatment should be dependent on the physical activity level of the patient. It has been reported that high-demand athletes with biceps degeneration perform better, with much less pain after either spontaneous rupture or surgical removal.[24] Biceps tenodesis, however, has potential advantages over biceps tenotomy. Tenodesis of the biceps helps to maintain the length-tension relationship of the tendon, which can prevent loss of flexion and supination power. Tenodesis may also prevent cramping in the muscle belly and avoid the cosmetically unpleasing Popeye deformity. Mariani et al[25] compared the results of surgical repair in patients with an acute rupture of the long head of the biceps and nonoperative treatment. Residual arm pain was infrequent in both groups, and the group treated without surgery was able to return to work earlier. On biomechanical testing, the nonsurgically treated group demonstrated a 21% loss in supination power and an 8% loss in flexion power. There was no loss of strength in either supination or flexion in the group treated with surgical repair.

The treatment algorithm of the biceps is not always straightforward. The majority of biceps tendon ruptures are associated with rotator cuff tears, and treatment should be directed toward the rotator cuff pathology before addressing the biceps tendon. On the rare occasion that an athlete's symptoms are localized to the biceps alone, a tenodesis or tenotomy is recommended. In athletes with bicipital degeneration associated with impingement, appropriate treatment includes a complete subacromial decompression and evaluation of the rotator cuff. Surgical options vary from benign neglect to synovectomy and partial tendon débridement to tenodesis or tenotomy. In the senior author's experience, the final decision to perform a biceps tenodesis is made after arthroscopic evaluation. In an athlete with anterior shoulder pain, associated tenderness in the bicipital groove, and arthroscopic evidence of greater than 50% involvement of the biceps tendon, an arthroscopic tenodesis is indicated.

SURGICAL TECHNIQUE: BICEPS TENODESIS

Several techniques for tenodesis of the biceps have been described that range from all open to arthroscopically assisted to all arthroscopic. Many of these techniques require expensive implants or involve creating large drill holes in bone. Presented in this chapter is a simple all-arthroscopic percutaneous intra-articular transtendon (PITT) technique.[26] This technique requires no specialized hardware and can be performed with a spinal needle, suture material, and standard arthroscopic equipment. The design of the percutaneous intra-articular transtendon technique is based on the premise of tenotomy with scarring in the bici-pital groove that occurs in cases of trauma or degeneration.

The patient is placed in the beach chair position, a standard posterior portal is established, and the arthroscope is placed into the glenohumeral joint. The anterior portal is made under direct visualization in the rotator interval just above the superior gleno-humeral ligament. It is helpful to locate this entrance point initially with a spinal needle prior to the introduction of a blunt trochar. A completed diagnostic arthroscopy is performed to rule out any associated shoulder pathology prior to evaluation of biceps tendon pathology. The extra-articular portion of the biceps can be visualized by placing a probe in the anterior portal and pulling the biceps into the glenohumeral joint. Additional tendon excursion can be obtained by elevating the arm forward with the elbow flexed.

Once biceps tendon pathology is confirmed, a spinal needle is placed from the anterior aspect of the shoulder through the deltoid and the transverse humeral ligament into the bicipital groove. Under direct visualization, the spinal needle is then placed through the biceps tendon (Fig. 24-3), and a no. 1 poly-diaxone monofilament suture (PDS; Ethicon, Cornelia, GA) is threaded into the glenohumeral joint and pulled out the ante-rior portal with a grasper. A second spinal needle is then placed in the same location piercing the biceps tendon near the first suture. The second PDS is then pulled out the anterior portal with a grasper (Fig. 24-4). A no. 2 braided, nonabsorbable poly-ester suture (Surgidac, United States Surgical, Norwalk, CT) is tied to one strand of the PDS and pulled through the puncture wound in the front of the shoulder through the biceps tendon and out the anterior portal (Fig. 24-5). The end of the Surgidac that is out the anterior portal is tied to the remaining PDS, and the PDS is pulled back into the anterior portal through the biceps tendon and then out the puncture site on the anterior aspect of the shoulder. This creates a mattress type suture that attaches the biceps to the transverse humeral ligament (Fig. 24-6). This process is completed a second time, providing extra fix-ation to the transverse humeral ligament. Using different colored sutures can be helpful to simplify suture management.

The biceps can then be cut proximal to the sutures with arthroscopic scissors or a narrow biter, and the remaining stump

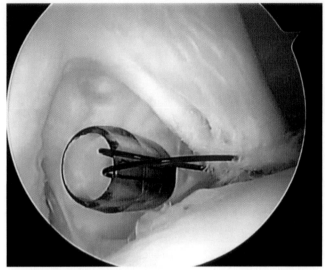

Figure 24-4 Photograph of two polydiaxone monofilament sutures passed through the diseased tendon. Both strands have been retrieved and pulled out the anterior cannula. (From Sekiya LC, Elkousy HA, Rodosky MW: Arthroscopic biceps tenodesis using the percutaneous intra-articular transtendon technique. Arthroscopy 2003;19:1137–1141.)

is débrided with a motorized shaver back to a stable rim on the superior labrum (Fig. 24-7). The arthroscope is then removed from the posterior portal and directed into the subacromial space through the same skin incision. A lateral acromial working portal is localized first with a spinal needle and then established under direct visualization. The subacromial space is evaluated, and, if needed, a decompression or rotator cuff repair can be performed. Care must be taken to avoid cutting the previously placed sutures transfixing the biceps tendon. The biceps sutures

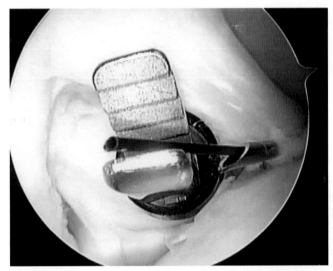

Figure 24-3 Arthroscopic photograph showing a spinal needle piercing the biceps tendon. A polydiaxone monofilament suture is threaded through the needle and a grasper is used to bring the suture out the anterior cannula. (From Sekiya LC, Elkousy HA, Rodosky MW: Arthroscopic biceps tenodesis using the percutaneous intra-articular transtendon technique. Arthroscopy 2003;19:1137–1141.)

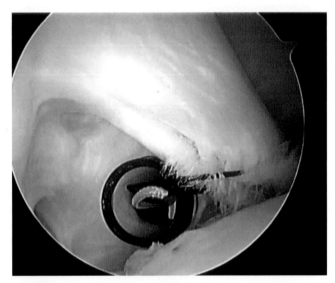

Figure 24-5 The polydiaxone monofilament suture is tied to the nonabsorbable polyester braided suture as it is being shuttled through the biceps tendon. (From Sekiya LC, Elkousy HA, Rodosky MW: Arthroscopic biceps tenodesis using the percutaneous intra-articular transtendon technique. Arthroscopy 2003;19:1137–1141.)

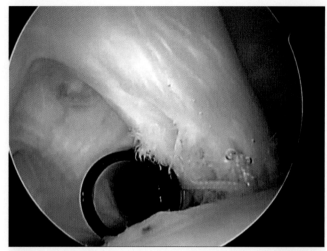

Figure 24-6 Arthroscopic photograph showing the mattress pattern of braided nonabsorbable sutures passed through the biceps tendon. Tendon is now sutured to the transverse humeral ligament. (From Sekiya LC, Elkousy HA, Rodosky MW: Arthroscopic biceps tenodesis using the percutaneous intra-articular transtendon technique. Arthroscopy 2003;19:1137–1141.)

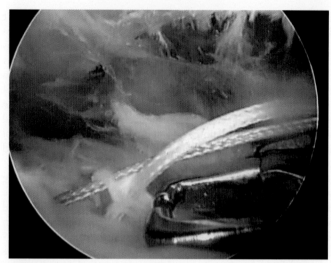

Figure 24-8 Loose sutures are shown in the subacromial space. A suture grasper is being used to pull the sutures out of the lateral cannula. (From Sekiya LC, Elkousy HA, Rodosky MW: Arthroscopic biceps tenodesis using the percutaneous intra-articular transtendon technique. Arthroscopy 2003;19:1137–1141.)

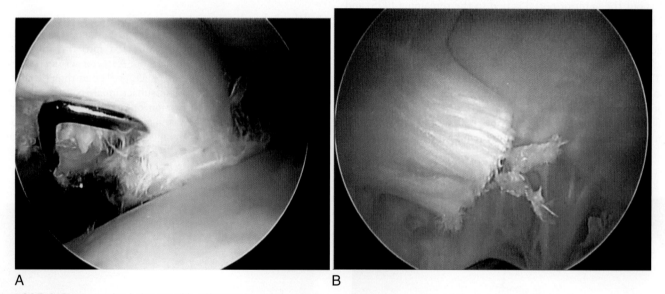

A   B

Figure 24-7 A, Biceps tendon being cut with arthroscopic scissors. **B,** The remaining stump of the biceps tendon attached to the superior labrum. (From Sekiya LC, Elkousy HA, Rodosky MW: Arthroscopic biceps tenodesis using the percutaneous intra-articular transtendon technique. Arthroscopy 2003;19:1137–1141.)

are located in the subacromial space (Fig. 24-8) and subsequently retrieved through the lateral portal. They are then sequentially tied using standard arthroscopic knot-tying techniques, thereby completing the soft-tissue tenodesis (Fig. 24-9).

POSTOPERATIVE REHABILITATION

Postoperative management of biceps tenodesis is dependent on any associated procedures that were performed. In the case of a concomitant rotator cuff tear, postoperative rehabilitation is focused on protecting the rotator cuff tear. Passive range of motion is initiated, followed by active range of motion for 6 weeks before strengthening exercises are allowed. In cases in which an isolated tenodesis was performed, passive pendulum and active wrist and elbow exercises are started immediately. Gentle shoulder passive range of motion is initiated at 1 week after surgery, and a sling is used for 4 weeks. Active biceps flexion is avoided for 6 weeks. By 8 weeks, active range of motion and gentle strengthening of the shoulder can progress. The patient should be on a home exercise program by 3 to 4 months, and full recovery with unrestricted activity is expected by 4 to 6 months after surgery.

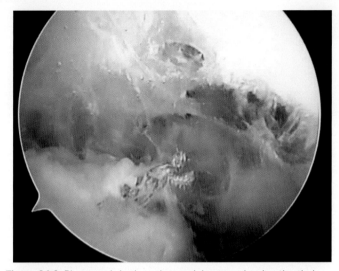

Figure 24-9 Photograph in the subacromial space showing the tied sutures of the completed percutaneous transtendon intra-articular biceps tenodesis. (From Sekiya LC, Elkousy HA, Rodosky MW: Arthroscopic biceps tenodesis using the percutaneous intra-articular transtendon technique. Arthroscopy 2003;19:1137–1141.)

COMPLICATIONS

Few complications occur in the treatment of biceps tendon disorders. Infection and neurovascular injury can occur with any surgery but are quite rare. Complications of spontaneous rupture of the biceps include shortening of the lateral biceps muscle belly causing a cosmetic defect. Although the functional deficit may be minimal, patients can complain of cramping of the muscle during elbow flexion. Postoperative stiffness is also a potential complication of any shoulder procedure.

CONCLUSIONS

Recommended treatment of disorders of the biceps tendon is a subject of controversy. Biceps tendonopathy can be a significant source of shoulder pain that is more debilitating than the loss of the tendon. Although some inherent humeral head stability is achieved by the long head of the biceps, it is difficult to characterize in vivo. Treatment must be individualized based on patient age, symptoms, and level of function. In most cases, treatment of the biceps is dependent on coexisting shoulder pathology. We recommend arthroscopic tenodesis in patients with chronic biceps inflammation recalcitrant to conservative therapy or in cases in which the structural integrity of the tendon is compromised such that there is little potential for healing.

REFERENCES

1. Cone RO, Danzig L, Resnick D, et al: The bicipital groove: Radiographic, anatomic, and pathologic study. AJR Am J Roentgenol 1983;141:781–788.
2. Cooper DE, Arnoczky SP, O'Brien SJ, et al: Anatomy, histology, and vascularity of the glenoid labrum. An anatomical study. J Bone Joint Surg Am 1992;74:46–52.
3. Clark JM, Harryman DT 2nd: Tendons, ligaments, and capsule of the rotator cuff. Gross and microscopic anatomy. J Bone Joint Surg Am 1992;74:713–725.
4. Andrews JR, Carson WG Jr, McLeod WD: Glenoid labrum tears related to the long head of the biceps. Am J Sports Med 1985;13:337–341.
5. Rodosky MW, Harner CD, Fu FH: The role of the long head of the biceps muscle and superior glenoid labrum in anterior stability of the shoulder. Am J Sports Med 1994;22:121–130.
6. Pagnani MJ, Deng XH, Warren RF, et al: Role of the long head of the biceps brachii in glenohumeral stability: A biomechanical study in cadavera. J Shoulder Elbow Surg 1996;5:255–262.
7. Itoi E, Newman SR, Kuechle DK, et al: Dynamic anterior stabilisers of the shoulder with the arm in abduction. J Bone Joint Surg Br 1994;76:834–836.
8. Warner JJ, McMahon PJ: The role of the long head of the biceps brachii in superior stability of the glenohumeral joint. J Bone Joint Surg Am 1995;77:366–372.
9. Yamaguchi K, Riew KD, Galatz LM, et al: Biceps activity during shoulder motion: An electromyographic analysis. Clin Orthop 1997;336:122–129.
10. Yamaguchi K, Bendra R: Disorders of the biceps tendon. In Iannotti J, Williams G (eds): Disorders of the Shoulder: Diagnosis and Management. Philadelphia, Williams & Wilkins, 1999, pp 159–190.
11. Neer CS 2nd: Anterior acromioplasty for the chronic impingement syndrome in the shoulder: A preliminary report. J Bone Joint Surg Am 1972;54:41–50.
12. Petersson CJ: Spontaneous medial dislocation of the tendon of the long biceps brachii. An anatomic study of prevalence and pathomechanics. Clin Orthop 1986;211:224–227.
13. Claessens H, Snoeck H: Tendinitis of the long head of the biceps brachii. Acta Orthop Belg 1972;58:124–128.
14. O'Donoghue DH: Subluxing biceps tendon in the athlete. Clin Orthop 1982;164:26–29.
15. Curtis AS, Snyder SJ: Evaluation and treatment of biceps tendon pathology. Orthop Clin North Am 1993;24:33–43.
16. Walch G, Nove-Josserand L, Boileau P, et al: Subluxations and dislocations of the tendon of the long head of the biceps. J Shoulder Elbow Surg 1998;7:100–108.
17. Snyder SJ, Karzel RP, Del Pizzo W, et al: SLAP lesions of the shoulder. Arthroscopy 1990;6:274–279.
18. Snyder SJ, Banas MP, Karzel RP: An analysis of 140 injuries to the superior glenoid labrum. J Shoulder Elbow Surg 1995;4:243–248.
19. Bennett WF: Specificity of the Speed's test: Arthroscopic technique for evaluating the biceps tendon at the level of the bicipital groove. Arthroscopy 1998;14:789–796.
20. Bell RH, Noble JS: Biceps disorders. In Hawkins RJ, Misamore GW (eds): Shoulder Injuries in the Athlete: Surgical Repair and Rehabilitation. New York, Churchill Livingstone, 1996, pp 267–282.
21. Gerber C, Hersche O, Farron A: Isolated rupture of the subscapularis tendon. J Bone Joint Surg Am 1996;78:1015–1023.
22. Middleton WD, Reinus WR, Totty WG, et al: Ultrasonographic evaluation of the rotator cuff and biceps tendon. J Bone Joint Surg Am 1986;68:440–450.
23. Erickson SJ, Fitzgerald SW, Quinn SF, et al: Long bicipital tendon of the shoulder: Normal anatomy and pathologic findings on MR imaging. AJR Am J Roentgenol 1992;158:1091–1096.
24. Eakin CL, Faber KJ, Hawkins RJ, et al: Biceps tendon disorders in athletes. J Am Acad Orthop Surg 1999;7:300–310.
25. Mariani EM, Cofield RH, Askew LJ, et al: Rupture of the tendon of the long head of the biceps brachii. Surgical versus nonsurgical treatment. Clin Orthop 1988;228:233–239.
26. Sekiya LC, Elkousy HA, Rodosky MW: Arthroscopic biceps tenodesis using the percutaneous intra-articular transtendon technique. Arthroscopy 2003;19:1137–1141.

CHAPTER
25 Rotator Cuff Disorders

J. Winslow Alford, Gregory Nicholson, and Anthony A. Romeo

In This Chapter

INTRODUCTION

- The past 3 decades have witnessed a revolution in our understanding of and treatment options for disorders of the rotator cuff and associated subacromial pathology. Several concepts have emerged as central tenets of the evaluation and management of these disorders.

- Rotator cuff disease is a true syndrome with a constellation of signs and symptoms that are associated with an alteration of normal anatomy. The incriminating anatomic structure or precipitating event that initiates the cascade of events leading to rotator cuff disease may relate not only to pathoanatomy of the anterior acromion and coracoacromial arch, but may also include traumatic events, repetitive overhead activity, or glenohumeral joint imbalance, such as that associated with posterior capsular tightness.

- Poor biologic health of the rotator cuff tissue may hinder the ability of tendon tissue to recover from small injuries.

- An appreciation of the complexity of shoulder anatomy, physiology, and biomechanics is an important part of evaluating and treating patients with suspected disorders of the rotator cuff and subacromial space.

- A thorough understanding of rotator cuff disease is important not only to the orthopedist who may provide surgical treatment, but also to the primary care physicians, physical therapists, and athletic trainers who are well positioned to diagnose and treat these disorders early in the spectrum of disease progression.

RELEVANT ANATOMY AND BIOMECHANICS

Accurate diagnosis and effective treatment of rotator cuff disease relies on an appreciation of shoulder anatomy and biomechanics. Structures that contribute to normal function will also influence pathologic conditions of the rotator cuff. An awareness of the discerning features of a patient's history and physical examination, and an understanding of potential contributions from surrounding structures will assist in developing a differential diagnosis and formulating an effective treatment plan.

The rotator cuff is formed from the coalescence of the tendinous insertions of the subscapularis, supraspinatus, infraspinatus, and teres minor muscles into one continuous band near their insertions on the greater and lesser tuberosities of the proximal humerus. This arrangement suggests that the muscles of the cuff function in concert. In fact, the name "rotator" cuff may be a misnomer; the major function of the rotator cuff is to depress and stabilize the humeral head, effectively compressing the glenohumeral joint to provide a stable fulcrum for arm movement.[1-3]

Abduction strength, although powered by the deltoid, requires a stable fulcrum provided by a functioning rotator cuff. Glenohumeral stability in mid-range relies on functioning rotator cuff muscles that, along with scapular stabilizers[4] and the deltoid,[5] permit balanced muscle pull and concavity compression. As passive restraints to glenohumeral translation are lax in mid-range, joint stability in this position is provided by dynamic stabilizers. A more complete discussion of glenohumeral joint stability is presented in other chapters. With respect to rotator cuff pathomechanics, specifically large rotator cuff tears, it is important to appreciate the effect of transverse plane force coupling in which the anterior generated subscapularis force and anterior supraspinatus are balanced by the posterior supraspinatus, infraspinatus, and teres minor. Balancing these forces with only partial repair of large tears, when complete repair is not possible, is thought to provide a more stable fulcrum for shoulder motion, leading to functional improvement.[1,3]

The concept of functional linking of force couples was popularized by Burkart[6] who described the phenomenon of the cuff acting as a single functional unit, with individual forces balancing one another to produce the desired functional effect. The rotator cuff cable is a normal thickening in the intact cuff that is seen arthroscopically from the articular, undersurface side of the cuff (Fig. 25-1). This thickening in the capsule and overlying tendon extends from its insertion just posterior to the biceps tendon to the inferior border of the infraspinatous tendon[6,7] and is thought to allow the forces across the rotator cuff to be dispersed in a manner similar to a suspension bridge. In this sense, the rotator cable transfers the stress from the supraspinatus and infraspinatus muscles to the terminal insertions of the cable, by directing the force along its length. This organization of force

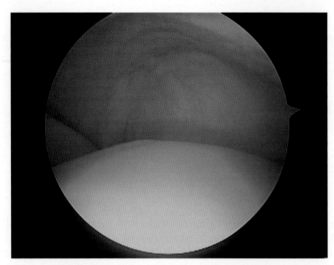

Figure 25-1 Normal anatomy: rotator cuff cable.

distribution explains why some patients can maintain reasonable shoulder function in the setting of a painful full-thickness tear of considerable size, if normal balanced kinematics patterns are maintained.[8]

There is considerable debate regarding the role of the biceps tendon as a humeral head depressor. Reports of the biomechanical properties[9] and clinical behavior[10] of the long head of the biceps may suggest its role as a humeral head depressor, but careful clinical analyses have demonstrated that its role as a humeral head depressor may be less than previously thought.[9] The tendon of the long head of the biceps traverses the glenohumeral joint at the rotator cuff interval. At the interval, the cuff is reinforced by the coracohumeral ligament, with extensions to the biceps-restraining sling at the upper biceps groove and to the rotator cuff cable.[11] The upper insertion of the subscapularis combines with the superior glenohumeral ligament at their insertion on the upper portion of the lesser tuberosity and continues laterally, forming the floor of the bicipital groove. The supraspinatus combines with the coracohumeral ligament inferiorly to form the roof of the groove. A confluence of these structures forms a ring around the biceps, providing stability.[12] Inflammation in this region will produce anterolateral pain similar to rotator cuff impingement, but is often discernible by tenderness directly over the biceps tendon in several arm positions. In the setting of a tear of the subscapularis or a supraspinatus tear that extends into the rotator cuff interval, the integrity of this restraining mechanism is often compromised, and biceps stability must be carefully assessed. Although the rotator cuff interval is a normally appearing gap between the anterior supraspinatus and the superior edge of the subscapularis, the two tendon edges are confluent near the insertion of the myotendinous unit onto the humerus. The "critical zone" in this region, located within the supraspinatus tendon insertion just posterior to the biceps tendon, is a common location for rotator cuff pathology.

It is thought that the quality of the blood supply to the cuff insertion on the greater and lesser tuberosity is a factor in the development of rotator cuff disease, particularly in the critical zone. The suprascapular artery is a primary vascular supply to the supraspinatus tendon, and the microvascular structure of the supraspinatus tendon suggests this region has a tenuous blood supply and an associated limited capacity for intrinsic repair.[13] This is a common location of partial-thickness and full-thickness degenerative rotator cuff tears.

Pathologic changes in the subacromial space can be both a cause and an effect of rotator cuff disease. For example, a hooked type III acromion, a thickened calcified coracoacromial ligament, or an excrescence on the anterolateral corner of the acromion can cause abrasion of the bursa and supraspinatus tendon, resulting in the inflammation and pain characteristic of early impingement syndrome. Alternatively, a large retracted rotator cuff tear in which the force coupling has failed will permit superior migration of the humeral head, which may articulate with the coracoacromial arch. Over time, this pathologic articulation results in rotator cuff arthropathy. Normal balanced kinematics rely on a functioning rotator cuff to allow for proper scapulohumeral articulation and concentric glenohumeral articulation against a stable fulcrum.

Pathogenesis of Cuff Disease

The pathogenesis of rotator cuff disease is multifactorial, including static and structural causes. Dynamic events combine with biologic factors to create a pathologic condition. The effect of aging on the rotator cuff tissue, especially at the insertion of the tendons, has been demonstrated by fiber thickening and granulation tissue. Combined with a tenuous blood supply, the local biologic environment may not be conducive to intrinsic repair, but it is more likely that cuff disease begins with a combination of static structural conditions and dynamic events.[14] In the end, the most consistent risk factor for the development of a rotator cuff tear is advancing age.

Static and Dynamic Causes

Structural abnormalities of the coracoacromial arch may cause abnormal compression of the cuff, leading to cuff disease, but dynamic events may also contribute to cuff injury in the setting of normal subacromial anatomy. Secondary changes in the subacromial morphology may occur as a result of dynamic events and may contribute to the progression of disease. This interrelationship between dynamic and static causes of rotator cuff pathology can be inconsistent. Primary structural abnormalities do not always lead to cuff pathology, and not all structural abnormalities are primary.

Static structural causes of cuff disease are related to the coracoacromial arch morphology. Changes or abnormalities in the arch can lead to focal regions of increased compression at the point where the rotator cuff articulates with the arch. For example, an acromion with an anterior hook, or a lateral slope, can pinch the cuff tendon. An os acromiale or nonunion of an acromial fracture will compress the underlying cuff by changing the shape of the acromion and by promoting the regional growth of osteophytes. Coracoacromial ligament ossification or hypertrophy changes the flexibility and shape of the anterior scapulohumeral articulation, causing abnormal compression of the cuff in provocative positions.

Dynamic events that lead to rotator cuff injury in the setting of normal subacromial anatomy may be due to high-energy traction to the arm causing an acute traumatic tear of the rotator cuff tendon or an avulsion of the tuberosities. Without a clear traumatic event, however, an injury to the rotator cuff is usually caused by either external or internal impingement. External impingement occurs when the bursal side of the rotator cuff is compressed against the coracoacromial arch. Internal impingement exists when the articular side of the cuff is pinched between the posterior superior glenoid and an eccentrically articulating humeral head.

A common cause of external impingement is muscle weakness, which allows for a superior orientation of the humeral head, causing the cuff to abrade on the undersurface of the acromion and coracoacromial ligament. A type II superior labrum anterior to posterior (SLAP) tear can allow excessive humeral head motion toward the coracoacromial arch. Weak scapular stabilizers can aggravate these problems by placing the acromion at an angle that promotes contact with the underlying cuff tendon. A tight posterior capsule will cause the humeral head to ride superior, as is seen in overhead athletes with glenohumeral internal rotation deficit.[15–17]

The theory of internal impingement and its role in causing articular-side rotator cuff tears and superior labral lesions is controversial. Internal impingement occurs with the arm in the cocked position of 90 degrees abduction and full external rotation.[18] In throwers and overhead athletes, this position brings the articular surface of the rotator cuff insertion against the posterosuperior glenoid rim. Repeated forceful contact between the undersurface of the rotator cuff and the posterosuperior glenoid and labrum is said to cause posterior superior labral lesions. With time, undersurface partial-thickness rotator cuff tears follow. Despite contact between these two structures occurring physiologically, the theory holds that repetitive contact with excessive force can produce injury. There are, however, many patients with this constellation of pathologic findings who are not overhead athletes,[19] and most throwers do not develop the condition despite achieving the position regularly.[20] Burkhart et al[15–17] have developed a comprehensive evaluation of arthroscopic findings, patient outcomes, and biomechanical experimental data to indicate that the so-called internal impingement found in throwers is caused by a complex syndrome related to scapular dyskinesis and kinetic chain abnormalities, which result in scapular malposition, inferior medial border prominence, coracoid pain and malposition, and dyskinesis of scapular movement (i.e., the SICK scapula). This combination of pathomechanics initiates a cascade leading to type II SLAP tears and partial thickness rotator cuff tears.

CLINICAL FEATURES AND EVALUATION

Rotator cuff disease presentation varies depending on the cause and classification of the cuff pathology. Cuff pathology ranges from traumatic rotator cuff tears, articular side partial thickness tears associated with "internal impingement" in a thrower or overhead athlete, or a classic impingement process with an insidious onset resulting from repetitive overhead activities, each with vastly different presentations. The presentation of a patient with a traumatic tear will relate the onset of symptoms to a specific traumatic event, and often the high-energy nature of the mechanism causes other injuries to the shoulder or other parts of the body. Often this is the result of abrupt force on the arm, as when trying to support oneself during a fall. An overhead athlete or thrower with articular side rotator cuff tendon pathology will describe a gradual onset of weakness and pain associated with throwing, often at the beginning of a season or as a result of a more strenuous training regimen. Throwers with internal impingement-derived cuff pathology report a gradual increase in pain and loss of performance (e.g., fast-ball velocity) as glenohumeral joint imbalance and/or scapular dyskinesis worsens.

In contrast, patients progressing along the spectrum of cuff impingement syndrome toward a true cuff tear have a different presentation. Due to a combination of subacromial morphology and repetitive overhead activity combined with intrinsic features of the cuff tissue (e.g., poor vascular supply[13]), these patients experience an insidious onset of pain and weakness, which is first noted and worse with overhead activities or while sleeping directly on their affected shoulder. In these patients, the initial symptom is pain. Overt weakness evolves with increased pain as a cuff tear develops and may worsen if the tear propagates. In large chronic untreated tears, patients experience both pain and weakness, but due to the debilitation of a nonfunctioning cuff, often their complaints are more of weakness than of pain.

When evaluating a patient with suspected or known rotator cuff disease, a thorough shoulder evaluation, as described in Chapter 16, is required. Most patients will have tenderness at the anterolateral aspect of the humerus at the insertion of the supraspinatus tendon and positive impingement signs as described by Neer[21] and Hawkins and Kennedy.[22] It is important to carefully evaluate the biceps tendon for tenderness and stability, especially in the setting of a subscapularis tear, which is often associated with biceps sling injury.[23]

Strength testing of the rotator cuff tendons should isolate each tendon to the extent possible. A patient with a large tear resulting in a loss of force coupling across the humeral head may only be able to shrug the shoulder in an effort to abduct. Specific weakness or pain elicited with resisted internal rotation, abduction, or external rotation may be found with isolated tears of the subscapularis, supraspinatus, or infraspinatus, respectively. The subscapularis is responsible for internal rotation of the shoulder and can be tested in isolation. The "belly press" or Napoleon test[24,25] requires that the patient press his or her hand into the belly. During this maneuver, the examiner must maintain a straight position of the patient's wrist and prevent shoulder posterior extension, which is a common compensation in the setting of a subscapularis tear. Alternatively, a patient with a large subscapularis tear would be unable to lift the hand of the affected shoulder off his or her back, thereby failing a so-called lift-off test. Anterior instability is not typical of isolated subscapularis tears.[26]

The supraspinatus is more difficult to test in isolation, but in a position of slight abduction and forward elevation, resistance to a downward force applied to the elbow is mostly generated by the supraspinatus. The infraspinatus functions as an external rotator as well as a head depressor and therefore is tested in isolation by resisting an internal rotation force applied to the wrist, with the patient's elbow bent at 90 degrees and held at the side.

Routine views used to evaluate the shoulder with suspected impingement or a rotator cuff tear include a true anteroposterior, axillary lateral, and scapular outlet. Radiographs are helpful in revealing the bony anatomy of the shoulder joint, specifically the acromial morphology,[27] and the relative position of the humeral head and glenoid, which provides information of the cuff integrity and function. In addition, plain radiographs can assess for other shoulder pathology or fractures, which may contribute to a patient's symptoms. For example, the axillary lateral may reveal an os acromiale, which can be a primary source of pain and often causes cuff impingement.

Shoulder arthrography, either plain film or with magnetic resonance imaging, can be used for evaluating the integrity of the rotator cuff. However, small defects in the capsule at the rotator cuff interval will allow extravasation into the subacromial space even in the setting of normal tendons, potentially leading to a false-positive plain radiograph arthrography. The advantages of magnetic resonance arthrography include the ability to visualize the cuff tissue directly and to inspect other potential contributing pathology such as a SLAP tear or biceps tendonitis. For that reason, we recommend magnetic resonance imaging as the procedure of choice for evaluating the rotator cuff.

Recent work[28] has identified dynamic ultrasonography as an accurate evaluation of the rotator cuff. Using arthroscopic findings as the gold standard, accuracy rates of 87% were reported for both magnetic resonance imaging and ultrasonography for diagnosis of rotator cuff tears. Magnetic resonance imaging was more accurate in diagnosing partial-thickness tears. Accurate ultrasound evaluations are technician dependent. In a similar study[29] comparing ultrasonography and magnetic resonance arthrography, ultrasonography offered accurate results for the large tears, but its sensitivity decreased proportionally with the size of the tears. Magnetic resonance arthrography correctly diagnosed 43 of 44 (98%) tears, with only one false-negative diagnosis of tendinosis made for a partial tear on the bursal side. Magnetic resonance imaging remains the gold standard for evaluation of rotator cuff pathology. The presence of a small full-thickness or a partial-thickness asymptomatic rotator cuff tear is not necessarily significant because it is known that a significant portion of the population has asymptomatic rotator cuff tears, with higher prevalence with advanced age, especially after the age of 60.

Prevalence

In one study, 23% of 411 asymptomatic volunteers with normal shoulder function were found to have full-thickness rotator cuff tears diagnosed by ultrasonography. In this study, 13% of volunteers between 50 and 59 years old and 51% older than 80 years old had full-thickness asymptomatic tears.[30] Cadaver dissections have demonstrated rates up to 60% for partial-thickness or small full-thickness tears in cadavers older than 75 years of age at the time of death.[31] The natural history of various tears is affected by several factors, and therefore it is often unclear what causes certain asymptomatic tears to become symptomatic in certain patients.

Natural History

Yamaguchi et al[32] evaluated the asymptomatic shoulder of 44 patients with unilateral symptoms that were found to have bilateral rotator cuff tears in an effort to learn the natural history of asymptomatic rotator cuff tears. In this study, 23 (51%) of the previously asymptomatic patients became symptomatic over a mean of 2.8 years, and 9 of 23 patients who underwent repeat ultrasonography had tear progression. As these patients all had an existing rotator cuff tears, they may represent a population with intrinsic cuff weakness or anatomy prone to cuff pathology. Nonetheless, this study indicates that there is a considerable risk that the size and/or symptoms of an asymptomatic tear will progress without treatment.

Despite the fact that there is little correlation between structure, symptoms, and shoulder mechanics, there is a rational progression of cuff pathology from small, asymptomatic structural abnormalities to larger, full-thickness tears that cause pain and weakness when they reach sufficient size. The likelihood of progression of an untreated cuff tear depends on the tear characteristics (size, location, mechanism, chronicity), the biologic health of the torn tissue (vascularity, diabetic, smoker), the status of force coupling in the shoulder (i.e., intact rotator cuff cable), and the activity level of the patient. Many small symptomatic tears that present with pain as the predominant complaint can be effectively treated with oral anti-inflammatory

medication, selective use of corticosteroid injections, and rehabilitation of the shoulder to improve range of motion and to strengthen the muscles of the rotator cuff and periscapular stabilizers. When a small symptomatic tear is successfully "treated" nonoperatively, the tear persists as an asymptomatic tear rather than spontaneously healing to bone.

Left untreated, small painful tears with intact mechanics can enlarge and lead to progressive loss of balanced forces coupling due to violation of the rotator cuff cable. With this progression, the patient will begin to experience a significant loss of function in addition to shoulder pain. As the tear enlarges, fat atrophy and retraction of the tear progress.[33] Further enlargement of the tear may occur with a decrease in pain. With extreme tear enlargement and loss of coracohumeral and glenohumeral ligament integrity, the humeral head may rise into the subacromial space, articulate with the acromion, and in time lead to rotator cuff arthropathy. The likelihood of a patient progressing through these steps is unpredictable and based on multiple factors.

In the overhead athlete, there may be a more predictable course. Competitive throwing athletes execute many repetitions of highly demanding motions with complex mechanics. Any imbalance in the kinetic chain, including a weak subscapularis, inadequate scapular mobility and stabilization, and even throwing techniques that cause improper foot placement or arm position while throwing, can initiate the process of pathologic internal impingement. Recognized early, these problems can be corrected through rehabilitation and training.

Early symptoms in the throwing athlete include slow warm-ups and stiffness, with no pain. During this time, the shoulder will usually respond to rest. If the condition is allowed to progress, there will be cuff-associated pain at the initiation of the acceleration phase of throwing. Shoulder pain elicited on examination will often be alleviated with a relocation of the humeral head to articulate concentrically with the glenoid. Further progression of the condition can cause lesions requiring surgical repair, including posterior superior labral tears, anterior shoulder instability, and articular sided rotator cuff tears. These lesions should be suspected in a throwing athlete who is not responding to rest, rehabilitation, and appropriate nonoperative treatment.

TREATMENT OPTIONS

Nonoperative Management

Nonoperative treatment of rotator cuff disorders provides the possibility of avoiding the inherent risks of surgery. Failure of nonoperative treatment results in continued or recurrent symptoms and/or progression of pathology, leading to eventual surgical treatment, possibly after irreversible changes have occurred in the rotator cuff. When counseling patients regarding treatment options, it is helpful to characterize a cuff disorder with respect to the patient's age, the tear size, injury mechanism, chronicity, and muscle atrophy/fatty infiltration. Within this framework, the overall risk of irreversible changes to the cuff with continued nonoperative treatment is weighed against the potential for improvement with continued nonoperative treatment.

Tendonitis or partial-thickness tears are readily reversible conditions with surgical treatment and are unlikely to progress rapidly with nonoperative treatment. Therefore, a prolonged period of nonoperative treatment may be offered to a patient with little risk of progression of the pathology. In addition, nonoperative treatment of these conditions has been reported with success rates of 67%, with only 18% recurrence for an average of 2 years.[34] Small- to medium-sized tears (2 to 3 cm), existing tears with a recent loss of function, or tears of any size in a young (younger than 60 years old) active population are at risk of progression if they fail early nonoperative therapy. In this group, prolonged nonoperative treatment has a low success rate and carries a risk of leading to irreversible changes that may complicate the eventual surgical repair. In this group, early surgical treatment after a short course of nonoperative treatment is preferable. Patients older than 70 years of age with large chronic tears have already experienced irreversible changes in their cuffs that lead to functional loss and pain. Because of these irreversible changes in the cuff there is little risk associated with attempting prolonged nonoperative treatment to control a patient's pain.

It is estimated that between 70% and 80% of rotator cuff tendonitis will be successfully treated nonoperatively. In one series of 616 patients, 78% of patients treated within 4 weeks of symptoms onset had a successful outcome versus 67% in patients who had symptoms for 6 months or more. In this study, acromial morphology played a role as well, with the highest rates (91%) of successful nonoperative treatment in patients with a type I (flat) acromion, compared to 68% with type II and 64% with type III.[34] Nonoperative methods of treating rotator cuff tendonitis and impingement syndrome include corticosteroid injections, oral anti-inflammatory medication, activity modification, modalities of ultrasound and phonophoresis, and rehabilitation emphasizing stretching and strengthening the rotator cuff and scapular musculature. There are few controlled studies that provide objective data on these therapeutic options.

Corticosteroids have been shown to be effective in controlling symptoms associated with rotator cuff pathology, often eliminating the need for surgical treatment.[35] Corticosteroid injections control pain and improve function better than lidocaine injections alone. However, these injections carry an inherent risk of causing necrosis and fragmentation of the tendon tissue, potentially making surgical repair more difficult.[35] For this reason, corticosteroid injections into the subacromial space to treat rotator cuff tendonitis or symptomatic small tears should be used with discretion. We recommend a guideline of limiting a series of injections to three injections given at 3-month intervals.

Rehabilitation is a mainstay of nonoperative treatment of rotator cuff disorders. Following a brief (3-day) rest period to decrease acute inflammation and pain, the patient should engage in a stretching protocol to increase the range of motion, especially in patients who have lost internal rotation, as the tight posterior capsule can elevate the humeral head and cuff into the acromion. After improvement in range of motion is achieved, the patient may engage in regular light exercise to strengthen the muscles of the rotator cuff and scapular stabilizers in addition to deltoid and trapezius strengthening. Strengthening the rotator cuff and scapular stabilizers will improve shoulder kinematics, and a strong deltoid will improve abduction strength, providing a stable fulcrum is present. In order to benefit from a rehabilitation program, compliance with a regular program is essential. Insofar as supervised therapy improves compliance, there is benefit to supervised physical therapy. However, in one study of patients who had undergone arthroscopic subacromial decompression without rotator cuff repair, there was no difference in outcomes between the group in supervised therapy and the group in a self-directed program.[36] It may be that being enrolled in the study heightened patients' awareness of the protocols and increased their compliance.

Supervised physical therapy often uses other modalities such as ultrasound, phonophoresis, or iontophoresis to treat subacromial bursitis, cuff tendonitis, or small symptomatic cuff tears. Ultrasound therapy is a common physical therapy modality that is often applied to the nonoperative treatment of rotator cuff tendonitis and subacromial impingement. High-frequency ultrasound (1 to 3 MHz) creates a thermal and possibly mechanical effect that can increase blood flow to a focal area, theoretically augmenting a tissue's capacity to heal. Although there are no studies that demonstrate its effectiveness in the treatment of rotator cuff tendonitis or subacromial impingement symptoms, ultrasound is used frequently. In a prospective, randomized, double-blind, placebo-controlled study, 20 patients with subacromial bursitis were randomized to receive either sham or real ultrasound 3 times per week for 4 weeks.[37] There was no demonstrable benefit in the ultrasound group in terms of pain ratings, function, or time to recovery. In this small study with only 20 subjects, the authors concluded that there was no benefit to treatment of subacromial bursitis with ultrasound. It is possible that the therapeutic benefit was small and was not detected by low numbers of subjects in a short period of time. Phonophoresis is a technique that uses ultrasound to deliver medication directly into superficial tissues. It is postulated that the mechanical and thermal effects of ultrasound together increase tissue permeability and even cellular permeability. In a controlled study,[38] 47 patients were randomized to receive either corticosteroid phonophoresis or the identical ultrasound doses without corticosteroid. There were no differences found between the groups. Iontophoresis is another modality whereby physical properties of electric current is used to deliver medication directly to pathologic tissues, usually corticosteroids. Much recent work has been directed at determining the optimal physical parameters for maximal medication delivery. There is scant literature available regarding the clinical effectiveness of this treatment.

Surgical Treatment

Despite appropriate nonoperative care, patients often require surgical treatment. Surgical treatment of rotator cuff pathology requires a thorough understanding of the specific pathologic condition to be treated. Even with adequate imaging studies, an arthroscopic diagnostic evaluation of the glenohumeral joint and the subacromial space will help define the pathology, and provide an understanding of the involved anatomy. Arthroscopic findings will guide treatment, and intraoperative decisions often need to be made as anatomic details of the pathology are revealed.

Arthroscopic evaluation and treatment of subacromial bursitis and rotator cuff tears may be performed in the beach chair or lateral decubitus position. Use of the beach chair position prevents potential distortion of normal anatomy and allows the surgeon to frequently reposition and examine the arm during the procedure. The advantage of the lateral position is that the arm is distracted, which enlarges the subacromial space, potentially providing greater arthroscopic perspective to facilitate an accurate interpretation of the tear anatomy. As the lateral position holds the arm in a fixed abducted position, the arm should be removed from traction to allow for inspection in several positions. Care must be taken not to repair a cuff tear with the arm in excessive abduction, as this repair will be under additional tension when the arm is in a neutral position.

Diagnostic Arthroscopy

Surgical treatment of rotator cuff tendonitis or tears starts with a thorough diagnostic arthroscopy of the entire glenohumeral joint. With visualization of the glenohumeral joint from the posterior portal, a standard anterosuperior portal is placed within the rotator interval to allow outflow and instrumentation. The subscapularis insertion is evaluated in various degrees of arm rotation, with particular attention paid to its confluence with the glenohumeral ligament complex comprising the biceps sling. The biceps tendon is pulled into the joint and inspected for erythema or fraying, indicative of biceps tendonitis (Fig. 25-2A), or a torn biceps sling (Fig. 25-2B), which may suggest the need for a biceps tenodesis or tenotomy. The articular side of the supraspinatus is carefully inspected with the arm abducted, externally rotated, and forward elevated. The rotator cuff cable is identified (see Fig. 25-1), and an absorbable monofilament suture is passed through a spinal needle to mark focal irregularities or small tears in the articular side of the cuff tendon (Fig. 25-3A), which will facilitate bursal side inspection (Fig. 25-3B).

Subacromial Decompression

The subacromial space is entered posteriorly and a thorough bursectomy is performed. Visualization is maximized by maintaining hemostasis, through careful dissection using radiofrequency

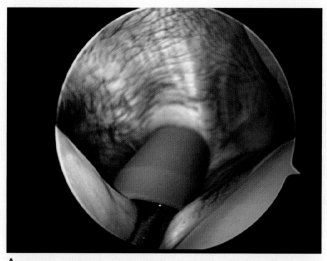

A

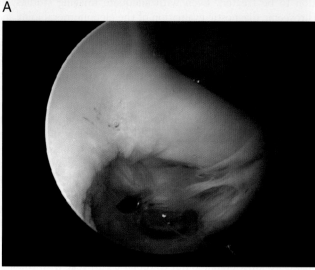

B

Figure 25-2 A, Biceps tendonitis. **B,** Torn biceps sling.

coagulation and careful fluid management in the setting of effective intraoperative blood pressure control. Besides providing visualization, complete bursal débridement removes a pain-producing structure.[39,40] If an acromioplasty is to be performed, the coracoacromial (CA) ligament insertion on the anterolateral corner of the acromion is identified and elevated with a radiofrequency device introduced from the lateral portal. It is advisable to use coagulation in the region of the acromial branch of the thoracoacromial artery, which runs in the substance of the CA ligament.[11] We recommend that radiofrequency dissection continue cautiously beyond the anterior and lateral edges of the acromion to but not beyond the fibers of the deltoid muscle in order to identify bone irregularities including an anterior hook or bone excrescence. Maintaining deltoid fascia integrity will help prevent extravasation of fluid into the surrounding soft tissues. A bur is introduced from the lateral portal and starting with the lateral edge and anterolateral corner, the anterior portion of the acromion is decompressed to a flat surface. The acromioplasty is then completed, working through the posterior portal via a cutting block technique viewing from the lateral portal.

The decision to perform a routine acromioplasty is a source of controversy. Gartsman and O'Connor[41] demonstrated no difference in outcomes in their series of 93 patients with primary rotator cuff tears and type II acromions who were prospectively randomized to undergo arthroscopic rotator cuff repair with or without acromioplasty. We often perform an acromioplasty when preparing an arthroscopic rotator cuff repair to maximize visualization, to ensure an absence of cuff impingement, and to reduce symptoms, as this has been a proven method for treating the pain associated with rotator cuff pathology.[42]

Arthroscopic Rotator Cuff Repair

If a repairable tear of the supraspinatus is identified, it is crucial to understand the anatomy of the tear and ensure the mobility of the tendon, remaining cognizant that large tears will be pulled medially and posteriorly. Dissection above the superior labrum, or through the rotator interval if necessary, will mobilize tendons and allow a low-tension reduction. Friable tendon edges are débrided carefully back to more intact tendon edge capable of holding suture. The footprint of the cuff is prepared by judicious use of a burr to expose fresh bone capable of evoking a healing response, taking care not to remove excessive (>1 mm) bone (Fig. 25-3C). To establish the working anterolateral accessory portal, dead man's[43] angle is determined with a spinal needle, and a 6-mm threaded cannula is inserted at that angle directly over the footprint to allow anchor insertion at that angle as well (Fig. 25-3D).

The various techniques of arthroscopic rotator cuff repair are not thoroughly reviewed here. For large U-shaped tears that have retracted to the glenoid (Fig. 25-4A), dissecting the tendon off the glenoid neck (Fig. 25-4B) and coracoid will mobilize the tendon for repair. It is advisable to place side-to-side margin convergence sutures to reestablish force couples and to convert the tear to a smaller C-shaped tear (Fig. 25-4C),[44,45] allowing for direct tendon to bone repair with anchors. With irregular L-shaped tears, it may be necessary to place and remove margin convergence sutures to determine that the location of the medial closure apex does not limit the ability to reduce the lateral tendon edge to bone. The location and total number of anchors should be planned before placing the first one, avoiding confluence of the anchor holes. Resorbable anchors have been shown to have adequate pull-out strength[46] in good quality bone, but we will occasionally use metal anchors in poor-quality bone.

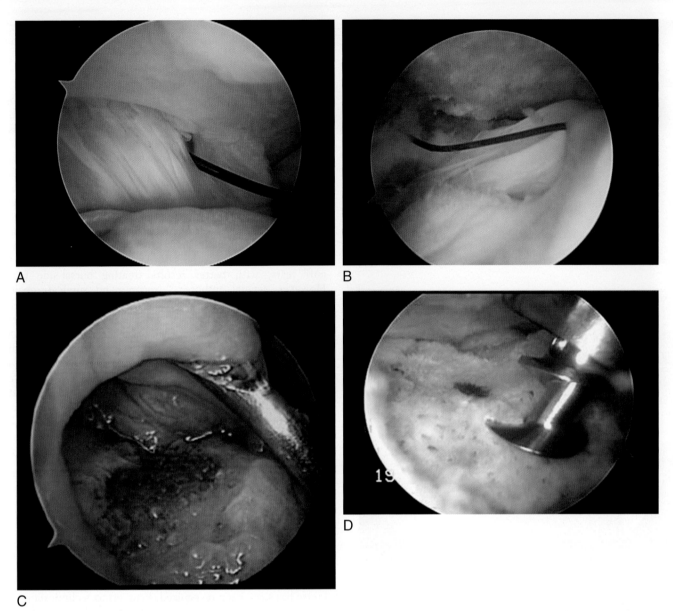

Figure 25-3 Four-part repair of rotator cuff: Crescent shaped. **A,** Marked tear articular side. **B,** Marked tear bursal side. **C,** Preparation of greater tuberosity. **D,** Placement of one anchor at "dead man's" angle.

Anchors loaded with multiple braided nonabsorbable sutures are our preference. Recent work has suggested that a double-row orientation of anchors and suture passage may improve healing by increasing the area of contact between the tendon and bone.[47]

Sutures are passed through tendon either directly or indirectly via a suture shuttle method using any number of commercially available devices. We routinely place anchors and pass sutures working posterior to anterior, as this provides the best visualization and the ability to reduce a posteriorly retracted cuff. Direct suture passage is performed by introducing a sharp-tipped grasping device via the posterior portal, penetrating the full thickness of the cuff 1 cm from the torn edge, taking care to avoid the articular surface of the humeral head that lies directly below the tendon edge. The desired suture can then be grasped and pulled directly through the tendon. Indirect suture passage uses an intermediary shuttle suture, which is passed through the cuff, retrieved through the working portal, tied to the desired suture, and then used to shuttle the suture through

the cuff. If anchors are placed in a "stacked" or double-row configuration, the medial sutures should pass through the tendon in a mattress stitch close to the musculotendinous junction.

Regardless of the surgeon's knot and suture selection, arthroscopic knot tying should follow principles of maintaining knot and loop security,[48] tension-free tissue reduction, and proper placement of the suture loop and knot. Loop security describes the degree to which the tension applied to the knot is actually transmitted to the tissue-bone interface; without secure loops, even the tightest knot will not have the desired effect on the repair. The task of arthroscopic knot tying is greatly facilitated by ensuring that all extraneous soft tissue is débrided, which will not only maximize visualization, but also prevent soft-tissue interposition and subsequent knot loosening. Sliding knots are appropriate in most situations where suture freely passes through tendon and anchor eyelet, but excessive abrasion may weaken sutures or damage tendon. Nonsliding knots can be used in all situations, but careful attention must be paid to ensure

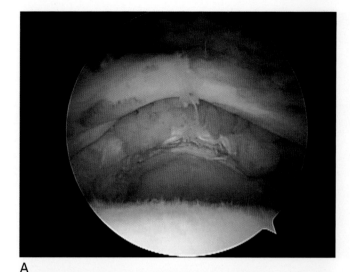

A

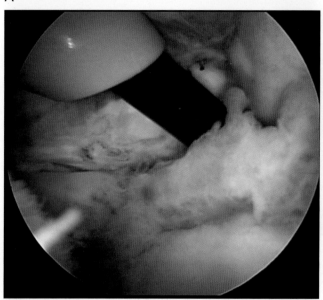

B

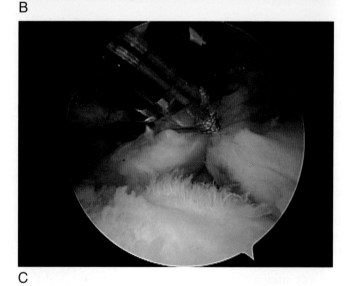

C

Figure 25-4 Massive tear. **A,** Retracted to glenoid. **B,** Release of adhesions between cuff and glenoid neck, above superior labrum. **C,** Side-to-side stitch closes U-shaped tear, allowing repair to greater tuberosity.

that the second and third throws seat the knot securely on tissue, preferably causing a slight indentation in the tendon tissue.

Partial-Thickness Tears

The treatment of partial-thickness tears is a controversial topic. Arthroscopic evaluation allows inspection of the cuff on both the articular and bursal sides, allowing accurate diagnosis of partial-thickness tears. This is especially true with respect to the articular-side tears, which cannot be fully appreciated without an arthroscopic evaluation of the glenohumeral joint. Early studies of arthroscopic débridement and acromioplasty alone as treatment of partial-thickness tears reported 76% to 89% good to excellent results.[49,50]

More recently, short-term pain relief has been reported following débridement and subacromial decompression of both articular- and bursal-side partial-thickness rotator cuff tears, with better results treating bursal-side tears.[51] However, several authors[52–54] recommend surgical repair of partial thickness tears, especially if they comprise 50% or more of the tendon thickness, with a lower threshold to repair bursal-side tears.[54] For bursal-side tears, even a more invasive, mini-open repair resulted in better outcomes than simple arthroscopic débridement and subacromial decompression alone.[55] Repair of articular-side partial-thickness rotator cuff tears can be performed arthroscopically by either completing the tear and using standard arthroscopic repair methods or by penetrating the intact portion with a suture anchor, pulling all sutures to the articular side, and passing sutures through the cuff by alternating between glenohumeral and subacromial visualization.[53,54]

Open/Mini-Open Rotator Cuff Repair

Prior to the advent of arthroscopic shoulder surgery, tears of the rotator cuff were identified and repaired with an open exposure of the subacromial space, requiring detachment of the anterior deltoid off the acromion, which required meticulous repair. Dehiscence of the deltoid from the acromion causes significant debilitation, and the value of minimizing deltoid intraoperative injury has since been recognized. In an effort to limit damage to the deltoid, mini-open techniques have been developed to allow open exposure to the subacromial space by splitting the deltoid without detachment from the acromion. We briefly describe the techniques of formal open exposure with deltoid repair and a less invasive mini-open deltoid-splitting technique.

Currently, the indications for considering formal open exposure include the inability to mobilize and repair a large retracted cuff tear arthroscopically or when performing a transfer of the latissimus or pectoralis as a salvage procedure. Even in the case of a formal open repair, a thorough arthroscopic evaluation of the shoulder is helpful to define the tear anatomy, mobilize the cuff, and identify other pathology. For open exposure of the supraspinatus tendon, every effort should be made to preserve the integrity of the deltoid attachment by using a mini-open approach that splits rather than detaches the deltoid. If necessary, the anterior 2 cm of the deltoid origin on the acromion may be elevated. Important anatomic features of the deltoid include its broad insertion on the periphery of the acromion. If detachment is necessary, it is critical to remove and maintain deep and superficial fascial planes of the deltoid to allow meticulous closure and full-thickness repair of both fascial layers directly to the acromion. Dehiscence of the anterior deltoid is a complication for which there is not a good solution, with predictably poor results following surgical repair.[56] For an open exposure of a sub-scapularis tear, a standard anterior approach through the deltopectoral interval is used.

The most serious risk involved with the mini-open deltoid split is damage to the axillary nerve. Anatomic studies have identified an average distance of 5 cm,[57] but a variable minimum between 4 and even 2 cm from the upper border of the deltoid muscle.[58] The subdeltoid bursa remains cephalad to the axillary nerve, at an average distance of 0.8 cm (range, 0.0 to 1.4 cm).[57] To minimize risk, the smallest exposure necessary to perform the repair should be used, and attempts should be made to limit that distance specifically to less than 4 cm. Furthermore, the split in the deltoid should remain above the boundry of the subdeltoid bursa. To prevent inadvertent propagation of the split with retractors, a stitch is placed through the bottom of the deltoid split at the beginning of the surgical procedure.

Whether the deltoid is detached or split, open exposure allows direct visualization of the subacromial space. Even in the setting of an open exposure of the cuff, an acromioplasty can be performed arthroscopically prior to open exposure because arthroscopy allows better visualization of the anteromedial acromion. During this arthroscopic subacromial decompression, a complete bursectomy and cuff tear preparation may be performed, depending on the arthroscopic skill of the surgeon. Direct open visualization of the subacromial space will allow further débridement of the bursa and preparation of both the cuff tear and the tendon footprint. Depending on the size, location, and chronicity of the tear, adhesions to the coracoid and glenoid (through a large tear) may be released to mobilize the cuff, although this is often easier to perform accurately using an arthroscopic technique.

After débridement of the bursa, preparation of the tear includes mobilization of the tendon to allow a low-tension reduction and repair directly to the footprint of the tendon through bone tunnels or with suture anchors. Whether bone tunnels or suture anchors are used, an effort is made to preserve bone at the insertion site. Bone preparation should expose but not remove cancellous bone, thereby stimulating a healing response, without compromising anchor fixation or bone tunnel strength. The fixation strength of transosseous sutures can be maximized by orienting tunnel exits 1 cm distal to the tuberosity and creating a healthy bone bridge approximately 1 cm thick. As tendon is reduced and repaired, an appropriate amount of tension may be estimated by comparing the repaired tendon to the adjacent intact tendon insertion in whatever position the arm is in at the time of repair.

POSTOPERATIVE REHABILITATION

Postoperative rehabilitation is conducted in phases. The first phase includes a 6-week period during which the patient is allowed passive range of motion only to allow tendon-to-bone healing to occur. During this phase, range-of-motion goals are 140 degrees of forward flexion, 40 degrees of external rotation with the arm at the side, and 60 degrees of abduction in neutral rotation. During this early phase, we do not allow the use of canes or pulleys, as these are active-assist devices.

Active motion begins during the next phase, from weeks 6 to 12, with a gradual increase in the range of motion. During this intermediate phase, gentle stretching is permitted at the end of motion ranges. Although active motion is allowed, no strengthening or resisted motion is allowed. At 8 weeks, isometric exercise with the arm at the side in a neutral position is allowed.

The third phase begins at 3 months following surgery and continues until maximal improvement is achieved. Full range of motion is a goal during this period. Strengthening is progressed from isometrics, to light resistive bands, to weights ranging from 1 to 5 pounds. In addition to rotator cuff muscles, it is important to strengthen scapular stabilizers and the deltoid. We recommend that strengthening work be performed only three times per week to avoid cuff tendonitis.

CRITERIA FOR RETURN TO SPORTS

The strengthening program that initiates at 3 months evolves to include plyometrics and sport-specific simulation training as the patient is able to tolerate. At 6 months, light throwing is allowed. Because a durable repair requires tendon-to-bone healing that can withstand dynamic loading, participation in collision sports or pitching from a mound is not permitted until 9 months. Full recovery and maximal performance gains are expected at 1 year, although functional improvement may continue well into the second postoperative year.

RESULTS AND OUTCOMES

The success of surgical treatment of rotator cuff pathology depends on the anatomy and classification of the tear, the biology of the tissue, the physiology of the tissue, the quality of the repair, and associated comorbidities as well as several medical and sociologic factors.[59] The results of arthroscopic repair of full-thickness tears appear to be at least equal to those of open repair with lower rates of complications such as infection, nerve injury, and deltoid detachment. Studies have demonstrated patient satisfaction to be as high as 98%, with low patient morbidity and pain.[60–62]

Massive retracted U-shaped tears can be mobilized and repaired via margin convergence, using side-to-side stitches to convert large U-shaped tears to smaller C-shaped tears, which are then repaired to bone in a standard fashion.[45] Patient satisfaction is reported to be as high as 100%, with 96% good to excellent results for arthroscopic repair of medium-sized tears (3 cm).[61,63] Even massive tears, which can only be partially repaired, provide significant pain relief and some improved function by reconstituting the balanced force couples transmitted through the rotator cuff cable.[64]

Durability of results appears to be related to the ability of a tendon to permanently heal to bone. A recent study demonstrated that improvement in the first year did not persist at 2 years if the tendon was not healed to bone.[65]

COMPLICATIONS

The major postoperative complication is failure of the tendon to heal, whether treated arthroscopically or open. There are many biologic, anatomic, and behavioral factors that relate to the likelihood that a tear will heal following repair. To increase the likelihood of healing, we recommend the surgeon employ the most biomechanically appropriate technique, with an attempt to maximize the area of contact between the tendon and bone.

Deltoid dehiscence is a rare but devastating complication of formal open treatment of rotator cuff tears. This can generally be avoided by not removing the lateral acromion and by performing a secure anatomic deltoid repair.[56] With partial deltoid dehiscence, arthrocutaneous fistulas may occur, for which early débridement and deltoid reattachment are recommended.

Infection occurs in less than 1% of patients. Infections can be due to *Staphylococcus aureus*, but are also associated with organisms such as *Proprionibacterium*, coagulase negative *Staphylococcus*, or *Peptostreptococcus*. Treatment of infections includes early detection, débridement, and proper antibiotics. In properly treated infected rotator cuff repairs, a good to excellent result can be expected in approximately one third of patients.

Shoulder stiffness is a potential complication that is minimized with an arthroscopic repair by avoiding the pain and morbidity associated with an incision and deltoid violation. Early postoperative loss of range of motion can usually be overcome with appropriate rehabilitation.

In one series, mini-open repair was associated with a 14% rate of stiffness compared to none in an all-arthroscopic group.

In this series, there was a trend for better motion in the arthroscopically treated group, although this difference did not reach statistical significance.[66] With proper patient compliance with a postoperative protocol that emphasizes early passive range of motion, prolonged stiffness following arthroscopic repair is rare.[67]

CONCLUSIONS

Rotator cuff disease is common in athletes and presents in a spectrum from rotator cuff tendonitis to full-thickness tears. An understanding of the underlying cause of the problem is important in developing an appropriate treatment plan. Nonoperative treatment is effective in most cases not involving full-thickness rotator cuff tears. Rotator cuff repair generally provides good results, but repair in high-level athletes has a more guarded prognosis.

REFERENCES

1. Burkhart SS, Nottage WM, Ogilvie-Harris DJ, et al: Partial repair of irreparable rotator cuff tears. Arthroscopy 1994;10:363–370.
2. Burkhart SS: Arthroscopic debridement and decompression for selected rotator cuff tears. Clinical results, pathomechanics, and patient selection based on biomechanical parameters. Orthop Clin North Am 1993;24:111–123.
3. Burkhart SS: Partial repair of massive rotator cuff tears: The evolution of a concept. Orthop Clin North Am 1997;28:125–132.
4. Magarey ME, Jones MA: Dynamic evaluation and early management of altered motor control around the shoulder complex. Man Ther 2003;8:195–206.
5. Lee SB, An KN: Dynamic glenohumeral stability provided by three heads of the deltoid muscle. Clin Orthop 2002;400:40–47.
6. Burkhart SS: Shoulder arthroscopy. New concepts. Clin Sports Med 1996;15:635–653.
7. Burkhart SS, Esch JC, Jolson RS: The rotator crescent and rotator cable: An anatomic description of the shoulder's "suspension bridge." Arthroscopy 1993;9:611–616. Erratum in Arthroscopy 1994;10:239.
8. Burkhart SS: Fluoroscopic comparison of kinematic patterns in massive rotator cuff tears. A suspension bridge model. Clin Orthop 1992;284:144–152.
9. McGough RL, Debski RE, Taskiran E, et al: Mechanical properties of the long head of the biceps tendon. Knee Surg Sports Traumatol Arthrosc 1996;3:226–229.
10. Eakin CL, Faber KJ, Hawkins RJ, et al: Biceps tendon disorders in athletes. J Am Acad Orthop Surg 1999;7:300–310.
11. Hulstyn MJ, Fadale PD: Arthroscopic anatomy of the shoulder. Orthop Clin North Am 1995;26:597–612.
12. Werner A, Mueller T, Boehm D, et al: The stabilizing sling for the long head of the biceps tendon in the rotator cuff interval. A histoanatomic study. Am J Sports Med 2000;28:28–31.
13. Lohr JF, Uhthoff HK: The microvascular pattern of the supraspinatus tendon. Clin Orthop 1990;254:35–38.
14. Sano H, Ishii H, Trudel G, et al: Histologic evidence of degeneration at the insertion of 3 rotator cuff tendons: A comparative study with human cadaveric shoulders. J Shoulder Elbow Surg 1999;8:574–579.
15. Burkhart SS, Morgan CD, Kibler WB: The disabled throwing shoulder: Spectrum of pathology. Part I: Pathoanatomy and biomechanics. Arthroscopy 2003;19:404–420.
16. Burkhart SS, Morgan CD, Kibler WB: The disabled throwing shoulder: Spectrum of pathology. Part II: Evaluation and treatment of SLAP lesions in throwers. Arthroscopy 2003;19:531–549.
17. Burkhart SS, Morgan CD, Kibler WB: The disabled throwing shoulder: Spectrum of pathology. Part III: The SICK scapula, scapular dyskinesis, the kinetic chain, and rehabilitation. Arthroscopy 2003;19:641–661.
18. Davidson PA, Elattrache NS, Jobe CM, et al: Rotator cuff and posterior-superior glenoid labrum injury associated with increased glenohumeral motion: A new site of impingement. J Shoulder Elbow Surg 1995;4:384–390.
19. Budoff JE, Nirschl RP, Ilahi OA, et al: Internal impingement in the etiology of rotator cuff tendinosis revisited. Arthroscopy 2003;19:810–814.
20. Burkhart SS, Parten PM: Dead arm syndrome: Torsional SLAP lesions versus internal impingement. Tech Shoulder Elbow Surg 2001;2:74–84.
21. Neer CS 2nd: Anterior acromioplasty for the chronic impingement syndrome in the shoulder: A preliminary report. J Bone Joint Surg Am 1972;54:41–50.
22. Hawkins RJ, Kennedy JC: Impingement syndrome in athletes. Am J Sports Med 1980;8:151–158.
23. Gerber C, Hersche O, Farron A: Isolated rupture of the subscapularis tendon. J Bone Joint Surg Am 1996;78:1015–1023.
24. Burkhart SS, Tehrany AM: Arthroscopic subscapularis tendon repair: Technique and preliminary results. Arthroscopy 2002;18:454–463.
25. Lo IK, Burkhart SS: The etiology and assessment of subscapularis tendon tears: A case for subcoracoid impingement, the roller-wringer effect, and TUFF lesions of the subscapularis. Arthroscopy 2003;19:1142–1150.
26. Gerber C, Krushell RJ: Isolated rupture of the tendon of the subscapularis muscle. Clinical features in 16 cases. J Bone Joint Surg Br 1991;73:389–394.
27. Kilcoyne RF, Reddy PK, Lyons F, et al: Optimal plain film imaging of the shoulder impingement syndrome. AJR Am J Roentgenol 1989;153:795–797.
28. Teefey SA, Rubin DA, Middleton WD, et al: Detection and quantification of rotator cuff tears. Comparison of ultrasonographic, magnetic resonance imaging, and arthroscopic findings in seventy-one consecutive cases. J Bone Joint Surg Am 2004;86:708–716.
29. Ferrari FS, Governi S, Burresi F, et al: Supraspinatus tendon tears: Comparison of US and MR arthrography with surgical correlation. Eur Radiol 2002;12:1211–1217.
30. Tempelhof S, Rupp S, Seil R: Age-related prevalence of rotator cuff tears in asymptomatic shoulders. J Shoulder Elbow Surg 1999;8:296–299.
31. Sakurai G, Ozaki J, Tomita Y, et al: Incomplete tears of the subscapularis tendon associated with tears of the supraspinatus tendon: Cadaveric and clinical studies. J Shoulder Elbow Surg 1998;7:510–515.

32. Yamaguchi K, Tetro AM, Blam O, et al: Natural history of asymptomatic rotator cuff tears: A longitudinal analysis of asymptomatic tears detected sonographically. J Shoulder Elbow Surg 2001;10:199–203.

33. Nakagaki K, Ozaki J, Tomita Y, et al: Fatty degeneration in the supraspinatus muscle after rotator cuff tear. J Shoulder Elbow Surg 1996;5:194–200.

34. Morrison DS, Frogameni AD, Woodworth P: Non-operative treatment of subacromial impingement syndrome. J Bone Joint Surg Am 1997;79:732–737.

35. Blair B, Rokito AS, Cuomo F, et al: Efficacy of injections of corticosteroids for subacromial impingement syndrome. J Bone Joint Surg Am 1996;78:1685–1689.

36. Anderson NH, Sojbjerg JO, Johannsen HV, et al: Self-training versus physiotherapist-supervised rehabilitation of the shoulder in patients treated with arthroscopic subacromial decompression: A clinical randomized study. J Shoulder Elbow Surg 1999;8:99–101.

37. Downing DS, Weinstein A: Ultrasound therapy of subacromial bursitis. A double blind trial. Phys Ther 1986;66:194–199.

38. Klaiman MD, Shrader JA, Danoff JV, et al: Phonophoresis versus ultrasound in the treatment of common musculoskeletal conditions. Med Sci Sports Exerc 1998;30:1349–1355.

39. Gotoh M, Hamada K, Yamakawa H, et al: Increased substance P in subacromial bursa and shoulder pain in rotator cuff diseases. J Orthop Res 1998;16:618–621.

40. Soifer TB, Levy HJ, Soifer FM, et al: Neurohistology of the subacromial space. Arthroscopy 1996;12:182–186.

41. Gartsman GM, O'Connor DP: Arthroscopic rotator cuff repair with and without arthroscopic subacromial decompression: A prospective, randomized study of one-year outcomes. J Shoulder Elbow Surg 2004;13:424–426.

42. Nicholson GP: Arthroscopic acromioplasty: A comparison between workers' compensation and non-workers' compensation populations. J Bone Joint Surg Am 2003;85:682–689.

43. Burkhart SS: The deadman theory of suture anchors: Observations along a south Texas fence line. Arthroscopy 1995;11:119–223.

44. Burkhart SS, Athanasiou KA, Wirth MA: Margin convergence: A method of reducing strain in massive rotator cuff tears. Arthroscopy 1996;12:335–338.

45. Burkhart SS, Danaceau SM, Pearce CE Jr: Arthroscopic rotator cuff repair: Analysis of results by tear size and by repair technique-margin convergence versus direct tendon-to-bone repair. Arthroscopy 2001;17:905–912.

46. Dejong ES, DeBerardino TM, Brooks DE, et al: In vivo comparison of a metal versus a biodegradable suture anchor. Arthroscopy 2004;20:511–516.

47. Lo IK, Burkhart SS: Double-row arthroscopic rotator cuff repair: Re-establishing the footprint of the rotator cuff. Arthroscopy 2003;19:1035–1042.

48. Lo IK, Burkhart SS, Chan KC, et al: Arthroscopic knots: Determining the optimal balance of loop security and knot security. Arthroscopy 2004;20:489–502.

49. Esch JC, Ozerkis LR, Helgager JA, et al: Arthroscopic subacromial decompression: Results according to the degree of rotator cuff tear. Arthroscopy 1988;4:241–249.

50. Snyder SJ, Pachelli, AF, Pizzo WD, et al: Partial thickness rotator cuff tears: Results of arthroscopic treatment. Arthroscopy 1991;7:1–7.

51. Park JY, Yoo MJ, Kim MH: Comparison of surgical outcome between bursal and articular partial thickness rotator cuff tears. Orthopedics 2003;26:387–390.

52. Fukuda H: The management of partial-thickness tears of the rotator cuff. J Bone Joint Surg Br 2003;85:3–11.

53. Lehman RC, Perry CR: Arthroscopic surgery for partial rotator cuff tears. Arthroscopy 2003;19:E81–E84.

54. Lo IK, Burkhart SS: Transtendon arthroscopic repair of partial-thickness, articular surface tears of the rotator cuff. Arthroscopy 2004;20:214–220.

55. Weber SC: Arthroscopic debridement and acromioplasty versus mini-open repair in the management of significant partial-thickness tears of the rotator cuff. Orthop Clin North Am 1997;28:79–82.

56. Sher JS, Iannotti JP, Warner JJ, et al: Surgical treatment of postoperative deltoid origin disruption. Clin Orthop 1997;343:93–98.

57. Beals TC, Harryman DT 2nd, Lazarus MD: Useful boundaries of the subacromial bursa. Arthroscopy 1998;14:465–470.

58. Kontakis GM, Steriopoulos K, Damilakis J, et al: The position of the axillary nerve in the deltoid muscle. A cadaveric study. Acta Orthop Scand 1999;70:9–11.

59. Romeo AA, Hang DW, Bach BR Jr, et al: Repair of full thickness rotator cuff tears. Gender, age, and other factors affecting outcome. Clin Orthop 1999;367:243–255.

60. Gartsman GM, Khan M, Hammerman SM: Arthroscopic repair of full-thickness tears of the rotator cuff. J Bone Joint Surg Am 1998;80:832–840.

61. Murray TF Jr, Lajtai G, Mileski RM, et al: Arthroscopic repair of medium to large full-thickness rotator cuff tears: Outcome at 2- to 6-year follow-up. J Shoulder Elbow Surg 2002;11:19–24.

62. Tauro JC: Arthroscopic rotator cuff repair: Analysis of technique and results at 2- and 3-year follow-up Arthroscopy 1998;14:45–51.

63. Bennett WF: Arthroscopic repair of isolated subscapularis tears: A prospective cohort with 2- to 4-year follow-up. Arthroscopy 2003;19:131–143.

64. Bennett WF: Arthroscopic repair of massive rotator cuff tears: A prospective cohort with 2- to 4-year follow-up. Arthroscopy 2003;19:380–390.

65. Galatz LM, Ball CM, Teefey SA, et al: The outcome and repair integrity of completely arthroscopically repaired large and massive rotator cuff tears. J Bone Joint Surg Am 2004;86:219–224.

66. Severud EL, Ruotolo C, Abbott DD, et al: All-arthroscopic versus mini-open rotator cuff repair: A long-term retrospective outcome comparison. Arthroscopy 2003;19:234–238.

67. Mansat P, Cofield RH, Kersten TE, et al: Complications of rotator cuff repair. Orthop Clin North Am 1997;28:205–213.

Disorders of the Acromioclavicular Joint

Theodore F. Schlegel and Patrick Siparsky

In This Chapter

INTRODUCTION

- AC joint disorders are among the most common causes of shoulder pain.

- Disorders involving this joint are often confused with other glenohumeral problems.

- The AC joint is susceptible to traumatic injury as well as a degenerative process from overuse.

- Successful treatment of AC disorders relies on an accurate diagnosis obtained through a detailed history, thorough physical examination, and a complete radiographic evaluation.

- For traumatic disorders, proper classification of the injury type will aid the clinician in employing a proper treatment algorithm.

- The majority of AC separations, including Grade III disorders, are usually successfully treated with a nonoperative program.

- High-grade AC separation (types IV, V, VI) and occasionally those occurring in the overhead throwing athlete can be expected to have a successful outcome following a "three-in-one" surgical reconstruction.

RELEVANT ANATOMY

Along with the sternoclavicular joint, the AC joint provides the only articulation between the upper extremity and the axial skeleton. This joint dissipates forces placed on the upper extremity and the axial skeleton. It is diarthrodial, consisting of the medial aspect of the acromion and the lateral aspect of the clavicle. Its unique anatomy allows movement between the clavicle and the scapula. During its development, the ends of the clavicle and acromion are fibrocartilage, creating an intra-articular disk that is subject to degeneration with use and aging. The

distal end of the clavicle does not ossify until around the age of 19, allowing for the possibility of a periosteal sleeve fracture in younger patients.

The stability of the joint is provided by two major ligamentous structures (Fig. 26-1). The AC ligaments are critical for anteroposterior stability.[1] The coracoclavicular (CC) ligament provides restraint of superior translation of the distal clavicle. The CC ligament consists of the trapezoid ligament and the conoid ligament. The trapezoid ligament is attached anterolaterally to the conoid ligament on the coracoid process, extending superiorly to the inferior aspect of the clavicle. The conoid ligament extends from the posteromedial margin of the coracoid process to the posterior inferior clavicular curve on the conoid tubercle.

CLINICAL FEATURES AND EVALUATION

Traumatic Acromioclavicular Separations

The most frequent cause of an AC separation is the application of a direct force, which frequently occurs during a fall onto the shoulder when the arm is adducted (Fig. 26-2). This commonly occurs in contact sports such as football and hockey or in recreational sports such as cycling when an individual goes over the handlebars of a bike. In these situations, the energy from the fall forces the acromion downward and medially, causing the AC ligaments to be damaged first, followed by a sequential disruption of CC ligaments in higher energy injuries.

AC injuries resulting from indirect trauma are less common. Typically, these injuries occur when landing on an outstretched arm. The force thrusts the humeral head superiorly into the acromion process, causing disruption of the AC ligaments. In these cases, it is rare to have a high-grade AC separation because the CC ligaments are not injured because this force decreases the CC space, thereby decreasing tension on the CC ligaments.

Chronic Disorders of Acromioclavicular Joint

Deterioration of the fibrocartilaginous disk that separates the two articular surfaces of the AC joint is thought to occur as early as the second decade of life.[2,3] The degeneration of the disk may be a natural process of aging. In elderly patients, radiographic changes of degeneration may occur in more than 50% of the population.[2,3] However, all patients with joint space narrowing may not be symptomatic. It is therefore critical to determine whether these changes are associated with any symptoms. Patients with a symptomatic AC joint may describe pain localized to the joint or may also experience pain that radiates into the neck with more strenuous activities.

The onset of these problems is often related to overhead activities such as throwing or weight lifting. The throwing

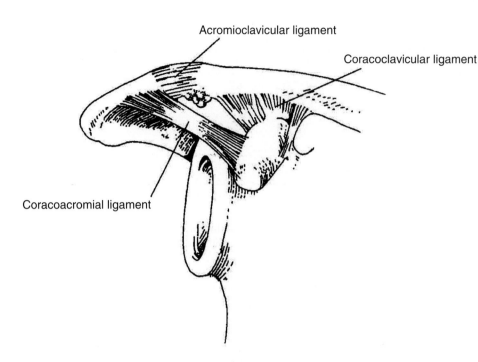

Acromioclavicular ligament

Coracoclavicular ligament

Coracoacromial ligament

Figure 26-1 Ligamentous structures of the acromioclavicular joint: acromioclavicular, coracoclavicular, and coracoacromial ligaments. (Adapted from Hawkins RJ, Bell SB, Lippitt LH: Atlas of Shoulder Surgery. Philadelphia, Mosby, 1996.)

motion may cause repetitive stress on the AC joint in the follow-through phase with horizontal cross-arm adduction. Weight lifters will often have excessive force on the AC joint with a bench press. This has been strongly implicated in the destruction of the articular cartilage. Cahill[4] reported 46 patients who were athletes, none of whom had an acute injury, but 45 lifted weights as part of their training.

Physical Examination

A complete physical examination should be performed, as described in Chapter 16, when evaluating disorders of the AC joint. In chronic disorders, there will frequently be a deformity secondary to a clavicle osteophyte or capsular hypertrophy. For acute injuries, the patient should be examined either standing or sitting since gravity tends to accentuate a deformity (Fig. 26-3). In these cases, the extent of the deformity may initially appear less severe because of acute soft-tissue swelling. Tender-

ness at the AC joint will often be elicited by direct palpation in both acute and chronic disorders. The range of motion of the shoulder may often be restricted secondary to AC pain. In both chronic and traumatic disorders, provocative maneuvers such as forced horizontal adduction will create pain.

In acute injuries, it is important to assess joint stability by gently applying pressure to the mid-clavicular area and evaluating motion in the superoinferior plane. Pain created by inferior traction to the affected extremity will be a common finding in high-grade AC separations. Each type of AC injury presents with a pattern of common findings on examination, including swelling and displacement. Type I injuries are characterized by minimal joint tenderness and swelling. There is no palpable displacement and pain is typically minimal. In type II injuries, superior displacement of the clavicle from the acromion can be seen and pain at the AC joint is common. Palpation of the CC interspace is not typically painful.

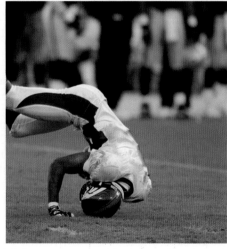

Figure 26-2 Direct trauma resulting in acromioclavicular joint injury.

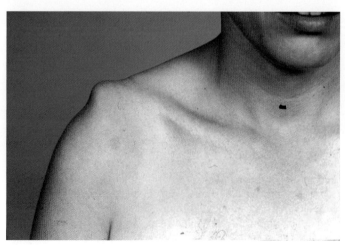

Figure 26-3 "Tenting" of the skin following acute acromioclavicular trauma.

Patients with type III injuries often present with the arm in adduction close to the body to limit pain in the AC joint. The distal portion of the clavicle may provide tenting of the skin from displacement. Pain is increased with abduction, and most motion will be uncomfortable. Unlike type II injuries, palpation of the AC joint, CC interspace, and superolateral clavicle produces pain. If the injured arm is adducted across the body, clavicular displacement becomes prominent from medial displacement of the acromion.

Type IV injuries often present like a more painful type III injury, with the additional pathology of trapezius puncture from a posteriorly displaced distal clavicle. On occasion, the clavicular displacement is extensive and tenting can be seen in the skin on the posterior aspect of the shoulder. In type IV injuries, the clavicle is often fixed posteriorly and difficult to manually reduce, causing pain.

Type V injuries are also like type III injuries, but they are characteristically denoted by severe deformity of the AC joint, often reflected by considerable drooping of the extremity compared to the contralateral normal side. Soft-tissue damage and clavicular displacement can cause significant pain, especially at the distal portion of the clavicle. A type V AC separation can often be difficult to differentiate from a type III injury. In both cases, the clavicle is high riding in relationship to the acromion. However, in a type V AC separation, the clavicle is often irreducible in relationship to the acromion even when the scapula and upper arm are manually elevated. The inability to reduce the clavicle is due to penetration through the deltotrapezial fascia, which can create a fixed deformity.

Type VI injuries are usually caused by acute trauma to the joint, such as a motor vehicle accident, and concomitant injuries should be suspected. This subcoracoid dislocation is often associated with neurovascular injury, of which paresthesias should be relieved with reduction of the dislocation. It should be noted that in each of the higher grade AC separations (types IV, V, and VI), all have some component of a fixed deformity that results in a poor outcome with nonoperative management.

Radiographic Evaluation

Accurate diagnosis is essential for the proper treatment of AC disorders. At a minimum, three radiographic views are required in most shoulder evaluations to ensure an adequate evaluation. The patient should be standing or sitting to fully appreciate any joint deformity. Radiographs of the affected shoulder are taken both perpendicular and parallel to the separation plane, along with an axillary view with the affected shoulder in 20 to 40 degrees of abduction (Fig. 26-4). Films should be taken at 50% intensity compared to those for investigating glenohumeral injury to avoid overpenetration. It is often beneficial to obtain a fourth view where the x-ray beam is angled 15 degrees in a cephalad direction.[5] This will eliminate the scapular spine superimposition of the AC joint in the anteroposterior radiograph (Fig. 26-5). These views should be used to assess for degenerative changes including joint space narrowing, translucency, cyst and/or osteophyte formation, and any accompanying deformity. In acute injuries, particular attention should be paid to assessing for fractures or any abnormal relationship of the clavicle to the acromion.

For traumatic injuries, weighted AP stress views of both joints obtained by attaching a 10- to 15-pound weight to the wrists while the patient is standing have been recommended to help differentiate between a partial or complete disruption. However, Bossart et al[6] demonstrated the lack of efficacy of this study. We have subsequently discontinued using this technique. Instead, we found that adding an anteroposterior radiograph with the arm adducted across the body and supported with the unaffected arm, as described by Basamania (unpublished data, 2006), provides more information regarding the instability of the injury. In grossly unstable joints, the acromion will slide medially under the distal end of the clavicle (Fig. 26-6).

Injury Classification

Two systems have been popularized for the classification of AC joint injuries. Tossy et al[7] proposed the division of AC injuries into three distinct groups. Type I injuries involve sprain of the AC ligaments, with no involvement of the CC ligaments. Type II injuries involve complete AC ligament rupture with sprain/partial tearing of the CC ligaments. Type III injuries require rupture of both the AC and CC ligaments and are therefore the most severe.

Rockwood and Young[8] further divided the type III injuries from the Tossy et al system in order to classify the more severe injuries in terms of severity and clinical outcome (Table 26-1).

Characteristic radiographic appearance for each AC injury type depends on injury severity. Use of the normal contralateral is necessary in all cases. Type I injuries show little radiographic change in joint space and no visible deformity. Type II injuries exhibit an increase in CC interval, typically less than 25% compared to normal. In type III injuries, the clavicle is superiorly displaced compared to the acromion, with between a 25% and 100% increase in the CC interval. If the clavicle is displaced 25% to 100% of clavicular width, but a concurrent increase in CC interval is not found, then a coracoid fracture should be suspected. Type IV injuries show posterior clavicular displacement compared to the acromion, most often seen on the axillary view. Type V injury characteristically reveals greater than 100% increase in CC interval. Severe displacement of the AC joint is also seen, extending two to three times the clavicular width. A type VI injury is rare; typical radiographs reveal a clavicle displaced inferior to the coracoid.

TREATMENT OPTIONS

Traumatic Injuries

It has been well accepted that type I and II AC separations should initially be treated nonoperatively. However, it should be noted that not all patients will fully recover following these seemingly benign injuries. Bergfeld et al[9] reported that 9% of type I and 23% of type II AC separations will have difficulties following nonoperative treatment. Similarly, it has been standard of care to treat type IV, V, and VI injuries operatively. Due to the severity of soft-tissue injury in these higher grade separations, nonoperative management has resulted in poor outcomes.[9]

The treatment of grade III AC separations remains controversial. Historically, the argument against nonoperative treatment has been based on retrospective studies that claim poor long-term results. Several authors claim that operative intervention is superior to nonoperative management due to findings indicating that surgical reduction of the joint will improve the subjective and objective long-term results.[10,11] These reports condemn nonoperative management (citing factors such as persistent deformity, AC arthritis, and residual weakness) as inadequate treatment of this injury.[12,13] For grade III AC separations, we generally recommend nonoperative management.[14] In a prospective evaluation of patients treated nonoperatively for AC separations, we followed a small group of recreational athletes

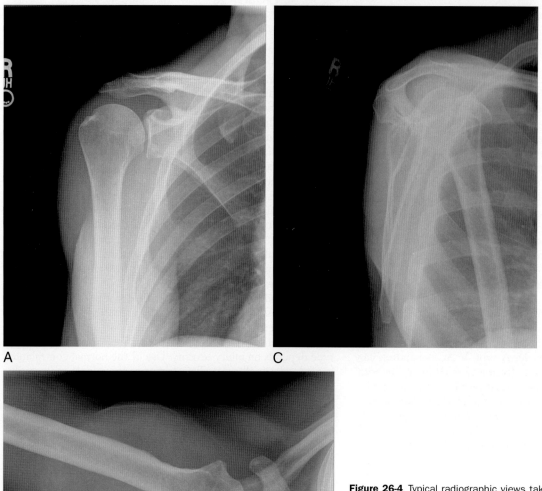

A

C

Figure 26-4 Typical radiographic views taken following an acute acromioclavicular injury. **A,** Anteroposterior. **B,** Axillary lateral. **C,** Scapular Y.

B

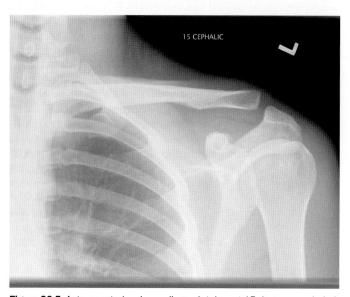

Figure 26-5 Anteroposterior view radiograph taken at 15 degrees cephalad.

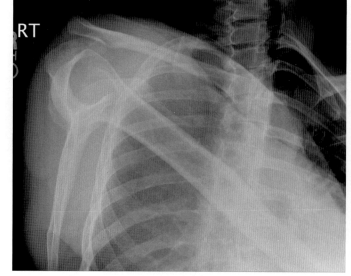

Figure 26-6 Cross-arm adduction view radiograph.

Table 26-1 Injury Classification of Acromioclavicular Joint Injuries

Type I

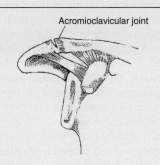

Acromioclavicular joint

AC ligament: strained
CC ligament: strained

Type II

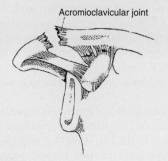

Acromioclavicular joint

AC ligament: ruptured
CC ligament: strained
≤25% displacement of CC distance.

Type III

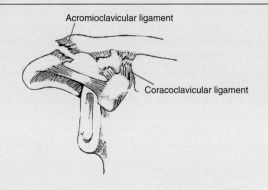

Acromioclavicular ligament

Coracoclavicular ligament

AC ligament: ruptured
CC ligament: ruptured
25%–100% displacement of CC interspace.

Type IV

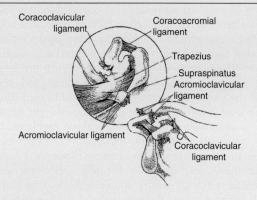

Coracoclavicular ligament

Coracoacromial ligament

Trapezius

Supraspinatus
Acromioclavicular ligament

Acromioclavicular ligament

Coracoclavicular ligament

AC ligament: ruptured
CC ligament: ruptured
Clavicle displaced posteriorly into trapezius.
25%–100% displacement of CC interspace.

Type V

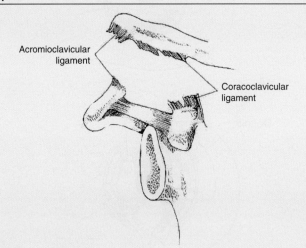

Acromioclavicular ligament

Coracoclavicular ligament

AC ligament: ruptured
CC ligament: ruptured
>100% displacement of CC interspace.
Deltotrapezial fascia often disrupted.

Type VI

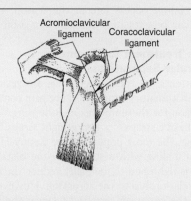

Acromioclavicular ligament

Coracoclavicular ligament

AC ligament: ruptured
CC ligament: ruptured
Inferior displacement of clavicle beneath coracoid.
Likely mechanism is severe hyperadduction with
   external rotation.

AC, acromioclavicular; CC, coracoclavicular.

with type III AC separations and found that the majority had acceptable results.[14] Patients were not given a specific treatment regimen other than rest, ice, and the use of nonsteroidal anti-inflammatory drugs. Patients demonstrated no limitation in range of motion or loss in rotational strength. However, there was, on average, a 17% deficit in bench press strength compared to the uninvolved extremity. Twenty percent believed their results were suboptimal, but none were severe enough to warrant surgery. Of these individuals, the perceived disability was fatigue with maximal overhead activities, such as lifting and climbing.

There is still considerable controversy regarding the management of high-grade AC separations in overhead athletes. There are very few studies in the literature that address this topic, particularly for the high-level thrower. Lemos[15] suggested operative management for high-level pitchers after a retrospective review of patients. McFarland et al[16] surveyed 42 orthopedic surgeons participating in the care of 28 professional baseball teams; 31% recommended immediate operative treatment. However, this same group of surgeons estimated that normal function and significant pain relief were achieved in 80% of their athletes with nonoperative management. We recently completed a retrospective review of National Football League quarterbacks with complete grade III AC separations. When the injury involved the dominant extremity, nonoperative management had variable success. If the player was treated in a Kenny-Howard sling full time for at least 3 weeks, missing an average of eight games, all were able to eventually return to play without problems. When the player was treated with a sling for comfort and early motion, the average time lost was only five games. However, a high percentage of these quarterbacks eventually underwent surgical reconstruction in the off season. In quarterbacks who had early surgery, all of them missed the remainder of the season but were able to return the following year without problems. From this review, it has been our opinion that if a quarterback has an injury to his dominant extremity early in the season, then a trial of nonoperative management is warranted. If he fails this treatment or if the injury occurs late in the season, then surgical reconstruction can be expected to result in a good outcome.

Nonoperative Treatment for Traumatic Acromioclavicular Separations

In all cases, patients are treated with ice, analgesics, and nonsteroidal anti-inflammatory drugs for acute pain control. Options for immobilization for these injuries include sling,[17,18] brace and harness,[19–21] adhesive straps,[22,23] figure-eight straps,[24] and a sling strap.[25] Of these, the most popular is the Kenny-Howard sling. This consists of a sling with a strap over the distal end of the clavicle, which is tightened to manually reduce the distal end of the clavicle in relationship to the acromion. However, for effective reduction, the patient is required to wear the sling continuously for the first 3 to 4 weeks. Removal of the strap leads to loss of joint reduction. The sling can also be problematic because the pressure of the strap can cause necrosis of the skin over the distal clavicle. One case of posterior interosseous nerve palsy caused by the sling has been reported in the literature.[26]

SURGERY

Open Distal Clavicle Resection

Traditionally, distal clavicle excisions have been performed using open techniques. These have been done in isolation for AC arthritis, as well as with concomitant surgeries for rotator cuff

pathology. In 1941, Gurd[27] and Mumford[28] independently described their results of excision of the distal end of the clavicle. Mumford recommended this operation for AC instability, particularly in those with arthritis of the joint.[28] Gurd[27] recommended his procedure in symptomatic type III AC separations. Technically speaking, excision of the distal end of the clavicle is referred to as the Mumford or Gurd operation only when this procedure is used for excision of the clavicle with associated instability. Nowadays, the distal clavicle excision is more routinely used for patients with arthritis. Patients with true AC instability are typically managed with a reconstructive procedure (described later in this chapter).

The operation is usually performed in the beach chair position. The arm is prepped and draped free. When this procedure is being done for isolated AC arthritis, a vertical incision approximately 2.5 to 3 cm in length is placed directly over the distal end of the clavicle (Fig. 26-7). An incision is made through the skin and dissection is carried out through the subcutaneous tissue. On incising the capsule by sharp dissection, a degenerative disk will often be identified along with articular cartilage changes on the distal end of the clavicle. After removing the disk and/or hypertrophic synovium, a subperiosteal dissection is then performed to expose the distal end of the clavicle. An attempt to preserve a thick fascial sleeve will be helpful at the time of closure.

A large Darrach retractor is placed underneath the clavicle to protect the underlying neurovascular structures. A sagittal saw is then used to make a perpendicular cut in order to remove approximately 1 to 1.5 cm of the distal clavicle (Fig. 26-8). Care

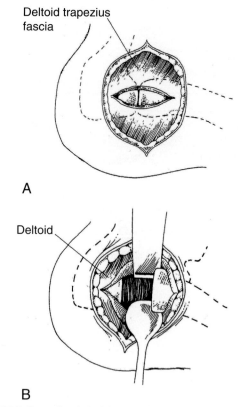

Deltoid trapezius fascia

A

Deltoid

B

Figure 26-7 Open distal clavicle resection. **A,** A vertical incision approximately 2.5 to 3 cm in length is placed directly over the distal end of the clavicle. **B,** A large Darrach retractor is placed underneath the clavicle to protect the underlying neurovascular structures. (Adapted from Hawkins RJ, Bell SB, Lippitt LH: Atlas of Shoulder Surgery. Philadelphia, Mosby, 1996.)

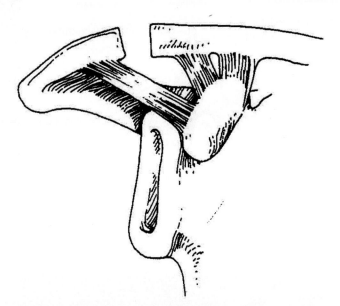

Figure 26-8 With a distal clavicle resection, approximately 1 to 1.5 cm of the distal clavicle is removed. (Adapted from Hawkins RJ, Bell SB, Lippitt LH: Atlas of Shoulder Surgery. Philadelphia, Mosby, 1996.)

should be taken to avoid excessive resection of the distal clavicle, as this will often lead to instability if the CC ligaments are disrupted. The completion of the cut can be done using osteotomes. Following the resection, a gloved finger should be able to remain between the clavicle and the acromion as the arm is brought into maximal adduction. This serves as a method to determine whether the distal clavicle has been sufficiently excised. It is not uncommon to find that more of the anterior portion of the clavicle has been removed, leaving more of the posterior clavicle, which can create pain from ongoing contact of the distal end of the clavicle with acromion (Fig. 26-9).

After thorough irrigation, the deltotrapezial fascia is reapproximated using no. 1 Vicryl sutures. The deep subcutaneous tissue is closed with interrupted 3-0 absorbable sutures. The skin is either closed with a running nylon suture or staples. Postoperatively, the patient is placed into a sling for comfort, passive range of motion is started between 0 and 2 weeks, active motion between 2 and 4 weeks, and a light strengthening program can begin at 4 weeks.

Arthroscopic Distal Clavicle Resection

With an increasing number of shoulder procedures being done completely arthroscopically, it is important for physicians treating these problems to have a method of addressing the degenerative AC joint using an all-arthroscopic technique. After performing a thorough diagnostic arthroscopy of the shoulder and addressing the associated pathology, preparations are made for distal clavicle excision.

The distal clavicle resection usually begins with the arthroscope in the posterior portal, using the lateral accessory portal for the working instruments. This procedure is often done in conjunction with a subacromial decompression. In most cases, the bursa has been excised and the acromion has been converted to a type I morphology. This allows visualization of the AC joint. The joint can be identified either by pushing on the end of the distal clavicle and looking for movement or by placing a spinal needle in the AC joint to identify the exact location. At this point, a shaver can be used to remove the underlying joint

capsule identifying the distal end of the clavicle. As noted with the open technique, there will often be a degenerative disk and/or degenerative changes of the articular cartilage overlying the clavicle.

Eventually, the working instruments will be brought to the anterior portal site to allow resection of the capsule and then bone. Synovial shavers are initially used to resect the soft tissue and then a round 4-0 bur is employed. As opposed to the open technique, the arthroscopic resection often will remove no more than a centimeter. This can be done by removing bone on both acromial and clavicular sides. Once an adequate amount of resection of the bone has been performed, the scope should be taken out of the posterior viewing portal and placed into the anterior portal. This will then allow visualization of the posterior aspect of the AC joint. A spinal needle is then used to identify the location for a direct posterior portal site, and once this is confirmed, a no. 11 scalpel blade can be used to make a skin incision. Blunt dissection is carried out to bring the shavers and bur into the posterior aspect of the AC joint. This is helpful to resect the bone posteriorly.

It is equally as problematic when using an arthroscopic technique as in the open technique if adequate posterior clavicle resection is not achieved. The other pitfall with the arthroscopic technique is often not taking enough of the soft tissue prior to bony resection, making assessment of the superior bone inadequate. This can be remedied by using an electric cautery wand to identify the end of the bone and the overlying capsule, particularly superiorly. Once an adequate resection has been performed, it is then possible to remove the scope from the anterior portal and place it in the direct posterior portal site to view the amount of anterior resection. An instrument such as an arthroscopic osteotome or probe can then be used to confirm an adequate amount of bony resection. Care is taken to preserve the

Supraspinatus

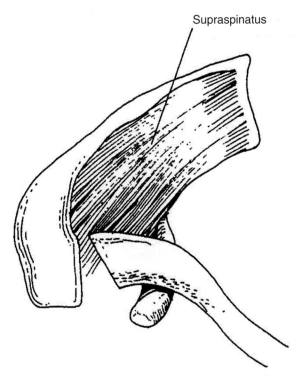

Figure 26-9 Contact between the distal end of clavicle and the acromion may cause pain. (Adapted from Hawkins RJ, Bell SB, Lippitt LH: Atlas of Shoulder Surgery. Philadelphia, Mosby, 1996.)

dorsal AC ligaments. This is one of the advantages of the arthroscopic technique. It is often thought to result in an earlier recovery.

In cases of osteolysis, there is rarely a need to resect any bone since this disorder leads to bone loss. In this pathologic entity, the joint usually has an inflammatory process that is best treated by resection of the inflamed joint tissue.

Postoperative care involves the use of a sling for comfort. Cryotherapy is also undertaken. Patients are able to work through the active and passive range-of-motion program more quickly than what is traditionally seen with an open procedure. Once pain subsides, progressive resisted exercises are initiated.

In our experience, the greatest advantage of the arthroscopic resection is that time lost can be reduced by nearly 4 weeks. By preserving the AC joint capsule and ligaments, the recovery time can be expected to be as short as 8 weeks.

Acromioclavicular Reconstruction

Indications for early surgery include a grossly unstable high-riding distal clavicle, fixed deformities, and occasionally in the overhead throwing athlete. Traditionally, these are addressed by performing a primary autogenous repair of the disrupted AC and CC ligaments. This is then supplemented with an absorbable no. 9 braided polydiaxone monofilament suture strand that is passed around the base of the coracoid and then through a drill hole in the anterior aspect of the clavicle, as described by Warren[29] (Fig. 26-10). This creates a strong absorbable construct lasting approximately 6 to 8 weeks, which is long enough to hold the clavicle in position while the autogenous tissue heals. In acute cases, the distal end of the clavicle may be preserved if there is a normal intra-articular disk and no evidence of arthritis.

Delayed AC reconstructions are recommended in patients who have a high-riding unstable dislocation that has failed non-operative treatment. Because of the difficulty in maintaining the

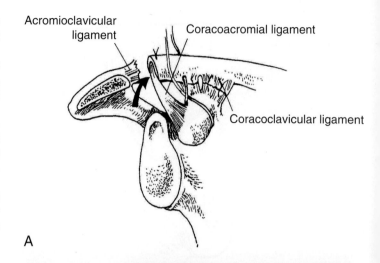

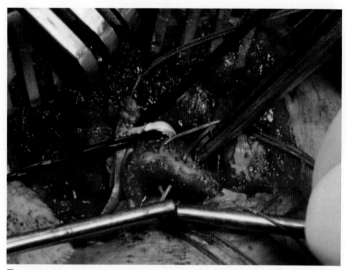

Figure 26-11 **A** and **B,** The reconstruction is performed using existing ligaments and supplemented with absorbable polydiaxone monofilament suture. (**A,** Adapted from Hawkins RJ, Bell SB, Lippitt LH: Atlas of Shoulder Surgery. Philadelphia, Mosby, 1996.)

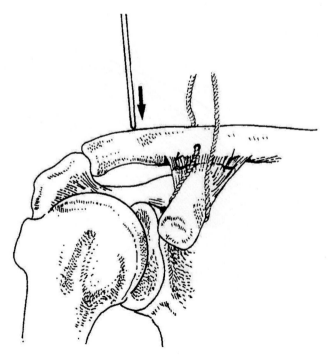

Figure 26-10 Acromioclavicular reconstruction. A vertical drill hole *(arrow)* is made through the anterior aspect of the clavicle. (Adapted from Hawkins RJ, Bell SB, Lippitt LH: Atlas of Shoulder Surgery. Philadelphia, Mosby, 1996.)

reduction in these situations, we have described a "three-in-one" repair (Fig. 26-11).[30] This technique employs a modified Weaver-Dunn reconstruction supplemented with either a palmaris or hamstring tendon as an autogenous graft. In chronic cases, we always resect approximately 1.5 cm of the distal end of the clavicle. This eliminates the possibility of postoperative pain in cases of degenerative arthritis or when there is partial loss of reduction of the distal clavicle. The coracoacromial ligament is then transferred into the medullary canal of the clavicle as part of the modified Weaver-Dunn reconstruction. A 3/8-inch drill is used to make a hole in the anterior aspect of the clavicle at the level of the coracoid to eventually pass a polydiaxone monofilament suture strand and palmaris/hamstring graft. It is important to keep the drill hole anterior so to better position the clavicle in relationship to the acromion as these structures are secured. If the drill hole is placed too posteriorly, it will have a tendency to pull the clavicle anteriorly in relationship to the acromion. Once these structures are around the coracoid, they are passed through the drill hole in the clavicle creating a figure-eight construct for both the polydiaxone monofilament suture and palmaris graft. With the clavicle reduced, it is now possible to maintain the reduction by tying the palmaris/hamstring graft using a surgeon's knot. This has been proved to be the strongest method to secure the autogenous tissue.[31] As with the acute surgeries, we protect the reconstruction with an absorbable suture strand. In the past, we used to braid the suture but found this extremely difficult to handle and tie this construct. We have now modified this braided technique after being shown a new method that we have nicknamed the Skyler Scroll after Dr. Skyler DeJong from West Point. This method creates a polydiaxone monofilament suture rope by taking three individual strands of polydiaxone monofilament suture and securing them at one end while rotating the group 30 times in a clockwise manner. After each of the three strands is created, the entire group is then rotated 40 times in a counterclockwise manner. Once the AC joint is reduced, the deltotrapezial fascial flaps are reapproximated as part of the repair. The skin is then closed with a running nylon stitch.

Postoperatively these patients are protected in a sling for a total of 4 weeks without any motion. We have learned that accelerated rehabilitation programs often lead to loss of reduction. At the 4-week mark, passive range of motion is employed for 2 weeks. An active range-of-motion program with terminal stretching then follows this for 2 weeks. At the 8-week mark, a light resisted strengthening program can be instituted, with return to the weight room at 3 months. The patient is released to all activities without restriction at 4 months.

CRITERIA FOR RETURN TO SPORTS

In general, patients are restricted from unlimited activities until they have a full pain-free range of motion with normal strength. With nonoperative treatment of acute AC separations, the time lost from participation depends on the grade of injury and the sport. On average, those with grade I injuries miss 1 week, those with grade II are out 2 to 4 weeks, and those with grade III AC separations can be expected to miss up to 6 weeks.

It has been our experience that in the athletic patient population, time lost can be significantly reduced when a corticosteroid injection is used acutely as an adjunct to the nonoperative program, immediately after these injuries occur (Fig. 26-12). We

have had experience with this form of treatment in the professional football player population.[32] With higher grade AC separations, time lost was dramatically reduced when the nonoperative program was augmented with injection. When an athlete returns to contact sports, an AC pad is helpful to limit recurrent injuries. In this select group, we have found the injections to be safe and have had no complications such as infection or progression to higher grade AC separations.

RESULTS AND OUTCOMES

The success rate of nonoperative treatment in grade I and II AC separations and chronic disorders is high. For this reason, it is critical to exhaust all options before recommending surgery. If surgery is necessary, a distal clavicle resection performed using either open or arthroscopic techniques can lead to good results. With open surgery, Cook and Heiner[33] and Tibone et al[34] reported a 95% success rate in an athletic population with a painful joint secondary to degenerative arthritis or as a result of traumatic arthritis from a first- or second-degree AC separation. The only complaint following treatment was that patients often were unable to regain maximal bench press strength. Recent studies evaluating the success of arthroscopic distal clavicle resection have demonstrated equally successful outcomes.[35-37] Kay et al[37] reported good and excellent long-term results in 100% of their patients. Martin et al[36] found no significant strength differences of the involved shoulder but did report that a small percentage of athletes had mild pain with strenuous overhead activities. Although the literature is scant on the subject, we have also found that arthroscopic débridement for osteolysis has a very high success rate.

For grade III AC separation, we have reported success in the majority of patients treated nonoperatively.[38] If an AC reconstruction is necessary, as is the case with higher grade injuries, good results have been achieved in 93% of the patients undergoing a Weaver-Dunn reconstruction.[39] In this series, the outcome was not affected by whether this was done acutely or in chronic injuries.[40]

COMPLICATIONS

The most frequent complication following distal clavicle resection is excess bone removal, which ultimately compromises the CC ligaments. In these situations, there is often a cosmetic deformity and pain. Although the case of pain is not fully understood, it is thought to be secondary to medial translation of the scapula in relation to the clavicle.

With AC reconstruction, loss of reduction is the most common problem. Although this leads to a deformity, it has been our experience that some of these patients still have a good functional outcome.

CONCLUSIONS

Successful treatment of AC disorders relies on an accurate diagnosis obtained through a detailed history, thorough physical examination, and a complete radiographic evaluation. The radiographic findings of degenerative arthritis alone are not enough to warrant treatment since this is commonly seen after the age of 40. The painful joint that is unresponsive to nonoperative management including injection will be expected to have a good outcome following a distal clavicle excision.

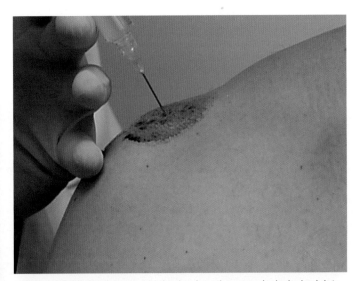

Figure 26-12 Corticosteroid injection into the acromioclavicular joint.

In traumatic AC separations, the majority of these injuries will respond to a nonoperative treatment regimen. In grade III AC separations including overhead throwers, we have recommended a trial of nonoperative management. For those with grade III separations who fail nonoperative treatment, along with high-grade AC separations (grades IV to VI), we have had success employing a "three-in-one" operative technique. The postoperative program should curtail any motion for the first 4 weeks to enhance the likelihood of maintaining the position of the distal clavicle in relationship to the acromion. Return to sports is allowed when the player has pain-free range of motion with good strength. In lower grade AC separations, this can occur within several weeks after the injury but will ultimately take as long as 4 months following surgery.

REFERENCES

1. Fukuda K, Craig EV, An KN, et al: Biomechanical study of the ligamentous system of the acromioclavicular joint. J Bone Joint Surg Am 1986;68:434–440.
2. Petersson CJ: Degeneration of the acromioclavicular joint. A morphological study. Acta Orthop Scand 1983;54:434–438.
3. Petersson CJ, Redlund-Johnell I: Radiographic joint space in normal acromioclavicular joints. Acta Orthop Scand 1983;54:431–433.
4. Cahill BR: Osteolysis of the distal part of the clavicle in male athletes. J Bone Joint Surg Am 1982;64:1053–1058.
5. Zanca P: Shoulder pain: Involvement of the acromioclavicular joint. (Analysis of 1,000 cases). Am J Roentgenol 1971;112:493–506.
6. Bossart PJ, Joyce SM, Manaster BJ, et al: Lack of efficacy of 'weighted' radiographs in diagnosing acute acromioclavicular separation. Ann Emerg Med 1988;17:20–24.
7. Tossy JD, Mead NC, Sigmond HM: Acromioclavicular separations: Useful and practical classification for treatment. Clin Orthop 1963; 28:111–119.
8. Rockwood CA, Young DC: Disorders of the acromioclavicular joint. In Matsen FA (ed): The Shoulder. Philadelphia, WB Saunders, 1990, pp 413–476.
9. Bergfeld JA, Andrish J, Clancy WG: Evaluation of the acromioclavicular joint following first- and second-degree sprains. Am J Sports Med 1978;6:153–159.
10. Kennedy DC, Cameron J: Dislocations of the acromioclavicular joint. J Bone Joint Surg Am 1954;36:202–208.
11. Warren-Smith CD, Ward MW: Operation for acromioclavicular dislocation. A review of 29 cases treated by one method. J Bone Joint Surg Am 1987;69:715–718.
12. Kennedy JC: Complete dislocation of the acromioclavicular joint: 14 years later. J Trauma 1968;8:311–318.
13. Imatani RJ, Hanlon JJ, Cady GW: Acute, complete acromioclavicular separation. J Bone Joint Surg Am 1975;57:328–332.
14. Schlegel TF, Burks RT, Marcus RL, et al: A prospective evaluation of untreated acute grade III acromioclavicular separations. Am J Sports Med 2001;29:699–703.
15. Lemos MJ: The evaluation and treatment of the injured acromioclavicular joint in athletes. Am J Sports Med 1998;26:137–144.
16. McFarland EG, Blivin SJ, Doehring CB, et al: Treatment of grade III acromioclavicular separations in professional throwing athletes: Results of a survey. Am J Orthop 1997;26:771–774.
17. Jones R: Injuries of Joints. London, Hoddard & Stoughton, 1917.
18. Watson-Jones R: Fractures and Joint Injuries. New York, Churchill Livingstone, 1982.
19. Currie DI: An apparatus for dislocation of the acromial end of the clavicle. BMJ 1924;(570).
20. Warner AH: A harness for the use of treatment of acromioclavicular separations. J Bone Joint Surg 1937;19:1132–1133.
21. Giannestras, NJ: A method of immobilization of acute acromioclavicular separations. J Bone Joint Surg 1944;26:597–599.
22. Rawlings G: Acromial dislocations and fractures of the clavicle. A simple method of support. Lancet 1939;2:789.
23. Thorndyke AG, Quigley TB: Injuries to the acromioclavicular joint: A plea for conservative treatment. Am J Surg 1942;55:250–261.
24. Usadel G: Zur Behandlung ter Luxatio Claviculae Supraacromialis. Arch Klin Chir 1940;200:621–626.
25. Howard NJ: Acromioclavicular and sternoclavicular joint injuries. Am J Surg 1939;46:284–291.
26. O'Neill DB, Zarins B, Gelberman RH, et al: Compression of the anterior interosseous nerve after use of a sling for dislocation of the acromioclavicular joint. A report of two cases. J Bone Joint Surg Am 1990;72: 1100–1102.
27. Gurd FB: The treatment of complete dislocation of the outer end of the clavicle: A hitherto undescribed operation. Ann Surg 1941;113: 1094–1098.
28. Mumford EB: Acromioclavicular dislocation. J Bone Joint Surg 1941; 23:799–802.
29. Warren LF, Field LD: Acromioclavicular joint separations. In Hawkins RJ, Misamore GW (eds): Shoulder Injuries in the Athlete: Surgical Repair and Rehabilitation. New York, Churchill Livingstone, 1996, pp 201–217.
30. Schlegel TF, Boublik M, Hawkins RJ: An Updated Approach to Acromioclavicular Injuries. Rosemont, IL, American Academy of Orthopaedic Surgeons, 2002.
31. Lee SJ, Nicholas SJ, Akizuki KH, et al: Reconstruction of the coracoclavicular ligaments with tendon grafts: A comparative biomechanical study. Am J Sports Med 2003;31:648–655.
32. Schlegel TF, Martin L, Keller J, et al: The use of corticosteroid injections for acute acromioclavicular separations. AOSSM Annual Meeting, 2005, Keystone, CO.
33. Cook DA, Heiner JP: Acromioclavicular joint injuries. Orthop Rev 1990;19:510–506.
34. Tibone J, Sellers R, Tonino P: Strength testing after third-degree acromioclavicular dislocations. Am J Sports Med 1992;20: 328–331.
35. Snyder SJ, Banas MP, Karzel RP: The arthroscopic Mumford procedure: An analysis of results. Arthroscopy 1995;11:157–164.
36. Martin SD, Baumgarten TE, Andrews JR: Arthroscopic resection of the distal aspect of the clavicle with concomitant subacromial decompression. J Bone Joint Surg Am 2001;83:328–335.
37. Kay SP, Dragoo JL, Lee R: Long-term results of arthroscopic resection of the distal clavicle with concomitant subacromial decompression. Arthroscopy 2003;19:805–809.
38. Schlegel TF, Boublik M, Hawkins RJ: Grade III AC separations in NFL quarterbacks. Paper presented at the AOSSM Annual Meeting, 2005, Keystone, CO.
39. Weaver JK, Dunn HK: Treatment of acromioclavicular injuries, especially complete acromioclavicular separation. J Bone Joint Surg Am 1972;54:1187–1194.
40. Weinstein DM, McCann PD, McIlveen SJ, et al: Surgical treatment of complete acromioclavicular dislocations. Am J Sports Med 1995;23:324–331.

Clavicle Fractures and Sternoclavicular Injuries

Carl J. Basamania, Elizabeth G. Matzkin, and George K. Bal

INTRODUCTION

- Clavicle fractures account for 1 of every 20 fractures[1] and most occur in men and women younger than the age of 25. Most commonly they are secondary to participation in contact or collision sports.

- Eighty percent of these fractures occur in the middle one third, 12% to 15% in the lateral one third, and 5% to 6% in the medial one third of the clavicle.[2]

- Most fractures of the clavicle unite by various treatment methods including benign neglect, sling, sling and swathe, figure-eight, Velpeau dressing, collar and cuff, external fixation, and open reduction and internal fixation with plates, screws, or intramedullary pins.

- Each treatment option has been shown to allow for fracture healing, nearly normal function, cosmesis, activity level, and satisfaction, but more recent studies have suggested that the satisfaction that patients achieve after fractures of the clavicle may not be as high as previously thought.[3–5]

- Many patients are left with some residual deformity and shortening. The ultimate goal of treatment is to restore the anatomy and allow rapid and safe return of the athlete to sports participation.

CLAVICLE

Clinical Features and Evaluation

Displaced fractures of the clavicle are easily diagnosed if the patient is seen soon after injury. Patients usually present with an obvious clinical deformity and a consistent history of some form of direct or indirect injury to the shoulder. The proximal frag-

ment is commonly displaced upward and backward and may be tenting the skin. Mobilization of the extremity elicits pain, and therefore the patient prefers to splint the involved extremity at the side in a forward and downward position due to the weight of the arm and pull of the pectoralis minor muscle. This position may accentuate the posterosuperior angulation seen in most clavicle fractures. The acute swelling and hemorrhage may hide the initial injury and deformity. In a fracture in close proximity to the acromioclavicular or sternoclavicular joints, the deformity may mimic a purely ligamentous injury.

Examination reveals tenderness to palpation over the fracture site and pain with any attempts at movement. There may be a significant amount of bruising over the fracture site, especially with severely displaced fractures. This indicates a tearing of the underlying soft tissues. Some patients may present with their heads tilted toward the injury, relaxing the pull of the trapezius. Alternatively, some may tilt their chin to the opposite side to decrease the pull of the sternocleidomastoid. A complete and thorough examination should rule out any associated injuries to the entire extremity, lungs, scapula, chest wall, and neurovascular structures.

Nondisplaced fractures or isolated fractures of the articular surfaces may not cause deformity and may be overlooked unless they are specifically sought for radiographically. If the diagnosis is in doubt, special radiographs or a repeat radiograph of the clavicle in 7 to 10 days may be indicated.

Radiographic Evaluation

In most cases, the diagnosis of a clavicular fracture is fairly obvious with the clinical deformity and confirmatory radiographs. Unfortunately, many physicians obtain only an anteroposterior radiograph of the shoulder when a clavicle fracture is suspected. Due to the unusual shape and orientation of the clavicle, it is difficult to adequately determine displacement and angulation on a single anteroposterior radiograph. This is due to the fact that the plane of the fracture is not perpendicular to the plane of the x-ray beam. The clavicle not only shortens, but it also becomes angulated inferiorly and rotated medially; therefore, the deformity is truly in three planes. It is extremely difficult, if not impossible, to characterize the true deformity with radiographs. For the most accurate radiographic evaluation of the fractured clavicle possible, at least two projections of the clavicle should be obtained: an anteroposterior view and a 45-degree cephalic tilt view. In the anteroposterior view, the proximal fragment is characteristically displaced upward and the distal fragment downward (Fig. 27-1A). In the cephalic tilt, the tube is directed from inferior, projecting upward. This view more accurately reveals the anteroposterior relationship of the two fragments and hence is the best view for assessment of

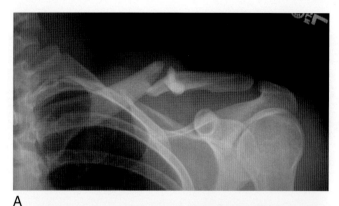

A

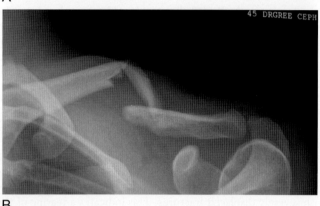

B

Figure 27-1 A, Preoperative anteroposterior radiograph of a patient with a middle third clavicle fracture. **B,** Preoperative 45-degree cephalic tilt radiograph of same patient.

displacement (see Fig. 27-1B).[6] An axillary view with the beam angled slightly cephalad can also help determine fracture displacement and can be useful in assessing possible nonunions.

Rowe[7] has recommended that with an anteroposterior radiograph, the film should include the upper third of the humerus, the shoulder girdle, and the upper lung fields to rule out any associated injuries. The fracture personality is also important to assess because it may give a clue to the presence of associated injuries. Normally the clavicular shaft fracture in the adult is slightly oblique; however, if there is significant comminution, this is indicative of significant force and neurovascular and pulmonary injuries must be ruled out.

Relevant Anatomy

The clavicle is the first bone in the body to ossify, around the fifth fetal week, but the medial physis does not fuse until young adulthood at ages 22 to 25. This is important in order to distinguish medial clavicle physeal injuries from fractures in this age group. The clavicle is an S-shaped bone that is anchored by strong ligamentous attachments on both its medial and lateral ends.

Muscular attachments to the clavicle include the sternocleidomastoid, pectoralis major, and subclavius muscles proximally and the deltoid and trapezius muscles distally. There are no muscular or ligamentous attachments on the middle section of the clavicle, and this supports the fact that most fractures occur in this area. There is thin coverage of the superior aspect of the clavicle by the platysma muscle. The supraclavicular nerves lie just below the platysma muscle, which give sensory innervation

to the overlying skin and after injury may result in painful neuroma. Below the clavicle lie the important neurovascular structures: the subclavian vessels and brachial plexus. These are protected by the clavipectoral fascia within the costoclavicular space. The medial cord of the brachial plexus (ulnar nerve) is located in the smallest portion of the costoclavicular space and can be compromised by fracture or healing callus.[8]

Behind the medial clavicle and the sternoclavicular joint, the internal jugular and subclavian veins join to form the innominate vein. Medially, the omohyoid fascia covers the internal jugular and subclavian veins. The myofascial layer also protects the subclavian and axillary veins at the middle and medial thirds behind the clavicle.[9]

Treatment Options

The concept of nonoperative treatment historically has consisted of bracing the shoulder girdle to raise the outer fragment upward, outward, and backward; depressing the inner fragment; maintaining the reduction; and enabling the ipsilateral elbow and hand to be used so that associated problems with immobilization can be avoided. Review of the literature indicates that immobilization of a clavicle fracture is virtually impossible to accomplish and shortening and deformity are often the results. Historically, clavicle shortening appeared to be inconsequential; however, more recent data indicate that this is one of the most significant predictors of an unsatisfactory outcome.[10,11] There are numerous methods to attempt to immobilize the clavicle, ranging from long-term recumbency,[12,13] various types of ambulatory treatment,[14] and numerous internal fixation methods.[15–25]

Partial immobilization can be performed by numerous bandaging methods such as a sling, sling and swathe, Velpeau dressing, figure-eight, or cuff and collar. These options are used to treat many middle third or shaft fractures. It is important to understand that the injury radiographs are predictive of the fracture healing results, and a completely displaced or shortened fracture is more likely to stay in this position regardless of the immobilization method used. A reduction maneuver may be performed and if crepitus between the two fractured ends of the clavicle are felt, then it may be more likely that the fracture will go on to union. If there is no crepitus felt, then soft tissue may be interposed and this may contribute to fracture nonunion.[25]

Operative treatment of clavicle fractures (external fixation or open reduction internal fixation) should be considered in the following cases:

1. Open fractures requiring débridement.
2. Neurovascular compromise that is progressive or nonresponsive to reduction maneuvers.
3. Displacement (angulation and comminution) that tents the skin.
4. Polytrauma patients that may need to use upper extremities for mobilization purposes.
5. The "floating shoulder" injury (clavicle and unstable scapular fracture with compromised acromioclavicular and coracoacromial ligaments).
6. Type II distal clavicular fractures.
7. Factors that render the patient unable to tolerate closed immobilization, such as with neurologic problems.[25]
8. Patients for whom the cosmetic lump over the healed clavicle is intolerable.
9. Relative indications are shortening of more than 15 to 20 mm and displacement greater than the width of the clavicle.

Medial clavicle fractures and physeal injuries are easily and best treated by nonoperative measures. One must also rule out sternoclavicular injuries in these cases, which may require additional treatment. Middle third clavicle fractures, which are the most common, can also be managed nonoperatively. The most concerning fractures of the midshaft of the clavicle are generally those that have absorbed the greatest energy. In the senior author's experience, these higher energy fractures tend to have a remarkably consistent pattern: shortened and comminuted with an anterior/inferior butterfly fragment. Soft-tissue injury and stripping are significant, leading to greater instability, all of which increase the risk of nonunion. It is our belief that these fractures are best treated with open reduction and internal fixation. Distal clavicle fractures, if nondisplaced, can be treated nonoperatively. If displaced, one must determine the integrity of the coracoclavicular ligaments. If the coracoclavicular ligaments or some portion of them remain attached to the medial clavicular fragment, then the coracoclavicular interval will be maintained and prevent further displacement of the fracture ends. If the coracoclavicular ligaments are not attached, then the medial fragment can displace, with an increased risk of nonunion. In unstable cases, operative stabilization of the coracoclavicular interval may be indicated.

Techniques

Open reduction and internal fixation can be performed by intramedullary devices or plate fixation. Plate fixation can be performed with a six- to eight-hole low-contact dynamic compression or reconstruction plate. Semitubular plates are less rigid and have a high risk of failure. The patient may be placed in a beach chair position. The fracture is exposed through a curvilinear incision. The platysma muscle is incised in line with its fibers, and care is taken to protect the branches of the supraclavicular nerve. The periosteum is sparingly stripped off the superior surface of the clavicle for plate application. Care must be taken when drilling and placing screws to avoid injury to the underlying subclavian vessels and thoracic cavity. A malleable retractor may be placed beneath the clavicle to protect the drill from unintentionally entering the thorax. The screw-plate fixation is performed using standard AO techniques. The plate does have the disadvantage of requiring a second operation to remove the hardware if its prominent position irritates the skin after healing. Also, the screw holes weaken the bone and protection is needed after hardware removal.

At our institution, intramedullary fixation is used for most of these fractures with a modified Hagie pin (Depuy Orthopaedics). We prefer this method for several reasons. First, the exposure for an intramedullary pin is much smaller than what is necessary for a formal open reduction and internal fixation with plates and screws. This preserves what remains of the soft-tissue envelope. The intramedullary pin allows for compression at the fracture site and load sharing, which has been shown to be advantageous in the healing of other long bone fractures. The intramedullary pins come in different sizes to allow for proper canal fill and can easily be removed under local anesthesia. Last, unlike plate and screw fixation, placement of the intramedullary pin allows us to avoid drilling in the direction of the lungs and neurovascular structures.

The patient is placed in a beach chair position on the operating table. A radiolucent shoulder-positioning device optimizes clavicle and shoulder visibility and an image intensifier or a C arm facilitates pin placement. A 2- to 3-cm incision in Langer's lines over the distal end of the medial fragment is made. Care

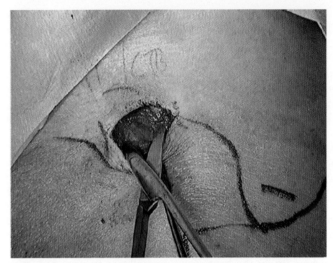

Figure 27-2 Incision over distal end of medial fragment. Splitting platysma muscle in line with its fibers.

is taken to prevent injury to the thin platysma muscle, which can be divided in line with its fibers using scissors (Fig. 27-2). The middle branch of the supraclavicular nerve, which is usually found directly beneath the platysma muscle near the midclavicle, should be identified and protected.

The proximal end of the medial clavicle is elevated through the incision using a towel clip, elevator, or bone-holding forceps. Once the appropriate sized drill is attached to the ratchet T handle or a power drill, the intramedullary canal is reamed and then tapped without penetrating the anterior cortex. Proper sizing is important. If the fit is too loose, the fixation will not be adequate, and if the fit is too tight, this may compromise the integrity of the bone. The C arm is used to assess the orientation of the drill (Fig. 27-3).

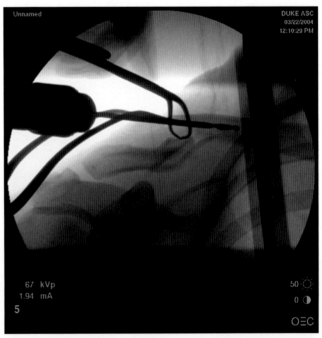

Figure 27-3 Drill positioned in medial fragment.

The lateral fragment is then elevated through the incision. The arm may be placed in external rotation to facilitate positioning of the lateral fragment canal. The same size drill used in the medial fragment is used to drill the intramedullary canal of the lateral fragment followed by the appropriate tap. Under C-arm guidance, the drill is advanced out through the posterolateral cortex of the clavicle, usually at the level of the coracoid.

While holding the distal fragment with a bone clamp, the nuts from the pin assembly are removed and the smaller trocar end of the DePuy clavicle pin are passed into the medullary canal of the lateral fragment. The pin should exit through the previously drilled hole in the posterolateral cortex. The pin tip can be felt subcutaneously, and a small incision is created over this area. The Jacobs chuck and T handle is attached to the end of the pin protruding laterally, and the pin is pulled in a retrograde fashion into the lateral fragment.

The shoulder and lateral fragment may be elevated by pushing up on the bent elbow to facilitate fracture reduction. The pin is then advanced into the medial fragment and the fracture reduced, ensuring that all threads of the pin are across the fracture site. Pin position and fracture reduction are then verified by the C arm or by obtaining a radiograph. The medial nut is then placed on the pin, followed by the smaller lateral nut. The two nuts are cold-welded together. The T-handle wrench is then placed on the medial nut and the pin backed out until the lateral nut is seen at the skin surface. A double-action pin cutter is used to cut the pin flush with the lateral nut. The pin is then advanced back in the medial fragment using the lateral wrench. The pin can generate considerable compression force, and care must be taken not to overreduce the fracture.

The common butterfly fragment may be cerclaged into a reduced position using no. 1 polydiaxone monofilament suture passed beneath the fragment and protected with a Crego elevator. The periosteum, platysma muscle, and skin are then reapproximated. Postoperative radiographs confirm reduction (Fig. 27-4).

Postoperative Rehabilitation
The patient is placed in a sling for comfort postoperatively but may remove it when comfort allows. The patient is allowed to resume daily living activities as soon as tolerated but is instructed to avoid strenuous activities such as pulling, lifting, or pushing and arm elevation higher than face level for 4 to 6 weeks. Sutures are removed at 7 to 10 days. Radiographs are obtained at the 4- to 6-week postoperative clinic visit. If the fracture appears clinically healed (nontender, palpable callus), the patient can advance to daily activities as tolerated. The patient should be seen at 8 to 12 weeks postoperatively. Once radiographs (anteroposterior and 45-degree cephalic tilt anteroposterior radiographs) show healing of the fracture, the pin is removed.

The pin can be removed in the office or in an ambulatory surgery setting. We typically use local anesthesia, which may be supplemented with IV sedation. Following pin removal, patients may resume activities of daily living as tolerated but are asked to refrain from strenuous or competitive sports for 6 weeks. If open reduction and internal fixation with plate and screws are performed, hardware removal is not routine, unless the plate and screws are prominent or are causing patient discomfort after evidence of fracture healing. This must be done through the initial incision in the operating room. Protection after plate removal is warranted for an extended period of time to avoid refracture.

Complications and Results
Complications of both plate and pin fixation include infection, hardware breakage, neurovascular compromise, refracture, malunion, and nonunion.[11,26-32]

Shen et al[27] treated 251 middle third clavicle fractures with a 3.5-mm reconstruction plate. Average time to union was 10 weeks with 7 nonunions, 14 malunions, and 5 infections; 28 had residual skin numbness and 171 eventually required plate removal. Overall, 94% were satisfied with the end result. Bostman et al[26] treated 103 middle third clavicle fractures with plate fixation and 24 (23%) had 1 or more complications, including infection, plate breakage, nonunion, and refracture after plate removal. Results of plate fixation have been favorable for both malunions and nonunions with or without bone grafting.[11,28]

Prior to the introduction of a specifically designed clavicle pin, the use of intramedullary devices has historically been fraught with complications, mostly secondary to pin migration.[29,30] More recently, intramedullary pin fixation using a specifically designed clavicle pin has had excellent results.[31,33] Boehme et al[33] treated 21 patients with a clavicle nonunion with a modified Hagie pin and bone grafting and showed healing in 20 of 21 of them. Wu et al[32] compared plate and intramedullary nail fixation with bone grafting in 33 patients with a middle third clavicular nonunion and noted a higher union rate and lower complication rate in the intramedullary group. Complications of the clavicle pin, in our experience, have been potential posterior skin breakdown from a prominent pin, possible skin numbness in the supraclavicular nerve distribution, and rarely nonunion.

Conclusions
Clavicle fractures are common and treatment historically has been conservative.

The ultimate goal of treatment is to achieve bone healing with minimal morbidity while avoiding loss of function and residual deformity. Nonoperative immobilization of the clavicle is nearly impossible and shortening is customary, resulting in altered biomechanics of the shoulder girdle. Recent studies indicate that displaced midshaft clavicle fractures have a higher nonunion rate (15% to 25%)[10,34] than previously thought, and as many as half of patients are symptomatic as long as 10 years after injury.[10] In view of this, we recommend operative intervention for displaced and shortened midshaft clavicle fractures, particularly in high-demand individuals and athletes. The clavicle pin offers an easy

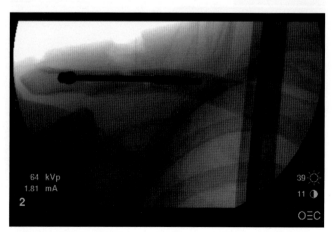

64 kVp
1.81 mA
2
39
11
O≡C

Figure 27-4 Postoperative reduction anteroposterior radiograph.

and safe method of treatment for most clavicle fractures with excellent results both cosmetically and functionally.

Sternoclavicular Joint

Relevant Anatomy

The S-C joint is the isolated articulating point for the upper extremity to the axial skeleton. The blood supply to the joint arises from the clavicular branch of the thoracoacromial arch, with contributions from the internal mammary and suprascapular arteries. The innervation of the S-C joint is from both the nerve to the subclavius and the medial suprascapular nerve. The joint ends are flattened, with poor congruity, and relatively little innate stability. The joint surface of the medial end of the clavicle is much larger than the corresponding joint surface of the sternum.[35] The superior portion of the clavicle is easily palpable in the sternal notch. A thick intra-articular disk is present, which improves the articular congruity. The disk is attached to the first rib and sternum inferiorly and superiorly to the superior border of the clavicle. The major ligaments supporting the joint are the anterior and posterior S-C ligaments. The costoclavicular ligaments run from the superior surface of the first rib to the inferior surface of the medial clavicle. The interclavicular ligament runs between the medial ends of both clavicles, attaching to the anterior surface of the sternum (Fig. 27-5). The epiphysis on the medial end of the clavicle is the last to ossify, at 18 to 20 years, and the last to close, at age 23 to 25.

Range of Motion

Motion of the S-C joint is directly linked to upper extremity motion. Fusion of the S-C joint has been shown to severely limit shoulder abduction. The sternum remains fixed as the clavicle moves in rotation, elevation, and levers anterior to posterior with upper extremity motion. The main resistance to rotation comes from the anterior and posterior S-C ligaments. The intra-articular disk resists superior translation of the medial end of the clavicle. The anterior capsule resists anterior translation. The posterior capsule is the most important restraint to posterior translation of the S-C joint.[36] The subclavius muscle functions as a dynamic stabilizer during activity.

Pathology
Degenerative Conditions

Osteoarthritis is the most common degenerative condition occurring in the S-C joint. It may occur as a primary process or secondary to injury/chronic instability. Other degenerative conditions include rheumatoid arthritis, gout, Reiter's syndrome, condensing osteitis, sternoclavicular hyperostosis, and psoriasis.[37]

Atraumatic Subluxation/Dislocation

Spontaneous instability of the S-C joint has been well described.[38] It most commonly occurs in young patients and is associated with ligamentous laxity in other joints. The patient is typically able to displace the medial end of the clavicle anteriorly with abduction or overhead motion. The condition is rarely symptomatic, and conservative treatment is usually acceptable. Attempting to operatively stabilize the joint in these patients is generally unsuccessful and should be avoided.

Trauma

Mechanisms of injury to the S-C joint can be viewed in two ways: direct blows and indirect force applied to the shoulder or upper back. As previously described, the medial epiphysis of the clavicle can persist into the mid-20s. Injuries to the epiphysis can mimic S-C joint injuries. Sprains and subluxations to the S-C joint can also be seen. These typically present as isolated pain and swelling. A spectrum of injuries can be grouped into three categories: type I (sprain), type II (subluxation), and type III (dislocation).[39] Recurrent subluxations can occur and should be treated similarly to the methods described in the following for traumatic dislocations. The two primary directions of dislocation are anterior and posterior.

Anterior dislocations occur more frequently than posterior. The most common mechanism is sports-related injuries. A compressive force is applied to the anterolateral shoulder, whether by a direct blow or traction, and the medial clavicle dislocates anteriorly. The injury presents with pain and swelling over the medial end of the clavicle. The patient will usually support the affected arm in internal rotation and resist any shoulder motion. The medial end of the clavicle can be palpated anterior to the sternum.

Posterior dislocations typically result from a direct blow to the medial end of the clavicle or compressive force applied to the posterolateral shoulder. This is seen most commonly in motor vehicle accidents and sports and crush injuries. There may be swelling over the S-C joint and a palpable defect where the medial clavicle would normally be felt. The patient will again resist any motion of the involved shoulder. More concerning symptoms can manifest with posterior dislocations because of pressure on the vital structures posterior to the joint. Shortness

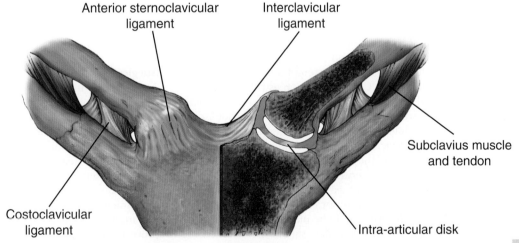

Figure 27-5 Anatomy of the sternoclavicular joint.

Anterior sternoclavicular ligament

Interclavicular ligament

Subclavius muscle and tendon

Costoclavicular ligament

Intra-articular disk

of breath, hoarseness, or difficulty swallowing can be seen. Venous congestion of the involved arm or neck may also be present.

Radiographic Evaluation

The S-C joint is difficult to visualize on plain chest or shoulder radiographs. The shadows from surrounding structures overlap the outlines of the joint. Several radiographic views have been described in a specific attempt to better visualize the S-C joint. The most familiar is the serendipity view, initially described by Rockwood and Wirth.[39] The view is obtained by placing the patient supine, with the x-ray cassette placed under the upper shoulders and neck. The x-ray beam is centered on the upper chest and tilted 40 degrees off of vertical. Plain tomography was originally described as the preferred way to visualize S-C joint injuries. When available, tomograms can be a simple, inexpensive way to evaluate the joint.

Computed tomography is now recognized as the most reliable way to identify abnormalities of the S-C joint. Fine-cut sections (1 to 2 mm) through the joint can easily define medial clavicle fractures, dislocations, or degenerative changes. Computed tomography should be performed to visualize any acute injury to the S-C joint. For posterior dislocations, compression of structures behind the medial end of the clavicle can be well seen on computed tomography. Efforts have been made to visualize structures of the S-C joint with magnetic resonance imaging. While not as well accepted as computed tomography for trauma, magnetic resonance imaging has been found to reliably identify damage to the intra-articular disk and supporting ligamentous structures.[40]

Treatment Options

Sprains (type I injuries) and subluxations (type II injuries) should be treated with ice and rest initially. A sling to prevent painful motion is useful. Persistent subluxations may require reduction by retracting the shoulders. Mild sprains should be protected for 1 to 2 weeks and then may gradually return to regular activity. More significant sprains or subluxations should be protected for 4 to 6 weeks. Occasionally, the subluxation may progress to chronic instability. Treatment for this eventuality is addressed in that section.

Medial clavicle epiphysis displacement must be considered when evaluating injuries to the S-C area in young patients. Most injuries can be treated conservatively, with the expectation that some remodeling of the deformity will occur. Symptomatic posterior deformities should be reduced. If the closed reduction is unsuccessful, an open reduction and possible internal fixation should be performed.[41]

The treatment of traumatic anterior dislocations is not clearly defined. There are reports of good outcomes with conservative management.[42] However, an initial attempt at closed reduction may reduce the deformity. Closed reduction usually requires IV sedation or general anesthesia. The patient is placed supine, with a towel or pad between the shoulders. The affected shoulder is pushed posterior, while manual pressure is used to reduce the medial end of the clavicle. The medial end of the clavicle is frequently unstable after the reduction. If a closed reduction cannot be maintained, conservative management is the best course. Operative stabilization is not recommended for the initial treatment of unstable anterior dislocations. If the reduction remains stable, the arm should be placed in a sling. Retraction and elevation of the shoulder should be avoided. A figure-eight wrap can be used to assist. These limitations should be followed for 6 to 8 weeks before activities progress.

Acute posterior dislocations need extremely careful evaluation. Associated intrathoracic injuries are commonly seen. Hoarseness or difficulty swallowing can indicate pressure on the trachea or esophagus. Venous congestion in the affected arm or jugular distention can indicate pressure on the great vessels. If these symptoms are present, a general or thoracic surgeon should be consulted. Computed tomography is indicated, possibly combined with arterial contrast, to evaluate the position of the medial clavicle and vascular structures. Attempted closed reduction should only be performed after careful preparation. Most authors agree that the reduction should be done in an operating room under general anesthesia. The positioning is the same as described for the reduction of anterior dislocations. Traction is then placed on the affected extremity, and the arm gradually extended. If the clavicle does not reduce easily, the skin over the area is cleaned, and the medial end of the clavicle grasped with a sharp towel clamp. Once the reduction is obtained, it is usually stable. Postreduction care is similar to that used for anterior dislocations, except that adduction of the affected extremity is the motion that should be avoided. This can be facilitated with a figure-eight harness.

If a closed reduction cannot be obtained, an operative reduction should be performed. An unreduced posterior dislocation can cause late intrathoracic complications from the posteriorly displaced medial clavicle.[43] The operative technique involves a curved incision over the S-C joint. Every effort should be made to preserve the intact anterior ligaments. The assistance of a thoracic surgeon should be considered if significant posterior displacement is present. Stabilization of the joint with pins or wires should be avoided, secondary to concerns of late migration.

Recurrent Instability

Recurrent instability or chronic dislocation of the S-C joint may result in persistent symptoms that require surgical treatment. The goals of the surgical reconstruction are the same as those for instability or persistent dislocation: to remove the degenerative, or damaged, end of the clavicular joint surface and stabilize the medial end of the clavicle. There were several procedures initially described for stabilization of the medial clavicle. These included subclavius tendon transfer, free fascia lata, and osteotomy of the medial clavicle. Arthrodesis of the S-C joint should not be performed because of the associated loss of motion. A recent biomechanical comparison suggests that a figure-eight free tendon graft reconstruction is stronger than using the intra-articular ligament or subclavius tendon.[44] The senior author advocates one of two reconstructive methods for S-C joint instability: free tendon transfer or transfer of the intra-articular ligament, as originally described by Rockwood et al.[45]

Surgical Technique

A curvilinear incision is made, based over the medial end of the clavicle and onto the sternum (Fig. 27-6). The attachment of the sternocleidomastoid muscle should be preserved and retracted medially. The anterior capsule is incised carefully to preserve the anterior capsular ligaments and intra-articular disk. The periosteal sleeve is elevated off of the medial clavicle, taking care to preserve it for later repair (Fig. 27-7). On exposure of the joint, care should also be used to preserve the inferior attachments of the intra-articular disk. Using a side-cutting bur, the medial end of the clavicle is resected, using caution to protect underlying structures (Fig. 27-8). Care should also be

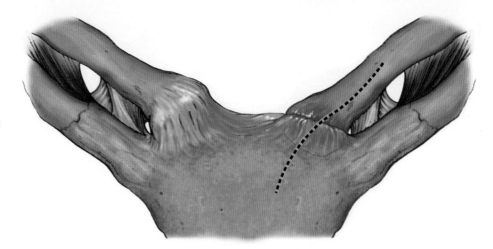

Figure 27-6 Incision for sternoclavicular joint reconstruction.

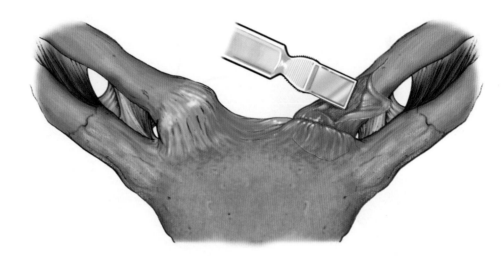

Figure 27-7 Preservation of periosteal sleeve.

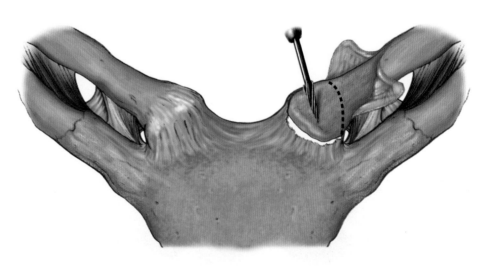

Figure 27-8 Resection of medial clavicle with side-cutting bur.

taken to avoid resecting too much bone and thus injuring the inferior costoclavicular ligaments and further destabilizing the medial clavicle. When using the intra-articular disk for reconstruction, the end of the clavicle must be hollowed with a bur (Fig. 27-9). Nonabsorbable sutures are woven into the ligament/disk and pulled into the medial clavicle, out through dorsal drill holes, and tied over a bone bridge (Fig. 27-10). If a free tendon graft (palmaris longus, semitendinosis, or allograft) is to

be used, drill holes are placed in the sternum and medial clavicle. The tendon is passed through these tunnels, tensioned, and sewn into place (Fig. 27-11). At the completion of either reconstruction, the periosteal sleeve is closed carefully over the repair.

Postoperative Care

Initial postoperative swelling and pain can be severe. The extremity should remain protected in a sling for 6 to 8 weeks.

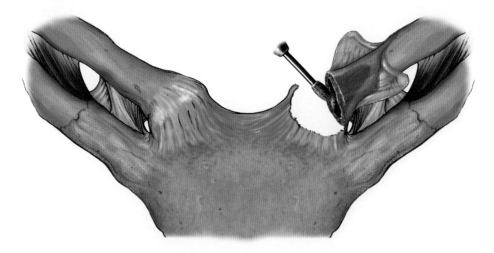

Figure 27-9 Preparation of medial clavicle for ligament transfer.

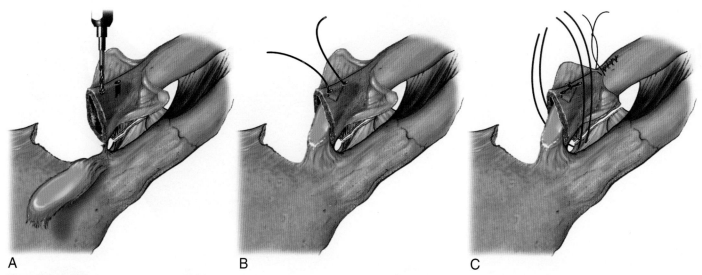

A   B   C

Figure 27-10 A–C, Intra-articular disk reconstruction. (From Spencer EE, Kuhn JE: Biomechanical analysis of reconstructions for sternoclavicular joint instability. J Bone Joint Surg [Am] 2004;86:98–105.)

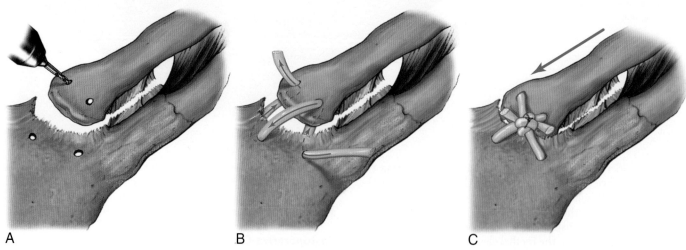

A   B   C

Figure 27-11 A–C, Sternoclavicular joint reconstruction with free soft-tissue graft. (From Spencer EE, Kuhn JE: Biomechanical analysis of reconstructions for sternoclavicular joint instability. J Bone Joint Surg [Am] 2004;86:98–105.)

Range-of-motion and strengthening exercises are slowly progressed. Activity restrictions should be enforced for 4 to 6 months. Recurrent instability can occur if activity is resumed too early.

Treatment for Arthritis

Symptomatic degenerative changes of the S-C joint are not usually associated with instability. Operative management should only be considered for persistently painful arthritis that is otherwise unresponsive. The goal of surgical treatment is to achieve pain relief by removing the degenerative end of the medial clavicle. The surgical technique is essentially the same as described previously, with the exception that no ligamentous reconstruction is necessary.[46] Postoperatively, for arthritic resections, a gradual return to full activity may begin after 8 weeks.

REFERENCES

1. Neer CS: Fractures of the clavicle. In DP RCaG (ed): Fractures in Adults. Philadelphia, JB Lippincott, 1984, pp 707–713.
2. Basamania C: Clavicle Fractures. In Delee J, Drez D (eds): Orthopaedic Sports Medicine, vol. 1. Philadelphia, Saunders, 2003, pp 958–969.
3. Eskola A, Vainionpaa S, Myllynen P, et al: Outcome of clavicular fracture in 89 patients. Arch Orthop Trauma Surg 1986;105:337–338.
4. Hicks J: Rigid fixation as a treatment for hypertrophic nonunion. Injury 1976;8:199–205.
5. McCandless DN, Mowbray MA: Treatment of displaced fractures of the clavicle. Sling versus figure-of-eight bandage. Practitioner 1979;223:266–267.
6. Widner LA, Riddervold HO: The value of the lordotic view in diagnosis of fractures of the clavicle. Rev Interam Radiol 1980;5:69–70.
7. Rowe CR: An atlas of anatomy and treatment of midclavicular fractures. Clin Orthop 1968;58:29–42.
8. Kay SP, Eckardt JJ: Brachial plexus palsy secondary to clavicular nonunion. Case report and literature survey. Clin Orthop 1986:219–222.
9. Abbott LC, Lucas DB: The function of the clavicle; its surgical significance. Ann Surg 1954;140:583–599.
10. Hill JM, McGuire MH, Crosby LA: Closed treatment of displaced middle-third fractures of the clavicle gives poor results. J Bone Joint Surg Br 1997;79:537–539.
11. McKee MD, Wild LM, Schemitsch EH: Midshaft malunions of the clavicle. J Bone Joint Surg Am 2003;85:790–797.
12. Bateman J: The Shoulder and Neck. Philadelphia, WB Saunders, 1978.
13. Quigley T: The management of simple fractures of the clavicle in adults. N Engl J Med 1950;243:286–290.
14. Conwell H: Fractures of the clavicle. JAMA 1928;90:838–839.
15. Breck LW: Partially threaded round pins with oversized threads for intramedullary fixation of the clavicle and the forearm bones. Clin Orthop 1958;4:227–229.
16. Jablon M, Sutker A, Post M: Irreducible fracture of the middle third of the clavicle. Report of a case. J Bone Joint Surg Am 1979;61:296–298.
17. Katznelson A, Nerubay J, Oliver S: Dynamic fixation of the avulsed clavicle. J Trauma 1976;16:841–844.
18. Lee H: Treatment of fracture of the clavicle by internal nail fixation. N Engl J Med 1946;234:222–224.
19. Lengua F, Nuss JM, Lechner R, et al: Treatment of fractures of the clavicle by closed pinning inside-out without back-and-forth. Rev Chir Orthop Reparatrice Appar Mot 1987;73:377–380.
20. Moore TO: Internal pin fixation for fracture of the clavicle. Am Surg 1951;17:580–583.
21. Murray G: A method of fixation for fracture of the clavicle. J Bone Joint Surg 1940;22:616–620.
22. Neviaser RJ, Neviaser JS, Neviaser TJ: A simple technique for internal fixation of the clavicle. A long term evaluation. Clin Orthop 1975;109:103–107.
23. Paffen PJ, Jansen EW: Surgical treatment of clavicular fractures with Kirschner wires: A comparative study. Arch Chir Neerl 1978;30:43–53.
24. Rush LV, Rush HL: Technique of longitudinal pin fixation in fractures of the clavicle and jaw. Mississippi Doctor 1949;27:332.
25. Zenni EJ Jr, Krieg JK, Rosen MJ: Open reduction and internal fixation of clavicular fractures. J Bone Joint Surg Am 1981;63:147–151.
26. Bostman O, Manninen M, Pihlajamaki H: Complications of plate fixation in fresh displaced midclavicular fractures. J Trauma 1997;43:778–783.
27. Shen WJ, Liu TJ, Shen YS: Plate fixation of fresh displaced midshaft clavicle fractures. Injury 1999;30:497–500.
28. Olsen BS, Vaesel MT, Sojbjerg JO: Treatment of midshaft clavicular nonunion with plate fixation and autologous bone grafting. J Shoulder Elbow Surg 1995;4:337–344.
29. Leppilahti J, Jalovaara P: Migration of Kirschner wires following fixation of the clavicle—A report of 2 cases. Acta Orthop Scand 1999;70:517–519.
30. Nordback I, Markkula H: Migration of Kirschner pin from clavicle into ascending aorta. Acta Chir Scand 1985;151:177–179.
31. Boehme D, Curtis RJ Jr, DeHaan JT, et al: The treatment of nonunion fractures of the midshaft of the clavicle with an intramedullary Hagie pin and autogenous bone graft. Instr Course Lect 1993;42:283–290.
32. Wu CC, Shih CH, Chen WJ, Tai CL: Treatment of clavicular aseptic nonunion: Comparison of plating and intramedullary nailing techniques. J Trauma 1998;45:512–516.
33. Boehme D, Curtis RJ Jr, DeHaan JT, et al: Non-union of fractures of the mid-shaft of the clavicle. Treatment with a modified Hagie intramedullary pin and autogenous bone-grafting. J Bone Joint Surg Am 1991;73:1219–1226.
34. Eskola A, Vainionpaa S, Myllynen P, et al: Surgery for ununited clavicular fracture. Acta Orthop Scand 1986;57:366–367.
35. Soames RW: Skeletal system. In Williams PL, Bannister LH, Berry MM, et al (eds): Gray's Anatomy, 38th ed. New York, Churchill Livingstone, 1995, pp 725–736.
36. Spencer EE, Kuhn JE, Huston LJ: Ligament restraints in anterior and posterior translation of the sternoclavicular joint. J Shoulder Elbow Surg 2002;11:43–47.
37. Ross JJ, Shamsuddin H: Sternoclavicular septic arthritis: Review of 180 cases. Medicine 2004;83:139–148.
38. Rockwood CA, Odor JM: Spontaneous atraumatic anterior subluxations of the sternoclavicular joint in young adults. Report of 37 cases. Orthop Trans 1988;12:557.
39. Rockwood CA, Wirth MA: Disorders of the sternoclavicular joint. In Rockwood CA, Matsen FA, Wirth MA, et al (eds): The Shoulder, 3rd ed. Philadelphia, WB Saunders, 2004, pp 597–653.
40. Benitez CL, Mintz DN, Potter HG: MR imaging of the sternoclavicular joint following trauma. Clin Imaging 2004;28:59–63.
41. Gobert R, Meuli M, Altermatt S, et al: Medial clavicular epiphysiolysis in children: The so-called sterno-clavicular dislocation. Emerg Radiol 2004;10:252–255.
42. Bicos J, Nicholson GP: Treatment and results of sternoclavicular joint injuries. Clin Sports Med 2003;22:359–370.
43. Noda M, Shiraishi H, Mizuno K: Chronic posterior sternoclavicular dislocation causing compression of a subclavian artery. J Shoulder Elbow Surg 1997;6:564–569.
44. Spencer EE, Kuhn JE: Biomechanical analysis of reconstructions for sternoclavicular joint instability. J Bone Joint Surg (Am) 2004;86:98–105.
45. Rockwood CA, Groh GI, Wirth MA, et al: Resection arthroplasty of the sternoclavicular joint. J Bone Joint Surg (Am) 1997;79:387–393.
46. Noble JS: Degenerative sternoclavicular arthritis and hyperostosis. Clin Sports Med 2003;22:407–422.

Scapulothoracic Disorders

John E. Kuhn

In This Chapter

INTRODUCTION

- The scapulothoracic articulation is an important, yet relatively unstudied component of upper extremity function, particularly in athletics.

- A variety of disorders have been described that affect the scapula directly. In addition, observations have been made in which the scapula functions abnormally in athletes with shoulder pain.

- For many of these observations, it is not known whether the scapulothoracic problem preceded the glenohumeral joint problem or vice versa, yet treating the scapulothoracic component of these disorders seems to be an important part of treating the athlete.

RELEVANT ANATOMY

Scapulothoracic Articulation

Seventeen muscles have their origin or insertion on the scapula (Table 28-1; Fig. 28-1) making it the command center for coordinated upper extremity activity. A number of muscles secure the scapula to the thorax, including the rhomboideus major and minor, the levator scapulae, the serratus anterior, the trapezius, the omohyoid, and the pectoralis minor. Scapular winging or scapulothoracic dyskinesia may occur as a result of dysfunction of these muscles. The rotator cuff muscles (supraspinatus, infraspinatus, subscapularis, and teres minor) provide dynamic stability and help to control activities of the glenohumeral articulation. Disorders of these muscles are common in athletes and are covered in other sections of this text. The series of muscles that join the humerus to the scapula provide power to the humerus and include the deltoid, the long head of the biceps, the short head of the biceps, the coracobrachialis, the long head of the triceps, and the teres major. Nearly every functional upper extremity movement has components of scapulothoracic and glenohumeral motion.

While at rest, the scapula is anteriorly rotated relative to the trunk approximately 30 degrees.[1,2] At rest, the medial border of the scapula is also rotated with the inferior pole diverging away from the spine approximately 3 degrees. When viewed from the side, the scapula is tilted forward about 20 degrees in the sagittal plane.[1] Deviations in this normal alignment conceivably could contribute to glenohumeral instability[3] and impingement[4-6] and likely contribute to scapulothoracic crepitus and bursitis. Interestingly, the resting scapular position may change with aging.[7]

Scapular Bursae

The location and orientation of the bursae about the scapulothoracic articulation have been known since Codman's time. Two major or anatomic bursae and four minor or adventitial bursae have been described (Table 28-2; Fig. 28-2). The major bursae are easily found,[8,9] whereas the adventitial bursae are not. These two major bursae are found in the space between the serratus anterior muscle and the chest wall and in the space between the subscapularis and the serratus anterior muscles.[8,10]

The superomedial angle and the inferior angle of the scapula are the most common anatomic regions involved in patients with scapulothoracic bursitis. When inflamed and symptomatic, the bursae are easily found; however, these bursae may be adventitious as they are not found reliably in cadavers.[8,11-13]

When scapulothoracic bursitis affects the inferior angle of the scapula, the inflamed bursa will be found between the chest wall and the serratus anterior muscle.[14-16] This bursa has been called the infraserratus bursa[14] and the bursa mucosa serrata.[16,17] The second and more common site of scapulothoracic bursitis occurs at the superomedial angle of the scapula. Codman[14] described the superomedial angle bursa as an infraserratus bursa lying between the upper and anterior portion of the scapula and the back of the first three ribs. O'Donoghue[18] agreed with Codman and described this bursa as a problem in athletes with pain and crepitus. Von Gruber,[17] on the other hand, described the bursa mucosa angulae superioris scapulae lying between the subscapularis and the serratus anticus muscles. A third major bursa, the scapulotrapezial bursa, was recognized by Williams et al,[9] lying between the superomedial scapula and the trapezius muscle. This bursa is not thought to be a source of scapulothoracic crepitus or bursitis and contains the spinal accessory nerve.

Codman[14] also recognized a third minor or adventitial bursa called the trapezoid bursa found over the triangular surface at the medial base of the spine of the scapula under the trapezius muscle, which he believed was another site of painful crepitus in scapulothoracic crepitus. Some believe that these minor bursae are not anatomic major bursae and develop in response to abnormal pathomechanics of the scapulothoracic

Table 28-1 Muscles with Origins or Insertions on the Scapula
Scapulohumeral Muscles
Long head of biceps
Short head of biceps
Deltoid
Coracobrachialis
Teres major
Long head of triceps
Scapulothoracic Muscles
Levator scapulae
Omohyoid
Rhomboid major
Rhomboid minor
Serratus anterior
Trapezius
Pectoralis minor
Rotator Cuff Muscles
Supraspinatus
Infraspinatus
Subscapularis
Teres minor

From Kuhn JE: The scapulothoracic articulation: Anatomy, biomechanics, pathology and management. In Iannotti JP, Williams GR Jr (eds): Disorders of the Shoulder: Diagnosis and Management. Philadelphia, Lippincott Williams & Wilkins, 1999, pp 817–845.

articulation.[8,11,13] This may help explain the variety of bursae and their different locations as described in these series.

WINGING OF THE SCAPULA

Winging of the scapula is one of the most common scapulothoracic disorders encountered in athletes. Winging can be divided into primary, secondary, and voluntary types. Primary scapular winging results from identifiable anatomic disorders that directly affect the scapulothoracic articulation. Secondary scapular winging usually is associated with some form of glenohumeral pathology. This type of winging will resolve as the glenohumeral pathology is addressed. Voluntary winging is quite rare and may have an underlying secondary gain concern or psychological cause. Primary winging is most commonly due to nerve injuries in athletes and is the focus of this review.

Serratus Anterior Palsy
Pathophysiology
The long thoracic nerve is the motor source for the serratus anterior muscle. It is found beneath the brachial plexus and clavicle and over the first rib. It then travels superficially along the lateral aspect of the chest wall, which makes the nerve susceptible to injury (Fig. 28-3). Blunt trauma or stretching of this nerve is particularly common in athletics and has been observed in tennis players, golfers, swimmers, gymnasts, soccer players, bowlers, weight lifters, ice hockey players, wrestlers, archers, basketball players, and football players.[19–22]

Evaluation
Patients with serratus anterior palsy will complain of pain as the other periscapular muscles fatigue as they are used to

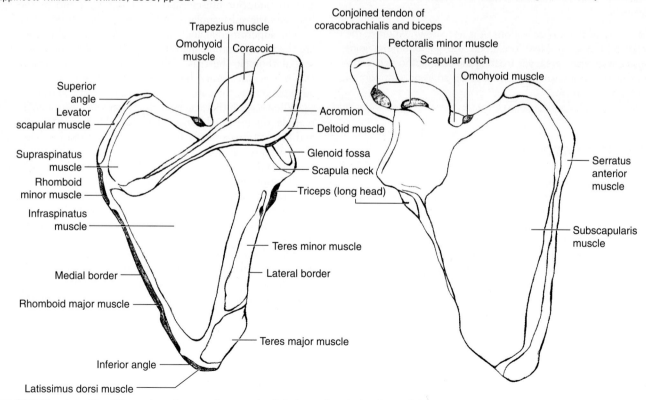

Figure 28-1 Muscles with origins or insertions on the scapula. Anterior and posterior views of the scapula demonstrate the multiple attachment sites for muscles of the scapula, making it the center for coordinated upper extremity motion. (From Kuhn JE: The scapulothoracic articulation: Anatomy, biomechanics, pathology and management. In Iannotti JP, Williams GR Jr [eds]: Disorders of the Shoulder: Diagnosis and Management. Philadelphia, Lippincott Williams & Wilkins, 1999, pp 817–845.)

Table 28-2 Bursae around the Scapula
Major/Anatomic Bursae
Infraserratus bursae: Between the serratus anterior and chest wall
Supraserratus bursae: Between the subscapularis and serratus anterior muscles
Minor/Adventitial Bursae
Scapulotrapezial bursae: Between the superomedial scapula and the trapezius
Superomedial angle of the scapula Infraserratus bursae: Between the serratus anterior and chest wall Supraserratus bursae: Between the subscapularis and serratus anterior
Inferior angle of the scapula Infraserratus bursae: Between the serratus anterior and chest wall
Spine of the scapula Trapezoid bursae: Between the medial spine of scapula and trapezius

From Kuhn JE, Hawkins RJ: Evaluation and treatment of scapular disorders. In Warner JJP, Iannotti JP, Gerber C (eds): Complex and Revision Problems in Shoulder Surgery. Philadelphia, Lippincott-Raven, 1997, pp 357–375.

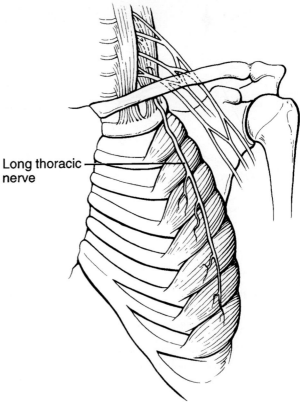

Figure 28-3 Location of the long thoracic nerve. Its superficial location along the chest wall makes it susceptible to injury. (From Kuhn JE, Hawkins RJ: Evaluation and treatment of scapular disorders. In Warner JJP, Iannotti JP, Gerber C [eds]: Complex and Revision Problems in Shoulder Surgery. Philadelphia, Lippincott-Raven, 1997, pp 357–375.)

compensate for the lost function. With a serratus anterior palsy, the scapula assumes a position of superior elevation and medial translation, and the inferior pole is rotated medially (Fig. 28-4). The patient will have difficulty with arm elevation above 120 degrees, which will magnify the degree of winging.[23,24]

Electromyography is recommended to confirm the diagnosis and follow the recovery of the injured long thoracic nerve. Because the majority of long thoracic nerve palsies will recover spontaneously, regular electromyographic examinations at 3-month intervals have been recommended to follow nerve recovery.[25,26]

Treatment
Nonoperative treatment with shoulder range-of-motion exercises is begun immediately after diagnosis in order to prevent glenohumeral stiffness. Many types of braces and orthotics have been developed, but their use is of questionable benefit.[22,25] In general, these braces attempt to hold the scapula against the

Figure 28-2 Bursae of the scapula. The location of both anatomic *(black)* and adventitial *(hatched)* bursae are shown. (From Kuhn JE, Hawkins RJ: Evaluation and treatment of scapular disorders. In Warner JJP, Iannotti JP, Gerber C [eds]: Complex and Revision Problems in Shoulder Surgery. Philadelphia, Lippincott-Raven, 1997, pp 357–375.)

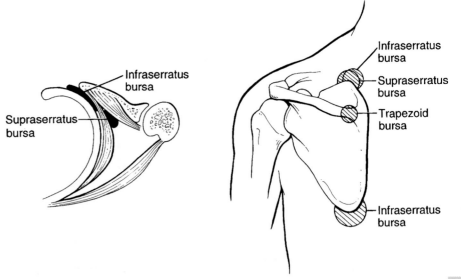

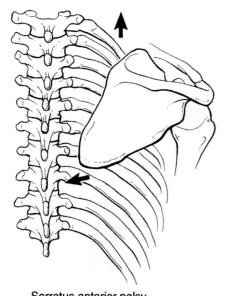

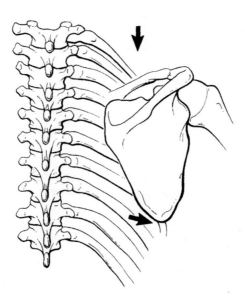

Serratus anterior palsy

Trapezius palsy

Figure 28-4 Resting location of the scapula with palsy of the serratus anterior, and trapezius palsy. (From Kuhn JE, Hawkins RJ: Evaluation and treatment of scapular disorders. In Warner JJP, Iannotti JP, Gerber C [eds]: Complex and Revision Problems in Shoulder Surgery. Philadelphia, Lippincott-Raven, 1997, pp 357–375.)

chest wall and may have some role if they provide symptom relief, despite their cumbersome nature.[24,26-28] Most long thoracic nerve injuries recover spontaneously within 1 year[20,23,24,26,27,29-38]; however some may take as long as 2 years.[23,39,40] Certainly, a trend for nerve recovery would be noted by at least 1 year.

There are few data in the literature regarding the results of neurolysis, nerve grafting, or repair of an injured long thoracic nerve.[41] Nevertheless, penetrating injuries should undergo nerve exploration and early repair. Neurorrhaphy may be indicated when the lesion can be localized.[26] Many patients with persistent impairment of the serratus anterior are able to compensate and not elect to have a surgical reconstruction.[26] In patients with

symptomatic serratus winging that persists for more than 1 year, surgical intervention may alleviate pain and improve function. While a number of procedures have been described for refractory serratus anterior palsy, transferring the sternocostal head of the pectoralis major with a fascia lata or hamstring graft extension has become the most popular[25,26,31,32,42-46] (Fig. 28-5). While this surgery has been shown to be very helpful for patients with permanent palsy of the serratus anterior, there are no data in athletes, and it is highly unlikely that athletes who require the use of their upper extremity would return to their previous level of competition following this surgery. Fortunately, most athletic injuries to the long thoracic nerve are neuropraxic and recover spontaneously.

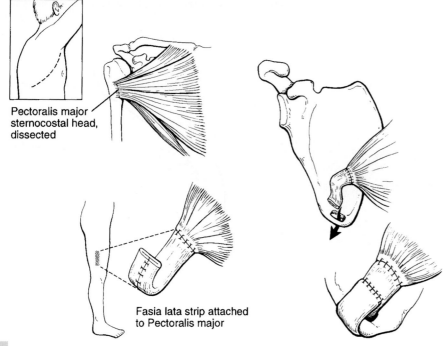

Pectoralis major sternocostal head, dissected

Fasia lata strip attached to Pectoralis major

Figure 28-5 Pectoralis major transfer for scapular winging. As described by Marmor and Bechtol,[114] the sternocostal head of the pectoralis major is sutured to a tubularized fascia lata graft and woven through a foramen made in the inferior angle of the scapula. (From Kuhn JE, Hawkins RJ: Evaluation and treatment of scapular disorders. In Warner JJP, Iannotti JP, Gerber C [eds]: Complex and Revision Problems in Shoulder Surgery. Philadelphia, Lippincott-Raven, 1997, pp 357–375.)

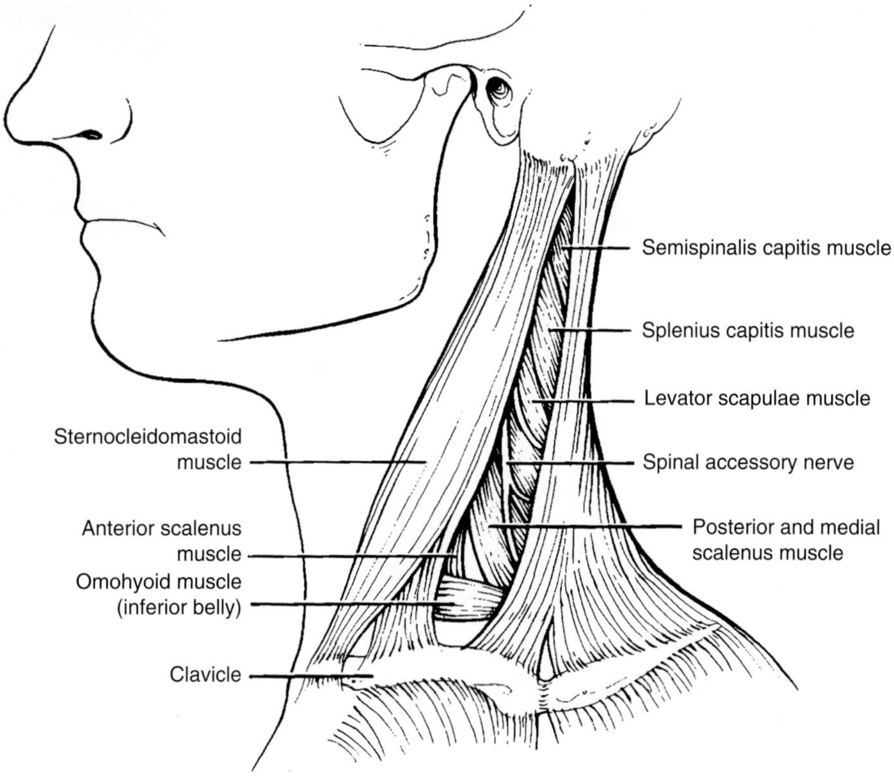

Figure 28-6 Location of the spinal accessory nerve. Its location in the posterior cervical triangle makes it susceptible to injury during surgical procedures in this area. (From Kuhn JE: The scapulothoracic articulation: Anatomy, biomechanics, pathology and management. In Iannotti JP, Williams GR Jr [eds]: Disorders of the Shoulder: Diagnosis and Management. Philadelphia, Lippincott Williams & Wilkins, 1999, pp 817–845.)

Trapezius Winging

Pathophysiology

The spinal accessory nerve, the only nerve to the large trapezius muscle, is superficial, lying in the subcutaneous tissue on the floor of the posterior cervical triangle. Its superficial location makes it susceptible to injury[47,48] (Fig. 28-6). Injury to this nerve results in painfully disabling alterations in scapulothoracic function as well as significant deformity.[47-55] This nerve can be injured by blunt trauma,[55-57] stretching of the nerve,[55] and penetrating trauma that includes surgical biopsy of lymph nodes in the posterior cervical triangle[50,53,54] and radical neck dissection.[58-60] In athletes, stretching and blunt trauma injuries are most common,[56] particularly in contact sports like wrestling.

Evaluation

Patients will attempt to compensate for a palsy of the trapezius by straining other muscles of the shoulder girdle, including the levator scapulae and the rhomboid muscles which can lead to disabling pain and spasm.[57] Patients can also develop pain from a stiff shoulder, shoulder subacromial impingement, and radiculitis from traction on the brachial plexus as the shoulder girdle droops.

Upon examination, patients will have difficulty when attempting to shrug their shoulder and will have weakness in forward elevation and abduction of the arm. The patient will assume a position with the shoulder depressed and the scapula translated laterally with the inferior angle rotated laterally (see Fig. 28-4). The diagnosis is confirmed by electromyography.

Treatment

The initial treatment for patients with trapezius winging is nonoperative. The arm can be placed in a sling to rest the other periscapular muscles. Physical therapy is helpful to maintain glenohumeral motion, preventing shoulder stiffness.[61] In cases

caused by blunt trauma, serial electromyographic analysis should be performed at 1- to 3-month intervals to follow the returning function of the nerve. In cases caused by penetrating trauma or when there is no evidence of nerve function on electromyographic analysis, neurolysis and/or nerve grafting can be performed.[50,54,62-64] The results of these procedures have been variable; however, the success rate seems to be improved if neurolysis is performed before 6 months.[57]

Patients who have had symptoms in excess of 1 year are unlikely to benefit from continued nonoperative treatment,[53] and surgery can be offered. Historically, a variety of procedures have been described for the treatment of trapezius winging,[49,65,66] but the Eden-Lange procedure[67-69] is the most popular. In this procedure, the levator scapulae, rhomboideus minor, and rhomboideus major muscles are transferred laterally (Fig. 28-7). The levator scapulae substitutes for the upper third of the trapezius; the rhomboid major substitutes for the middle third of the trapezius; and the rhomboid minor substitutes for the lower third of the trapezius. By moving these muscle insertions laterally, their mechanical advantage is improved and winging is eliminated. Bigliani et al[57] recently reported their results using this procedure in 23 patients with trapezius scapular winging, with excellent and good results in 87%. Significant improvement in pain was seen in 91% of these patients, and 87% had significant improvement in function.[57] This procedure, while effective at improving function for activities of daily living, would be unlikely to return a competitive athlete back to a high level of performance.

SCAPULOTHORACIC CREPITUS

Pathophysiology

Symptomatic scapulothoracic crepitus has been described by a number of different authors and has been called the snapping

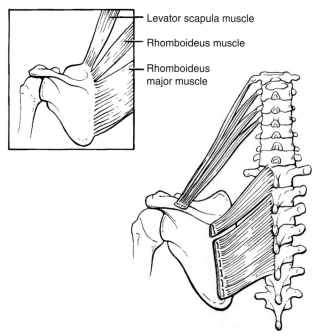

Levator scapula muscle
Rhomboideus muscle
Rhomboideus major muscle

Figure 28-7 Eden-Lange procedure for trapezius palsy. In this procedure, the levator scapulae is transferred laterally to function as the upper trapezius, while advancement of the rhomboid major and minor compensates for the loss of the middle and lower trapezius. (From Kuhn JE: The scapulothoracic articulation: Anatomy, biomechanics, pathology and management. In Iannotti JP, Williams GR Jr [eds]: Disorders of the Shoulder: Diagnosis and Management. Philadelphia, Lippincott Williams & Wilkins, 1999, pp 817–845.)

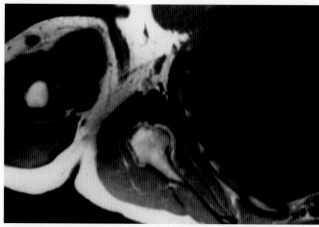

Figure 28-8 Osteochondroma of the scapula causing scapulothoracic crepitus. Note the increased signal in the bursa surrounding this osteochondroma of the scapula. (From Kuhn JE: The scapulothoracic articulation: Anatomy, biomechanics, pathology and management. In Iannotti JP, Williams GR Jr [eds]: Disorders of the Shoulder: Diagnosis and Management. Philadelphia, Lippincott Williams & Wilkins, 1999, pp 817–845.)

Table 28-3 Causes of Scapulothoracic Crepitus
Interposed Tissue
Muscle Atrophy[15] Fibrosis[15,17,76] Anatomic variation[77]
Bone Rib osteochondroma[78] Scapular osteochondroma[76,79,80] Rib fracture[15,76] Scapular fracture[81] Hooked superomedial angle of the scapula[79,82] Luschka's tubercle[15,81,83] Reactive bone spurs from muscle avulsion[67,84,85]
Other soft tissue Bursitis[86,87] Tuberculosis[15] Syphilitic lues[15]
Abnormalities in Scapulothoracic Congruence
Scoliosis[88,89]
Thoracic kyphosis[11]

From Kuhn JE, Hawkins RJ: Evaluation and treatment of scapular disorders. In Warner JJP, Iannotti JP, Gerber C (eds): Complex and Revision Problems in Shoulder Surgery. Philadelphia, Lippincott-Raven, 1997, pp 357–375.

scapula,[15] the grating scapula,[43] the rolling scapula,[11] the washboard syndrome,[70] the scapulothoracic syndrome,[71] and the scapulocostal syndrome.[72] Boinet[73] was the first to describe this disorder in 1867. Mauclaire,[74] some 37 years later, classified scapulothoracic crepitus into three groups: *froissement* was considered physiologic and was described as a gentle friction sound, *frottement* was a louder sound with grating and was usually pathologic, and *craquement* was a loud snapping sound and was always pathologic. These noises are thought to occur from two sources, from either anatomic changes in the tissue interposed between the scapula and the chest wall or incongruence in the scapulothoracic articulation (Table 28-3). In reviewing Milch,[15] *frottement* (the lower volume crepitus) may suggest soft-tissue pathology or bursitis while *craquement* may suggest bony pathology as the source of symptomatic scapulothoracic crepitus. Codman[14] writes that he was able to make his own scapula "sound about the room without the slightest pain," and was likely demonstrating *froissement*. In every instance, the air-filled thoracic cavity will amplify these noises, acting like a resonance chamber of a string instrument.[75]

A number of pathologic conditions that could lead to crepitus that affect the muscle in the scapulothoracic articulation include atrophied muscle,[15] fibrotic muscle,[15,17,76] and anomalous muscle insertions.[77] With regard to bony pathology, the most common source of scapulothoracic crepitus is an osteochondroma, arising from either the ribs[78] or the scapula[76,79,80] (Fig. 28-8). Malunited fractures of the ribs or scapula are also capable of creating painful crepitus.[15,76,81] Abnormalities of the superomedial angle of the scapula, including a hooked superomedial angle[79,82] and a Luschka's tubercle (which originally was described as an osteochondroma but has subsequently come to mean a prominence of bone at the superomedial angle[15,81,83]), have also been implicated as sources for scapulothoracic crepitus. Others[67,84,85] implicate reactive spurs of bone that are created by repeated small periscapular muscle avulsions.

Any bony pathology that causes scapulothoracic crepitus is capable of forming a reactive bursa around the area of pathology.[86,87] In fact, at the time of resection of bony pathology, a bursa is frequently seen. Bursae can become inflamed and painful in the absence of bony pathology and may, by themselves, become a source of crepitus.

Other soft-tissue pathologies that have been implicated in scapulothoracic crepitus include tuberculosis lesions in the scapulothoracic region and syphilitic lues,[15] which are exceedingly rare in athletes. However, it is not uncommon for athletes to have abnormalities in congruence of the scapulothoracic articulation that could lead to scapulothoracic crepitus. Both thoracic kyphosis[11] and scoliosis,[88,89] have been identified as sources of scapulothoracic crepitus. In many sports, particularly swimming, thoracic kyphosis is common[90,91] and may be the most likely source of scapulothoracic crepitus.

Evaluation

When evaluating the athlete, it is important to know the primary sport and training in which the athlete participates. Athletes who participate in sports that require repetitive overhead activity are commonly affected by scapulothoracic crepitus.[13] There may be a familial tendency toward developing symptoms.[11] Patients may relate a history of mild trauma that precipitates symptoms,[92] and scapulothoracic crepitus may be bilateral in some patients.[10] If scapular winging or fullness is identified on inspection of the resting scapula, the examiner should consider a space-occupying lesion, such as an osteochondroma. It is helpful to ask the patient with symptomatic scapulothoracic crepitus to point to the location of the pain. He or she will generally point to the superomedial angle or the inferior angle. Palpation or auscultation while the patient moves the shoulder may help to identify the source and location of the periscapular crepitus.[10,93] Supplemental radiographs, which include tangential views of the lateral scapula, computed tomography, or magnetic resonance imaging may be helpful in identifying bony pathology.

Treatment

It is important to recognize that scapulothoracic crepitus is not necessarily a pathologic condition. Up to 35% of normal asymptomatic people can demonstrate scapulothoracic crepitus,[94] including Codman.[14] Therefore, scapular crepitus could potentially be used for secondary gain in patients with hidden agendas or psychiatric conditions. However, if the athlete presents with pain, winging, or other disorders of the scapulothoracic articulation, the scapulothoracic crepitus is considered to be pathologic.

Most athletes with scapulothoracic crepitus can successfully be treated nonoperatively, particularly if the crepitus is related to soft-tissue abnormalities, altered posture, or scapulothoracic dyskinesia.[10,15] Nonoperative treatment includes postural exercises designed to prevent sloping of the shoulders.[10,95] A figure-eight clavicle fracture brace may be a useful tool to remind patients to maintain upright posture. Exercises to strengthen periscapular muscles are also important.[10,13,15] Oral nonsteroidal anti-inflammatory drugs as well as local modalities such as heat, massage, phonophoresis, ultrasound, and the application of ethyl chloride to trigger points may also prove useful.[10,13,15] Injectable local anesthetics and corticosteroids into the painful area have also been recommended.[11,13,15,42,92] Caution must be used, as there is a risk of creating a pneumothorax.[92] Using these means, most athletes are expected to improve significantly.[13,42] However, for those who fail, a number of operations have been described. Athletes with clearly defined bony pathology such as an osteochondroma generally require surgical treatment.[15]

Resection of the bony pathology is usually necessary to alleviate symptoms with a high likelihood of success.[13,76,96]

Historically, some authors have used muscle plasty operations to treat scapulothoracic crepitus.[74,92] This is thought to be inadequate, however, because the muscle flap may atrophy with time and symptoms could return.[15] The most popular method for the surgical treatment of scapulothoracic crepitus involves a partial scapulectomy, which has been performed on the medial border of the scapula[97] and more commonly on the superomedial angle.[11,15,82,85,93,98,99]

Surgery

The surgical technique for the resection of the superomedial angle of the scapula begins with the patient in the prone position (Fig. 28-9). An incision following Langer's lines is made slightly lateral to the medial border of the scapula, from the superior angle to the scapular spine. The subcutaneous tissue is undermined, exposing the spine of the scapula. Following the spine of the scapula, the periosteum is incised and a plane is developed between the superficial trapezius and the underlying scapula and supraspinatus. Next a plane is developed between the supraspinatus and the rhomboids and levator scapulae muscles along the medial border of the scapula starting at the spine of the scapula. The supraspinatus is elevated in a subperiosteal plane from the supraspinatus fossa. The medial scapulothoracic muscles are dissected from the medial border of the scapula and the dissection in this subperiosteal plane is carried around the medial border and to the subscapularis fossa, elevating the serratus and subscapularis with the rhomboids and levator. The superomedial angle of the scapula is resected with an oscillating saw. It is important to avoid progressing too far laterally as the scapular notch is at risk with the potential for injury to the dorsal scapular artery and the suprascapular nerve. After resecting the bone, the reflected muscles fall back into place, and the medial border of the supraspinatus is repaired to the rhomboid/levator flap with permanent no. 2 polyester suture. Inferiorly, the periosteum is repaired back to the spine of the scapula using suture passed through drill holes. Postoperatively, the patient is placed in a sling and begins passive motion immediately. Active motion is begun at 6 weeks, and resistance exercises follow at 8 to 12 weeks.

Complications associated with partial scapulectomy include postoperative hematoma, pneumothorax, and mild residual winging. In younger patients, bone may try to form again, but this rarely produces symptoms. The exposure and potential for complications have led some to perform this procedure arthroscopically.[100]

The reported results for this procedure are generally good.[11,15,82,98] However, it must be remembered that athletes typically do not require surgical intervention; as such, there are few data in the literature regarding the effect of superomedial angle resection of the scapula on athletic performance. It is also important to note that the bone resected is not pathologic and appears normal histologically, which has prompted some to perform bursectomies and avoid a partial scapulectomy.[16,101,102]

SCAPULOTHORACIC BURSITIS

When scapulothoracic crepitus is accompanied by pain, an inflamed scapulothoracic bursa is typically found. It is important to realize that, while these two conditions are frequently found

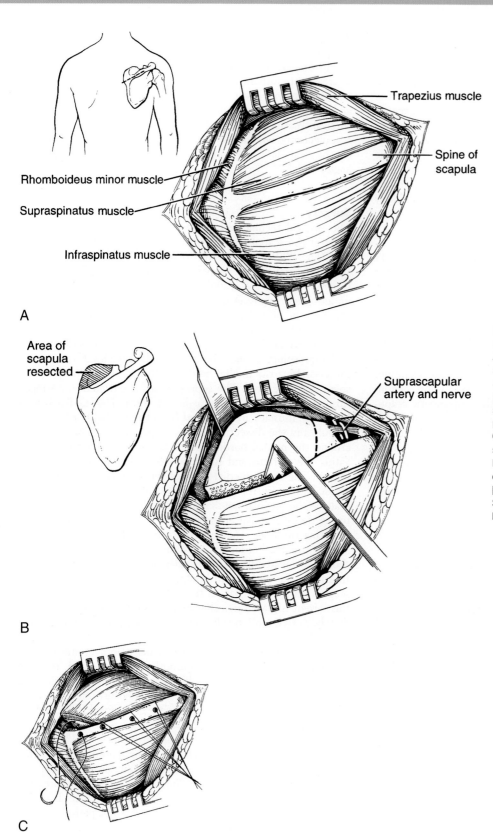

Trapezius muscle

Spine of scapula

Rhomboideus minor muscle

Supraspinatus muscle

Infraspinatus muscle

A

Area of scapula resected

Suprascapular artery and nerve

B

C

Figure 28-9 Surgical approach for excision of superomedial angle of the scapula. **A,** Trapezius is elevated from the spine of the scapula. **B,** The supraspinatus, rhomboids, and serratus are elevated in a subperiosteal plane from the medial border, and the superomedial scapula is resected while protecting the suprascapular nerve and artery. **C,** The supraspinatus is sutured back to the spine of the scapula. (From Kuhn JE, Hawkins RJ: Evaluation and treatment of scapular disorders. In Warner JJP, Iannotti JP, Gerber C [eds]: Complex and Revision Problems in Shoulder Surgery. Philadelphia, Lippincott-Raven, 1997, pp 357–375.)

together, an athlete may have crepitus without pain and another may have scapulothoracic bursitis without crepitus. As described previously, symptomatic scapulothoracic bursitis seems to affect two areas of the scapula: the superomedial angle and the inferior angle. These bursae, when inflamed, are thought to be adventitious.[8,11,13]

Evaluation

Patients with scapulothoracic bursitis generally complain of pain with activity and may have audible and palpable crepitus of the scapulothoracic articulation. Usually the scapular crepitus associated with bursitis is of a much lesser quality and nature than that described with bony pathology. Periscapular fullness is frequently appreciated in thinner athletes. This may become significant enough to produce subtle scapular winging. Scapular winging has been identified in 50% of patients with a snapping scapula and no bony abnormalities.[13] Infrequently, patients may describe minor trauma as a predisposing event,[93,101] but most have a history of repetitive overhead activities in work or athletics.[16,42,101] The repetitive motion may irritate soft tissues until inflammation occurs and chronic bursitis develops. The bursa may undergo scarring and fibrosis, which may be the source of crepitus. Scapulothoracic bursitis in athletes may have its roots in postural abnormalities and scapulothoracic dyskinesia. In the evaluation of athletes with scapulothoracic crepitus, local anesthetic injected into the bursa may relieve pain and serve as a diagnostic aid.[18]

Treatment

Nonoperative measures (rest, analgesics, and nonsteroidal anti-inflammatory drugs) are the mainstay of treatment for scapulothoracic bursitis. Physical therapy to improve posture, heat, and local steroid injections has also been recommended.[16,42] Efforts to strengthen periscapular muscles and stretching are frequently added.[16,42] For patients who continue to have symptoms despite conservative treatment, surgery may be considered.

As recognized by Sisto and Jobe,[16] baseball pitchers may be at risk of bursitis at the inferior angle of the scapula. They described an open procedure for resecting a bursa at the inferior angle of the scapula in four pitchers. Pitchers with this problem have difficulty pitching and tend to have pain during the early and late cocking phases as well as during acceleration (Fig. 28-10). While all pitchers had a palpable bursal sac ranging in size from 1 to 2 cm, best seen with the arm abducted to 60 degrees and elevated forward 30 degrees, only one of the four patients presented with scapulothoracic crepitus. All four pitchers failed conservative therapy and underwent a bursal excision via an oblique incision just distal to the inferior angle of the scapula. The trapezius muscle, and then the latissimus dorsi muscle, were reflected medially, exposing the bursa. The bursa was sharply excised and any bony prominence on the inferior pole of the scapula or ribs was removed. The wounds were closed routinely over a drain, and a compression dressing was applied. Physical therapy, stressing motion, was begun after 1 week and progressed to allow gentle throwing at 6 weeks with progression to full speed pitching as symptoms allowed. After this procedure, all were able to return to their former level of pitching.

Open excision of symptomatic superomedial scapulothoracic bursae have been described by many authors.[42,101–103] In most of these reports, dissection is carried out until a plane is developed between the serratus anterior and the chest wall. The thickened bursa is resected and any bony projections removed. With this technique, more than 80% of patients with symptomatic scapulothoracic bursitis had good or excellent results.

Resection of the symptomatic scapulothoracic bursa has been performed endoscopically as well.[8,10,104–107] Ciullo and Jones[10] have the largest endoscopic series to date with 13 patients who underwent subscapular endoscopy after failing a conservative treatment program for symptomatic scapulothoracic bursitis. Débridement was performed for fibrous adhesions found in the bursa between the subscapularis and serratus muscles as well as the bursa between the serratus and chest wall. In addition, débridement or scapuloplasty of changes at the superomedial angle or inferior angle was performed. All 13 patients returned to their preinjury activity level, except for physician-imposed restrictions in a few patients, limiting the assembly line use of vibrating tools.[10]

Matthews et al[106] have described the technique for scapulothoracic endoscopy. Patients can be placed in the prone or lateral position; however, the lateral position is preferred, as it allows arthroscopic evaluation of the glenohumeral joint and the subacromial space. In addition, if the arm is extended and maximally internally rotated, the scapula will fall away from the thorax, improving access to the bursae.

Three portals are used, placed at least 2 cm from the medial border of the scapula in the region between the scapular spine and the inferior angle. For the middle portal, a spinal needle is inserted into the bursa between the serratus anterior and the chest wall. This needle should be inserted midway between the scapular spine and the inferior angle, at least three finger breadths medial to the medial border of the scapula to avoid

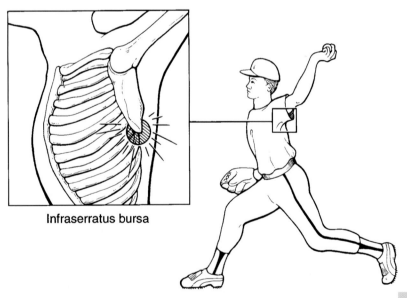

Figure 28-10 Bursa at the inferior angle of the scapula in throwers. This is an infraserratus bursa, which has been described in baseball pitchers, where an excision of the bursa has allowed a return to throwing. (From Kuhn JE, Hawkins RJ: Evaluation and treatment of scapular disorders. In Warner JJP, Iannotti JP, Gerber C [eds]: Complex and Revision Problems in Shoulder Surgery. Philadelphia, Lippincott-Raven, 1997, pp 357–375.)

Infraserratus bursa

injury to the dorsal scapular artery and nerve. The bursa under the serratus anterior can be distended with fluid before a stab wound is made in the skin and the blunt obturator and endoscope are inserted. Deep penetration may traverse the serratus entering the axillary space and should be avoided.

Once this initial middle portal has been established, a superior portal placed three finger breadths medial to the vertebral border of the scapula just below the spine will penetrate the interval between the rhomboideus major and rhomboideus minor. This portal will allow access to the superomedial angle of the scapula. Portals placed superior to the scapular spine jeopardize the dorsal scapular nerve and artery, the spinal accessory nerve, and the transverse cervical artery and should be avoided. A third inferior portal can be made in a similar fashion at the inferior angle of the scapula.

In the bursa between the serratus anterior and chest wall, landmarks are generally absent except the ribs. A motorized shaver and electrocautery are required to perform the bursectomy and obtain hemostasis. The arthroscopic pump should be kept at low pressure throughout the procedure. After completing the bursectomy, the portals are closed in a standard fashion and the patient is placed in a sling for comfort. Physical therapy, beginning with active range of motion, is initiated as tolerated by the patient. Early results suggest this condition can be treated successfully using the arthroscope with minimal risk.[10,103,107]

SCAPULOTHORACIC DYSKINESIS

Abnormalities in scapulothoracic motion are now receiving much more attention in the literature. Burkhart et al[108] recently described a condition known as the SICK scapula. The acronym SICK stands for *s*capula malposition, *i*nferior medial border prominence, *c*oracoid pain and malposition, and dys*k*inesis of scapular movement. The scapula assumes an abnormal position at rest characterized by a position that is inferior, protracted, and tilted anteriorly. Tenderness is typically found on the medial edge of the coracoid, and the pectoralis minor is thought to be in spasm. The authors recognized this pattern in throwing athletes with shoulder pain.

Myers et al[109] studied this concept by measuring scapulothoracic motion in a population of throwing athletes and compared this to scapulothoracic motion in a control population. They showed that throwing athletes demonstrated significantly increased upward rotation, internal rotation, and retraction of the scapula during humeral elevation, implying that throwing athletes may develop these adaptations for more efficient performance of the throwing motion. Su et al[110] have demonstrated that scapular kinematics may be altered in symptomatic swimmers, an effect that is magnified with fatigue associated with a practice.

Evaluation

Patients with scapulothoracic dyskinesis will not typically direct the physician toward the scapula and will commonly complain of pain in the glenohumeral joint. Inspection of the scapulae from the back will demonstrate asymmetry at rest, with the affected shoulder frequently depressed, the scapula protracted and tilted forward. Mild scapular winging may be present with the posterior angle and the medial border of the scapula prominent. Patients will frequently have pain to palpation at the medial coracoid, the insertion of the pectoralis minor. Asking the patient to elevate the arm in the frontal plane and in the scapular plane will reveal asymmetry of scapulothoracic motion. In the presence of rotator cuff pathology, this may be related to decreased firing of the middle and lower trapezius.[111]

Treatment

Treatment of scapulothoracic dyskinesis is with exercises and modalities of physical therapy. Kinetic chain–based rehabilitation programs have been recommended,[112,113] as many of the patients with scapulothoracic kinematic abnormalities will have weakness in the core stabilizers of the trunk. This work is currently in its infancy. Clearly much more work is needed to clearly define pathologic scapulothoracic kinematics and their effect on other shoulder pathologies.

CONCLUSIONS

A variety of scapulothoracic conditions can affect the athlete's shoulder. These include winging of a variety of forms, crepitus and bursitis, and dyskinesia of the scapulothoracic articulation. Scapular winging in athletes most commonly results from a long thoracic nerve neuropraxic injury and will recover spontaneously. Scapulothoracic crepitus and scapulothoracic bursitis are two related conditions but may be found independently in athletes with periscapular pain. In general, treatment for athletes is nonoperative and requires postural exercises designed to prevent sloping of the shoulders[10,95] and periscapular muscle strengthening.[10,13,15] A figure-eight harness may be a useful tool to remind patients to maintain upright posture. Local modalities, nonsteroidal anti-inflammatory drugs, and local injections have also been recommended.[10,11,13,15,42,92] In athletes with refractory symptoms, surgical correction may be considered; however, there are only a few reports in the literature for this select population and thus it is difficult to predict outcomes with regard to returning to sport. Scapular dyskinesia is only now under study as a source of shoulder pathology, and early results suggest the effects of scapular dyskinesia may be of critical importance. Clearly more work is needed to gain a complete understanding of scapulothoracic problems in the athlete.

REFERENCES

1. Laumann U: Kinesiology of the shoulder joint. In Kolbel R, Helbig B, Blauth W, et al (eds): Shoulder Replacement. Berlin, Springer-Verlag, 1987, pp 23–31.
2. Steindler A: Kinesiology of the Human Body under Normal and Pathological Conditions. Springfield, IL, Charles C Thomas, 1955.
3. von Eisenhart-Rothe R, Matsen FA 3rd, Eckstein F, et al: Pathomechanics in atraumatic shoulder instability: Scapular positioning correlates with humeral head centering. Clin Orthop 2005;433:82–89.
4. Endo K, Ikata T, Katoh S, Takeda Y: Radiographic assessment of scapular rotational tilt in chronic shoulder impingement syndrome. J Orthop Sci 2001;6:3–10.
5. Hebert LJ, Moffet H, McFadyen BJ, Dionne CE: Scapular behavior in shoulder impingement syndrome. Arch Phys Med Rehabil 2002;83:60–69.
6. Lewis JS, Wright C, Green A: Subacromial impingement syndrome: The effect of changing posture on shoulder range of movement. J Orthop Sports Phys Ther 2005;35:72–87.
7. Endo K, Yukata K, Yasui N: Influence of age on scapulo-thoracic orientation. Clin Biomech (Bristol, Avon) 2004;19:1009–1013.
8. Kolodychuk LB, Regan WD: Visualization of the scapulothoracic articulation using an arthroscope: A proposed technique. Orthop Trans 1993–1994;17:1142.

9. Williams GR Jr, Shakil M, Klimkiewicz J, Ianotti JP: The anatomy of the scapulothoracic articulation. Clin Orthop 1999;357:237–246.

10. Ciullo JV, Jones E: Subscapular bursitis: Conservative and endoscopic treatment of "snapping scapula" or "washboard syndrome." Orthop Trans 1992–1993;16:740.

11. Cobey MC: The rolling scapula. Clin Orthop 1968;60:193–194.

12. Colas F, Nevoux J, Gagey O: The subscapular and subcoracoid bursae: Descriptive and functional anatomy. J Shoulder Elbow Surg 2004;13:454–458.

13. Percy EL, Birbrager D, Pitt MJ: Snapping scapula: A review of the literature and presentation of 14 patients. Can J Surg 1988;31:248–250.

14. Codman EA: The anatomy of the human shoulder. In Codman EA (ed): The Shoulder, Supplemental Edition. Malabar, FL, Kreiger Publishing, 1984, pp 1–31.

15. Milch H: Snapping scapula. Clin Orthop 1961;20:139–150.

16. Sisto DJ, Jobe FW: The operative treatment of scapulothoracic bursitis in professional pitchers. Am J Sports Med 1986;14:192–194.

17. Von Gruber W: Die Bursae mucosae der Inneren Aschselwand. Arch Anat Physiol Wissenschaft Med 1864;358–366.

18. O'Donoghue DH: Treatment of Injuries to Athletes. Philadelphia, WB Saunders, 1962, pp 14–144.

19. Fiddian NJ, King RJ: The winged scapula. Clin Orthop 1984;185:228–236.

20. Gregg JR, Labosky D, Harty M: Serratus anterior paralysis in the young athlete. J Bone Joint Surg Am 1979;61:825–832.

21. Leffert RD: Pectoralis major transfers for serratus anterior paralysis. Orthop Trans 1992–1993;16:761.

22. Vastamaki M, Kauppila LI: Etiologic factors in isolated paralysis of the serratus anterior muscle: A report of 197 cases. J Shoulder Elbow Surg 1993;2:240–243.

23. Foo CL, Swann M: Isolated paralysis of the serratus anterior. J Bone Joint Surg Br 1983;65:552–556.

24. Johnson JTH, Kendall HO: Isolated paralysis of the serratus anterior muscle. J Bone Joint Surg Am 1955;37:563–574.

25. Iceton J, Harris WR: Results of pectoralis major transfer for winged scapula. J Bone Joint Surg Br 1987;69:108–110.

26. Leffert RD: Nerve injuries about the shoulder. In: Rowe CR (ed): The Shoulder. New York, Churchill Livingstone, 1988, pp 435–454.

27. Foucar HO: The "clover leaf" sling in paralysis of the serratus magnus. BMJ 1933;2:865–866.

28. Wolfe J: The conservative treatment of serratus palsy. J Bone Joint Surg Am 1941;23:959–961.

29. Berkheiser EJ, Shapiro F: Alar scapula. Traumatic palsy of the serratus magnus. JAMA 1937;108:1790–1793.

30. Duncan MA, Lotze MT, Gerber LH, Rosenberg SA: Incidence, recovery, and management of serratus anterior muscle palsy after axillary node dissection. Phys Ther 1983;63:1243–1247.

31. Fery A: Results of treatment of anterior serratus paralysis. In Post M, Morrey BF, Hawkins RJ (eds): Sugery of the Shoulder. St. Louis, CV Mosby, 1990, pp 325–329.

32. Gozna ER, Harris WR: Traumatic winging of the scapula. J Bone Joint Surg Am 1979;61:1230–1233.

33. Hauser CU, Martin WF: Two additional causes of traumatic winged scapula occurring in the armed forces. JAMA 1943;121:667–668.

34. Horowitz MT, Tocantins LM: An anatomic study of the role of the long thoracic nerve and the related scapular bursae in the pathogenesis of local paralysis of the serratus anterior muscle. Anat Rec 1938;71:375–385.

35. Ilfeld FW, Holder HG: Winged scapula: Case occurring in soldier from knapsack. JAMA 1942;120:448–449.

36. Overpeck DO, Ghormley RK: Paralysis of the serratus magnus muscle caused by lesions of the long thoracic nerve. JAMA 1940;114:1994–1996.

37. Potts CS: Isolated paralysis of the serratus magnus: Report of a case. Arch Neurol Psychiatry 1928;20:184–186.

38. Prescott MU, Zollinger RW: Alar scapula an unusual surgical complication. Am J Surg 1944;65:98–103.

39. Goodman CE, Kenrick MM, Blum MV: Long thoracic nerve palsy: A follow-up study. Arch Phys Med Rehabil 1975;56:352–355.

40. Leffert RD: Neurological problems. In Rockwood CA, Matsen FA (eds): The Shoulder, vol 2. Philadelphia, WB Saunders, 1990, pp 750–773.

41. Skillern PG: Serratus magnus palsy with proposal of a new operation for intractable cases. Ann Surg 1913;57:909–915.

42. McCluskey GM III, Bigliani LU: Scapulothoracic disorders. In Andrews JR, Wilk KE (eds): The Athlete's Shoulder. New York, Churchill Livingstone, 1994, pp 305–316.

43. Neer CS II: Less frequent procedures. In Neer CS II (ed): Shoulder Reconstruction. Philadelphia, WB Saunders, 1990, pp 421–485.

44. Noerdlinger MA, Cole BJ, Stewart M, Post M: Results of pectoralis major transfer with fascia lata autograft augmentation for scapula winging. J Shoulder Elbow Surg 2002;11:345–350.

45. Post M: Pectoralis major transfer for winging of the scapula. J Shoulder Elbow Surg 1995;4:1–9.

46. Steinmann SP, Wood MB: Pectoralis major transfer for serratus anterior paralysis. J Shoulder Elbow Surg 2003;12:555–560.

47. Kauppila LI: Iatrogenic serratus anterior paralysis. Long term outcome in 26 patients. Chest 1996;109:31–34.

48. Kauppila LI: The long thoracic nerve: Possible mechanisms of injury based on autopsy study. J Shoulder Elbow Surg 1993;2:244–248.

49. Dewar FP, Harris RI: Restoration of function of the shoulder following paralysis of the trapezius by fascial sling fixation and transplantation of the levator scapulae. Ann Surg 1950;132:1111–1115.

50. Dunn AW: Trapezius paralysis after minor surgical procedures in the posterior cervical triangle. South Med J 1974;67:312–315.

51. Hoaglund FT, Duthie RB: Surgical reconstruction for shoulder pain after radical neck dissection. Am J Surg 1966;112:522–526.

52. Langenskiold A, Ryoppy S: Treatment of paralysis of the trapezius muscle by the Eden-Lange operation. Acta Orthop Scand 1973;44:383–388.

53. Olarte M, Adams D: Accessory nerve palsy. J Neurol Neruosurg Psychiatry 1977;40:1113–1116.

54. Woodhall B: Trapezius paralysis following minor surgical procedures in the posterior cervical triangle. Results following cranial nerve suture. Ann Surg 1952;136:375–380.

55. Wright YA: Accessory spinal nerve injury. Clin Orthop 1975;108:15–18.

56. Hirasawa Y, Sakakida K: Sports and peripheral nerve injury. Am J Sports Med 1983;11:420–426.

57. Bigliani LU, Perez-Sanz JR, Wolfe IN: Treatment of trapezius paralysis. J Bone Joint Surg Am 1985;67:871–877.

58. Bocca E, Pignataro O: A conservation technique in radical neck surgery. Ann Otol Rhinol Laryngol 1967;76:975–978.

59. Roy PH, Bearhs OH: Spinal accessory nerve in radical neck dissections. Am J Surg 1969;118:800–804.

60. Spira E: The treatment of the dropped shoulder. A new operative technique. J Bone Joint Surg Am 1948;30:229–233.

61. Pianka G, Hershman EB: Neurovascular injuries. In Nicholas JA, Hershman EB (eds): The Upper Extremity in Sports Medicine. St. Louis, CV Mosby, 1990, pp 691–722.

62. Anderson R, Flowers RS: Free grafts of the spinal accessory nerve during radical neck dissection. Am J Surg 1969;118:769–799.

63. Harris HH, Dickey JR: Nerve grafting to restore function of the trapezius muscle after radical neck dissection. (A preliminary report). Ann Otol Rhinol Laryngol 1965;74:880–886.

64. Norden A: Peripheral injuries to the spinal accessory nerve. Acta Chir Scand 1946;94:515–532.

65. Hawkins RJ, Willis RB, Litchfield RB: Scapulothoracic arthrodesis for scapular winging. In Post M, Morrey BF, Hawkins RJ (eds): Surgery of the Shoulder. St. Louis, CV Mosby, 1990, pp 356–359.

66. Ketenjian AY: Scapulocostal stabilization for scapular winging in fascioscapulohumeral muscular dystrophy. J Bone Joint Surg Am 1978;60:476–480.

67. Eden R: Zur Behandlung der Trapeziuslahmung mittelst Muskelplastick. Dtsch Z Chir 1924;184:387–389.

68. Lange M: Die Behandlung der Irrepairablem Trapeziuslahmung. Langenbecks Arch Klin Chir 1951;270:437–439.

69. Lange M: Die Operative Behandlung der Irrepairablem Trapeziuslahmung. Tip Fakult Mecmausi 1959;22:137–141.

70. Cohen JA: Multiple congenital anomalies. The association of seven defects including multiple exostoses, Von Willebrand's disease, and bilateral winged scapula. Arch Int Med 1972;129:972–974.

71. Moseley HF: Shoulder Lesions, 2nd ed. New York, Hocher Publishing, 1933.

72. Shull JR: Scapulocostal syndrome: Clinical aspects. South Med J 1969;62:956–959.

73. Boinet W: Societe Imperiale de Chirurge (2nd series) 1867;8:458.

74. Mauclaire M: Craquements sous-scapulaires pathologiques traites par l'interposition musculaire interscapulo-thoracique. Bull Mem Soc Chir Paris 1904;30:164–168.

75. Bateman JE: The Shoulder and Neck, 2nd ed. Philadelphia, WB Saunders, 1978.

76. Milch H: Partial scapulectomy for snapping scapula. J Bone Joint Surg Am 1950;32:561–566.

77. Ssoson-Jaroschewitsch JA: Uber Skapularkrachen. Arch Klin Chir 1923;123:378.

78. DeMarquay J: Exostosis of Rib. In Dictionare de Medicine et de Chirugie Pratique, 1868.

79. Milch H, Burman MS: Snapping scapula and humerus varus: Report of six cases. Arch Surg 1933;26:570–588.

80. Parsons TA: The snapping scapula and subscapular exostoses. J Bone Joint Surg Br 1973;55:345–349.

81. Steindler A: Traumatic Deformities and Disabilities of the Upper Extremity. Springfield, IL, Charles C Thomas, 1946, pp 112–118.

82. Richards RR, McKee MD: Treatment of painful scapulothoracic crepitus by resection of the superomedial angle of the scapula. Clin Orthop 1989;247:111–116.

83. Von Luschka H: Uber ein Costo-scaplular-gelenk des Menschen. Vierteljahrshefte Prakt Heilk 1870;107:51–57.

84. Roldan R, Warren D: Abduction deformity of the shoulder secondary to fibrosis of the central portion of the deltoid muscle. (Proceedings of the American Academy of Orthopaedic Surgeons). J Bone Joint Surg Am 1972;54:1332.

85. Strizak AM, Cowen MH: The snapping scapula syndrome. J Bone Joint Surg Am 1982;64:941–942.

86. Cuomo F, Blank K, Zuckerman JD, Present DA: Scapular osteochondroma presenting with exostosis bursata. Bull Hosp Jt Dis 1993;52:55–58.

87. Shogry ME, Armstrong P: Case Report 630: Reactive bursa formation surrounding an osteochondroma. Skel Radiol 1990;19:465–467.

88. Gorres H: Ein Fall von Schmerzhaften Skapularkrachen durch Operation Geheilt. Dtsch Med Wochenschr 1921;472:897–898.

89. Volkmann J: Uber Sogenannte Skapularkrachen. Klin Wochenschr 1922;37:1838–1839.

90. Hellstrom M, Jacobsson B, Sward L, et al: Radiologic abnormalities of the thoraco-lumbar spine in athletes. Acta Radiol 1990;31:127–132.

91. Wojtys EM, Ashton-Miller JA, Huston LJ, Moga PJ: The association between athletic training time and the sagittal curvature of the immature spine. Am J Sports Med 2000;28:490–498.

92. Butters KP: The scapula. In Rockwood CA, Matsen FA (eds): The Shoulder. Philadelphia, WB Saunders, 1990, pp 335–366.

93. Arntz CT, Matsen FA III: Partial scapulectomy for disabling scapulothoracic snapping. Orthop Trans 1990;14:252.

94. Grunfeld G: Beitrag zur Genese des Skapularkrachens und der Skapulargerausche.

95. Michele A, Davies JJ, Krueger FJ, Lichtor JM: Scapulocostal syndrome (fatigue-postural paradox). NY J Med 1950;50:1353–1356.

96. Morse BJ, Ebrahem NA, Jackson WT: Partial scapulectomy for snapping scapula syndrome. Orthop Rev 1993;22:1141–1144.

97. Cameron HU: Snapping scapulae. A report of three cases. Eur J Rheumatol Inflamm 1984;7:66–67.

98. Kouvalchouk JF: Subscapular crepitus. Orthop Trans 1985;9:587–588.

99. Wood VE, Marchinski L: Congenital anomalies of the shoulder. In Rockwood CA, Matsen FA (eds): The Shoulder. Philadelphia, WB Saunders, 1990, pp 98–148.

100. Harper GD, McIlroy S, Bayley JI, Calvert PT: Arthroscopic partial resection of the scapula for snapping scapula: A new technique. J Shoulder Elbow Surg 1999;8:53–57.

101. McCluskey GM III, Bigliani LU: Surgical management of refractory scapulothoracic bursitis. Orthop Trans 1991;15:801.

102. Nicholson GP, Duckworth MA: Scapulothoracic bursectomy for snapping scapula syndrome. J Shoulder Elbow Surg 2002;11:80–85.

103. Lehtinen JT, Macy JC, Cassinelli E, Warner JJ: The painful scapulothoracic articulation: Surgical management. Clin Orthop 2004;423:99–105.

104. Bizousky DT, Gillogly SD: Evaluation of the scapulothoracic articulation with arthroscopy. Orthop Trans 1992–1993;16:822.

105. Gillogly SD, Bizouski DT: Arthroscopic evaluation of the scapulothoracic articulation. Orthop Trans 1992–1993;16:196.

106. Matthews LS, Poehling GC, Hunter DM: Scapulothoracic endoscopy: Anatomical and clinical considerations. In McGinty JB, Caspari RB, Jackson RW, Poehling GG (eds): Operative Arthroscopy, 2nd ed. Philadelphia, Lippincott-Raven, 1996, pp 813–820.

107. Pavlik A, Ang K, Coghlan J, Bell S: Arthroscopic treatment of painful snapping of the scapula by using a new superior portal. Arthroscopy 2003;19:608–612.

108. Burkhart SS, Morgan CD, Ben Kibler WB: The disabled throwing shoulder: Spectrum of pathology. Part III: The SICK scapula, scapular dyskinesis, the kinetic chain, and rehabilitation. Arthroscopy 2003;19:641–661.

109. Myers JB, Laudner KG, Pasquale MR, et al: Scapular position and orientation in throwing athletes. Am J Sports Med 2005;33:263–271.

110. Su KP, Johnson MP, Gracely EJ, Karduna AR: Scapular rotation in swimmers with and without impingement syndrome: Practice effects. Med Sci Sports Exerc 2004;36:1117–1123.

111. Cools AM, Witvrouw EE, Declercq GA, et al: Scapular muscle recruitment patterns: Trapezius muscle latency with and without impingement symptoms. Am J Sports Med 2003;31:542–549.

112. Kibler WB, McMullen J: Scapular dyskinesis and its relation to shoulder pain. J Am Acad Orthop Surg 2003;11:142–151.

113. Rubin BD, Kibler WB: Fundamental principles of shoulder rehabilitation: Conservative to postoperative management. Arthroscopy 2002;18(9 Suppl 2):29–39.

114. Marmor L, Bechtol CO: Paralysis of the serratus anterior due to electrical shock relieved by transplantation of the pectoralis major muscle. A case report. J Bone Joint Surg Am 1983;45:156–160.

In This Chapter

INTRODUCTION

- An increased awareness of peripheral nerve injuries about the shoulder and their effect on athletic function is reflected in the growing body of published reports on the subject.

- These injuries have a varied presentation, with associated acute trauma demanding on-field decision making or athletes with chronic symptoms presenting in the clinic after failure of previous diagnostic attempts.

- These injuries present a significant challenge to medical personnel attempting to provide athletes with full and safe participation in competitive activities.

- In this chapter, we discuss the presentation, diagnosis, and management of commonly encountered nerve injuries about the shoulder. These include the burner/stinger syndrome, suprascapular nerve entrapment and surgical techniques used in its treatment, and axillary, long thoracic, spinal accessory, and musculocutaneous nerve injuries.

- Less commonly encountered conditions, such as the Parsonage-Turner and thoracic outlet syndromes, are beyond the scope of this chapter but are mentioned in the context of a complete diagnostic workup.

PERIPHERAL NERVE INJURY

The pathophysiology of peripheral nerve injury has been studied in great detail. Seddon[1] developed the classification system most commonly used today, defining three progressive patterns of injury severity. This has been further modified by Sunderland[2] to include five levels of injury. The mildest form, neurapraxia, involves an interruption of axonal function without frank disruption of the axon. The prognosis for recovery is favorable, with complete functional return expected within weeks to months.

Axonotmesis involves loss of continuity of the axon, with varying degrees of injury to the endoneurium and perineurium. Prognosis for recovery varies greatly due to varying degrees of nerve tissue injury. Wallerian degeneration takes place, and the nerve must regenerate from the site of injury at the rate of 1 mm/day, with recovery of end-organ function possibly taking months. Neurotmesis involves complete disruption of the nerve, including the axon, endoneurium, perineurium, and epineurium, although the outermost nerve sheath may or may not be intact. The prognosis for recovery is very poor, and nerve repair or grafting may be indicated.

The differential diagnosis of peripheral nerve injury about the shoulder includes cervical spine instability, cervical spine fracture, herniated cervical disk, cord concussion/contusion, transient quadriplegia, acute brachial plexitis (Parsonage-Turner syndrome), rotator cuff tear or tendonitis, clavicular fracture, acromioclavicular joint injury, glenohumeral subluxation/dislocation, glenohumeral arthritis, adhesive capsulitis, thoracic outlet syndrome, scapular fracture, and proximal humerus fracture. Each of these must be considered in the evaluation of the athlete with shoulder-related complaints.

TRANSIENT BRACHIAL PLEXOPATHY (BURNER/STINGER SYNDROME)

Clinical Features and Evaluation

The "burner" or "stinger" is one of the most frequently encountered conditions evaluated by athletic team medical personnel. The majority of these injuries occur in American football, in which as many as 65% of collegiate squad members have reported one or more episodes during a 4-year career.[3,4] The syndrome is so frequently encountered by and familiar to athletes that it may often go unreported to team staff.

An athlete with a burner usually presents after a traumatic event with a complaint of pain, numbness, burning, tingling, or stinging pain radiating from the shoulder down the arm, possibly into the hand, most often unilaterally. The athlete may also complain of weakness in the shoulder, elbow, or hand of the affected upper extremity. He or she may be holding the affected extremity by his or her side or be noticed to shake the hand or arm as if it is "asleep" or "dead." More ominous signs may include holding the neck in a flexed position to alleviate pressure on the cervical nerve roots or a complaint of bilateral or lower extremity symptoms. This may suggest the possibility of spinal cord involvement instead of nerve root or plexus injury. Pain localized to the trapezius may be present, but neck pain is usually not a complaint, and its presence, especially if severe, requires medical personnel to initiate spinal precautions and to perform a detailed workup for spinal injury.

The physical examination should focus on the spine and affected extremity of the athlete. Careful attention to the results will help differentiate a relatively benign condition from a more severe injury. Most athletes will have a normal physical examination by the time they arrive on the sideline. Clinical observation of the athlete is followed by palpation for tenderness and deformity along the spine, shoulder, and extremity, facilitated by removal of clothing and protective gear as needed. Spinal examination should then test active flexion, extension, lateral bending, and rotation and, if normal, may include provocative tests such as Spurling's compression maneuver or axial manual traction. The shoulder/extremity examination should concentrate on sensation, motor testing, and reflexes. The upper trunk of the brachial plexus, most often involved in burner syndrome, is evaluated by sensory examination of the C5 and C6 dermatomes, and strength testing of the deltoid, biceps, and rotator cuff. Weak shoulder abduction may be present, even after pain cessation. Deep tendon reflex testing of the biceps (C5), brachioradialis (C6), and triceps (C7) should then be performed. The lower trunk is less frequently involved. Sensory examination is performed with attention to the C7, C8, and T1 dermatomes, and motor testing should concentrate on the intrinsic muscles of the hand, including grip strength and finger abduction.

Relevant Anatomy and Pathophysiology

The exact mechanism of burner syndrome is debated and likely represents varying levels of injury location and severity. The injury location can vary from nerve root, which is thought to be less common in athletic injuries,[5] to peripheral nerve injury, as described previously. The injury level likely is a function of the position of the neck, arm, and shoulder at the time of impact. It is thought to result from a compression or traction (pinchstretch) injury to either the cervical nerve root or the brachial plexus, most frequently the upper trunk.[6]

There are three commonly described mechanisms of injury in burner syndrome, occurring in isolation or combination. Forceful neck extension and lateral bending can cause neural foraminal narrowing, leading to compression of the cervical nerve roots.[6,7] A traction injury may occur from forceful depression of the ipsilateral shoulder, as occurs in blocking, tackling, or wrestling, with the nerve roots fixed proximally.[3] This injury mechanism may be enhanced with lateral bending of the neck to the contralateral side. A third mechanism may be a direct blow to the anterolateral neck at Erb's point (Fig. 29-1), located superior and deep to the clavicle, lateral to the sternocleidomastoid. At this point, the brachial plexus is most superficial and susceptible to injury.

The relationship of cervical stenosis to burner syndrome has been extensively reviewed. The Torg ratio is determined by measuring the distance from the midpoint of the posterior aspect of the vertebral body to the nearest point on the corresponding spinolaminar line and dividing this value by the anteroposterior diameter of the vertebral body on a lateral radiograph.[8] Meyer et al[6] concluded that there was a relationship between cervical stenosis, defined as a Torg ratio less than 0.8, and the occurrence of stingers or nonparalyzing extension/compression injuries, although the clinical significance of the Torg ratio continues to be debated.[9]

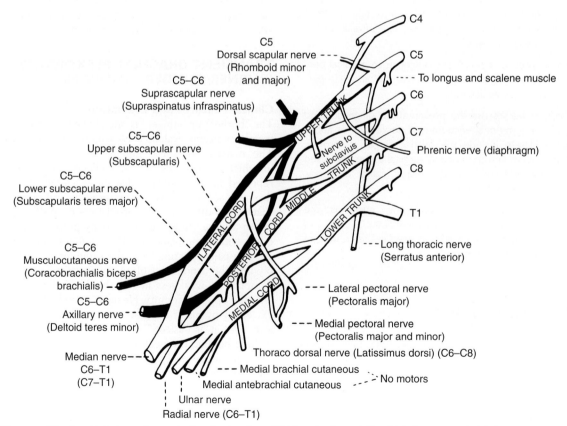

Figure 29-1 Diagram of the brachial plexus demonstrating the location of Erb's point *(arrow)*. Brachial plexus stretch injuries may result from traction at this point. (From Torg JS: Athletic Injuries to the Head, Neck and Face, 2nd ed. St. Louis, Mosby-Year Book, 1991.)

Criteria for Return to Sports

If the athlete's sensory and motor symptoms resolve within seconds or minutes and there is no associated neck pain, range-of-motion limitation, or findings consistent with other more significant injuries to the neck or shoulder, then the player may safely return to competition. Full motor strength is an absolute requirement for return to sports. Paresthesias usually resolve within seconds to minutes and motor symptoms within 24 hours. Persistence of symptoms, including paresthesias, weakness, limited range of motion of the neck or extremity, or pain, requires removal from participation and further evaluation. Persistent or recurrent episodes require complete neurologic workup, including cervical spine radiographs and possibly magnetic resonance imaging (MRI) or computed tomography myelography to assess for cord or root compression. If symptoms persist for more than 2 to 3 weeks, electromyography (EMG) may be useful in determining the extent of injury. However, electromyographic changes may persist for several years after injury and should not be used as a criterion for return to sports. Abnormal findings on these studies require a case-by-case evaluation for return to sports.

A physical rehabilitation program that emphasizes neck and trunk strengthening should be instituted on return to competition. The use of a neck roll, collar, or molded thermoplastic neck-shoulder-chest orthosis,[4] in conjunction with well-fitted shoulder pads, has been shown to decrease the recurrence and severity of episodes in athletes with a history of stingers.

SUPRASCAPULAR NERVE ENTRAPMENT

Clinical Features and Evaluation

Injury to the suprascapular nerve has been associated with multiple sports, including baseball, football, tennis, swimming, volleyball, and weight lifting.[10] Direct trauma to the neck or scapula may cause injury to the suprascapular nerve, and crutch use has been implicated,[11] as has heavy labor. The athlete with suprascapular nerve palsy may present with an often vague range of symptoms or even be asymptomatic.[12] Pain over the posterolateral shoulder or easy fatigability with overhead activities may be reported, or painless weakness of external rotation with or without spinati muscle atrophy may be noted. Compression of the nerve at the suprascapular or spinoglenoid notch is a commonly reported mechanism of injury in the athlete and is discussed in detail.

The physical examination plays a critical role in discerning the site of suprascapular nerve injury. Clinical observation of the athlete's shoulder girdle is important. More proximal injury, as seen with suprascapular notch compression, may result in atrophy of both the supraspinatus and infraspinatus, whereas more distal compression at the spinoglenoid notch will result in isolated infraspinatus weakness and atrophy (Fig. 29-2). Tenderness over the course of the nerve may be present but is often difficult to localize. Weakness of shoulder abduction or external rotation with vague posterolateral shoulder pain may be the only significant examination finding, although a decreased range of motion, specifically adduction, may be noted due to pain.

Plain radiographs of the shoulder are routinely negative. EMG and nerve conduction velocity (NCV) studies play a particularly useful role in the diagnosis and localization of a suspected suprascapular nerve injury. As with most nerve injuries, these studies are generally more useful if obtained in the subacute phase of injury, at least 3 to 4 weeks after onset of symptoms. However, careful clinical correlation with study results

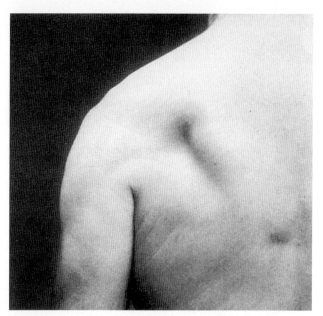

Figure 29-2 Suprascapular neuropathy resulting in infraspinatus atrophy. (From Jobe FW: Operative Techniques in Upper Extremity Sports Injuries. St. Louis, Mosby, 1996.)

must be used, as both false-negative and false-positive nerve findings have been described.[13] MRI may be useful in demonstrating atrophic muscle degeneration of the spinatii or to reveal the presence of a compressive lesion along the course of the nerve. Most commonly, this will be a ganglion cyst, often seen in association with a superior labral tear (Fig. 29-3).

Relevant Anatomy and Pathophysiology

At Erb's point, the suprascapular nerve branches from the upper trunk of the brachial plexus, with contributions from C5 and C6. The nerve then travels below the transverse scapular

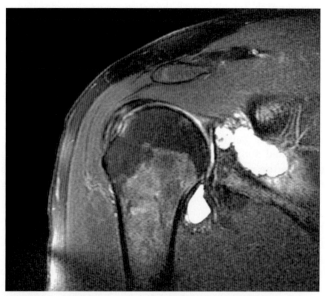

Figure 29-3 Magnetic resonance imaging of the right shoulder demonstrating a ganglion in the spinoglenoid notch compressing the infraspinatus branch of the suprascapular nerve.

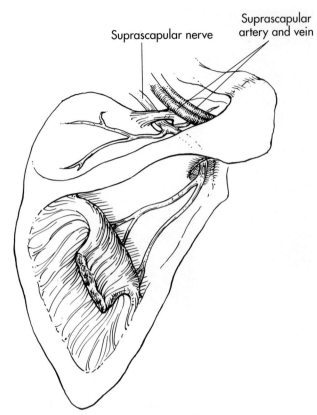

Suprascapular nerve

Suprascapular artery and vein

Figure 29-4 Anatomy of the suprascapular nerve. (From Jobe FW: Operative Techniques in Upper Extremity Sports Injuries. St. Louis, Mosby, 1996.)

ligament as it crosses the suprascapular notch to enter the supraspinatus fossa (Fig. 29-4), while the suprascapular artery usually travels above the ligament. The nerve traverses the supraspinatus fossa, giving motor branches to the supraspinatus, with variable minor sensory contributions to the glenohumeral and acromioclavicular joints and occasionally to the skin.[14] The nerve then angles around the spine of the scapula at the spinoglenoid notch, traveling with the artery under the spinoglenoid ligament.[15] The motor branches to the supraspinatus are approximately 3 cm from the origin of the long head of the biceps, while the motor branches to the infraspinatus average 2 cm from the posterior glenoid rim.[16]

Like other nerves, the suprascapular nerve is susceptible to injury from compression, traction, or direct trauma. Vascular microtrauma has also been postulated to cause nerve dysfunction. The most commonly reported mechanism of injury is compression by a ganglion cyst, usually at the suprascapular or spinoglenoid notch. A thickened or calcified ligament may also compress the nerve. A ganglion cyst is often associated with a tear in the glenohumeral joint capsule or labrum, with fluid being forced through the tear and then being trapped outside the joint.

Treatment Options

Treatment of the acute injury to the suprascapular nerve is similar to that for most nerve injuries about the shoulder. Relative rest and pain control are followed with progressive range-of-motion and strengthening exercises as tolerated. More chronic cases are managed depending on the duration of symptoms and the mechanism of injury, although the exact duration of symptoms is frequently difficult to determine. MRI can be used to evaluate for a compressive lesion. If a compressive lesion or cyst is noted on imaging, the patient can be observed for 2 to 3 months, followed by surgical decompression if symptoms continue (see "Surgery"). An athlete with symptoms associated with repetitive overhead activity, as seen with volleyball, tennis, or baseball players, should be followed for 6 to 12 months with observation, activity restriction, and periscapular therapy, after confirming the absence of a compressive lesion. Periodic EMG/NCV studies can follow the electrophysiologic nerve recovery. Surgical intervention with this overuse mechanism of injury has demonstrated variable results at best,[17] and function usually returns by 12 months. As with other painful nerve injuries about the shoulder, Parsonage-Turner syndrome (acute brachial neuritis) must be considered and, if present, should be managed conservatively with pain control, observation, and therapy.

Surgery

The suprascapular nerve can be approached either with an open technique or arthroscopic technique. If the lesion is proximal and both the supraspinatus and infraspinatus are involved, then the entire nerve should be released, but most importantly the transverse scapular ligament must be released. If only the infraspinatus is involved or if there is a structural lesion in the spinoglenoid notch such as a paralabral cyst, then the nerve may be simply decompressed at the spinoglenoid notch. Associated labral tears should be repaired using standard techniques.

Open Decompression

The suprascapular nerve can be approached either by the direct approach, splitting the trapezius, or by an extensile approach, elevating the trapezius from the spine of the scapula. The transverse scapular ligament is found 2.5 to 3 cm medial to the acromioclavicular joint at the medial border of the coracoid process. With a direct superior approach, the skin is incised in line with Langer's lines medial to the acromioclavicular joint in a typical Saber style. The trapezius muscle is split in line with its fibers for approximately 5 cm. The supraspinatus muscle is retracted posteriorly, and the suprascapular notch and transverse ligament are palpated. The suprascapular artery can either be retracted out of the way or ligated and the transverse scapular ligament is then released. A neurolysis can then be performed. If the ligament is ossified, which can be seen on computed tomography scan, then a small rongeur can be used to remove the bone and decompress the nerve. This approach is cosmetic but limits access to the posterior course of the nerve at the spinoglenoid notch.

For open suprascapular nerve decompression, the authors prefer to use the extensile approach. This allows access to the entire nerve if necessary. An incision is made along the spine of the scapula and the trapezius is elevated and reflected anteriorly. This gives access to the entire supraspinatus fossa. The supraspinatus muscle is retracted posteriorly and the transverse scapular ligament is palpated, visualized, and released as described. By working on either side of the supraspinatus muscle belly, the suprascapular nerve can be visualized over most of its course and can be followed to the spinoglenoid notch. By extending the incision inferiorly and splitting the posterior deltoid, the suprascapular nerve can be traced to its terminal arborization into the motor branches that supply the infraspinatus muscle. The suprascapular nerve runs just at the base of the scapular spine in the spinoglenoid notch. Often there is a thickened band of connective tissue called the spinoglenoid ligament that can tether the nerve in this region. If present, this should be released as well. Since this approach uses extensile, internervous planes, closure is simply done by repairing the trapezius back to the spine of the scapula using nonabsorbable sutures.

Arthroscopic Decompression

An arthroscopic approach is a more sophisticated way of addressing the suprascapular nerve and is our preference when there is an associated intra-articular lesion, such as a SLAP (superior labrum anterior to posterior) tear or labral tear. It is our preferred method for treating spinoglenoid neuropathy due to paralabral cysts, and, furthermore, it is becoming our preferred method for decompressing the nerve at the suprascapular and spinoglenoid notches. It does require advanced arthroscopic skills but offers a less invasive and more cosmetic approach with better overall visualization and access. Moreover, concomitant intra-articular pathology can be addressed easily.

Arthroscopic Release at the Suprascapular Notch

We prefer to use the beach chair position. The arthroscope is placed in an anterolateral portal and accessory anterior and posterior portals are used. The view is initially into the subacromial space. The coracoid process must be visualized and the dissection is then carried medially. Arthroscopic retractors are helpful to retract the supraspinatus muscle belly posteriorly. The dissection is carried along the posterior aspect of the coracoid process. The coracohumeral and coracoclavicular ligaments are identified and at the base of the coracoid the suprascapular notch is identified. The artery is cauterized using radiofrequency ablation, and the ligament is released using hand-held arthroscopic tissue punches (Fig. 29-5). The nerve can be probed to ensure there is no compression. It can be seen passing deep to the supraspinatus.

Arthroscopic Release at Spinoglenoid Notch or Cyst Decompression

This is our preferred technique for treating paralabral cysts. Again the beach chair position is used. Standard anterior and posterior portals are created. A transrotator cuff portal as used

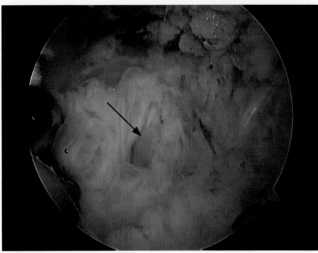

Figure 29-6 Arthroscopic view of right shoulder spinoglenoid notch cyst immediately following perforation (arrow) and decompression. The suprascapular nerve is deep and medial to the cyst wall.

for SLAP repairs is created. The arthroscope is placed laterally through the transcuff portal. This gives excellent visualization. If there is a labral tear, it is repaired with suture anchors using standard technique. Some have advocated working through the labral tear to access the cyst, but we have found this to be quite difficult and furthermore it is virtually impossible to visualize the suprascapular nerve. Therefore, we have gone to performing a capsulotomy, releasing the posterosuperior capsule at the periphery of the labrum until the fibers of the supraspinatus are identified. The supraspinatus muscle is then elevated superiorly using a retractor, which is placed from our anterior portal. With careful and meticulous dissection, the cyst itself can invariably be demonstrated and resected. The typical ganglion cyst fluid is seen when the cyst is perforated (Fig. 29-6). The suprascapular nerve runs 2.5 to 3 cm medial to the superior aspect of the glenoid at the base of the supraspinatus fossa (Fig. 29-7). It can be traced posteriorly from there until it passes through the

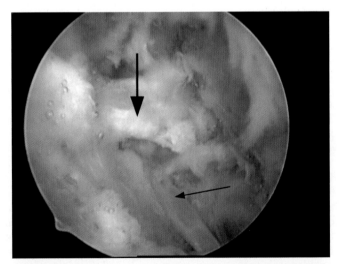

Figure 29-5 Arthroscopic view of right shoulder suprascapular notch demonstrating the transverse scapular ligament (large arrow) traveling over the suprascapular nerve (small arrow). The suprascapular artery above the ligament has been coagulated.

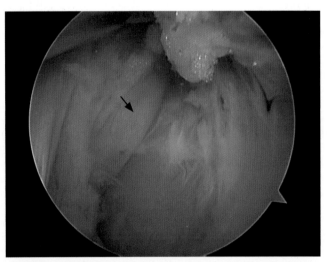

Figure 29-7 Arthroscopic view of right shoulder spinoglenoid notch demonstrating the infraspinatus branch of the suprascapular nerve (arrow) after débridement of the compressive cyst.

spinoglenoid notch. Using hand-held basket punches and arthroscopic probes, a careful neurolysis can be performed.

Results and Outcomes

The results of both operative and nonoperative treatment of suprascapular nerve injuries are not easily interpreted. The duration of symptoms is often difficult to assess, and the diagnosis may be incorrect or incomplete with respect to associated intra-articular pathology. Several studies have reported on the results of both operative and nonoperative treatment.[10,13,17] In a recent meta-analysis of the literature, Zehetgruber et al[18] found suprascapular nerve entrapment to be rare, occurring mainly in patients younger than 40 years of age. Isolated infraspinatus atrophy was most often associated with a ganglion cyst, whereas a history of trauma was usually associated with ligamentous compression of the nerve. Surgical treatment seems to give reliable pain relief, with persistent atrophy of the spinatii muscle, a common but well-tolerated finding.

Postoperative Rehabilitation

Postoperatively patients are immobilized in a sling for comfort. Early motion is encouraged. If a labral tear was repaired, then the athlete is protected for 4 weeks before resuming active motion. Strengthening begins at 6 weeks. Throwing and overhead activities generally commence at 4 to 5 months postoperatively.

Criteria for Return to Sports

While the athlete remains symptomatic, full athletic function should be avoided, especially when the injury mechanism is one of overuse. Patients undergoing surgical intervention for persistent symptoms demonstrate excellent pain relief, and although the spinatii often demonstrate persistent atrophy, return to full competitive activity can still be expected.[19]

AXILLARY NERVE INJURY

Clinical Features and Evaluation

Axillary nerve injury is a relatively common peripheral nerve injury in the athlete, particularly in contact sports.[20] Shoulder dislocation or direct trauma to the deltoid muscle can result in axillary nerve injury and subsequent deltoid or teres minor muscle paralysis. When injury does occur, the athlete often presents not with an obvious motor deficit, but rather may complain of easy fatigability of the shoulder with overhead activity or resisted shoulder abduction.[21] However, the athlete may note weakness of shoulder external rotation, forward flexion, or abduction. Sensation over the lateral aspect of the shoulder may or may not be intact, even in the face of motor weakness.

The quadrilateral space of the shoulder may be a site of compression of the axillary nerve[22] and posterior humeral circumflex vessels, with subsequent injury and dysfunction (Fig. 29-8). The athlete may complain of a vague, poorly localized ache over the lateral or posterior shoulder, often aggravated by activity, especially forward flexion, abduction, and external rotation, as seen in overhead sports such as throwing. A history of unsuccessful shoulder surgery for the pain is not uncommon.

The physical examination should, as stated previously, concentrate on the cervical spine, shoulder, and extremity involved. Observation of the shoulder girdle may demonstrate deltoid and/or teres minor atrophy if the injury is long-standing. A detailed neurovascular examination should always be performed, with special attention paid to sensation to light touch

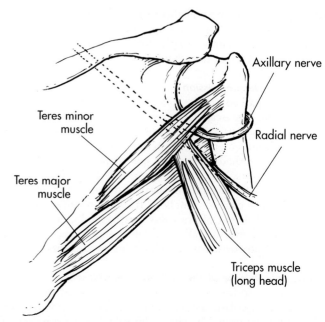

Figure 29-8 The boundaries of the quadrilateral space as viewed from behind. (From Jobe FW: Operative Techniques in Upper Extremity Sports Injuries. St. Louis, Mosby, 1996.)

over the lateral shoulder. Point tenderness is often present over the quadrilateral space[22] if neurovascular compression is present, and this may be accentuated by testing in the FABER (forward flexion, abduction, and external rotation) position.[22] Weakness of external rotation due to teres minor involvement may be present, and deltoid dysfunction may be noted in testing shoulder abduction, forward flexion, or extension.

With respect to diagnostic testing, plain radiographs of the shoulder are a necessity to rule out associated bony injury, especially in the traumatic injury setting. Cervical spine radiographs may also be indicated. EMG and NCV studies are useful to confirm the diagnosis and determine the severity of injury but will likely not be positive until 3 or more weeks after injury. The intermittent compression of quadrilateral space syndrome may result in normal EMG and NCV studies. Magnetic resonance imaging may demonstrate muscle substance changes in chronic cases.

With regard to quadrilateral space syndrome, associated arterial occlusion of the posterior humeral circumflex artery can be diagnosed with arteriography.[22] Historically, the study will be normal with the affected shoulder in adduction but will demonstrate a filling defect with the shoulder in the FABER position (Fig. 29-9). However, magnetic resonance arthrography has demonstrated positive findings in asymptomatic patients, and its value is unclear.[23]

Relevant Anatomy and Pathophysiology

The axillary nerve originates from the posterior cord of the brachial plexus, directly behind the coracoid process and conjoined tendon, with contribution from the C5 and C6 cervical nerve roots. It courses along the anterior inferolateral border of the subscapularis tendon and then passes near the inferior shoulder capsule,[24] receiving a sensory branch from the anterior capsule. The nerve then passes with the posterior humeral circumflex artery through the quadrilateral (quadrangular) space, formed by the long head of the triceps medially, the humeral

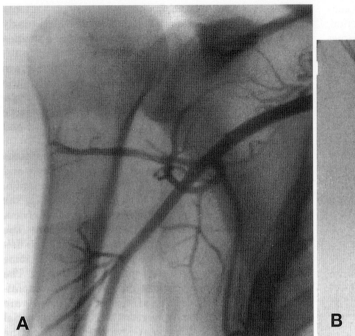 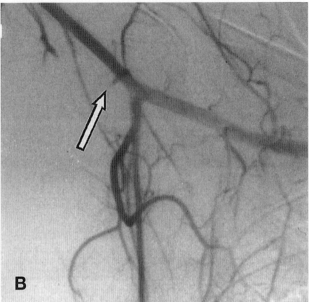

Figure 29-9 An angiogram of a patient with quadrilateral space syndrome. **A,** Digital subtraction angiogram with arm in adduction reveals patent posterior humeral circumflex artery. **B,** Angiogram of same patient with the arm in abduction reveals complete occlusion of the posterior humeral circumflex artery *(arrow)*, confirming the diagnosis. (From Safran MR: Nerve injury about the shoulder. Am J Sports Med 2004;32:803–819, 1063–1076.)

shaft laterally, the teres minor superiorly, and the teres major inferiorly. At this point, it branches into an anterior and posterior branch along the posterior humeral surgical neck. The anterior branch innervates the middle and anterior deltoid, traveling an average of 6 cm distal to the lateral edge of the acromion.[5] The posterior branch divides into the upper lateral brachial cutaneous sensory branch and the nerve to teres minor. The posterior deltoid is variably innervated by the anterior, or less frequently, the posterior branch.[5]

The axillary nerve is relatively fixed at the posterior cord and the deltoid, thus leaving it susceptible to traction injury in anterior shoulder dislocation or proximal humeral fracture. The proximity to the shoulder capsule also makes the nerve susceptible to injury during arthroscopic or open shoulder surgery. Direct injury to the nerve from impact to the anterolateral shoulder has also been reported.[21] The factors that may increase the likelihood of axillary nerve injury with shoulder dislocation include age older than 40 years, unreduced dislocation longer than 12 hours, or higher energy mechanisms of injury.[20]

Treatment Options

The treatment of an axillary nerve injury is a function of the mechanism of injury. Timely shoulder reduction and management of bony injury must be addressed when present, and the athlete should be reassured that the prognosis for recovery of function is good. Even with persistent weakness of the deltoid, return to competitive sports can be expected,[20] although athletes with significant overhead demands may note decreased function. Nonoperative treatment is the mainstay of management of these injuries, particularly in the first 3 to 6 months after injury.[25]

Surgery

In the symptomatic athlete with incomplete clinical or EMG/NCV evidence of recovery after 3 to 6 months, surgery may be indicated. This may include decompression of the quadrilateral space in the presence of a positive arteriogram, neurolysis, or nerve grafting and results in more predictable functional return if undertaken within the first year after injury. Tendon transfer may also be considered for refractory cases, but return to competitive activity may not be possible.

Criteria for Return to Sports

As with other injuries about the shoulder, maintenance of motion is key during the recovery period. Passive, active-assisted, and active range-of-motion exercises should be instituted early. Sport-specific rehabilitation begins when symptoms allow. Residual weakness of the deltoid and teres minor is often well tolerated but may result in easy fatigability of the shoulder. Therefore, a maintenance program of posterior capsular stretching and rotator cuff and periscapular strengthening should be instituted.

LONG THORACIC NERVE INJURY (MEDIAL SCAPULAR WINGING)

Clinical Features and Evaluation

Although relatively uncommon, traction injury to the long thoracic nerve has been recognized in athletes participating in numerous sports. Some of the activities previously associated with this injury include archery, backpacking, baseball, basketball, bowling, football, golf, gymnastics, hockey, rifle sports, shoveling, soccer, tennis, volleyball, weight lifting, and wrestling.[26] The athlete may present with medial winging of the scapula during shoulder forward flexion but more often may note only vague shoulder pain or easy fatigability, especially with overhead activity. Onset of symptoms is often insidious but may be associated with trauma, often a result of depression of the shoulder girdle from a direct blow to the top of the shoulder or a traction injury to the arm.[27] Symptom onset may follow the trauma by several weeks. Acute brachial neuritis should be considered when significant pain precedes the onset of dysfunction, as the long thoracic nerve is often involved in Parsonage-Turner syndrome.

As with any complaint of shoulder pain or dysfunction, the physical examination should include evaluation of the cervical spine, shoulder, and extremity involved. Observation of the shoulder girdle may demonstrate medial winging of the scapula at rest. This involves medial and posterior translation of the inferior angle of the scapula (Fig. 29-10), which can be accentuated with resisted forward flexion of the shoulder, as demonstrated by the wall push-up. Forward flexion may be weak, and serratus anterior muscle atrophy may be noted in the thin, muscular patient. Scapular dyskinesia will be evident,[28] with possible associated impingement symptoms. Relief of the impingement symptoms may be noted with stabilization of the medial scapular border by the examiner while testing forward flexion and abduction. Complete serratus anterior paralysis may limit forward flexion to 110 degrees.[29] Confirmation of the diagnosis with EMG and NCV studies may useful to determine the severity of injury.

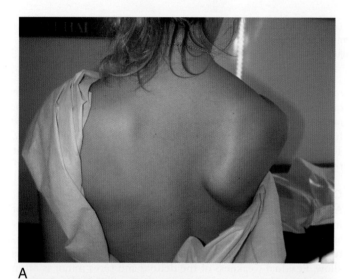

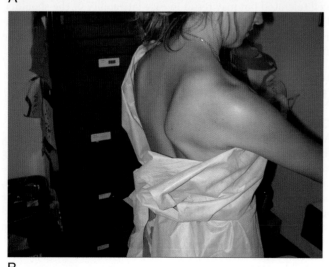

Figure 29-10 Photographs of patient with right long thoracic neuropathy demonstrating medial scapular winging, as seen from behind **(A)** and laterally **(B)**.

Relevant Anatomy and Pathophysiology

The long thoracic nerve originates from the ventral rami of the C5, C6, and C7 cervical nerve roots. There are variable contributions from the intercostal nerves and, less frequently, the C8 cervical nerve root. The individual contributing roots variably pass through or between the middle and anterior scalene muscles, before joining and traveling anterior to the posterior scalene muscle. The nerve then travels deep to the clavicle and variably the first or second rib before exiting the thoracic wall in the midaxillary line. The nerve innervates the serratus anterior muscle slips. The serratus anterior muscle arises from the anterolateral surface of the first eight ribs and inserts into the medial scapular border, functioning to stabilize and protract the scapula during abduction or forward flexion of the shoulder.

In sports, repetitive stretching of the nerve, as may occur in overhead activity, has been implicated in the dysfunction of the serratus anterior muscle.[29] As with brachial plexus injuries, shoulder depression and contralateral neck bending may further contribute to neurapraxia of the long thoracic nerve. Compression from multiple locations along the nerve as well as direct trauma to the anterolateral chest wall may also contribute to injury.

Treatment Options

As with many sports-related nerve injuries about the shoulder, conservative treatment should be the mainstay. The aggravating activity must be curtailed to allow recovery, which can be expected usually within 9 months.[29] Application of a canvas brace may stabilize the scapula enough to prevent stretching of the serratus anterior during recovery but it is insufficient to allow full return to activity.[30]

Surgery

Surgical treatment of isolated long thoracic nerve injury is rarely necessary and is aimed at restoring scapular stability. For severe dysfunction of 6 months' duration or longer, neurolysis may play a role.[31] For refractory cases of longer than 12 to 24 months' duration, transfer of the sternal head of the pectoralis major to the scapula has been shown to provide excellent restoration of scapular function.[32] Scapulothoracic fusion may stabilize the scapula but has been shown to result in significantly decreased function.[33]

Criteria for Return to Sports

Exercises to maintain range of motion should be instituted early, followed by progressive strengthening of the rotator cuff and periscapular muscles. Maintenance of motion is vital during the recovery period, with passive, active-assisted, and active range-of-motion exercises playing a key role. Sport-specific rehabilitation begins when symptoms allow, usually within 6 months of injury. A maintenance program of rotator cuff and periscapular strengthening should be instituted, as with other shoulder injuries.

SPINAL ACCESSORY NERVE INJURY (LATERAL SCAPULAR WINGING)

Clinical Features and Evaluation

The diagnosis of an injury to the spinal accessory nerve in the athlete is often missed due to its rarity, thus potentially delaying its treatment.[34] A history of surgery in the area of the posterior neck, such as a cervical lymph node biopsy, or of penetrating trauma may lead to consideration of the diagnosis.

Blunt trauma to the posterior neck or traction may also result in injury to the accessory spinal nerve.[35] The most common presentation is a painful shoulder or neck, especially with activities that involve using the involved extremity above eye level. Loss of motion or early fatigue may be a secondary complaint. The athlete may note shoulder asymmetry, and rotator cuff impingement symptoms are often present.

Examination of the athlete with a spinal accessory nerve injury will reveal a depressed, or sagging, shoulder on the involved side. The supraclavicular recess may be relatively deepened due to trapezius atrophy. Lateral winging of the scapula, involving lateral rotation of the inferior scapular angle, may be elicited with resisted forward flexion but will not be as dramatic as the medial winging of long thoracic nerve palsy. Inability to elevate the acromion with a shoulder shrug may also indicate trapezius dysfunction. This may result in examination findings of rotator cuff tendonopathy. The levator scapulae and rhomboids may be prominent and palpable due to spasm in their effort to compensate for the weak trapezius. As with many nerve injuries about the shoulder, EMG and NCV studies may be useful in confirming the diagnosis and determining the severity of injury after 4 to 6 weeks of observation.

Relevant Anatomy and Pathophysiology

The spinal accessory, or 11th cranial, nerve exits the skull through the jugular foramen, innervating the sternocleidomastoid and traveling across the posterior cervical triangle to innervate the trapezius. The trapezius arises from the ligamentum nuchae to the lower thoracic vertebrae and inserts into the lateral clavicle, the acromion, and the scapular spine. It functions to stabilize, elevate, and retract the scapula. The trapezius receives innervation not only from the spinal accessory nerve but also the ventral rami of the C2, C3, and C4 spinal nerve roots, possibly preventing complete denervation atrophy after accessory nerve injury. Scapulohumeral dyskinesia may result in depression of the acromion, with resultant subacromial impingement symptoms.

Treatment Options

The treatment of spinal accessory nerve injury depends on the mechanism history. A closed injury, either from a direct blow or trauma, can be observed for a minimum of 6 months. If the patient remains symptomatic with continued pain, sagging of the shoulder, or weakness on forward flexion, surgical exploration with neurolysis, direct repair, or nerve grafting can be considered, especially if EMG/NCV findings confirm dysfunction. In the face of penetrating or operative trauma to the nerve, consideration of surgical exploration should be given after 6 weeks, with the best results reported for surgical intervention within 6 months.[34] It is imperative that shoulder range of motion be maintained during the observation period.

Surgery

As stated previously, local surgical exploration may be beneficial with associated "open" trauma. When symptomatic trapezius weakness continues for more than 12 months, regardless of the injury mechanism, reconstructive surgical intervention should be considered. Tendon transfer procedures, most notably the Eden-Lange procedure with transfer of the levator scapulae and rhomboids, have a good prognosis for return of functional activities of daily living.[36] Prognosis for return to sports, however, is less favorable. Scapulothoracic fusion is an acceptable salvage procedure and may be considered the primary reconstructive option

in patients with heavy demands on the shoulder. Prognosis for return to competitive athletic activity is very poor, however.

Criteria for Return to Sports

Full functional return of trapezius strength is a prerequisite for return to vigorous overhead athletic activity. Many patients may be able to compensate for mild to moderate weakness of the nondominant shoulder, allowing adequate daily activity function and return to less demanding athletic activity. Although shoulder range of motion and strengthening exercises can maximize available function, it is unlikely that the other periscapular muscles can compensate for significant trapezius paralysis, especially if the dominant extremity is involved. Shoulder function may not be sufficient to allow return to competitive activity with persistent trapezius weakness, even after reconstructive surgery.[36]

MUSCULOCUTANEOUS NERVE INJURY

Clinical Features and Evaluation

Isolated musculocutaneous nerve injury in the athlete is rare. It has been reported in weight lifters[37] and rowers[38] and has been associated with strenuous, sustained physical activity. The athlete presents with paresthesias of the lateral forearm, with or without painless weakness of the biceps. The history may often reveal recent surgery to the anterior shoulder, or a direct blow to the anterior chest in the area of the coracoid. Rarely, history of a recent anterior glenohumeral dislocation may be elicited.

The examination must differentiate between isolated musculocutaneous nerve dysfunction and injury to the brachial plexus or C5 or C6 nerve roots. Observation may reveal an atrophied or flaccid biceps, and reflex testing should demonstrate an absent biceps reflex with an intact brachioradialis reflex. The sensory changes will be isolated to the lateral and radial forearm, with sparing of the C6 dermatome of the radial hand. Relative weakness of elbow flexion and forearm supination may also be present.

Relevant Anatomy and Pathophysiology

The musculocutaneous nerve arises from the posterior cord of the brachial plexus, with contributions from the C5 and C6 nerve roots. It enters the coracobrachialis approximately 5 cm distal to the coracoid,[13] although smaller branches may enter earlier. It then exits the tendon approximately 7 cm distal to the coracoid before entering the biceps and brachialis muscles, providing motor innervation to these.[39] The nerve leaves the brachialis and enters the deep brachial fascia above the elbow crease to continue as the lateral antebrachial cutaneous nerve, providing sensory innervation to the anterolateral forearm.

The most common mechanism of injury is associated with anterior shoulder surgery, usually due to vigorous medial retraction of the conjoined tendon near the coracoid, although anterior arthroscopic portal placement may also injure the nerve.[40] This combined motor-sensory dysfunction may be differentiated from the isolated dysesthesias in the lateral forearm that may occur with compression of the musculocutaneous nerve as it enters the deep brachial fascial compartment at the elbow.

Treatment Options

Since most injuries are related to stretching of the nerve, observation of the athlete for a period of 4 to 6 weeks usually results in evidence of recovery. However, continued weakness or paresthesias after 4 weeks can be further evaluated with EMG/NCV studies to determine the level and severity of injury.

Surgery

If clinical and/or electrophysiologic recovery is not noted, surgical exploration within the first 6 months after injury may be indicated. Surgical treatment may include decompression, neurolysis, and nerve grafting or may include nerve transfer using branches of the proximal ulnar nerve. For cases evaluated more than 1 year after injury, tendon transfer procedures may be indicated to supplement weak elbow flexion.

Criteria for Return to Sports

Return to sports-related activity should be customized to the individual athlete. The prognosis for return of full function after postsurgical traction injury or direct blow trauma to the nerve is good, and athletic participation can be allowed. However, if the nerve injury is associated with repetitive or sustained sport-specific activity, modification of the athlete's mechanics may be necessary to prevent recurrence.

CONCLUSIONS

An athlete presenting with pain about the shoulder can pose a significant diagnostic challenge to the athletic medical staff. The etiologies of the symptoms vary from minor to career ending. The examination of the athlete includes a detailed examination of the spine, shoulder, and upper extremity, and nerve injuries must be considered in the wide differential diagnosis. A thorough understanding of the presentation, anatomy, and pathophysiology of nerve injuries about the shoulder of the athlete is imperative for accurate and timely diagnosis and treatment. Prompt management of both bony and soft-tissue injuries may prevent or minimize the long-term impact of these injuries on the athlete.

REFERENCES

1. Seddon JH: Surgical Disorders of the Peripheral Nerves. Baltimore, Williams & Wilkins, 1972.
2. Sunderland S: The anatomy and physiology of nerve injury. Muscle Nerve 1990;13:771–784.
3. Clancy WG Jr, Brand RL, Bergfeld JA: Upper trunk brachial plexus injuries in contact sports. Am J Sports Med 1977;5:209–216.
4. Markey KL, Di Benedetto M, Curl WW: Upper trunk brachial plexopathy. The stinger syndrome. Am J Sports Med 1993;21:650–655.
5. Bateman JE: Nerve injuries about the shoulder in sports. J Bone Joint Surg Am 1967;49:785–792.
6. Meyer SA, Schulte KR, Callaghan JJ, et al: Cervical spinal stenosis and stingers in collegiate football players. Am J Sports Med 1994;22:158–166.
7. Levitz CL, Reilly PJ, Torg JS: The pathomechanics of chronic, recurrent cervical nerve root neurapraxia. The chronic burner syndrome. Am J Sports Med 1997;25:73–76.
8. Torg JS, Naranja RJ Jr, Palov H, et al: The relationship of developmental narrowing of the cervical spinal canal to reversible and irreversible injury of the cervical spinal cord in football players. J Bone Joint Surg Am 1996;78:1308–1314.
9. Brigham CD, Warren R: Head to head on spear tackler's spine: Criteria and implications for return to play. J Bone Joint Surg Am 2003;85:381–383.
10. Martin SD, Warren RF, Martin TL, et al: Suprascapular neuropathy. Results of non-operative treatment. J Bone Joint Surg Am 1997;79:1159–1165.
11. Shabas D, Scheiber M: Suprascapular neuropathy related to the use of crutches. Am J Phys Med 1986;65:298–300.
12. Holzgraefe M, Kukowski B, Eggert S: Prevalence of latent and manifest suprascapular neuropathy in high-performance volleyball players. Br J Sports Med 1994;28:177–179.
13. Post M: Diagnosis and treatment of suprascapular nerve entrapment. Clin Orthop 1999;368:92–100.
14. Ajmani ML: The cutaneous branch of the human suprascapular nerve. J Anat 1994;185:439–442.
15. Plancher KD, Peterson RK, Johnston JC, et al: The spinoglenoid ligament. Anatomy, morphology, and histological findings. J Bone Joint Surg Am 2005;87:361–365.
16. Warner JP, Krushell RJ, Masquelet A, et al: Anatomy and relationships of the suprascapular nerve: Anatomical constraints to mobilization of the supraspinatus and infraspinatus muscles in the management of massive rotator-cuff tears. J Bone Joint Surg Am 1992;74:36–45.
17. Antoniou J, Tae SK, Williams GR, et al: Suprascapular neuropathy. Variability in the diagnosis, treatment, and outcome. Clin Orthop 2001;386:131–138.
18. Zehetgruber H, Noske H, Lang T, et al: Suprascapular nerve entrapment. A meta-analysis. Int Orthop 2002;26:339–343.
19. Ringel SP, Treihaft M, Carry M, et al: Suprascapular neuropathy in pitchers. Am J Sports Med 1990;18:80–86.
20. Perlmutter GS, Apruzzese W: Axillary nerve injuries in contact sports: Recommendations for treatment and rehabilitation. Sports Med 1998;26:351–361.
21. Perlmutter GS, Leffert RD, Zarins B: Direct injury to the axillary nerve in athletes playing contact sports. Am J Sports Med 1997;25:65–68.
22. Cahill BR, Palmer RE: Quadrilateral space syndrome. J Hand Surg [Am] 1983;8:65–69.
23. Mochizuki T, Isoda H, Masui T, et al: Occlusion of the posterior humeral circumflex artery: Detection with MR angiography in healthy volunteers and in a patient with quadrilateral space syndrome. AJR Am J Roentgenol 1994;163:625–627.
24. Price MR, Tillett ED, Acland RD, et al: Determining the relationship of the axillary nerve to the shoulder joint capsule from an arthroscopic perspective. J Bone Joint Surg Am 2004;86:2135–2142.
25. Lester B, Jeong GK, Weiland AJ, et al: Quadrilateral space syndrome: Diagnosis, pathology, and treatment. Am J Orthop 1999;28:718–722, 725.
26. Mendoza FX, Main WK: Peripheral nerve injuries of the shoulder in the athlete. Clin Sports Med 1990;9:331–342.
27. Warner JJ, Navarro RA: Serratus anterior dysfunction. Recognition and treatment. Clin Orthop 1998;349:139–148.
28. Kibler WB, McMullen J: Scapular dyskinesis and its relation to shoulder pain. J Am Acad Orthop Surg 2003;11:142–151.
29. Gregg JR, Labosky D, Harty M, et al: Serratus anterior paralysis in the young athlete. J Bone Joint Surg Am 1979;61:825–832.
30. Marin R: Scapula winger's brace: A case series on the management of long thoracic nerve palsy. Arch Phys Med Rehabil 1998;79:1226–1230.
31. Disa JJ, Wang B, Dellon AL: Correction of scapular winging by supraclavicular neurolysis of the long thoracic nerve. J Reconstr Microsurg 2001;17:79–84.
32. Connor PM, Yamaguchi K, Manifold SG, et al: Split pectoralis major transfer for serratus anterior palsy. Clin Orthop 1997;341:134–142.
33. Bunch WH, Siegel IM: Scapulothoracic arthrodesis in facioscapulohumeral muscular dystrophy. Review of seventeen procedures with

three to twenty-one-year follow-up. J Bone Joint Surg Am 1993; 75:372–376.

34. Kretschmer T, Antoniadis G, Braun V, et al: Evaluation of iatrogenic lesions in 722 surgically treated cases of peripheral nerve trauma. J Neurosurg 2001;94:905–912.

35. Cohn BT, Brahms MA, Cohn M: Injury to the eleventh cranial nerve in a high school wrestler. Orthop Rev 1986;15:590–595.

36. Bigliani LU, Compito CA, Duralde XA, et al: Transfer of the levator scapulae, rhomboid major, and rhomboid minor for paralysis of the trapezius. J Bone Joint Surg Am 1996;78:1534–1540.

37. Braddom RL, Wolfe C: Musculocutaneous nerve injury after heavy exercise. Arch Phys Med Rehabil 1978;59:290–293.

38. Mastaglia FL: Musculocutaneous neuropathy after strenuous physical activity. Med J Aust 1986;145:153–154.

39. Flatow EL, Bigliani LU, April EW: An anatomic study of the musculocutaneous nerve and its relationship to the coracoid process. Clin Orthop 1989;244:166–171.

40. Speer KP, Bassett FH 3rd: The prolonged burner syndrome. Am J Sports Med 1990;18:591–594.

In This Chapter

INTRODUCTION

- Traumatic muscle ruptures about the shoulder girdle are rare. However, these injuries do occur and are typically avulsion injuries to either the pectoralis major or rotator cuff muscles.

- Rupture of one of these muscles can lead to substantial functional disability.

- Pectoralis major ruptures most commonly occur during weight-lifting activities and in response to external trauma, such as during high-impact contact sports.

- Isolated subscapularis tendon tears are relatively rare and usually occur in conjunction with other injuries about the shoulder.

- The purpose of this chapter is to review the relevant anatomy, presentation, and management of traumatic muscle injuries of the pectoralis major and subscapularis muscles.

RUPTURE OF THE PECTORALIS MAJOR

Relevant Anatomy

The pectoralis major is a triangle-shaped muscle that arises from the clavicle, sternum, ribs, and external oblique fascia (Fig. 30-1). The muscle has two heads: clavicular and sternal. As these various origins converge to their insertion at the lateral aspect of the bicipital groove, the muscle twists. Ultimately, the superior fibers insert distally and the inferior fibers insert proximally. These fibers terminate in a flat tendon that is approximately 4 to 5 cm wide. This tendon consists of two laminae, one anterior to the other. The main function of the pectoralis major is to adduct and internally rotate the humerus. The pectoralis major is innervated by the medial (C8–T1) and lateral (C5–C7) pectoral nerves; the muscle receives its blood supply from the pectoral branch of the axillary artery.

Clinical Features and Evaluation

Rupture of the pectoralis major is a relatively rare injury; approximately 200 case outcomes have been described in the literature.[1-3] Few of these reports have more than 20 patients, and to date, there have been no prospective studies that have examined clinical outcomes following surgical repair. The first case report dates back to 1822 and was described by Patissier.[4] Most patients sustain a rupture of the pectoralis major while participating in sports. Weight lifting is the most common activity associated with acute pectoralis tendon rupture. Other sports, including football, rugby, wrestling, rodeo riding, and windsurfing have also been reported to have caused pectoralis tendon injury.[5] The injury usually occurs in skeletally mature males in the third, fourth, and fifth decades of life; there have been no cases reported in a female.

Pectoralis major ruptures are classified as complete or incomplete and usually involve the humeral attachment of either the sternal or clavicular head. Most cases reports describe a complete rupture in an individual participating in athletics. Incomplete tears or complete tears involving the musculotendinous junction or muscle belly have also been reported.[6]

Patients with an acute tear of the pectoralis major often present with some inciting event, whether it be weight lifting or a direct blow to the chest. Many patients will report an audible pop and pain that is described as tearing or burning in nature. In most cases, an immediate disability is noted. As most reported cases are associated with bench pressing, the mechanism of injury is thought to be indirect. A forceful eccentric muscle contraction of the pectoralis major muscle in response to a large, acutely applied load results in the muscle injury. Incomplete or complete tears that involve the muscle belly or musculotendinous junction can also be caused by eccentric muscle contraction, but can also occur following direct trauma to the chest wall. Avulsion injuries of the clavicular and sternal heads may also occur in older individuals.[7]

Physical Examination

A complete physical examination is essential in evaluating patients who are suspected of having a pectoralis major rupture. The patient is examined with a bare chest; symmetry between the two pectoralis muscle bellies is assessed. Patients will often present with a splinted ipsilateral upper extremity often supported by the opposite hand. Ecchymosis may be present in the axilla on the affected side. Physical examination usually demonstrates an obvious defect in the anterior axillary border. Acutely, it can be very difficult to distinguish between complete and incomplete tears because of the local swelling, edema, and ecchymosis in the upper thorax and axillary area. In subacute or chronic injuries, complete tears will often have a bulge where the muscle belly has retracted, a characteristic webbed appearance of the axillary fold, and obvious cosmetic deformity (Fig. 30-2). These findings can be accentuated by having the

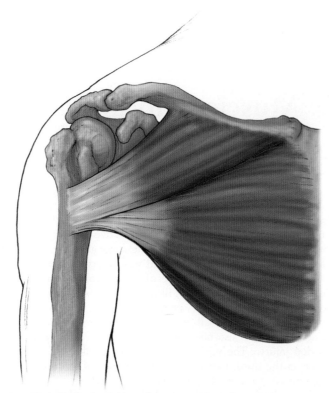

Figure 30-1 Anatomic drawing of the pectoralis major muscle demonstrating its origins from the clavicle and sternum and its insertion onto the humerus.

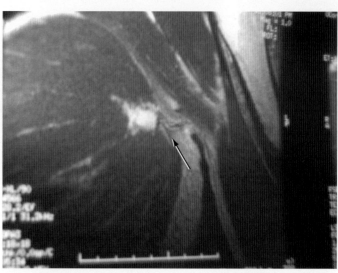

Figure 30-3 Magnetic resonance image demonstrating avulsion of the pectoralis muscle tendon off the humeral insertion (*arrow*).

patient actively contract the muscle by placing both arms in the forward flexed position and having the patient press his or her palms together in front of the abdomen. A great deal of discomfort with minimal movement about the shoulder is present and weakness is noted when the patient tries to adduct and internally rotate the shoulder.

Imaging

Radiographs of the chest (posteroanterior, lateral) and shoulder (anteroposterior, axillary) should be obtained as bony avulsion

type fractures involving the proximal humerus can occur. Typically, radiographs are without significant findings. Magnetic resonance imaging is the gold standard diagnostic imaging modality in detecting pectoralis muscle injury. Connell et al[8] found magnetic resonance imaging to be optimal in evaluating the location, size, and degree of the tear Acute injuries often show a high signal intensity near the humeral cortex, due to periosteal stripping off the humerus as the tendon is avulsed from its insertion[9] (Figs. 30-3 and 30-4). Chronic injuries are more associated with muscle retraction and dense scarring at the lateral border of the pectoralis major.

Treatment Options

Distinguishing between incomplete and complete tears, as well as the location of the tear, is crucial. Most authors agree that partial ruptures of the pectoralis major tendon and intramuscular strain or crush injuries can be successfully treated without surgery. These injuries typically have less pain, swelling, and

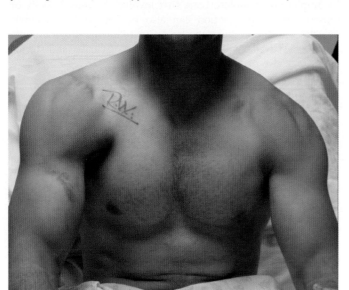

Figure 30-2 A patient with an acute pectoralis major muscle rupture. Notice the webbed appearance of the axillary fold on the right side.

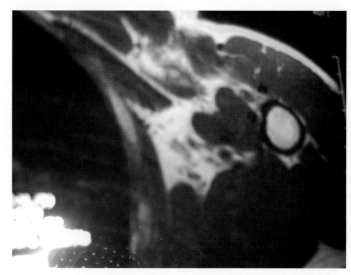

Figure 30-4 Axial magnetic resonance image demonstrating avulsion of the pectoralis muscle tendon off the humeral insertion (*hatch marks*).

ecchymosis and lack the physical examination characteristics that were previously outlined. Initial management should consist of rest, cryotherapy, and sling wear; activity is increased according to patient tolerance. For the most part, these injuries heal without a significant strength loss. It is important to stress the idea of gradual rehabilitation and patients often will not return to heavy lifting for at least 8 to 12 weeks.

Both surgical and nonsurgical approaches have been described in the literature for the treatment of complete rupture of the pectoralis major. Nonsurgical management of complete tears is usually applied in those cases in which an intramuscular injury has occurred. Complete tears of the pectoralis tendon are generally managed operatively. Park and Espiniella[10] reviewed 29 patients and found that only 58% of patients with rupture of the pectoralis major tendon treated by nonoperative means had good results, while nearly 90% in the same series had good to excellent results after surgery. Other studies have also shown poor results after nonoperative management.[11] The goal of surgery is to restore strength, function, and cosmesis. The authors recommend operative repair of the pectoralis major for the active patient who wishes to return to his or her previous level of function; this includes participation in sport. It is clear that the clinical results after surgery are significantly better than those that follow nonoperative treatment. We also recommend surgery for patients who are not satisfied with their function despite extensive rehabilitation.

Surgical Technique: Pectoralis Tendon Repair

Patients indicated for pectoralis tendon repair are positioned in the supine position, with the torso flexed to approximately 45 degrees. Regional anesthesia (interscalene block) is used and should be supplemented with local anesthetic injections at the inferior-most portion of the wound. Following a full prepping and sterile draping of the operative arm, a deltopectoral approach is used. The cephalic vein should be identified and spared if possible. A deep retractor is placed beneath the distal deltoid to facilitate visualization of the humeral insertion of the pectoralis major. The lateral free tendon end is identified and retracted. The muscle belly should be mobilized and freed from any adhesions or residual hematoma. The humeral insertion of the pectoralis lies just lateral to the biceps tendon. The authors' preferred approach uses suture anchors for fixation of the damaged tendon to the humerus. Alternatively, a bone trough can be fashioned and used to reinsert the torn pectoral tendon (Figs. 30-5 through 30-7). Pectoralis repair is preferable in the acute setting, but repair up to 2 years following injury has been described. Chronic cases occasionally require tendon reconstruction with autograft or allograft tissue. This tissue is woven into the distal muscle and sutured in place, and repair to bone is accomplished as described previously, with suture anchors or a bone trough.

Postoperative Rehabilitation

Patients are kept in a sling for approximately 6 weeks. Passive range-of-motion exercises, including pendulum and Codman exercises, are started immediately. Patients are encouraged to begin active elbow, wrist, and hand exercises immediately following the surgical repair. Isometric abduction and external rotation exercises are employed during this early phase. At 6 weeks after surgery, active, active-assisted, and terminal end range stretch passive range-of-motion exercises are begun. At this point, the patient may start to use the extremity for activities of daily living. A weight limit of 20 pounds is suggested for the operative extremity through the first 12 weeks following surgery. Progressive upper extremity strengthening begins in earnest at 6 weeks postoperatively. In general, most patients are cleared for noncontact sports at 4 months; avid weight lifters and contact athletes are held from full participation for 6 months.

Results and Outcomes

In general, because pectoralis major ruptures typically occur in young athletic patients, most surgeons advocate surgical repair in order to regain strength and optimal function. Several studies have shown the advantages of surgical intervention. Wolfe et al[12] found that surgically treated patients showed comparable torque and work measurements, while conservatively treated individuals demonstrated a marked deficit in both peak torque and work repetition. Schepsis et al[13] retrospectively reviewed 17 patients with distal pectoralis major rupture to compare acute and chronic injuries as well as conservative versus operative management. Both subjective and objective results were better in the acute group versus the chronic group, and these patients fared significantly better than patients treated nonoperatively.

RUPTURE OF THE SUBSCAPULARIS TENDON

Relevant Anatomy

The subscapularis arises from the deep surface of the scapula anteriorly and its broad tendon inserts onto the lesser tuberosity of the humeral head (Fig. 30-8). It also acts as a dynamic stabilizer of the shoulder. It is one of the four rotator cuff muscles and is the only one that is an internal rotator of the shoulder. The subscapularis forms the upper border of the quadrangular space, which contains the axillary nerve and posterior humeral circumflex artery.

Clinical Features and Evaluation

Isolated subscapularis muscle tears are uncommon. However, these are significant injuries because they are often difficult to diagnose and can lead to prolonged disability. These injuries typically occur in an older population, although younger patients are more commonly affected in the traumatic setting. The exact mechanism of injury is poorly described in the literature, but it is thought that the typically affected patient falls on an outstretched arm or experiences a traumatic external rotation of an adducted arm. Deutsch et al[14] described a series of 14 shoulders in 13 patients with surgically confirmed isolated subscapularis tears and found that the injuries were a result of violent, traumatic events such as falls, direct blows, or forceful boxing punches. Traumatic hyperextension or external rotation accounted for 11 of the 14 injuries.

Most patients will present with pain, swelling, and disability about the affected shoulder joint. It is important to do a thorough physical examination, looking for other injuries because, as described previously, these injuries are rarely isolated. Weakness of internal rotation along with increased passive external rotation is present. There are a number of tests that are applicable in both diagnosing isolated tears as well as other associated injuries. Gerber et al[15] described a "lift-off" test that is performed by bringing the arm passively behind the body into maximum internal rotation away from the small of the back. If the patient is able to maintain the internal rotation, the test is negative for subscapularis rupture. If the patient cannot maintain maximal internal rotation and the hand drops straight back,

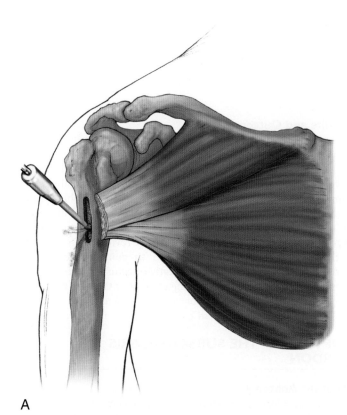

Figure 30-5 A–C, The classic pectoralis tendon repair technique. The tendon is mobilized and tagged with several nonabsorbable sutures that are then used to attach the ruptured tendon to the humerus, using a bone trough medially and drill holes laterally.

A

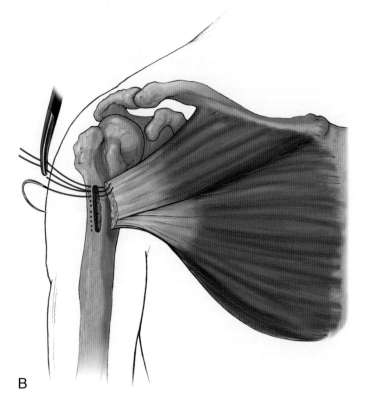

B

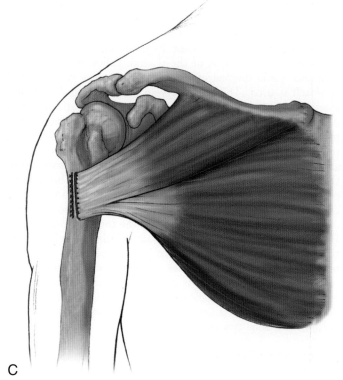

C

Figure 30-6 A–C, The authors' preferred technique of pectoralis tendon repair. This method requires a preparation of a bony bed at the humeral insertion using a bur followed by tendon attachment to bone using double-loaded suture anchors.

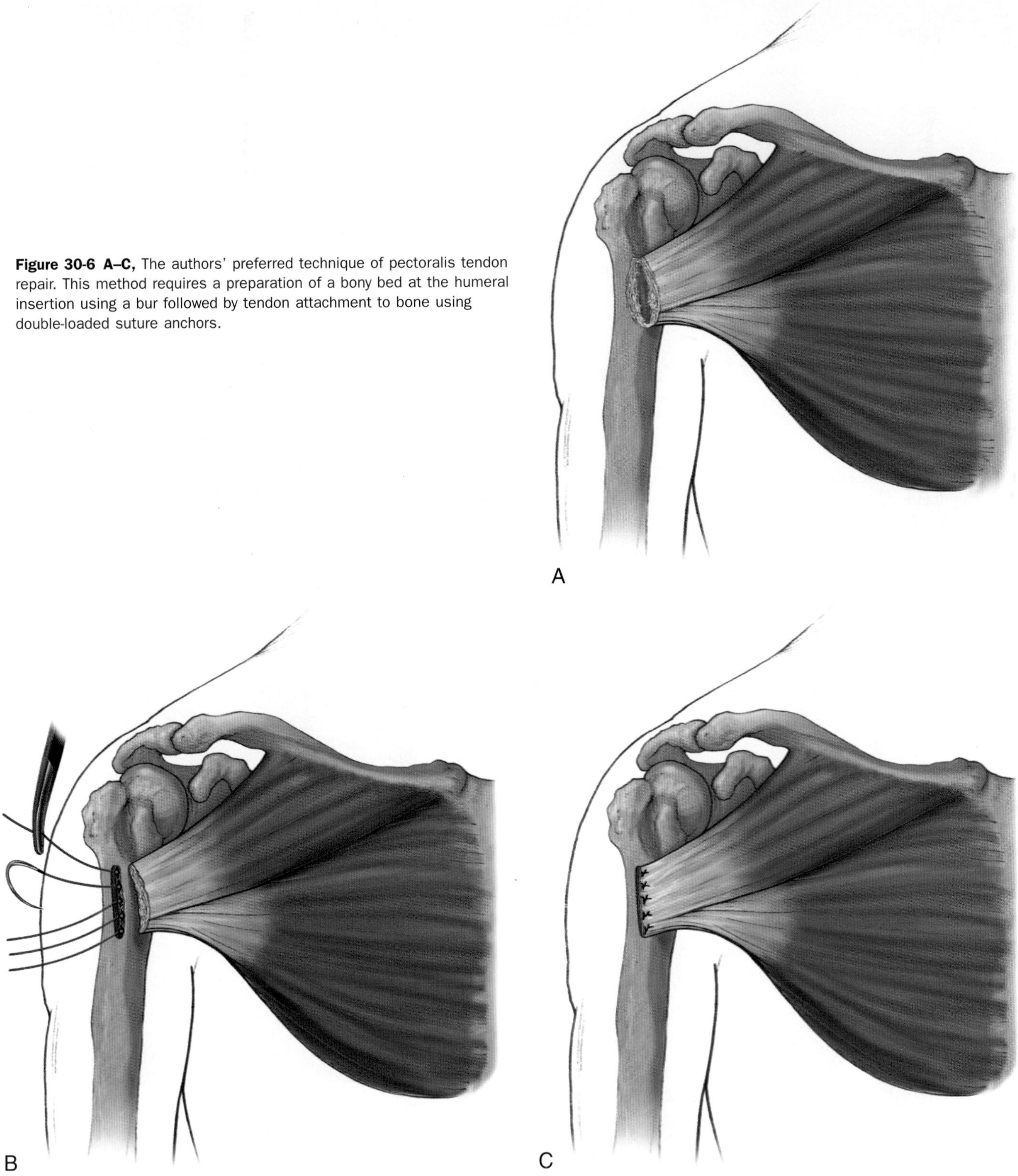

A

B

C

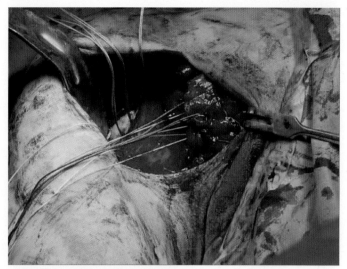

Figure 30-7 Intraoperative photograph demonstrating mobilization of the ruptured pectoralis tendon.

then the test is considered positive. If the resistance is weak and the hand drops back more than 5 degrees but not all the way to the spine, it is called a weak test. In the study by Gerber et al[15] of 16 patients, 13 tests were positive and three were weak. In the same report, they also describe a "belly press test" for instances in which the patient cannot get the hand behind the back to perform the lift-off test. In the belly press test, the patient sits upright and presses the abdomen with the hand flat and attempts to keep the arm in maximum internal rotation. If active internal rotation is strong, the elbow stays in front of the trunk (Fig. 30-9A). If the function of the

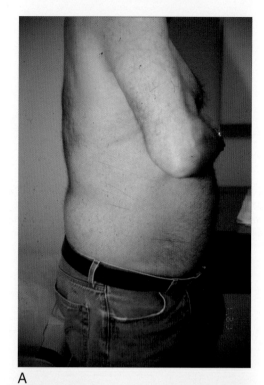

A

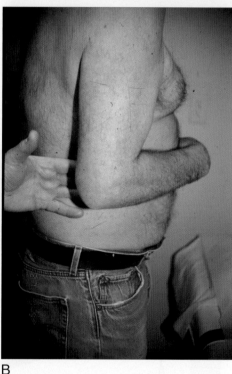

B

Figure 30-9 A, Belly press test as described by Gerber et al.[15] The patient in this figure has a negative test. Active internal rotation by the subscapularis is intact; thus, the elbow remains anterior to the patient's torso during the test. **B,** Positive belly press test. The injured subscapularis cannot internally rotate the humerus during the maneuver; thus, the elbow falls posterior to the torso.

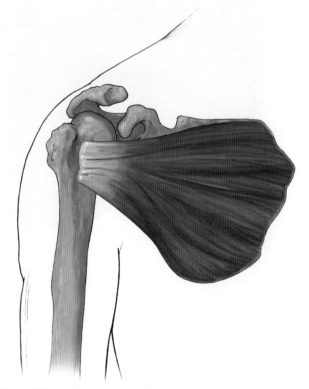

Figure 30-8 Anatomy drawing of the subscapularis muscle demonstrating its origin and insertion.

subscapularis is impaired, then, the elbow falls behind the trunk (Fig. 30-9B). The patient exerts pressure on the abdomen by extension of the shoulder. This test was positive for all eight patients with complete subscapularis tears for whom the study was performed.

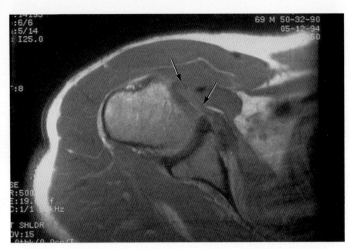

Figure 30-10 Axial magnetic resonance imaging demonstrating an acute subscapularis tear.

Lesions of the biceps tendon have been reported in the traumatic setting of subscapularis tears. The Speed test and Yergason test may be helpful in diagnosing bicipital subluxation or dislocation in the setting of a subscapularis tear. Anterior instability can also be associated with subscapularis tears and can be diagnosed clinically by the apprehension test. Most reported cases of subscapularis tears are associated with supraspinatus tears. We cannot overemphasize the importance of a complete physical examination of the shoulder, even when a diagnosis seems apparent.

Plain radiographs including anteroposterior, lateral, and axillary views of the shoulder will usually not be helpful in diagnosing isolated subscapularis tears. However, they can be crucial in diagnosing avulsion fractures of the lesser tuberosity, subacromial pathology, and dislocation when present. Magnetic resonance imaging is the gold-standard imaging modality in confirming this diagnosis. Deutsch et al[14] emphasized the importance of high-contrast axial plane images that permit visualization of the subscapularis tendon as it inserts onto the lesser tuberosity, as well as the appearance of the long head of the biceps tendon in the bicipital groove. When the biceps tendon is dislocated medially out of its groove, this is nearly pathognomonic for subscapularis injury. Axial magnetic resonance imaging of the shoulder demonstrating an acute subscapularis tear is shown in Figure 30-10. The normal insertion onto the lesser tuberosity is completely disrupted.

Treatment Options
When diagnosing a subscapularis tear, it is important to distinguish between isolated tears and tears associated with other injuries. When tears occur in conjunction with anterior instability, the subscapularis should be repaired during anterior stabilization. Tears associated with lesser tuberosity avulsions, biceps tendon subluxation or dislocation, and other injuries to the rotator cuff also require treatment of all injured structures. There are no reports describing conservative management of symptomatic isolated tears. We recommend primary repair of all isolated injuries.

Surgical Technique: Subscapularis Repair
Patients indicated for subscapularis tendon repair are positioned in the beach chair position. Regional anesthesia (interscalene

block) is used and should be supplemented with local anesthetic injections at the inferior-most portion of the wound. An arm holder is used for upper extremity positioning. Following a full prepping and sterile draping of the operative arm, a deltopectoral approach is used. The cephalic vein should be identified and retracted. A deep retractor is placed beneath the deltoid laterally and the pectoralis tendon medially to facilitate visualization of the anterior shoulder. The subdeltoid bursa and hematoma are removed. The ruptured lateral free edger of the subscapularis tendon should be within the field of view. If the tendon is not immediately visualized, the surgeon should carefully dissect medially along the glenoid neck, posterior to the conjoined tendon and inferior to the coracoid process. Once the tendon has been identified and tagged, the muscle is mobilized to ensure that the lateral tendon edge reaches the lesser tuberosity of the humerus (Fig. 30-11).

The lesser tuberosity is gently prepared using a bur; suture anchors are used to reattach the free subscapularis tendon to the lesser tuberosity. The rotator interval should also be closed using nonabsorbable sutures.

Alternatively, subscapularis repair can be performed arthroscopically. The method is similar. Suture anchors are placed in the lesser tuberosity, the tendon is mobilized, the sutures are passed through the tendon, and arthroscopic knots are tied.

Postoperative Rehabilitation
Patients are kept in a sling for approximately 6 weeks. Passive range-of-motion exercises, including pendulum and Codman's exercises are started immediately. Patients are encouraged to begin active elbow, wrist, and hand exercises immediately following the surgical repair. Isometric abduction and external rotation exercises are employed during this early phase. While passive internal rotation can also be started immediately, no active range-of-motion exercises are started until 6 weeks following surgery. At 6 weeks after surgery, active, active-assisted, and terminal end range stretch passive range-of-motion exercises are begun. At this point, the patient may start to use the extremity for activities of daily living. A weight limit of 20 pounds is suggested for the operative extremity through the first 12 weeks following surgery. Progressive upper extremity strengthening begins in earnest at 6 weeks postoperatively.

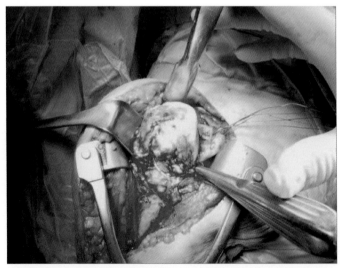

Figure 30-11 Intraoperative photograph demonstrating mobilization of the subscapularis before reinsertion on the lesser tuberosity.

Results and Outcomes

The management of isolated traumatic subscapularis tears has only been addressed in a few studies, most of which are limited by the number of patients. Gerber et al[15] reported on 16 patients treated surgically and found that 82% of the patients assessed their postoperative functional shoulder score as good and that the capacity of the patients to work in their original occupation had increased from 59% preoperatively to 95% postoperatively.

In the study by Deutsch et al,[14] with an average follow-up of 2 years, an improvement in preoperative symptoms, including pain with activities of daily living, pain with attempted sports activities, and weakness of the extremity was reported in 100% of the shoulders tested. All patients returned to their previous employment, and 12 of 13 patients returned to their previous sports activities. Other authors have also reported favorable results after operative treatment.[16-18]

REFERENCES

1. Bak K, Cameron EA, Henderson IJ: Rupture of the pectoralis major: A meta-analysis of 112 cases. Knee Surg Sports Traumatol Arthrosc 2000;8:113–119.
2. Kretzler HH, Richardson AB: Rupture of the pectoralis major muscle. Am J Sports Med 1989;17:453–458.
3. McEntire JE, Hess WE, Coleman SS: Rupture of the pectoralis major muscle. J Bone Joint Surg (Am) 1972;54:1040–1046.
4. Patissier P: Traite des Maladies des Artisans. Paris, 1822, pp 162–165.
5. Dunkelman NR, Collier F, Rook JL, et al: Pectoralis major muscle rupture in windsurfing. Arch Phys Med Rehabil 1994;75:819–821.
6. Zeman SC, Rosenfeld RT, Lipscomb PR: Tears of the pectoralis major muscle. Am J Sports Med 1979;7:343–347.
7. Berson BL: Surgical repair of pectoralis major rupture in an athlete. Am J Sports Med 1979;7:348–351.
8. Connell DA, Potter HG, Sherman MF, et al: Injuries of the pectoralis major muscle: Evaluation with MR imaging. Radiology 1999;210:785–791.
9. Shubin Stein BE, Potter HG, Wickiewicz TL: Repair of chronic pectoralis major ruptures. Tech Shoulder Elbow Surg 2002;3:174–179.
10. Park JY, Espiniella JL: Rupture of pectoralis major muscle: A case report and review of the literature. J Bone Joint Surg (Am) 1970;52:577–581.
11. Liu J, Wu JJ, Chang Cy, et al: Avulsion of the pectoralis major tendon. Am J Sports Med 1992;20:366–368.
12. Wolfe SW, Wickiewicz TL, Cavanaugh JT: Ruptures of the pectoralis major muscle: An anatomic and clinical analysis. Am J Sports Med 1992;20:587–593.
13. Schepsis AA, Grafe MW, Jones HP, et al: Rupture of the pectoralis major muscle: Outcome after repair of acute and chronic injuries. Am J Sports Med 2000;28:9–15.
14. Deutsch A, Altchek DW, Veltri DM, et al: Traumatic tears of the subscapularis tendon: Clinical diagnosis, MRI findings, and operative treatment. Am J Sports Med 1997;25:13–22.
15. Gerber C, Hersche O, Farron A: Isolated rupture of the subscapularis tendon: Results of operative repair. J Bone Joint Surg Am 1996;78:1015–1023.
16. Gerber C, Krushell RJ: Isolated ruptures of the tendon of the subscapularis muscle. J Bone Joint Surg Br 1991;73:389–394.
17. McAuliffe TB, Dowd GS: Avulsion of the subscapularis tendon: A case report. J Bone Joint Surg 1987;69:1454–1455.
18. Edwards TB, Walch G, Sirraux F, et al: Repair of tears of the subscapularis. J Bone Joint Surg Am 2005; 87:725–730.

Pediatric Shoulder

T. Bradley Edwards and K. Mathew Warnock

In This Chapter

Clavicle fracture
Proximal humerus fracture
Glenohumeral dislocation/instability
Acromioclavicular (AC) and sternoclavicular (SC) dislocation/instability
Little leaguer's shoulder
Internal impingement
Scapular winging

INTRODUCTION

- Although once considered rare, increasing participation of children in sports has increased the frequency of pediatric shoulder injuries.

- The majority of pediatric shoulder injuries involve fractures of the shoulder girdle, both physeal and extraphyseal.

- The increasing level of competition within organized pediatric athletics, however, has led to a rise in the occurrence of overuse-type injuries.

- Most pediatric shoulder problems, whether traumatic or related to overuse, can be successfully treated nonoperatively.

RELEVANT ANATOMY AND PHYSIOLOGY

The principal anatomic factor differentiating pediatric shoulder injuries from adult shoulder injuries is the presence of open physes. The proximal humerus is formed by the coalescence of three ossification centers (humeral head, greater tuberosity, lesser tuberosity) occurring between 5 and 7 years of age. The remaining proximal humeral physis between the epiphysis and metaphysis contributes 80% of the longitudinal growth to the humerus and completely closes between 19 and 22 years of age.[1] The proximal humeral physis is commonly involved in both traumatic and overuse pediatric shoulder injuries.

The clavicle, one of the most frequently fractured bones in childhood, forms via intramembranous ossification. The medial physis of the clavicle is the last to fuse in the body between 22 and 27 years of age and provides 80% of the longitudinal growth of the clavicle.[1] The scapula is similarly formed by intramembranous ossification and is largely protected from injury during sports participation by its close proximity to the thorax and protective muscular covering.

Physeal biomechanics play a role in the type of injuries observed in pediatric athletes. In early childhood, the cartilaginous nature of the physis protects the ossified portions of the bone by helping absorb forces. When this absorptive capacity is overcome, residual forces are transmitted to the metaphysis resulting in a torus type fracture. In later childhood, the resiliency of the physis is reduced, and, by virtue of its relative biomechanical weakness, the physis becomes the most likely site of fracture.[1] The physis is susceptible to not only acute fracture, but also stress fracture from overuse.

The soft tissues of the shoulder girdle are grossly identical to those observed in adults. In our experience, we have noted, however, that the amount of physiologic laxity present in children exceeds that observed in adults. This observation becomes important when evaluating a patient for glenohumeral instability, particularly when evaluating pediatric patients with multidirectional hyperlaxity. As these patients complete adolescence, much of this hyperlaxity will resolve, in many cases resulting in resolution of shoulder symptoms.

RELEVANT BIOMECHANICS

The biomechanics of throwing are well described and have been divided into wind-up, cocking, acceleration, and follow-through.[2] Large forces are generated during throwing with peak angular velocity rates exceeding 7000 degrees per second occurring during the acceleration phase.[3] The forces generated during throwing have unique implications in the immature athlete. The effects of competitive throwing on a skeletally immature proximal humerus are usually adaptive and protective but in some cases become pathologic.

As the arm enters late cocking and transitions to early acceleration, a large external rotation torsional moment is placed on the arm. As the soft tissues of the shoulder (rotator cuff, capsuloligamentous structures) reach maximal limits of external rotation, the remaining forces are transmitted to the humerus. These torsional forces preferentially affect the weaker physis. With repetitive throwing, these forces result in an adaptive and protective remodeling of the proximal humerus.

Previously, throwers were thought to have increased external rotation and decreased internal rotation in their dominant shoulder as a result of lax anterior soft tissue and a tight posterior capsule. More recently, however, it has been recognized that osseous change in the form of increased humeral retroversion is largely responsible for this phenomenon.[4] The torsional forces occurring with repetitive throwing introduce remodeling of the proximal humerus through the open physis resulting in more humeral retroversion (Fig. 31-1). This remodeling provides two benefits. First, increased external rotation is advantageous to pitching mechanics, allowing for greater throwing velocity. Second, increased humeral retroversion effectively moves the

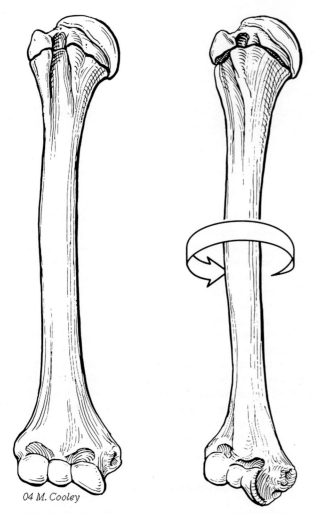

04 M. Cooley

Figure 31-1 The torsional forces occurring with repetitive throwing introduce remodeling of the proximal humerus through the open physis resulting in more humeral retroversion.

greater tuberosity further away from the posterior superior glenoid rim, minimizing the mechanical contact now referred to as internal impingement (Fig. 31-2).

Unrestricted throwing by skeletally immature patients may create a pathologic effect. The repetitive forces acting on the physis may cause what is effectively a stress fracture. This phenomenon has been well described and tagged with the moniker "little leaguer's shoulder."[5]

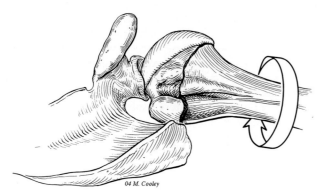

04 M. Cooley

Figure 31-2 Increased humeral retroversion effectively moves the greater tuberosity further away from the posterior superior glenoid rim minimizing the mechanical contact now referred to as internal impingement.

FRACTURES, DISLOCATIONS, AND INSTABILITY

Clavicle Fractures

Clavicle fractures are among the most common injuries observed in childhood sports. These injuries usually result from a fall onto the shoulder during activity. These fractures most often occur in the midshaft of the clavicle but may also be observed at the terminal portions of the bone.

Clinical Features and Evaluation

Pain, swelling, and deformity are the common presenting features of a clavicle fracture. Physical examination of the shoulder girdle is usually limited by pain in the acute setting. Particular attention is paid to skin and soft tissues overlying the area of injury to ensure that fracture fragments do not jeopardize these structures. Additionally, a thorough neurovascular examination is performed to evaluate for compromise caused by displaced fracture fragments.

Physical examination is always followed by radiographic examination of the clavicle. In cases with midshaft deformity, a simple anterior posterior radiograph of the clavicle is sufficient. In cases with lateral deformity, a 20-degree cephalic tilt acromioclavicular joint view is added.[1] In cases with medial deformity, a sternoclavicular joint view is added (serendipity view).[1] Fractures of the medial and lateral clavicle most commonly occur through the physis and may appear radiographically as a dislocation of the sternoclavicular or acromioclavicular joints. In cases of medial clavicle fractures presenting with signs of neurovascular compromise, difficulties breathing or swallowing, or posterior displacement on plain radiography, computed tomography should be performed as part of the evaluation.

Treatment and Results

Treatment of clavicle fractures in pediatric patients is largely nonoperative. Clavicle fractures generally do not require reduction because of the remarkable ability to remodel in the pediatric and adolescent age group. Children up to age 17 years have shown the ability to remodel clavicle fractures with as much as 90 degrees of angulation and as much as 4 cm of overlap.[6]

The vast majority of middle third clavicle fractures are best treated nonoperatively. Nonoperative treatment of clavicle fractures in the pediatric age group is sling immobilization. Reduction maneuvers are seldom necessary or helpful. Figure-eight strapping is often uncomfortable and unnecessary. Shortening and malunion generally do not occur in children, and the clinical results are usually excellent, with most fractures healing successfully with nonoperative treatment (Fig. 31-3).

In the skeletally immature patient, operative management is indicated in open fractures or when the clavicle impinges on the subclavian vessels or brachial plexus causing neurologic or vascular compromise. "Floating shoulder," a concomitant fracture of the clavicle and scapula, is a relative indication for operative management; however, this severe injury is very rare in childhood athletics, only occurring with severe trauma such as might be seen in junior motor cross.

Occasionally, in adolescents who are approaching or who have reached skeletal maturity, operative management is indicated. These patients often have comminuted fractures or large butterfly fragments, and many have considerable shortening of the clavicle. Highly competitive athletes nearing skeletal maturity, especially those who use their arm for overhead sports or throwing, may benefit from open reduction and internal fixation.

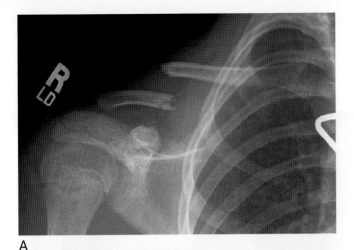

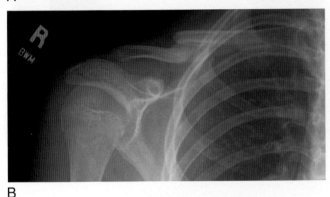

Figure 31-3 A, Displaced midshaft clavicle fracture in a skeletally immature patient. **B,** Complete healing of the fracture 6 weeks later.

Medial clavicle fractures are usually physeal injuries that successfully remodel in pediatric patients. The best treatment for these injuries is nonoperative. Patients with a posteriorly displaced medial clavicle fracture who have difficulty swallowing or breathing or signs of neurovascular compromise may require operative reduction. Operative reduction is performed under general anesthesia in the operating room with a thoracic surgeon available in case of vascular complications.

The distal clavicle, like the medial clavicle, has tremendous potential for remodeling. Most pediatric distal clavicle fractures can be treated nonoperatively. Some distal clavicle injuries in children are, however, actually periosteal sleeve avulsion injuries.[1] In these injuries, the lateral clavicle rips through the thick periosteal sleeve that surrounds the distal clavicle. The acromioclavicular and coracoclavicular ligaments are strongly attached to the periosteum of the distal clavicle. In cases of severe displacement, management involves operative reduction, placing the clavicle back into the thick periosteal sleeve, and repairing the periosteum with sutures.

Rehabilitation after clavicle fracture should begin as soon as pain permits. Initially, pendulum exercises are begun followed by isometric exercises of the triceps, biceps, deltoid, and rotator cuff muscles. Normal activities of daily living are permitted, and active range of shoulder motion is begun 4 to 6 weeks after injury. Strengthening begins when there is radiographic evidence of healing and the patient has regained full range of shoulder motion. When strength has returned to normal, a return to non-contact sports is permitted. Contact sports are permitted when there is adequate radiographic and clinical evidence of healing and sufficient remodeling, usually around 3 months after injury.

Generally, results of treatment of clavicle fractures in children are excellent without residual dysfunction.

Proximal Humerus Fractures

Proximal humeral fractures in children are relatively common and may involve the growth plate or be strictly metaphyseal. Most of these fractures occur as a result of a fall during activity, although rarely insignificant trauma will cause a proximal humeral fracture through a preexisting benign bone cyst. Physeal fractures with varus displacement have been reported in skeletally immature gymnasts.[7] Proximal humeral physeal fractures have tremendous remodeling potential. This fact combined with a wide arc of shoulder motion allows for good shoulder function despite significant fracture displacement.

Clinical Features and Evaluation

Proximal humerus fractures generally present with pain and deformity. The deformity is often obvious with the arm held in internal rotation. Physical examination consists of palpation, which causes pain at the fracture site, and neurovascular examination. Further examination is usually limited by pain. Radiographs are always obtained including perpendicular views of the proximal humerus and of the entire humerus. Fractures are usually obvious on radiographs; however, certain nondisplaced physeal fractures may have normal-appearing radiographs. In this circumstance, diagnosis of nondisplaced physeal fracture is largely clinical.

Treatment and Results

Most proximal humeral fractures can be treated nonoperatively. Metaphyseal and physeal fractures that are nondisplaced or minimally angulated are generally stable and heal quite well with immobilization followed by early pendulum exercises. Displaced fractures often have a bayonet apposition with shortening. These fractures generally heal with minimal residual deformity, especially in younger children. Patients who are approaching skeletal maturity with more limited remodeling potential may require closed reduction with or without internal fixation. Dameron and Rockwood[8] have proposed guidelines for managing pediatric proximal humeral fractures. Nonoperative treatment is indicated in patients younger than 5 years of age with less than 70 degrees of angulation and as much as 100% displacement and in patients 5 to 12 years of age with less than 40 degrees of angulation and 50% displacement. Patients older than 12 years of age have more limited remodeling potential and should be treated more aggressively in cases of moderate to severe angulation and displacement.

Nonoperative treatment consists of early pendulum exercises as soon as the fracture is stable. Formal rehabilitation is generally begun 3 to 4 weeks after the initial injury when the fracture shows early signs of consolidation. Early passive motion exercises are followed by active range of motion exercises. Subsequent physical therapy focuses on strengthening of the rotator cuff, trapezius, and deltoid muscles. Full return to sports is usually allowed between 3 and 6 months.

In patients approaching skeletal maturity with moderate to severely displaced proximal humeral fractures, reduction should be performed to avoid potential deformity and functional limitation. Specifically, high-level athletes involved with overhead sports or throwing may require operative treatment. These patients require a near anatomic reduction in order to regain full shoulder motion and return to their same level of play. We emphasize, however, that operative treatment should generally be reserved for patients with little or no growth remaining who are unlikely to remodel significantly displaced fractures.

Reduction of proximal humeral fractures is generally carried out with the patient under anesthesia. A reduction of maneuver of longitudinal traction, abduction, and external rotation will usually reduce the fracture. Fluoroscopic examination is helpful to assess adequacy of reduction and stability. If the fracture is unstable, percutaneous fixation with Kirschner wires is used (Fig. 31-4). The wires can be left protruding externally allowing for removal in clinic at about 4 weeks postoperatively. Rarely,

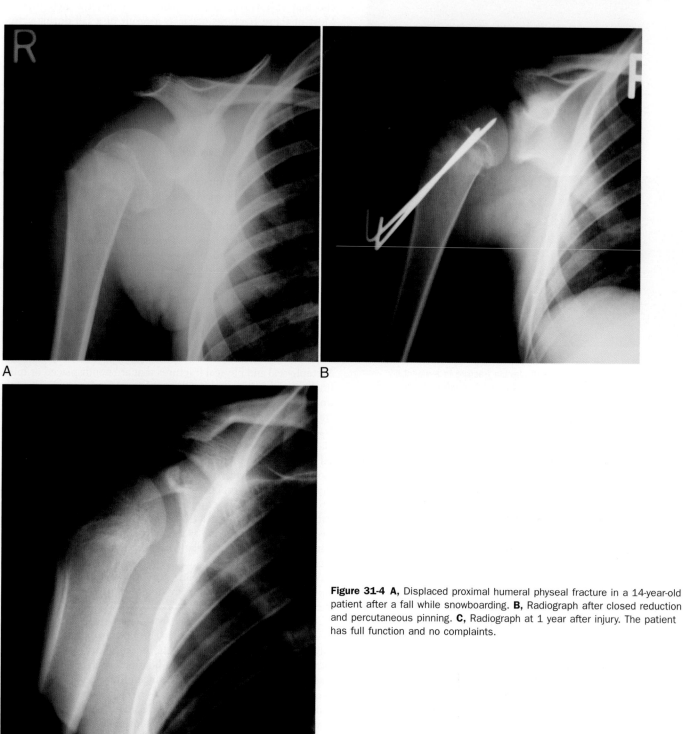

Figure 31-4 A, Displaced proximal humeral physeal fracture in a 14-year-old patient after a fall while snowboarding. **B,** Radiograph after closed reduction and percutaneous pinning. **C,** Radiograph at 1 year after injury. The patient has full function and no complaints.

closed reduction is not possible because of soft-tissue incarceration. In this scenario, open reduction is necessary. After surgery, rehabilitation consists of the same regimen used for nonoperative treatment of proximal humerus fractures with full return to sports expected between 3 and 6 months postoperative.

Glenohumeral Dislocations/Instability
Traumatic dislocations of the shoulder in young skeletally immature patients are rare. However, traumatic dislocations are seen in adolescents, and recurrent instability in these patients is a common problem. Anterior dislocations are far more common than posterior and inferior dislocations.

Clinical Features and Evaluation
Anterior shoulder dislocations present with pain, swelling, and deformity. The acromion often appears prominent, and the posterolateral portion of the shoulder may appear flattened. The arm is generally supported and held in an abducted and externally rotated position. Pain is present with movement of the shoulder. The humeral head is usually palpable anterior to the glenoid. Posterior shoulder dislocations present with the arm at the side and the forearm internally rotated. A painful loss of external rotation and inability to supinate the forearm is commonly seen in posterior dislocations. In athletic events, posterior dislocations are often associated with posteriorly directed force acting on the outstretched arm. Inferior shoulder dislocations present with the arm abducted, the elbow flexed, and the hand above the head and may result from a hyperabduction force acting on the arm.

Evaluation of the neurologic and vascular status of the arm is an essential part of the physical examination both initially and after reduction. The remainder of the physical examination is limited in acute dislocations. In patients with initial or recurrent glenohumeral instability presenting in the subacute phase, complete physical examination including stability examination is usually possible (details of shoulder examination for instability are covered in Chapter 16).

With acute shoulder dislocation, two perpendicular radiographic views of the shoulder are obtained. These are used to identify the presence of any fractures as well as the direction of the dislocation. Postreduction radiographs confirm the reduction and help identify any associated injuries. In the subacute setting, we use an anteroposterior radiograph and a glenoid profile radiograph, as described by Bernageau et al[9,10] to identify osseous abnormalities consistent with instability. In patients with suspected instability (no clear history of dislocation) and normal radiographs, we obtain secondary imaging with magnetic resonance arthrography to confirm the presence of instability lesions, that is, labral injury.

Treatment and Results
The treatment of acute shoulder dislocations includes sedation or an intra-articular lidocaine injection followed by reduction using one of the standard reduction techniques. Care must be used during the reduction maneuver to prevent a proximal humerus fracture.

Considerable debate exists over proper management of adolescent first-time shoulder dislocations. While some authors recommend surgical stabilization after an initial instability episode to prevent recurrence, new research suggests that a brief period of immobilization in external rotation after reduction of a traumatic anterior dislocation reduces the incidence of recurrent instability.[11,12]

In the absence of early immobilization in external rotation, the incidence of recurrent shoulder instability after an acute traumatic shoulder dislocation in young patients is extremely high. These patients may benefit from surgery after a traumatic first-time shoulder dislocation. Details of operative treatment of recurrent shoulder instability are detailed in preceding chapters.

Atraumatic Shoulder Instability
Atraumatic shoulder instability is the most common type of instability seen in skeletally immature patients. Rehabilitation should be the mainstay of treatment for nearly all these cases. The goal of treatment is to increase the dynamic stabilization force of the shoulder joint by strengthening the rotator cuff musculature. Second, the scapular stabilizers should be strengthened to maintain proper positioning of the glenoid in relation to the humeral head. Neuromuscular control should also be emphasized during rehabilitation to improve shoulder proprioception. A minimum of 12 months of aggressive rehabilitation and avoidance of provocative maneuvers should be achieved before surgical management should be considered. Most patients will eventually improve with the passage of time. Voluntary dislocators comprise a unique group that should almost universally be treated nonoperatively.[13]

Acromioclavicular and Sternoclavicular Dislocations/Instability
Since the joint capsule and ligaments in a child are much stronger than the physis, sternoclavicular and acromioclavicular dislocations are extremely rare in the pediatric population. Acromioclavicular separations are generally not seen until adolescence at which time they can be treated like adult injuries (see Chapter 26). Skeletally immature patients may appear to have an acromioclavicular separation, but most of these injuries are actually physeal fractures.

Injuries to the lateral clavicle and acromioclavicular joint are different in children compared to adults. The pediatric distal clavicle has a thick periosteal tube that is continuous with the acromioclavicular joint. The acromioclavicular joint is rarely dislocated in children because the weak link is the physis, not the ligamentous attachments. The acromioclavicular and coracoclavicular ligaments are tightly connected to the periosteum encasing the distal clavicle. Injuries to this area most commonly result in physeal fractures with the distal clavicle splitting out of the periosteal sleeve. True dislocations of the sternoclavicular joint in children and adolescents are very rare. Medial clavicular injuries usually affect the medial physis of the clavicle.

OVERUSE INJURIES

Proximal Humeral Epiphyseolysis
Proximal humeral epiphyseolysis, more commonly known as little leaguer's shoulder, is an overuse injury occurring exclusively in skeletally immature throwing athletes and almost exclusively in baseball pitchers.[5,14] During repetitive throwing, torsional forces act on the arm, externally rotating the humerus distally, while the proximal portion is secured at the glenohumeral joint via the capsuloligamentous structures. These forces result in remodeling of the proximal humerus through the weakest osseous point, the proximal humeral physis. When throwing becomes excessive, this remodeling phenomenon may become pathologic resulting in a stress fracture through the proximal humeral physis.

Clinical Features and Evaluation

Individuals presenting with proximal humeral epiphyseolysis are nearly always high level little league baseball pitchers between 10 and 14 years of age.[14] They report progressive onset of pain that occurs only with throwing activities. They also commonly report loss of velocity and/or control of their pitches. They usually are able to participate in hitting activities without exacerbation of symptoms.

Physical examination findings may demonstrate mild tenderness over the proximal humeral physis with deep palpation. A provocative maneuver of abduction, external rotation, and extension may produce pain in the dominant shoulder. Alternatively, examination may not reveal any pathologic findings. Mobility examination usually demonstrates greater external rotation and less internal rotation of the dominant shoulder compared to the nondominant shoulder. This discrepancy in the arc of motion between the two shoulders is a result of physiologic remodeling and is a nonspecific finding in pitchers.[4]

Radiographic examination serves to confirm the diagnosis of proximal humeral epiphyseolysis, which is suspected initially largely based on the history. Proximal humeral radiographs demonstrate widening of the physis, usually most readily apparent on the anteroposterior view. Comparative radiographs of the contralateral proximal humerus are helpful in confirming the pathologic condition of the physis (Fig. 31-5).

Treatment and Results

Treatment of proximal humeral epiphyseolysis involves a period of selective rest and activity modification. After diagnosis of proximal humeral epiphyseolysis, repetitive throwing activities are halted for a period of 3 months. During this time, painless activities such as hitting are allowed. Often pitchers are allowed to play first base, enabling continuation of hitting while minimizing throwing activities. After 3 months of activity restrictions, gradual resumption of throwing is allowed, preferably using a progressive throwing program under the supervision of a qualified athletic trainer or physical therapist. Provided symptoms do not recur, full return to pitching is usually possible within 6 months of initiation of treatment. Recurrence of pain with throwing is treated with prolongation of throwing restrictions until symptoms subside.

Appropriate treatment of proximal humeral epiphyseolysis nearly always results in successful return to throwing activities. Rarely, a patient may have continued symptoms preventing pitching until reaching a more skeletally mature age. We have never observed a case of permanent physeal damage or early physeal closure caused by proximal humeral epiphyseolysis.

Internal Impingement

Internal impingement, or posterosuperior glenoid impingement, is the contact that occurs between the greater tuberosity and the posterosuperior aspect of the glenoid rim during abduction, external rotation, and extension of the arm (Fig. 31-6).[15,16] This contact is physiologic, occurring in nearly all individuals including the skeletally immature. In the throwing athlete, the repetitive nature of this contact can result in pathologic glenohumeral lesions including partial thickness rotator cuff tears and/or superior labral tears.

In the skeletally immature throwing athlete, symptomatic internal impingement is uncommon with proximal humeral epiphyseolysis predominating as the cause of pain. When symptomatic internal impingement occurs in pediatric athletes, it usually results from poor pitching mechanics. Davidson et al[17]

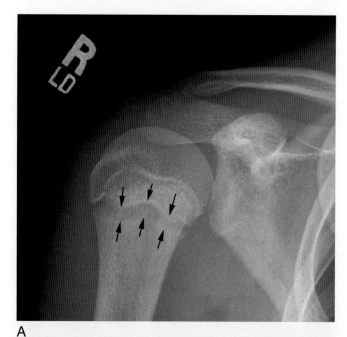

A

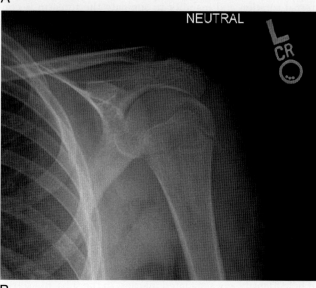

B

Figure 31-5 A, Radiograph showing physeal widening *(arrows)* of the throwing shoulder of a 12 year old. **B,** Contralateral normal physis.

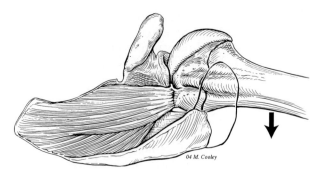

Figure 31-6 Mechanism of internal impingement.

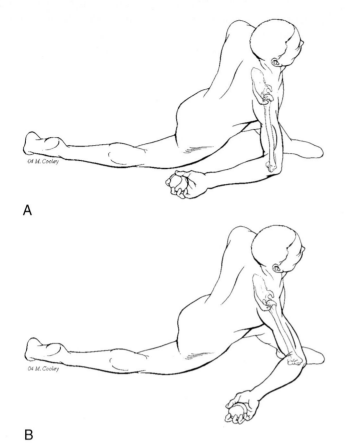

Figure 31-7 A, Hyperangulation occurs from the arm being in excessive extension and/or the scapula being in excessive protraction during late cocking and early acceleration and may result in symptomatic internal impingement. **B,** Throwing with the arm in the plane of the scapula prevents hyperangulation and minimizes internal impingement.

reported the role of *hyperangulation* of the arm during throwing in the development of symptomatic internal impingement. This hyperangulation can occur from the arm being in excessive extension and/or the scapula being in excessive protraction during late cocking and early acceleration (Fig. 31-7). Although some authors maintain that underlying anterior glenohumeral instability is the etiology of symptomatic internal impingement, this has not been scientifically substantiated in the pediatric or adult population as most of these patients lack evidence of anterior capsulolabral injury on imaging studies or during arthroscopy.[16]

Clinical Features and Evaluation

Symptomatic internal impingement occurs only in throwing athletes including participants in baseball, tennis, volleyball, team handball, and javelin. The athlete's chief complaint is typically shoulder pain during throwing activities that is usually relieved by rest. Pitchers commonly report loss of velocity and/or control of their pitches. Nonthrowing activities are usually unaffected. Frequently, symptoms begin after an increase in frequency of throwing activities.

Physical examination demonstrates pain with abduction, external rotation, and extension of the involved shoulder; no apprehension occurs with this maneuver. The pain is relieved by eliminating the extension component of the maneuver. Rotator cuff testing is usually unremarkable in pediatric patients as they

usually lack rotator cuff pathology associated with internal impingement. Poor control of the scapula as evidenced by scapular winging during glenohumeral elevation is usually present in skeletally immature individuals with symptomatic internal impingement. This type of scapular winging results from fatigued or poorly conditioned scapular retractors and not from neurologic deficit. Additionally, individuals will have increased external rotation and decreased internal rotation of the dominant shoulder compared to the nondominant shoulder as a result of physiologic remodeling.[3]

Walch et al[16] described a variety of findings in individuals with symptomatic internal impingement using various imaging modalities and diagnostic arthroscopy in a skeletally mature population. Plain radiography demonstrates changes (sclerosis, geodes, cysts) on the greater tuberosity in 67% of patients and lesions of the posterosuperior glenoid in 33% of patients (Fig. 31-8). Computed tomography demonstrates posterosuperior glenoid changes in 70% of patients. Arthrography demonstrates partial thickness tearing of the supraspinatus and/or infraspinatus in 50% of adult patients, although this probably occurs much less frequently in pediatric patients. Magnetic resonance imaging shows an abnormal signal at the insertion of the rotator cuff in 95% of adult patients. Labral pathology has been identified in most adult patients with symptomatic internal impingement undergoing arthroscopy including a torn or frayed posterior superior labrum in 83% and frank labral disinsertion in 72%. The arthroscopic hallmark of the diagnosis is the "kissing lesion." During arthroscopy, the arm is positioned in abduction, external rotation, and extension, incurring contact in the area of the labral and rotator cuff lesions (Fig. 31-9).

In our practice, we obtain radiographs on all pediatric patients presenting with shoulder pain at the time of initial evaluation including an anteroposterior view and a glenoid profile view as described by Bernageau et al.[9] We only obtain secondary imaging with magnetic resonance arthrography in patients with suspected symptomatic internal impingement who have failed all reasonable nonoperative treatment to evaluate them

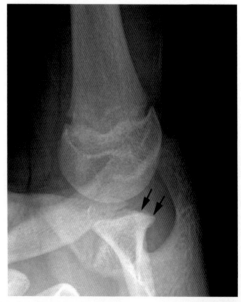

Figure 31-8 Posterior glenoid changes *(arrows)* in an adolescent pitcher with symptomatic internal impingement. This same individual also has physeal changes consistent with proximal humeral epiphyseolysis.

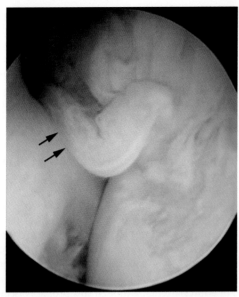

Figure 31-9 Arthroscopic view (looking from the anterior portal) of the contact that occurs between the posterior superior glenoid labrum and the supraspinatus tendon. This patient has a partial thickness supraspinatus tear *(arrows)* as a result.

for mechanical lesions (labral tears, partial thickness rotator cuff tears).

Treatment and Results

In the pediatric population, almost all cases of symptomatic internal impingement can be treated successfully with nonoperative interventions. A period of relative rest combined with a specific physical therapy regimen addressing the pathomechanics of internal impingement is employed. This physical therapy regimen attempts to minimize hyperangulation by strengthening the scapular retractors (trapezius, rhomboids, levator scapulae), controlling scapular protraction, strengthening the subscapularis, and controlling external rotation and extension during throwing activities. Posterior capsular stretching is used to address any posterior capsular tightness. Therapeutic modalities and nonsteroidal anti-inflammatory medications are used as indicated. As symptoms subside, a progressive throwing program, preferably under the supervision of a qualified athletic trainer or physical therapist, is initiated. Attempts are made to correct mechanical deficiencies in the throwing motion to avoid recurrence of symptoms. Successful return to throwing activities may be possible in as little as 6 weeks in mild cases but may take up to 6 to 9 months in more severe cases.

Operative treatment is rarely indicated in the skeletally immature patient with symptomatic internal impingement. In select individuals with symptomatic labral tears from internal impingement with persistent pain after appropriate nonoperative treatment and correction of faulty pitching mechanics, arthroscopic labral repair can be considered with or without an associated anterior capsulorrhaphy to control hyperangulation. Although this arthroscopic treatment has been reported successful in as many as 85% of adult patients, results in the pediatric population are unknown.[18]

Scapular Winging

Traditionally, scapular winging is related to an injury of the long thoracic nerve resulting in serratus anterior paralysis. While this injury pattern occurs in the pediatric population, it is quite rare; more commonly, scapular winging in skeletally immature athletes is caused by overuse and/or poor conditioning of the scapular retractors (trapezius, rhomboids, levator scapulae). Scapular winging leads to hyperangulation (excessive extension angle occurring between the humerus and scapula), which in turn leads to symptomatic internal impingement. The athletes most commonly presenting with scapular winging are those participating in baseball pitching and swimming.

Clinical Features and Evaluation

Most athletes with scapular winging present with findings of internal impingement as described previously caused by overuse and/or poor conditioning of the scapulothoracic musculature. Symptoms, generally shoulder pain, occur almost exclusively with overhead and throwing activities. Rarely, athletes with scapular winging report a direct blow to the thorax just beneath the axilla resulting from a fall onto an object (commonly a piece of equipment in gymnasts) or during contact sports. In this second scenario, blunt injury to the long thoracic nerve causes paralysis of the serratus anterior muscle with resultant scapular winging.

Scapular winging is observed on clinical examination by the examiner standing behind the patient as he or she actively forward flexes the shoulder. Subtle scapular winging may be observed only as asymmetry of the scapula during forward flexion. Having the patient push against a fixed object (wall or closed door) will also demonstrate scapular winging.

Plain radiography is performed and may reveal findings consistent with internal impingement as described previously in patients with scapular winging emanating from overuse/poor conditioning. Additionally, magnetic resonance arthrography may show labral tears and/or partial thickness rotator cuff tears in these patients. In patients with scapular winging resulting from an injury to the long thoracic nerve, imaging studies are usually normal. Electromyography and nerve conduction studies will usually demonstrate decreased potentials in the serratus anterior muscle in this second group of patients.

Treatment and Results

Nonoperative treatment is initially indicated in all pediatric patients presenting with scapular winging. Physical therapy concentrating on strengthening of the periscapular and trunk musculature is nearly always successful. Surgical treatment of patients with long thoracic nerve palsy has been reported (nerve exploration, pectoralis major transfer), although we have no experience with this in the pediatric population. Even in cases of electromyographically proven long thoracic nerve palsy, physical therapy and observation usually result in resolution of symptoms in children, although complete resolution may take an average of 9 months.[19]

CONCLUSIONS

The presence of an open proximal humeral physis leads to some clinical problems unique to the pediatric shoulder. The majority of these injuries result from overuse, and they are becoming more common as children more frequently concentrate on one or two sports and spend increased time participating in them, with fewer seasonal breaks. Most of these problems can be successfully treated nonoperatively.

REFERENCES

1. Curtis RJ Jr, Dameron TB Jr, Rockwood CA Jr: Fractures and dislocation of the shoulder in children. In Rockwood CA Jr, Wilkins KE, King RE (eds): Fractures in Children, 3rd ed. Philadelphia, Lippincott, 1991, pp 829–919.

2. Tullos HS, King JW: Lesions of the pitching arm in adolescents. JAMA 1972;220:264–271.

3. Dillman CJ, Fleisig GS, Andrews JR: Biomechanics of pitching with emphasis upon shoulder kinematics. J Orthop Sports Phys Ther 1993;18:402–408.

4. Crockett HC, Gross LB, Wilk KE, et al: Osseous adaptation and range of motion at the glenohumeral joint in professional baseball pitchers. Am J Sports Med 2002;30:20–26.

5. Dotter WE: Little leaguer's shoulder: A fracture of the proximal humeral epiphyseal cartilage of the humerus due to baseball pitching. Guthrie Clinic Bull 1953;23:68–72.

6. Wilkes JA, Hoffer MM: Clavicle fractures in head-injured children. J Orthop Trauma 1987;1:55–58.

7. Dalldorf PG, Bryan WJ: Displaced Salter-Harris type I injury in a gymnast: A slipped capital humeral epiphysis? Orthop Rev 1994;23:538–541.

8. Dameron TB Jr, Rockwood CA Jr: Fractures and dislocation of the shoulder. In Rockwood CA Jr, Wilkins KE, King RE (eds): Fractures in Children. Philadelphia, Lippincott, 1984, pp 589–607.

9. Bernageau J, Patte D, Bebeyre J, et al: Intérêt du profil glénoïdien dans les luxations récidivantes de l'épaule. Rev Chir Orthop 1976;62(Suppl II):142–147.

10. Edwards TB, Boulahia A, Walch G: Radiographic analysis of bone defects in chronic anterior shoulder instability. Arthroscopy 2003;19:732–739.

11. DeBerardino TM, Arciero RA, Taylor DC, et al: Prospective evaluation of arthroscopic stabilization of acute, initial anterior shoulder dislocations in young athletes: Two- to five-year follow-up. Am J Sports Med 2001;29:586–592.

12. Itoi E, Hatakeyama Y, Kido T, et al: A new method of immobilization after traumatic anterior dislocation of the shoulder: A preliminary study. J Shoulder Elbow Surg 2003;12:413–415.

13. Huber H, Gerber C: Voluntary subluxation of the shoulder in children: A long term follow-up study of 36 shoulders. J Bone Joint Surg Br 1994;76:188–122.

14. Carson WG Jr, Gasser SI: Little leaguer's shoulder: A report of 23 cases. Am J Sports Med 1998;26:575–580.

15. Jobe CM, Sidles J: Evidence for a superior glenoid impingement upon the rotator cuff. J Shoulder Elbow Surg 1993;2:S19.

16. Walch G, Boileau P, Noel E, et al: Impingement of the deep surface of the supraspinatus tendon on the posterosuperior glenoid rim: An arthroscopic study. J Shoulder Elbow Surg 1992;1:238–245.

17. Davidson PA, Elattrache NS, Jobe CM, et al: Rotator cuff and posterior-superior glenoid labrum injury associated with increased glenohumeral motion: A new site of impingement. J Shoulder Elbow Surg 1995;4:384–390.

18. Levitz CL, Dugas J, Andrews JR: The use of arthroscopic capsulorrhaphy to treat internal impingement in baseball players. Arthroscopy 2001;17:573–577.

19. Gregg JR, Labosky D, Harty M, et al: Serratus anterior paralysis in the young athlete. J Bone Joint Surg Am 1979;61:825–832.

32 Shoulder Rehabilitation

Tracy Spigelman and Tim Uhl

In This Chapter

Adjacent joints
Pain control
Restoring range of motion
Dynamic stability
Neuromuscular control
Strengthening
Interval training

INTRODUCTION

- The shoulder is a complex system and is second only to the knee to being commonly injured in athletic endeavors.

- Shoulder rehabilitation is often carried out by a licensed therapist or certified athletic trainer, but the physician often oversees the process and makes recommendations of progression.

- Rehabilitation progression depends on the severity and nature of the injury determined by the physical examination or surgical procedures.

- The rehabilitation process is typically laid out in three primary phases.

- The underlying principles of shoulder rehabilitation drive the intervention undertaken (Table 32-1).

The first principle of appropriate rehabilitation is that a complete and accurate diagnosis must be made that identifies not only the problem but the cause of the problem as well. This is particularly critical in the shoulder as there are several microtraumatic injuries from high demand tasks such as throwing.[1-3] It is critical that the clinician considers the entire body in the examination of all shoulder injuries, particularly in an activity such as throwing, because the shoulder can be the victim of another dysfunctioning component of the kinetic chain.[4] If the rehabilitation program only addresses shoulder symptoms, the precipitating issue will not be identified and treated adequately. Understanding of this complex anatomic and biomechanical system is critical to making the correct diagnosis and properly rehabilitating the shoulder. The nature of many sports medicine rehabilitation programs is that the goal of the program is to return the athlete to the exact same event that caused the injury. Therefore, a comprehensive understanding of the sport's biomechanical demands and pathomechanics that can lead to a microtraumatic injury must be addressed to get the athlete back to the sport activity when designing a rehabilitation program.[5]

The rate at which the return can take place depends on respecting the physiologic healing restraints and the tissue state of irritability. After an acute traumatic event or surgical intervention, the physiologic healing restraints of the injured tissue must be considered when prescribing rehabilitation activities.[5] The exercise progression must be adequate to facilitate healing but not overload a tissue. Overloading tissue can produce pain and substitution patterns that are difficult to resolve later in the rehabilitation process. Often the demands of the total exercise program prescribed are not completely appreciated until the day after. Providing the patient with variations of an exercise and considering the total volume of exercises prescribed can help prevent flare-ups. The final, and probably most important, principle to any rehabilitation program is open and honest communication between all parties, particularly between the patient, physician, and rehabilitation specialists. The exchange of concerns and findings will enhance the process of recovery. Nothing is more frustrating to a patient than to get conflicting information from caregivers. In those patients undergoing surgical rehabilitation, the operating surgeon has the best information as to quality of tissue and repair, which will dictate the rehabilitation program.

Once the complete and accurate diagnosis has been made and the recommendation from the physician to start rehabilitation is given, the patient needs to enter into the appropriate phase of the rehabilitation program. There are three basic phases of rehabilitation: acute, prefunctional, and functional (Table 32-2). The primary goals of the acute phase are to decrease pain and increase motion. Restoration of upper extremity neuromuscular control and dynamic stability of the glenohumeral joint is the primary goal during the prefunctional phase. In the functional phase, the goal is to regain full endurance and power in order to return the athlete to sport participation.[2] The nature of the injury, deficits found, and the goals of the individual patient will determine which phase is most appropriate for the patient. It is not uncommon for athletes with chronic overuse problems, which are typically degenerative and not inflammatory conditions,[6] to focus on the functional phases during their rehabilitation.

ACUTE PHASE

During the acute phase, rehabilitation focuses on decreasing the multiple components of inflammation and restoring normal motion, while protecting the injured area from further damage.[5] The patient is often requested to go through a relative rest period to minimize inflammation and in some cases may actually be immobilized for a short period of time. It is critical that maintenance of strength, endurance, and mobility of the rest of the body is addressed along with cardiovascular conditioning during this period.[2,5]

Table 32-1 Principles of Rehabilitation
1. Complete an accurate diagnosis with appreciation of etiology
2. Understand anatomic and biomechanical concepts of the shoulder complex
3. Respect physiologic healing of injured tissue
4. Maintain open communication lines among the sports medicine team members

Adjacent Joints

To minimize loss of function and maintain conditioning, exercising the noninvolved extremities is essential. This benefits the immobilized tissues by cross-education training, which helps maintain muscular strength on the untrained limb.[7] Surgical patients with an immobilized shoulder are commonly prescribed active range of motion (ROM) exercise of the hand, wrist, and elbow to minimize distal swelling, facilitate venous return, and prevent stiffness.[8] In addition, proximal joints of the scapula, cervical, thoracic, and lumbar spine should be exercised along with the lower extremity.[4] The neuromuscular system uses the proximal trunk as a base of support for distal motion.[9] Initiating a core strengthening and stretching program will activate the normal neuromuscular system and potentially minimize losses due to the relative rest period.[10] Loss of muscular strength can occur as soon as 3 days in a trained individual and significant cardiovascular decreases have been noted within 14 days.[11]

Pain Control

Medical management of this phase is typically carried out with nonsteroidal anti-inflammatory agents, although some concerns exist that this may delay healing.[12] Physical therapy modalities such as electrical stimulation and ultrasound are often recommended to control inflammation.[8] However, only cryotherapy and compression have been demonstrated with good scientific evidence to be effective in controlling inflammation.[13] Cryotherapy continuously for 3 days after arthroscopic surgery of the shoulder has been found to decrease the use of pain medication.[14]

Positioning of the injured extremity is critical to facilitate healing and minimize discomfort. After injury to a rotator cuff tendon or surgical intervention, a resting position of neutral rotation, 20 to 40 degrees of abduction, and 20 to 30 degrees of flexion minimize the load of the rotator cuff tendon and facilitates blood flow through the poorly vascularized rotator cuff tendon.[15] A reclined position of 30 to 45 degrees with the elbow supported to prevent shoulder extension is recommended to address the common complaint of patients who are unable to find a comfortable sleep position.[15,16] Historically, traumatic shoulder dislocations were immobilized in a sling and swathe with the arm internally rotated.[16] Protzman[17] suggests that time of immobilization did not have a significant bearing on redislocation rate. Recently, a position of external rotation at 45 degrees for 3 weeks has been advocated by some to diminish redislocation rates and promote labral compression onto the glenoid by the tension of the subscapularis.[18]

Diminishing pain and swelling minimizes the inhibitory effect on the neuromuscular system.[19] The dynamic neuromuscular system is critical to the stability of the shoulder[2,20] and is primarily supplied by the rotator cuff and periscapular musculature. Without adequate pain control, muscular re-education will be delayed and normal movement patterns will be difficult to reestablish in this acute phase.[19,21] Exercises or activities that elicit pain should be modified to reduce the negative and inhibitory effects.

Table 32-2 Outline of the Three Healing Phases and Suggested Rehabilitation Interventions That Are Appropriate for Each Level

	Acute Phase	*Prefunctional Phase*	*Functional Phase*	
	1. Control pain 2. Increase motion 3. Protect healing structures	1. Re-establish neuromuscular control 2. Encourage tissue remodeling along lines of functional stress 3. Restore normal motion	1. Expose tissue to loads specific to sport demands 2. Interval return to sport activities	Goals
	Immobilization (relative rest) Cryotherapy Electrical stimulation Manual therapy	Heat/cold modalities Ultrasound Electrical stimulation Massage Biofeedback	Heat/cold modalities Massage	Modalities
	PROM AAROM Isometrics Neuromuscular training Adjacent joint motion Cardiovascular exercises	AROM Proprioceptive neuromuscular facilitation Manual therapy Closed chain kinetics Mirroring sports motions Cardiovascular exercise	Overload resistive exercises Sport-specific drills Isokinetic exercises Plyometrics Power exercises Interval programs	Therapeutic Exercise
Healing Progression	AROM to at least 90 degrees with minimal pain and without scapular substitution 75% of PROM reestablished	Full AROM with minimal pain and coordinated scapulohumeral rhythm 70%–80% of opposite side's strength	Completes interval program without symptoms Strength, endurance, and power of the upper extremity can withstand the demands of the sport activity	Criteria to Progress
Time				

AAROM, active assisted range of motion; AROM, active range of motion; PROM, passive range of motion.

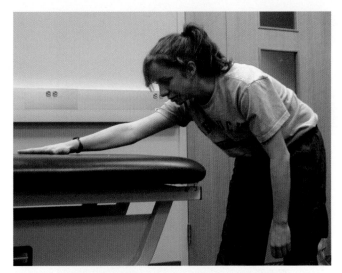

Figure 32-1 Illustration of forward bow exercise with hand stabilized and the body moving away from the stable hand.

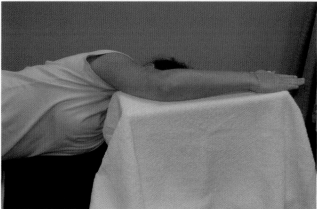

Figure 32-3 Arm sliding along elevated surface to allow a greater range of motion while minimizing the load of the arm.

Therapeutic Exercise

Passive ROM is often the initial exercise routine after significant shoulder injury or surgery. Passive ROM is prescribed during the inflammatory phase of healing to increase joint surface nutrition, prevent adhesions from forming, minimize stress to healing tissue, and decrease pain.[8] Passive ROM is an exercise that takes the joints through a partial or complete ROM by some external source. This source can be from another individual, use of the healthy arm, or through a machine. Theoretically, passive ROM involves no volition of the dynamic system, but electromyographic studies indicate low to minimal activity present in the involved shoulder musculature.[22] This low demand of muscle activity may place gentle stress on healing tissue collagen fibers to help with alignment, strength, and blood flow but not overload healing tissues.[5] Passive exercises such as pendulum, supine passive elevation, and standing forward bow (Fig. 32-1) have all been found to activate the rotator cuff musculature by less than 10% of maximal voluntary isometric contraction, a common reference used to standardize electromyographic studies.[22]

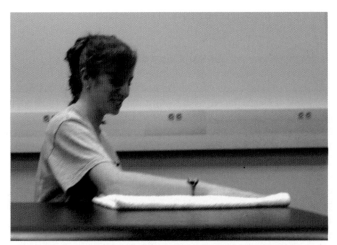

Figure 32-2 Arm sliding along horizontal surface with a towel under the hand to diminish friction and load on the upper extremity while activating the shoulder musculature.

Exercises are progressed from passive to active assisted ROM exercises to incrementally increase tissue demand and engage the neuromuscular system. In some cases, patients can start in this phase if minimal tissue protection is appropriate. Our goal is to start with low-demand and progress to high-demand activities. A common mistake made by rehabilitation specialists is to rush through this exercise level because it seems "too easy" for the patient. This is a critical step in the rehabilitation program to reestablish neuromuscular control of the shoulder girdle and to prevent substitution patterns from developing.[1] If an exercise is too stressful, the motivated patient will focus on the goal of lifting the arm overhead 30 times and develop a substitution pattern of his or her upper trapezius, which may lead to further problems in the later phases.[4]

Active assisted ROM exercise is defined as movement through a partial or complete range that involves voluntary effort of the involved limb but is performed with external assistance.[23] There are several examples of external assistance exercises from which to choose. Based on our electromyographic research, we have found assistive elevation tasks that minimize gravitational loads on the arm such as table slides (Fig. 32-2) and side-lying elevation (Fig. 32-3) are less demanding than exercises performed against gravity, such as rope and pulley– or stick-assisted elevation exercises.[24] These active assisted ROM exercises indicate greater electromyographic activity than passive ROM but typically less than active ROM exercises.[22] Therefore, active assisted ROM can be initiated before active and resistive exercises, without taxing new tissue. The goal is to engage the neuromotor system to facilitate the reestablishment of normal patterns of upper limb motion.

Criteria to Progress

Once patients demonstrate good neuromuscular control of active assisted ROM, they typically are ready to progress to the next phase of the program. A general guideline for this is active elevation to at least 90 degrees in the plane of the scapula with no substitution and minimal pain. Passive ROM should be well established and have at least reached 140 degrees of elevation and external rotation of 30 degrees in most cases.[2,5]

PREFUNCTIONAL PHASE

The initial inflammatory phase has typically resolved, and the proliferative phase of healing is ongoing as patients enter this phase of rehabilitation. The tissue is less irritable and is now ready for more demanding activity. Reestablishing dynamic control of the shoulder girdle by activating both feedforward (voluntary motor program) and feedback (sensorimotor reflexive responses) neuromotor systems is a goal of this phase and important in prevention of future injuries.[20] Exercises during this phase will certainly strengthen the shoulder musculature but also will emphasize activities to compress and centralize the humeral head on the glenoid.[10]

Restoring Full Range of Motion

Normal motion is an important component of the prefunctional phase because most overhead sports require excessive external rotation to perform successfully at high levels. Restoring full ROM requires movement through the terminal ranges of motion.[3] This is achieved through voluntary or active movement (active ROM) with static passive overpressure, which may result in increased joint compression along with stimulation of afferent joint and muscle receptors.[6,25] Stimulation of these receptors may produce protective guarding but is necessary to reestablish afferent input. Care should be taken, however, not to damage the newly arranged collagen fiber. By applying these stresses, the collagen tissue will adapt to the stresses that they will be subjected to in the future.[26] Joint mobilization techniques and static stretching techniques are effective measures to regain complete passive and active ROM.

Restoring Dynamic Stability

Restoring dynamic stability of the glenohumeral joint primarily involves increased joint concavity/compression[27] by engaging the periscapular muscles to stabilize and control scapular motion while allowing the rotator cuff to compress the humeral head into the glenoid. Closed kinetic chain exercises can facilitate dynamic stability by increasing glenohumeral congruency and stimulate joint receptors through functional ranges of motion. These types of exercises can stimulate motor activation[20,28] and improve joint position sense,[29,30] which enhances dynamic stability. Dynamic stability is also enhanced by progressive resistive strengthening exercises. Incorporation of light resistive elastic bands or dumbbells that target rotator cuff and scapular musculature has been demonstrated to increase shoulder strength.[31] Gradual progression to higher resistive exercises such as prone horizontal abduction (Fig. 32-4) or rows places higher demands

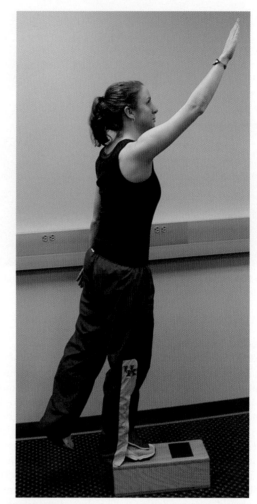

Figure 32-5 Kinetic chain step-up with arm elevation.

on the trapezius and rhomboid muscles to regain the scapular strength and endurance necessary in overhead sports.[32] Incorporation of greater loads through this phase with closed kinetic chain exercises, such as rhythmic stabilization with a ball, facilitates more demand on the shoulder musculature while simulating sports such as football and wrestling.[20] Incorporating sport-specific tasks involving the entire body facilitates dynamic stability and helps recreate normal neuromuscular control of the upper extremity.

Restoring Neuromuscular Control

Neuromuscular control of a joint entails two components, a feedforward and feedback motor response. Feedforward motor programs are associated with voluntary movements that occur without afferent input. These motor programs have been found to incorporate not simply the prime movers of the limb but actually incorporate the entire body.[9,33] This is necessary to provide a stable base for the distal limb to move on. As we are trying to return the athlete to normal motor patterns, we attempt to recreate these movement patterns during the rehabilitation of the athlete. This is accomplished by activating proximal trunk and hip extensor musculature just before activating the prime arm elevation musculature in order to retrain normal arm elevation movement patterns (Fig. 32-5). This technique is a primary principle of proprioceptive neuromuscular facilitation techniques that are commonly used in this rehabilitation phase.

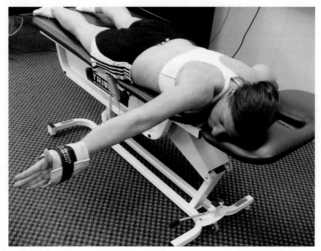

Figure 32-4 Prone horizontal abduction, found to place large demands on lower and mid-trapezius musculature.

The feedback component is necessary to stabilize the joint to unexpected perturbations. Athletes often have to stabilize the shoulder complex in response to an unexpected external stimulus, such as catching themselves from a fall or attempting to grasp an opponent who is trying to evade them. These types of exercises, called rhythmic stabilization, are often incorporated into the closed chain dynamic stability exercises described previously, by placing the hand on an unstable surface and disturbing the surface. This requires the athlete to contract shoulder girdle musculature and stabilize the joint and his or her body to prevent losing his or her balance (Fig. 32-6). Development of full strength and endurance of the rotator cuff and scapular muscles is the key to maintaining dynamic stability and regaining neuromuscular control in the shoulder.[25]

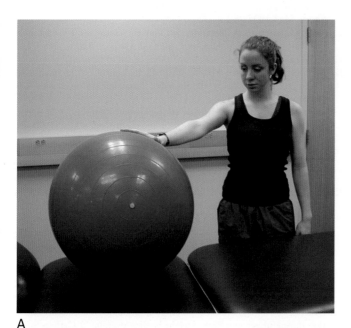

A

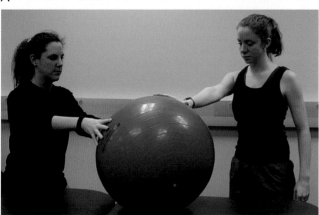

B

Figure 32-6 A and **B,** Rhythmic stabilization with ball perturbation.

Criteria to Progress

Progression into the final phase should depend on physiology of healing and the individual functional response during the prefunctional phase. Certainly, we should expect nearly full active and passive ROM for most patients. No observable substitution patterns should be present with active ROM and sport-specific motions. Strength should be approaching 70% to 80% of the opposite side by isometric or dynamic testing.

FUNCTIONAL PHASE

The functional phase of rehabilitation focuses on return to play. Rehabilitation exercises introduced in this phase should continue to stress the static and dynamic restraints by increasing velocity and torque demands. Emphasis on ballistic sport-specific exercises that incorporate eccentric and plyometric activities are recommend during the functional phase.[4,32] These types of exercises prepare the shoulder for the demands required to return to full sport participation.[34] The athlete should also begin an interval training program to gradually reintroduce proper biomechanics and demands of the sport to the body. During interval training, the coach should be involved in evaluating and providing feedback to the athlete about proper mechanics of the skill being performed.[2,4]

Progressive resistive open kinetic chain exercises incorporating heavier dumbbells or requiring performance at a faster rate increase demands at the shoulder joint because the distal segment is not fixed. These exercises add to the eccentric forces placed on the rotator cuff musculature. Another way to increase the stress on the static and dynamic stabilizers is with plyometric exercises.[2] The objective of plyometrics is to use elastic properties of the muscle to increase concentric power, prestretching the tissue with an eccentric action followed quickly with a concentric action. The shorter the period is between eccentric and concentric phases, the better.[35] Weighted ball overhead plyometric activities simulate demands of the act of throwing and are a good indicator that the athlete is able to progress to interval sport activities.[34]

Interval Training Program

Return to any overhead sport requires that the athlete is gradually exposed to the sport demands. Much of the functional phases is focused on sport-specific activities that are created for the individual's needs. Incorporating the coach and a certified athletic trainer is very helpful at this point to ensure that proper biomechanics of the task are being met. The goal is to return the athlete to play with correct mechanics, thus preventing recurrence of the same injury. There are several excellent resources for a variety of sports interval training programs available in the literature.[2,36]

Return to Play Criteria

The final, and often most difficult, task of the physician is to determine when it is safe to return an athlete to sport. Return to play criteria should include objective physical parameters specific to the sport demands. Nothing replaces experience in making this decision, but we have attempted to give some general suggestions of minimal requirements for most overhead athletic activities in Table 32-3.

Table 32-3 Suggested Minimal Requirements for Most Overhead Athletic Activities

Criteria	Assessment
Range of motion	Full active arm elevation in both frontal and sagittal planes. External rotation equal or greater than opposite arm for dominant arms. Internal rotation should be within 10% of opposite arm internal rotation.
Strength	Normal (5/5) with manual muscle testing of the rotator cuff, deltoid, and scapular musculature. If isokinetic testing is available, assessment at a safe position of 45 degrees abduction in the plane of the scapula is suggested for internal (25% of body weight) and external rotation (15% of body weight) with an external-to-internal rotation ratio of 66%.
Endurance	Completion of interval program; isokinetic testing at 300 degrees/sec; limited fatigue
Quality of pain	Athlete describes only minimal "fatigue" after exercises but no sharp pain, night pain, or increase in pain the following day.
Quality of motion	Coordinated scapular-thoracic motion; no substitutions; no hesitation
Quality of attitude	Confident without hesitation; positive; eager to return to play

REFERENCES

1. Pink M, Jobe FW: Shoulder injuries in athletes. Clin Manag 1991;1:39–47.
2. Wilk KE, Meister K, Andrews JR: Current concepts in the rehabilitation of the overhead throwing athlete. Am J Sports Med 2002;30:136–151.
3. Bigliani LU, Codd TP, Conner P, et al: Shoulder motion and laxity in the professional baseball player. Am J Sports Med 1997;25:609–613.
4. Pappas AM, Zawacki RM, McCarthy CF: Rehabilitation of the pitching shoulder. Am J Sports Med 1985;13:223–235.
5. Uhl TL: Rehabilitation after shoulder injury and surgery. In Baker CL, Flandry F, Henderson JM (eds): Hughston Clinic Sports Medicine. Baltimore, Williams & Wilkins, 1995, pp 291–298.
6. Almekinders LC, Temple JD. Etiology, diagnosis, and treatment of tendonitis: An analysis of the literature. Med Sci Sports Exerc 1998;30:1183–1190.
7. Yue G, Cole KJ: Strength increases from the motor program: Comparison of training with maximal voluntary and imagined muscle contractions. J Neurophysiol 1992;67:1114–1123.
8. Prentice WE: Therapeutic Modalities in Sports Medicine, 3rd ed. St. Louis, Mosby, 1994.
9. Cordo PJ, Nashner LM: Properties of postural adjustments associated with rapid arm movements. J Neurophysiol 1982;47:287–308.
10. Borsa PA, Livingston B, Kocher MS, Lephart SP: Functional assessment and rehabilitation of shoulder proprioception for glenohumeral instability. J Sport Rehabil 1994;3:84–104.
11. Convertino VA, Bloomfield SA, Greenleaf JE: An overview of the issues: Physiological effects of bed rest and restricted physical activity. Med Sci Sports Exerc 1997;29:187–190.
12. Prisk V, Huard J: Muscle injuries and repair: The role of prostaglandins and inflammation. Histol Histopathol 2003;18:1243–1256.
13. Merrick MA, Knight KL, Ingersol CD, Potteiger JA: The effects of ice and compression wraps on intramuscular temperature at various depths. J Athl Train 1993;28:241–245.
14. Speer KP, Warren RF, Horowitz L: The efficacy of cryotherapy in the postoperative shoulder. J Shoulder Elbow Surg 1996;5:62–68.
15. Itoi E, Tabata S: Conservative treatment of rotator cuff tears. Clin Orthop 1992;275:165–173.
16. Bankart AS, Cantab MC: Recurrent or habitual dislocation of the shoulder-joint. Clin Orthop 1993;291:3–6.
17. Protzman RB: Anterior instability of the shoulder. J Bone Joint Surg Am 1980;62:909–918.
18. Itoi E, Hatakeyama Y, Kido T, et al: A new method of immobilization after traumatic anterior dislocation of the shoulder: A preliminary study. J Shoulder Elbow Surg 2003;12:413–415.
19. Roe C, Brox J, Bohmer A, Vollestad N: Muscle activation after supervised exercises in patients with rotator tendinosis. Arch Phys Med Rehabil 2000;81:67–72.
20. Lephart SM, Pincivero DM, Giraldo JL, Fu FH: The role of proprioception in the management and rehabilitation of athletic injuries. Am J Sports Med 1997;25:130–137.
21. Wilk KE, Arrigo CA, Andrews JR: Current concepts: The stabilizing structures of the glenohumeral joint. J Orthop Sports Phys Ther 1997;25:364–379.
22. McCann PD, Wootten ME, Kadaba MP, Bigliani LU: A kinematic and electromyographic study of shoulder rehabilitation exercises. Clin Orthop 1993;288:179–188.
23. Kisner K, Colby L: Introduction to therapeutic exercise. In: Therapeutic Exercise—Foundations and Techniques, 3rd ed. Philadelphia, FA Davis, 1996, pp 3–23.
24. Gaunt B, Uhl TL, Humphrey L, et al: Electromyography of shoulder and scapular musculature during exercise strengthening progression. J Orthop Sports Phys Ther 2006 (in review).
25. Riemann BL, Lephart SM: The sensorimotor system, part I: The physiological basis of functional joint stability. J Athl Train 2002;37:71–79.
26. Woo SL-Y, Gomez MA, Siters TJ, et al: The biomechanical and morphological changes in the medial collateral ligament of the rabbit after immobilization and remobilization. J Bone Joint Surg Am 1987;69:1200–1211.
27. Lippitt SB, Vanderhooft JE, Harris SL, et al: Glenohumeral stability from concavity-compression: A quantitative analysis. J Shoulder Elbow Surg 1993;2:27–35.
28. Uhl TL, Carver TJ, Mattacola CG, et al: Shoulder musculature activation during upper extremity weight-bearing exercise. J Orthop Sports Phys Ther 2003;33:109–117.
29. Ubinger ME, Prentice WE, Guskiewicz KM: Effect of closed kinetic chain training on neuromuscular control in the upper extremity. J Sport Rehabil 1999;8:184–194.
30. Rogol IM, Ernst G, Perrin DH: Open and closed kinetic chain exercises improve shoulder joint reposition sense equally in healthy subjects. J Athl Train 1998;33:315–318.
31. Wang C-H, McCure P, Pratt N, Nobilini R: Stretching and strengthening exercises: Their effects on three-dimensional scapular kinematics. Arch Phys Med Rehabil 1999;80:923–929.
32. Swanik KA, Swanik CB, Lephart SM, Huxel K: The effect of functional training on the incidence of shoulder pain and strength in intercollegiate swimmers. J Sport Rehabil 2002;11:140–154.
33. Zattara M, Bouisset S: Posturo-kinetic organisation during the early phase of voluntary upper limb movement. 1. Normal subjects. J Neurol Neurosurg Psychiatry 1988;51:956–965.
34. Cordasco F, Wolfe IN, Wootten ME, Bigliani LU: An electromyographic analysis of the shoulder during a medicine ball rehabilitation program. Am J Sports Med 1996;24:386–392.
35. Stone JA, Partin NB, Lueken JS, et al: Upper extremity proprioceptive training. J Athl Train 1994;29:15–18.
36. Axe MJ, Konin J: Distance based criteria interval throwing program. J Sport Rehabil 1992;1:326–336.

33 Physical Examination and Evaluation

Grant L. Jones and Champ L. Baker, Jr.

INTRODUCTION

- The keys to diagnosing elbow injury are a comprehensive history and physical examination of the elbow and the surrounding anatomy, such as the shoulder, wrist, hand, and cervical spine, to rule out possible causes of referred pain.

- A detailed history can help to narrow the differential diagnosis.

- Many specialized tests exist for confirming the diagnosis of specific pathologic entities about the elbow.

- Diagnostic tests, such as radiography, computed tomography (CT), and magnetic resonance imaging (MRI) can help in making a diagnosis or ruling out potential disorders.

HISTORY

Taking a comprehensive history helps the physician to develop a differential diagnosis. The examiner should determine whether a single traumatic event or repetitive traumatic episodes caused the symptoms. Acute injuries to be considered include ulnar collateral ligament (UCL) rupture, medial epicondyle avulsion, biceps rupture, loose-body formation, acute wrist extensor or flexor origin muscle strain or tendon rupture, and acute subluxation of the ulnar nerve. Chronic injuries include UCL strain or rupture, valgus extension overload, musculotendinous strains, tendonopathies, and osteochondral defects that can progress to degenerative changes.[1,2]

The examiner should inquire about the location of the pain. Dividing the elbow into four anatomic regions (lateral, medial, anterior, and posterior) helps to narrow the range of differential diagnoses.[1-7] Symptoms in the lateral region of the elbow indicate radiocapitellar chondromalacia, osteochondral loose bodies, radial head fractures, osteochondritis dissecans lesions, or posterior interosseous nerve entrapment. Symptoms in the medial region can indicate UCL sprain or rupture, a medial epicondyle avulsion fracture, ulnar neuritis, ulnar nerve subluxation, medial epicondylitis, osteochondral loose bodies, valgus extension overload syndrome, or pronator teres syndrome. The differential diagnoses for symptoms of the anterior region include anterior capsular sprain, distal biceps tendon strain or rupture, brachialis muscle strain, and coronoid osteophyte formation. Finally, symptoms in the posterior region can indicate valgus extension overload, posterior osteophytes with impingement, triceps tendonitis, triceps tendon avulsion, olecranon stress fracture, osteochondral loose bodies, or olecranon bursitis.[1,2]

The examiner should ask the patient about the presence and character of the pain, swelling, and locking and catching episodes. Sharp pain radiating down the medial portion of the forearm with paresthesia in the fifth and the ulnar-innervated half of the fourth digit indicates ulnar neuritis or cubital tunnel syndrome. When these symptoms are associated with a snapping or popping sensation, ulnar nerve subluxation might be the underlying cause. Pain that occurs in the posteromedial portion of the elbow with intense throwing and is associated with localized crepitation might indicate valgus extension overload syndrome.[8,9] Pain localized in the posterior region of the elbow at the triceps tendon insertion or poorly localized, deep, aching pain in the posterior region of the elbow at the triceps insertion can signal triceps tendonitis. Poorly localized, deep, aching pain in the posterior region of the elbow can also be associated with an olecranon stress fracture.[1,2,10] Sharp pain in the lateral region associated with locking or catching can be the result of loose bodies in the radiocapitellar joint from a radial head fracture or osteochondritis dissecans lesions of the capitellum.[11,12] Acute, sharp pain in the anterior region of the elbow can be caused by an acute rupture of the biceps tendon. Persistent, aching pain in the anterior region can indicate inflammation involving the anterior capsule.

A patient whose symptoms are related to throwing or to an occupational stress should be asked to reproduce the position that causes the symptoms. Pain during the early cocking phase of throwing might be the result of biceps or triceps tendonitis. Pain during the late cocking phase caused by valgus stresses on the medial region of the elbow can indicate UCL incompetency or ulnar neuritis. A thrower who reports pain in the posterior region of the elbow during the late cocking and acceleration phases and reports an inability to "let the ball go" might have valgus extension overload syndrome. Pain during the late acceleration or follow-through phases may signal a flexor-pronator tendonopathy due to forceful wrist flexion and forearm pronation during these phases. In the skeletally immature patient, pain in the lateral region of the elbow during the late acceleration and follow-through phases often indicates radio-capitellar joint injuries, such as osteochondritis dissecans lesions.

PHYSICAL EXAMINATION

Inspection

Careful inspection of the elbow joint and surrounding areas is the next step in evaluating the elbow. First, the examiner should note atrophy or hypertrophy of muscle groups of the arm or forearm and should obtain girth measurements. Hypertrophy of the forearm musculature often is present in the dominant extremity of the throwing athlete and should be considered a normal variant. Atrophy of arm and forearm musculature, however, could be the result of an underlying neurologic disorder.

Next, the examiner should measure the carrying angle of the elbow with the arm extended and the forearm supinated (Fig. 33-1). The normal carrying angle is 11 degrees in men and 13 degrees in women.[13] An increase in the carrying angle is termed cubitus valgus. Often, this angle increases from 10 to 15 degrees in throwing athletes because of adaptive remodeling from repetitive valgus bony stress.[9,14] A progressive cubitus valgus deformity can also be caused by a nonunited lateral condylar fracture, which can lead to a tardy ulnar nerve palsy.[15] Cubitus varus, a decrease in the carrying angle, can be the result of a malunited supracondylar humeral fracture or a previous growth plate disturbance caused by trauma or inflammation.

Inspection of the four mentioned elbow regions should be performed next.[16] First, on the lateral aspect, the soft spot, a

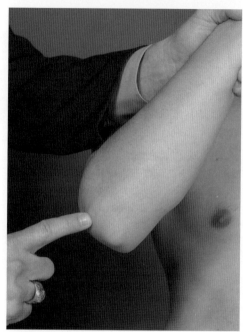

Figure 33-2 Palpate the lateral "soft spot" for swelling from a joint effusion or synovial proliferation.

triangular region defined by the lateral epicondyle, olecranon, and the radial head, is evaluated. Swelling or fullness in this region can indicate joint effusion, synovitis, or bony deformity (Fig. 33-2). Next, inspection of the posterior region is performed. Swelling or a prominence in this region may indicate an olecranon bursitis, an olecranon traction spur, or nodules from gout or rheumatoid arthritis. The olecranon may also appear prominent as a result of a defect in the distal triceps tendon when there is a distal triceps tendon rupture. Swelling or fullness medially may indicate an avulsion fracture of the medial epicondyle, a UCL injury, a subluxated ulnar nerve, or, in the more chronic situation, an enthesophyte in the wrist flexor-pronator origin on the medial epicondyle. The anterior region should be inspected for any deformity. A more proximal position of the distal end of the biceps muscle belly compared with that of the contralateral muscle may be indicative of a distal biceps tendon rupture. A deformity in the more proximal portion of the lateral biceps muscle ("Popeye" deformity) is indicative of a rupture of the long head of the tendon proximally, whereas a medial deformity in the proximal portion of the muscle belly suggests a rupture of the short head.[17,18] Finally, the skin should be inspected for erythema, which can be a sign of an infectious or inflammatory process.

Palpation

The examiner palpates the medial and lateral epicondyles and views them from a posterior angle. When the elbow is in full extension, these landmarks normally form a straight line (Fig. 33-3). With the elbow in 90 degrees of flexion, however, they form an equilateral triangle. Any alignment abnormality can indicate fracture, malunion, unreduced dislocation, or growth disturbances involving the distal end of the humerus.[19] The examiner should palpate all four regions of the elbow (anterior, medial, posterior, and lateral) in an orderly fashion. Beginning with the anterior structures, the distal biceps tendon is palpated anteromedially in the antecubital fossa with the patient's

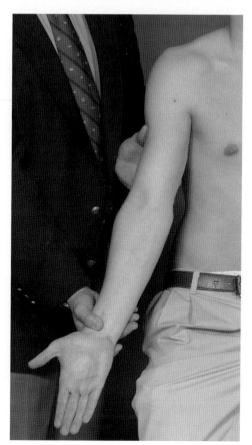

Figure 33-1 Observe the carrying angle of the elbow with the arm extended and forearm supinated.

lacertus fibrosus, which can be confused with the biceps tendon. Deep, poorly localized tenderness can be caused by anterior capsulitis or coronoid hypertrophy due to hyperextension injuries or repetitive hyperextension stress.[6] Next, the examiner should feel the brachial artery pulse deep to the lacertus fibrosus, which is just medial to the biceps tendon. Finally, one should conduct Tinel's test in the area of the lacertus fibrosus, which is a common site of median nerve compression.[21] A positive Tinel sign can indicate pronator syndrome.

Next, the clinician should palpate the structures in the medial region of the elbow, beginning with the supracondylar ridge. If a congenital medial supracondylar process is present in this area, it gives rise to a fibrous band (ligament of Struthers) that inserts on the medial epicondyle. This band can compress the brachial artery and median nerve and result in neurovascular symptoms with strenuous use of the extremity. The examiner should palpate the medial epicondyle and flexor-pronator mass. Tenderness at the origin of the flexor-pronator mass on the epicondyle suggests an avulsion fracture in adolescents or medial epicondylitis in adults. Flexor-pronator strains produce pain anterior and distal to the medial epicondyle. The UCL also is present in this area as it courses from the anteroinferior surface of the medial epicondyle to insert on the medial aspect of the coronoid at the sublime tubercle (Fig. 33-4).[22] Palpation of the ligament can be facilitated by using the "milking maneuver."[23,24] During this maneuver, the patient grasps the thumb of the affected arm with the opposite hand. With the injured elbow flexed to greater than 90 degrees, a valgus stress is applied to the elbow by pulling on the thumb. This hyperflexion isolates the anterior bundle of the UCL, and the valgus stress places the anterior bundle under stretch. This elbow position facilitates the location and palpation of the tensioned ligament under the mass of the flexor-pronator origin. This position alone can elicit pain

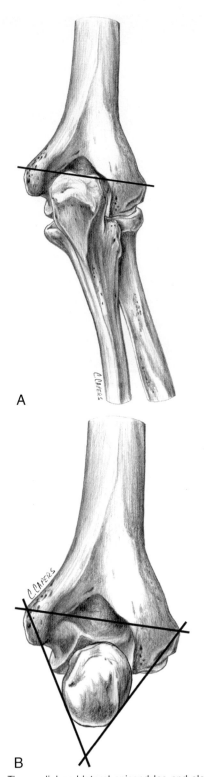

A

B

Figure 33-3 A, The medial and lateral epicondyles and olecranon form a straight line with the elbow in full extension. **B,** When the elbow is flexed to 90 degrees, these landmarks form an equilateral triangle.

forearm in supination and elbow in active flexion.[1] Tenderness in this area without a defect could indicate biceps tendonitis or a partial biceps tendon rupture.[20] Tenderness with a defect or decreased tension in the biceps tendon is consistent with a complete rupture. To avoid missing a distal biceps tendon rupture, it is imperative to make sure that one is not palpating an intact

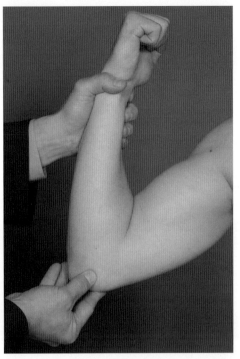

Figure 33-4 The examiner flexes the patient's elbow to 100 degrees to facilitate palpation of the ulnar collateral ligament (UCL) and to uncover the distal insertion of the anterior oblique portion of the UCL.

over the medial elbow as the anterior bundle is placed on stretch.

In the posteromedial area of the elbow, the ulnar nerve is easily palpable in the ulnar groove. An inflamed ulnar nerve is tender and can have a doughy consistency. The examiner should conduct Tinel's test in three areas: proximal to the cubital tunnel (zone I), at the level of the cubital tunnel where the fascial aponeurosis joins the two heads of the flexor carpi ulnaris (zone II), and distal to the cubital tunnel where the ulnar nerve descends to the forearm through the muscle bellies of the flexor carpi ulnaris (zone III).[25] A positive test produces paresthesia in the fifth digit and ulnar-innervated half of the fourth digit and suggests a diagnosis of ulnar neuritis due to entrapment, trauma, or subluxation. The clinician also should test the nerve for hypermobility. The examiner brings the patient's elbow from extension to terminal flexion as he or she palpates the nerve to determine whether it subluxates or completely dislocates over the medial epicondyle (Fig. 33-5).[26]

In the posterior region of the elbow, the clinician evaluates the olecranon bursa for swelling or fluctuation, which would indicate olecranon bursitis. One should also palpate this region for any palpable osteophytes on the subcutaneous border of the olecranon that could contribute to the overlying bursitis. The medial subcutaneous border is then palpated for tenderness that could be caused by a stress fracture in a throwing athlete.[27] Next, the triceps insertion is examined (Fig. 33-6); tenderness here indicates triceps tendonitis or an avulsion injury if there is an associated defect. Finally, the clinician palpates the posterior,

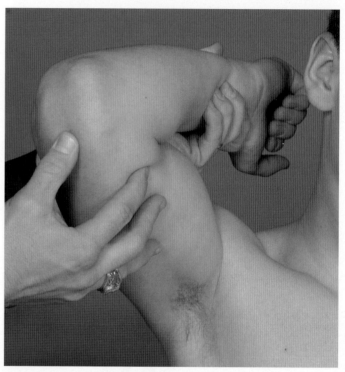

Figure 33-6 Tenderness over the triceps tendon insertion on the olecranon might indicate triceps tendonitis or triceps avulsion injury.

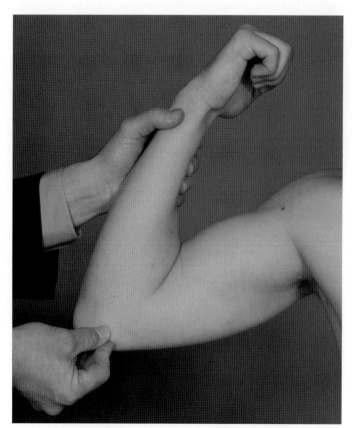

Figure 33-5 As the patient's elbow is brought from extension to flexion, the examiner might feel the ulnar nerve subluxate or dislocate anteriorly over the medial epicondyle as in this subject who has a hypermobile nerve.

medial, and lateral aspects of the olecranon in varying degrees of flexion to detect osteophytes or loose bodies. Palpation of the posteromedial olecranon can reveal an osteophyte and swelling, which are present in the throwing athlete with valgus extension overload syndrome.[8]

Examination of the lateral region of the elbow begins with palpation of the lateral epicondyle. Tenderness directly over the lateral epicondyle is typical of lateral epicondylitis (Fig. 33-7). Tenderness approximately 4 cm distal to the lateral epicondyle over the wrist extensor muscle mass is present in a patient with radial tunnel syndrome, which is a compressive neuropathy of the radial nerve as it travels from the radial head to the supinator muscle.[25] Finally, tenderness distal to the location of the radial tunnel can be due to compression of the posterior interosseous nerve as it descends beneath the arcade of Frohse and the supinator muscle.

The radial head and radiocapitellar joint distal to the lateral epicondyle are palpated next. Pronation and supination of the forearm enhance this evaluation. Tenderness or crepitation in this area could indicate fracture or dislocation of the radial head, osteochondritis dissecans, or Panner's disease in the adolescent athlete, or articular fragmentation and bony overgrowth with possible progression to loose-body formation in the young adult athlete.[1,28] Finally, palpation of the lateral recess, or soft spot, is performed to evaluate elbow joint effusion.

Range of Motion

Range of motion of the elbow occurs about two axes: (1) flexion and extension and (2) pronation and supination. The normal arc of flexion and extension ranges from 0 to 140 degrees of flexion,[29] but the functional arc about which most activities of daily living are performed ranges from 30 to 130 degrees (Fig.

33-8).[30,31] The examiner must compare the range of motion to that of the contralateral extremity to account for normal individual variance. An athlete who has pitched many innings may have a flexion contracture on the dominant side that increases as the season progresses and can decrease between seasons. Injuries that cause loss of extension include capsular strain, flexor muscle strain, intra-articular loose bodies, and an intra-articular fracture. In a recent study, lack of full extension in an acute situation was found to be 97% sensitive in diagnosing a significant bone or joint injury; therefore, if a patient has full extension of the elbow after an acute injury, there is a very low likelihood of a significant bone or joint injury.[32] Injuries that cause abnormal lack of flexion include loose bodies, capsular tightness, triceps strain, anterior osteophytes, and coronoid hypertrophy.

To measure pronation and supination, the examiner has the patient flex the elbows to 90 degrees while holding pencils in each hand (Fig. 33-9). The examiner must immobilize the humerus in a vertical position when evaluating forearm rotation because patients tend to adduct or abduct the shoulder to compensate for loss of forearm pronation or supination. Acceptable norms for full pronation and supination are 70 and 85 degrees, respectively.[19] The functional arc of motion is 50 degrees for both pronation and supination.[19] Loss of pronation or supination can be caused by loose bodies, radiocapitellar osteochondritis, radial head subluxation, radial head fractures, or motor nerve entrapment lesions resulting in weakness of the biceps, pronator teres, pronator quadratus, or supinator muscles.[1] The examiner also should assess the wrist because wrist injury can cause loss of forearm rotation.

When testing range of motion, the examiner also should note the presence or absence of crepitus. He or she must test both

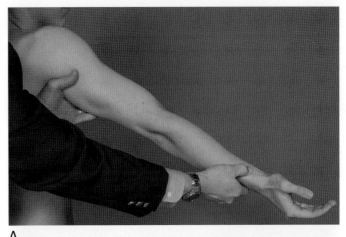

A

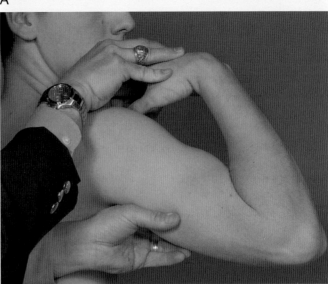

B

Figure 33-8 The normal arc of extension (**A**) and flexion (**B**).

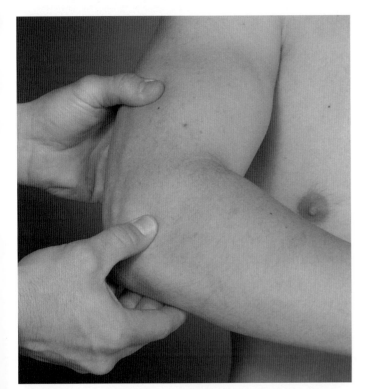

Figure 33-7 Lateral epicondylitis causes tenderness over the lateral epicondyle.

active and passive range of motion because crepitus might not be present on passive range of motion and might be unveiled only through active range of motion. In addition, the clinician should compare active and passive range of motion; if motion is full on passive testing but limited on active testing, pain or paresis might be the limiting factor rather than a mechanical block. Finally, the quality of the endpoint should be noted. Firm endpoints often mean that there is a bony block to motion such as loose bodies, osteophytes, or other joint incongruities. Soft endpoints, on the other hand, most likely are a result of soft-tissue contractures, such as flexion contractures seen in baseball pitchers.

Strength Testing

It is important to examine the strength of elbow, wrist, and hand muscle groups when evaluating an elbow disorder to assess for a neurologic problem or tendon injury. Biceps brachii muscle strength testing is best conducted against resistance with the forearm supinated and the shoulder flexed from 45 to 50 degrees (Fig. 33-10). Triceps strength testing, on the other hand, is best performed with the shoulder flexed to 90 degrees and

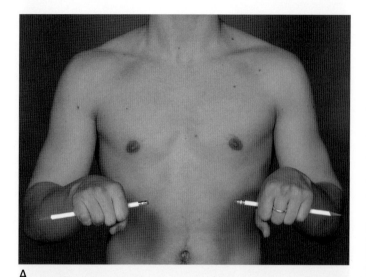

A

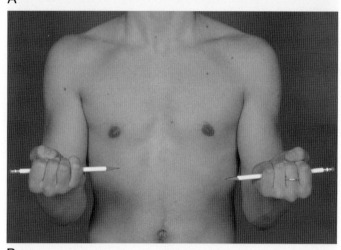

B

Figure 33-9 While the patient holds pencils in each hand and flexes the elbows to 90 degrees, measure pronation (**A**) and supination (**B**). Due to a previous fracture in the distal radius, this patient demonstrates a slight loss of pronation in the left extremity compared with the right extremity.

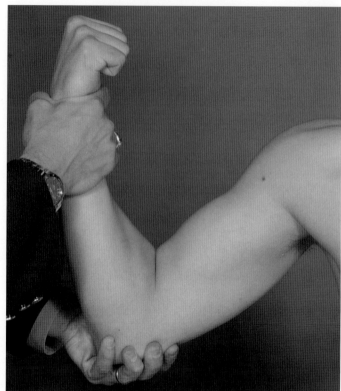

Figure 33-10 Biceps muscle strength is assessed with the forearm supinated and the shoulder flexed from 45 to 50 degrees. The examiner applies resistance to flexion.

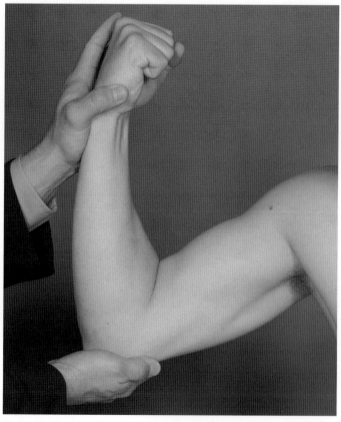

Figure 33-11 Triceps muscle strength is best tested with the shoulder flexed to 90 degrees and the elbow flexed from 45 to 90 degrees.

the elbow flexed from 45 to 90 degrees (Fig. 33-11).[1] Elbow extension strength is normally 70% of flexion strength.[29] Pronation, supination, and grip strength are best studied with the elbow in 90 degrees of flexion and the forearm in neutral rotation. Supination strength is approximately 15% greater than pronation strength, and the dominant extremity is from 5% to 10% stronger than the nondominant extremity.[29]

Finally, the examiner tests the forearm musculature and hand intrinsic strength. The extensor carpi radialis longus musculotendinous unit is best studied with the elbow flexed to 30 degrees and resistance applied to wrist extension.[1] However, the extensor carpi radialis brevis musculotendinous unit is best isolated by providing resistance to wrist extension with the elbow in full flexion. The clinician studies the extensor carpi ulnaris muscle by resisted ulnar deviation of the wrist. Weakness in the wrist, finger, and thumb extensors may indicate a posterior interosseous nerve palsy. Weakness of the flexor pollicis longus and flexor digitorum profundus muscles of the index finger is present in an entrapment palsy of the anterior interosseous nerve, which branches from the median nerve approximately 5 cm distal to the medial epicondyle.[33] Finally, weakness in the hand intrinsics can indicate ulnar nerve entrapment at the cubital tunnel.

Reflexes

Reflexes are evaluated to rule out potential sources of referred pain, such as cervical radiculopathy. An increased response to stimulation can indicate an upper motor neuron lesion, whereas a decreased response can signify a lower motor lesion. The examiner tests the C5 nerve root by the biceps reflex, the C6 nerve root by the brachioradialis reflex, and C7 nerve root by the triceps reflex.

Sensory Examination

Next, the examiner should conduct a comprehensive sensory examination to assess for a cervical radiculopathy or a peripheral neuropathy. Light touch and pinprick sensation are both assessed. Diminished sensation in the fifth and ulnar-innervated half of the fourth digits can signify an ulnar neuropathy. However, many entrapment neuropathies of the elbow and forearm, such as anterior interosseous neuropathy, pronator syndrome, posterior interosseous neuropathy, and radial tunnel syndrome, do not have abnormal objective sensory examinations.

Stability Testing

Either an acute traumatic event or a chronic overload syndrome can result in valgus instability of the elbow. Attenuation or rupture of the anterior oblique bundle of the UCL causes this pattern of instability.[1,2] The elbow is examined with patient in either the seated or supine position and the shoulder in maximal external rotation.[2] The manual valgus stress test is performed with the elbow flexed 20 to 30 degrees to unlock the olecranon tip from the olecranon fossa while stabilizing the humerus (Fig. 33-12). Valgus stress is then applied to the elbow with the forearm in maximal pronation. Any increased opening or reproduction of the patient's pain with valgus stress may be indicative of injury to the UCL.[2] Often only pain can be elicited without any detectable opening when performing this test when the patient is awake due to patient guarding and the fact that even with complete sectioning of the anterior bundle of the UCL in cadaveric studies, there is only minimal valgus opening that may not be clinically detectable.[34]

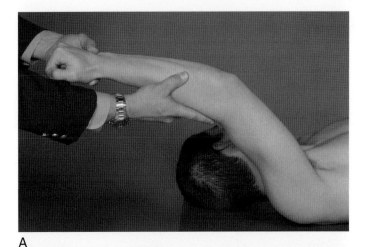

A

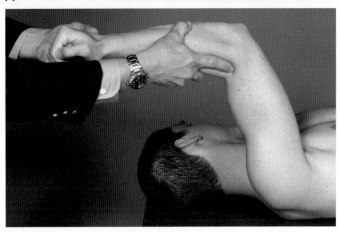

B

Figure 33-13 The lateral pivot-shift test. The examiner supinates the elbow, applies a valgus moment and axial compression, and moves the elbow from full extension (**A**) to flexion (**B**).

Posterolateral rotatory instability is essentially a rotational displacement of the ulna and radius on the humerus that causes the ulna to supinate away from the trochlea.[35] O'Driscoll[35] describes four principal physical examination tests to diagnose this form of instability. The most sensitive is the lateral pivot-shift apprehension test. The patient is placed in the supine position with the affected extremity overhead, and the patient's wrist and elbow are grasped as the ankle and knee are held when examining a knee. The elbow is supinated with a mild force at the wrist, and a valgus moment and compressive force are applied to the elbow during flexion (Fig. 33-13). This results in an apprehension response with reproduction of the patient's symptoms akin to the anterior apprehension test of the shoulder. The next test is the lateral pivot-shift test or posterolateral rotatory instability test, which reproduces the actual subluxation and the clunk that occurs with reduction. This can usually be accomplished only with the patient under general anesthesia or occasionally after injecting local anesthetic into the elbow. The pivot-shift maneuver causes posterolateral subluxation or dislocation of the radius and ulna off the humerus that reaches a maximum at 40 degrees of flexion, creating a posterolateral prominence over the dislocated radial head and a dimple between the radius and capitellum. As the elbow is flexed past

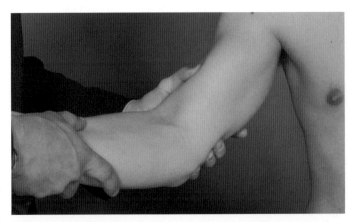

Figure 33-12 Valgus stress testing is accomplished with the patient's elbow flexed from 20 to 30 degrees and his or her arm secured between the examiner's arm and trunk.

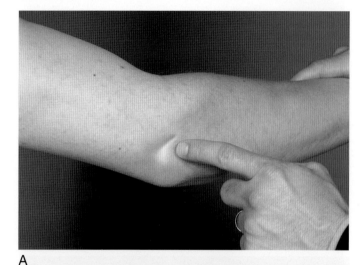

A

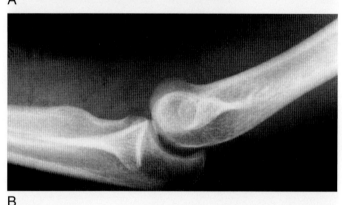

B

Figure 33-14 **A,** A positive test for posterolateral rotatory subluxation of the elbow. The posterolateral dislocation of the radiohumeral joint produces an osseous prominence and an obvious dimple in the skin just proximal to the dislocated radial head. **B,** Lateral radiograph made simultaneously with the photograph. The radiohumeral joint is dislocated posterolaterally, and there is rotatory subluxation of the ulnohumeral joint. The semilunar notch of the ulna is rotated away from the trochlea. (From Hyman J, Breazeale NM, Altchek DW: Valgus instability of the elbow in athletes. Clin Sports Med 2001;20:25–45.)

40 degrees, reduction of the ulna and radius together on the humerus occurs suddenly and produces a palpable and visible snap (Fig. 33-14). The third test is the posterolateral drawer test, which is a rotatory version of the Lachman test of the knee. During the test, the lateral side of the forearm subluxates away from the humerus, pivoting around the medial collateral ligament. The final test is the "stand-up test" in which the patient's symptoms are reproduced as he or she attempts to stand up from the sitting position by pushing on the seat with the hand at the side and the elbow fully supinated.

Provocative and Special Tests
Lateral
Stress to the extensor carpi radialis longus and brevis muscles reproduces the discomfort associated with lateral epicondylitis. To create this stress, the patient fully extends the elbow and resists active wrist and finger extension (Fig. 33-15). Pain at the lateral epicondyle with this maneuver indicates lateral epicondylitis. This is the most sensitive provocative maneuver for this disorder. Passive flexion of the wrist with the elbow

extended can also cause discomfort as it stretches the extensor tendons. Finally, the "chair test" can also aid in the diagnosis.[36,37] In this test, the patient raises the back of a chair with the elbow in full extension, the forearm pronated, and the wrist dorsiflexed (Fig. 33-16). As the patient attempts to lift the chair, he or she exhibits apprehension in anticipation of pain.

The most sensitive test for radial tunnel syndrome is resisted supination with the supinator and extensor carpi radialis brevis muscles in the stretched position (pronation and wrist flexion), which produces pain approximately 4 to 5 cm distal to the lateral epicondyle.[38] Resisted third-digit extension can also cause pain in this area in patients with radial tunnel syndrome; however, this maneuver also causes similar pain in patients with lateral epicondylitis. Another indicator of radial tunnel syndrome is the pronator-supinator sign.[39] The test is positive if direct tenderness over the radius at 5 cm distal to the lateral epicondyle is markedly greater in full supination than in pronation due to the fact that the radial nerve is located in this position in full supination but moves medially and distally with pronation. Passive pronation of the forearm to its end range with elbow extension also can recreate the symptoms of radial tunnel syndrome by causing a tightening of the origin of the extensor carpi radialis brevis muscles over the nerve.[40] Recently, a neural tension test has been described to aid in the diagnosis of radial tunnel syndrome.[41] In this test, the radial nerve is placed under tension, which causes pain distal to the lateral epicondyle if the patient has radial tunnel syndrome. This nerve tension is created with shoulder girdle depression, forearm pronation, elbow extension, wrist and finger flexion, and shoulder abduction while the patient is in the supine position.

Finally, the clinician tests for damage to the articular surface of the radiocapitellar joint. With the patient's elbow extended,

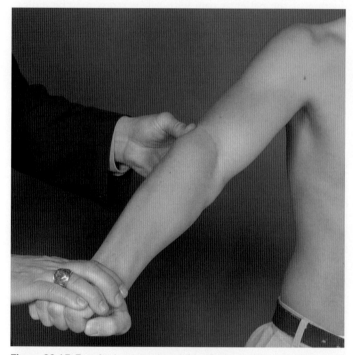

Figure 33-15 Test for lateral epicondylitis. Stress to the origin of extensor carpi radialis brevis and longus tendons, which is created by resisting active wrist extension with the elbow fully extended, elicits pain at the lateral epicondyle.

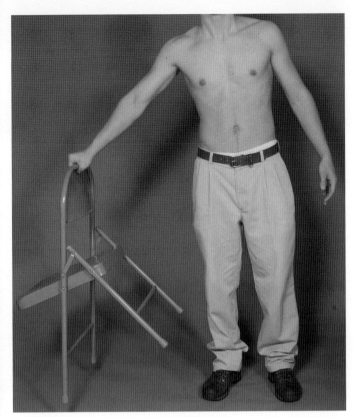

Figure 33-16 The "chair test." While holding the elbow in full extension, pronating the forearm, and dorsiflexing the wrist, the patient lifts the back of a chair. The test elicits apprehension in patients with lateral epicondylitis.

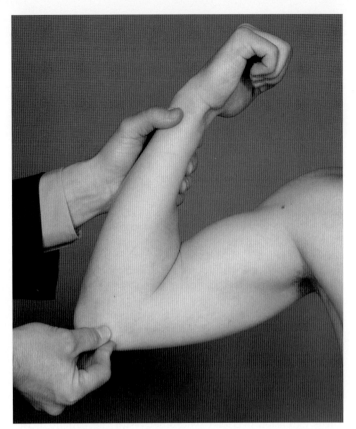

Figure 33-18 Elbow flexion test for ulnar nerve compression. With the patient's wrist neutral and forearm supinated, the examiner flexes the patient's elbow to 135 degrees as he or she applies digital pressure over the cubital tunnel.

the examiner applies an axial load to the joint while supinating and pronating the forearm repeatedly. Pain with this maneuver is a positive radiocapitellar compression test.

Medial

The most sensitive indirect maneuver for the diagnosis of medial epicondylitis is resisted forearm pronation, which is positive in 90% of patients with this disorder (Fig. 33-17).[39] A positive test

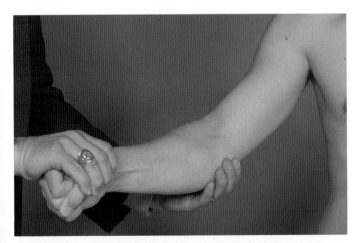

Figure 33-17 Resisted forearm pronation elicits pain at the medial epicondyle in patients who have medial epicondylitis.

elicits pain at the flexor-pronator muscle mass origin on the medial epicondyle. The second most sensitive maneuver is resisted palmar flexion, which is positive in 70% of patients.[39] Passive extension of the wrist and fingers also can elicit pain at the medial epicondyle in these patients.

The most sensitive and specific provocative test maneuver for diagnosing ulnar nerve compression at the elbow is the elbow flexion test conducted with direct pressure over the cubital tunnel.[33] With the patient's wrist in neutral and forearm supinated, the examiner flexes the elbow to 135 degrees and applies digital pressure over the cubital tunnel for a period of 3 minutes or until the symptoms are elicited (Fig. 33-18).[42] A positive test results in paresthesia or dysesthesia in the fifth and ulnar-innervated half of the fourth digit. A simple nerve compression test and Tinel's test also are used to aid in making the diagnosis. Positive findings with these tests without the use of electrodiagnostic studies have been shown to accurately predict the success rate of an ulnar nerve transposition procedure.[43]

Anterior

Vague anterior elbow or proximal forearm pain can be caused by entrapment of the median nerve at many sites. First, as discussed previously, the median nerve can become compressed under the ligament of Struthers. In this case, resisted flexion of the elbow between 120 and 135 degrees of flexion elicits the symptoms.[25] Active elbow flexion with the forearm in pronation, which tightens the lacertus fibrosus, causes symptoms in patients with compression of the nerve by the lacertus fibrosus.[25]

If resisted pronation of the forearm combined with flexion of the wrist reproduces the symptoms, the nerve may be compressed as it passes through the pronator teres muscle.[25] Finally, if resisted flexion of the superficialis muscle of the third digit results in pain in this area, the nerve may be entrapped in the superficialis arch.[25]

Anterior elbow pain also can be due to biceps or brachialis tendonitis. These diagnoses are suggested when resisted forearm supination and elbow flexion produce increased pain. The clinician should also assess for the tension on the distal biceps tendon with resisted flexion and supination because decreased tension could be the result of a distal biceps tendon tear. Finally, a new clinical test has been described for the diagnosis of complete distal biceps tendon ruptures, the passive pronation-supination test (Warren Harding, MD, personal communication, 2004). With an intact biceps tendon, the biceps' muscle belly rises visibly and palpably in the arm with passive supination, returns to a normal position with return to the neutral position, and then flattens and moves to a more distal position with pronation. In an unpublished study of patients with MRI-documented complete biceps tendon avulsions, Harding found that the muscle belly did not rise and fall with passive supination and pronation of the forearm.

Posterior

The valgus extension overload test and valgus extension snap maneuver consistently produce discomfort in patients with valgus extension overload syndrome.[1] With the patient in the seated position, the examiner applies a moderate amount of valgus stress to the elbow as he or she moves the elbow from 30 degrees of flexion to full extension. This maneuver simulates posteromedial olecranon impingement and recreates the pain that the athlete experiences during the late acceleration phase of throwing.

A modified Thompson test has been described to help diagnose a complete distal triceps tendon tear.[44] This test is performed with the elbow flexed to 90 degrees and the arm abducted to eliminate the effect of gravity on elbow extension. The examiner squeezes the triceps muscle belly and observes the elbow for extension motion. If there is no motion, a complete tear is present.

Imaging Studies
Plain Radiography

Plain radiographs may be ordered to supplement the information obtained during the history and physical examination. They enable the clinician to gather formative information on bone, joint positioning, and the presence or absence of soft-tissue swelling, loose bodies, ectopic ossification, and foreign bodies. Standard radiographic views include anteroposterior and lateral projections, which can be supplemented by oblique and axial views as necessary.[45] An anteroposterior view is taken with the arm in full extension and the forearm supinated (Fig. 33-19). This position allows good visualization of the medial and lateral epicondyles, the radiocapitellar joint, and the trochlear articulation with the medial condyle. The lateral radiographic view should be taken with the elbow flexed to 90 degrees and the forearm in neutral rotation and the beam should be reflected distally to account for the normal valgus position of the elbow (Fig. 33-20). The lateral projection provides visualization of the radiocapitellar and ulnotrochlear articulations, the distal

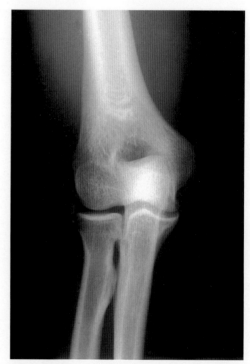

Figure 33-19 Anteroposterior radiographic view.

humerus, and the olecranon and coronoid processes. Fat pad signs are visualized on the lateral view and indicate capsular distention or joint effusion, and, if present, intra-articular abnormalities should be suspected. The presence of the anterior fat pad sign sometimes is normal, whereas the presence of the posterior fat pad sign is always abnormal.

If an injury to the radiocapitellar joint is suspected, the clinician should order a radiocapitellar view, which is obtained with the elbow positioned as for a lateral projection, but with the beam angled 45 degrees anteriorly (Fig. 33-21). This provides an unobstructed view of the proximal radius and capitellum and is useful in making the diagnosis of osteochondral fractures of the capitellum or injuries to the radial head and neck.

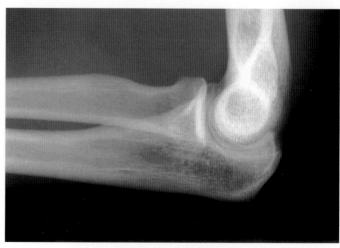

Figure 33-20 Lateral radiographic view.

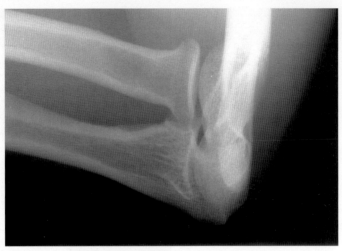

Figure 33-21 Radial head radiographic view.

The axial view is often helpful in evaluating injury in the throwing athlete. For this view, the elbow is flexed to 110 degrees with the forearm flat on the cassette, and the beam is directed perpendicular to the cassette (Fig. 33-22). This allows visualization of the posterior compartment, specifically visualization of the articulation of the posterior olecranon and the humerus. The clinician should closely evaluate this view for a posteromedial osteophyte, which occurs with valgus extension overload syndrome. The reverse axial projection, which provides better visualization of the olecranon and trochlea, is taken with the elbow in maximal flexion and the arm flat on the cassette.[45]

Stress Radiography

Stress views can be obtained in patients with suspected ligament disruption or elbow instability. The examiner applies varus or valgus stress to the elbow during radiography and assesses the films for any asymmetrical widening of the joint. A gravity stress view is obtained with the patient supine and the arm abducted to 90 degrees from the body; the beam is centered on the elbow. With maximal supination of the forearm, a valgus stress is applied to the elbow. Static views that demonstrate an increase in joint space of more than 2 mm are considered abnormal.[45]

Cain et al[2] suggest obtaining anteroposterior views with 0, 5, 10, and 15 N of valgus stress applied to each elbow at 25 degrees. An increase in opening with increasing stress compared with the contralateral uninjured side is indicative of UCL injury. Dynamic evaluation under fluoroscopy can be helpful in identifying subtle abnormalities; however, instability is often not well visualized with these dynamic views.

Computed Tomography

CT provides excellent osseous detail and can be used to evaluate the elbow for loose bodies not evident on plain films, osteochondral defects, articular congruity, trabecular irregularities, and fractures for displacement (Fig. 33-23).[45] Images are acquired in 1-mm intervals and can be reformatted into coronal, sagittal, or three-dimensional images to help with surgical planning.

CT arthrography may be indicated to detect intra-articular loose bodies, to evaluate capsular topography in patients with capsular contractures or tears, and to evaluate the articular-bearing surfaces.[45] It may be the diagnostic modality of choice to examine these entities in patients in which an MRI is contraindicated (e.g., patients with loose metal fragments in

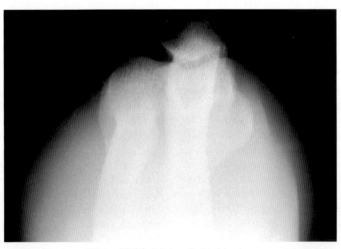

Figure 33-22 Axial radiographic view.

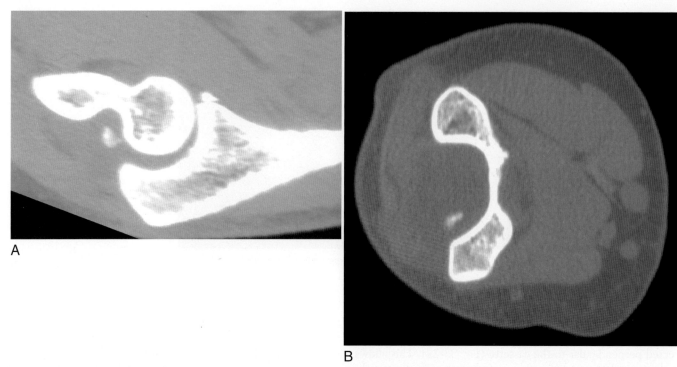

Figure 33-23 This 34-year-old woman had a traumatic elbow dislocation. After reduction, sagittal computed tomography scan reconstruction (**A**) shows a small coronoid fracture and posterior olecranon fossa intra-articular bone fragment, also seen in axial image (**B**).

their eye orbits or perispinal region or in those with pacemakers). Timmerman et al[46] compared CT arthrography with nonenhanced MRI in 25 baseball players for the ability to correctly diagnose UCL injuries and discovered that CT arthrography had a sensitivity of 86% and specificity of 91% compared to nonenhanced MRI, which had sensitivity of 57% and specificity of 100%. Both techniques were 100% sensitive for complete tears; however, partial tears were more accurately diagnosed by CT arthrogram.

Magnetic Resonance Imaging

MRI is the modality of choice for the evaluation of soft-tissue structures, such as ligaments, tendons, and muscles, and has largely replaced arthrography as the study of choice for intra- and periarticular soft-tissue structures. MRI is used to evaluate capsuloligamentous or musculotendinous disruption as well as intra-articular abnormalities, such as epiphyseal fractures or chondral defects (Fig. 33-24). Images are obtained in 1- to 3-mm intervals with formats in sagittal, coronal, and axial planes. Nonenhanced MRI can be used to evaluate tendons such as the biceps and triceps when physical examination is equivocal. MRI may be helpful to evaluate for partial-thickness distal biceps tendon ruptures (Fig. 33-25) when physical examination reveals an intact tendon but a patient has pain in the distal biceps tendon area with associated weakness.[20] T1-weighted images demonstrate a replacement of the normal low signal intensity in the distal biceps tendon with intermediate signal intensity, and T2-weighted images reveal high signal edema surrounding the distal biceps tendon and its insertion. MRI can also aid in the diagnosis of tendonopathy and partial tears involving the wrist extensor and pronator-wrist flexor tendon origins seen in patients with lateral and medial epicondylitis, respectively. The changes that accompany tendinosis manifest as either intermediate to low signal intensity on T1-weighted images in cases of fibroblastic proliferation or high signal intensity in cases of

fibroblastic proliferation with mucoid degeneration.[47] Attrition on both T1- and T2-weighted images with high signal intensity is consistent with a partial tear of the tendon's origin. Discontinuity on both T1- and T2-weighted images with high signal intensity of the free ends is indicative of a complete tear (Fig. 33-26).

Saline-enhanced MRI direct arthrogram has been shown to be the most accurate study to evaluate UCL injuries (Fig. 33-27).[48] Schwartz et al[48] reported 92% sensitivity and 100% specificity with diagnosing UCL injury using this modality. Sensitivity was higher for complete tears (95%) than for partial tears (86%). Saline is injected through the lateral soft spot into the joint, and saline extravasation through the UCL indicates a full-thickness tear. MRI can also be used to identify disorders associated with UCL injury, such as posteromedial impingement changes. A recent study, however, cautions against diagnosing UCL injuries and associated disorders based solely on MRI findings.[49] Sixteen asymptomatic professional baseball players with no history of injury to their elbows underwent MRI. UCL abnormalities (thickening, signal heterogeneity, or discontinuity) were present on 87% of players' dominant elbows, and findings consistent with posteromedial impingement were present in 13 of 16 subjects.[49]

Finally, MRI can also be used to evaluate for subtle avulsion fractures or stress fractures that may not be evident on plain radiographs (Fig. 33-28). Using a combination of radiographs and MRI scans, Salvo et al[50] were able to identify eight avulsion fractures of the sublime tubercle of the ulna in 33 consecutive patients treated for UCL injuries. Regarding stress injury to bone, Schickendantz et al[27] reported on a series of seven professional baseball players with proximal ulnar osseous stress injury detected on MRI with normal plain radiographs. Poorly defined, patchy areas of low signal intensity in the proximal posteromedial olecranon continuous with the cortex were seen on all of the T1-weighted images. All short tau inversion recovery

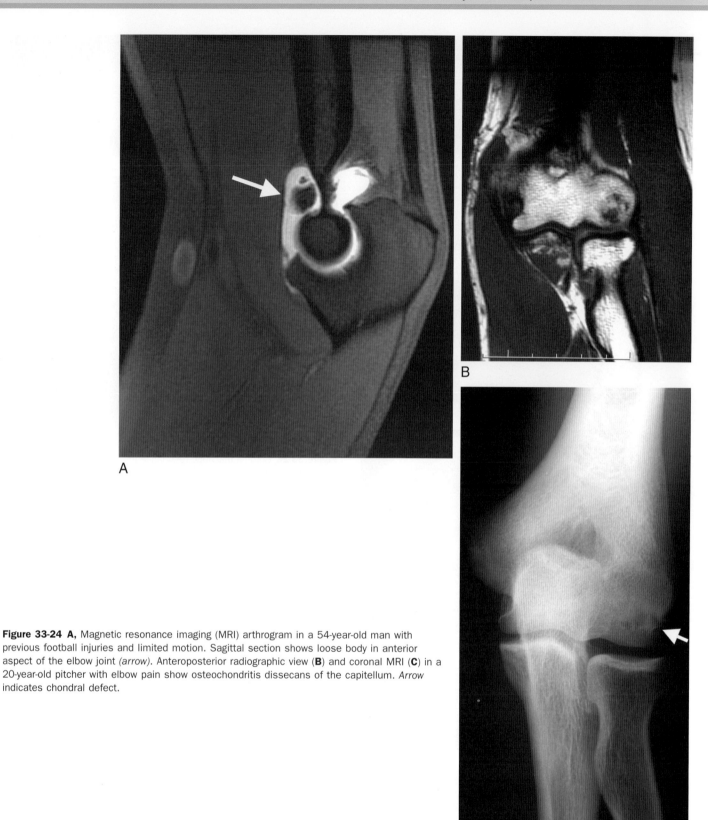

Figure 33-24 A, Magnetic resonance imaging (MRI) arthrogram in a 54-year-old man with previous football injuries and limited motion. Sagittal section shows loose body in anterior aspect of the elbow joint *(arrow)*. Anteroposterior radiographic view (**B**) and coronal MRI (**C**) in a 20-year-old pitcher with elbow pain show osteochondritis dissecans of the capitellum. *Arrow* indicates chondral defect.

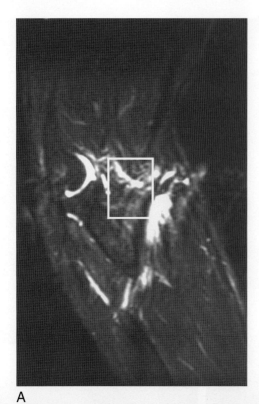

A

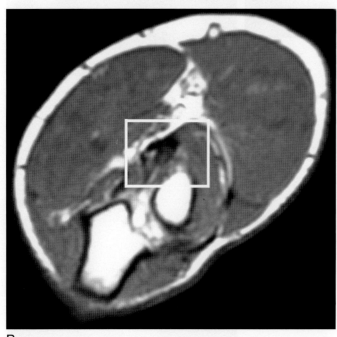

B

Figure 33-25 Sagittal (**A**) and axial (**B**) images show a complete distal biceps tendon avulsion off the radius.

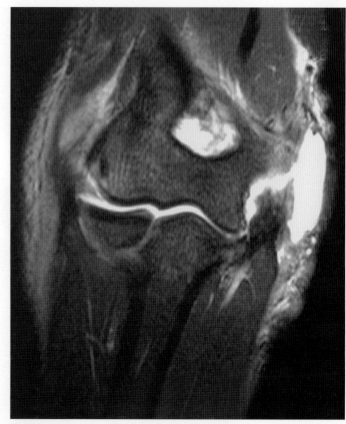

Figure 33-26 Coronal magnetic resonance image shows traumatic combined proximal ulnar collateral ligament disruption and common flexor origin disruption in a 17-year-old wrestler after a second elbow dislocation.

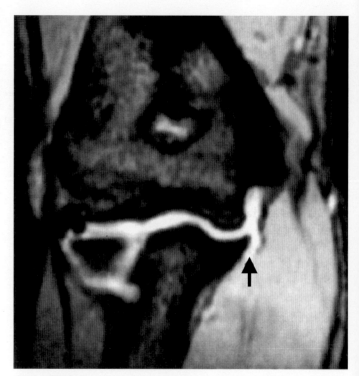

Figure 33-27 Contrast coronal magnetic resonance image reveals complete ulnar collateral ligament disruption. Arrow indicates positive capsular T sign.

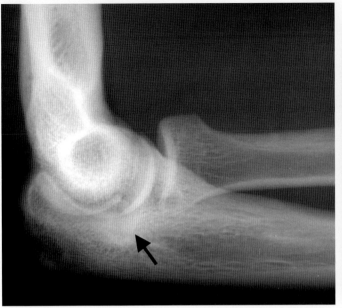
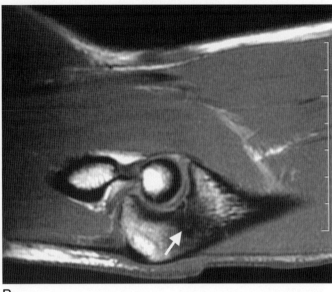

A   B

Figure 33-28 Lateral radiographic view (**A**) and lateral magnetic resonance image (**B**) show posterior olecranon stress fracture in a teenage pitcher with posteromedial impingement. Arrows indicate area of stress.

images showed areas of high signal intensity in the posteromedial olecranon.

CONCLUSIONS

A comprehensive history and physical examination of the elbow and surrounding joints are the most important part of the evaluation of elbow disorders. The examiner can use additional diagnostic tests, such as plain radiographs, CT, and MRI, to confirm the diagnosis or further narrow the scope of potential diagnoses. Because the elbow is a very complex joint with multiple different potential disorders, it is imperative to perform a very thorough examination and to conduct every portion of the examination to avoid missing a diagnosis.

REFERENCES

1. Andrews JR, Whiteside JN, Buettner CM: Clinical evaluation of the elbow in throwers. Oper Tech Sports Med 1996;4:77–83.
2. Cain EL, Dugas JR, Wolf RS, et al: Elbow injuries in throwing athletes: A current concepts review. Am J Sports Med 2003;31:621–635.
3. Slocumb DB: Classification of elbow injuries from baseball pitching. Tex Med 1968;64:48–53.
4. Jobe FW, Nuber GN: Throwing injuries of the elbow. Clin Sports Med 1986;5:621–635.
5. Dehaven KE, Evarts CM: Throwing injuries of the elbow in athletes. Orthop Clin North Am 1973;4:801–808.
6. Barnes DA, Tullos HS: An analysis of 100 symptomatic baseball players. Am J Sports Med 1978;6:62–67.
7. Bennett GE: Elbow and shoulder lesions of baseball players. Am J Surg 1959;98:484–492.
8. Wilson FD, Andrews JR, Blackburn TA, et al: Valgus extension overload in the pitching elbow. Am J Sports Med 1983;11:83–87.
9. King JW, Brelsford HJ, Tullos HS: Analysis of the pitching arm of the professional baseball pitcher. Clin Orthop 1969;67:116–123.
10. Parr TJ, Burns TC: Overuse injuries of the olecranon in adolescents. Orthopedics 2003;26:1143–1146.
11. Kobayashi K, Burton KJ, Rodner C, et al: Lateral compression injuries in the pediatric elbow: Panner's disease and osteochondritis dissecans of the capitellum. J Am Acad Orthop Surg 2004;12:246–254.
12. Yadao MA, Field LD, Savoie FH 3rd: Osteochondritis dissecans of the elbow. Instr Course Lect 2004;53:599–606.
13. Beals RK: The normal carrying angle of the elbow. Clin Orthop 1976;19:194–196.
14. Andrews JR, Wilks KE, Satterwhite YE, et al: Physical examination of the thrower's elbow. J Orthop Sports Phys Ther 1993;17:296–304.
15. Flynn JC, Richards JF, Saltzman RI: Prevention and treatment of non-union of slightly displaced fractures of the humeral condyle in children. An end-result study. J Bone Joint Surg Am 1975;57:1087–1092.
16. Coleman WW, Strauch RJ: Physical examination of the elbow. Orthop Clin N Am 1999;30:15–20.
17. Shah AK, Pruzansky ME: Ruptured biceps brachii short head muscle belly: A case report. J Shoulder Elbow Surg 2004;13:562–565.
18. Cope MR, Ali A, Bayliss NC: Biceps rupture in bodybuilders: Three case reports of rupture of the long head of the biceps at the tendon-labrum junction. J Shoulder Elbow Surg 2004;13:580–582.
19. Volz RE, Morrey BF: The physical examination of the elbow. In Morrey BF (ed): The Elbow and Its Disorders. Philadelphia, WB Saunders, 1985, pp 62–72.
20. Vardakas DG, Musgrave DS, Varitimidis SE, et al: Partial rupture of the distal biceps tendon. J Shoulder Elbow Surg 2001;10:377–379.
21. Gessini L, Jandolo B, Pietrangeli A: Entrapment neuropathies of the median nerve at and above the elbow. Surg Neurol 1983;19:112–116.
22. O'Driscoll SW, Jaloszynski R, Morrey BF, et al: Origin of the medial collateral ligament. J Hand Surg [Am] 1992;17:164–168.
23. Veltri DM, O'Brien SJ, Field LD, et al: The milking maneuver: A new test to evaluate the MCL of the elbow in the throwing athlete [Abstract]. J Shoulder Elbow Surg 1995;4:S10.
24. Hyman J, Breazeale NM, Altchek DW: Valgus instability of the elbow in athletes. Clin Sports Med 2001;20:25–45.

25. Eversmann WW: Entrapment and compressive neuropathies. In Green DP (ed): Operative Hand Surgery. New York, Churchill Livingstone, 1993, pp 1341–1385.

26. Childress HM: Recurrent ulnar-nerve dislocation at the elbow. Clin Orthop 1975;108:168–173.

27. Schickendantz MS, Ho CP, Koh J: Stress injury of the proximal ulna in professional baseball players. Am J Sports Med 2002;30:737–741.

28. Birk GT, DeLee JC: Osteochondral injuries: Clinical findings. Clin Sports Med 2001;20:279–286.

29. Boone DC, Azen SP: Normal range of motion of joints in male subject. J Bone Joint Surg Am 1979;61:756–759.

30. Morrey BF, Askew LJ, An K-N, et al: A biomechanical study of normal functional elbow motion. J Bone Joint Surg Am 1981;63:872–877.

31. Askew LJ, An K-N, Morrey BF, et al: Functional evaluation of the elbow: Normal motion requirements and strength determinations. Orthop Trans 1981;5:304–305.

32. Docherty MA, Schwab RA, Ma OJ: Can elbow extension be used as a test of clinically significant injury? South Med J 2002;95:539–541.

33. Wright TW: Nerve injuries and neuropathies about the elbow. In Norris TR (ed): Orthopaedic Knowledge Update: Shoulder and Elbow. Rosemont, IL, American Association of Orthopedic Surgeons, 1997, pp 369–377.

34. Callaway GH, Field LD, O'Brien SJ, et al: The contribution of medial collateral ligaments to valgus stability of the elbow: A biomechanical study [Abstract]. J Shoulder Elbow Surg 1995;4:S58.

35. O'Driscoll SW: Classification and evaluation of recurrent instability of the elbow. Clin Orthop 2000;370:34–43.

36. Plancher KD, Halbrecht J, Lourie GM: Medial and lateral epicondylitis in the in the athlete. Clin Sports Med 1996;15:283–305.

37. Gardner RC: Tennis elbow: Diagnosis, pathology, and treatment: Nine severe cases treated with a new reconstructive operation. Clin Orthop 1970;72:248–253.

38. Lister GD, Belsole RB, Kleinert HE: The radial tunnel syndrome. J Hand Surg [Am] 1979;4:52–59.

39. Gabel GT, Morrey BF: Tennis elbow. Instr Course Lect 1998;47:165–172.

40. Portilla Molina AE, Bour C, Oberlin C, et al: The posterior interosseous nerve and the radial tunnel syndrome: An anatomical study. Int Orthop 1998;22:102–106.

41. Ekstrom RA, Holden K: Examination of and intervention for a patient with chronic lateral elbow pain with signs of nerve entrapment. Phys Ther 2002;11:1077–1086.

42. Buehler MJ, Thayer DT: The elbow flexion test. A clinical test for cubital tunnel syndrome. Clin Orthop 1988;233:213–216.

43. Greenwald D, Moffitt M, Cooper B: Effective surgical treatment of cubital tunnel syndrome based on provocative clinical testing without electrodiagnostics. Plast Reconstr Surg 1999;104:215–218.

44. Viegas SF: Avulsion of the triceps tendon. Orthop Rev 1990;19:533–536.

45. Chen AL, Youm T, Ong BC, et al: Imaging of the elbow in the overhead throwing athlete. Am J Sports Med 2003;31:466–473.

46. Timmerman LA, Schwartz ML, Andrews JR: Preoperative evaluation of the ulnar collateral ligament by magnetic resonance imaging and computed tomography arthrography. Evaluation in 25 baseball players with surgical confirmation. Am J Sports Med 1994;22:26–32.

47. Miller TT: Imaging of elbow disorders. Orthop Clin North Am 1999;30:21–36.

48. Schwartz ML, Al-Zahrani S, Morwessel RM, et al: Ulnar collateral ligament injury in the throwing athlete: Evaluation with saline-enhanced MR arthrography. Radiology 1995;197:297–299.

49. Kooima CL, Anderson K, Craig JV, et al: Evidence of subclinical medial collateral ligament injury and posteromedial impingement in professional baseball players. Am J Sports Med 2004;32:1602–1606.

50. Salvo JP, Rizio L, Zvijac JE, et al: Avulsion fracture of the ulnar sublime tubercle in overhead throwing athletes. Am J Sports Med 2002;30:426–431.

In This Chapter

INTRODUCTION

- The incidence of overuse elbow injuries is increasing at an alarming rate, particularly in the young overhead athlete population.

- With increasing frequency, injuries that were once limited to the elite professional are now being treated in the young adolescent. Awareness of these trends on the part of the treating physicians, trainers, therapists, and parents is crucial to injury prevention.

- This chapter is designed to review the injuries that occur to the elbow that cause instability, along with the evaluation and treatment of these injuries. As a related topic, elbow arthroscopy techniques and indications are reviewed.

ELBOW INSTABILITY

Relevant Anatomy

The elbow articulation allows two major motions: flexion-extension through the ulnohumeral and radiocapitellar joints and pronation-supination through the proximal radioulnar joint. The osseous configuration confers up to 50% of the stability of the joint when in full extension, but stability is increasingly reliant on soft tissues with increasing flexion. Disruption of the bony architecture as a result of fractures or dysplasias can affect the stability of the elbow and subsequently alter the motion and stresses placed on the soft-tissue supports. As an example, some fractures of the coronoid process can lead to significant elbow instability and increased stress on the radial head. The radial head is an important secondary restraint to valgus load that becomes the primary restraint with injury to the UCL. Thus, if the radial head is fractured, it is important to check the UCL for injury.

The soft-tissue stabilizers are the joint capsule, ligaments, and musculotendinous units.[1] The major ligaments of the elbow are the UCL (ulnar collateral ligament) and the lateral collateral ligament (LCL) complex (Fig. 34-1). The UCL has two clinically important bundles: the anterior bundle and the posterior bundle. The LCL complex is the primary restraint to varus and posterolateral rotatory stress. The lateral UCL, connecting the lateral epicondyle of the humerus to the supinator crest of the lateral side of the ulna, is the most important stabilizer for posterolateral rotatory instability. The annular ligament stabilizes the proximal radioulnar joint[1] and functions as a secondary restraint to posterolateral rotatory stress along with the common extensor origin, anterior and posterior capsules, and the radial collateral ligament, which is the portion of the LCL between the lateral epicondyle and the annular ligament.[2]

Epidemiology

The elbow is the second most common joint that is dislocated in adults, with most dislocations occurring in the posterolateral direction.[3] The annual incidence is 6 to 8 dislocations per 100,000 people. Elbow dislocations account for 11% to 28% of elbow injuries.[1] Although simple elbow dislocations are typically managed with closed reduction and early range of motion, a small percentage of patients continue to have instability symptoms, many of these due to posterolateral rotatory instability. The exact percentage is not known.

Medial instability can occur secondary to an elbow dislocation that was traumatic or can be secondary to chronic overuse. Although medial instability is rarely symptomatic in the non-overhead athlete, it can be problematic in activities of daily living or recreation and warrants investigation in such individuals. In the overhead athletic population, UCL injury is rarely the result of a frank dislocation but rather due to chronic overuse. Acute medial elbow instability can occur in overhead athletes but occurs more commonly in contact or tumbling sports. In football, UCL injuries can be an acute injury, but, as documented in a report by Kenter et al,[4] even in the National Football League, UCL injuries that are acute rarely require operative intervention even in overhead athletes (e.g., the quarterback). It is similarly believed that an acute UCL injury to a baseball thrower also can be treated nonoperatively if it is secondary to trauma and the player has not previously had medial-side elbow pain. Chronic injuries are becoming an increasingly concerning problem, even in the high school baseball athlete, as we have seen a significant increase in the number of high school athletes seeking medical attention for medial-side elbow pain, secondary to UCL tears.

Acute Dislocation

Elbow dislocation usually occurs from a fall on an outstretched hand. It is theorized that valgus and axial load occur while the forearm is in supination (Hildebrand) and the elbow may be

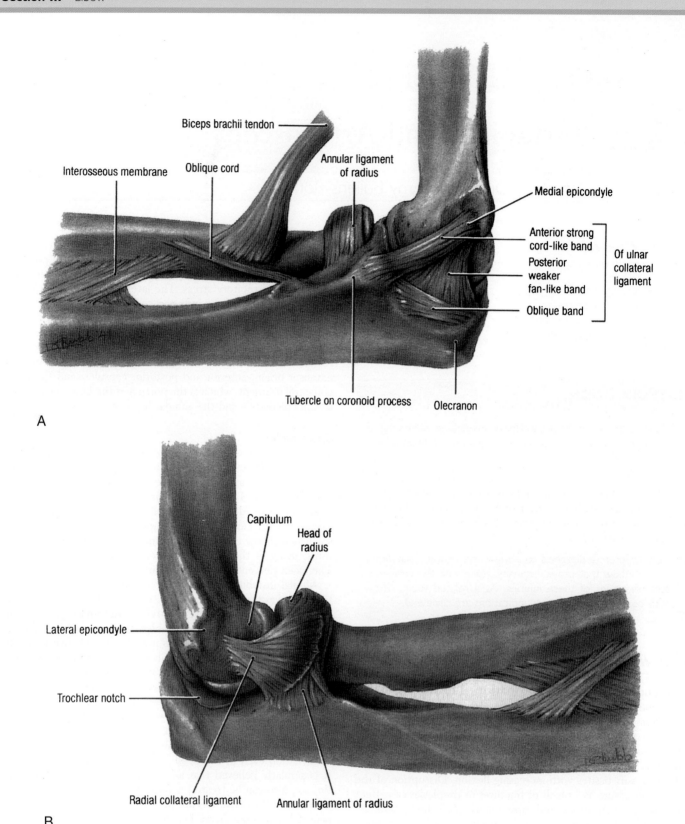

Biceps brachii tendon

Interosseous membrane

Oblique cord

Annular ligament of radius

Medial epicondyle

Anterior strong cord-like band

Posterior weaker fan-like band

Oblique band

Of ulnar collateral ligament

Tubercle on coronoid process

Olecranon

A

Capitulum

Head of radius

Lateral epicondyle

Trochlear notch

Radial collateral ligament

Annular ligament of radius

B

Figure 34-1 A, The medial ligamentous structures of the elbow. Note the anterior band of the ulnar collateral ligament, which is the main stabilizer to a valgus stress. **B,** The lateral collateral ligament complex. (From Agur AMR, Lee MJ: Grant's Atlas of Anatomy, 10th ed. Philadelphia, Lippincott, Williams & Wilkins, 1999.)

slightly flexed or hyperextended. Elbow dislocations are classified by direction of dislocation as posterior, lateral, anterior, or divergent and also as simple or complex, depending on whether fractures are also present. Posterior or posterolateral dislocations are most common.

Elbow dislocations occur during a variety of sporting activities, both contact and noncontact. The effect of the injury on the athlete's return to play depends on the sport and position as well as associated injuries. Some sports are more commonly associated with elbow dislocations. A recent study highlighted the increase in elbow dislocations associated with winter sporting activities since snowboarding has become more popular. Snowboarders had 17 elbow dislocations (simple or complex) of 64 elbow injuries compared to 8 elbow dislocations of 152 elbow injuries in skiers.[5]

Treatment of acute simple elbow dislocations begins with a good history and examination of the affected extremity. While obtaining the history, the mechanism of injury, previous injury to the affected extremity, symptoms of numbness, paresthesias, weakness, and excessive pain should be sought. Physical examination should involve inspection, palpation (elbow, forearm, shoulder, wrist, and hand) as well as a thorough neurologic and vascular examination of the affected extremity and comparison to the unaffected extremity before reduction. Reduction should be performed with adequate sedation and should be followed by a postreduction radiograph showing concentric reduction. There are many techniques to reduce posterior elbow dislocations, but the most common method is by longitudinal traction of the forearm with the elbow held in about 30 degrees of flexion while an assistant is holding countertraction on the upper arm. If any medial or lateral translation is present, it is corrected first, then the olecranon is pushed distally with the thumb of the person performing the reduction. Once the elbow is reduced, it is fully flexed. Prior to splinting, the elbow should be taken through a range of motion to determine the stable arc of motion. Checking for instability of the UCL should be performed and the forearm should be pronated and supinated while the elbow is flexed and extended. If there is isolated damage to the UCL, then the elbow will be more stable with the forearm in supination. If the LCL complex is damaged without damage to the UCL being present, then the elbow will be more stable with the forearm in pronation. If both ligaments are damaged, then the elbow is best splinted with the forearm in neutral.[1] The elbow should be splinted, and then an early range-of-motion program begun as early as 3 days postreduction. In some cases, a hinged brace can be employed with increasing degrees of extension allowed as the healing process progresses.[1] It is rare for a simple elbow dislocation to be irreducible by closed means or for immediate surgical repair or reconstruction of the ligaments to be required.

There has been a recent trend to shortening the immobilization period even further. In a study performed at the Naval Academy, 20 posterior elbow dislocations were treated on postreduction day 1 with an active range-of-motion protocol. They were seen on nearly a daily basis for a supervised range-of-motion program and supplemental modalities such as cryotherapy, electrical stimulation, and compression bandages to reduce swelling for 2 weeks. These patients achieved their final range of motion in 19 days. All patients achieved range of motion within 5 degrees of the unaffected elbow. Only 15% had heterotopic ossification on follow-up radiographs, none of which were clinically significant. No early redislocations occurred. One patient had a redislocation 15 months later in a contact injury and was treated with the same protocol without further incident. No other cases of instability occurred.[6]

Common sequelae of acute simple elbow dislocations include loss of motion of the affected elbow, heterotopic ossification, and recurrent instability. Loss of motion is the most frequent complaint, with loss of 10 to 20 degrees of extension not uncommon.[3] Heterotopic ossification can occur in as many as 55% of patients.[1] Degenerative changes were also found after dislocation in some patients.[3] Neurovascular injuries can occur in simple dislocations and must be identified in the initial assessment in order to avoid potentially disastrous complications. The brachial artery can become entrapped as can the median or ulnar nerves. Treatment is exploration of the affected structures immediately upon discovery of the problem.

Return to play is based on sport-specific and position-specific requirements. In the early postdislocation period, a noncontact athlete may be able to perform at competition level with a hinged brace for protection. In contact sports, even a hinged brace may not be enough protection. Certain minimal goals should be achieved before return to play in any sport. These include return of range of motion, normal neurovascular examination, and relative stability through the functional range of motion for the sport. Soft-tissue healing is generally adequate to begin ligament-stressing exercise by 6 weeks after the injury. Return to contact sports with a brace can be considered after stability is restored but should be individually based. As a general rule, we do not like to remove a protective brace from an athlete during a competition season. If an athlete suffers an elbow dislocation and we begin bracing for sport activity, we continue the brace until the end of the season. If the elbow is stable after the season is over, bracing is not required for further participation in subsequent seasons.

MEDIAL INSTABILITY

Medial elbow pain in the overhead athlete should be taken seriously by both the player and health care team. Medial instability secondary to UCL injury should be suspected and ruled out. Chronic medial instability can be caused by chronic overuse due to repetitive intrinsic stress such as muscular contraction or extrinsic stress due to tensile overload.[7] This can lead to microtears in the UCL that, if not given appropriate time to heal, can lead to attenuation and medial instability.

Relevant Anatomy
The UCL is the primary restraint to valgus stress, with the radial head being a secondary restraint. The UCL has two components: the anterior bundle and the posterior bundle. The anterior bundle is the primary restraint to valgus stress to the elbow when it is at 30, 60, or 90 degrees of flexion.[8] Its origin is the anteroinferior aspect of the medial epicondyle of the humerus and its insertion is the medial portion of the coronoid process, an area called the sublime tubercle.[9] Its mean length is 27.1 ± 4.3 mm and mean width, in one study, is 4.7 ± 1.2 mm.[8] An unpublished study done at our institution, regarding the anterior bundle of the UCL, showed that the mean proximal width of the ligament is 6.8 ± 1.4 mm and mean distal width is 9.2 ± 1.6 mm. Also noted in this cadaveric study was a mean distance of 2.8 mm from the proximal edge of insertion of the ligament into the ulna to the ulnar articular cartilage edge.[10]

Biomechanics of the Ulnar Collateral Ligament and Pitching
The majority of stress present in the UCL occurs during the late cocking and early acceleration phases of throwing.[11–13] The baseball pitch occurs with the elbow flexed from 90 to 120 degrees during the acceleration phase of throwing, after which the elbow rapidly extends.[14] The elbow is then subjected to distraction stress during extension in the release phase. The UCL accounts for 54% of the valgus stability during elbow flexion of 90 degrees and resists 78% of distraction during the release phase.[15] The static torque experienced by the UCL in the course of overhead throwing is nearly the same as the ultimate strength of the lig-

ament itself.[12] Tensile stress occurs in the medial compartment subjecting the UCL, flexor-pronator mass, ulnar nerve, and medial epicondyle apophysis in the skeletally immature athlete to tremendous stress. Shear stress occurs in the posterior compartment subjecting the olecranon and olecranon fossa/trochlea to injury. Compression laterally occurs during throwing, which subjects the radiocapitellar joint to injury. Thus, if the medial elbow is chronically unstable, other areas of the elbow can have clinical findings as well, such as chondromalacia and osteophyte formation as a result of microinstability. Subtle laxity may present with symptoms of ulnar neuritis or flexor-pronator tendonitis. All cases of elbow pain in the throwing athlete should be checked for UCL laxity as an underlying cause.[13]

History

Overhead athletes presenting with medial elbow pain need a very detailed history taken for diagnostic as well as educational purposes. Information on onset of symptoms, the phase of throwing in which the symptoms occur, training changes, previous injuries to the elbow or shoulder, changes in velocity and accuracy, which types of pitches are painful, the number of innings pitched in recent seasons, and associated symptoms such as nerve and vascular symptoms should all be collected.[7,13,16] Eighty-five percent of patients have pain in the acceleration phase and less than 25% have any pain in the deceleration phase.[13,17] In some patients, the offending pitch can be identified as causing an acute rupture of the UCL, but more often the pain comes on gradually and becomes more persistent and painful over time. Ulnar nerve symptoms such as paresthesias in the fourth and fifth digits are present in nearly one fourth of patients; some authors have found ulnar neuritis in as many as 40%.[7,11] Nineteen percent have accompanying posterior elbow pain as noted in one study.[11] Any history of previous treatment such as therapy, injections, and surgery is essential to interpreting current signs and symptoms as well as radiographic studies.

Physical Examination

Physical examination should begin with an inspection of the elbow for any deformity, limitation of motion, swelling, or bruising. Carrying angle averages 11 degrees in men and 13 degrees in women. Some asymptomatic professional throwers can have carrying angles exceeding 15 degrees. Elbow flexion contractures are seen in 50% of professional throwers as well. Neither finding is necessarily indicative of an injury but is important to note nonetheless.[13,18]

Palpation of the elbow should include all bony prominences as well as the UCL, flexor-pronator origin, ulnar nerve, and other soft-tissue structures. The UCL is best palpated with the elbow in 50 to 70 degrees of flexion.[13] Point tenderness is most common 1 to 2 cm distal to the medial epicondyle.[7] Palpation of the ulnar nerve for tenderness, subluxation, and Tinel's sign as well as distal motor and sensory examination should be performed to evaluate for ulnar neuritis or neuropathy.[13] Palpation of pulses should also be performed.

Testing the elbow for medial laxity is best performed with the elbow flexed at 30 degrees, forearm pronated, and the wrist passively flexed (Fig. 34-2). The patient can also be placed supine with the arm abducted and the shoulder maximally external rotated. This position provides the examiner with the easiest position to hold the patient's arm and prevents shoulder rotation from clouding the examination. The pronation and wrist flexion, when done passively, relax the flexor-pronator mass and make the medial aspect of the elbow easier to palpate for joint

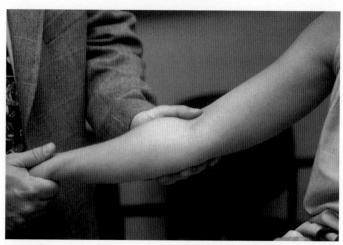

Figure 34-2 Clinical evaluation of the ulnar collateral ligament. The elbow is placed in 30 degrees of flexion and full pronation with the wrist passively flexed. The examiner places a valgus stress and assesses the end feel, the amount of valgus opening, and any pain elicited.

opening. This also decreases any potential dynamic stabilization that occurs.[13] Andrews tests the laxity in the position described with the patient seated, then tests the stability also with the patient supine, the forearm supinated, and elbow flexed at 30 degrees. The test is then repeated with the patient prone with the elbow flexed 30 degrees and the forearm pronated. The Milking maneuver is also performed by grasping the patient's thumb and flexing the elbow to 90 degrees using the thumb to provide valgus stress. This was originally described with the patient grasping his or her own thumb with the opposite hand, but not all patients can perform this maneuver and the examiner needs to be able to simulate it in those patients who cannot. Valgus extension overload can be tested by repeatedly forcefully extending the elbow while placing a valgus stress on it. A positive test occurs when the patient has pain at the posteromedial olecranon tip as the elbow reaches full extension.[7,13,19]

Radiographic Studies

Radiographic studies are necessary in the evaluation of a throwing athlete with medial elbow pain. Anteroposterior, lateral, two oblique, an oblique axial with the elbow in 110 degrees of flexion, and stress views of both the affected and the unaffected extremity comprise a thorough radiographic examination.[13] The oblique axial view is helpful for visualizing posteromedial osteophytes. The standard anteroposterior, lateral and two oblique views may appear normal or may show signs of chronic injury to the medial elbow such as medial osteophytes or calcifications within the ligament.[8] Stress radiographs should be obtained bilaterally to compare the patient's overall ligamentous laxity. A difference of 2 mm is considered diagnostic of medial elbow instability.[8]

In the past, computed tomography arthrography was used frequently to check for UCL tears. Its sensitivity is 86% and specificity is 91%. Saline-enhanced magnetic resonance imaging is now the gold standard, with sensitivity of 92% and specificity of 100% (Fig. 34-3).[20] Magnetic resonance imaging also has the added benefit of diagnosing other potential injuries such as injuries to the flexor-pronator origin. It was previously believed that the T sign of dye on a contrast study was diagnostic of UCL injury. Recent data suggest that the proximal fibers of the UCL insertion onto the sublime tubercle and the capsular fibers may

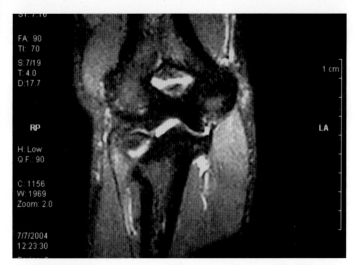

Figure 34-3 Contrast-enhanced magnetic resonance imaging of the elbow. Note the contrast extravasated distal to the elbow joint on the medial side. The ulnar collateral ligament is noted to have a tear in its midsubstance.

insert up to 3 mm distal to the articular surface, making the T sign a less-than-perfect diagnostic finding.[10]

Treatment Options

Once the diagnosis of UCL injury is made, the decision regarding treatment is made with careful consideration of the athlete's demands on the injured area (sport and position played), previous treatment of the injury (rest and rehabilitation done appropriately), and the degree of ligament injury. The vast majority of partial ligament injuries should be treated initially with conservative treatment. Complete injuries in nonthrowing athletes or low-demand throwing athletes may also be treated with a trial of conservative care. Nonoperative treatment consists of a period of rest, anti-inflammatory medi-cation, and therapy modalities such as cryotherapy to decrease pain. Range-of-motion exercises of the elbow and strengthening exercises of the flexor-pronator muscles should be performed during the rest period. Bracing may be used if necessary. In throwing athletes, shoulder strengthening should also be performed to prevent any shoulder injury from occurring when returning to throwing. After a period of "active rest," a throwing program should be instituted. Generally, the program takes about 3 months to complete if done properly.[13,14] Some authors recommend a brace be worn at night in the "active rest" period and a hyperextension brace be worn in the throwing program. With this protocol, one study shows that 42% of players will return to play at the same level in 24 to 25 weeks. In the patients with an acute injury, 44% returned without the need for surgical treatment.[14] It is very important to note that nonoperative treatment does not include any injections into the ligament or elsewhere in the elbow.[13]

Operative treatment is reserved for the overhead athlete with a complete tear or a partial tear that has failed nonoperative treatment. Select other athletes (e.g., gymnasts, wrestlers) may also be unable to return to their sports of choice and may also be considered for reconstruction. There are several different methods of reconstructing the UCL. These include the docking technique, the muscle-splitting approach using bone tunnels, and a suture anchor technique. Although UCL repair

has not met with favorable results in overhead athletes, all the currently employed reconstruction techniques have enjoyed significant clinical success with high rate of return in elite athletes. Our preference is to use a modification of Jobe's original technique, including ulnar nerve transposition to a subcutaneous location beneath a leash of flexor-pronator fascia. This preference is born out of nearly 2 decades of experience at our institution with predictably good results. It is not, however, considered by us to be the only way to achieve the expected goal. This is simply the technique with which we are most acquainted and comfortable.

Author's Preferred Surgical Technique

The patient is placed supine on the operating table and general anesthesia is used. The elbow is examined under anesthesia and then placed on an arm board. We use a tourniquet inflated to 250 mm Hg. Until 3 years ago, we performed elbow arthroscopy through an anterolateral portal prior to beginning the UCL reconstruction. We abandoned performing the elbow arthroscopy because we did not change anything in our surgical technique based on the findings during the arthroscopy.

The procedure begins with a medial incision centered over the medial epicondyle approximately 10 cm in length. Identification of the medial antebrachial cutaneous nerve is performed, and it is protected using a vessel loop for retraction. The ulnar nerve is then dissected from the cubital tunnel and release of the nerve is taken proximally to the arcade of Struthers and distally into the flexor carpi ulnaris muscle mass (Fig. 34-4). The medial intermuscular septum is excised distally to prevent tenting of the nerve after transposition. The anterior band of the UCL is exposed by elevating the flexor muscle mass from the ligament at its attachment to the sublime tubercle (Fig. 34-5). The ligament is then incised longitudinally, from the apex of the sublime tubercle toward its origin on the medial epicondyle in line with the fibers (Fig. 34-6). This splitting of the native ligament allows direct visualization of the origin and insertion of the ligament, as well as excision of any bony osteophytes or previously avulsed bony fragments.

If valgus extension overload is also present, we perform a vertical incision in the posterior capsule proximal to the fibers of

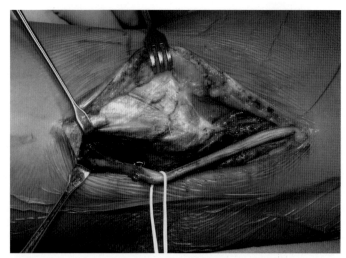

Figure 34-4 Surgical exposure of the medial elbow, including isolation of the ulnar nerve. Note the preservation of the motor branch to the flexor musculature. At the time of ulnar nerve dissection, the medial intermuscular septum is excised.

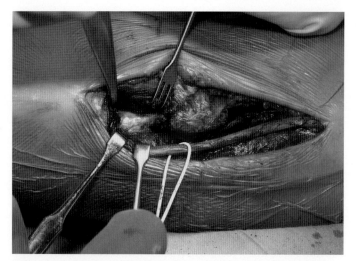

Figure 34-5 The flexor-pronator mass is elevated off the underlying ulnar collateral ligament. This allows visualization of the entire length of the anterior band of the ligament. Note also the tear in the proximal portion of the ligament.

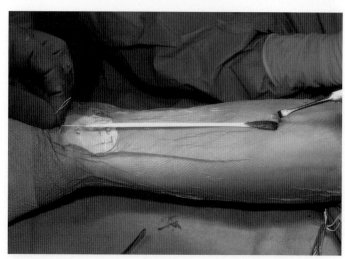

Figure 34-7 The palmaris longus graft is harvested using two small incisions at the distal forearm and one incision at the level of the muscle-tendon junction.

the posterior band. This exposes the olecranon tip for inspection and removal of any offending osteophytes. The osteophytes are removed with a small osteotome and a high-speed bur. The capsule is then closed with absorbable suture.

Graft harvest is then performed. We prefer the ipsilateral palmaris longus tendon if it is present and of sufficient size (Fig. 34-7). If it is not, then the contralateral gracilis tendon is our next choice. The palmaris is harvested with three small transverse incisions in the volar forearm with the most distal incision at the proximal wrist crease. Care should be taken to avoid harvesting the flexor carpi radialis or median nerve, which are in close proximity.

Next, the ulnar tunnels are drilled using a 9/64-inch drill bit (palmaris graft) or 5/32-inch drill bit (gracilis graft). The ulnar tunnels are drilled 3 to 4 mm distal to the articular surface. The first tunnel begins just at the posterior aspect of the sublime

tubercle and is directed laterally and slightly posteriorly. The second tunnel begins at the anterior aspect of the sublime tubercle and is directed posteriorly. The two tunnels are connected to each other with curved curets and irrigated. Two tunnels are then drilled in the medial epicondyle of the humerus, converging at the origin of the native UCL. The first tunnel is drilled proximally to distally, and the second medially to distally with a 1-cm bridge between the two tunnels. The tunnels are then curetted and irrigated. Suture loops are then passed through the three tunnels. The distal portion of the native ligament is closed with nonabsorbable suture to enhance the stability, leaving the proximal portion of the native ligament open to allow graft passage. The graft is brought on the table, and a tendon-gathering stitch is placed in each end of the graft in order to allow tensioning. One of the graft ends is passed through the ulnar tunnel using a suture loop. The ends of the graft are then passed in a figure-eight fashion through the humeral tunnels, and the proximal portion of the native ligament is closed (Fig. 34-8).

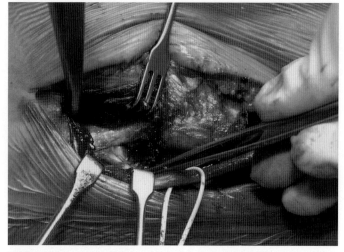

Figure 34-6 The ulnar collateral ligament is split longitudinally to expose the underlying lateral elbow articulation. This allows the surgeon exposure of the undersurface of the ligament, which is the location of most pathology. Also, the visualization facilitates drilling of the humeral and ulnar tunnels.

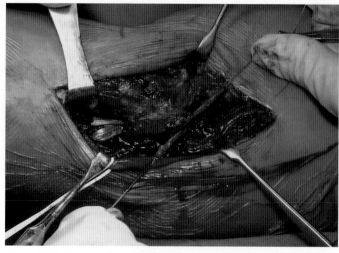

Figure 34-8 The graft is passed in figure-eight fashion through the ulnar and humeral tunnels.

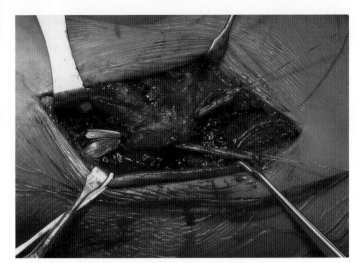

Figure 34-9 The graft is tensioned with the elbow in 30 degrees of flexion and neutral rotation. The limbs of the graft are then tied to one another above the medial epicondyle of the humerus.

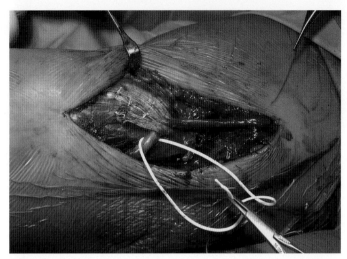

Figure 34-11 The ulnar nerve is transposed beneath a leash of flexor fascia in a subcutaneous fashion. After transposition, the cubital tunnel is closed to prevent the ulnar nerve from returning to its previous location.

The graft is tensioned with the elbow in 30 degrees of flexion and the valgus stress on the elbow removed. While holding this position and holding the tension on the graft ends, which are crossed above the medial epicondyle, the graft is sutured to itself with multiple nonabsorbable sutures (Fig. 34-9). The limbs of the graft spanning the humeral-ulnar course of the ligament are then sutured to one another using permanent suture to add more tension to the graft (Fig. 34-10).

The ulnar nerve is transposed anteriorly using a fascial sling from the flexor-pronator muscle mass (Fig. 34-11). The cubital tunnel is closed and the split in the flexor carpi ulnaris fascia is closed distally with one stitch to prevent propagation of the split and herniation of the muscle. The skin is closed and the elbow placed in a well-padded posterior splint flexed to 90 degrees for 5 to 7 days. The patient then is placed in a hinged range-of-motion brace and follows a supervised rehabilitation program. The patient will begin a throwing program at 16 weeks, and will be able to return to competition at an average of nearly 9 months.

Results

After nonoperative treatment of UCL injuries in overhead athletes, the return to play rate is 42%.[14] UCL repair may have a better return to play rate (50% to 63%) than nonoperative treatment, but it does not approach the rate of return of reconstructive treatment.[17,21] This decreased chance to return to play is especially true for the attenuated and partial ligament tears, which are not amenable to repair but could theoretically be imbricated. UCL reconstruction fares much better with reported return to play rates being 80% to 92%.[11,12,22] The rate of return to play at the same or higher level is not as good for high school baseball players, averaging 74%. The reason for the lower rate of return to play in the high school athlete may be only secondary to other issues with adolescents such as loss of interest in the sport or decreased opportunity to play at the next level (e.g., a senior high school player being injured and not being recruited for college or drafted).[23]

POSTEROLATERAL ROTATORY INSTABILITY

Posterolateral rotatory instability was a phrase coined by O'Driscoll et al[24] in 1991 after describing the clinical entity as we know it today. Since then, interest and knowledge of the topic has grown. It is thought that this condition usually arises after traumatic dislocation of the elbow and clinically presents along a wide spectrum of instability. The affected structure is the LCL complex of the elbow, with specific injury to the lateral UCL. The degree of injury to the lateral side of the elbow that is necessary to cause instability is currently still under investigation. As stated earlier in this chapter, elbow dislocations are relatively common injuries and yet this type of instability was only recognized in the past 2 decades. It is still unknown how common this condition is and what the predisposing factors are that cause instability after elbow dislocation. The percentage of elbow dislocations that later have posterolateral rotatory instability is still unknown.

Relevant Anatomy

As noted at the beginning of the chapter, the elbow joint is a very congruous joint with bony anatomy accounting for the

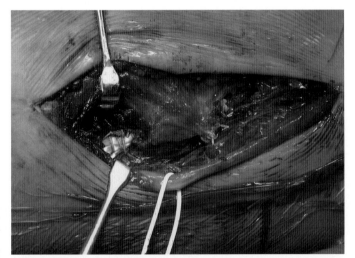

Figure 34-10 The graft is sewn to itself and the underlying native ulnar collateral ligament. This provides additional tension to the graft.

majority of the stability of the elbow. The LCL complex is thought to have four major components: lateral UCL, radial collateral ligament (RCL), annular ligament, and accessory LCL. It appears to have a Y-shaped configuration.[25] Proximally, the complex originates as a broad band from the lateral humeral epicondyle.[26] Some authors refer to this as the superior band.[25] Distally, the ligament may continue as one band or split into two bands, the anterior band being the radial collateral ligament and the posterior band being the lateral UCL.[25,26] The annular ligament stabilizes the proximal radioulnar joint and the accessory collateral ligament is a band from the ulna to the annular ligament.[26] The insertion point of the lateral UCL is the supinator crest of the ulna.

Cadaveric studies have shown that the entire LCL complex provides stability to the elbow. Sectioning of the radial collateral ligament does cause an increase in external rotation when the elbow is passively flexed and extended and causes an increase in varus laxity with the elbow ranged from 10 to 120 degrees. However, subluxation did not occur when the radial collateral ligament was sectioned because the lateral UCL and the coronoid prevented subluxation in those situations. When the lateral UCL was sectioned, gross instability with joint subluxation occurred to rotation.[25]

The common extensor origin also provides some dynamic stability to the lateral side of the elbow. Maintenance of the integrity of the proximal radioulnar joint is also necessary for posterolateral rotatory instability to occur as both the radial head and the ulna rotate and subluxate. If the proximal radioulnar joint is disrupted, then the ulna will not subluxate with the radial head, causing solely radial head instability.[24,26,27] O'Driscoll et al also believe that the posterolateral capsule provides some stability.[2,24]

A study of 62 elbow dislocations and fracture-dislocations showed that 52% of injuries to the lateral UCL complex occurred as a proximal soft-tissue avulsion off the lateral humeral epicondyle. Twenty-nine percent sustained a midsubstance rupture. Eight percent had a proximal bony avulsion that was large enough to repair by osteosynthesis and 2% had a similar injury off the ulna. Only 5% had distal soft-tissue avulsion off the ulna.[2]

Concomitant rupture of the common extensor origin was seen in 62% of fracture-dislocations and 80% of pure dislocations.[2] Though these injuries were more severe than the average elbow injuries because they required treatment secondary to inability to obtain or maintain closed reduction, a study of elbow dislocations that were able to be reduced found that 14 of 18 elbows where the lateral side was explored showed injury to the common extensor origin.[28] It is O'Driscoll's opinion that damage to the supporting structures on the lateral side of the elbow (RCL, common extensor origin, anterior and posterior capsules) may cause posterolateral rotatory instability in the situation where the lateral UCL is torn.

History

Most patients present to the office complaining of lateral elbow pain or discomfort combined with sensation of snapping, catching, or locking. They may be able to express the feeling that the elbow is slipping out of place with the forearm in supination and the elbow slightly flexed. Some more severe cases may present with the history of multiple dislocation episodes. Seventy-five percent of patients younger than 20 years old will have a history of traumatic dislocation. Older patients may have a history of varus/extension stress. Still others may have other history such

as lateral epicondylar release or cubitus varus deformity from childhood trauma.[7,26,29]

Physical Examination

Primarily, the elbow should be palpated for tenderness and inspected for deformity and range-of-motion deficits. Testing for other types of instability including valgus instability should be performed. The pivot-shift maneuver should be done by standing at the head of the patient with the patient lying supine and the arm extended above his or her head. The forearm should be maximally supinated, the elbow should begin extended, then the axial load is applied, and the elbow is slowly flexed. Many patients will have pain or apprehension with this maneuver but may not have noticeable subluxation in the office. Often the subluxation is only felt with the patient under general anesthesia.[26,29,30]

Other provocative maneuvers include having the patient push up from a prone or wall position with the forearms in maximal pronation, then repeat with forearms maximally supinated. The patient will have symptoms with maximal supination. Another method is to have the patient push up from a seated position in a chair with the arm maximally supinated.[26]

Radiographic Studies

Standard practice is to obtain anteroposterior and lateral radiographs to look for evidence of previous trauma (e.g., heterotopic ossification, fracture deformity). Usually these radiographs are normal. Stress views can be obtained with the arm held in the pivot-shift position if the patient can tolerate it. Magnetic resonance imaging and computed tomography are of very limited value.[7,26]

Arthroscopy

Diagnostic arthroscopy can show evidence of posterolateral rotatory instability with two signs. First, the radial head can be demonstrated to subluxate when a pivot-shift maneuver is performed. Second, a drive-through sign can be seen by driving from the lateral gutter from the posterolateral portal and going into the ulnohumeral joint (i.e., driving through the radiocapitellar joint).[26]

Treatment

The first line of treatment is prevention of the problem. Although it is unknown how many elbow dislocations will later develop posterolateral rotatory instability, recognition of damage to lateral structures in a dislocated elbow and treating it accordingly are the first steps in prevention. If an elbow dislocation has evidence of damage to the lateral structures, then stabilizing the elbow with the forearm in pronation is helpful to prevent future lateral instability problems.[27,31] Unfortunately, elbows with significant medial instability as well may not be stable in pronation.

Once chronic posterolateral rotatory instability is diagnosed, there are no conservative measures that appear to treat this condition. Surgical reconstruction of the LCL complex is the only treatment with known clinical success. The method of surgical treatment in chronic cases is usually ligament reconstruction with a tendon graft obtained from palmaris longus or a piece of triceps tendon.[26,29,30] Occasionally, the ligament is only attenuated and can be imbricated.[26,29] The reconstruction of the ligament complex can be performed via bone tunnels similar to the method of UCL reconstruction described earlier in the chapter or with anchors and bone tunnels.[29,30] Recently arthroscopic capsular plication and ligament imbrication has been performed in some centers with some success.[26]

Rehabilitation and Results

The rehabilitation protocols are still evolving for this condition. Different surgeons are still using slightly different recommendations. Postoperatively, the elbow is immobilized at 70 to 90 degrees of flexion in full pronation from 2 to 6 weeks, depending on the surgeon. Full range of motion is begun from 3 to 6 weeks. Some surgeons require that the patient wear a hinged elbow brace until 3 months postoperatively for protection of the reconstruction. Return to play is allowed at 6 to 9 months postoperatively.[26,29,30]

Complications of the procedure that have been reported include recurrent instability, loss of motion, and injury to the lateral antebrachial cutaneous nerve.[7,30] A potential risk to the posterior interosseous nerve is present, especially with the arthroscopic technique. There are very few studies with long-term follow-up or a significant patient sample size from which to report results. O'Driscoll et al[24] found 90% satisfactory outcomes in the patients without significant degenerative changes. Olsen and Sojbjerg[30] had 89% good to excellent results using their technique with suture anchors and bony trough in the ulna and a triceps graft; 83% returned to preinjury activity level and 94% were satisfied with the outcome.

It is important to note that the natural history of posterolateral rotatory instability is not known.[7] If a patient is symptomatic but not surgically reconstructed, it is unknown whether degenerative changes or worsening of the symptoms will result.

ELBOW ARTHROSCOPY

Elbow arthroscopy is becoming a more common procedure as surgeons become more familiar with the techniques of arthroscopy and the indications for the use of arthroscopy in elbow surgery expand. The equipment necessary to perform elbow arthroscopy is similar to that of other arthroscopic procedures. A 4.0-mm, 30-degree arthroscope and a 2.7-mm short-barreled arthroscope are necessary to perform a thorough procedure. Standard 3.5- and 4.5-mm shavers and burs and graspers are often needed. A gravity or inflow pump and, depending on positioning, a bean bag, a traction setup, and a post are needed. In some cases, osteotomes and mallets may be used as well. Generally, an experienced arthroscopist has all these tools available.

Indications for performing elbow arthroscopy are constantly evolving. Well-accepted indications include diagnostic arthroscopy, removal of loose bodies, excision of osteophytes, synovectomy in patients with inflammatory arthropathies, treatment of osteochondritis desiccans of the capitellum, radial head excision, treatment of lateral epicondylitis, treatment of arthrofibrosis, septic arthritis, resection of plica, and assisting in fracture reduction.[32] A newer indication includes treatment of posterolateral rotatory instability.[26]

Contraindications to elbow arthroscopy are significant distortion of normal anatomy, bony ankylosis, and severe fibrous ankylosis. Caution should be used in cases of previous ulnar nerve transposition, as anterior medial portals and some posterior portals place this structure at risk.

Positioning in the operating room is mostly surgeon preference. There are three main ways in which a patient may be positioned: supine with the arm on a table or suspended from a boom, prone with the arm over a post, or lateral decubitus with the arm over a post. Supine positioning has the advantage of ease of transitioning to an open procedure. The disadvantage to supine positioning is that the surgeon is often working with the instruments directed upward, which can be awkward, and the arm may swing back and forth while working. The advantages to prone positioning are the ease of working in the posterior compartment, the ease of manipulating the joint, and the improved scope mobility. Disadvantages to the prone position are the lack of flexion that can be obtained in that position, difficulty in working in the anterior compartment, and difficulty in repositioning the patient for a subsequent open procedure. Advantages to the lateral position are the relative ease to convert to supine, good posterior visualization, and other benefits similar to those of prone positioning. A disadvantage to the lateral position is some difficulty in accessing the anterior compartment.

The procedure starts with elevation of the extremity and inflation of the tourniquet. Ten to 15 milliliters of sterile fluid is injected into the elbow from the "soft spot" in the lateral elbow (between the lateral epicondyle, radial head, and olecranon). There are several portals that can be used in elbow arthroscopy. The anterolateral portal can be used as the initial portal. The location of the portal is 2 to 3 cm distal and 1 cm anterior to the lateral epicondyle.[33] The structure that is most at risk with this portal placement is the radial nerve, which is 2 to 10 mm away from the portal.[34] The proximal lateral portal is also used as the initial portal by some because it is farther away from the neurovascular structures. The proximal lateral portal is located approximately 2 cm proximal to the lateral epicondyle along the anterior surface of the distal humerus.[34] The posterior antebrachial cutaneous nerve may be the closest structure to the portal at 0 to 14 mm away and the radial nerve is on average 10 mm away.[34] The anteromedial portal is generally made under direct visualization. The location is 2 cm distal and 2 cm anterior to the medial epicondyle.[33] The most at-risk major structure there is the median nerve, which is 5 to 13 mm away (lateral) from the cannula.[34] The proximal medial portal is thought to be safer than the anteromedial portal and is located 2 cm proximal to the medial epicondyle and just anterior to the intermuscular septum.[35] Again, the median nerve is at risk but is farther away at 7 to 20 mm.[34] The ulnar nerve is not at risk except for possible subluxating ulnar nerve or history of transposition. The direct lateral portal is located between the lateral epicondyle, radial head, and olecranon, in the soft spot.[33] This is a safe portal. If work is going to be performed in the lateral compartment of the elbow, two portals need to be made laterally. One should be about 1 cm distal so there is enough room to work in this space. The posterolateral portal is placed under direct visualization with the elbow in 30 to 45 degrees of flexion. The portal should be 3 cm proximal to the olecranon tip at the lateral edge of the triceps tendon.[33] This portal has relatively low risk. The direct posterior portal is placed under spinal needle localization. It may be placed either directly through the triceps tendon or just medial to it, 3 cm proximal to the olecranon tip. The ulnar nerve is at risk if the portal is placed medial to the tendon. Care must be taken to cut away from the nerve and use the nick-and-spread technique.[33]

Results and Outcomes

An early study of results following elbow arthroscopy showed that the best results followed loose body removal, with up to 89% of patients significantly improved, and the results for treatment of chondromalacia were less favorable.[33,36] A follow-up study by Andrews et al[37] confirmed that the best results occurred after treatment of mechanical problems such as loose bodies. Treatment of capitellar OCD has also been found to have good short-term results with 13 of 16 adolescent athletes returning to their sports after surgery.[38] Treatment of osteophytes with posterior elbow impingement showed 100% good to excellent results in one study of 21 patients at nearly 3 years of follow-up.[39] Treatment of arthrofibrosis, while beneficial, shows moderately impressive results with 79% rated as good to excellent; although the average flexion contracture was still more than 10 degrees postoperatively, the average gain of extension was 18 degrees.[40] The results of arthrofibrosis surgery are good overall, but it is more risky to perform.

Complications

Reported complications of elbow arthroscopy include compartment syndrome, septic arthritis, superficial infection, drainage from portal sites, and neurovascular injuries. In one study, the most common immediate complication was transient nerve palsy; it occurred in 12 of 473 patients. Four were superficial radial nerve, five ulnar nerve, one posterior interosseous nerve, one anterior interosseous nerve, and one medial antebrachial cutaneous nerve palsies. All palsies resolved within 6 weeks except one, which resolved in 6 months. Factors that were found to increase risk included rheumatoid arthritis, contractures, and capsular releases. No permanent nerve injuries were found in 473 procedures. No compartment syndromes or hematomas

occurred. The most common delayed complication was prolonged drainage from the portal site (defined as drainage for longer than 5 days), which occurred in 5% of patients. Increased risk factors for this drainage included not suturing the portals or using simple stitches. The anterolateral and direct lateral portals were the most common portals affected. Superficial infections occurred in 2% of patients. Septic arthritis occurred in nearly 1% of patients. This was increased in patients who had steroids injected into the elbow at the end of the procedure. Seven of 473 procedures had persistent loss of motion between 5 and 15 degrees.[32]

Reported severe nerve injuries include posterior interosseous nerve transection during capsulectomy, and complete transection of the median and radial nerves in a patient with posttraumatic elbow contracture.[41,42] Kim also reported two transient median nerve palsies.[43]

Risk factors for neurovascular injuries include rheumatoid arthritis and arthrofibrosis. Rheumatoid arthritis increases the risk of injury secondary to the thin and friable capsule and loss of normal intra-articular landmarks. Arthrofibrosis increases risk secondary to decreased capsular distention and the process of capsular release as well as the increased complexity of the procedure. Kelly et al[32] believe that the use of retractors in the anterior part of the elbow while performing capsular release and arthroscopic identification of the nerves decrease the risk of serious nerve injury.

REFERENCES

1. Hildebrand KA, Patterson SD, King GJW: Acute elbow dislocations: Simple and complex. Orthop Clin North Am 1999;30:63–79.
2. McKee MD, Schemitsch EH, Sala MJ, O'Driscoll SW: The pathoanatomy of lateral ligamentous disruption in complex elbow instability. J Shoulder Elbow Surg 2003;12:391–396.
3. Eygendaal D, Verdegaal SHM, Rosing PM et al: Posterolateral dislocation of the elbow joint: Relationship to medial instability. J Bone Joint Surg Am 2000;82:555–560.
4. Kenter K, Behr CT, Warren RF, et al: Acute elbow injuries in the National Football League. J Shoulder Elbow Surg 2000;9:1–5.
5. Takagi M, Sasaki K, Kiyoshige Y: Fracture and dislocation of snowboarder's elbow. J Trauma 1999;47:77–81.
6. Ross G, McDevitt ER, Chronister R, Ove PN: Treatment of simple elbow dislocation using an immediate motion protocol. Am J Sports Med 1999;27:308–311.
7. Lee ML, Rosenwasser MP: Chronic elbow instability. Orthop Clin North Am 1999;30:81–89.
8. Hyman J, Breazeale NM, Altchek DW: Valgus instability of the elbow in athletes. Clin Sports Med 2001;20:25–45.
9. Salvo JP, Rizio L, Zvijac JE, et al: Avulsion fracture of the ulnar sublime tubercle in overhead throwing athletes. Am J Sports Med 2002;30:426–431.
10. Ostrander R, Dugas J, Kingsley D: Anatomy of the anterior bundle of the ulnar collateral ligament (unpublished data, 2006).
11. Thompson WH, Jobe FW, Yocum LA, et al: Ulnar collateral ligament reconstruction in athletes: Muscle-splitting approach without transposition of the ulnar nerve. J Shoulder Elbow Surg 2001;10:152–157.
12. Rohrbough JT, Altchek DW, Hyman J, et al: Medial collateral ligament reconstruction of the elbow using the docking technique. Am J Sports Med 2002;30:541–548.
13. Cain EL, Dugas JR, Wolf RS, Andrews JR: Elbow injuries in throwing athletes: A current concepts review. Am J Sports Med 2003;31:621–635.
14. Rettig AC, Sherrill C, Snead DS, et al: Nonoperative treatment of ulnar collateral ligament injuries in throwing athletes. Am J Sports Med 2001;21:15–17.
15. Andrews JR, Heggland EJH, Fleisig GS, Zheng N: Relationship of ulnar collateral ligament strain to amount of medial olecranon osteotomy. Am J Sports Med 2001;29:716–721.
16. Dugas JR, Weiland AJ: Vascular pathology in the throwing athlete. Hand Clin 2000;16:477–485.
17. Conway JE, Jobe FW, Glousan RE, et al: Medial instability of the elbow in throwing athletes: Treatment by repair or reconstruction of the ulnar collateral ligament. J Bone Joint Surg Am 1992;74:67–83.
18. King JW, Brelsford HJ, Tullos HS: Analysis of the pitching arm of the professional baseball pitcher. Clin Orthop 1969;67:116–123.
19. Wilson FD, Andrews JR, Blackburn TA, et al: Valgus extension overload in the pitching elbow. Am J Sports Med 1983;11:83–88.
20. Schwartz ML, Al-Zahrani S, Morwessel RM, et al: Ulnar collateral ligament injury in the throwing athlete: Evaluation with saline-enhanced MR arthrography. Radiology 1995;197:297–299.
21. Azar FM, Andrews JR, Wilk KE, Groh D: Operative treatment of ulnar collateral ligament injuries of the elbow in athletes. Am J Sports Med 2000;28:16–23.
22. Andrews JR, Timmerman LA: Outcome of elbow surgery in professional baseball players. Am J Sports Med 1995;23:407–413.
23. Petty DH, Andrews JR, Fleisig GS, Cain EL: Ulnar collateral ligament reconstruction in high school baseball players: Clinical results and injury risk factors. Am J Sports Med 2004;32:1158–1164.
24. O'Driscoll SW, Bell DF, Morrey BF: Posterolateral rotatory instability of the elbow. J Bone Joint Surg Am 1991;73:440–446.
25. Seki A, Olsen BS, Jensen SL, et al: Functional anatomy of the lateral collateral ligament complex of the elbow: Configuration of Y and its role. J Shoulder Elbow Surg 2002;11:53–59.
26. Yadao MA, Savoie FH, Field LD: Posterolateral rotatory instability of the elbow. Instructional Course Lecture 2004;53:607–614.
27. O'Driscoll SW: Elbow dislocations. In Morrey BF (ed): The Elbow and Its Disorders, 3rd ed. Philadelphia, WB Saunders, 2000, pp 409–420.
28. Josefsson PO, Johnsell O, Wendeberg B: Ligamentous injuries in dislocations of the elbow joint. Clin Orthop 1987;221:221–225.

29. Lee BPH, Teo LHY: Surgical reconstruction for posterolateral rotatory instability of the elbow. J Shoulder Elbow Surg 2003;12:476–479.

30. Olsen BS, Sojbjerg JO: The treatment of recurrent posterolateral instability of the elbow. J Bone Joint Surg Br 2003;85:342–346.

31. Cohen MS, Hastings H: II. Acute elbow dislocation: Evaluation and management. J Am Acad Orthop Surg 1998;6:15–33.

32. Kelly EW, Morrey BF, O'Driscoll SW: Complications of elbow arthroscopy. J Bone Joint Surg Am 2001;83:25–34.

33. Andrews JR, Carson WG: Arthroscopy of the elbow. Arthroscopy 1985;1:97–107.

34. Stothers K, Day B, Regan WR: Arthroscopy of the elbow: Anatomy, portal sites, and a description of the proximal lateral portal. Arthroscopy 1995;11:449–457.

35. Poehling GG, Whipple TL, Sisco L, Goldman MS: Elbow arthroscopy: A new technique. Arthroscopy 1989;5:22–24.

36. Ogilvie-Harris DJ, Schemitsch E: Arthroscopy of the elbow for removal of loose bodies. Arthroscopy 1993;9:5–8.

37. Andrews JR, St Pierre RK, Carson WG Jr: Arthroscopy of the elbow. Clin Sports Med 1986;5:653–662.

38. Baumgarten TE, Andrews JR, Satterwhite YE: The arthroscopic classification and treatment of osteochondritis dissecans of the capitellum. Am J Sports Med 1998;26:520–523.

39. Ogilvie-Harris DJ, Gordon R, MacKay M: Arthroscopic treatment for posterior impingement in degenerative arthritis of the elbow. Arthroscopy 1995;11:437–443.

40. Timmerman LA, Andrews JR: Arthroscopic treatment of posttraumatic elbow pain and stiffness. Am J Sports Med 1994;22:230–235.

41. Jones GS, Savoie FH: Arthroscopic capsular release of flexion contractures (arthrofibrosis) of the elbow. Arthroscopy 1993;9:277–283.

42. Haapaniemi T, Berggren M, Adolfsson L: Complete transection of the median and radial nerves during an arthroscopic release of posttraumatic elbow contracture. Arthroscopy 1999;15:784–787.

43. Kim SJ, Kim HK, Lee JW: Arthroscopy for limitation of motion of the elbow. Arthroscopy 1995;11:680–683.

35 Overuse Injuries, Tendonosis, and Nerve Compression

Laurence Laudicina and Thomas Noonan

In This Chapter

INTRODUCTION

- Overuse injuries of the elbow are best diagnosed by a thorough history and physical examination.

- Most overuse injuries of the elbow can be treated with conservative means.

- Some conditions may prove recalcitrant to such treatment.

- Less invasive surgical techniques have evolved.

- Avoidance of iatrogenic injury caused by surgical intervention, especially for nerve compression disorders, remains paramount.

LATERAL TENDONOSIS/EPICONDYLITIS (TENNIS ELBOW)

Clinical Features and Evaluation

Lateral epicondylitis or tendonosis is usually an overuse injury, although it may be precipitated by minor elbow trauma. The condition is typically due to repetitive flexion/extension or pronation/supination with the elbow near extension. It generally presents as lateral-side elbow pain and tenderness directly over the lateral epicondyle (at the extensor origin), and just distal to it. Pain is elicited at the lateral epicondyle extensor insertion with passive wrist flexion and with resisted wrist and digital extension. The elbow is extended for both provocative maneuvers.[1]

Relevant Anatomy

Lateral epicondylitis (tennis elbow) occurs secondary to repetitive microtrauma involving extensor carpi radialis brevis, sometimes also involving the extensor carpi radialis longus and extensor carpi ulnaris (Fig. 35-1). Microscopic changes in the extensor carpi radialis brevis have been described as angiofibroblastic hyperplasia and hyaline degeneration (Fig. 35-2).[2]

Treatment Options

The mainstay of treatment is nonoperative and can include activity modification, nonsteroidal anti-inflammatory drugs, counterforce brace, physical therapy with stretching and strengthening, ultrasound therapy, ionto-/phonophoresis[3,4] as well as activity modification and sport technique refinement such as modifying racquet grip size and string tension. Limited corticosteroid injections may also be considered. Trephination of tissue and bone in conjunction with percutaneous injection has provided anecdotal relief. Laser therapy and extracorporeal shock wave therapy have recently been suggested as treatments, although significant benefit has yet to be demonstrated.[5–7] Corticosteroid injections have demonstrated short-term benefit, while physical therapy has demonstrated long-term benefit.[8]

Surgery

Surgery is generally reserved for cases not relieved by conservative means and persisting for longer than 6 months. Several techniques have been described (Figs. 35-3 and 35-4). Generally, open excision of the torn abnormal origin and granulation tissue with repair of the extensor carpi radialis and extensor digitorum communis is performed. Decortication of the lateral epicondyle with a rongeur, bur, or pick is typically preferable to lateral epicondylectomy.[9,10]

Arthroscopy has been recently described to delineate concurrent intra-articular pathology. The undersurface of the lateral pathology is débrided via an anterolateral portal and visualized through an anteromedial portal.[11] Percutaneous release has also been described.[12]

Complications of surgical treatment can include residual pain, posterolateral instability, and posterior interosseous nerve injury.

Postoperative Rehabilitation

A postoperative posterior splint at 90 degrees of elbow flexion and neutral rotation is removed within 2 weeks. Progressive range-of-motion exercises are followed by progressive resistance exercises once full range of motion is achieved. Residual or recurrent pain is treated with decreased activities, anti-inflammatory drugs, scar massage, ultrasound therapy, and cryotherapy.

Criteria for Return to Sports

Little or no residual pain, full range of motion, full strength, and ability to tolerate activities in a progressive manner are appropriate return to activity criteria. Initially, a counterforce brace should be used during activities.

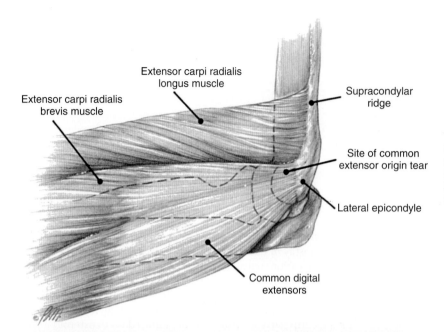

Extensor carpi radialis
longus muscle

Extensor carpi radialis
brevis muscle

Supracondylar
ridge

Site of common
extensor origin tear

Lateral epicondyle

Common digital
extensors

Figure 35-1 Lateral elbow anatomy with common extensor origin. (From Froimson A: Tennis elbow. In Green DP, Hotchkiss RN, Pederson WC [eds]: Green's Operative Hand Surgery, 4th ed. New York, Churchill Livingstone, 1999, p 684.)

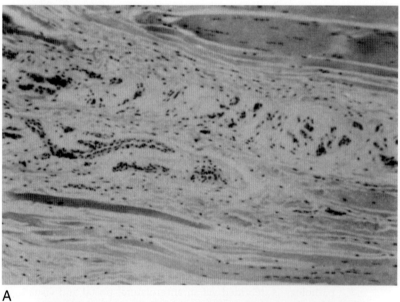

A

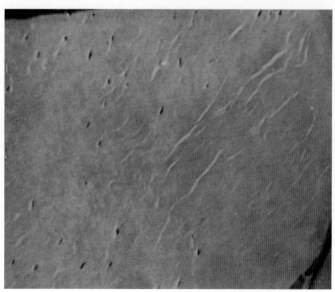

B

Figure 35-2 A, Angiofibroblastic hyperplasia demonstrating vascular proliferation. **B,** Focal hyaline degeneration. (From Morrey B, Regan W: Elbow and forearm: Section B: Tendinopathies about the elbow. In DeLee J, Drez D, Miller, MD [eds]: DeLee and Drez's Orthopaedic Sports Medicine: Principles and Practice. Philadelphia, WB Saunders, 2003, p 1222.)

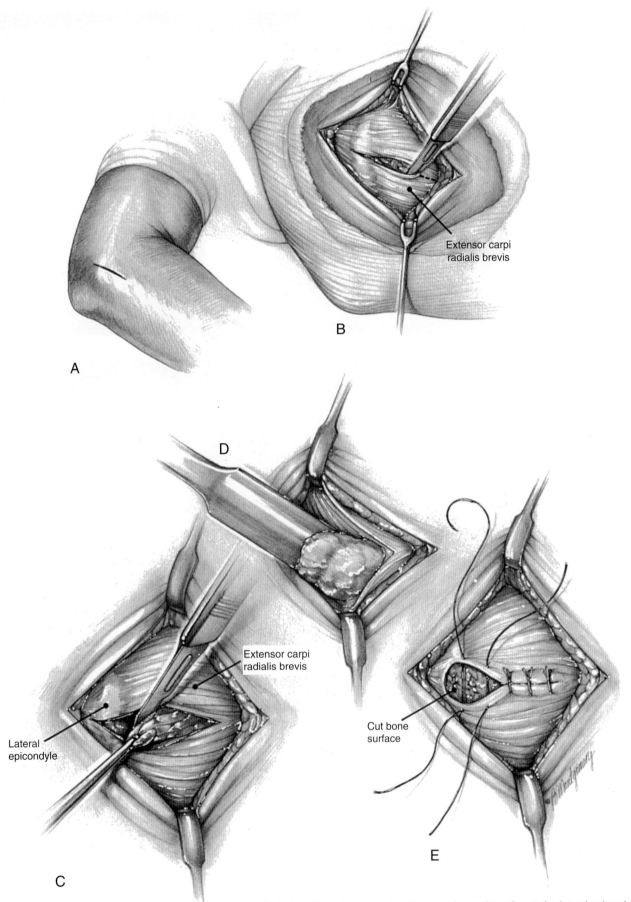

Figure 35-3 Lateral elbow extensor tendon débridement and repair. **A,** Longitudinal incision directly over extensor insertion at the lateral epicondyle. **B,** Common extensor tendon longitudinally incised. **C,** Necrotic, degenerative tendon and granulation tissue excised. **D,** Lateral epicondyle decorticated with osteotome, rongeur, bur, or pick. **E,** Common extensor tendon reapproximated over lateral epicondyle. (From Froimson A: Tennis elbow. In Green DP, Hotchkiss RN, Pederson WC [eds]: Green's Operative Hand Surgery, 4th ed. New York, Churchill Livingstone, 1999, p 686.)

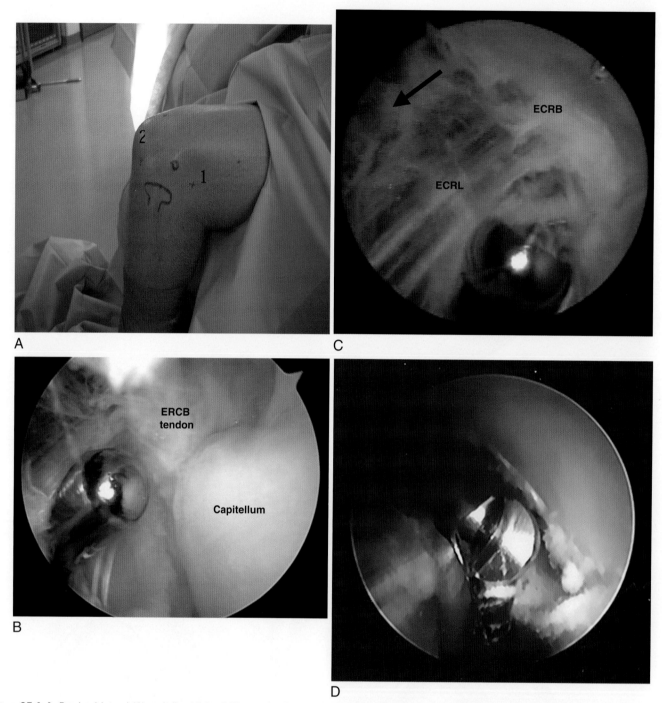

Figure 35-4 A, Proximal lateral (1) and direct lateral (2) portals. **B,** An arthroscopic shaver is used to débride the extensor carpi radialis brevis (ECRB) tendon at the insertion. **C,** Fatty degenerative changes *(arrow)* in the extensor carpi radialis brevis tendon overlying the extensor carpi radialis longus (ECRL). **D,** A hooded bur is used to decorticate the lateral epicondyle. (From Murphy K, Lehman R: Arthroscopic management of lateral epicondylitis. In Miller M, Cole B [eds]: Textbook of Arthroscopy. Philadelphia, WB Saunders, 2004, pp 355–357.)

MEDIAL EPICONDYLITIS/TENDONOSIS (GOLFER'S ELBOW)

Clinical Features and Evaluation

Medial epicondylitis is usually an overuse injury, although it may be precipitated by minor elbow trauma. Repetitive pronation and valgus with the elbow near extension is the typical mechanism. It presents with medial elbow pain, pain with active wrist flexion, and weakness of grip with tenderness over the medial epicondyle at the flexor-pronator origin. Provocative maneuvers include pain with passive wrist extension and elbow extension and pain with resisted wrist and digital flexion and forearm pronation.

Relevant Anatomy

The flexor-pronator mass inserts at the medial epicondyle (Fig. 35-5). Ulnar collateral ligament injury is differentiated by valgus stress testing with pain localized to the ligament. Mild ulnar neuropathy may also be concurrent with medial epicondylitis.

Treatment Options

The mainstay of treatment is nonoperative and involves nonsteroidal anti-inflammatory drugs, counterforce brace, physical therapy with stretching and strengthening, ultrasound therapy, ionto-/phonophoresis, and activity modification and sport technique refinement. Injections may be considered; however, care should be taken and multiple injections are to be avoided due to the proximity of the ulnar nerve and ulnar collateral ligament. Injections should remain anterior to the medial epicondyle to avoid the ulnar nerve.[1]

Surgery

Surgical intervention is reserved for refractory cases with symptoms persisting longer than 6 months to 1 year despite persistent conservative management. Precise localization of the maximal point of tenderness preoperatively is important (Fig. 35-6). The origin of the pronator teres and flexor carpi radialis are exposed. Torn, scarred, and abnormal tissue is excised. Normal tissue is left intact to avoid iatrogenic injury to the ulnar collateral ligament. Care must be taken to protect the medial antebrachial cutaneous nerve branches. Avoid medial epicondylectomy and consider nerve transposition if significant preoperative neuropathy exists.[9]

Postoperative Rehabilitation

Postoperative care is slower than that of lateral epicondylitis and may require as long as 6 months. A posterior elbow splint is placed in 90 degrees of elbow flexion and neutral forearm rotation for 3 weeks. Range of motion is progressively increased followed by progressive strength and endurance exercises at approximately 6 weeks.

Criteria for Return to Sport

Little or no residual pain, full range of motion, full strength (within 85% of the contralateral side), and ability to tolerate activities in a progressive manner are appropriate return to activity criteria. A counterforce brace should be used during initial sporting activities.

Complications

Persistent ulnar neuropathy, ulnar nerve injury, iatrogenic medial instability, and elbow stiffness are recognized complications. All are fortunately rare.[13]

OLECRANON BURSITIS (MINER'S OR STUDENT'S ELBOW)

Clinical Features and Evaluation

Olecranon bursitis involves inflammation of the superficial olecranon bursa and may be considered acute, chronic, or septic. It has been termed miner's or student's elbow. Nonseptic bursitis is most commonly seen in football and hockey and other contact sports that may involve a direct fall onto a partially flexed elbow. Painless swelling of the bursa after a direct blow is the most common presentation. Recurrent episodes may be the result of less trauma than the initial insult. Septic bursitis is more commonly seen in mat sports such as wrestling or gymnastics, and clinical suspicion should leave a low threshold for aspiration and analysis of warm, erythematous or painful bursitis. The most common organism is *Staphylococcus aureus*. Chronic cases may replace the bursa with fibrous tissue and

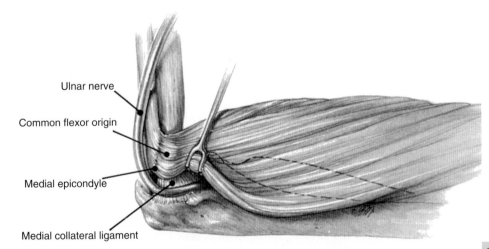

Figure 35-5 Medial elbow anatomy demonstrating the common flexor insertion and ulnar nerve. (From Froimson A: Tennis elbow. In Green DP, Hotchkiss RN, Pederson WC [eds]: Green's Operative Hand Surgery, 4th ed. New York, Churchill Livingstone, 1999, p 685.)

Ulnar nerve

Common flexor origin

Medial epicondyle

Medial collateral ligament

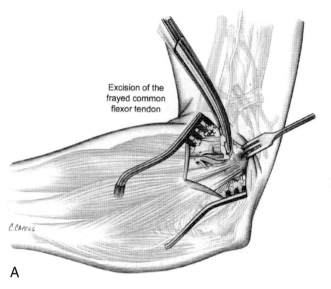

Excision of the
frayed common
flexor tendon

C. CAPERS

A

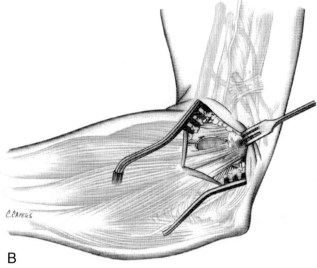

C. CAPERS

B

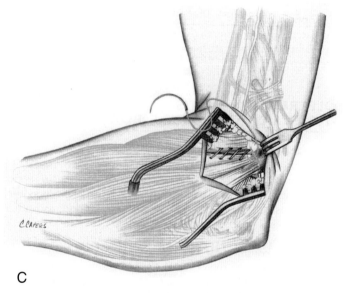

C. CAPERS

C

Figure 35-6 Medial epicondylitis operative débridement. **A,** Excision of the frayed, degenerative common flexor origin. **B,** Normal tissue of the flexor pronator origin left intact. **C,** Reapproximation of the flexor pronator origin following decortication. (From Dlabach JA, Baker CL: Lateral and medial epicondylitis in the overhead athlete. Op Tech Orthop 2001;11:52.)

can prove difficult to resolve by conservative means (Fig. 35-7).

Relevant Anatomy
The subcutaneous bursa is most often involved in olecranon bursitis. Intratendinous and subtendinous bursae have been described but are rarely involved. With recurrent episodes, trabeculae and villiform and fibrous masses may be palpable in the subcutaneous bursa. An olecranon bone spur may be present in chronic recurrent cases.

Treatment Options
Compression and cryotherapy can help minimize swelling following traumatic acute olecranon bursitis. Protective covering and doughnut padding are important to prevent recurrent trauma and subsequent swelling, fibrous tissue formation, and progression to chronic bursitis. Aspiration may be considered for severe bursa distension interfering with elbow function and is recommended if there is suspicion of infection. Cell count, crystal analysis, and Gram stain should be performed. A purulent aspiration may be lavaged and injected with 0.5 g methicillin in 10 mL saline. Aspiration is performed with sterile technique and followed by compressive dressing for 36 to 48 hours.[1]

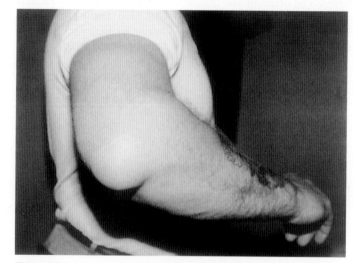

Figure 35-7 Olecranon bursitis clinical appearance. (From Baker CL, Cummings PD: Arthroscopic management of miscellaneous elbow disorders. Op Tech Sports Med 1998;6:16–21.)

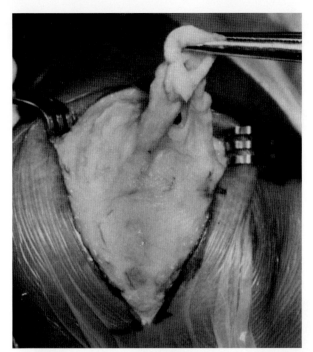

Figure 35-8 The thickened, scarred olecranon bursa is excised through an incision centered lateral to the midline. (From Morrey B, Regan W: Elbow and forearm: Section B: Tendinopathies about the elbow. In DeLee J, Drez D, Miller, MD [eds]: DeLee and Drez's Orthopaedic Sports Medicine: Principles and Practice. Philadelphia, WB Saunders, 2003, p 1234.)

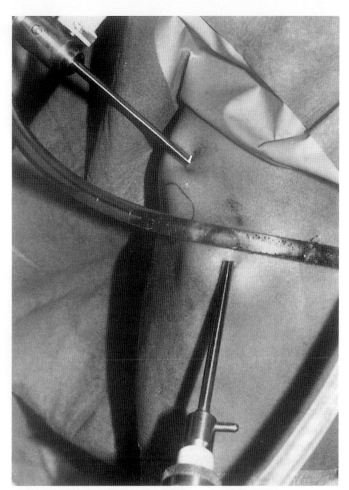

Figure 35-9 Portal placement for olecranon bursectomy. The arthroscope is in the proximal central portal; the shaver is in the lateral portal. (From Baker CL, Cummings PD: Arthroscopic management of miscellaneous elbow disorders. Op Tech Sports Med 1998;6:16–21.)

Surgery

Surgical intervention is considered for cases that do not respond to nonoperative therapy or prevent function and performance (Fig. 35-8). Septic bursitis that does not respond to aspiration and antibiotics should undergo open incision and drainage. A longitudinal incision directly over the midline or slightly lateral (to avoid the ulnar nerve) is performed, carefully dissecting the bursa in its entirety (Fig. 35-9). Meticulous skin handling and closure followed by compressive dressing and 7 to 10 days of elbow splinting help prevent wound-healing problems and recurrence. Protective padding should be used for return to activities. Endoscopic débridement has also been described.

OLECRANON STRESS FRACTURE

Clinical Features and Evaluation

The insidious onset of posterior elbow pain during the acceleration phase of throwing and point tenderness over the olecranon or pain with valgus stress should raise suspicion for an olecranon stress fracture (Fig. 35-10). Repetitive impaction of the olecranon against the olecranon fossa as in valgus extension overload or triceps traction during the deceleration phase of throwing may cause stress reaction. Plain radiographs may show the stress fracture, but computed tomography, bone scan, and magnetic resonance imaging may be more definitive studies.

Relevant Anatomy

Transverse olecranon stress fractures are due to triceps traction and extension forces, while oblique fractures are due to olecranon impaction on the medial wall of the olecranon fossa due to valgus extension overload. Ulnar collateral ligament injury, often partial, may be concurrent with olecranon stress fracture. Epiphyseal injury should also be considered in the skeletally immature gymnast, wrestler, or weight lifter.[14]

Treatment Options

Initial nonoperative treatment involves rest from throwing with lifting restrictions and may require as long as 6 months. Once point tenderness resolves and radiographic union is present, reconditioning may commence. Gradual progression through rotator cuff, scapulothoracic, biceps, and triceps exercises; plyometrics; and eventually an interval throwing program is appropriate.

Surgery

Should symptoms fail to resolve with nonoperative means or if lengthy healing times cannot be tolerated, operative intervention is indicated. A single large cannulated screw across the fracture site placed percutaneously through the triceps tendon is most appropriate (Fig. 35-11). The screw only needs to be removed if local soft-tissue irritation persists after the fracture is well healed. A titanium screw may cause less artifact should magnetic resonance imaging be required at some point in the postoperative course.[15,16]

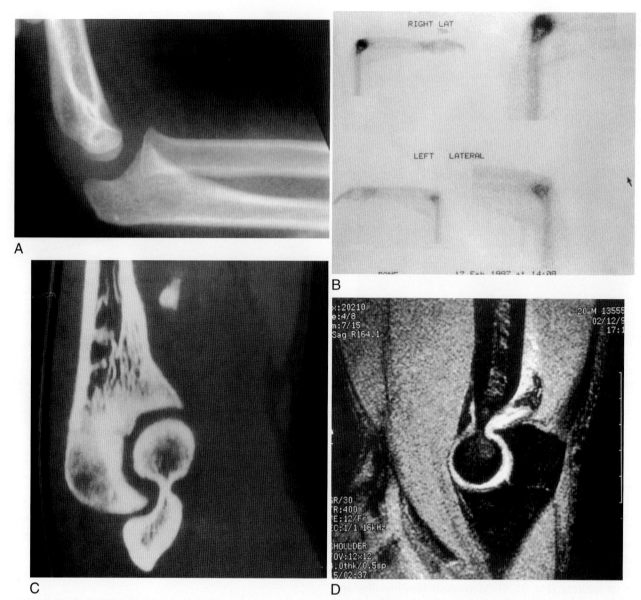

Figure 35-10 Radiographic appearance of olecranon stress fracture. **A,** Plain film lateral view. **B,** Bone scan. **C,** Computed tomography scan. **D,** Magnetic resonance imaging. (From Jones R, Miller R: Bony overuse injuries about the elbow. Op Tech Orthop 2001;11:58.)

VALGUS EXTENSION OVERLOAD/POSTERIOR MEDIAL OSTEOPHYTE

Valgus extension overload can occur during the acceleration phase of throwing (Fig. 35-12). Posterior elbow pain during acceleration is characteristic. Flexion contracture, pain with forced extension, and tenderness of the posterior joint line is typical. A posterior medial osteophyte results from repetitive stress to this area. The osteophyte can be excised through open or arthroscopic techniques (Figs. 35-13 and 35-14). Evaluation for medial instability is also important clinically, under anesthesia and arthroscopically, as posteromedial bone resection may unmask underlying medial instability. Care should be taken not to create iatrogenic medial instability by overzealous resection of the posteromedial olecranon.[17]

NERVE COMPRESSION SYNDROMES

Ulnar Nerve Compression
Clinical Features and Evaluation
The ulnar nerve is most commonly compressed at the elbow. Medial elbow pain with radiating paresthesias to the small and ring fingers is a common presentation in these patients. Examination may reveal decreased ulnar sensation, a positive Tinel's sign at the cubital tunnel, reproduction of symptoms with prolonged elbow flexion, and, in severe cases, weakness of the ulnar intrinsics (flexor carpi ulnaris, interossei, adductor). Subluxation of the ulnar nerve can also occur.[1] Segmental nerve conduction velocity may prove more sensitive than standard motor conduction velocity testing.[18]

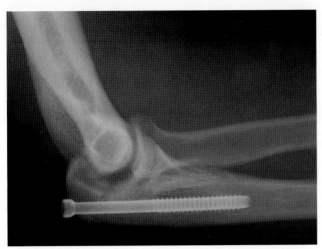

Figure 35-11 Percutaneous screw fixation of an olecranon stress fracture. (From Morrey B, Regan W: Elbow and forearm: Section B: Tendinopathies about the elbow. In DeLee J, Drez D, Miller, MD [eds]: DeLee and Drez's Orthopaedic Sports Medicine: Principles and Practice. Philadelphia, WB Saunders, 2003, p 1246.)

Relevant Anatomy

The ulnar nerve passes through the cubital tunnel at the medial elbow. Several potential sites of compression include the aponeurosis of the flexor carpi ulnaris, arcade of Struthers, or cubital tunnel retinaculum (Fig. 35-15). Ulnar neuropathy may be the result of mechanical irritation due to medial collateral ligament deficiency in an athlete.

Treatment Options

Nonsurgical Typical nonoperative treatment involves cessation of aggravating activities, elbow padding, elbow extension splints at night, and evaluation for valgus overload.

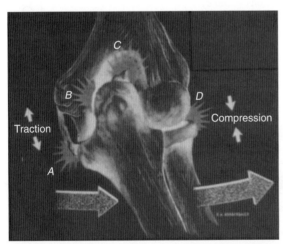

Figure 35-12 Biomechanical forces on the elbow during throwing. Traction on the medial collateral ligament *(A)*; posteromedial olecranon stress *(B)*; olecranon fossa stress *(C)*; compression stress on the radiocapitellar joint *(D)*. (From Morrey B, Regan W: Elbow and forearm: Section B: Tendinopathies about the elbow. In DeLee J, Drez D, Miller, MD [eds]: DeLee and Drez's Orthopaedic Sports Medicine: Principles and Practice. Philadelphia, WB Saunders, 2003, p 1272.)

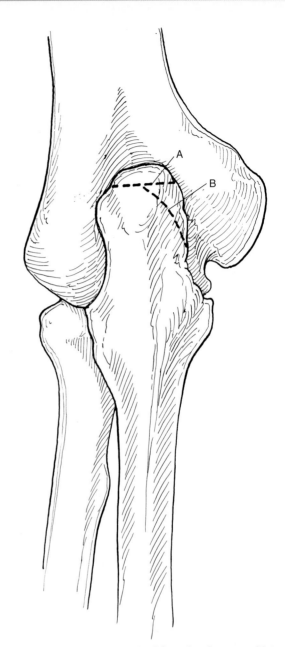

Figure 35-13 Osteophytes are excised from the olecranon with two osteotomies: transverse (A) and oblique (B). (From Miller M, Howard R, Plancher K: Surgical Atlas of Sports Medicine, Saunders 2003, p 439.)

Surgery Surgical techniques for ulnar nerve compression include decompression as well as submuscular, subcutaneous, and intramuscular transposition techniques. Submuscular techniques have generally achieved better results.[19,20]

Posterior Interosseous and Radial Nerve

Clinical Features and Evaluation

Posterior interosseous compression syndrome can present with vague elbow pain, weakness of the wrist and finger extensors, and lack of sensory changes.

Radial tunnel syndrome presents with dorsal lateral forearm pain at night. Passive pronation with wrist flexion and resisted

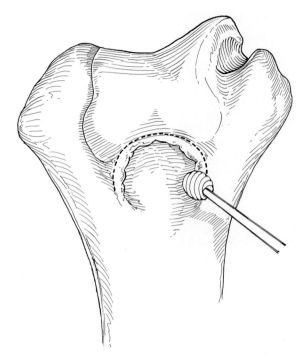

Figure 35-14 Osteophytes are débrided from the olecranon fossa. (From Miller M, Howard R, Plancher K: Surgical Atlas of Sports Medicine. Philadelphia, WB Saunders, 2003, p 439.)

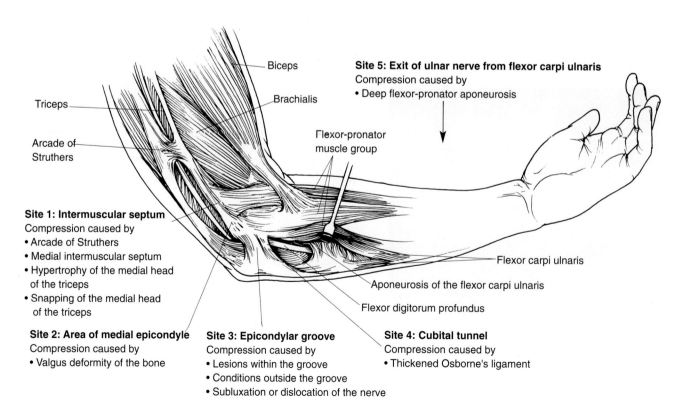

Site 5: Exit of ulnar nerve from flexor carpi ulnaris
Compression caused by
• Deep flexor-pronator aponeurosis

Biceps

Brachialis

Flexor-pronator muscle group

Triceps

Arcade of Struthers

Flexor carpi ulnaris

Aponeurosis of the flexor carpi ulnaris

Flexor digitorum profundus

Site 1: Intermuscular septum
Compression caused by
• Arcade of Struthers
• Medial intermuscular septum
• Hypertrophy of the medial head of the triceps
• Snapping of the medial head of the triceps

Site 2: Area of medial epicondyle
Compression caused by
• Valgus deformity of the bone

Site 3: Epicondylar groove
Compression caused by
• Lesions within the groove
• Conditions outside the groove
• Subluxation or dislocation of the nerve

Site 4: Cubital tunnel
Compression caused by
• Thickened Osborne's ligament

Figure 35-15 Potential ulnar nerve compression sites. (From Posner M: Compressive ulnar neuropathies at the elbow. I. Etiology and diagnosis. J Am Acad Orthop Surg 1998;6:283.)

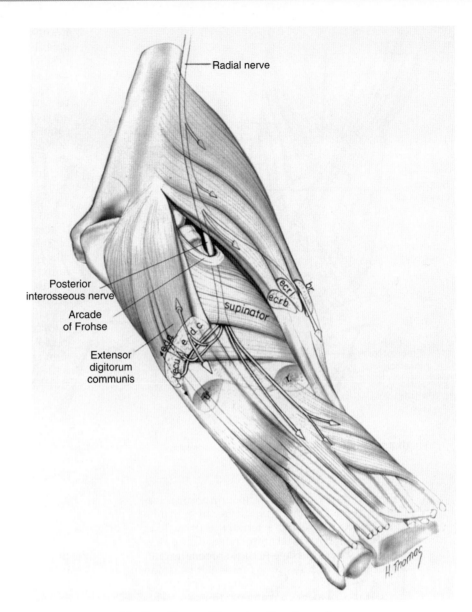

Figure 35-16 Potential radial nerve compression sites. ecrb, extensor carpi radialis brevis; ecrl, extensor carpi radialis longus. (From Spinner M: Injuries to the Major Branches of the Forearm, 2nd ed. Philadelphia, WB Saunders, 1978.)

forearm supination with wrist extension aggravate symptoms. Pain with resisted middle finger extension during elbow extension (Maudsley's test) can distinguish radial tunnel syndrome from lateral epicondylitis.[21]

Relevant Anatomy

The radial nerve divides proximal to the elbow joint into the posterior interosseous nerve and superficial radial nerve. The supinator muscle's two heads can compress the posterior interosseous nerve as it passes distally (Fig. 35-16). Nerve conduction velocity studies are generally diagnostic.

Treatment Options

For posterior interosseous nerve compression, cessation of aggravating activities and conservative means should provide relief. Surgical decompression may be considered for recalcitrant cases.

For radial tunnel syndrome, injection of the radial tunnel should eliminate pain and produce a temporary wrist drop. If rest and nonsteroidal anti-inflammatory drugs do not relieve symptoms, surgical decompression may be considered.[22]

Median Nerve (Pronator Syndrome)
Clinical Features and Evaluation

Repetitive pronation/supination activities can aggravate symptoms. Symptoms are similar to carpal tunnel syndrome with paresthesias of the radial digits and weakness or atrophy of the thenar muscles. However, Phalen's test is negative and percussion at the volar elbow and forearm reproduces symptoms. Anterior interosseous nerve compression can result in vague anterior forearm pain and the loss of thumb to finger pinch. Bilateral anterior interosseous nerve compression present for at least 3 months is known as Parsonage-Andrew-Turner syndrome.

Relevant Anatomy

Pronator syndrome involves compression of the median nerve at the elbow by the bicipital aponeurosis, pronator teres, flexor digitorum superficialis, medial supracondylar process, and/or ligament of Struthers (Fig. 35-17).

Treatment Options

If rest and nonsteroidal anti-inflammatory drugs do not relieve symptoms, surgical decompression may be considered if debilitating symptoms persist despite extended conservative management.[14]

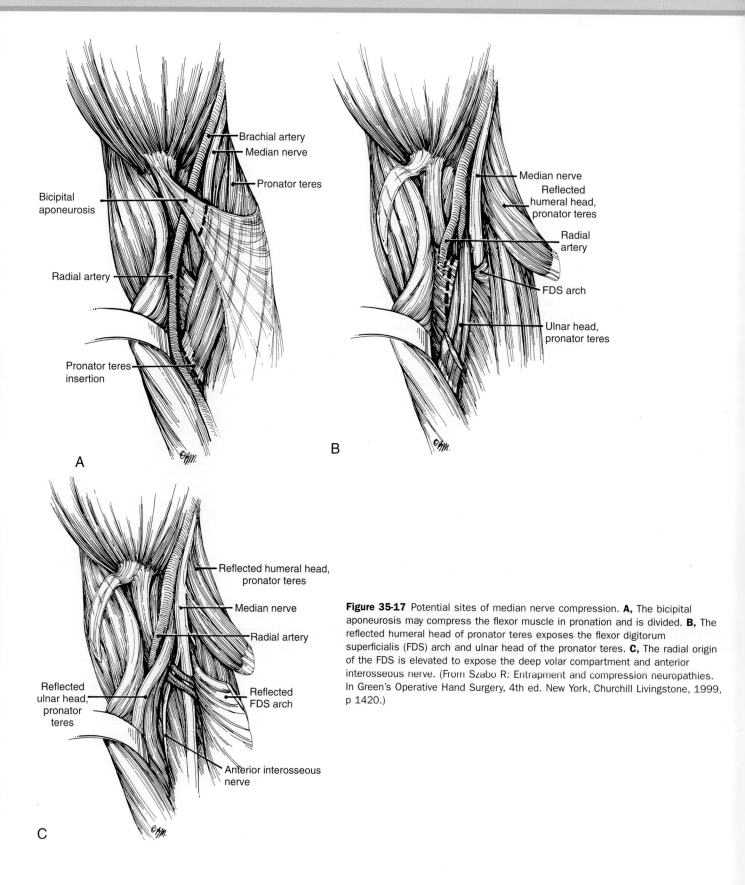

Brachial artery
Median nerve
Pronator teres
Bicipital aponeurosis
Radial artery
Pronator teres insertion

A

Median nerve
Reflected humeral head, pronator teres
Radial artery
FDS arch
Ulnar head, pronator teres

B

Reflected humeral head, pronator teres
Median nerve
Radial artery
Reflected ulnar head, pronator teres
Reflected FDS arch
Anterior interosseous nerve

C

Figure 35-17 Potential sites of median nerve compression. **A,** The bicipital aponeurosis may compress the flexor muscle in pronation and is divided. **B,** The reflected humeral head of pronator teres exposes the flexor digitorum superficialis (FDS) arch and ulnar head of the pronator teres. **C,** The radial origin of the FDS is elevated to expose the deep volar compartment and anterior interosseous nerve. (From Szabo R: Entrapment and compression neuropathies. In Green's Operative Hand Surgery, 4th ed. New York, Churchill Livingstone, 1999, p 1420.)

REFERENCES

1. Morrey B, Regan W: Elbow and forearm: Section B: Tendinopathies about the elbow. In DeLee J, Drez D, Miller, MD (eds): DeLee and Drez's Orthopaedic Sports Medicine: Principles and Practice. Philadelphia, WB Saunders, 2003, pp 1221–1235.

2. Kraushaar B, Nirschl R: Current concepts review—tendonosis of the elbow. Clinical features and findings of histological immunohistochemical and electron microscopy studies. J Bone Joint Surg (Am) 1999;81:259–278.

3. Nirschl R, Rodin D, Ochiai D, et al: Iontophoretic administration of sodium dexamethasone phosphate for acute epicondylitis: A randomized, double-blind, placebo controlled study. Am J Sports Med 2003;31:189–195.

4. Runeson L, Haker E: Iontophoresis with cortisone in the treatment of lateral epicondylalgia (tennis elbow): A double-blind study. Scand J Med Sci Sports 2002;12:136–142.

5. Simunovic Z, Trobonjaca T, Trobonjaca Z: Treatment of medial and lateral epicondylitis—tennis and golfer's elbow—with low level laser therapy: A multicenter double-blind, placebo-controlled clinical study on 324 patients. J Clin Laser Med Surg 1998;16:145–151.

6. Haake M, Konig I, Decker T, et al: Extracorporeal shock wave therapy in the treatment of lateral epicondylitis: A randomized multicenter trial. J Bone Joint Surg Am 2002;84:1982–1991.

7. Speed C, Nichols D, Richards C, et al: Extracorporeal shock wave therapy for lateral epicondylitis: A double blind randomized controlled trial. J Orthop Res 2002;20:895–898.

8. Smidt N, van der Windt D, Assendelft W, et al: Corticosteroid injections, physiotherapy, or a wait and see policy for lateral epicondylitis: A randomized controlled trial. Lancet 2002;359:657–662.

9. Teitz C, Garrett W, Miniaci A, et al: Tendon problems in athletic individuals. Instructional course lecture. J Bone Joint Surg Am 1997; 79:138–152.

10. Jobe F, Ciccotti M: Lateral and medial epicondylitis of the elbow. J Am Acad Orthop Surg 1994;2:1–8.

11. Baker C, Murphy K, Gottlob C, et al: Arthroscopic classification and treatment of lateral epicondylitis: Two-year clinical results. J Shoulder Elbow Surg 2000;9:475–482.

12. Grundberg A, Dobson J: Percutaneous release of the common extensor origin for tennis elbow. Clin Orthop 2000;376:137–140.

13. Dlabach JA, Baker CL: Lateral and medial epicondylitis in the overhead athlete. Op Tech Orthop 2001;11:46–54.

14. Garrick J: Sports Medicine 3 Orthopaedic Knowledge Update. Rosemont, IL, American Academy of Orthopaedic Surgeons, 2004.

15. Nuber G, Diment M: Olecranon stress fractures in throwers: A report of two cases and review of the literature. Clin Orthop 1992;278:58–61.

16. Schickendantz M, Ho C, Koh J: Stress injury of the proximal ulna in professional baseball players. Am J Sports Med 2002;30:737–741.

17. Azar F, Andrews J, Wilke K, et al: Operative treatment of ulnar collateral ligament injuries of the elbow in athletes. Am J Sports Med 2000;28:16–23.

18. Azreili Y, Weimer L, Lovelace R, et al: The utility of segmental nerve conduction studies in ulnar mono-neuropathy at the elbow. Muscle Nerve 2003;27:46–50.

19. Posner M: Compressive ulnar neuropathies at the elbow. I. Etiology and diagnosis. J Am Acad Orthop Surg 1998;6:289–297.

20. Nikitins M, Ch'ng S, Rice N: A dynamic anatomical study of ulnar nerve motion after anterior transposition for cubital tunnel syndrome. Hand Surg 2002;7:177–182.

21. Fairbank S, Corelett R: The role of the extensor digitorum communis muscle in lateral epicondylitis. J Hand Surg (Br) 2002;27:405–409.

22. Lorei M, Hershman E: Peripheral nerve injuries in athletes: Treatment and prevention. Sports Med 1993;16:130–147.

SUGGESTED READING

Gabel G: Acute and chronic tendinopathies at the elbow. Curr Opin Rheumatol 1999;11:138–143.

Miller M, Cole B: Textbook of Arthroscopy. Philadelphia, WB Saunders, 2004.

Miller M, Cooper D, Warner J: Review of Sports Medicine and Arthroscopy, 2nd ed. Philadelphia, WB Saunders, 2002.

36 Tendon Ruptures

William M. Isbell

In This Chapter

INTRODUCTION

- Distal biceps tendon ruptures are more common than triceps ruptures.

- In athletes, triceps tendon ruptures are most commonly seen in professional football players, particularly linemen.

- Nonoperative treatment of a complete distal biceps tear results in significant loss of supination strength, while nonoperative treatment of a complete triceps tendon tear results in loss of elbow extension strength.

- Partial tears of both biceps and triceps ruptures can be treated nonoperatively. If pain and/or weakness persist, surgical repair is undertaken.

Ruptures of the tendons of the elbow joint are relatively rare. Rupture of the distal biceps tendon accounts for most of these injuries. The distal biceps tendon is ruptured most commonly in the dominant extremity of patients in their 40s to 60s and is more common in men than women.[1] The mechanism of injury is thought to occur from traumatic extension of a flexed elbow with a maximally contracted biceps. Degradation or degeneration of the tendon may play some role in its rupture. Other theories that have been advanced for the cause of biceps rupture have included hypovascularity of the tendon, mechanical failure of the tendon, and impingement of the surrounding structures on the tendon leading to its failure.[2]

Compared to the number of patients presenting with biceps rupture, the number of patients with triceps rupture is small. The largest number of triceps tendon ruptures has been reported in professional football players.[3] The mechanism of injury involves an eccentric load to a contracting triceps. Several risk factors have been identified for this injury including anabolic steroids, renal dialysis, lupus, and hyperparathyroidism.[4-8] Tendinosis of the triceps tendon is thought to play some role, with the weakened tendon often progressing from a partial tear to a complete rupture.

BICEPS RUPTURE

Clinical Features and Evaluation

Patients who present to the orthopedic clinic after sustaining a rupture of the biceps tendon often complain of feeling a sudden pop at the elbow. Frequently, there is the onset of significant swelling and pain, followed by a reduction in pain and increasing ecchymosis. These patients may or may not have a palpable defect at the elbow. There is detectable weakness with resisted supination and flexion of the elbow. In some patients, with resisted elbow flexion, the muscle belly may be seen retracting proximally forming a mass in the arm much larger than that of the contralateral biceps (Fig. 36-1). Plain radiographs are usually obtained but have a limited role in making the diagnosis. MRI is helpful to determine the location of the tear as well as the degree to which the tendon is torn. It is also useful to evaluate for tendinosis and the quality of the ruptured tissue.

Relevant Anatomy

The biceps muscle lies in the anterior compartment of the arm. Its proximal origin of the short head is at the coracoid, and its proximal origin of the long head is intra-articular at the glenoid. The distal biceps tendon attaches at the radial tuberosity, the most common site of its rupture. It is innervated by the musculocutaneous nerve, which originates at cervical roots 5, 6, and 7. The biceps is the strongest supinator of the forearm. This supination force increases as the elbow is flexed. With the brachialis, the biceps acts as an elbow flexor as well. When the elbow is flexed with a supinated forearm, the biceps is more active than when the forearm is in a pronated position.[9]

Treatment Options

Treatment of injuries of the distal biceps tendon depends on the degree to which the tendon is torn and whether it is acutely or chronically ruptured. There is no universally established treatment for partial ruptures of the biceps tendon. If some tendon remains attached, frequently the initial treatment is conservative. In the initial phase, reducing swelling and re-establishing range of motion are paramount. The patient gradually progresses to strengthening once the pain has subsided and motion has been regained. If there is persistent pain and weakness, the partially ruptured tendon is débrided and reattached anatomically to the radial tuberosity. Simple débridement of the tendon has not been shown to effectively reduce pain following partial ruptures.[10]

The results of surgical repair of acute, complete ruptures of the biceps are far more favorable than those of chronic repairs, as one might expect. However, not all patients require repair of a completely ruptured tendon. Low demand and elderly patients

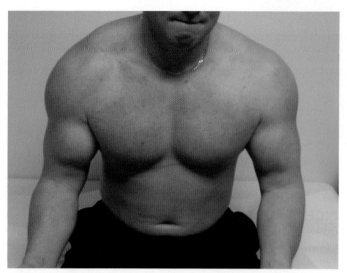

Figure 36-1 Patient flexing the elbows after right distal biceps tendon rupture, showing retraction of the affected muscle belly into arm.

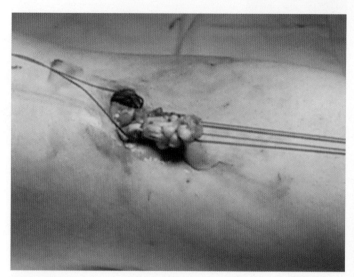

Figure 36-2 Tendon of ruptured distal biceps taken out through a transverse incision in the flexion crease of the elbow.

without significant pain are often treated conservatively for these ruptures, especially if it involves the nondominant arm. However, in most patient populations, the benefit of greater strength and function make acute repair the best choice. The primary reason to fix these complete tears is the restoration of supination strength.

Many techniques have been described for the repair of distal biceps ruptures using a single or a double incision. The most commonly used technique is that of Boyd and Anderson, using two incisions for the anatomic repair. Single-incision techniques have been shown to have higher incidences of posterior interosseous nerve complications, but newer techniques using suture anchors have shown some promise in reducing these complications.[11]

Surgery

Biceps Tendon Repair (Modified Boyd-Anderson[12])

In the case of an acute rupture, a transverse incision is made over the flexion crease of the elbow. Dissection is carried down to the level of the ruptured tendon. Careful attention is made to retract the lateral antebrachial cutaneous nerve laterally. The ruptured tendon is bluntly freed from any adhesions or scar. Its end is tagged with two nonabsorbable locking stitches (Fig. 36-2). A tunnel is created between the radius and ulna with blunt dissection. A curved clamp can aid in this dissection. With the curve of the clamp going medially around the radius, a small posterolateral incision is made at the tip of the clamp. Through this incision, the radial neck and tuberosity are exposed while keeping the forearm in maximal pronation, thereby protecting the posterior interosseous nerve. Once the radial tuberosity is exposed, a trough is created in the tuberosity with a bur. Three holes are drilled in the radius adjacent to the trough. The tagged tendon is then passed through the interval between the radius and ulna once again with a curved clamp pointing away from the ulna and following the curve of the radius (Fig. 36-3). The suture limbs are then passed through the trough and out the holes in the radius and tied over the top of the bony bridge. The incisions are then closed in two layers, and the elbow is placed into a well-padded posterior splint.

Chronically ruptured biceps tendons may be repaired directly, provided that the tendon of the biceps has not retracted significantly or that the muscle itself has not shortened significantly. It is recommended that these repairs be performed through two incisions to reduce the risk of injury to the radial nerve. If the native tendon is significantly retracted or if the quality of the chronically ruptured tendon is poor, the repair may be augmented with either autograft or allograft tendon. The semitendinosus is a good choice for this augmentation because of its similarity in size to that of a native biceps tendon.

Postoperative Rehabilitation

The patient's arm is immobilized in 90 degrees of flexion for 2 weeks. At the time of suture removal, the patient is placed into a hinged elbow brace. Range of motion is progressed to full over the next 4 weeks. At 6 to 8 weeks postoperatively, gentle strengthening of the biceps is begun. Any aggressive strengthening is avoided until at least 12 weeks postoperatively. The patient is allowed to return to competitive activities when full

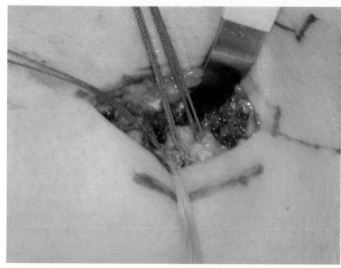

Figure 36-3 Posterolateral incision with tagged biceps tendon pulled into position to be anchored into the radial tuberosity.

range of motion is obtained and strength is close to that of the opposite side, somewhere around 4 to 6 months postoperatively.

Results

The results of nonoperative treatment of distal biceps ruptures have been shown to result in a loss of as much as 50% of supination strength at the elbow. Morrey et al have shown a return of 97% of flexion strength and 95% of supination strength in patients who had repairs of distal biceps ruptures.[13] D'Alessandro et al[14] showed similar excellent results in a group of 10 athletes who underwent distal biceps repair. All the athletes in this group returned to full unlimited activity, with the only deficit seen being a decrease in endurance of 20% compared with the opposite side in functional testing. The repair of chronic ruptures has shown less favorable results. Weakness following chronic repair has been reported as high as 50%[15] (similar to that of nonoperative repair) and as little as 13% in other cases.[16]

TRICEPS RUPTURE

Clinical Features and Evaluation

Patients with distal triceps tendon ruptures often present with a history of a direct blow to the elbow or forced elbow flexion while the triceps was contracted. Oftentimes, these patients have a history of corticosteroid injections for presumed olecranon bursitis.[4] There are usually pain and swelling at the elbow with some limitation of range of motion and weakness with resisted extension. In patients with a complete rupture, there is usually a palpable defect in the distal triceps. Using a modification of the T. Campbell Thompson Test for Achilles tendon ruptures, the elbow may be flexed over the examination table and the triceps muscle belly squeezed, resulting in no elbow extension when the triceps tendon is torn.[17] Lateral radiographs of the elbow may show a small piece of bone pulled off with the triceps tendon. Occasionally there is a large piece of bone similar to that of an olecranon fracture. Magnetic resonance imaging is useful to delineate between partial and complete tears as well as to localize the tear itself (Fig. 36-4).

Relevant Anatomy

The triceps is named for its three heads. The origin of the lateral head is the posterolateral aspect of the humerus, the origin of the long head is the infraglenoid tubercle of the scapula, and the medial head originates from the spiral groove of the humerus. The insertion of the triceps is the olecranon. The function of the triceps is to extend the elbow, and the long head aids in shoulder adduction and arm extension. The innervation of the triceps is the radial nerve, which originates at cervical roots 6, 7, and 8.

Treatment Options

There is no consensus regarding what percentage of the triceps tendon must be torn before repair is warranted. In general, most partial tears of the tendon may initially be treated conservatively. Treatment focuses on swelling reduction, pain relief, and restoration of range of motion. Contact athletes may return to play after partial tears in a hinged brace with an extension block. However, there are reported cases of complete ruptures of partial tears following a return to contact sports.[3]

Complete ruptures of the triceps tendon have been shown to cause significant disability, not only in athletes, but also in chronically ill patients in whom the triceps is very important for transfers and mobilization.[5] There have been reports of repairs of both acute and chronic ruptures of the triceps tendon. The cornerstone of the surgical treatment of these ruptures is repair of the tendon to the bone of the olecranon. Occasionally large bony avulsions of the triceps are treated like an olecranon fracture with screw or tension band fixation.

Surgery

Triceps Tendon Repair

The repair is accomplished through a posterior approach to the elbow with a direct midline incision, curving around the tip of the olecranon. Dissection is carried through the subcutaneous tissue to the triceps muscle and tendon below (Fig. 36-5). The dissection medially is done carefully to prevent injury to the ulnar nerve (in chronic cases, the nerve may be encapsulated in scar requiring decompression and transposition). Once the torn tendon is dissected free, a nonabsorbable suture is placed through the tendon with a locking stitch. Two bone tunnels are drilled in the olecranon. These may be placed parallel to or crossing each other. The sutures are then tied down through these bone tunnels while the elbow is in extension (Fig. 36-6). Particular attention is made not to place the knot medially

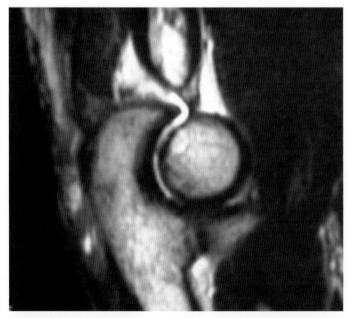

Figure 36-4 Magnetic resonance imaging showing a rupture of the triceps tendon off the olecranon.

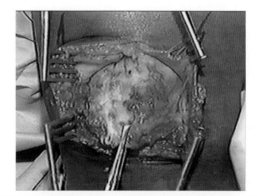

Figure 36-5 A complete rupture of the distal triceps mobilized for repair.

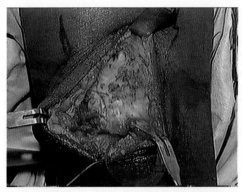

Figure 36-6 Distal triceps rupture being repaired through drill holes in the olecranon.

(adjacent to the ulnar nerve) to prevent irritation or too superficially, which will cause pain when resting the elbow on a hard surface. The incision is closed in two layers. The elbow is immobilized in a well-padded posterior splint in 45 degrees of flexion.

Postoperative Rehabilitation

After repair of a distal triceps rupture, the arm is immobilized in 45 degrees of flexion for 2 weeks. At the time of suture removal, the elbow is put into a hinged elbow brace and active and passive range-of-motion exercises are begun. At 6 weeks postoperatively, gentle strengthening is begun. Aggressive resistive strengthening is avoided until 3 months postoperatively. Athletes may return to competitive play between 4 and 6 months postoperatively if range of motion has returned and strength is similar to that of the opposite side. Additional protection for contact athletes may be provided by a hinged elbow brace.

Results

Excellent results have been reported with both early and delayed repairs of complete ruptures of the triceps. In the largest series reported, 10 of 11 professional football lineman who had early repair of a complete rupture of the triceps returned to play at least 1 year of football following repair. All the players were found to have full range of motion, no pain, and no discernible weakness 1 year following repair. Ten players with partial tears were identified. The tears of one of these players progressed to a complete tear when he returned to play. The remaining nine players were able to finish out their season with a partial tear. Six of these players healed their partial tears and required no further intervention, and three players underwent repair of partial tears in the off season.[3]

CONCLUSIONS

Ruptures of the tendons about the elbow may be uncommon injuries, but they will be encountered in a sports medicine practice. Complete ruptures of both the distal biceps tendon and the triceps tendon are best treated with early anatomic repair followed by early restoration of range of motion and delayed strengthening. Partial ruptures of either of these tendons may be initially treated conservatively with pain and swelling reduction and restoration of motion. However, in highly active patients, these partial tears may continue to be symptomatic or progress to complete tears, requiring repair.

REFERENCES

1. Friedmann E: Rupture of the distal biceps brachii tendon: Report on 13 cases. JAMA 1963;184:60–63.
2. Siler JG III, Parker LM, Chamberland PD, et al: The distal biceps tendon: Two potential mechanisms involved in its rupture—Arterial supply and mechanical impingement. J Shoulder Elbow Surg 1995; 4:149–156.
3. Mair SD, Isbell WM, Gill TJ, et al: Triceps tendon ruptures in professional football players. Am J Sports Med 2004;32:431–434.
4. Lambert MI, St. Clair Gibson A, Noakes TD: Rupture of the triceps tendon associated with steroid injections. Am J Sports Med 1995;23:778.
5. Mankin HJ: Rickets, osteomalacia, and renal osteodystrophy. J Bone Joint Surg Am 1974;56:101, 352–386.
6. Martin JR, Wilson CL, Matthews WH: Bilateral rupture of ligament patellae in case of disseminated lupus erythematosus. Arthritis Rheum 1958;6:548–552.
7. Preston FS, Adicaff A: Hyper parathyroidism with avulsion of three major tendons: Report of a case. N Engl J Med 1962;266:968–971.
8. Sallender JL, Ryan GM, Borden GA: Triceps tendon rupture in weight lifters. J Shoulder Elbow Surg 1984;7:151–153.
9. Basmajian JV, Latif A: Integrated actions and functions of the chief flexors of the elbow: A detailed electromyographic analysis. J Bone Joint Surg Am 1957;39:1106–1118.
10. Bourne MH, Morrey BF: Partial rupture of the distal biceps tendon. Clin Orthop 1985;193:189–194.
11. Ozyurekoglu T, Tsai TM: Ruptures of the distal biceps brachii tendon: Results of three surgical techniques. Hand Surg 2003;8:65–73.
12. Boyd HD, Anderson LD: A method for reinsertion of the distal biceps brachii tendon. J Bone Joint Surg Am 1961;43:1041–1043.
13. Morrey BG, Askew LJ, An KN, Dobyns JH: Rupture of the distal tendon of the biceps brachii: A biomechanical study. J Bone Joint Surg Am 1985;67:418–421.
14. D'Alessandro DF, Shields CL Jr, Tibone JE, Chandler RW: Repair of distal biceps tendon ruptures in athletes. Am J Sports Med 1993;21:114–119.
15. Boucher PR, Morton KS: Rupture of the distal biceps brachii tendon. J Trauma 1967;7:626–632.
16. Hang DW, Bach BR Jr, Bojchuk J: Repair of chronic distal biceps brachii tendon rupture using free autogenous semitendinosis tendon. Clin Orthop 1996;323:188–191.
17. Viegas SF: Avulsion of the triceps tendon. Orthop Rev 1990; 19:533–536.

CHAPTER
37 Pediatric Elbow

C. David Geier, Jr. and George A. Paletta, Jr.

In This Chapter

INTRODUCTION

- The widespread participation in organized sports among skeletally immature athletes has led to an increase in elbow injuries among this population in recent years. Children and adolescents are competing at earlier ages, and single-sport specialization often requires these athletes to participate throughout the year.

- As the frequency and intensity of these athletes' participation have increased, the cause of elbow injuries has shifted from macrotrauma, including fractures and dislocations, to repetitive microtrauma.

- Athletic elbow injuries are seen in both overhead sports, such as baseball and tennis, and sports requiring the elbow to serve as a weight-bearing joint, as in gymnastics.

- Treatment of elbow injuries in these athletes requires a thorough knowledge of the anatomy and bony development of the adolescent elbow, an understanding of the natural history of its disorders, and a grasp of the expected outcomes with conservative and operative management.

RELEVANT ANATOMY

The growth and development of the human skeleton can be divided into three general stages. The first, childhood, ends with the appearance of the secondary centers of ossification. Adolescence ends with the fusion of the secondary ossification centers to their respective long bones. Finally, young adulthood terminates with the completion of all bone growth and the achievement of the final adult musculoskeletal form.[1] Characteristic patterns of elbow injury occur during each stage of elbow growth and development. The injury patterns are influenced greatly by the sport played and the resulting forces applied to the athlete's upper extremity. In each stage of development,

the elbow has a characteristic weak link that is susceptible to injury.

Skeletal growth and development of the male and female elbow occur at characteristic times.[1-4] At birth, the distal humerus is a single epiphysis comprised of both condyles and epicondyles with one physis. Over the course of the first decade, the epiphysis differentiates into two epiphyses (the capitellum and trochlea) and two apophyses (the medial and lateral epicondyles). The radial head and olecranon epiphyses also develop secondary growth centers during this period. The appearance of the secondary centers of ossification follows a characteristic pattern. The capitellum appears at age 1 to 2. At roughly 2-year intervals, the other centers appear. The appearance of the radial head at age 3 is followed by the medial epicondyle at age 5, the trochlea at age 7, the olecranon at age 9, and the lateral epicondyle at age 10 in females and age 11 in males. Fusion of these secondary ossification centers occurs in a sequential, age-dependent order in the early teens in girls and mid-teens in boys. The capitellum, trochlea, and olecranon close at approximately age 14, while the medial epicondyle closes at 15, and the radial head and lateral epicondyle fuse at 16 years of age.

LITTLE LEAGUER'S ELBOW

The term *little leaguer's elbow* refers to a group of elbow problems in the young throwing athlete.[4-7] The injuries include medial epicondyle fragmentation and avulsion, delayed or accelerated apophyseal growth of the medial epicondyle, delayed closure of the medial epicondylar apophysis, osteochondrosis and osteochondritis of the capitellum, osteochondrosis and osteochondritis of the radial head, hypertrophy of the ulna, olecranon apophysitis, and delayed closure of the olecranon apophysis.

Repetitive overuse injuries in the adolescent elbow can be categorized based on the pattern of applied forces. These categories include medial tension, lateral compression, and posterior shear or traction injuries. Medial epicondyle apophysitis, medial epicondyle avulsion fractures, and ulnar collateral ligament injuries comprise medial tension overload injuries. Lateral compression injuries include Panner's disease and osteochondritis dissecans (OCD) of the capitellum. Olecranon apophyseal injury and avulsion of the olecranon fall within the realm of posterior shear or traction injuries.

CLINICAL FEATURES AND EVALUATION

A thorough clinical history and physical examination along with routine radiography are critical for the diagnosis of adolescent elbow pathology.[2,4] Necessary historical information includes the age, handedness, sport, and position of the athlete as well as the level of competition and the amount of practice and playing time per week. The onset, duration, quality, and anatomic location of elbow symptoms must be elicited. Whether sports participation affects the symptoms is critical to address. The specific motions and positions that precipitate the elbow complaints, such as medial pain in the late cocking and acceleration phases of throwing, should be sought. Previous treatments should be noted. The duration of symptoms and the acute or chronic nature of the injury are important for making the diagnosis. A single traumatic episode suggests an acute traumatic condition such as an avulsion fracture of the medial epicondyle, while an insidious onset of chronic pain implies an overuse syndrome such as medial epicondylar apophysitis.

The physical examination includes inspection and palpation of the elbow, motion assessment, stability testing, and neurologic and vascular evaluation. Bony hypertrophy, flexion contracture, and carrying angle are important to note. The presence of tenderness at the epicondyles, olecranon, radial head, and collateral ligaments should be recorded. Any ulnar nerve subluxation should be recorded. The ulnar collateral ligament is tested with valgus stress and external rotation of the arm, while the lateral ligaments are stressed with varus and internal rotation.

Basic imaging includes at least anteroposterior and lateral radiographs. Often oblique views and stress films are helpful. Common lateral elbow radiographic findings include lucent areas in the capitellum or loose bodies in the anterior or lateral compartments that suggest OCD of the capitellum or radial head. Enlargement, beaking, and fragmentation of the medial epicondyle or an avulsion of the epicondyle are common observations on the medial side of immature elbows. Posterior findings, including osteophytes or loose bodies, are often seen with repetitive impingement of the olecranon. It is critical to evaluate comparison views of the opposite elbow when assessing equivocal radiographic findings of the symptomatic elbow.

Magnetic resonance imaging is becoming more popular for evaluation of pediatric elbow injuries. Young patients often have difficulty cooperating sufficiently to obtain a magnetic resonance imaging, but in older adolescents, it can be helpful for defining developing apophyses and epiphyses, joint capsules, ligaments, and soft tissues that are not well seen on plain radiographs.

MEDIAL EPICONDYLAR APOPHYSITIS

Repetitive tensile stress from the flexor-pronator mass and the ulnar collateral ligament on the medial epicondyle can lead to medial epicondylar apophysitis and ultimately a stress fracture of the medial epicondylar apophysis.[1,3,8] Throwing athletes with this disorder will often complain of progressively worsening medial elbow pain with activity. The characteristic triad includes medial epicondyle pain, a decrease in throwing distance or velocity, and a decrease in throwing effectiveness.[1,4] The valgus stress placed on the elbow in the late cocking or early acceleration phases causes an exacerbation of the pain with repetitive throwing.

Physical examination reveals tenderness at the medial epicondyle. Valgus stress often reveals pain, but obvious instability is not present. Radiographs often appear normal. A comparison with the opposite elbow will sometimes demonstrate widening of the apophysis. Occasionally fragmentation or hypertrophy of the medial epicondyle is present.

Conservative management of medial epicondylar apophysitis usually results in complete resolution of symptoms with no lasting functional deficit. Eliminating repetitive valgus stress on the elbow by stopping all throwing activities, often for at least 6 weeks, as well as ice and nonsteroidal anti-inflammatory medications will usually provide symptomatic relief. Physical therapy focusing on range of motion, muscle stretching, and strengthening can be helpful. Evidence of radiographic healing is not necessary to allow a return to activity, as long as the athlete gradually increases his throwing in a supervised program that emphasizes proper mechanics.

MEDIAL EPICONDYLE AVULSION FRACTURES

Medial epicondyle avulsions are acute injuries that usually result from a single tensile force applied to the medial elbow of adolescent athletes.[1–4,6,9,10] Failure of the medial epicondylar apophysis results from an acute valgus stress coupled with a violent contraction of the flexor-pronator muscle mass. The player will present with acute onset of medial pain after a throw. The pain is severe enough to prevent him or her from returning to play. It usually occurs in the late cocking or early acceleration phases of throwing, and the athlete will often feel or hear a pop. Ulnar nerve paresthesias may occur after the injury. Chronic medial elbow symptoms occasionally precede the event.

Physical examination reveals discrete tenderness to palpation at the medial epicondyle, edema, and occasionally ecchymosis. The last 15 degrees of elbow extension are limited due to pain, which can make stability testing difficult. Ulnar collateral ligament injury is possible in this setting, although it is less likely given the fact that the physis of the medial epicondyle is the weak link in the developing elbow. Coexisting ulnar collateral ligament rupture and medial epicondyle avulsion is unusual. The occurrence of a spontaneously reduced elbow fracture-dislocation should be kept in mind.

Radiographs will usually show a minimally displaced avulsion fracture (Fig. 37-1). Findings are often subtle, requiring comparison elbow views or stress radiographs. While rare, the avulsed fragment can be displaced by the flexor-pronator mass, sometimes into the elbow joint, as often seen in elbow dislocations.

The appropriate treatment for these fractures is a matter of some debate. Stress fractures and nondisplaced fractures are usually treated nonoperatively, while fractures in which the fragment is displaced or incarcerated in the joint are treated operatively if the fragment cannot be reduced by closed manipulation. Ulnar nerve dysfunction often mandates exploration along with open reduction and internal fixation of the fracture.

Nonoperative management of minimally displaced medial epicondyle fractures is based on the observation that fractures displaced less than 3 to 5 mm will develop an asymptomatic fibrous union. Ulnar nerve symptoms and valgus instability must be absent. Whether this approach is adequate for the young throwing athlete is not fully understood. If a nonoperative approach is chosen, the elbow should be immobilized in 90 degrees of flexion and moderate pronation in a long-arm splint for as long as 2 to 3 weeks.[2,3,8,11] A hinged elbow brace can then be used to regain range of motion. When the fracture site is nontender and there is radiographic evidence of healing, flexor-pronator strengthening is started, and a gradual return to

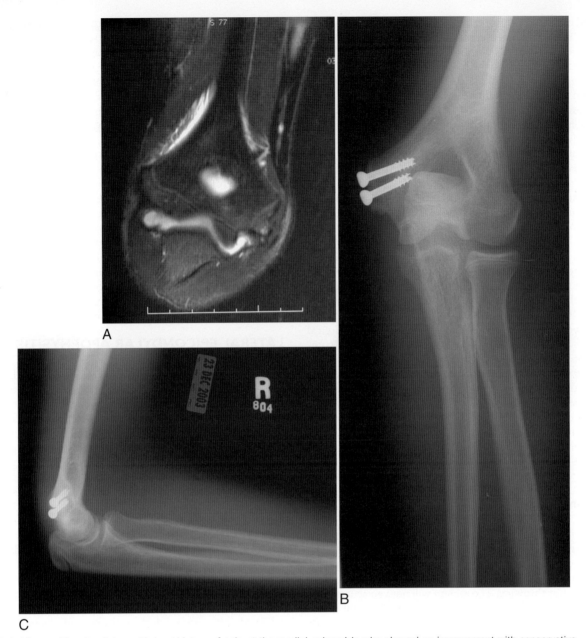

Figure 37-1 A 15-year-old male pitcher with long history of pain at the medial epicondyle who showed no improvement with conservative management. **A,** Magnetic resonance arthrography demonstrates edema in the medial epicondyle, consistent with a nondisplaced avulsion injury. **B** and **C,** Anteroposterior and lateral postoperative radiographs showing two cancellous screws across the fracture.

throwing is initiated in a supervised program when the athlete is asymptomatic.[2,3]

Many authors advocate an operative treatment of these fractures, especially with more than 2 mm of displacement, rotation or incarceration of the fragment, valgus instability, or ulnar nerve symptoms.[3,10,12,13] Young overhead throwing athletes may be prone to developing radiocapitellar degenerative changes if displaced fractures are treated nonoperatively,[12] so accepting less displacement may be indicated in these patients.

Surgical management consists of open reduction and internal fixation using one or two cancellous screws (see Fig. 37-1B and C). Valgus stability is determined intraoperatively after fixation is achieved, with exploration and possible repair of the ulnar collateral ligament necessary if instability still exists. If the fragment is too small for adequate fixation, it should be excised, and the ulnar collateral ligament and possibly the flexor-pronator muscles primarily repaired.[2,3,10] Postoperatively, the elbow is placed in a hinged-elbow orthosis for 6 weeks, with early range-of-motion and strengthening exercises started immediately if the fixation is adequate. When radiographs show fracture union and the athlete is asymptomatic, a gradual return to activity is allowed.

ULNAR COLLATERAL LIGAMENT INJURIES

Ulnar collateral ligament injuries, especially the chronic attritional tears seen in the skeletally mature, are uncommon in the juvenile and adolescent thrower.[12] If a rupture is present, it most likely is the result of an acute event.[9,14] The thrower will complain of the acute onset of pain and inability to continue throwing. The physical examination will reveal tenderness to palpation distal to the medial epicondyle. Jobe's valgus stress test may demonstrate pain and instability. Radiographs are needed to rule out the presence of a medial epicondyle fracture. Stress films are often helpful to demonstrate instability. Greater than 2 mm of medial opening compared to the uninjured side is strongly suggestive of a tear. Magnetic resonance arthrography with gadolinium contrast can also help demonstrate the presence of an ulnar collateral ligament tear.[15]

The treatment for an ulnar collateral ligament tear in the juvenile or adolescent thrower begins with conservative measures before proceeding to operative intervention, if necessary. A brief period of immobilization, nonsteroidal anti-inflammatory medications, and ice are used to control the initial pain. Physical therapy to regain motion and maintain strength and a hinged elbow brace to prevent valgus stress on the elbow are used for approximately 6 weeks. At this point, stability of the elbow is reassessed. If a complete tear and instability are present in a young thrower who wants to continue throwing sports, surgical treatment is advised. Athletes who do not demonstrate a complete tear or instability but continue to have medial elbow pain with activity for at least 3 months are also offered surgery. If an avulsion of the ligament is observed, direct repair may be possible. Reconstruction using autograft tendon such as the palmaris longus, as is commonly performed in adults, is more commonly the procedure of choice. Premature closure of the medial epicondylar apophysis is possible, but this is not significant clinically, as the longitudinal growth of the distal humerus is not affected.

AVULSION OF THE OLECRANON

An avulsion fracture of the tip of the olecranon results from an acute overload failure of the olecranon apophysis. It occurs more commonly in older adolescents than in juvenile or young adolescent throwers. The injury occurs in the acceleration or follow-through phases of throwing. The athlete will note an acute onset of severe pain at the olecranon. Physical examination will reveal tenderness to palpation at the tip of the olecranon and pain with active extension. Full active extension of the elbow is often not present. Radiographs will demonstrate avulsion of the tip of the olecranon. This diagnosis may be difficult in younger throwers in whom the secondary ossification center of the olecranon is not visible. If more than 2 mm of displacement of the fracture exists, open reduction and internal fixation using a tension band or cannulated screw technique is recommended.

OLECRANON APOPHYSEAL INJURY

Repetitive throwing places stress on the olecranon apophysis due to powerful contraction of the triceps during the acceleration phase of throwing. The resulting tensile stress can lead to olecranon apophyseal injury.[2,8,11,12] A traction apophysitis, similar to that which occurs at the medial epicondyle, occurs as a result of the traction force applied by the triceps. Throwers often complain of acute or chronic pain at the posterior tip of the elbow, swelling, and decreased range of motion. Tenderness to palpation at the olecranon tip and pain with resisted extension are seen on physical examination. Radiographs will show widening, fragmentation, or sclerosis of the olecranon physis compared to

the uninvolved elbow. Normal radiographs, however, do not rule out the presence of this disorder, so a high index of suspicion must be maintained when appropriate signs and symptoms exist. Comparison views of the opposite elbow are important to differentiate this entity from a stress fracture of the olecranon, which can be seen in the older adolescent athlete whose olecranon apophysis has already closed.

Treatment of olecranon apophyseal injury depends on the duration and severity of symptoms, as well as the degree of separation of the apophysis. The initial management consists of conservative measures to decrease the athlete's symptoms, such as ice, nonsteroidal anti-inflammatory drugs, activity modification, and physical therapy. Good results are usually seen in 4 to 6 weeks. The persistence of symptoms or failure of the olecranon apophysis to close as seen on radiographs within 3 to 6 months of conservative treatment implies the need to consider operative management. Fixation can be achieved with a single cancellous screw (Fig. 37-2A and B). A short period of immobilization followed by physical therapy to resume active flexion and passive extension begins postoperatively. Active extension should be restricted for 6 weeks.

LATERAL EPICONDYLAR APOPHYSITIS

Lateral epicondylitis in the adolescent is similar to the analogous disorder in adults. It is more commonly seen in the athlete who participates in racquet sports due to repetitive wrist extension. While medial epicondylitis is more common in the throwing athlete, lateral symptoms can occur due to the eccentric activity of the wrist extensors and traction forces applied to the lateral apophysis during the follow-through phase of throwing.[2] Improper technique or equipment can exacerbate the microtrauma to the apophysis.[9] The athlete will give a history of pain at the lateral epicondyle or the extensor muscle origin that is aggravated by activity. On examination, pain may be reproduced with resisted wrist and finger extension. If the symptoms are attributable to an apophysitis, point tenderness will be present at the lateral epicondyle rather than the muscle origin, as in a tendonitis. Radiographs are usually normal but can show widening or fragmentation of the lateral epicondylar apophysis.

In the vast majority of cases, successful treatment can be achieved with nonsurgical measures. Ice, nonsteroidal anti-inflammatory drugs, and activity modification should decrease symptoms. When the athlete is more comfortable, physical therapy for stretching and strengthening are instituted. Correcting improper techniques and poorly fitting equipment is essential. A counterforce brace can be used to try to alter the pull of the extensor muscles on the apophysis. Surgical treatment is rarely indicated.

PANNER'S DISEASE

Panner's disease is a focal lesion or osteochondrosis of the subchondral bone and overlying articular cartilage of the capitellum that begins as degeneration or necrosis followed by regeneration or recalcification of the capitellar ossification center.[2,3,8,14,16,17] It is the most common cause of lateral elbow pain in young children, characteristically occurring in children younger than 10 years old. In the vast majority of cases, it is a benign, self-limiting process. The appearance, size, and contour of the capitellum and the overlying cartilage are usually restored. Collapse of the subchondral bone is rare.[17-19] The distinction between Panner's disease and osteochondritis dissecans is important because they

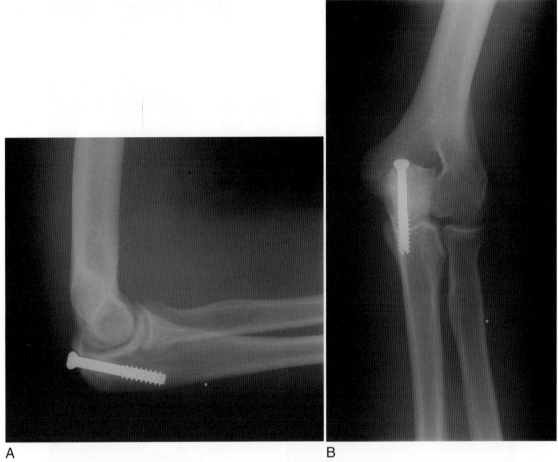

A   B

Figure 37-2 A 16-year-old male high school pitcher with posterior elbow pain with throwing and persistence of the olecranon apophysis. Lateral **(A)** and anteroposterior **(B)** postoperative radiographs show closure of the apophysis 6 months after single cancellous screw fixation.

have markedly different natural histories and therefore, different treatment options.

Children with Panner's disease complain of dull, aching pain of the lateral elbow that is increased with activity and relieved with rest. They may complain of joint stiffness or loss of motion. Physical examination may reveal tenderness at the radiocapitellar joint, a flexion contracture of 20 degrees or less, and crepitus. Radiographs often show an irregular capitellum that appears smaller than that on the opposite side. Areas of fissuring or fragmentation can be seen. Involvement can be found in the anterior capitellum or in the entire ossific center.[3,20]

Conservative management of Panner's disease, including activity modification, avoidance of valgus stress to the elbow, ice, nonsteroidal anti-inflammatory drugs, and exercises to maintain range of motion, is usually sufficient. Arthroscopic treatment for this disorder has been described,[16] but surgical treatment is rarely necessary. Symptoms may persist for many months, but the long-term prognosis is excellent.[3,20]

OSTEOCHONDRITIS DISSECANS

OCD of the capitellum is a condition in which a focal injury to the subchondral bone causes a loss in structural support for the overlying articular cartilage. The articular cartilage and subchondral bone then undergo degeneration and fragmentation, often resulting in alteration of the capitellar articular surface

congruency and even the development of loose bodies. Although the term OCD implies an inflammation of the osteochondral articular surface, a true inflammatory process has not been proven to exist.[3,20] The exact cause of OCD is unknown, but it is commonly thought to be related to a combination of repetitive microtrauma in the face of a tenuous blood supply to the capitellum.[2,3,21,22]

Unlike Panner's disease, which affects children younger than 10 years old, OCD usually causes lateral elbow pain in adolescents between ages 11 and 16. It is seen in the elbows of throwing athletes, which sustain repetitive valgus stress and lateral compression and in those of gymnasts whose elbows function as weight-bearing joints and thus are subjected to repetitive compressive loads and shear forces.[23] The athlete will present complaining of poorly localized, progressive lateral elbow pain. Pain is often exacerbated with activity and relieved with rest. Mechanical symptoms such as locking, clicking, and catching can occur if a fragment has become unstable or a loose body is present. Physical examination often reveals tenderness to palpation in the anterolateral elbow, swelling, and crepitus. Loss of extension and forearm rotation can be seen. The active radiocapitellar compression test, consisting of pronation and supination with the elbow in full extension, often provokes symptoms.[3]

Radiographs classically demonstrate radiolucency or rarefaction of the capitellum with flattening and irregularity of the articular surface (Fig. 37-3A). The lesion will often be seen as a

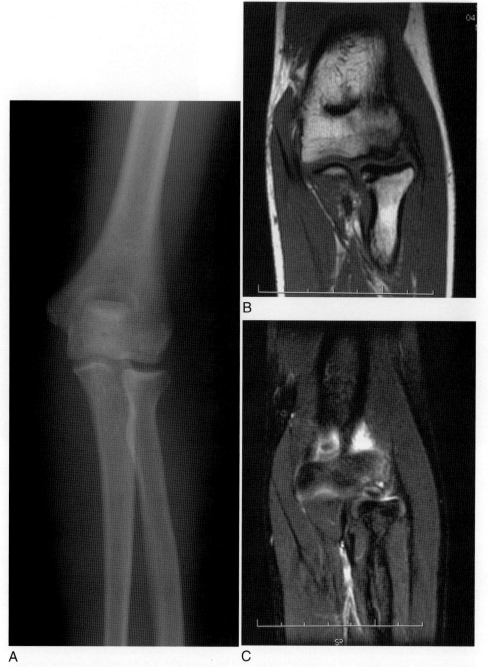

Figure 37-3 A 13-year-old female gymnast with lateral elbow pain but no mechanical symptoms. **A,** Anteroposterior radiograph demonstrates the osteochondritis dissecans (OCD) lesion in the capitellum. **B** and **C,** T1- and T2-weighted magnetic resonance images showing marrow edema and disruption of the subchondral plate. The fluid deep to the base of the lesion suggests that this is an unstable lesion.

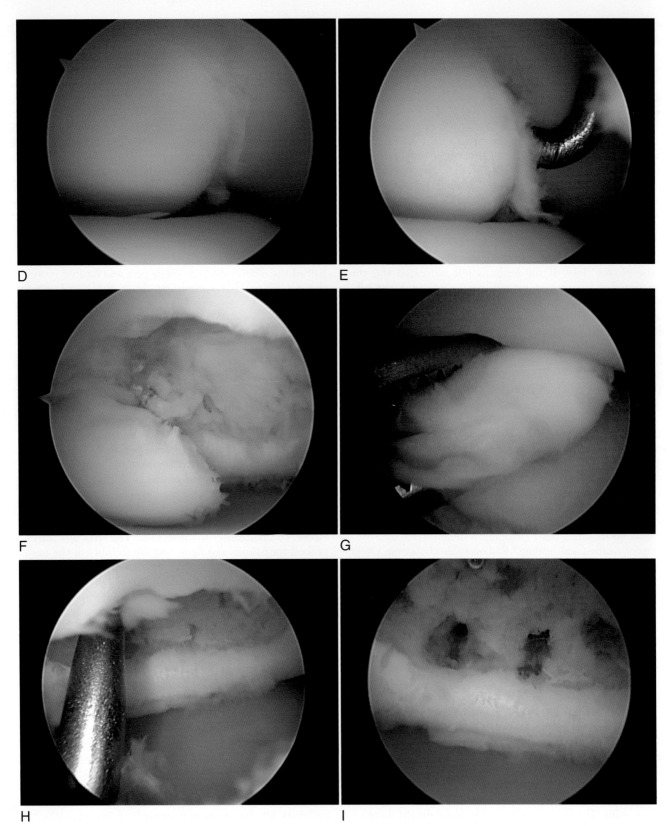

Figure 37-3—Cont'd D, Arthroscopy demonstrates the nondisplaced, unstable OCD lesion in the capitellum. **E,** A probe placed in the fissure on the medial side of the lesion proves this to be unstable. **F,** The crater of the lesion is seen after the unstable flap of cartilage has been detached. **G,** The cartilaginous piece is manually removed with an arthroscopic grasper. **H,** A microfracture awl is directed into the base of the lesion. **I,** Bleeding is demonstrated from the multiple microfracture sites after the tourniquet has been deflated.

focal sclerotic rim surrounding a radiolucent crater. Anteroposterior radiographs with the elbow in 45 degrees of flexion can be helpful.[24] In advanced OCD, collapse of the articular surface, loose bodies, enlargement of the radial head, subchondral cysts, and osteophyte formation can be seen. However, plain radiographs are often nondiagnostic in this condition, especially in the early stages of the disease.

Magnetic resonance imaging can be useful in diagnosing OCD in its earlier stages and assessing the status of the articular cartilage.[25,26] Low signal changes on T1-weighted images in the capitellum can suggest early OCD lesions.[24] Fluid between a fragment and the capitellum seen on T2-weighted images indicates a detached fragment (Fig. 37-3B and C).

The natural history of a capitellar osteochondritis dissecans lesion is hard to predict. There are no reliable criteria to predict which lesions will heal and which will collapse and cause later joint incongruity. If healing is to occur, it will occur by the time that the physes close. If the lesion is left untreated and the elbow continues to experience repetitive microtrauma, the subchondral bone may eventually collapse. The joint incongruity can cause articular cartilage damage, loose body formation, and degenerative joint changes.[1-3,27] Therefore, appropriate treatment of OCD lesions in the young athlete is not only critical for return to competition but also for long-term acceptable elbow function with normal everyday activities.

A useful classification of capitellar OCD is based on the stability of the subchondral bone and its overlying articular cartilage. The combination of clinical, radiographic, and arthroscopic findings can be used to classify lesions into three types.[17] Type Ia lesions have intact articular cartilage and no loss of subchondral bone stability. Type Ib lesions are intact but unstable, having intact articular cartilage but unstable subchondral bone potentially at risk of collapse. The treatment of these type I lesions is initially nonsurgical, emphasizing rest, ice, nonsteroidal anti-inflammatory drugs, and early range-of-motion exercises. Activity should be modified until radiographs demonstrate evidence of revascularization and healing.[1] Radiographic changes in OCD often persist for several years, so the decision to return an athlete to sports is based on resolution of symptoms. Conservative treatment of OCD of the capitellum is not always successful.[14,26,28] Surgical indications for type I lesions include radiographic evidence of lesion progression, such as capitellar collapse, or failure of nonsurgical management to relieve symptoms after a 6-month period. The preferred surgical treatment involves arthroscopic evaluation; débridement, if necessary; and drilling or microfracture of the lesion.

Type II lesions are open and unstable, with cartilage fracture and collapse or partial displacement of the subchondral bone. These are often flap lesions that should be treated surgically, usually with débridement and drilling the bed of the lesion.[18,27,29] If the fragment is large and has adequate subchondral bone backing, open reduction and internal fixation can be attempted.[30]

Type III lesions are completely detached loose bodies within the elbow joint. The most accepted surgical treatment involves arthroscopy or arthrotomy with excision of the loose bodies, débridement, and drilling the bed of the lesion.[1,18,31,32] Type IV lesions have accompanying radial head involvement. These

"bipolar" lesions often lead to severe degenerative changes with likely poor long-term outcomes.

Few long-term studies of OCD lesions have been published. Ruch et al[32] presented the results of 12 adolescents who had undergone arthroscopic débridement. They noted that at an average follow-up of 3.2 years 92% of the patients were highly satisfied with minimal symptoms.[32] McManama et al[18] reviewed the results of 14 athletes who underwent arthrotomy, excision of loose bodies, and curettage of the lesion beds. Of those 14 athletes, 12 returned to competitive activity without restrictions. Many authors believe that the beneficial short-term results will deteriorate over time if repetitive loads are continually placed on incongruous joints. Jackson et al[31] observed that in gymnasts with OCD lesions that required surgery, return to competition was unlikely. Bauer et al[25] showed that at an average follow-up of 23 years, radiographic evidence of degenerative changes and reduced range of motion were present in more than half of the elbows studied. While pain and limited motion were the most common complaints, little functional impairment resulted.

SURGERY

For arthroscopic treatment of OCD lesions, we prefer to place the patient in the prone position with the elbow draped over a padded arm board. Portals are carefully made in standard fashion to avoid neurovascular injury. We base our decision regarding portal placement on the pathology observed and the angle at which the appropriate instruments can approach the lesion. We use anteromedial and anterolateral portals to visualize the anterior compartment, followed by proximal posterolateral, direct posterior, and direct lateral or anconeus portals for work in the posterior compartment.

The OCD lesion is visualized and probed in order to plan treatment. Loose bodies observed in the assessment of each elbow compartment are removed. The articular cartilage is probed for fissures and flaps, and the stability of the underlying subchondral bone is assessed. If a ballotable area without an unstable flap is noted, drilling with a Kirschner wire is performed. Areas of cartilage surface fraying can be débrided with a shaver if necessary. If an unstable flap of cartilage is lifted with the probe, inspection for attached subchondral bone is necessary. If sufficient subchondral bone is seen on the base of the lesion, internal fixation using cannulated screws can be attempted. In our experience, subchondral bone is rarely found on the flap of cartilage. If no subchondral bone is seen attached to the lesion, fixation efforts are unlikely to be successful. The articular surface is débrided back to a stable rim of cartilage. Microfracture of the subchondral bone in the lesion bed is performed. The tourniquet is deflated to ensure adequate bleeding from the microfracture sites (Fig. 37-3D through I).

The portal incisions are closed with a nylon suture. A sterile soft dressing is applied, and the patient's upper extremity is placed in a standard sling for comfort. Early range-of-motion exercises are begun in the immediate postoperative period. Strengthening is delayed until approximately 12 weeks postoperatively. Return to sports such as baseball or gymnastics is not permitted for at least 6 to 12 months.

REFERENCES

1. Pappas AM: Elbow problems associated with baseball during childhood and adolescence. Clin Orthop 1982;164:30–41.
2. DeFelice GS, Meunier MJ, Paletta GA: Elbow injuries in children and adolescents. In Altchek DW, Andrews JR (eds): The Athlete's Elbow. New York, Lippincott Williams & Wilkins, 2001, pp 231–248.
3. Rudzki JR, Paletta GA: Juvenile and adolescent elbow injuries in sports. Clin Sports Med 2004;23:581–608.
4. Bradley JP, Petrie RS: Elbow injuries in children and adolescents. In DeLee JC, Drez D, Miller MD (eds): DeLee & Drez's Orthopaedic Sports Medicine: Principles and Practice, 2nd ed. Philadelphia, Saunders, 2003, pp 1249–1264.
5. Augustine SJ, McCluskey GM, Miranda-Torres L: Little league elbow. In Baker CL, Plancher KD (eds): Operative Treatment of Elbow Injuries. New York, Springer, 2002, pp 69–77.
6. Gugenheim JJ, Stanley RF, Woods GW, et al: Little league survey: The Houston study. Am J Sports Med 1976;4:189–200.
7. Larson RL, Singer KM, Bergstrom R, et al: Little league survey: The Eugene study. Am J Sports Med 1976;4:201–209.
8. DaSilva MF, Williams JS, Fadale PD, et al: Pediatric throwing injuries about the elbow. Am J Orthop 1998;27:90–96.
9. Jobe FW, Nuber G: Throwing injuries of the elbow. Clin Sports Med 1986;5:621–636.
10. Woods GW, Tullos HS: Elbow instability and medial epicondyle fractures. Am J Sports Med 1977;5:23–30.
11. Gill TJ, Micheli LJ: The immature athlete. Common injuries and overuse syndromes of the elbow and wrist. Clin Sports Med 1996;15:401–423.
12. Ireland ML, Andrews JR: Shoulder and elbow injuries in the young athlete. Clin Sports Med 1988;7:473–494.
13. Case SL, Hennrikus WL: Surgical treatment of displaced medial epicondyle fractures in adolescent athletes. Am J Sports Med 1997;25:682–686.
14. Norwood LA, Shook JA, Andrews JR: Acute medial elbow rupture. Am J Sports Med 1981;9:16–19.
15. Chen AL, Youm T, Ong BC, et al: Imaging of the elbow in the overhead throwing athlete. Am J Sports Med 2003;31:466–473.
16. Ruch DS, Poehling GG: Arthroscopic treatment of Panner's disease. Clin Sports Med 1991;10:629–636.
17. Petrie RS, Bradley JP: Osteochondritis dissecans of the humeral capitellum. In DeLee JC, Drez D, Miller MD (eds): DeLee & Drez's Orthopaedic Sports Medicine: Principles and Practice, 2nd ed. Philadelphia, WB Saunders, 2003, pp 1284–1293.
18. McManama GB, Micheli LJ, Berry MV, et al: The surgical treatment of osteochondritis of the capitellum. Am J Sports Med 1985;13:11–21.
19. Baumgarten TE, Andrews JR, Satterwhite YE: The arthroscopic classification and treatment of osteochondritis dissecans of the capitellum. Am J Sports Med 1998;26:520–523.
20. Kobayashi K, Burton KJ, Rodner C, et al: Lateral compression injuries in the pediatric elbow: Panner's disease and osteochondritis dissecans of the capitellum. J Am Acad Orthop Surg 2004;12:246–254.
21. Cain EL, Dugas JR, Wolf RS, et al: Elbow injuries in throwing athletes: A current concepts review. Am J Sports Med 2003;31:621–635.
22. Schenck RC, Athanasiou KA, Constantinides G, et al: A biomechanical analysis of articular cartilage of the human elbow and a potential relationship to osteochondritis dissecans. Clin Orthop 1994;299:305–312.
23. Peterson RK, Savoie FH, Field LD: Osteochondritis dissecans of the elbow. Instr Course Lect 1999;48:393–398.
24. Takahara M, Shundo M, Kondo M, et al: Early detection of osteochondritis dissecans of the capitellum in young baseball players. Report of three cases. J Bone Joint Surg Am 1998;80:892–897.
25. Bauer M, Jonsson K, Josefsson PO, et al: Osteochondritis dissecans of the elbow. A long-term follow-up study. Clin Orthop 1992;284:152–160.
26. Takahara M, Ogino T, Sasaki I, et al: Long term outcome of osteochondritis dissecans of the humeral capitellum. Clin Orthop 1999;363:108–115.
27. Schenck RC, Goodnight JM: Osteochondritis dissecans. J Bone Joint Surg Am 1996;78:439–456.
28. Takahara M, Ogino T, Fukushima S, et al: Nonoperative treatment of osteochondritis dissecans of the humeral capitellum. Am J Sports Med 1999;27:728–732.
29. Byrd JW, Jones KS: Arthroscopic surgery for isolated capitellar osteochondritis dissecans in adolescent baseball players: Minimum three-year follow-up. Am J Sports Med 2002;30:474–478.
30. Harada M, Ogino T, Takahara M, et al: Fragment fixation with a bone graft and dynamic staples for osteochondritis dissecans of the humeral capitellum. J Shoulder Elbow Surg 2002;11:368–372.
31. Jackson DW, Silvino N, Reiman P: Osteochondritis in the female gymnast's elbow. Arthroscopy 1989;5:129–136.
32. Ruch DS, Cory JW, Poehling GG: The arthroscopic management of osteochondritis dissecans of the adolescent elbow. Arthroscopy 1998;14:797–803.

SECTION IV
Wrist and Hand

Physical Examination and Evaluation

Michael R. Boland

In This Chapter

INTRODUCTION

- The history is important in directing the examination of the wrist and hand.

- When inspecting or examining the wrist, it is best to divide the wrist into four basic areas for assessment: radial, dorsal, ulnar, and palmar.

- Special examination tests are available to test for wrist instability and impaction syndromes.

- Plain radiographs are the mainstay of diagnostic imaging of the wrist and hand.

- Specific radiographic views are available for many wrist problems.

- Computed tomography and magnetic resonance imaging scans are often used when further studies are necessary.

Injuries to the wrist and hand are common in all sports. About 10% of all athletic injuries involve the wrist and hand.[1] The incidence of wrist problems is much higher in contact sports and is seen in as many as 85% of participants in gymnastics.[2] The function of the wrist in athletic endeavors is twofold. The primary motion is from a position of radial deviation/extension to ulnar deviation/flexion. This motion assists in the power of throwing activities where the wrist is cocked into radial deviation/extension, accelerates through a neutral position into ulnar deviation/flexion, and then recovers back to a neutral position. For example, basketball free-throw shooting involves an extension-flexion arc of about 120 degrees in the shooting hand.[1] In baseball, the arc of motion is approximately 94 degrees.[3] The second function of the wrist is to position the hand in space, along with positioning the forearm in various degrees of pronation and supination. The function of the hand in sports is to grasp objects such as rackets, balls, or clubs.

Wrist anatomy is complex, but functionally the extensor carpi radialis longus and extensor carpi radialis brevis are the cocking muscles of the wrist, with flexor carpi ulnaris the primary accelerator. The flexor carpi radialis and extensor carpi ulnaris are primarily dynamic stabilizers of the wrist. These four primary motors of the wrist (extensor carpi radialis longus and extensor carpi radialis brevis act together) sit at four corners of a quadrilateral pulling the wrist into the distal radius like a hot air balloon is held against the ground by guide ropes. The true collateral ligaments of the wrist assist in holding the carpus against the radius. These include the radioscaphocapitate ligament on the volar side and the dorsal radiocarpal ligament on the dorsal side, the former coming from a relatively radial volar position and the latter coming from a dorsal ulnar direction. The hand and carpus are slung up to the distal radius. At the distal radioulnar joint, the ulnar head holds up the distal radius during pronation and supination of the wrist. The distal radius is held against the distal ulna by the ligaments within the triangular fibrocartilage. The ligaments from the ulna to the carpus are relatively loose.

Joint anatomy within the hand is relatively uniform. Each interphalangeal and metacarpophalangeal joint contains a volar plate to prevent translation of the joint, two collateral ligaments, and a flimsy dorsal capsule.

Injuries to the wrist and hand can be summarized as being either traumatic in nature or from overuse. Overuse injuries occur due to either compression or stretch tension when the wrist is moved outside its primary range of motion. An example is ulnar-side wrist pain in tennis players who use a western grip, which places the wrist into extreme ulnar deviation. These athletes are prone to tendonitis of the first and second dorsal compartments due to stress and compression problems of the triangular fibrocartilage. Traumatic injuries include fractures, dislocations, and ligament tears, all of which are common in collision or contact sports.

CLINICAL FEATURES AND EVALUATION

Evaluation of the hand and wrist in athletes requires a careful history followed by a specific examination. Many radiographic techniques have been described to assist in the visualization of the wrist and hand, and these should be obtained when looking for specific problems. Table 38-1 shows the radiographic views that are available and summarizes when they should be used.

The history should begin with an evaluation of the specific sport and level at which the patient participates. This often directly affects the management of the wrist or hand problem.

Table 38-1 Summary of Radiologic Views

Radiograph	When to Use	Reasons for Use
Posteroanterior	Routine view	Standard radiograph looking at contours of distal radius and ulna for fractures; alignment of proximal and distal rows
Oblique wrist	Routine view	Helpful in looking at distal radius fractures with displacement in ulnar columns
Lateral	Routine view	Important for proper carpal alignment looking for dorsal and volar intercollating instability deformities
Radial deviation	Instability series	Scaphoid should flex and thus the ring sign should be present; look for scapholunate widening
Ulnar deviation	Instability series	Also for scapholunate widening, ulnar impaction, and instability; increases relative ulnar variance, important in ulnar impaction syndromes
Clenched fist	Impaction and stability series	Can increase the scapholunate and lunotriquetral gap when there is ligament injury
Posteroanterior in pronation	Impaction series	Increased ulnar plus impaction
Scaphoid view	Special view	Look for scaphoid fractures
Carpal tunnel view	Special view	Look for hamate and scaphoid tubercle fractures
Pisotriquetral view	Special view	Shows pisotriquetral osteoarthritis and hamate fractures

For example, a lineman in football can often play wearing a cast, but a quarterback needs a nearly complete range of wrist motion. The history important in decision making is how the problem started, how the problem is affecting the patient's sporting endeavor currently, what the general health of the patient is with particular reference to joint-related diseases, previous upper extremity injury, and what treatment the patient has had prior to presentation.

After obtaining a general sports history, the first question should be how did this problem begin? A differential should be obtained between traumatic and spontaneous origin of onset. A specific history of the mechanism of injury should be obtained when there has been a traumatic event. The most common event causing wrist injury in athletes is a direct fall onto an outstretched hand. Finger injuries and fractures are often caused by a direct blow to the end of the finger, or getting the finger caught in another object such as an opponent's jersey. Sudden flexion of the distal interphalangeal joint will cause a mallet finger, whereas sudden extension creates a flexor digitorum profundus tendon avulsion (jersey finger) or avulsion fracture. A radial deviation injury to the thumb may result in an ulnar collateral ligament tear.

With injuries of insidious onset, overuse is usually the pertinent factor. With these injuries, a description of technique can be helpful in elucidating the origin of the problem.

With wrist injuries, pain is the usual presenting factor. Table 38-2 gives a differential diagnosis of wrist pain.

This differential diagnosis is very helpful when assessing wrist problems. The patient will generally point to the location of pain as either being radial, dorsal central, ulnar, or palmar wrist pain. As with any pain, aggravating and relieving factors are important, particularly the specific position that the wrist is in when pain occurs. The presence of a click or catch is uncommon but helpful when considering mechanical problems within the wrist joint itself or secondary to instability.

Following wrist or hand injuries, specific tingling and/or numbness can occur. Postural changes occur in the cervical spine and shoulder region causing compression of the thoracic outlet leading to an escalation in pain and often nonspecific tingling or numbness below the elbow region. Pain associated with this problem is often generalized, involving the entire upper extremity. The specific site of numbness and tingling can be indicative of carpal or cubital tunnel syndrome. Patients with cubital

Table 38-2 Wrist Pain: Differential Diagnoses

Radial	Intersection syndrome
	de Quervain's tenosynovitis
	Wartenberg's radial neuritis
	Radial styloid/scaphoid impingement
	Scaphoid fracture
	STT problems
	Thumb CMC joint problems
Dorsal central	Scapholunate ligament tear
	Carpal boss
	Ganglion
	Lunotriquetral ligament tear
	Kienböck's disease
	CMC joint instability (other than thumb)
	Tendonitis of the second to fifth extensor compartments
	Distal radius fracture
Ulnar	Distal radioulnar joint osteoarthritis
	Distal radioulnar joint instability
	Triangular fibrocartilage tear
	Extensor carpi ulnaris tendonitis
	Triquetral avulsion fracture
	Ulnar lunate impaction
	Ulnar triquetral impaction
	Cubital tunnel syndrome
Palmar	Carpal tunnel syndrome
	Hook of hamate fracture
	Wrist flexor tenosynovitis
	STT problems
	Scaphoid tubercle fracture

CMC, carpometacarpal; STT, scaphotrapeziotrapezoid.

tunnel syndrome often present with ulnar-side wrist pain and clumsiness of the hand.

When looking specifically at the hand, the site of pain and swelling is important, as is any deformity. Examples include abnormal radial or ulnar deviation in a proximal interphalangeal dislocation, or the presence of a boutonniere or mallet deformity when the central slip or common distal tendon of the extensor mechanism has been injured.

The site and quality of wrist pain can help direct the differential diagnosis. Pain secondary to instability occurs with weight bearing, such as lifting a heavy object or pushing oneself up from a chair. Pain because of impingement or impaction occurs in certain positions. Post-traumatic arthritic pain increases with activity and is often greatest after activity.

PHYSICAL EXAMINATION

While history taking is very important in the evaluation of wrist and hand problems, physical examination is the cornerstone of diagnosis. It should be directed toward the type of injury suspected. Physical examination should follow a methodical and reproducible pattern.

Examination should begin with the patient sitting directly opposite the examiner with the patient undressed from the mid-humerus down and the hands placed upon a small examination table, directly in front of the examiner. Visual inspection should be performed, assessing for deformity and swelling. Swelling of an interphalangeal joint can be easily seen with direct inspection in comparison with other interphalangeal joints and in particular the opposite extremity. Visual inspection of the fingers for a mallet or a boutonniere deformity is performed. Hand fractures will cause radial and ulnar deviation deformities and swelling. The examiner particularly needs to look for abnormal rotation of the affected digit. The more proximal a fracture, the less angulation or displacement is acceptable. Visual inspection of the wrist and distal radioulnar joint may show swelling of the radiocarpal or snuff box regions, a prominence of the distal ulna, or swelling around the distal radioulnar joint with ulnar-side wrist problems.

When inspecting or examining the wrist, it is best to divide the wrist into four basic areas for assessment: radial, dorsal, ulnar, and palmar. Physical examination should then follow this regional approach.[4] The differential diagnosis listed in Table 38-2 is very helpful in looking for and ruling out specific wrist conditions.

If physical examination is the mainstay of diagnosis in the wrist and hand, then palpation of specific tenderness and in particular the maximum site of tenderness is the key to a diagnosis. Structures of the wrist and hand are readily palpated.[5] The joint to be palpated will be directed by the history of injury and by the presence of deformity and swelling. Palpation of a thumb or finger joint needs to include palpation of radial collateral ligament origin and insertion, ulnar collateral ligament origin and insertion, insertion of tendons in the region of the joints (such as the central slip of the extensor tendon), and palpation over the volar aspect, in particular the volar plate. The metacarpophalangeal joint of the thumb requires specific palpation of the preceding structures and the volar sesamoid bones on the radial and ulnar aspects.

Wrist
Radial Side
The best way to palpate the wrist for tenderness is to work regionally, proximally to distally. If there is radial-side wrist pain, palpation should begin proximally with tapping over the radial nerve for radial neuritis as it passes beneath the brachioradialis. This is over the radial border of the radius at the junction between the middle and distal thirds of the radius. As one moves distally, there is a prominence over the dorsal and radial aspect of the radius approximately 8 cm from the radial styloid. This is where the long tendons to the thumb cross the wrist extensors, the site of intersection syndrome. All extensor tendons pass through a fibrous tunnel and can be subject to tenosynovitis. Tenosynovitis in the first dorsal compartment is known as de Quervain's disease. Swelling over the first dorsal compartment and tenderness associated with it is an indicator of this problem. Next, one should palpate the radiocarpal joint and over the radial styloid. Tenderness here is an indicator of styloid scaphoid impingement. Classic scaphoid fracture tenderness is in the anatomic snuff box, but tubercle scaphoid fractures are tender more volarly over the scaphoid. Problems of the scaphotrapeziotrapezoid joint and thumb carpometacarpal joint, such as chondromalacia and occasionally carpometacarpal instability, cause tenderness specifically over these joints and are best felt on the volar aspect. The scaphotrapeziotrapezoid joint is palpated by feeling the scaphoid tubercle and rolling the examining digit into the crevice just distal to that tubercle. Carpometacarpal tenderness is best palpated by providing longitudinal traction to the thumb and palpating down the metacarpal distally until a crevice is felt over the joint.

Dorsal Side
If the wrist pain is dorsal and central, then one needs to palpate over the second to fifth dorsal compartments looking for tendonitis. The soft spot bordered by extensor digitorum communis, extensor carpi radialis brevis, and extensor pollicis longus on the dorsum of the wrist is the site of most dorsal wrist ganglions and tenderness over this point is indicative of a ganglion or a scapholunate ligament tear (Fig. 38-1). Dorsal wrist ganglions are usually associated with grade I to II dorsal scapholunate ligament disruption. The distal radius should be palpated, and tenderness may represent a distal radius fracture.

Ulnar Side
Ulnar-side wrist pain has been called the back pain of the upper extremity. However, as with examination of other regions of the wrist, a methodical examination can usually determine the cause of ulnar-side wrist pain. This should begin with palpation of the distal radioulnar joint proper, the region where the ulnar head meets the sigmoid notch of the radius. Tenderness at this point is often indicative of post-traumatic osteoarthritis and distal radioulnar instability. A tear of the triangular fibrocartilage complex is tender more distally at the region of the ulnar carpal joint. The sixth dorsal compartment (the compartment for the extensor carpi ulnaris) should be palpated proximally to distally, and swelling or tenderness in this region is an indication of tendonitis of the extensor carpi ulnaris. Impaction syndromes occur between the ulna and lunate, resulting in tenderness more in the region of ulnar carpal joint. Ulnar styloid triquetral impaction is felt more medially, directly over the ulnar styloid (Fig. 38-2). It should be noted that patients with ulnar-side wrist problems often have cubital tunnel syndrome and Tinel's sign should be part of a routine examination of the ulnar side of the wrist.

Palmar Side
If the patient has palmar-side wrist pain, the patient is likely to have one of the following conditions: carpal tunnel syndrome,

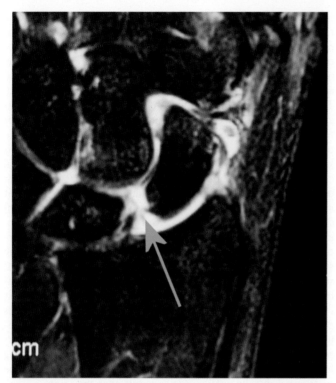

Figure 38-1 Magnetic resonance imaging showing an acute tear of the scapholunate ligament *(arrow)*.

hook of hamate fracture, flexor tenosynovitis, a scaphoid tubercle fracture, or scaphotrapeziotrapezoid joint problems. Direct compression of the median nerve with a flexed wrist (Phalen's compression test), which reproduces the tingling in the hand, is a reliable sign for carpal tunnel syndrome. When looking for Tinel's sign over the median nerve, one should start in the prox-

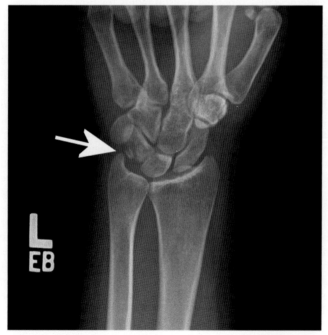

Figure 38-2 Radiograph of a patient with ulnar styloid triquetral impaction. Note the length of the ulna in relation to the radius (ulnar positive variance). Arrow indicates prominent ulnar styloid.

imal volar forearm and work distally toward the wrist. Often Tinel's sign is in the distal third of the forearm, not just over the carpal tunnel itself. Specific tenderness over the hook of the hamate or the scaphoid tubercle can be indicative of fractures in this region.

Range of Motion

Once a thorough inspection and palpation has taken place, the patient should be asked to put the forearm, wrist, and hand joints through a range of motion. Usually this can be done quickly by asking the patient to place the palm of the hand up toward the ceiling to look for supination, then the palms downward for full pronation. Full wrist dorsiflexion can be examined by placing the entire volar surfaces of the hands against one another as in a religious prayer position and then asking the patient to elevate both elbows. Wrist palmar flexion is evaluated with the reverse prayer position by placing the dorsal aspect of each hand against its opposite and lowering the elbows toward the floor. Next one should assess active radial and ulnar deviation. Then the patient is asked to do a full power grip, followed by full-spanning finger and thumb extension. Finally, the range of motion of the thumb is examined by asking the patient to touch the base of the volar aspect of the small finger. The patient should be able to at least touch the metacarpophalangeal crease at the base of the small finger for full thumb range of motion. Any lack of range of motion is measured with a goniometer and documented. Obviously, a lack of motion in any direction is indicative of stiffness of wrist or hand joints. Lack of range of motion is a major cause of morbidity in athletes. Certain sports require a full range of wrist motion, such as the shooting hand in basketball. The supporting nonshooting hand can have a markedly reduced range of motion and the basketball player may still be functional.

Wrist Instability and Impaction

Specific tests are available for assessing wrist stability. This should start at the distal radioulnar joint. Anteroposterior translational force is placed on the distal radioulnar joint in full pronation, in neutral, and in full supination.

If scapholunate ligament instability is suspected, then one should perform the Watson shift test. This is done by placing a thumb over the scaphoid tubercle and moving the hand from radial to ulnar deviation. The test is positive when the scaphoid tubercle does not become prominent or flex during radial deviation.[6] If the Watson test is painful, this is likely due to scaphotrapeziotrapezoid joint pathology and is indicative of a positive grind test due to the scaphoid moving in relation to the trapezoid and trapezium.

Lunotriquetral instability is assessed by performing a Ballottement test, whereby one holds the pisiform and triquetrum in a pinch grasp with one hand and the scaphoid and lunate in a pinched grasp of the opposite. An anteroposterior force is then placed between the two.

Mid-carpal instability is assessed by grasping the proximal row of the wrist with one hand and the distal with another and then placing an anteroposterior force. An associated clunk is indicative of mid-carpal instability.

Ulnar impaction syndromes are assessed by ulnarly deviating the wrist and then rotating the forearm. Pain with this maneuver indicates ulnar impaction and is often associated with a triangular fibrocartilage tear. Painful radial deviation of the wrist is an indicator of a possible radioscaphoid impaction syndrome.

Wrist Tendonitis

Tendonitis of the wrist occurs due to excessive tension involving any of the wrist compartments. The most common of these is tendonitis of the first dorsal compartment (de Quervain's disease). This is examined by placing tension on the tendons within the first compartment. These tendons are extensor pollicis brevis and abductor pollicis longus. Finkelstein's test is performed by asking the patient to grasp a fully flexed thumb, followed by application of a radial deviation force. The patient should have significant pain over the radial aspect of the wrist for a positive test. This test can be positive for extensor pollicis longus tendonitis if the pain is caused during ulnar deviation and with wrist flexion. Forced radial deviation with wrist flexion creates tension in the extensor carpi ulnaris tendon, and if the patient gets significant ulnar-side wrist pain in this position, then extensor carpi ulnaris tendonitis may be present.

Hand Injuries

If a metacarpophalangeal or interphalangeal joint injury is suspected, then that particular joint should be placed into radial and ulnar deviation and hyperextension. This evaluates collateral ligament and volar plate injury, respectively. The most important collateral ligament injury in the hand is a Stener lesion, with an ulnar collateral ligament tear of the metacarpophalangeal joint of the thumb. The importance of this is that if it is not surgically corrected, then permanent instability will result. A Stener lesion occurs when the ulnar collateral ligament avulses from the proximal phalanx and gets caught on the superficial side of the adductor aponeurosis (Fig. 38-3).

The hand examination is completed by examining the long tendons. Extensor pollicis longus and flexor pollicis longus are examined by actively flexing and extending the interphalangeal joint of the thumb, but if the extensor pollicis longus injury is more proximal than the dorsal thumb extensor hood, then this is examined by placing the palm of the hand on a flat tabletop and asking the patient to lift the thumb off the tabletop. The extensor pollicis longus tendon can be palpated to assess its potency. The long flexor tendons to the fingers are examined as follows: the flexor digitorum profundus is examined by grasping the proximal interphalangeal joint and holding it in extension. The patient is then asked to flex the distal interphalangeal joint. Because the profundus tendon is essentially a mass action muscle, by holding all fingers in full extension (except for the digit to be examined), the intact superficialis tendon should still be able to flex that finger.

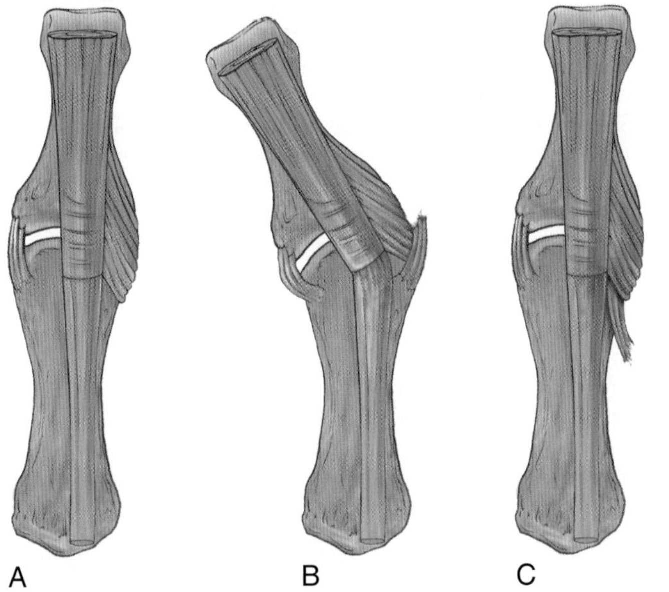

IMAGING

Plain Radiographs

Plain radiographs are essential in the evaluation of any sports-related wrist and hand injury. Three standard radiographs of the involved part should be obtained. For example, if the proximal interphalangeal joint is involved, then anteroposterior, oblique, and true lateral views should be obtained. The radiograph is centered over the involved part. When evaluating the radiograph, it should be noted that the radiograph taken is centered on the involved or injured part.

Specific radiographs of the wrist are summarized in Table 38-1. For all wrist problems, a routine series of posteroanterior, lateral, and oblique radiographs should be taken. In the posteroanterior view, the ring sign (Fig. 38-4) at the distal scaphoid should not be present and there should be easily defined carpal arches at the radiocarpal and mid-carpal joints. When specifically looking at the lunate, cystic change can occur in ulnar lunate impaction syndrome and sclerosis or collapse in Kienböck's disease. The normal finding on a posteroanterior radiograph is that the ulna is slightly shorter than the radius, there is a slight ulnar negative variance, and the slope of the distal radius relative to the shaft of the radius is about 14 degrees volar. On a lateral radiograph, the first step is to look at overall carpal alignment where the radius, lunate, capitate, and third

Figure 38-3 A complete tear of the ulnar collateral ligament of the thumb can result in a Stener lesion. **A,** The ulnar collateral ligament is normally covered by the adductor aponeurosis. **B,** With significant radial deviation, the ulnar collateral ligament tears distally and is displaced outside the aponeurosis. **C,** After the stress is released, the torn ulnar collateral ligament remains outside the aponeurosis in a position far from its insertion. This cannot heal and requires surgery to restore stability.

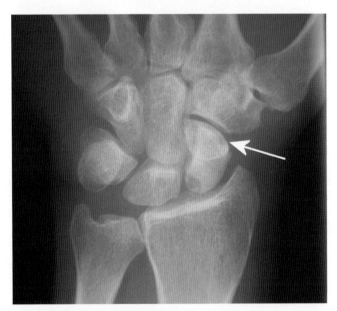

Figure 38-4 Scaphoid ring sign *(arrow)*. The distal scaphoid is seen on end, due to abnormal flexion of the bone in a volar direction, as a result of chronic scapholunate instability.

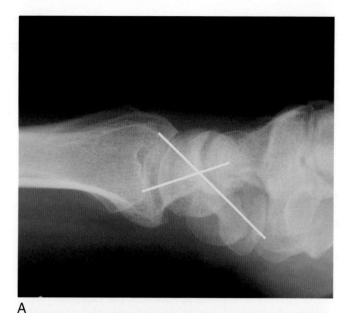

A

B

Figure 38-5 **A,** Lateral radiograph of a patient with chronic scapholunate instability, resulting in a dorsal intercollating segment instability deformity. The angle between the scaphoid and lunate is greater than 65 degrees. **B,** Magnetic resonance imaging in a patient with chronic scapholunate instability with the lunate *(arrow)* angulated.

the scaphoid is best appreciated by finding the distal pole and tubercle and following them in a proximal and dorsal direction. In dorsal intercollating segment instability, a line drawn through the midpole of the lunate will point distally in a dorsal direction, and the angle between the midpole of the scaphoid and the lunate will be greater than 65 degrees (Fig. 38-5). In volar intercollating segment instability, the lunate scaphoid angle will be less than 30 degrees. A dorsal intercollating segment instability deformity indicates probable scapholunate instability, and volar intercollating segment instability indicates probable lunotriquetral instability.

In looking for impaction or instability problems, ulnar deviation, radial deviation, clenched fist, and posteroanterior clenched fist views can be helpful (see Table 38-1). Special scaphoid, carpal tunnel, or pisotriquetral views are useful when considering other specific conditions.

Other imaging including radioisotope scanning, ultrasonography, and wrist arthrography have now been generally superseded by computed tomography and magnetic resonance imaging, and the author rarely uses these in his practice.

Computed tomography is very useful when looking for occult fractures of the carpal bones or a carpometacarpal fracture dislocation. Magnetic resonance imaging is useful in looking for a wrist ganglion, ligament tears, triangular fibrocartilage tears, Kienböck's disease, and occult scaphoid fractures.

CONCLUSIONS

Wrist and hand problems are common in the sporting arena. Evaluation of these problems requires a careful history with particular attention to the initiating factor, be it traumatic or spontaneous. Attention should be paid to how the injury is affecting the athlete at the time of presentation. The specific site and associated factors of pain will help guide the examiner to the site of specific pathology. With hand and digital injuries, the site of pathology is usually obvious. With the wrist, the site of pathology should be divided into radial, dorsal, ulnar, and palmar aspects.

Specific examination of the anatomic part involved should then be performed. An exposed upper extremity should then be inspected. Palpation should be specific to the region involved. Tests for range of motion, instability, and impaction should then be done.

Plain radiographs are still the mainstay of imaging in the wrist and hand. When further studies are needed, magnetic resonance imaging and computed tomography are most commonly used.

After careful evaluation of the wrist or hand problem, the clinician should be able to come to a specific diagnosis. This allows for decision making with regard to treatment options; observation, bracing or splinting, hand therapy, or open or arthroscopic surgery can be tailored to the specific diagnosis. Details of such management are provided in subsequent chapters of this text.

metacarpal are generally in a straight line. This line will be broken in a perilunate dislocation, with the lunate sitting anterior to the capitate. A true lateral radiograph aligns the tubercle of the scaphoid and pisiform. With this alignment, the radius and ulna should be overlapping totally; if they are not, consider distal radioulnar joint subluxation or dislocation. The outline of

REFERENCES

1. Rettig AC: Athletic injuries of the wrist and hand: Part 1, traumatic injuries of the wrist. Am J Sports Med 1998;31:1038–1048.
2. Buterbaugh JA, Brown TR, Horn PC: Ulnar sided wrist pain in athletes. Clin Sports Med 1998;17:567–583.
3. Pappas AM, Morgan WJ, Schulz LA, et al: Wrist kinematics during pitching—A preliminary report. Am J Sports Med 1995;23:312–315.
4. Cooney WP, Bishop AT, Linscheid RL: Physical examination of the wrist.

In Cooney WP, Linscheid RL, Dobyns JH (eds): Wrist Diagnosis and Operative Treatment. St. Louis, Mosby Year-Book, 1998, pp 236–261.
5. Linscheid RL, Dobyns JH: Physical examinations of the wrist. In Linscheid RL, Dobyns JA (eds): Physical Examinations of the Musculoskeletal System. Chicago, Yearbook Medical Publishers, 1987, pp 80–94.
6. Watson HK, Ashmead D, Makhlof V: Examination of the scaphoid. J Hand Surg [Am] 1988;13:657–660.

39 Carpal Fractures

Steven D. Maschke and Jeffrey N. Lawton

In This Chapter

INTRODUCTION

- Hand and wrist injuries account for 3% to 9% of all athletic injuries; these are being seen more frequently as recreational and competitive sports participation increases.[1,2]

- The human wrist consists of eight carpal bones arranged in two rows, stabilized by numerous volar and dorsal ligaments that function synergistically to provide stability and pain-free range of motion.

- Most athletic activities involve the extremes of wrist range of motion. Therefore, physicians must identify carpal injuries early in order to prevent long-term functional decline and select operative procedures, when appropriate, that do not limit the required sport-specific wrist range of motion.

- Carpal fractures are often misdiagnosed as "wrist sprains" leading to delays in diagnosis and treatment. These delays may limit the options for both conservative and operative interventions leading to (1) longer treatment protocols, (2) more significant operative procedures, (3) extended loss of sports participation, and (4) permanent functional decline with decreased athletic performance.

- Scaphoid fractures account for the majority of carpal fractures. Hook of the hamate fractures occur with increased frequency in stick-handling sports. Appropriate diagnosis requires a high index of suspicion for each fracture type with expeditious treatment optimizing long-term outcomes. Newer percutaneous and arthroscopically assisted procedures allow improved outcomes and early return to play due to less operative morbidity.

SCAPHOID

Relevant Anatomy

The unique anatomy of the scaphoid leads to a predisposition for significant functional sequelae of malunited fractures while increasing the risks for fracture nonunion and avascular

necrosis. First, the scaphoid is positioned anatomically as a link between the proximal and distal carpal rows. Fracture leads to uncoupling of the distal and proximal fragments, resulting in altered load distribution and abnormal wrist kinematics. The distal fragment flexes and the proximal fragment extends leading to the commonly described "humpback" deformity. The resultant scaphoid shortening and/or angular malunion or nonunion often progresses to carpal collapse resulting in significant functional disability and wrist degeneration.[3]

Second, the scaphoid has a precarious vascular supply. Branches from the radial artery enter the dorsal ridge of the scaphoid either at or distal to the anatomic waist of the bone. These dorsal branches provide 70% to 80% of the entire intraosseous blood supply and 100% of the vascularity to the proximal pole.[4] This retrograde blood supply accounts for the direct correlation between proximal fractures and the increasing risk of delayed healing, nonunion, and avascular necrosis. Thus, successful management of scaphoid fractures demands restoring precise anatomy and choosing appropriate treatments based on fracture location and configuration.

Clinical Features and Evaluation

Scaphoid fractures account for 60% to 70% of all carpal fractures.[1,2] Athletes are at increased risk due to the extremes of wrist positions and forces at injury. The annual incidence of scaphoid fractures in collegiate football players is estimated to be as high as 1%.[5] The mechanism of injury is most often a fall on the outstretched hand, placing the wrist in extreme dorsiflexion and radial deviation.[6]

Athletes present with pain localized to the radial side of the wrist either following an acute trauma or, not uncommonly, at the conclusion of the athletic season. Often, the athlete provides a history of recurrent, nagging "wrist sprains." Clinical and radiographic evaluation must be systematically performed to identify the presence of a scaphoid fracture and define the parameters known to guide appropriate treatment and affect long-term outcomes. Paramount to this endeavor is a high index of suspicion for scaphoid fracture in any athlete presenting with radial-side wrist pain. History centers on (1) the acute event, with emphasis placed on the timing and energy of injury and (2) history of upper extremity trauma or wrist pain/swelling. Time from injury to presentation has significant implications with regard to success of treatment and length of time to fracture union. Several studies have documented substantially increased risk of delayed healing and nonunion in fractures where treatment is initiated later than 4 weeks after injury.[1,2,6,7] Defining the energy of injury, documenting previous wrist pain/swelling, and correlating these with radiographic findings allow the differentiation of an acute fracture versus an exacerbation of a previous scaphoid nonunion. It is critical that these two diagnoses remain separate with appropriate treatment initiated for each specific diagnosis.

Physical examination of the entire upper extremity is undertaken to diagnose concomitant upper extremity injuries and establish the clinical suspicion for a scaphoid fracture. The athlete will often demonstrate painful wrist motion, radial-side swelling, and decreased grip strength. Focused examination of the involved wrist helps the athlete define the location and quality of the pain and allows the examiner to grade the current functional impact of the injury with respect to wrist strength and range of motion. Tenderness localized to the anatomic snuff box and pain with wrist dorsiflexion/radial deviation increase the clinical suspicion for a scaphoid fracture.

Radiographic evaluation confirms the diagnosis and defines the fracture configuration and geometry. Routine radiographs of the wrist include posteroanterior, true lateral, and scaphoid (30 degrees of supination and ulnar deviation) views.[6,8] These initial images identify established fracture nonunions, displaced/angulated fractures, and concomitant wrist injuries. However, plain radiographs are notorious for missing acute nondisplaced scaphoid fractures and are often the cause for delay in diagnosis and treatment (Fig. 39-1). Seven percent of patients with clinical evidence of scaphoid injury and negative plain radiographs will have a scaphoid fracture.[9] Therefore, further imaging is often required to establish the diagnosis. Bone scintigraphy has been the gold standard for evaluating patients with clinical suspicion of fracture and no radiographic evidence of injury.[8,9] All fractures should have increased tracer uptake at 3 days after injury and most are apparent within the initial 24 hours.[8] However, false positives are expected given this modality's high sensitivity but relatively low specificity.[9] Therefore, magnetic resonance imaging is gaining favor as a first-line imaging modality in the diagnosis of occult scaphoid fractures.[9] Studies have shown equivalent sensitivity with superior specificity compared to bone scintigraphy.[9] Magnetic resonance imaging has the additional advantages of (1) excellent soft-tissue evaluation including the scapholunate ligament,[8] (2) ability to assess proximal pole vascularity, (3) identification of fracture location and configuration, (4) no radiation exposure, and (5) speed of examination.[9]

Radiographs further establish fracture location (distal third, waist, or proximal third) and define stability based on radiographic evidence of fracture displacement and/or angulation. Computed tomography is used when fracture displacement remains uncertain given its superior definition of cortical integrity and bony anatomy.[6,8] By definition, displaced scaphoid fractures have at least 1 mm of cortical offset and an increased intrascaphoid angle greater than 30 degrees.[1,2,6] Therefore, a high index of clinical suspicion, thorough history and physical examination, and appropriate imaging allow early identification of scaphoid injuries and accurate determination of fracture location, geometry, and time from injury to presentation.

Treatment Options

Management of acute scaphoid fractures is guided by fracture location, displacement, and time from injury to presentation.[1,2,6] Athletes require additional consideration as to sport and position as well as the athlete's specific wishes regarding return to play. Restoring precise anatomy and achieving solid fracture union are the primary goals of any treatment.

The importance of restoring precise anatomy cannot be overstated. Displacement is the hallmark of unstable fractures. Several studies evaluating closed treatment of fractures with greater than 1 mm of cortical offset have revealed nonunion rates ranging from 46% to 92%.[10] Fracture nonunion and/or malunion often lead to painful wrist instability and debilitating degenerative arthritis.[3] Therefore, we perform open reduction and internal fixation on all acute displaced scaphoid fractures. Alternatively, arthroscopic reduction with percutaneous fixation may be employed.[11]

The treatment of nondisplaced scaphoid fractures is more controversial. Historically, cast immobilization was initiated for all nondisplaced fractures, with 6 weeks in a long-arm cast followed by an additional 6 weeks or longer in a short-arm thumb spica cast.[7,12,13] The prolonged periods of immobilization coupled with the continued risk of fracture nonunion spurred the development of more aggressive treatment regimens. Today, the selection of an appropriate treatment algorithm is guided by fracture location and individualized to the patient's vocational, recreational, and athletic demands.

Distal third fractures of the scaphoid occur infrequently and involve the tuberosity in isolation or the entire distal third of the bone. Fractures occurring in this location maintain an adequate blood supply and have a high propensity to heal.[1,7] Successful union is most often achieved with 6 weeks of immobilization in a short-arm thumb spica cast.[7]

Proximal third fractures account for 20% of scaphoid fractures and are plagued by higher rates of nonunion and avascular necrosis. Casting has been the standard of care, often requiring as long as 6 months of strict immobilization to achieve successful healing.[1,13] Considerable disagreement as to the appropriate type and duration of immobilization continues.[6,14] Current recommendations consist of 6 weeks in a long-arm thumb spica cast followed by immobilization in a short-arm thumb spica cast until clinical and radiographic fracture union.[2] Few patients can afford such lengthy periods of immobilization. Prolonged casting often leads to significant muscle atrophy, stiffness, and contractures requiring extended periods of rehabilitation prior to return to work or sport.[1] Therefore, we recommend consideration of early operative intervention for all proximal scaphoid fractures occurring in active individuals. We use a dorsal approach and perform our fixation either open or percutaneously based on the need for fracture reduction.

The vast majority of scaphoid fractures (70% to 80%) are nondisplaced fractures through the anatomic waist.[1] Treatment

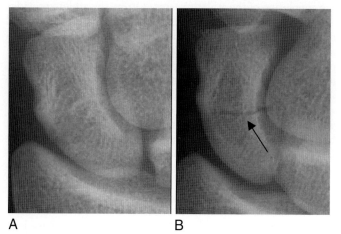

Figure 39-1 A, Occult scaphoid fracture: Initial presentation. **B,** Scaphoid waist fracture: Two-week follow-up *(arrow)*.

options include (1) cast immobilization until radiographic union, (2) cast treatment plus application of playing splints, or (3) immediate internal fixation.

Cast immobilization is an effective and appropriate treatment when initiated early for nondisplaced scaphoid waist fractures. Studies have shown 95% rates of union following 8 to 10 weeks of cast immobilization initiated within 4 weeks of injury.[12,15] Fractures showing no radiographic evidence of healing after 6 to 8 weeks of appropriate immobilization should be considered for internal fixation to minimize the risks of both prolonged casting and fracture nonunion.[1,16] Athletes must be appropriately counseled regarding the anticipated 3 months out of competition prior to initiating cast immobilization. Few athletes are willing to undergo this prolonged regimen, and, thus, alternatives have been sought for nondisplaced scaphoid waist fractures in the athletic population.

Cast immobilization with the application of a playing splint and immediate return to competition have been described.[2] The specific athletic event and the level of competition determine whether playing casts/splints are permitted. Review of this treatment regimen has revealed increased rates of fracture nonunion and subsequent operative intervention.[2] Athletes must be informed of the increased risks with this treatment protocol, and we currently do not implement this as a preference in our practice.

Advances in surgical technique and internal fixation have revolutionized the operative repair of scaphoid fractures. Absolute indications for immediate internal fixation include displaced fractures, nonunions, and fractures associated with carpal instability.[1] Relative indications include delayed presentation (greater than 4 weeks), proximal pole fractures, and malunions.[1] Immediate internal fixation for nondisplaced fractures of the scaphoid waist remains controversial, but this approach is gaining more widespread acceptance.[1,2,6,13,16] Recent studies comparing immediate operative repair versus cast immobilization reveal equivalent rates of fracture healing with dramatically reduced times to return to work and sport.[1,2,6,13,16] We advise our athletes about the risks and benefits of all treatment regimens and advocate immediate internal fixation of nondisplaced scaphoid waist fractures in those desiring an expeditious return to competition.

Surgery

Operative fixation of scaphoid fractures is increasing in popularity with advances in intraoperative imaging, surgical approaches/instrumentation, and trends toward less invasive surgical procedures. Currently, acute scaphoid fractures can be repaired via open volar or dorsal approaches, percutaneous techniques, or arthroscopically assisted procedures.[1,6,11] Fracture location and geometry as well as surgeon skill and experience guide the appropriate selection for operative repair.

Common to all operative techniques is the use of biplanar fluoroscopy to confirm fracture reduction and appropriate guidewire/screw insertion as well as the use of headless compression screws specifically designed for scaphoid fixation. Precise restoration of anatomy and compression of the fracture surfaces are paramount to achieving successful healing. Appropriate screw placement requires critical evaluation. Biomechanical and clinical studies have shown superior loads to failure, stiffness, and strength with central screw placement resulting in decreased times to fracture union.[16] Ideally, contact sport athletes are immobilized postoperatively in a short-arm thumb spica cast until radiographic confirmation of bony union, while noncontact athletes may be placed in a removable splint,

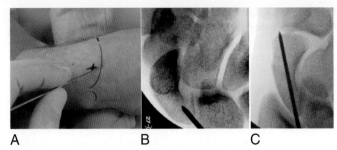

Figure 39-2 Dorsal, percutaneous, scaphoid stabilization. **A,** Placement of guidewire. **B,** Fluoroscopic image of starting point for insertion. **C,** Final guidewire placement.

allowing immediate range-of-motion exercises and potentially earlier return to competition.

Minimally invasive techniques have been developed to reduce operative morbidity and expedite fracture healing and rehabilitation (Figs. 39-2 and 39-3). Both percutaneous and arthroscopic procedures are currently in practice.[1,6,11,13] Cannulated, headless compression screws allow insertion via minimal incisions, and biplanar fluoroscopy confirms accurate, central screw placement. Both techniques are best suited for nondisplaced or minimally displaced scaphoid fractures.[1,6] Athletes are immobilized in a postoperative cast and may immediately return to competition if permitted; alternatively, some must delay return until confirmed fracture healing and cast removal. Taras et al[13] reported return to athletics averaging 5.4 weeks with successful union achieved in all patients undergoing percutaneous scaphoid fixation. These techniques are best reserved for surgeons experienced in wrist arthroscopy and operative scaphoid repair. Compromising accurate reduction and central screw placement, for the sake of a percutaneous approach, must be avoided.

Open reduction and internal fixation remains the treatment of choice for displaced, unstable scaphoid fractures.[6] The operative approach is determined by fracture location. The volar approach preserves the vital dorsal blood supply and allows easy access to middle and distal third fractures. The dorsal approach provides exposure of proximal third fracture and is reserved for this indication as the vascular leash is maintained. Direct visualization of fracture reduction and guidewire placement is correlated with biplanar imaging to confirm anatomic reduction and central screw placement.

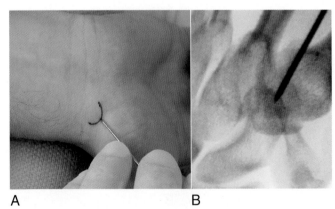

Figure 39-3 Volar, percutaneous, scaphoid stabilization. **A,** Placement of guidewire. **B,** Fluoroscopic image of volar starting point.

Technique: Volar Open Reduction/Internal Fixation

The volar approach to the wrist begins with a 4- to 5-cm curvilinear incision extending from the scaphoid tuberosity along the radial border of the flexor carpi radialis tendon. The flexor carpi radialis tendon sheath is exposed and longitudinally incised allowing ulnar retraction of the tendon. Commonly, the superficial palmar branch of the radial artery is encountered, requiring ligation. The volar capsule is obliquely incised exposing the radioscaphocapitate and long radiolunate ligaments. These ligaments are critical to wrist stability and are either partially divided or completely transected and tagged for later repair. The fracture is visualized and cleared of clot and debris. Preliminary reduction, usually by wrist extension, is achieved and fluoroscopic imaging obtained to confirm reduction and correction of the "humpback" deformity. Careful scrutiny of the scapholunate angle on lateral fluoroscopy is critical. The scaphotrapezial joint is entered and 2 to 3 mm of volar trapezium excised to allow accurate guidewire and screw placement. A compression jig or free-hand technique is used to centrally place the guidewire. Biplanar imaging confirms accurate wire placement and a second Kirschner wire may be inserted to control rotation and displacement during drilling, tapping, and screw insertion. Screw placement/length and fracture reduction and stability are confirmed with biplanar imaging and both Kirschner wires removed (Fig. 39-4). The volar radiocarpal ligaments and capsule are reapproximated and repaired using 3-0 permanent figure-eight sutures. The wound is closed in layers and a sterile dressing is applied. A short-arm volar thumb spica splint is applied. The patient is seen at 1 week postoperatively for splint removal and application of a short-arm thumb spica cast.

Postoperative Rehabilitation

Immobilization is continued until radiographic confirmation of fracture healing. Computed tomography is the gold standard for defining fracture union and can be obtained on patients prior to discontinuation of immobilization. The average time to fracture union following operative repair ranges from 5 to 7 weeks.[12,13] Therapy is instituted immediately following cast removal with emphasis on wrist and digital range of motion followed by strengthening.

Criteria for Return to Play

The athlete's return to play is individualized, dependent on progress in healing, sport, position, and level of competition. All scaphoid fractures must be protected with a cast or splint until radiographic confirmation of fracture healing.[6] The goal of splint/cast immobilization is to limit wrist hyperextension upon potential impact. Noncontact sport athletes can immediately return to competition following stable internal fixation with a short-arm thumb spica cast/splint. Contact athletes and those undergoing conservative management should remain out of competition until confirmed fracture union. Athletes must demonstrate painless, full wrist range of motion and near normal strength prior to allowing unprotected athletic participation.

Results and Outcomes

Cast immobilization of a nondisplaced scaphoid fracture initiated within 4 weeks of injury has a greater than 90% chance of achieving fracture union.[15] Conservative treatment of fractures with 1 mm or greater displacement is complicated by nonunion rates ranging from 46% to 92%.[10] Immediate operative repair for both displaced/unstable fractures as well as nondisplaced scaphoid waist and proximal third fractures leads to fracture union rates exceeding 90%.[2,12] Early diagnosis and treatment with anatomic reduction and appropriate immobilization optimize long-term results.

Complications

Scaphoid fracture nonunions and malunions alter carpal kinematics potentially leading to radiocarpal and midcarpal osteoarthritis.[4] These degenerative changes often lead to chronic pain, limited motion, and diminished function.[1,2,4,6] Athletes with symptomatic malunions and nonunions require thorough evaluation and consideration of scaphoid reconstruction. Athletes with an incidental finding of a scaphoid fracture nonunion and/or malunion present a treatment dilemma. The patient must understand the natural history of these clinical entities with either observation or operative intervention instituted at the conclusion of the season on an individualized basis.

HOOK OF THE HAMATE

Anatomy

The hamulus, or hook of the hamate, protrudes into the palm surrounded by critical soft-tissue structures. The hook serves as the origin of the flexor and opponens digiti minimi muscles and forms the ulnar border of the carpal tunnel and radial border of Guyon's canal.[1] The deep motor branch of the ulnar nerve courses around the base of the hook with the superficial sensory branch remaining in close contact with the tip. The hook also functions as a pulley for the superficial and deep flexor tendons to the small and ring fingers, especially during ulnar deviation involved with power grip. Therefore, fracture and/or fracture nonunion of the hook of the hamate jeopardize injury to any or all of the previously mentioned structures.

The vascular anatomy of the hamate hook has been extensively evaluated.[17] Vessels penetrate the radial base as well as the ulnar tip with relatively poor vascular anastomoses between the two.[7,17] This resultant vascular watershed predisposes even nondisplaced hook fractures to nonunion.[1,17,18]

Clinical Features and Evaluation

Hook of the hamate fractures account for only 2% to 4% of all carpal fractures.[1] Athletes participating in stick-handling sports account for the vast majority of these injuries and are most at risk of long-term complications secondary to missed or delayed diagnosis.[1,2,19,20] The mechanism of injury is either (1) direct

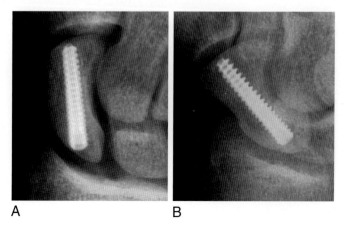

Figure 39-4 Postoperative radiographs: Percutaneous scaphoid stabilization. **A,** Scaphoid view. **B,** Oblique view.

A   B

impact via the handle of a club, racquet, or bat or (2) shearing forces arising from the hypothenar muscles as well as the flexor tendons to the ring and small fingers. The nondominant hand is most commonly involved in golf and baseball, whereas the dominant hand is more common in tennis and racquetball.[1]

Early diagnosis is critical to successful management of hook of the hamate fractures. The majority of these injuries will proceed to nonunion if left untreated.[20] Fracture nonunion predisposes the athlete to (1) chronic ulnar-side wrist pain, (2) ulnar nerve paresthesias/motor weakness, and/or (3) flexor tenosynovitis with potential flexor tendon rupture. Diagnosis begins with a detailed history focusing on the mechanism and timing of injury. Ulnar wrist pain occurring during stick-handling sports is almost pathognomonic for hook fracture. Athletes with symptoms directed at the carpal tunnel, Guyon's canal, or ulnar-side digital flexors require critical evaluation for established nonunion of the hamate's hook. Tenderness to palpation over the hook, painful grip, pain with resisted small/ring finger flexion, and a high index of suspicion further aid in the diagnosis.

Radiographic evaluation confirms suspected diagnoses. Routine anteroposterior, lateral, and oblique wrist radiographs often do not reveal the fracture.[1,17,21] Subtle radiographic signs on anteroposterior projections include (1) absence of the hook, (2) lack of cortical density, and (3) sclerosis.[1] Special projections can be useful in establishing the diagnosis. The carpal tunnel view may allow imaging of the hamate hook but requires wrist dorsiflexion often unattainable in patients with wrist injuries (Fig. 39-5).[17] Computed tomography is the gold standard for confirming the presence of hook of the hamate fracture and should be obtained in any athlete with ulnar-side wrist pain and negative plain radiographs (see Fig. 39-5).[1,2,17] A high index of suspicion for fracture and appropriate radiographic evaluation allow prompt diagnosis, early management, and avoidance of long-term complications.

Treatment Options

Appropriate management of hook of the hamate fractures aims to eliminate the risk of long-term complications and return the athlete to his or her preinjury level of play. Treatment options include cast immobilization, fragment excision, and open reduction and internal fixation.[1,17] The choice of management is guided by time from injury to presentation, displacement, and accompanying nerve/tendon pathology.[1,17] Athletes must be appropriately counseled regarding the potential complications arising from untreated fractures and fracture nonunions.

Displaced fractures compromise the intricate anatomy and encroach on the vital soft-tissue structures adjacent to the hamate's hook. Neurovascular and tendinous structures are at risk and must be preserved.[1,19,20,22] Therefore, all displaced fractures require immediate fragment excision.

Nondisplaced fractures are treated based on the timing from injury to presentation. Acute fractures are defined as those diagnosed and treated within 7 days of injury. Whalen et al[23] managed six acute fractures in short-arm casts incorporating the fourth and fifth metacarpophalangeal joints. Successful union was achieved in all acute injuries, with healing times averaging 8 to 12 weeks. Other studies document high rates of nonunion following cast immobilization that is initiated greater than 7 days from injury.[10,17,24] Thus, cast immobilization is a viable treatment option only for fractures diagnosed and immobilized within 7 days of injury.[1,23] Athletes must be informed of the 3 to 4 months out of competition required for successful conservative management. Fractures presenting more than 7 days from injury require operative intervention.

Operative management consists of fragment excision versus open reduction and internal fixation. Indications for surgery include (1) displaced fractures, (2) fractures accompanied by ulnar nerve paresthesias or tendinous pathology, (3) fractures diagnosed later than 7 days from injury, and (4) athletes unwilling to undergo prolonged immobilization of acute injuries.[1,17,24] Open reduction and internal fixation have been described. The small size of the fragment and precarious vascular supply adds complexity and uncertainty to this procedure.[1,10] Thus, excising the fractured hook remains the gold standard among operative procedures.[1,24,25] A volar approach is used, with care to identify and protect the surrounding neurovascular and tendinous structures. The fragment is subperiosteally excised, and the bone edges smoothed to prevent ulnar nerve irritation or tendon fraying. The wrist is immobilized postoperatively to protect the operative wound.

Postoperative Rehabilitation

Following fragment excision, the wrist is immobilized for 10 to 14 days to protect wound healing. Athletes undergoing prolonged immobilization require hand therapy following cast removal to regain full, painless wrist range of motion.

Criteria for Return to Play

Stable fracture healing and painless full wrist range of motion are required following cast immobilization or open reduction and internal fixation prior to return to play. Athletes undergoing fragment excision may return to competition as tolerated following successful wound healing. The majority of athletes prefer to wear well-padded gloves for several months after treatment to protect the hypothenar eminence from irritation inflicted by their racquet, club, or bat.[1,21]

Results and Outcomes

The vast majority of athletes return to their previous level of sports participation following hook of the hamate excision.[10,19,24] The time to return to full athletics averages 8 weeks with nearly normal grip strength regained within 3 months of fragment excision.[2,20] Associated nerve or tendon injury prolongs the time course for return to athletics and complicates the surgical repair and postoperative rehabilitation.[22]

Complications

The surrounding soft-tissue structures can be irritated and damaged by the fractured hamate hook or callous from a hypertrophic nonunion. Ulnar nerve compression is common and presents as paresthesias extending into the ring and small fingers.[21] The flexor tendons to the small and ring fingers can be abraded by the fractured hook, developing painful

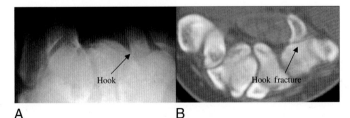

A   B

Figure 39-5 Hook of the hamate. **A,** Carpal tunnel view: hook (arrow). **B,** Computed tomography image: hook fracture (arrow).

tenosynovitis.[19,22] Untreated, these tendons are at risk of rupture.[19,22] All complications must be promptly identified and treated appropriately along with fragment excision. Early diagnosis is critical in avoiding the late sequelae of hook fracture and nonunion.

OTHER CARPAL FRACTURES

Significant forces transmitted through the wrist from a fall or collision can potentially fracture any of the eight carpal bones. Unlike the previously discussed injuries, the remaining carpal fractures are more straightforward with regards to diagnosis and treatment. Athletes presenting with significant wrist pain, swelling, or deformity require a precise physical examination with palpation of each carpal bone followed by appropriate radiographs. Subtle fractures may be difficult to identify on plain radiographs. Computed tomography can significantly aid in the diagnosis of occult fractures occurring in the setting of wrist pain/swelling and negative plain radiographs.

Dorsal triquetral fractures require specific mention as they are the second most common carpal fracture in athletes.[1] These injuries arise from either bony impaction occurring with extreme wrist dorsiflexion and ulnar deviation or from bony avulsion via the strong dorsal capsular ligaments.[1,10] Plain radiographs demonstrate the injury on the lateral film. Immobilization for 4 weeks with protected athletic participation leads to excellent clinical results and early return to play.[1,10]

Fractures of the other carpal bones are rare and most often occur in high-energy trauma. These injuries require immobilization and referral to a hand surgery specialist. Excellent outcomes and return to play are expected following appropriate treatment.

CONCLUSIONS

Early diagnosis is critical in the appropriate diagnosis of carpal fractures. Scaphoid fractures are most common, and plain radiographs may not reveal the acute fracture. Magnetic resonance imaging or computed tomography is often required. Treatment of scaphoid fractures has evolved, and operative intervention is commonly employed. This generally allows for earlier return to sports. When diagnosed acutely and treated appropriately, a good outcome is usually achieved.

REFERENCES

1. Geissler WB: Carpal fractures in athletes. Clin Sports Med 2001; 20:167–188.
2. Rettig AC: Athletic injuries of the wrist and hand—part 1: Traumatic injuries of the wrist. Am J Sports Med 2003;31:1038–1048.
3. Mack GR, Bosse MJ, Gelberman RH, et al: The natural history of scaphoid non-union. J Bone Joint Surg Am 1984;66:504–509.
4. Gelberman RH, Menon J: The vascularity of the scaphoid bone. J Hand Surg 1980;5:508–513.
5. Zemel NP, Stark HH: Fractures and dislocations of the carpal bones. Clin Sports Med 1986;5:709–724.
6. Cooney WP: Scaphoid fractures: Current treatment and techniques. Instr Course Lect 2003;52:197–208.
7. Burge P: Closed cast treatment of scaphoid fractures. Hand Clin 2001;17:541–552.
8. Plancher KD: Methods of imaging the scaphoid. Hand Clin 2001; 17:703–721.
9. Fowler C, Sullivan B, Williams L, et al: A comparison of bone scintigraphy and MRI in the early diagnosis of occult scaphoid waist fracture. Skeletal Radiol 1998;27:683–687.
10. Melone CP: Fractures of the wrist. In Nicholas JA, Hershman EB (eds): The Upper Extremity in Sports Medicine, 2nd ed. St. Louis, Mosby, 1995, pp 401–448.
11. Slade JF, Geissler WB, Gutow AP, et al: Percutaneous internal fixation of selected scaphoid non-unions with an arthroscopically assisted dorsal approach. J Bone Joint Surg Am 2003;85:20–31.
12. Saeden B, Tornkvist H, Ponzer S, et al: Fracture of the carpal scaphoid: A prospective, randomized 12 year follow up comparing operative and conservative treatment. J Bone Joint Surg Br 2001;83: 230–234.
13. Taras JS, Sweet S, Shum W, et al: Percutaneous and arthroscopic screw fixation. Hand Clin 1999;15:467–473.
14. McAdams TR, Spisak S, Beaulieu CF, et al: The effects of pronation and supination on the minimally displaced scaphoid fracture. Clin Orthop 2003;411:255–259.
15. Cooney WP, Dobyns JH, Linscheid RL: Non-union of the scaphoid: Analysis of the results from bone grafting. J Hand Surg Am 1980;5:343–354.
16. Chan KW, McAdams TR: Central screw placement in percutaneous screw scaphoid fixation: A cadaveric comparison of proximal and distal techniques. J Hand Surg Am 2004;29:74–79.
17. Walsh JJ, Bishop AT: Diagnosis and management of hamate hook fractures. Hand Clin 2000;16:397–403.
18. Failla JM: Hook of the hamate vascularity: Vulnerability to osteonecrosis and non-union. J Hand Surg Am 1993;18:1075–1079.
19. Stamos BD, Leddy JP: Closed flexor tendon disruption in athletes. Hand Clin 2000;16:359–365.
20. David TS, Zemel NP, Mathews PV: Symptomatic, partial union of the hook of the hamate fracture in athletes. Am J Sports Med 2003;31:106–111.
21. Murray PM, Cooney WP: Golf-induced injuries of the wrist. Clin Sports Med 1996;15:85–108.
22. Milek MA, Boulas HJ: Flexor tendon ruptures secondary to hamate hook fractures. J Hand Surg Am 1990;15:740–744.
23. Whalen JL, Bishop AT, Linscheid RL: Non-operative treatment of acute hamate hook fractures. J Hand Surg Am 1992;17:507–511.
24. Stark HH, Chao E, Zemel NP, et al: Fracture of the hook of the hamate. J Bone Joint Surg Am 1989;71:1202–1207.
25. Aldridge JM, Mallon WJ: Hook of the hamate fractures in competitive golfers: Results of treatment by excision of the fractures hook of the hamate. Orthopedics 2003;26:717–719.

In This Chapter

INTRODUCTION

- Athletic soft-tissue injuries of the wrist may be acute or degenerative in nature.

- Injuries of the TFCC are a frequent source of ulnar side wrist pain.

- Wrist arthroscopy is often employed to repair or débride TFCC tears.

- The preferred treatment of acute disruption of the scapholunate ligament is open repair.

- Chronic scapholunate injuries are more difficult to treat and often require a salvage procedure.

- Other wrist soft-tissue problems include tendonitis, de Quervain's disease, and intersection syndrome.

TRIANGULAR FIBROCARTILAGE COMPLEX INJURIES

Clinical Features and Evaluation

One of the most common complaints about the wrist is ulnar side wrist pain. Injuries to the TFCC usually occur as the result of a hyperextension, ulnar deviation, and axially loading force and can also be found in association with distal radius fractures. However, not all disruptions of the TFCC are traumatic in nature, as inflammatory and degenerative conditions can also lead to TFCC pathology. Patients presenting with TFCC injuries may report ulnar side wrist pain, occasional clicking, loss of grip strength, and pain with pronation and supination. The mechanical symptoms may improve with rest and are worsened with loading. A complete history including any history of trauma or repetitive use injury should be taken and a complete examination of the wrist should be performed. Traumatic injuries may present with a pop and immediate pain and swelling, and chronic injuries may be indolent in nature. On inspection of the injured wrist, prominence of the distal ulna may indicate distal radial ulnar joint (DRUJ) instability or a significant TFCC injury. On physical examination, the TFCC may be palpated midway between the extensor carpi ulnaris (ECU) and flexor carpi ulnaris (FCU) tendons, in the soft recess just distal to the ulnar styloid. The piano key test is performed by balloting the distal ulna in an anteroposterior direction indicating a DRUJ or TFCC injury.

Findings are always compared to the contralateral wrist and should be compared on multiple positions of forearm rotation. Comparison between wrists is important because (in young women in particular) physiologic laxity may exist. Additional ulnar side structures to be examined include the lunotriquetral interval, which is located between the fourth and fifth extensor compartments, one fingerbreadth distal to the DRUJ, with the wrist in 30 degrees of flexion. The ECU tendon must also be examined for subluxation or tendonitis along the distal ulna and its insertion into the base of the fifth metacarpal. Tenderness may be elicited with the TFCC grind or compression test, which can be performed by ulnar deviation of the wrist while applying an axial load and rotating the forearm. The differential diagnosis of ulnar side wrist pain includes ECU subluxation, lunotriquetral ligament injury, pisotriquetral arthritis, hook of the hamate fracture, ulnar artery thrombosis, ulnar neuropathy, and ulnar impaction. Radiographic imaging for TFCC injuries should begin with posteroanterior and lateral views of the wrist, but plain films are usually normal. Arthrography was the previous gold standard but has been replaced in many centers by magnetic resonance imaging or magnetic resonance arthrography. On a T2-weighted magnetic resonance image, the synovial fluid will have a bright signal that outlines a TFCC tear, while a normal TFCC should be homogeneously dark throughout.

The Palmer classification[1] of TFCC injuries divides injuries into types I (traumatic) and II (degenerative; Fig. 40-1). Type I injuries are subclassified into type A, B, C, and D depending on the location of the lesion. A type IA lesion is a tear in the horizontal portion of the TFCC near the attachment to the radius. A type IB lesion is a traumatic avulsion of the TFCC off its attachment to the distal ulna and may be associated with a fracture of the ulnar styloid. This lesion may be associated with DRUJ instability since the TFCC is the major stabilizer of the DRUJ. It may also be associated with ECU subluxation. A type IC lesion involves a peripheral avulsion from the insertions of the ulnolunate and ulnotriquetral ligaments. A type ID injury is a traumatic avulsion of the TFCC from its radial attachment at the distal aspect of the sigmoid notch.

Degenerative lesions of the TFCC are a result of chronic loading to the TFCC (i.e., ulnar impaction syndrome) and are

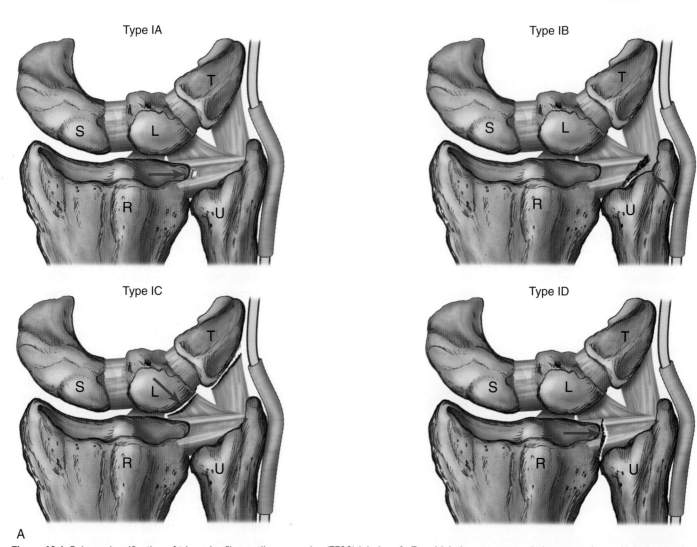

Type IA   Type IB

Type IC   Type ID

A

Figure 40-1 Palmer classification of triangular fibrocartilage complex (TFCC) injuries. **A,** Type I injuries are traumatic in nature. A type IA lesion involves a perforation near the radius. A type IB lesion is an avulsion of the TFCC from the ulnar attachment. A type IC lesion is an avulsion of the ulnar ligaments. A type ID lesion is an avulsion from the distal radius.

subclassified A, B, C, D, and E. Ulnar impaction syndrome is a degenerative condition usually associated with a length imbalance between the distal radius and ulna (i.e., the ulna is longer than the radius). This syndrome can present in a wide age range depending on the predisposing condition. Conditions that predispose to this syndrome include Madelung's deformity, premature closure of the radial physis secondary to trauma, naturally positive ulnar variance, malunions of distal radius fractures leading to shortening of the distal radius, or excision of the radial head with distal forearm instability (i.e., Essex-Lopresti injury). On physical examination, symptoms can be reproduced with an axial load applied to an ulnar deviated wrist and extremes of pronation and supination. A posteroanterior radiograph of the affected wrist will typically reveal a positive ulnar variance or ulnar styloid index. The ulnar styloid index is equal to the ulnar styloid length minus the ulnar variance divided by the ulnar head width. An index greater than 0.22 is considered elevated. Radiographs may also reveal sclerotic or cystic changes between the lunate and ulnar styloid. Magnetic resonance imaging of the wrist may reveal edema on the ulnar side of the lunate. This can be confused with Kienböck's disease, but findings on the ulnar aspect of the lunate are not characteristic of Kienböck's disease.

Arthroscopy may reveal a TFCC tear or a lunotriquetral ligament tear. TFCC tears secondary to degenerative change are classified according to the presence or absence of a TFCC tear and/or chondromalacia. Type IIA lesions involve wear of the horizontal portion of the TFCC without perforation. Type IIB involves wear of the TFCC plus lunate or ulna chondromalacia. Type IIC involves perforation of the TFCC and chondromalacia. Type IID lesions are TFCC perforation, chondromalacia, and lunotriquetral ligament perforation. Type IIE lesions are the final stage of ulnar impaction syndrome including TFCC perforation, chondromalacia, lunotriquetral ligament perforation, and ulnocarpal arthritis.

Relevant Anatomy
The TFCC has three major functions: First, it is considered the primary stabilizer of the DRUJ; second, it transmits approximately 20% of the load across the wrist; and third, it supports the ulnar carpus. Palmer and Werner[2] described the TFCC as the triangular fibrocartilage proper, the palmar and dorsal radioulnar ligaments, the ulna collateral ligament, the subsheath of the ECU tendon and the ulnolunate and ulnotriquetral ligaments (Fig. 40-2). Volar and dorsal branches of the anterior

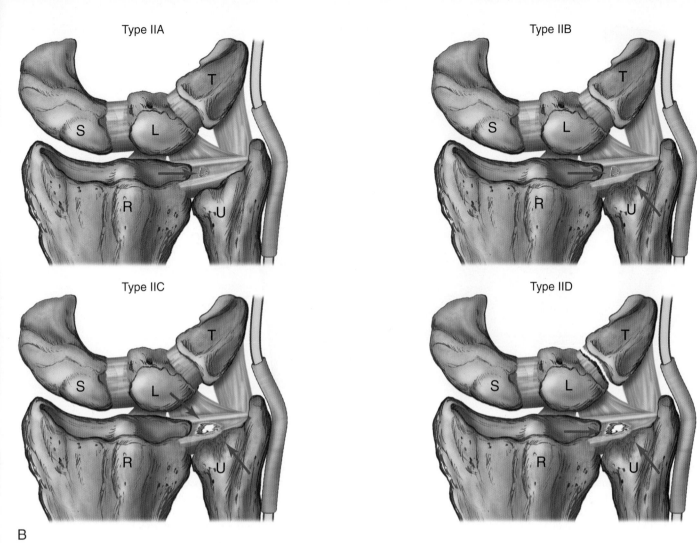

Type IIA

Type IIB

Type IIC

Type IID

B

Figure 40-1—cont'd B, A type II lesion is a degenerative lesion. A type IIA lesion is TFCC wear without perforation. A type IIB lesion involves TFCC wear and lunate or ulnar chondromalacia. A type IIC lesion involves TFCC perforation. A type IID lesion involves TFCC perforation, chondromalacia, and lunotriquetral ligament perforation. L, lunate; R, radius; S, schaphoid; T, triquetrum; U, ulna. (From Palmer AK, Werner FW: The triangular fibrocartilage complex of the wrist—Anatomy and function. J Hand Surg [Am] 1981;6:153–162.)

interosseous artery supply the TFCC. The central portion of the TFCC is relatively avascular, while the peripheral portion is well vascularized. This pattern is analogous to the knee menisci and explains why central tears are débrided and peripheral tears may by repaired.

The relationship between the distal radius and distal ulna is important in the transmission of forces across the wrist. When the variance is neutral, 80% of a load will be transmitted through the radius and 20% through the ulna. A positive ulnar variance leads to increased load sharing by the ulna and the opposite is also true; decreased ulnar variance leads to decreased load sharing across the ulna. Ulnar variance is measured on a posteroanterior neutral rotation radiograph of the wrist and is equal to the difference between a line drawn across the lunate fossa of the distal radius and another line drawn across the top of the ulnar head.

Treatment Options

Initial treatment of acute TFCC injuries is immobilization for 6 to 8 weeks. Significant instability of the DRUJ and ECU sub-luxation should be ruled out. Peripheral tears are expected to heal because of their vascularity, and central tears may become asymptomatic despite not healing. Indications for wrist arthroscopy include a proven or suspected TFCC injury with ulnar wrist symptoms that interfere with activities. Patients should have failed 3 to 4 months of conservative management including rest, immobilization, and anti-inflammatory medications.

Surgery

Wrist arthroscopy has gained a prominent role in the diagnosis and treatment of wrist disorders. It may used in the débridement and repair of TFCC tears, débridement of intercarpal ligament tears, visualization of scaphoid and distal radius fractures, removal of loose bodies, débridement of articular injuries, excision of ganglion cysts, radial and ulnar styloidectomy, synovectomy, and débridement of septic joints. The Palmer classification of TFCC injuries serves as a guide to surgical treatment. Type IA lesions, isolated central tears of the TFCC, can be treated with limited arthroscopic débridement of the tear. It has been

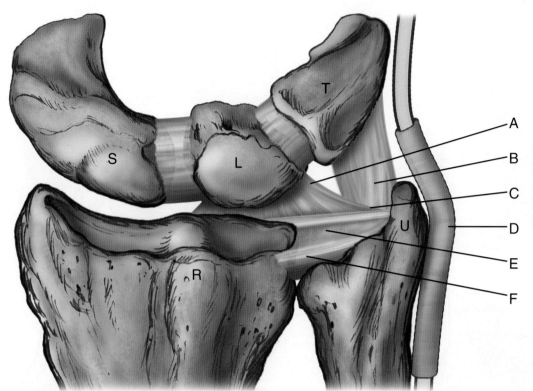

Figure 40-2 Anatomy of the triangular fibrocartilage complex (TFCC). Ulnolunate ligament (A); ulnotriquetral ligament (B); palmar radioulnar ligament (C); ECU sheath (D); triangular fibrocartilage proper (E); dorsal radioulnar ligament (F). L, lunate, R, radius; S, scaphoid; T, triquetrum; U, ulna.

reported that 80% to 85% of patients have had a good result with limited débridement. Type IB lesions, a peripheral detachment from the ulnar styloid, are often diagnosed by a diagnostic arthroscopy. The pathognomic sign is the "trampoline" sign, which is the loss of the normal tautness of the TFCC when probed. Type IB lesions can be associated with ECU subluxation, which, if present, requires an open repair of the ECU subsheath in addition to an arthroscopic or open repair of the TFCC. In the acute setting of DRUJ instability associated with an ulnar styloid fracture, an open repair of the fracture may be required. This scenario is often associated with displaced distal radius fractures. After repair, 85% to 90% of patients have good to excellent results.[3] A type IC lesion, a distal avulsion of the ulnolunate and ulnotriquetral ligaments, theoretically can be repaired because it is peripheral and well vascularized. A type ID lesion, avulsion of the TFCC from the sigmoid notch, is most commonly associated with a distal radius fracture and may be repaired by open or arthroscopic techniques. The preferred treatment for type ID lesions remains controversial.

Degenerative tears of the TFCC are related to chronic overloading of the ulnar side of the wrist. These lesions are the result of ulnar impaction. Diagnostic arthroscopy is the best method to stage the ulnar impaction lesion. The primary goal in treating ulnar impaction is unloading the ulnar head. This is usually done by an ulnar shortening procedure such as a shortening osteotomy, partial ulnar head resection, or ulnar salvage procedures. Arthroscopy will reveal TFCC wear and chondromalacia associated with type IIA and IIB lesions. They can be treated with TFCC débridement arthroscopically, followed by an open or arthroscopic Feldon ulnar shortening procedure (distal ulnar head resection)[4] or an ulnar shortening procedure proximal to the wrist. Type IIC lesions, including TFCC perforation and chondromalacia, are treated with arthroscopic débridement of the TFCC and/or an ulnar shortening procedure. Type IID and

IIE lesions are the end stage of ulnar impaction syndrome. Arthroscopic débridement of the TFCC and ulnar shortening may be performed. The assessment of the integrity of the lunotriquetral ligament is the primary indication for arthroscopy. If the lunotriquetral ligament is unstable after ulnar shortening osteotomy, the lunotriquetral joint can be pinned or a lunotriquetral fusion can be performed. Lesions with ulnocarpal arthritis are treated with a Bower's distal ulna resection[5] or Suave-Kapandji procedure,[6] if the surgeon thinks that a distal ulnar resection will be sufficient.

Surgical Technique: Wrist Arthroscopy

Regional anesthesia is generally used and a tourniquet is placed. After the patient has been placed under anesthesia, an examination of the wrist should be performed. The patient is placed supine and the wrist is then placed under 10 to 15 pounds of distraction force. Distraction towers are available commercially for this purpose. Arthroscopes are between 2 and 3 mm and a 30-degree arthroscope is the most commonly used. Arthroscopic portals are named in relation to the extensor tendon compartments. There are five radiocarpal portals, two midcarpal portals, one STT (scapho-trapezio-trapezoid) portal, and two DRUJ portals. Portals are named for their relationship to the extensor compartments. The 3-4 portals are the primarily visualization portals, the 4-5 portals are work portals, and the 6-R and 6-U portals are used as outflow portals or working portals for the ulnar wrist. The portals can be used interchangeably. Portals used depend on the pathology present. Following the 12-degree volar tilt of the radius, an 18-gauge needle is introduced into the third to fourth interval, distal to Lister's tubercle, and the joint is injected with 5 to 7 mL of normal saline. A skin incision is made and a blunt trocar is introduced into the joint (Fig. 40-3). From the 3-4 portal, 70% of the joint can be examined including the radial styloid, scaphoid, scapholunate ligament, radial

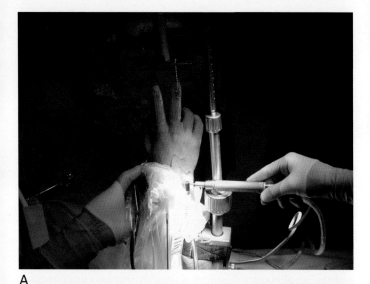

A

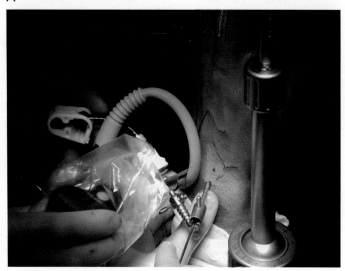

B

Figure 40-3 A, Arthroscopic setup. **B,** Portals. Cannula is placed in 3-4 portal. Midcarpal portal is marked 1 cm distal to 3-4 portal.

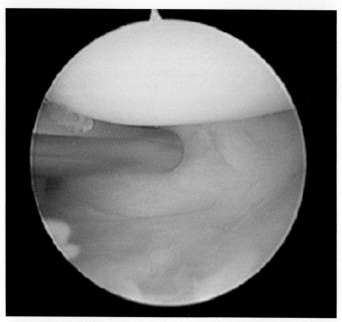

Figure 40-4 Trampoline sign. A probe is inserted to test the tautness of the triangular fibrocartilage complex (TFCC). The TFCC is relatively firm when probed. If it is not firm, the TFCC should be closely examined for a perforation.

attachment of the TFCC, extrinsic ligaments, and tautness of the TFCC. An ulnar portal such as the 6-R or 4-5 is made when needed to improve visualization. A shaver can be introduced to remove synovitis that is present. A probe is inserted to test for a flap tear, the tautness of the TFCC (trampoline sign), and the integrity of the intercarpal ligaments (Fig. 40-4). From the ulnar portal, the lunate, triquetrum, lunotriquetral ligament, TFCC, ulnolunate ligament, and ulnotriquetral ligament can be examined if the arthroscopic portal is switched. For resection of an unstable flap, a punch is used and the edges can be débrided with a shaver. Alternatively, a bipolar or monopolar electrocautery can débride the tissue. Only unstable portions are débrided. If chondromalacia is present indicating a type II lesion, a distal ulna resection can be performed arthroscopically using a bur. Once the radiocarpal joint has been examined from the radiocarpal and ulnar portals, the midcarpal joint must be examined. The radial midcarpal portal is 1 cm distal to portal 3/4. From this portal, the scapholunate and lunotriquetral articulations, distal scaphoid, proximal capitate, and proximal hamate

can be examined. After wrist arthroscopy has been completed, the wrist should be re-examined and clicks present secondary to TFCC injury should not be present. The portals are closed with a nylon suture. The wrist is placed in a splint for 1 week to support the extensor tendons and then intermittently for 3 weeks with restrictions on grasping and repetitive activities.

Postoperative Rehabilitation

For TFCC lesions in which only a débridement is performed, the wrist is placed in a splint for 1 week and then used intermittently as needed for the next 3 weeks. At 1 week, range-of-motion exercises are started with restrictions on lifting and repetitive motions. Repaired TFCC lesions should be immobilized in either a splint or cast for 4 to 6 weeks and then range-of-motion exercises are begun with restrictions on lifting and repetitive motion.

Return to Sports

Patients may return to athletics once they have demonstrated progress in strength and range of motion of the affected extremity. For débridement, this is typically at 4 to 6 weeks. Three months is typically the minimum after a repair. One to 3 months of a supervised physical therapy program is normally required. A protective splint should be worn while participating in athletic activities. The protective splint may be discontinued once full strength and range of motion have been obtained.

Complications

Complications of wrist arthroscopy involve injury to superficial nerves during portal placement. The dorsal cutaneous branch of the ulnar nerve can be injured during the placement of the 6-U portal. The superficial radial and lateral antebrachial cutaneous nerves may be injured during placement of the 1-2 portal.

SCAPHOLUNATE INSTABILITY

Clinical Features and Evaluation

Scapholunate instability is the most common carpal instability pattern, either alone or in conjunction with another instability pattern or distal radius fracture. The most common mechanism of injury is a fall on an outstretched wrist with hyperextension, ulnar deviation, and supination of the wrist. Patients will often have pain and swelling with acute injuries. Those presenting with chronic injuries may report pain and popping with loading of the wrist. Patients may also complain of weak grip, limited motion, and point tenderness over the dorsal aspect of the scapholunate interval. Diagnosis is often delayed because the injury is thought only to be a sprained wrist. On physical examination, patients will have tenderness located over the anatomic snuffbox and dorsally over the scapholunate interval. The Watson scaphoid shift test is the provocative maneuver for scapholunate ligament injury (Fig. 40-5). The examiner places his or her thumb over the distal pole of the scaphoid and the other hand moves the wrist in an ulnar to radial direction, which elicits pain or a palpable clunk. Imaging consists of posteroanterior and lateral radiographs of the injured wrist. Injuries may be static or dynamic. Static injuries will be seen on radiographs. On the posteroanterior wrist, the scapholunate interval may be greater than 3 mm (positive Terry Thomas sign), the scaphoid will appear shortened (positive cortical ring sign), and the lunate will be extended (Fig. 40-6). On the lateral film, the normal scapholunate angle is 30 to 60 degrees. A scapholunate angle greater than 70 degrees suggests scapholunate instability[7] (Fig. 40-7). In cases of dynamic instability a load must be applied to generate abnormal findings. A clenched-fist anteroposterior radiograph of the wrist can be obtained to accentuate the scapholunate diastasis. Magnetic resonance imaging is a noninvasive modality that can be used to evaluate wrist ligaments, although it is thought to be technique and interpreter dependent. Arthroscopy can also be used to diagnose scapholunate injury. Geissler et al,[8] devised a classification system to standardize arthroscopic observation of injury to the intercarpal ligaments. Grade I lesions involve attenuation or hemorrhage of the involved ligament. Grade II lesions involve attenuation or hemorrhage of the interosseous ligament with intercarpal step-off and a slight gap is present between carpal bones. Grade III lesions involve a step-off in carpal alignment and a probe may be passed between carpal bones. Grade IV lesions involve a step-off in carpal alignment and there is gross instability in which the arthroscope may be passed between carpal bones. During a diagnostic arthroscopy, a positive "drive through" sign is a grade IV lesion in which the arthroscope can be passed through the scapholunate interval into the midcarpal joint.

Relevant Anatomy

The interosseous scapholunate ligament, the dorsal scapholunate ligament, and the palmar radioscaphoid ligament are involved in scapholunate instability. Isolated transection of the interosseous scapholunate ligament has been shown not to reproduce instability in cadavers. Scapholunate disassociation results from injury to the scapholunate interosseous ligament and the palmar radioscaphoid ligament.[9]

Treatment Options

Treatment of scapholunate instability depends on when the injury is diagnosed. Partial tears of the interosseous scapholunate ligament can be treated with cast immobilization for 6 to 10 weeks to allow healing. Patients with partial tears that remain symptomatic after immobilization may undergo arthroscopic débridement of the tear with some relief of symptoms. Complete tears of the scapholunate ligament should be treated surgically.

Acute Scapholunate Injuries

Injuries of the scapholunate ligament usually involve an avulsion of the ligament off the scaphoid. Closed reduction and cast immobilization are no longer used in the treatment of complete scapholunate ligament tears because there are no data supporting the success of this method. Even when an anatomic reduction could be achieved, it was rarely maintained. Closed reduction and percutaneous pinning of the scapholunate ligament have also been abandoned because of inability to maintain reduction. The preferred treatment of acute scapholunate ligament injuries is open reduction and direct repair of the scapholunate ligament. Through a dorsal approach, the joint is reduced and the scapholunate ligament is directly repaired using sutures through bone tunnels or suture anchors. Some authors also advocate reinforcement of the repair with dorsal capsulodesis (Blatt procedure). After open reduction and internal fixation of the scapholunate ligament, the wrist is kept in a thumb spica cast for 2 to 3 months, followed by 1 month in a short arm cast, followed by a protective splint and physical therapy.

Return to Sports

Patients may return to athletics once they have demonstrated progress in strength and range of motion of the affected extremity. One to 3 months of a supervised physical therapy program is normally required after cast removal. A protective splint should be worn while participating in athletic activities. The protective splint may be discontinued once full strength and range of motion have been obtained.

Treatment of Chronic Injuries without Degenerative Changes

Chronic instability is defined as a scapholunate ligament injury that has been present for more than 3 months. These injuries are more difficult to deal with. Over time, the scapholunate ligament becomes scarred and the edges contract so a direct repair is no longer feasible. Subacute injuries that do not have cartilage wear secondary to the injury have a joint that remains reducible, but as time progresses and fibrosis develops, the joint becomes irreducible and this influences the chosen treatment. When the scapholunate joint remains reducible, a soft-tissue reconstruction (Blatt procedure) may be performed to prevent rotatory subluxation of the scaphoid. The Blatt procedure[10] involves a proximally based flap of dorsal capsule off the ulnar side of the distal radius, approximately 1 cm wide, which serves as a check-rein to volar rotation of the scaphoid. The scaphoid then is reduced and held in place by a Kirschner wire. The flap is inserted into the distal pole of the scaphoid. The flap of tissue is then secured by a pullout wire over a button on the volar surface of the wrist or with a suture anchor. The wrist is kept in a thumb spica for 2 months, followed by active range-of-motion exercises. The Kirschner wire is removed at 3 months and intercarpal motion is allowed. Other options for treatment of reducible injuries include free tendon grafts, bone-ligament-bone grafts, or other types of capsulodesis using dorsal wrist capsule.

Normal intercarpal mechanics cannot be restored when the scapholunate joint cannot be reduced; therefore, treatment of

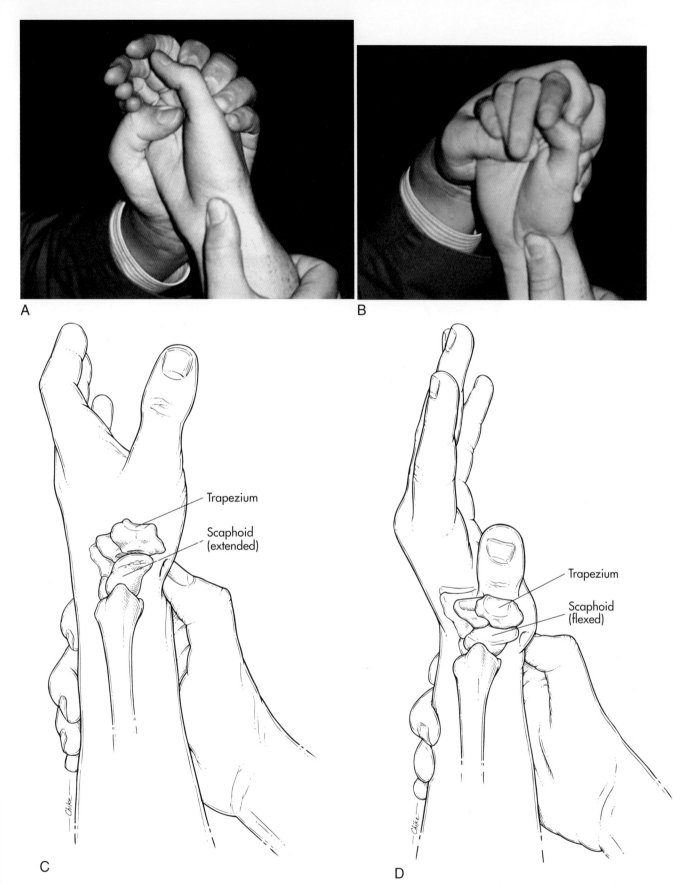

Figure 40-5 Watson's scaphoid shift test. **A** and **B,** Clinical photographs of Watson's scaphoid shift test. **C** and **D,** Diagram of Watson's scaphoid shift test. (From Cooney WP, Linscheid RL, Dobyns JH: The Wrist. St. Louis, Mosby, 1997, p 258.)

Figure continues

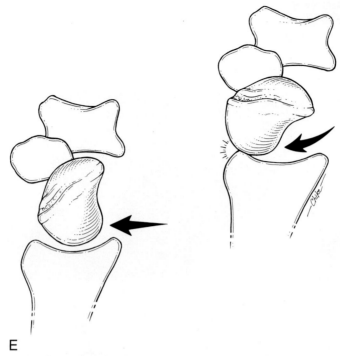

Figure 40-5—cont'd E, Diagram of a positive test.

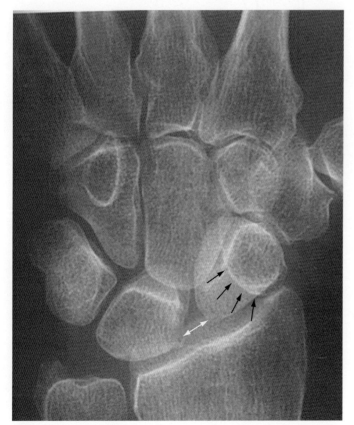

Figure 40-6 Radiographic findings of scapholunate injury on a posteroanterior radiograph. Scapholunate interval of 3 mm or greater *(white arrow)*. Flexed scaphoid appears as a cortical ring *(black arrows)*.

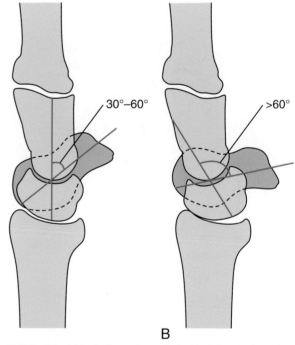

A   B

Figure 40-7 Radiographic findings of scapholunate injury on lateral radiograph. **A,** Normal scapholunate angle is 30 to 60 degrees. This angle can be measured by a line bisecting the lunate and a line following the longitudinal axis of the scaphoid. **B,** A scapholunate angle greater than 60 degrees suggests injury to the scapholunate ligament.

the injury focuses on salvage procedures. The STT arthrodesis, also known as the triscaphoid arthrodesis, has commonly been used in the treatment of irreducible chronic scapholunate instability. The goal is to realign the radioscaphoid joint to minimize future degenerative change. Unfortunately, cases of joint deterioration after a lengthy reduced level of symptoms do occur and the incidence is unclear. Both range of motion and grip strength are lost after fusion. A meta-analysis of STT arthrodesis reported in the literature revealed nonunion rates of approximately 13%.[11] Although scapholunate arthrodesis seems like the

most logical treatment for this injury, nonunion rates are as high as 50%.[11]

Treatment of Chronic Instability with Arthritic Change

Patients with long-standing scapholunate instability who have developed arthritis will not have relief of symptoms with the previously mentioned procedures. The most common type of wrist arthritis is the SLAC (scapholunate advanced collapse) pattern described by Watson and Ballet[12] (Fig. 40-8). Stage I

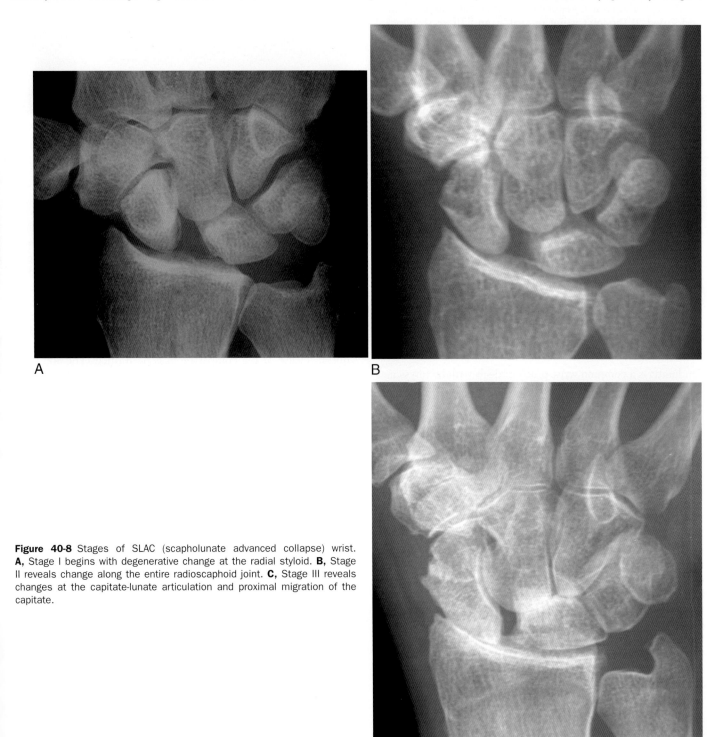

Figure 40-8 Stages of SLAC (scapholunate advanced collapse) wrist. **A,** Stage I begins with degenerative change at the radial styloid. **B,** Stage II reveals change along the entire radioscaphoid joint. **C,** Stage III reveals changes at the capitate-lunate articulation and proximal migration of the capitate.

begins with degenerative change between the radial styloid and distal pole of the scaphoid. Stage II reveals change along the entire radioscaphoid joint. Stage III reveals arthritic change of the capitate-lunate joint and proximal migration of the capitate. As the capitate continues to migrate proximally, pancarpal arthrosis develops. Patients will often present with decreased grip strength and stiffness with extension and radial deviation. In stage I disease, radial styloidectomy will decrease symptoms associated with impingement of the scaphoid on the radial styloid, but the underlying instability will lead to further deterioration. If the joint is reducible, a dorsal capsulodesis can be performed. If the joint is not reducible, an STT or scaphocapitate (SC) fusion can be performed in addition to the radial styloidectomy. In stage II disease, the arthritic radioscaphoid joint must be eliminated. This can be accomplished with either a proximal row carpectomy or a scaphoid excision and four-corner fusion (lunate-capitate-hamate-triquetrum), which is also known as the SLAC procedure. A proximal row carpectomy is considered by many to be contraindicated if arthritic change is present on the proximal capitate. Both the SLAC procedure and proximal row carpectomy will lead to decreased grip strength and range of motion compared to the normal wrist. After proximal row carpectomy, patients retain approximately 52% of motion and 67% of grip strength compared to the normal wrist.[13] Although stage II disease may be treated with a variety of procedures, proximal row carpectomy was found to retain the most motion.[14] Patients with stage III disease may be treated with either the SLAC procedure or total wrist arthrodesis. A proximal row carpectomy is contraindicated if arthritic change is present on the proximal capitate. The ideal position for wrist arthrodesis is 10 degrees of extension and neutral or slight ulnar deviation.

TENDONITIS

Tendonitis is a common wrist problem dealt with by physicians. Patients may present with pain and swelling of the involved tendons. History often reveals overuse as the inciting event, and patients report that the pain worsens with use of the inflamed tendon. Physical examination often reveals swelling and tenderness of the involved tendon. Radiographs are most often negative.

de Quervain's Disease

de Quervain's disease involves a stenosing tenosynovitis of the first dorsal wrist compartment, which contains the abductor pollicis longus and the extensor pollicis brevis. Patients often present with radial side wrist pain that is worsened with movement of the thumb. It is more common in the fourth and fifth decades and in females. Patients often report a history of repetitive activities involving thumb abduction and ulnar deviation of the wrist. On physical examination, Finkelstein's test will be positive (Fig. 40-9). This test is performed by fully adducting the thumb and then the wrist, which will reproduce the patient's pain. The differential diagnosis includes intersection syndrome and carpometacarpal arthritis. Patients with intersec-

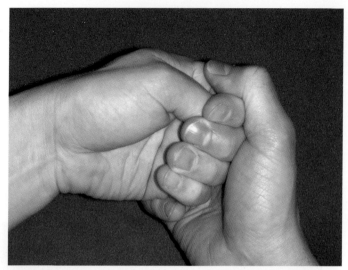

Figure 40-9 Finkelstein's test. The thumb is fully adducted and the wrist is ulnar deviated, which will reproduce the patient's symptoms.

tion syndrome report pain 4 cm proximal to the wrist joint. Patients with carpometacarpal arthritis may have evidence of arthritis on radiographs. Patients are treated conservatively with a combination of splinting, anti-inflammatory medications, and avoidance of the inciting activity. Corticosteroid injections can be used with 50% to 80% success. It has been shown that patients receiving an injection did not receive any additional benefit from splinting after the injection.[15] The first dorsal compartment can be injected with 0.5 mL 1% lidocaine and 1 mL dexamethasone. When conservative measures fail, surgical release of the first dorsal compartment may be performed. A dorsal release of the compartment is performed. The abductor pollicis longus can often have multiple slips, and the extensor pollicis brevis may sometimes have its own subsheath so care must be taken to release all slips and subsheaths. Some authors report that surgical cases have an increased incidence of these minor anatomic differences. Care must be taken not to injure the radial sensory nerve. The patients are placed in a soft dressing for 10 to 14 days and then strengthening and range-of-motion exercises are begun.

Intersection Syndrome

Intersection syndrome is a stenosing tenosynovitis of the second extensor compartment. Patients often report radial side wrist pain 4 cm proximal to the wrist joint. This syndrome is often found in lifting and rowing athletes. On physical examination, an audible squeak may be heard and there may be palpable crepitus. Conservative management includes modifying activities, splinting in extension, anti-inflammatory medication, and corticosteroid injection of the second dorsal compartment. In cases that fail conservative management, surgical release of the second dorsal compartment can be performed, but this is rarely necessary.

REFERENCES

1. Palmer AK: Triangular fibrocartilage complex lesions: A classification. J Hand Surg [Am] 1989;14:594–606.

2. Palmer AK, Werner FW: The triangular fibrocartilage complex of the wrist—Anatomy and function. J Hand Surg [Am] 1981;6:153–162.

3. Zachee B, De Smet L, Fabry G: Arthroscopic suturing of TFCC lesions. Arthroscopy 1993;9:242–243.

4. Feldon P, Terrono AL, Belsky MR: Wafer distal ulnar resection for triangular fibrocartilage tears and/or ulna impaction syndrome. J Hand Surg [Am] 1992;17:731–737.

5. Bowers WH: Distal radioulnar joint hemiarthroplasty, the hemiresection technique. J Hand Surg [Am] 1985;10:169–178.

6. Nakamura R, Tsunoda K, Wantanabe K, et al: The Suave-Kapandji procedure for chronic dislocation of the distal radial ulnar joint with destruction of the articular surface. J Hand Surg [Br] 1992;17:127–132.

7. Dobyns JH, Linscheid RL, Chao EYS, et al: Traumatic instability of the wrist. Intr Course Lect 1975;24:182–199.

8. Geissler WB, Freeland AE, Savoie FH, et al: Intercarpal soft tissue lesions associated with an intraarticular fracture of the distal end of the radius. J Bone Joint Surg [Am] 1996;78:357–365.

9. Mayfield JK: Mechanism of carpal injuries. Clin Orthop 1980;149:45–59.

10. Blatt G: Capsulodesis in reconstructive hand surgery: Dorsal capsulodesis for unstable scaphoid and volar capsulodesis following excision of the distal ulna. Hand Clinics 1987;3:81–101.

11. Seigal JM, Ruby LK: A critical look at intercarpal arthrodesis: Review of literature. J Hand Surg [Am] 1996;21:717–723.

12. Watson HK, Ballet FL: The SLAC wrist: Scapholunate advanced collapse pattern of degenerative arthritis. J Hand Surg [Am] 1984;9:358–365.

13. Culp RW, McGulgan FX, Turner MA, et al: Proximal row carpectomy: A multicenter study. J Hand Surg [Am] 1993;1A:19–25.

14. Krakauer JD, Bishop AT, Cooney WP: Surgical treatment of scapholunate advances collapse. J Hand Surg [Am] 1994;19:751–759.

15. Weiss AP, Akelman E: Treatment of de Quervain's disease. J Hand Surg [Am] 1994;19:595–598.

Hand Injuries

Arthur C. Rettig, Dale S. Snead, and Lance A. Rettig

In This Chapter

INTRODUCTION

- The energy transmitted to the hand that causes injuries in athletics is often relatively low; thus, the fracture patterns are generally simple and minimal soft-tissue injury is involved.

- The goal of treating hand fractures is to allow the athlete to participate in a safe fashion but to prevent the development of malunion, nonunion, joint stiffness, and tendon adhesions.

- Treatment is determined by the sport, position played, and timing of the injury in relationship to the season.

- The high demand on the upper extremity in sports makes the hand very susceptible to a variety of injuries.[1]

- Fractures of the metacarpals and phalanges frequently result in the loss of playing time and altered performance. Sports-related activities are the most common cause of phalangeal fractures in 10- to 49-year-olds.

- There are a variety of ways to treat fractures of the metacarpals and phalanges. In many cases, treatment can allow the athlete to return to competition safely and quickly.

EPIDEMIOLOGY

Injuries to the fingers or hand can occur from a direct blow, a crush injury, or a laceration. A direct blow causes most phalangeal and metacarpal fractures. This typically results in a transverse fracture. Spiral fractures occur secondary to a torsional type injury. Intra-articular fractures occur secondary to an axial load. These are the most common fracture patterns seen in the hand.

Basketball players injure the PIP joint more frequently. Baseball players are more likely to sustain an injury of the distal phalangeal joint and distal phalanx. Football players usually sustain a crush injury resulting in a metacarpal or proximal phalanx fracture.

A study performed at the Cleveland Clinic evaluated 113 hand and wrist injuries; 96 of these injuries were fractures and 97 of the injuries occurred in football, with metacarpal fractures being most common at 40% (38 fractures). DeHaven and Lintner[2] described hand injuries based on 3431 cases treated at the University of Rochester. Hand injuries represented 5% (171 cases) of those treated, again the most common injury to the hand involved fracture. There were 102 fractures in this study representing 60% of the hand injuries, with the majority occurring in football. Of the 102 fractures, 72 were of the phalanx and 27 involved the metacarpals. A study by Dawson and Pullos[3] looked at baseball and softball injuries in a suburban 150-bed hospital over a 3.5-month period. There were 153 injuries and fractures represented 6% of the injuries. Interestingly, a greater percentage of injuries occurred when a larger softball was used. The number of people seen for hand injuries represented 2.2% of the emergency department visits. Stein and Ellasser[4] reported on significant hand injuries that occurred in a professional football team over a 15-year period. There were 46 major injuries, almost equally split among offense and defense. Fingers were the most commonly injured area of the body. Rettig[5] performed a study over a 1-year period noting 213 injuries in 207 athletes. These 207 patients represented approximately 3% of the new patient visits seen at the center during this time period. Of these injuries, 125 were fractures. The greatest number of hand injuries occurred during football, and the majority of injuries occurred during competition.

CLINICAL FEATURES AND EVALUATION

Metacarpal and phalangeal fractures often present with swelling, ecchymosis, and gross deformity. Passive flexion can falsely create a normal-appearing alignment of the digits. Having the patient actively flex each digit allows a more accurate check of rotation. This is a crucial part of the evaluation despite the discomfort that it may cause the athlete. A missed rotational deformity can be devastating.[6] It is useful to compare the injured extremity with the unaffected side when evaluating for a rotational deformity. At full flexion, all digits should point toward the tubercle of the scaphoid.

Radiography

Many fractures of the hand are overlooked or misinterpreted because of failure to obtain appropriate radiographs. Short spiral fractures may appear relatively nondisplaced on an anteroposterior view, yet are significantly displaced on an oblique view. Fractures of the hand must be evaluated with appropriate

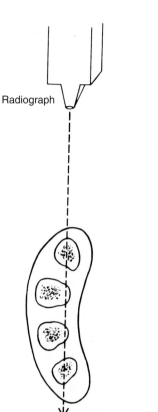
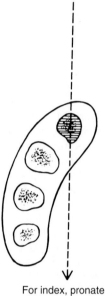
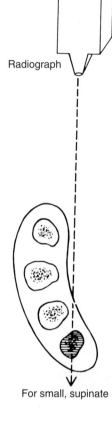

Radiograph   Radiograph   Radiograph

Lateral radiograph   For index, pronate   For small, supinate

Figure 41-1 Axial relationships of metacarpals illustrating that a lateral radiograph of the hand requires slight pronation and slight supination for independent visualization of index and small metacarpals. (From Hastings, Rettig, Strickland: Management of Extra-articular Fractures of the Phalanges and Metacarpals. Philadelphia, Elsevier, 1992.)

radiographs and include at a minimum posteroanterior, lateral, and oblique views. It is important to know that a true lateral radiograph is a lateral view of the third metacarpal only and an oblique view of the other digits. The hand must be rolled into 30 degrees of supination to obtain a lateral view of the index metacarpal and 20 to 30 degrees of pronation to obtain a lateral view of the ring and small fingers (Fig. 41-1). A Brewerton view is helpful for evaluation of fractures at the base of the proximal phalanx.[7]

METACARPAL FRACTURES

Metacarpal Neck Fractures

Metacarpal neck fractures account for as many as 36% of all fractures of the hand.[8] Metacarpals are weakest at the metacarpal neck and are often fractured by a direct blow, torsion, or bending load applied to the digit distally. Most metacarpal neck fractures affect the ring and little fingers. The most famous of these is the Boxer's fracture (although rarely seen in boxers), a fracture of the fifth metacarpal neck. Fractures at this level occur secondary to the instability of the ulnar digits and because the metacarpal head is already in 15 degrees of flexion.

Treatment of these injuries is usually splinting and early range of motion (ROM). If angulation is greater than 50 degrees, closed reduction and casting or operative fixation may be necessary.[9,10] A prospective study by Lowdon[11] found no relationship between residual angulation and the presence of symptoms.

Metacarpal Shaft Fractures

Metacarpal fractures are the most commonly seen hand fractures.[12] Due to the low forces involved in athletic activities, com-

pared to motor vehicle accidents, most fractures are stable. Metacarpals are connected to one another via the transverse intermetacarpal ligament (Fig. 41-2). This is important when there is a fracture of a single metacarpal. Fractures of the middle and ring metacarpals are more stable because there are two transverse intermetacarpal ligaments supporting these bones. Rotational and shortening deformities are more likely to be seen in the index and small finger fractures.

The more distal the fracture is, the greater amount of angulation that can be accepted (Fig. 41-3). The ulnar aspect of the hand is more susceptible to fractures due to its greater mobility when compared to the radial aspect of the hand, and for the same reason, more angulation can be tolerated in the ulnar digits. Between 30 and 40 degrees of angulation can be accepted in the ring and small fingers.[13] Carpometacarpal motion at the index and long fingers is minimal; therefore, the amount of angulation that is tolerated by these digits is less. The amount of angulation that can be accepted in the index and long fingers is 15 degrees.[13] Dorsal angulation of these fractures affects the biomechanics of the digit. This angulation weakens the intrinsic muscles, resulting in metacarpal phalangeal joint hyperextension and weakness of the central slip as it extends the PIP joint.

A closed reduction maneuver, as described by Jahss,[14] is performed by first disimpacting the fracture by longitudinal traction. The metacarpophalangeal (MCP) and PIP joints are then fully flexed, and a dorsally directed pressure is applied to the proximal phalanx through the flexed PIP joint. The digit should not be immobilized in the Jahss position, but in the safe position (metacarpal phalangeal joints flexed, fingers extended), using an ulnar or radial gutter splint. This allows the extensor

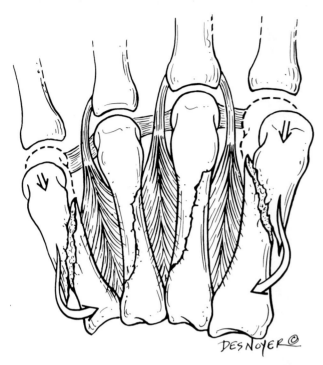

Figure 41-2 A spiral fracture of the metacarpal tends to be more unstable in the border digits, where only one side of the metacarpal is supported by a deep intermetacarpal ligament. (From Hastings, Rettig, Strickland: Management of Extra-articular Fractures of the Phalanges and Metacarpals. Philadelphia, Elsevier, 1992.)

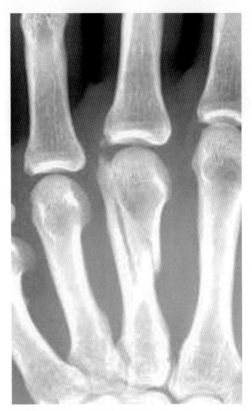

Figure 41-4 Radiograph of a displaced metacarpal fracture.

mechanism to act as a tension band. The splint is continued for 10 to 14 days, and the affected finger is buddy taped to an adjacent finger. It is important to repeat radiographs early in the treatment to prevent any unrecoverable displacement. When treating metacarpal fractures the patient is told to expect that (1) the knuckle contour may be lost permanently, (2) there will be some residual deformity of the digit, (3) if the finger heals in a more flexed position, there is a greater likelihood of refracture with less trauma, and (4) there may be a residual bump on the dorsum of the hand.

Nondisplaced fractures of the index and long fingers and minimally displaced fractures of the ring and small fingers can usually be treated by external immobilization alone. If crepitus is present, a cast is used for the first 2 weeks. Splinting for a total of 4 to 6 weeks is sufficient to heal most fractures.

Surgery

Various methods can be used to treat failed closed reductions or comminuted fractures in which a closed reduction would not be possible (e.g., intra-articular fractures). Open reduction internal fixation is often necessary if there is entrapment of soft tissues, irreducibility of the fracture, or the fracture is a result of high-energy trauma.[15] It is important to rule out any rotational deformity because a slight misalignment at the base is greatly magnified at the tip of the finger. Rotational deformity is an indication for surgery. Dorsal angulation greater than 10 to 15 degrees in the index and long fingers or 30 to 40 degrees in the ring and small fingers or greater than 5 mm of shortening (Fig. 41-4) are other parameters of fractures of metacarpals that call for surgical treatment. Intra-articular extension of a fracture is also generally treated operatively.

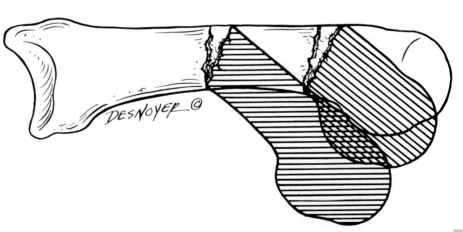

Figure 41-3 Effect of fracture level on metacarpal head displacement. (From Hastings, Rettig, Strickland: Management of Extra-articular Fractures of the Phalanges and Metacarpals. Philadelphia, Elsevier, 1992.)

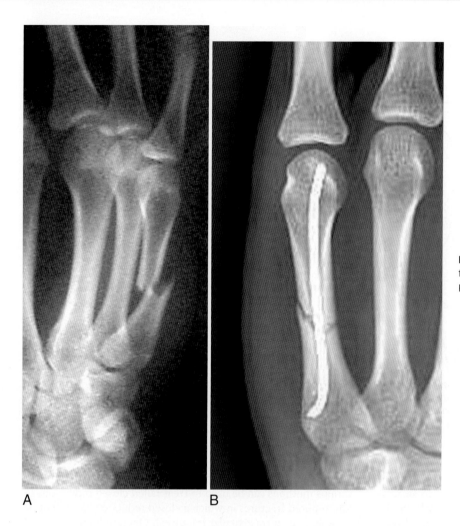

A   B

Figure 41-5 A, Radiograph of a midshaft metacarpal fracture. **B,** Radiograph after closed reduction percutaneous pinning of metacarpal fracture.

Many arrangements of Kirschner (K)-wire fixation have been described.[16–18] This can consist of crossed K wires, intramedullary wires, or transverse K wires[16–18] (Fig. 41-5). The downside of using K wires is that it does not allow for immediate ROM. The use of a single dorsal plate provides the greatest stability and will allow early ROM.[19,20] Interfragmentary screws alone may be chosen when the fracture is greater than twice the diameter of the shaft.[21] Incisions should not be made directly over the metacarpal in order to minimize adhesions.

The average return to sports is approximately 14 days in football for metacarpal injuries and is independent of nonoperative or operative fixation. This time frame is very sport specific and position dependent. For example, a football lineman will be able to return more quickly than a receiver. However, the receiver will return sooner than a person involved in a racquet sport.

Fractures of the Metacarpal Base

There are certain fractures of the first and fifth metacarpal that deserve to be mentioned. There are essentially two types of intra-articular fractures involving the thumb: a Bennett fracture and a Rolando fracture.

A Bennett fracture involves a portion of the base of the first metacarpal that is displaced by the pull of the abductor pollicis longus tendon (Fig. 41-6). Rolando fractures are more comminuted and affect both sides of the first metacarpal base.

Treatment of both of these fractures consists of operative fixation, either closed reduction and percutaneous fixation[22,23] or open reduction and screw fixation.[15] With either treatment, return to sports can be as rapid as 1 week, if return to play in a cast is possible. Complete recovery from this type of injury takes 4 to 6 weeks.

A similar fracture is also seen in the fifth metacarpal (Fig. 41-7). This is the so-called baby Bennett fracture, which becomes displaced by the pull of the extensor carpi ulnaris tendon.[24] Treatment and return to play are similar for fractures at the base of the first metacarpal.

PHALANGEAL FRACTURES

Phalangeal fractures are usually stable due to the adhering soft-tissue envelope. The diaphysis is thicker on the radial and ulnar borders than on the anterior/posterior borders. This thickening is continued laterally by osteocutaneous ligaments called Cleland's and Grayson's ligaments. These ligaments anchor the bone at the mid-portion of the diaphysis and stabilize the bony shaft to the envelope. Occasionally these structures can become trapped in the fracture site and prevent reduction of the fracture. The flexor and extensor tendons provide both stability and induce deforming forces. The flexor tendons are stronger and can cause a dorsal angulation of the fracture. Healing in this position can result in the extensor tendons being weakened and functioning with an extensor lag. The extensor tendons can also

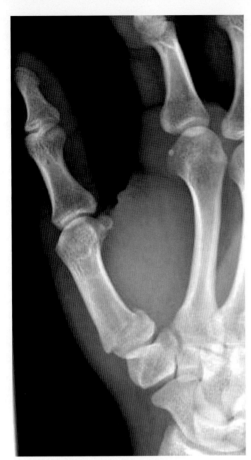

Figure 41-6 Radiograph of a first metacarpal fracture (Bennett fracture).

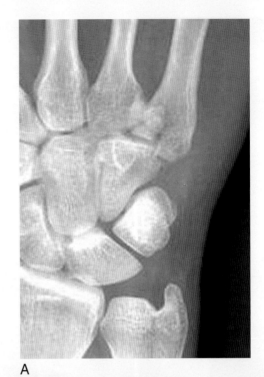

A

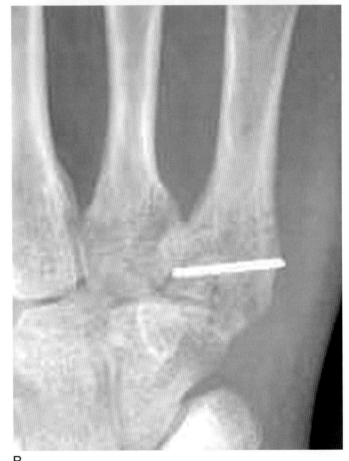

B

Figure 41-7 A, Radiograph of a fifth metacarpal fracture (baby Bennett fracture). **B,** Radiograph after reduction.

cause a volar angulation of the bone, which will limit flexion of the digit.

It is important to remember that fractures of the proximal phalanx displace with volar angulation. The proximal fragment is flexed by the bony insertion of the interossei into the base of proximal phalanx. The distal fragment is pulled into hyperextension by the central slip through the PIP joint.

Base of the Proximal Phalanx Fractures

Fractures at the base of the proximal phalanx usually occur in a transverse direction with dorsal impaction and apex volar angulation. This fracture is seen more commonly in teenagers. It can usually be treated with an orthosis in the safe position; however, fracture instability can occur. Burkhalter[25] described an immobilization method whereby the MCP joint is flexed and active motion of the PIP joint is allowed. For unstable fractures, the use of closed reduction percutaneous pinning, open reduction with internal fixation with screws or a plate and screws or external fixation is often used. In displaced fractures, the finger will rest in the position of abduction.[26] Of surgical importance, it is often difficult to place pins in the proximal phalanx from a distal to proximal direction. However, it is much easier to place the pins from a proximal to distal direction through the dorsal portion of the metacarpal head into the proximal phalanx fracture.[13] This aids in maintaining the metacarpal phalangeal joint in the safe position (30 to 40 degrees of flexion). Immediate

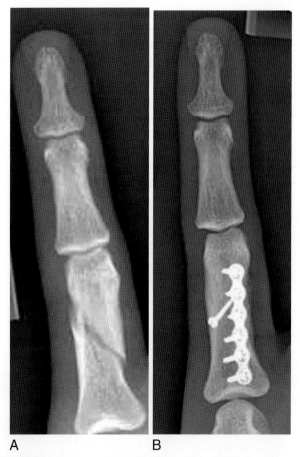

A   B

Figure 41-8 **A,** Radiograph of a proximal phalanx fracture.
B, Radiograph after reduction.

thus creating "ice cream on the tip of a cone" effect. Intra-articular fractures that are nondisplaced (<1 mm) or minimally displaced dorsal or volar chip avulsions may be treated with splinting and early ROM. Radiographs must be checked frequently to ensure that there has been no change in the fracture position.[28] Surgical indications include displacement of the joint surface of greater than 3 mm, fractures involving greater than 40% of the articular surface, or comminuted fractures with large fragments. Occasionally pins are placed across the PIP joint. Rotational alignment is crucial, especially in children. If the fracture fragment is large, then screw fixation can be entertained, but the surgeon must be careful not to devascularize the condyle during the operative approach. Return to sports can be expected at 4 to 6 weeks.

Middle Phalanx Fractures

The middle phalanx (MP) is usually protected from a fracture by its hard cortical nature. Also, the distal and PIP joints help to absorb the blow. When fractures do occur, they usually are from a direct blow and create an oblique or transverse fracture. There are forces acting on the MP, which are dependent on where the fracture occurs, that will cause angulation of the phalanx. If the fracture occurs distal to the flexor digitorum profundus insertion, this will cause a volar apex angulation of the fracture due to the pull of the flexor tendon on the proximal fragment. If the fracture occurs proximal to this location, angulation will be dorsal secondary to the pull of the central slip on the proximal portion of the MP and the flexor tendon distally[29] (Fig. 41-9).

For nondisplaced fractures, early return to sports with buddy taping is permitted. Three weeks of continuous splinting is usually necessary.[30,31] If volar angulation is greater than 30 degrees, this must be corrected in order to avoid an extensor lag or a swan neck deformity. Also, angulation should be less than 10 degrees in the anterior/posterior plane, shortening less than 2 mm, and bone apposition greater than 50% if nonoperative

interphalangeal joint motion is begun, and K wires are removed at 3 weeks and protection for another 3 weeks in a splint is recommended.

Midshaft Proximal Phalanx Fractures

With midshaft proximal phalanx fractures, there is minimal soft-tissue disruption; thus, the fractures are usually stable. Rotational stability is conveyed by the fibro-osseous tendon sheath, specifically the A-2 pulley. Nondisplaced fractures are treated with buddy taping the injured finger to the adjacent digit and early ROM. Displaced fractures are reduced by traction and digital flexion, causing a tension band effect through the dorsal mechanism. ROM is initiated by 3 weeks with progression to full motion by 4 to 6 weeks. For unstable fractures, closed reduction and internal fixation, open reduction with screws and/or plate and screws, or external fixation can be used for stabilization[27] (Fig. 41-8). Return to sports can be anticipated at 2 to 4 weeks.

Condylar Fractures of the Proximal Phalanx

Fractures involving the condyles (unicondylar or bicondylar) often require surgery to restore the articular surface. These fractures frequently rotate and are difficult to hold in a reduced position due to the phalanx narrowing in the subcondylar area,

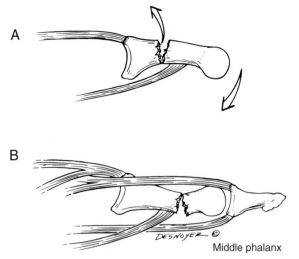

A

B

Middle phalanx

Figure 41-9 **A,** Fracture proximal to flexor digitorum superficialis insertion, dorsal angulation. **B,** Fracture distal to flexor digitorum superficialis insertion, volar angulation. (From Hastings, Rettig, Strickland: Management of Extra-articular Fractures of the Phalanges and Metacarpals. Philadelphia, Elsevier, 1992.)

treatment is employed. Closed reduction and percutaneous pinning, screws, or plate and screws may be chosen when operative intervention is necessary.[32,33]

Distal Phalanx Fractures

More than half of all fractures of the hand occur at the distal phalanx.[34] The distal phalanx of the long finger is most commonly involved, followed by the thumb.[35] Unique to the distal phalanx is the tuft. The tuft anchors specialized skin and the complex nail matrix and plate. Fibrous septae radiate from the bone to the skin to form a dense meshwork that stabilizes the fracture and prevents displacement. Most injuries occur as a result of a direct blow or a crushing injury.

With a nondisplaced fracture, it is important to protect only the distal phalanx (e.g., a tip protector or splint) and to allow PIP motion. A tip protector should extend distal to the tip to protect this area from external trauma. Occasionally displaced fractures require closed reduction and pinning (Fig. 41-10). Usually a wire is placed across the distal interphalangeal joint for approximately 3 weeks.

Displaced fractures or fractures beneath the nail plate suggest that there has been damage to the nail fold. In this instance, some recommend that even if the nail plate is intact, it should be removed and the nail bed repaired. If a subungal hematoma is present, it is not only beneficial to relieve this pressure, and, in the case of hematomas involving greater then 50% of the nail plate, some recommend removal of the nail plate and repair of the nail bed.

These fractures can have significant morbidity with as many as 31% of the fractures still nonunited and 70% of patients with residual tenderness at 6 months. Most injuries that involve the distal phalanx will allow the athlete to return to sports rapidly with splinting.

LIGAMENTOUS INJURIES OF THE HAND

- Ligamentous injuries about the hand are among the most common injuries in athletes.
- Many of the ligamentous injuries about the joints of the hand are incomplete and do not compromise stability. These injuries tend to heal with minimal protection and result in good functional recovery.
- A subset of injuries with complete ligamentous disruption can result in joint instability and compromise function. It is paramount that these types of destabilizing ligamentous injuries are recognized and treated promptly.

THUMB LIGAMENT INJURIES

The MCP joint of the thumb is a condyloid type joint.[36] The osteoarticular anatomy of the thumb MP joint provides minimal intrinsic stability.[37] The lateral static stabilizers include the proper collateral ligaments and accessory collateral ligaments. Dynamic stability is provided by the abductor and adductor aponeurosis. The proper and accessory collateral ligaments originate from the lateral condylar region of the metacarpal and insert on the volar aspect of the proximal phalanx and the volar plate, respectively.[36] Palmar support is provided by a fibrocartilaginous volar plate, which is further supported by thenar intrinsic muscles. Smith and others emphasized the importance of the dorsal capsule and the accessory collateral ligaments as static stabilizers of the MP joint.[38,39]

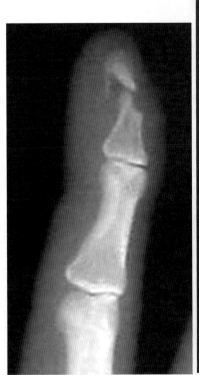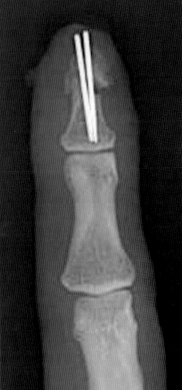

Figure 41-10 A, Radiograph of a distal phalanx fracture. **B,** Radiograph after reduction.

A   B

Ulnar Collateral Ligament Injuries

UCL injuries (skier's or gamekeeper's thumb) of the thumb MP joint are seen among athletes participating in ball-handling and contact sports. UCL injuries have been recognized to be more common than radial collateral ligament (RCL) injuries of the thumb.[40–42] Ulnar MCP joint injuries are most commonly caused by an abrupt forced radial deviation of the thumb. Athletes usually report a fall onto the outstretched hand with the thumb abducted. Disruption of the UCL usually occurs at its distal insertion on the proximal phalanx.[43] Mid-substance tears, although uncommon, can occur. Associated injuries with UCL tears include volar plate and dorsal capsular disruptions. Avulsion fracture at the ulnar base of the proximal phalanx may occur (Fig. 41-11). Complete tears of the UCL can have interposition of the adductor aponeurosis (termed a Stener lesion), whereby the distally avulsed ligament cannot reasonably reapproximate its insertion onto the proximal phalanx.[44]

Clinical Features and Evaluation

Athletes with UCL injuries usually present with global swelling of the thumb MP joint and point tenderness along the ulnar joint line. In the case of UCL injuries without associated fracture, it is important to distinguish partial versus complete tears. Determination of complete (grade III) and partial (grade I/II) UCL disruptions is largely clinical with the use of a stress test of the thumb MP joint in full extension and 30 degrees of flexion. Loss

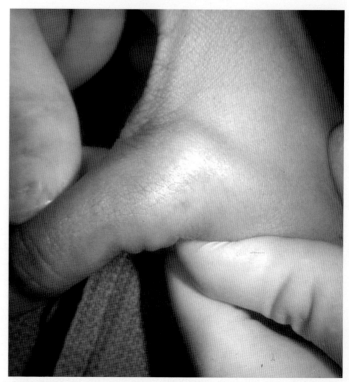

Figure 41-12 Significant clinical ulnar-side instability of the thumb middle phalanx joint is demonstrated with loss of endpoint and excessive laxity with radial stress testing.

of a firm endpoint with radial stress of the MP joint in full extension and greater than 30 degrees of laxity compared to the contralateral side in both extension and flexion are suggestive of a complete UCL tear (Fig. 41-12). Athletes with partial tears demonstrate pain with radial stress but have a firm endpoint and minimal to moderate laxity. The presence of a palpable mass on the ulnar side of the proximal MP joint can suggest a Stener lesion. The use of a local anesthetic block is useful in the evaluation of patients with significant pain or guarding.

Radiographic evaluation should include posteroanterior, oblique, and lateral views to assess for fracture and joint congruency. With complete UCL disruption, occasionally volar subluxation occurs as a result of an associated dorsal capsular injury. Stress radiographs confirm a complete tear of the UCL when greater than one third subluxation of the proximal phalanx on the metacarpal head is present.[45] It is always important to compare these results to stress radiographs of the contralateral thumb. In certain cases, MRI evaluation of the thumb to assess for a complete tear of the UCL or the presence of a Stener lesion may be a helpful adjunct (Fig. 41-13).[46]

Treatment Options

Acute partial tears are managed with a hand-based thumb spica splint or cast for 4 weeks. The cast or orthosis is placed with the MCP joint in slight flexion and neutral alignment. Active ROM is initiated 4 weeks after injury with continued splint wear for an additional 2 weeks. Some authors have advocated cast immobilization in the case of complete tears.[47] The thumb UCL plays a significant role in the athlete's ability to provide pinch grip. It is for this reason, along with the unpredictability of nonoperative management, that anatomic repair is generally indicated for complete disruption of the UCL in the athlete.

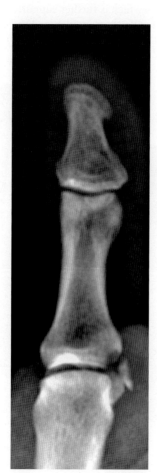

Figure 41-11 A frontal plane radiograph of a 43-year-old master swimmer who sustained an avulsion fracture of the ulnar proximal phalanx after hitting the pool wall with the thumb in abduction.

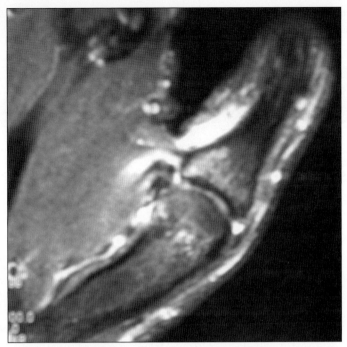

Figure 41-13 Magnetic resonance imaging of the thumb demonstrates a complete disruption of the ulnar collateral ligament with distal avulsion of the ligament.

Surgery: Acute Ulnar Collateral Ligament Repair

A curvilinear incision is made centered over the ulnar aspect of the thumb MP joint. The distal limb skin incision is completed along the mid-axial line of the proximal phalanx. The incision is extended proximally over the dorsoulnar aspect of the joint. Blunt dissection is undertaken within the subcutaneous tissues to identify branches of the superficial radial nerve, which are carefully protected (Fig. 41-14). The adductor aponeurosis is identified and released longitudinally just volar to the extensor

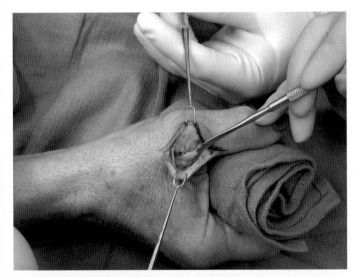

Figure 41-14 The intraoperative photograph demonstrates the approach for repair of the thumb ulnar collateral ligament and a branch of the superficial radial nerve (Freer). Dissection within the subcutaneous tissues should be done with care to avoid injury to branches of the superficial radial nerve, which commonly traverse the surgical field.

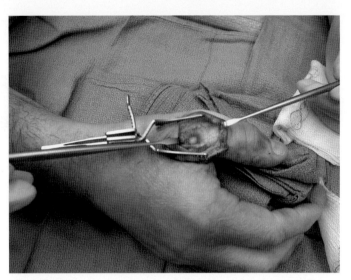

Figure 41-15 In this intraoperative photograph of acute repair of the ulnar collateral ligament, the ligament was found to be avulsed from the proximal phalanx.

pollicis longus. The aponeurosis is reflected volarly to expose the ulnar side of the MP joint. The UCL is identified and most commonly found to be avulsed from the proximal phalanx (Fig. 41-15). An arthrotomy of the MP joint is completed and the articular cartilage examined. If there is a small bony fragment still attached to the ligament, it is excised. If the fragment is greater than 15% of the articular surface, attempts should be made to fix the fragment with wire or mini screws. Midsubstance tears can be repaired in an end-to-end fashion. Although pull-out suture technique has been described with good results, we have routinely used bone anchors to secure the avulsed ligament.[48] In preparation for placement of the suture anchors, the ulnar volar and dorsal aspect of the proximal phalanx is exposed. Two drill holes are placed into the volar-ulnar and dorsoulnar base of the proximal phalanx (Fig. 41-16). The mini suture anchors, metallic or biodegradable, are placed into the predrilled holes. Most of the mini anchors come prethreaded with a 2-0 Ethibond suture. The distally avulsed ligament is then reapproximated to its insertion via the suture anchors (Fig. 41-17). Sutures are placed to repair the dorsal capsule and reapproximate the volar plate to the most distal aspect of the repaired ligament. A gentle radial stress is applied to assess the adequacy of repair. The adductor aponeurosis is then reattached. The skin is sutured and the hand placed in a thumb spica splint.

For the "weekend athlete," the thumb is immobilized in a hand-based thumb spica cast for 4 weeks postoperatively. ROM exercises are permitted at 1 month with continued protection in an orthosis. Splint wear is discontinued at 6 weeks for most activities. Depending on the sport, protection is recommended for 3 months postoperatively. If the repair is considered adequate, athletes may be converted to a thumb spica orthosis after 2 weeks of cast immobilization as described by Lane.[49] This has resulted in a quicker return to sports with good long-term functional outcome. Following repair, the athlete may return to play in a protective playing cast at 2 to 3 weeks. Athletes participating in sports requiring significant pinch strength, such as the throwing hand of a quarterback, may require 6 to 9 weeks prior to return.

Chronic thumb UCL injuries may occur after a missed Stener lesion, failed treatment of an acute complete disruption, or

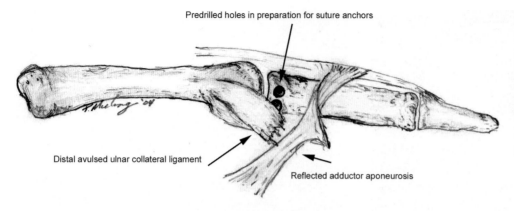

Predrilled holes in preparation for suture anchors

Distal avulsed ulnar collateral ligament

Reflected adductor aponeurosis

Figure 41-16 The illustration demonstrates the location of the predrilled holes in preparation for placement of mini bone suture anchors. Attempts are made to place the anchors just distal to the articular surface on the volar-ulnar and dorsoulnar aspect of the proximal phalanx.

progressive attenuation. Complete ruptures of the UCL less than 2 months after injury can usually be addressed by careful excision of scar and reinsertion of the retracted ligament.[45] Chronic UCL injuries have been treated by using a scarred capsule to create a new ligament, adductor advancement, or reconstruction with a free tendon graft.[45,50,51] The postoperative rehabilitation is similar to that for acute repair. However, an additional 1 to 2 weeks of immobilization is recommended. MP arthrodesis may also be considered to address chronic UCL insufficiency.

Radial Collateral Ligament Injuries

Although RCL tears are less common than UCL ruptures, they can become a debilitating injury if unrecognized. Among 100 collateral ligament repairs of the thumb, Melone et al[45] identified 40 serious radial-side ligament injuries. The mechanism of injury is an adduction force across the MCP joint. Proximal and distal disruption of the RCL occurs with equal frequency.[52] Stener lesions do not occur after complete disruptions of the RCL because of the anatomy of the abductor aponeurosis.

Athletes may present with ecchymosis, pain, and swelling along the radial side of the MP joint. Dorsoradial pain with prominence of the thumb metacarpal head may be seen in complete RCL tears. The prominence occurs as the proximal phalanx shifts volarward and into pronation because of dorsal

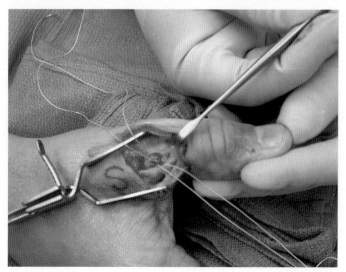

Figure 41-17 Bone anchors have been placed into the proximal phalanx. The prethreaded suture on the anchors is then utilized to secure the avulsed UCL ligament back to its insertion.

capsule disruption and an intact UCL. Three views of the thumb should be obtained. Lateral radiographs may demonstrate volar subluxation of the proximal phalanx. It is important to differentiate partial (grade I/II) from full-thickness (grade III) tears. An ulnar stress is applied to the thumb MP joint in full extension and 30 degrees of flexion and compared to the uninjured thumb. The absence of a firm endpoint with ulnar stress and greater than 30 degrees of instability compared to the contralateral side suggest a complete tear. Stress radiographs are consistent with a complete tear when more than one third ulnar subluxation on the metacarpal head is present.[45]

Partial RCL tears are treated with immobilization in a hand-based thumb spica cast or splint for approximately 4 weeks. Mobilization of the MP joint is initiated at 1 month with continued splinting for an additional 2 weeks. Athletes are protected with splint or taping for 10 to 12 weeks after injury. Both immobilization and early repair have been advocated for the treatment of complete ruptures of the RCL.[45,52,53] Physical examination findings consistent with a complete rupture and/or the presence of MP joint subluxation are indications for exploration and repair of the ligament. The postoperative management and return to sports is similar to that for acute repair of the UCL. Chronic RCL injuries can be surgically addressed with mobilization of the scarred ligament or reconstruction with a free tendon graft.

VOLAR PLATE INJURIES IN THE THUMB METACARPOPHALANGEAL JOINT

Dislocation of the thumb MP joint most commonly occurs dorsally. The injury is secondary to a sudden hyperextension load. On-field examination of these injuries may demonstrate a mild to moderate hyperextension deformity of the proximal phalanx and dimpling within the palm (Fig. 41-18). The injuries can be classified into simple and complex. Complex dislocations are irreducible by closed methods. Radiographs demonstrating interposition of the sesamoid bones between the metacarpal head and proximal phalanx is suggestive of a complex dislocation. Simple MP joint dislocations result in proximal disruption of the volar plate. Concomitant injuries include sesamoid fracture and varying degrees of collateral ligament injuries. In reducing the joint, it is important to avoid longitudinal traction with the possibility of converting a simple dislocation into an irreducible one. After regional anesthesia is administered, closed reduction is attempted by flexion of the wrist and axial loading of the proximal phalanx onto the metacarpal head with gentle MP flexion. The majority of MP dislocations are easily reducible

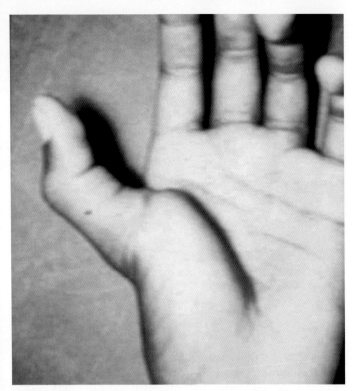

Figure 41-18 A clinical picture of a complex dorsal dislocation of the thumb middle phalanx joint in an 18-year-old football player who sustained a significant hyperextension load. There is noted hyperextension of the middle phalanx joint and adduction of the thumb metacarpal.

and stable after reduction. The collateral ligaments should be assessed after reduction. If postreduction radiographs demonstrate concentric reduction and the joint is stable, then the thumb is immobilized for 3 weeks. If the joint is found to be clearly stable, then a more abbreviated period of immobilization could be considered depending on the specific requirements of the sport.

Complex dislocations are irreducible and require open reduction. The volar plate, flexor pollicis longus, and sesamoids have all been found to block reduction at the time of surgical exploration. The joint is approached through a volar, dorsal, or lateral approach. Once the interposed tissue has been removed, the joint is usually found to be stable. The MP joint may be pinned in 20 to 30 degrees of flexion in cases of instability after congruent reduction. Four weeks of immobilization is recommended following open reduction. Volar MP dislocations of the thumb are much less common. They are sometimes associated with concomitant injury to the extensor mechanism and the dorsal capsule requiring open repair.

THUMB CARPOMETACARPAL LIGAMENTOUS INJURIES

Acute dislocation of the thumb carpometacarpal (CMC) joint without fracture is a rare injury with few reported cases in the literature.[54] Injury to the volar ligament usually occurs as the thumb metacarpal dislocates dorsally after an axial load onto the flexed thumb. Complete and partial tears occur following a dislocation or subluxation event. Athletes with partial tears present with post-traumatic pain in the absence of clinical insta-

bility or radiographic subluxation on stress views. These injuries are managed with 4 weeks of immobilization in a thumb spica cast or splint. The thumb interphalangeal joint should be included to limit axial loading of the thumb. If concentric reduction of the CMC joint is obtained after complete dislocation, the patient is placed into a cast with repeat radiographs obtained in 1 week. Cast immobilization is continued an additional 3 weeks if radiographs demonstrate reduction. Closed reduction and percutaneous pinning of the CMC joint are indicated for persistent radiographic subluxation or clinical instability. Open reduction and percutaneous pinning are indicated if the metacarpal base is not well seated on the trapezium after a closed reduction attempt. Athletes who have continued symptoms following closed management may be indicated for volar ligament reconstruction of the thumb CMC joint, as described by Eaton and Littler.[55]

PROXIMAL INTERPHALANGEAL JOINT LIGAMENT INJURIES

Ligamentous injuries about the PIP joints are among the most common hand injuries in sports. Stability of the PIP joint is provided by the bicondylar articular anatomy, ligamentous support, extensor tendon apparatus, and the flexor tendon retinacular system.[56] The key to stability is the relationship of the ulnar and radial collateral ligaments and volar plate. The lateral stabilizers of the joint include the accessory and proper RCLs and UCLs. The ligaments originate from the lateral aspect of each condyle. The proper and accessory collateral ligaments pass in an oblique manner to insert on the volar third of the MP and the volar plate, respectively. The volar plate serves as the floor of the joint and inserts into the palmar region of the MP. Check-rein ligaments are attached to the proximal region of the volar plate preventing hyperextension of the PIP joint. With the strong collateral ligament attachments on both sides of the volar plate, a three-sided box configuration is present to stabilize the PIP joint.

Collateral ligament injuries are frequently seen in athletes participating in ball-handling sports. RCLs are the most commonly injured. The majority of tears occur through the proximal region of the collateral ligament.[57] The athlete may not recall the specific time of the injury and often will present in a delayed fashion. Patients complain of joint-line pain, swelling, and stiffness of the injured digit. Stability of the joint is assessed through a dynamic and passive examination. The ability to flex and extend the injured digit through a full arc ROM suggests adequate joint stability. Passive stability of the collateral ligaments should be assessed with the PIP joint in full extension and 30 degrees of flexion. Glickel et al[37] have classified collateral ligament injuries of the PIP joint into three categories based on the degree of laxity. Athletes with grade I sprains have pain with stress of the ligament but no laxity. Clinical examination of grade II injuries demonstrates mild to moderate laxity on stress examination. A firm endpoint is noted on passive examination and no instability with active ROM is noted. Grade III injuries demonstrate significant laxity on stress examination. More than 20 degrees of angulation on lateral stress examination may indicate complete disruption of the proper collateral ligament[57] (Fig. 41-19).

Grade I and II PIP joint collateral sprains are treated with early ROM and buddy taping. Most athletes may return to play with protective buddy taping. It is important to educate the athlete about the possibility of prolonged soreness, swelling, and stiffness in these types of injuries. The majority of grade III

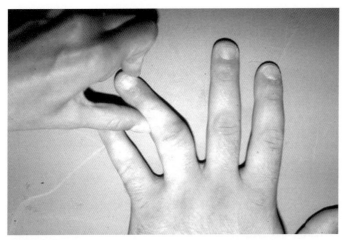

Figure 41-19 Stress examination of the ring finger proximal interphalangeal joint in a 25-year-old recreational flag football player demonstrates significant laxity (30 degrees) of the radial collateral ligament. This examination finding is suggestive of a grade III radial collateral ligament injury.

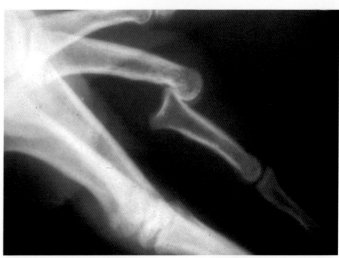

Figure 41-20 Lateral radiograph of a digit with a volar dislocation of the proximal interphalangeal joint.

injuries are managed with buddy taping, early ROM, and a short period of protection in a dorsal blocking splint with the PIP joint in 30 degrees of flexion. The indication for surgical repair of the ligament is instability on active ROM, nonanatomic joint reduction, or chronic pain. Consideration may be given to surgical repair of significant injuries to the RCL of the index finger because of the restraints required for lateral pinch.

PROXIMAL INTERPHALANGEAL JOINT DISLOCATION

There are three types of PIP joint dislocations: dorsal, lateral, and volar. Dorsal dislocations of the PIP joint are frequently seen in athletes playing ball-handling sports. The injuries often occur when a ball or object hits the tip of the digit. The mechanism of injury is an axial load with an associated hyperextension force. The majority of dorsal dislocations result in distal avulsion of the volar plate. Pure ligamentous dislocations usually have varying degrees of collateral ligament injuries. The injuries are often reduced by the player, coach, or trainer. Radiographs of the injured digit should be taken to evaluate for fracture and congruent joint reduction. If the joint is stable following reduction, early ROM is instituted with the injured digit buddy taped for 3 weeks. Return to play may be possible with protective buddy taping. If some instability exists and radiographs demonstrate congruent reduction, the patient may be placed into a dorsal blocking splint with the joint in 30 degrees of flexion for approximately 7 to 10 days.

Lateral dislocations usually indicate complete disruption of the collateral ligament and portions of the volar plate. These injuries are most often amenable to nonsurgical management similar to dorsal dislocations of the PIP joint.

Volar dislocations of the PIP joint are rare injuries (Fig. 41-20). The mechanism of injury is a longitudinal compression load across a partially flexed MP. This injury may result in a straight volar dislocation or one with a rotatory component. Straight volar dislocations are more likely to have a severe injury to the central slip.[58] With rotatory volar dislocation, the middle phalangeal condyle may become entrapped between the central slip and the lateral band as it displaces palmarly. This results in only partial tearing of the central slip along with disruption of the collateral ligament. The majority of these injuries can be reduced by closed methods. With both the MCP and PIP joints flexed, gentle traction is applied.[59] In the case of volar rotatory dislocation, avoidance of straight longitudinal traction is important because of the buttonhole entrapment of the MP. After congruent reduction of a rotatory dislocation, athletes who demonstrate full active extension may return to play with buddy taping and ROM as tolerated. Straight volar dislocations and extensor lag after reduction of a volar rotatory dislocation should be managed as an acute boutonniere injury (see "Closed Tendon Injuries").

PROXIMAL INTERPHALANGEAL JOINT FRACTURE DISLOCATIONS

Injuries to the PIP joint, especially those that involve a fracture, require a true lateral view of the joint to assess this area. This is necessary to ensure concentric reduction of the joint. If the volar fragment of the MP is greater than 30% to 40% of the articular surface, the joint is often rendered unstable. Treatment varies from dorsal block splinting to closed reduction, open reduction to external fixation. No splinting is necessary in nondisplaced fractures. Dorsal block splinting is used in a displaced fracture that reduces concentrically with the finger in a flexed position.[60] If concentric reduction is not obtained, then closed reduction and pinning of the PIP joint for 10 to 14 days, followed by dorsal block splinting, may be necessary.[61] If the fracture fragment is large, open reduction and internal fixation may be beneficial.[62,63] Comminuted fractures involving the PIP joint often require external fixation. Return to sports after operative fixation generally occurs in 6 to 8 weeks with protective splinting.

LIGAMENT INJURIES OF THE DISTAL INTERPHALANGEAL JOINT OF THE DIGITS AND INTERPHALANGEAL JOINT OF THE THUMB

The distal joints of the thumb and fingers have ligamentous anatomy similar to that of the PIP joint. Dislocations within these joints are less common in part because of the adjacent insertions of the extensor mechanism and flexor tendon. However, there is a higher propensity for open injuries because of the relationship of the soft-tissue envelope to the joint. These injuries are most commonly seen in ball-handling sports. Athletes may present in a delayed fashion with pain and stiffness of the digit after self-reducing the dislocation. Subluxations or dislocations usually occur dorsally or lateral. Closed reduction is usually possible after placement of a digital block. The dislocation is reduced by applying longitudinal traction and flexing the joint. After reduction, anteroposterior and lateral radiographs are taken. If congruent reduction is obtained, the collateral ligaments are assessed. If the joint is stable, a dorsal blocking splint is applied to the injured joint in 20 degrees of flexion for approximately 2 weeks. Because instability of these injuries is rare, athletes may return to play with a protective splint. Irreducible dislocations are rare and are usually secondary to interposition of the volar plate or flexor tendons.[64] Open injuries should be managed with irrigation, débridement, and administration of antibiotics.

LIGAMENT INJURIES OF THE FINGER METACARPOPHALANGEAL JOINT

Unlike PIP joint injuries, dislocations and ligamentous injuries of the MP joint are uncommon. The location of the joint at the base of the digits and ligamentous restraints play an important role in the stability of the MP joint. Except for the absence of the check-rein structures, the ligamentous design of the MP joint is similar to that of the PIP joint already described. It is important to note that the volar plate of the MP joint is firmly attached distally to the proximal phalanx. The proximal metacarpal insertion is not anchored as well. Dorsally, a thin capsule is present but reinforced by overlying extensor tendons.

Dorsal dislocation of the MP joint is most commonly seen within the border digits. The mechanism of injury is usually a hyperextension force of the finger. The proximal membranous portion of the volar plate becomes detached and is interposed between the base of the proximal phalanx and the metacarpal head. Prior to closed reduction, the clinician must attempt to distinguish between simple and complex dislocations. Complex dorsal dislocations require open reduction. Athletes with simple dislocations present with the injured digit hyperextended 60 to 80 degrees. In complex dislocations, the injured digit is found to be in 10 to 15 degrees of extension and slight deviation toward the more central ray. Occasionally, puckering or dimpling within the palmar skin is seen. Closed reduction of simple MP dislocations is performed by flexing the wrist and applying a distally and volarly directed pressure to the base of the dislocated phalanx.[65,66] These injuries are managed with a dorsal blocking splint, permitting active flexion exercises. Complex dislocations require an open reduction, usually through a volar approach.

Collateral ligament injuries of the MCP joint are uncommon. The mechanism of injury is usually an ulnarly directed force on a flexed MCP joint. The injury most commonly occurs in the long, ring, and small fingers. Clinically, the athlete presents with pain and swelling along the radial side of the MCP joint. To assess for injuries of the proper collateral ligament, the MCP joint is brought into flexion and an ulnar directed stress is applied. A Brewerton view radiograph of the injured hand can be helpful to assess for avulsion fractures.[67] In cases of significant instability, consideration of direct primary repair of the ligament may be given to RCL injuries of the border digits[68] (Fig.

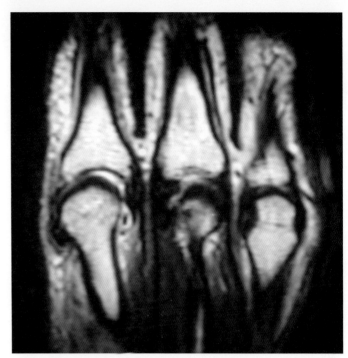

Figure 41-21 Magnetic resonance imaging of the hand in a 38-year-old indoor soccer player who sustained an ulnar-side stress to the index finger when he hit the retaining wall of the field. The imaging study demonstrates complete disruption of the radial collateral ligament of the index finger metacarpophalangeal joint with associated ulnar subluxation of the joint.

41-21). The majority of complete ligamentous injuries respond to a 2- to 3-week period of immobilization in slight flexion, followed by protective buddy taping. Most incomplete MCP joint collateral ligament injuries and complete tears in nonborder digits heal with immediate protective buddy taping, early ROM, and return to play.

LIGAMENT INJURIES OF THE CARPOMETACARPAL JOINT

The index and middle finger CMC joints are stable as a result of the articular relationships with the trapezoid and capitate, respectively. The stability affords minimal motion at the index and middle finger CMC joint. The ring and small finger CMC joints are more mobile, allowing 10 to 15 degrees of motion. Acute ligament injuries of the CMC joint are most commonly associated with subluxation or dislocation of the joint. The injuries are often high energy and associated with avulsion fractures of the base of the metacarpal and adjacent carpal bones. Athletes present with significant dorsal swelling and pain along the base of the metacarpal joints. Initially, minimal deformity may be present and the injury could go undiagnosed. The majority of subluxations or dislocations are dorsal. Injuries recognized acutely are easily reducible but unstable. These injuries are best managed with closed reduction and percutaneous pinning. The pins are maintained for 6 to 8 weeks postoperatively. Once the pins are removed, a gradual return to activities is permitted.

CLOSED TENDON INJURIES

- Closed tendon injuries of the hand are common in the athlete and may occur from direct trauma such as an impact from an opponent or a ball, from striking the ground, or during the course of grasping activities.

- As in many cases of sports-related hand injury, these problems are often neglected and are not seen by a physician until the end of the season when the athlete notes a significant disability.[1]
- Failure to initiate treatment in the acute stages may jeopardize the final result in certain cases. Every effort should be made to ensure early evaluation and treatment of these injuries.

MALLET FINGER

Disruption of the terminal extensor tendon at its insertion on the distal phalanx is one of the most common tendon injuries in sports. It is known as mallet finger, drop finger, or baseball finger. This is especially common in softball, baseball, and basketball and in football receivers.[1] The injury usually occurs when a ball or other object hits the tip of the finger resulting in a flexion force while the extensor is actively contracting. The mallet deformity also may result from a direct blow to the dorsum of the DIP joint or secondary to a hyperextension force at this joint.[69]

Anatomically the lateral bands merge and intertwine to form one tendon just distal to the dorsal tubercle of the proximal portion of the MP. This tendon forms a wide structure that inserts into the dorsal base of the distal phalanx, attaching to the dorsal part of the capsule and anterior ridge distal to the articular cartilage.[70]

McCue and Wooten[71] classify mallet finger pathology into five types: (1) tendon stretching, (2) tendon rupture, (3) rupture with avulsion fragment, (4) large fracture fragment, and (5) epiphyseal fracture. An alternate classification is by Doyle,[72] with four main types. Type I is a classic hyperflexion injury in which the tendon is avulsed or stretched, which may be accompanied by a small fragment of bone being avulsed from the base of the distal phalanx. Type II involves laceration in which the tendon is divided. Type III is quite rare and involves an abrasion with loss of skin and subcutaneous and tendinous tissue over the DIP joint. Type IV is a mallet fracture, which can be subdivided into (1) transepiphyseal, (2) hyperflexion injury with a fragment involving 20% to 50% of the articular surface, and (3) hyperextension injury in which the fragment involves 50% or more of the articular cartilage (Fig. 41-22). The hyperextension type is frequently accompanied by volar subluxation of the joint.

Mallet finger is readily detected on physical examination by the flexion posture of the DIP joint and the inability to actively extend the joint. Stability of the DIP joint should also be tested to evaluate possible involvement of the collateral ligaments, although this is rare. A true lateral radiograph is mandatory to determine the presence or absence of a fracture fragment and whether subluxation of the joint exists.

Most authors agree that treatment of closed injuries with or without fracture primarily involves simple splinting of the DIP joint in full extension (Fig. 41-23). The splint should maintain the DIP joint in full extension, allowing free PIP motion. The extensor mechanism is moderately lax at the MP, PIP, and DIP joints when the DIP joint is in extension. Allowing ROM at the PIP joint level minimizes stiffness of this joint and permits more normal use of the hand during treatment.

Splints may be applied to the volar or dorsal aspects of the joint and *should remain in place continuously* for a minimum of

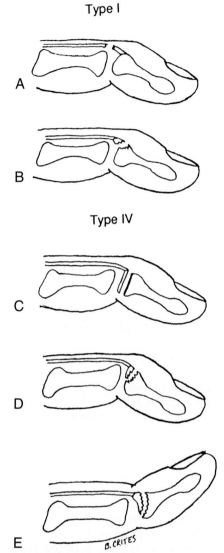

Figure 41-22 Divisions of type I mallet injury showing avulsion without *(A)* and with *(B)* bone fragment. Type IV mallet injury: Transepiphyseal *(C)*; hyperflexion with fragment involving 20% to 50% of the articular surface *(D)*; and hyperextension injury with 50% or greater articular surface, and often volar subluxation *(E)*. (From Hastings, Rettig, Strickland: Management of Extra-articular Fractures of the Phalanges and Metacarpals. Philadelphia, Elsevier, 1992.)

6 to 8 weeks. Excellent results have been reported using these methods. McFarlane and Hampole[73] have reported satisfactory results using a splinting program in mallet cases that presented as late as 3 months after injury.

In certain cases in which wearing a splint is not practical, such as in the health care professional, a single longitudinal K wire may be placed percutaneously across the DIP joint to maintain extension and allow continued function. This technique has limited application and is not usually recommended in the athlete. Continued participation in most sports is allowed during treatment of mallet finger as long as the finger is splinted appropriately. Injuries to the throwing hand of a baseball pitcher or football quarterback may result in some time loss from sport, although figure-eight taping to prevent full flexion may be employed.

Transepiphyseal fractures must be reduced anatomically and satisfactorily stable reduction may be maintained by external

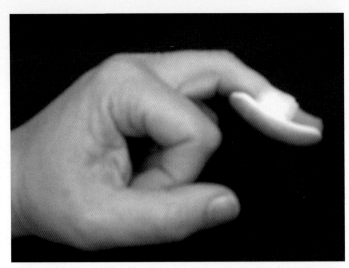

Figure 41-23 The Orthoplast splint maintains the distal interphalangeal joint in full extension and allows motion at the proximal interphalangeal joint.

splinting. If significant instability is present, soft-tissue interposition is frequently present and open reduction internal fixation using a longitudinal K wire is indicated. The K wire may be continued for 4 weeks, and then protection for sports is indicated for an additional 4 weeks.[71]

Conflict of opinion exists as to the treatment of hyperextension injuries in which a considerable size fracture fragment is present with volar subluxation of the joint. Lange and Engber[74] and Crawford[75] recommend open treatment when subluxation exists to restore joint congruity. They recommend placement of a transepiphyseal pin and fixation of the dorsal fragment with K wires or pull-out suture or wire. Dorsal extension block fixation technique has recently been proposed by Hofmeister et al[76] as another alternative of internal fixation. Wehbe and Schneider,[77] on the other hand, recommend closed treatment of mallet injuries including cases in which subluxation is present. They maintain that satisfactory remodeling occurs so that DIP joint function is adequate.

Chronic mallet injuries, if left untreated, may progress to a flexion deformity at the DIP joint and hyperextension deformity at the PIP joint (swan neck lesion). Delayed treatment of chronic mallet injury depends on the severity of the deformity and symptomatology and is beyond the scope of this chapter.

MALLET THUMB

Mallet thumb injuries are much less common than the mallet finger, but this lesion may also occur as a result of athletic activity. These injuries constitute 2% to 3% of all mallet injuries, and diagnosis is usually apparent by the inability to actively extend the interphalangeal joint of the thumb. Radiographs are usually within normal limits, although occasionally a small avulsion fracture is noted.

Most authors recommend[78] conservative treatment of this lesion. Din and Meggitt,[79] in 1983, recommended open repair because the extensor pollicis longus is thicker than the digital extensors, and they noted a significant gap between tendon ends at the time of exploration. Miura et al,[80] on the other hand, treated 25 of 35 mallet thumb injuries with extension splints and noted that satisfactory extension was present in 84%. These

authors also noted that patients who received treatment within 2 weeks following injury obtained more satisfactory results compared to those who were treated at later than 2 weeks.

Athletes can frequently continue to participate in their sport during treatment of mallet thumb. In ball-handling positions in football, the thumb may be taped to prevent full flexion during play and splinted in extension when not participating.

BOUTONNIERE INJURIES

Boutonniere injury involves rupture of the central slip of the extensor mechanism at its insertion into the base of the MP. Injuries may be due to either direct trauma to the dorsum of the PIP joint or an acute flexion force applied to the PIP joint with opposed active extension. The term boutonniere is derived from the French word for buttonhole, which refers to a split that occurs in the dorsal covering of the PIP joint where the central slip of the extensor mechanism avulses from its insertion. Late cases with a classic boutonniere deformity consisting of flexion of the PIP joint and hyperextension of the DIP joint are readily apparent on physical examination. However, the acute case can easily be missed.

Acutely, the athlete presents with swelling about the PIP joint with inability to actively extend the joint. Diagnosis may be confused with more common PIP joint sprain or even dislocation that has been reduced. Radiographs are frequently normal. However, a small avulsion at the dorsal base of the MP may be present in some cases. An effective diagnostic measure in acute cases is to perform a digital block, thus limiting pain and guarding, and to ask the patient to actively extend the PIP joint. If the patient is unable to do this, it is most likely due to rupture of the extensor mechanism.

The goal of treatment of an acute central slip injury is to prevent the late classic boutonniere deformity. If this lesion is untreated or splinted in flexion as is sometimes done for PIP joint sprains, the unopposed pull of the flexor digitorum sublimis along with swelling of the PIP joint will maintain a flexion deformity. The disrupted ends of the central slip will migrate proximally and the lateral bands will migrate volarly, thus giving a classic boutonniere posture (Fig. 41-24). Burton[81] has

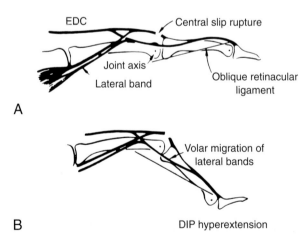

Figure 41-24 A, Rupture of the central slip of the extensor mechanism. **B,** Central slip rupture with volar migration of the lateral bands causing flexion of the proximal interphalangeal joint and hyperextension of the distal interphalangeal joint (DIP). EDC, extensor digitorum communis. (From Hastings, Rettig, Strickland: Management of Extra-articular Fractures of the Phalanges and Metacarpals. Philadelphia, Elsevier, 1992.)

described three stages of deformity: stage 1, dynamic imbalance that is fully correctable passively; stage 2, extensor tendon contracture that is not passively correctable but does not involve the joint structure; stage 3, fixed contracture with joint changes involving a collateral ligament and volar plate scarring and intra-articular adhesions.

Once the diagnosis of acute extensor disruption at the base of the MP is made, splinting of the PIP joint in full extension is begun. The DIP joint is allowed to be free, and active flexion of this joint is encouraged. Active DIP joint flexion with the PIP joint maintained in extension is encouraged as this helps to maintain the lateral bands in anatomic position dorsal to the PIP joint. Splinting should be continued for a period of 6 to 8 weeks. The athlete may continue to compete with the protective splint holding the joint in full extension or taping to prevent full flexion of the PIP joint during participation and splinting all other times.

If avulsion of a significant portion of the MP is present, open reduction and internal fixation may be indicated. The PIP joint is maintained in full extension by placement of a transarticular pin and the fragment is fixed by either a pull-out suture or small K wires. The transarticular pin may be removed in 10 days to 2 weeks. A protective splint with the PIP joint in extension should be worn for an additional 2 months.

Volar PIP joint dislocations result in rupture of the central slip along with collateral ligament rupture. In these cases, which are frequently irreducible by closed means, authors have recommended open reduction and repair of the central slip and transarticular pinning for 3 weeks.[82] If these dislocations can be reduced closed, they should be treated as an acute boutonniere injury with splinting to protect the central slip.

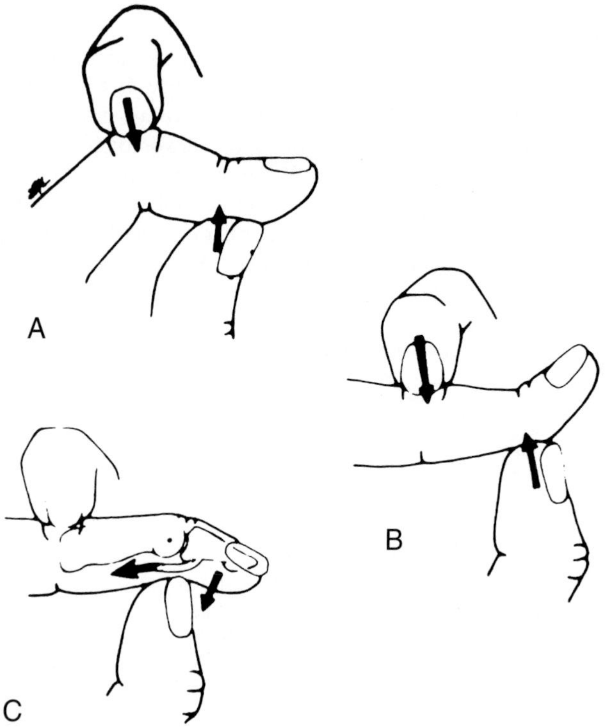

Frequently the physician is presented with boutonniere injuries that have been neglected or treated inappropriately. Treatment of chronic boutonniere deformity has been well documented and involves the use of dynamic splinting and in some cases the use of serial casts in order to decrease the flexion contracture of the PIP joint. Of most importance is a boutonniere exercise program in which the PIP joint is extended to a maximum degree, and active flexion at the DIP joint is instituted (Fig. 41-25). These exercises must be done regularly for long periods of time.

Surgery for the correction of chronic boutonniere deformity is very rarely indicated. In some cases, once full extension has been achieved passively, an Elliott type repair of the extensor mechanism may be performed followed by postoperative transarticular pin fixation for 3 weeks, and then rehabilitation.

It is important to carefully evaluate the finger to differentiate boutonniere from pseudoboutonniere injuries described by McCue and Wooten.[71] Pseudoboutonniere occurs if hyperextension injury results in rupture of the proximal attachment of the volar plate with fibrosis and occasional calcification leading to a flexion contracture at the PIP joint. This lesion is not usually accompanied by a hyperextension deformity at the DIP joint, and calcification may often be seen on lateral radiographs at the proximal volar plate attachment.

The pseudoboutonniere can frequently be treated just by simple splinting; however, in cases of greater than 45 degrees of flexion contracture, an open release of the proximal portion of the volar plate may be undertaken.

THUMB BOUTONNIERE

Traumatic boutonniere injuries to the thumb are rare but have been reported. These injuries occur due to trauma to the thumb with hyperflexion of the MP joint. The patient presents with an extensor lag at the MP joint with or without interphalangeal joint hyperextension.

Pathology involves rupture or attenuation of the insertion of the extensor pollicis brevis and stretching of the dorsal radial capsule. Treatment may include splinting with the MP joint extended. Cardon et al[83] has reported excellent results with surgical repair in which the extensor pollicis brevis is reattached to its insertion site and the dorsal radial capsule is imbricated.

EXTENSOR MECHANISM INJURIES AT THE METACARPOPHALANGEAL JOINT

Subluxation of Extensor Digitorum Communis

Traumatic dislocation or subluxation of the extensor tendon apparatus at the MCP joint is less common than other extensor injuries but can occur in the athlete. The injury has been reported by Elson[84] and described in detail by Kettelkamp et al[85] and Harvey and Hume.[86] The injury may be due to a direct blow to the flexed MCP joint or by a flexion ulnar deviation force exerted over the involved digit. The lesion involves tearing of the sagittal band of the extensor hood, usually on the radial side of the extensor tendon. The sagittal fibers function to keep the extensor tendons centered over the metacarpal head, and when a rupture occurs, the tendon dislocates or subluxates into the valley between metacarpal heads.[86] The long finger is the most commonly involved digit.

Figure 41-25 Three-stage exercise program for boutonniere deformity. **A,** The index finger of the opposite hand is placed on the dorsum of the involved proximal interphalangeal (PIP) joint. The uninjured thumb is placed on the flexor aspect of the distal interphalangeal (DIP) joint. **B,** The PIP joint is passively extended as tolerated. **C,** Patient actively flexes the DIP joint over the thumb of the opposite hand. (From Hastings, Rettig, Strickland: Management of Extra-articular Fractures of the Phalanges and Metacarpals. Philadelphia, Elsevier, 1992.)

On physical examination, the athlete presents with swelling about the MCP joint and inability to fully extend the digit at this joint. Once the MP joint is passively extended, the patient may maintain this position because it usually reduces the tendon. This helps differentiate the lesion from a radial neuropathy or extensor rupture.[71]

Treatment of this lesion in acute cases may involve simple splinting in extension for 4 weeks and intermittent splinting and ROM exercises for another 4 weeks.[87] If reduction cannot be maintained or there is a delay in diagnosis, primary suture of the defect in the radial sagittal band is indicated.[85] In late cases in which primary repair is not possible or the tissue is of poor quality, reconstruction of the radial retinaculum may be indicated.[88,89]

Boxer's Knuckle

Another extensor injury at the MCP joint has been described by Melone[90] and termed boxer's knuckle. This refers to a longitudinal tear in the extensor digitorum communis tendon or the sagittal bands overlying the metacarpal head, usually arising from a single event or repetitive direct trauma to this area such as seen in boxing. The long finger is most commonly involved due to its prominence in the fisted position, although the lesion may occur in other digits. The athlete presents with pain over the metacarpal head and frequently a defect is palpable in the extensor mechanism. There may be some weakness to full extension or an extensor lag. Melone[90] has found that disruption occurs with equal frequency in the ulnar and radial sagittal bands with splits in the central tendon being less common.

Once diagnosed, treatment usually involves exploration and side-to-side repair of the tear. In the boxer, care must be taken to place the incision in such a location as to avoid the prominence of the knuckle. The capsule should not be closed so that full flexion may be obtained postoperatively.

Following surgery, splinting is maintained for 6 weeks followed by an aggressive rehabilitation program. If the injury occurs in a boxer, he or she does not return to punching until full ROM and normal strength is obtained, which usually requires 4 months.

FLEXOR TENDON INJURIES

Avulsion of Flexor Tendon Profundus

Avulsion of the flexor digitorum profundus at its insertion on the distal phalanx is known as jersey finger. This is commonly seen in football, rugby, or flag football and usually results from grasping the pants or jersey of an opposing player. As the player pulls away, the finger is forcibly extended while the profundus continues to contract and avulsion may result. McMaster,[91] in 1933, showed experimentally that a normal tendon ruptures most commonly at its insertion, less commonly at the musculotendinous junction, and rarely in the substance of the tendon.

Although any digit may be involved in profundus avulsion, the ring finger is most commonly affected. This is likely because the insertion of the profundus in the ring is anatomically weaker than that of the surrounding fingers and frequently the small finger slips away when grasping an opponent's jersey, leaving the ring finger to bear the brunt of the forces.[92] Profundus avulsion injuries frequently go undetected in acute stages, resulting in a delay in diagnosis and treatment, which may adversely affect the end result.

On examination, the diagnosis may be apparent by the relative position of extension of the digit. The function of the pro-fundus and sublimis tendons must be specifically tested individually (Fig. 41-26). The amount of soft-tissue swelling should be noted and precise localization of the tenderness is very important in an attempt to identify the level of retraction of the avulsed tendon. Leddy and Packer[92] classified profundus avulsion into three main categories: type 1 in which the tendon retracts to the palm, type 2 in which the tendon retracts to the PIP level, and type 3 in which a bony fragment is avulsed with the tendon. It is important to try to ascertain by physical examination and radiograph studies which type is present.

Tendon nutrition has been studied extensively, and there appears to be a dual supply of nutrients to tendons within the sheath consisting of a vascular profusion and diffusion from synovial fluid from within the sheath.[93] Potenza,[94] in 1963, showed that diffusion of nutrients from the synovial fluid occurs and contributes significantly to tendon nutrition. The most important consideration in determining treatment of profundus avulsion are the level of tendon retraction, the remaining nutritional supply to the tendon, the length of time between diagnosis and treatment, and the presence of a bony fragment.[95]

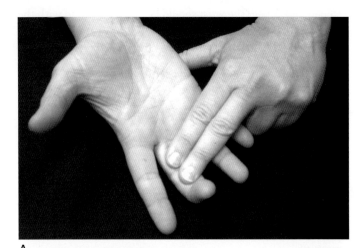

A

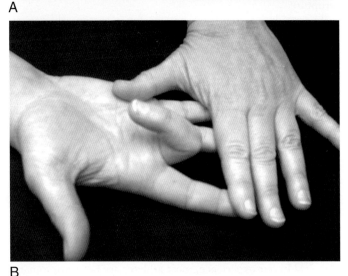

B

Figure 41-26 A, Testing of the flexor digitorum profundus. The intact profundus tendon actively flexes the distal interphalangeal joint. **B,** Testing the flexor digitorum superficialis, which actively flexes the proximal interphalangeal joint. The profundus unit is inactivated by passive extension of the other fingers.

Type 1 usually reflects the most severe injury as the blood supply from the vincular system is disrupted and the diffusion pathway is not functional. The tendon must be reinserted within 7 to 10 days following injury or it will become retracted and nonrepairable.

In type 2 injury, the tendon retracts to the PIP joint and is held there by a long vinculum attachment. Presumably because of the intact profusion to the vinculum and the fact that the tendon remains in its sheath, nutrition through profusion and diffusion is relatively intact. On examination, tenderness is usually maximal at the PIP joint and no palmar mass is palpable, thus differentiating it from type 1. Optimal treatment of type 2 is by early repair, but repair may be delayed 3 to 6 weeks or even as long as 3 months according to Leddy.[95] It should be remembered that it is possible for a type 2 to convert to a type 1 on a delayed basis, particularly in the case of an athlete completing the season prior to repair.

In type 3, the avulsed bony fragment is usually trapped by the A-4 pulley, preventing proximal retraction. Here tendon nutrition is preserved and delayed repair is usually possible. However, one should be aware of cases in which the fragment is trapped by the A-4 pulley but the tendon avulsed from the fragment, producing a type 1 situation.

Following repair, the wrist should be ulnarly splinted with the wrist slightly flexed and MCP joints in 50 to 60 degrees of flexion and interphalangeal joints in relative extension. Passive ROM exercises may be started within the first few days, and splinting continues for 4 to 5 weeks. If pull-out suture is used, it is removed at 4 weeks and intermittent splinting begun. Repair may also be performed by mini suture anchors, although the traditional pull-out wire is still favored by most.

If the athlete is involved in a sport in which grasping is not essential, return to competition within 2 weeks is possible with the use of a mitten-type splint or playing cast with the wrist in neutral or slight flexion with the digits flexed into the palm in the fisted position. The patient should not be allowed maximum gripping activities for 10 to 12 weeks after repair. This should always be explained in detail to the athlete and his or her family, as competing too soon after repair carries a definite risk of rerupture.

In considering treatment options for in-season athletes, all should be informed that best results are obtained from early repair regardless of the level of tendon retraction. At the high school level, we recommend early repair in most cases as career requirements are unknown and the goal is to restore normal DIP joint function. In higher levels of competition (college or professional), we discuss in detail the option for delayed repair in certain cases. Most professional athletes opt to be treated without early repair, while the collegiate athlete's desires vary according to career plans.

Many profundus avulsions are seen at a time remote from the injury. At this time, treatment options include delayed primary repair in types 2 and 3 if the injury is less than 3 months old, neglect in cases in which symptoms are minimal, excision of the retracted tendon in the palm if painful, arthrodesis of the DIP joint in cases in which the DIP is unstable or recurrent dorsal dislocation occurs, or a tendon graft through the intact sublimis.[92,96] In our experience, most athletes are not symptomatic enough to require any of the preceding procedures except occasionally excision of the tendon in the palm. The PIP joint usually functions quite normally in these patients, and the goal of independent profundus function in the ring finger is frequently not necessary except in musicians and other highly skilled professionals.

Rupture of the flexor profundus of the small finger in the palm has been reported by Stark et al,[97] secondary to nonunited hook of the hamate fractures. This should be considered in the differential diagnosis of athletes presenting with isolated small finger flexor digitorum profundus rupture particularly if the sport involves use of a bat, racquet, or golf club. In Stark et al[97] series, two cases of flexor tendon rupture in 62 cases of hook of the hamate fracture were noted. Bishop and Beckenbaugh[98] found a 25% incidence of tenosynovitis, tendon fraying, or rupture in a series of hook of hamate fractures. The tendon damage is produced as it glides against the rough bony surface of the fracture of the hook. Base fractures are more commonly associated with tendon injuries.

Diagnosis may be made clinically by demonstrating the inability to flex the DIP joint of the small finger as well as noting tenderness over the hook of the hamate. Fractures may be well demonstrated by supinated carpal tunnel views on radiographic examination or computed tomography scan. Tendon rupture may be apparent on magnetic resonance imaging. Treatment of the tendon rupture, if isolated to the flexor digitorum profundus of the small finger, may be accomplished by transfer of the flexor digitorum sublimis of the ring finger or side-to-side repair to the adjacent profundus to the ring. If multiple tendons are ruptured, primary repair may be considered, although frequently a bridge graft using flexor digitorum sublimis or free tendon graft is necessary.

Although quite rare, Schnebel et al[99] reported a case of isolated traumatic avulsion of the flexor digitorum sublimis in a college football player. Several previous cases were reported in the literature that were treated without surgical intervention, although in one case presenting with pain and loss of extension at the PIP joint, the sublimis was excised and synovectomy performed.

ROCK CLIMBER'S FINGER: INJURY TO THE PULLEY

The flexor tendon sheath is a continuous structure that includes a series of thickened fibrous tunnels called pulleys. These structures function to keep the flexor tendons adjacent to the bone during flexion/extension of the digit. Rupture of a pulley(s) may cause bowstringing of the tendon during flexion, which results in decreased power. The most important pulleys are the A-2, which attaches to the proximal phalanx, and the A-4, which attaches to the MP.

Injury to the pulley system occurs most commonly in rock climbers. Bollen[100] has noted bowstringing of variable degrees in 26% of 67 male competitive rock climbers. Rohrbough et al[101] found 26% of elite climbers had evidence of pulley rupture or attenuation. Most occurred doing a pocket-type hold of the rock, in which the DIP is flexed and PIP and MP are extended. In cadaver studies, it appears that rupture of the A-2, A-3, and A-4 pulleys is necessary for bowstringing to occur. Isolated A-2 ruptures result in pain but not instability.

Treatment is controversial. Bowers[102] recommends surgical repair and excision of scar as PIP flexion contracture is common. Other authors recommend taping and nonoperative treatment. Ring pulley supports may be effective in treatment of these injuries.

REFERENCES

1. McCue FC, Andrews JR, Hakala M, et al: The coach's finger. Am J Sports Med 1974;2:270–275.
2. DeHaven KE, Lintner DM: Athletic injuries: Comparison by age, sport, and gender. Am J Sports Med 1986;14:218–224.
3. Dawson WJ, Pullos N: Baseball injuries to the hand. Ann Emerg Med 1981;10:302–306.
4. Ellasser JC, Stein AH: Management of hand injuries in a professional football team. Review of 15 years experience with one team. Am J Sports Med 1979;7:178–182.
5. Rettig AC: Epidemiology of hand and wrist injuries in sports. Clin Sports Med 1998;17:401–406.
6. Burkhalter WE, Reyes FA: Closed treatment of fractures of the hand. Bull Hosp Jt Dis 1984;44:145–162.
7. Kaye JJ, Lister GD: Another use of the Brewerton view. J Hand Surg 1978;3:603.
8. Holst-Nielsen F: Subcapital fractures of the four ulnar metacarpal bones. Hand 1976;8:290–293.
9. Heim U, Pfeiffer KM, Meuli HC: [Results of 332 AO-osteosyntheses of the hand skeleton]. Handchirurgie 1973;5:71–77.
10. Sloan JP, Dove JP, Maheson AN, et al: Antibiotics in open fractures of the distal phalanx. J Hand Surg [Br] 1987;12:123–124.
11. Lowdon IMR: Fracture of the metacarpal neck of the little finger. Injury 1986;17:189–192.
12. Green DP, O'Brien ET: Fractures of the thumb metacarpal. South Med J 1972;65:807–814.
13. Flatt AE: Fractures. The Care of Minor Hand Injuries, 3rd ed. St. Louis, CV Mosby, 1972.
14. Jahss SA: Fractures of the metacarpals. A new method of reduction and immobilization. J Bone Joint Surg 1938;20:178–186.
15. Ford DJ, El-Hadidi S, Lunn PG, et al: Fractures of the metacarpals: Treatment by A.O. screw and plate fixation. J Hand Surg [Br] 1987;12:34–37.
16. Brown PW: The management of phalangeal and metacarpal fracture. Surg Clin North Am 1973;53:1393–1437.
17. Edwards GS Jr, O'Brien ET, Heckman MM: Retrograde cross pinning of transverse metacarpal and phalangeal fractures. Hand 1982;14:141–148.
18. Gonzalez MH, Igram CM, Hall RF Jr: Flexible intramedullary nailing for metacarpal fractures. J Hand Surg [Am] 1995;20:382–387.
19. Mann RJ, Black D, Constine R, et al: A quantitative comparison of metacarpal fracture stability with five different methods of internal fixation. J Hand Surg [Am] 1985;10:1024–1028.
20. Vanik RK, Weber RC, Matloub HS, et al: The comparative strengths of internal fixation techniques. J Hand Surg [Am] 1984;9:216–221.
21. Hastings H II, Cohen MS: Screw fixation of the diaphysis of the metacarpals. In Blair WF (ed): Techniques in Hand Surgery. Baltimore, Williams & Wilkins, 1996, pp 246–254.
22. Howe LM: Fractures of the hand. Scand J Plast Reconstr Hand Surg 1993;27:317–319.
23. Kahler DM: Fractures and dislocations of the base of the thumb. J South Orthop Assoc 1995;4:69–76.
24. Lilling M, Weinberg H: The mechanism of dorsal fracture dislocation of the fifth carpometacarpal joint. J Hand Surg 1979;4:340–342.
25. Burkhalter WE: Closed treatment of hand fractures. J Hand Surg [Am] 1989;14:390–393.
26. Freeland AE, Jabaley ME: Screw fixation of the diaphysis for phalangeal fractures. In Blair WF (ed): Techniques in Hand Surgery. Baltimore, Williams & Wilkins, 1996, pp 192–201.
27. Hastings H II: Unstable metacarpal and phalangeal fracture treatment with screws and plates. Clin Orthop 1987;214:37–52.
28. Bloem JJ: The treatment and prognosis of uncomplicated dislocated fractures of the metacarpals and phalanges. Arch Chir Neerl 1971;23:55–65.
29. McNealy RW, Lichtenstein ME: Fractures of the metacarpals and phalanges. West J Surg Obstet Gynecol 1935;43:156–161.
30. Strickland JW, Steichen JB, Kleinman WB, et al: Factors influencing digital performance after phalangeal fracture. In Strickland JW,
31. Strickland JW, Steichen JB, Kleinman WB, et al: Phalangeal fractures: Factors influencing digital performance. Orthop Rev 1982;11:39–51.
32. Dabezies EJ, Schutte JP: Fixation of metacarpal and phalangeal fractures with miniature plates and screws. J Hand Surg 1986;11:283–288.
33. Green DP, Anderson JR: Closed reduction and percutaneous pin fixation of fractured phalanges. J Bone Joint Surg 1973;55:1651–1654.
34. Schneider LH: Fracture of the distal phalanx. Hand Clin 1988;4:537–547.
35. Butt WD: Fractures of the hand. I. Description. CMAJ 1962;86:731–735.
36. Eaton RG: Joint Injuries of the Hand. Springfield, IL, Charles C Thomas, 1971, pp 51–66.
37. Glickel SZ, Barron OA, Eaton RG: Dislocation and ligament injuries in the digits. In Green DP (ed): Surgery of the Hand, 4th ed. New York, Churchill Livingstone, 1991, pp 772–781.
38. Heyman P, Gelberman RH, Duncan K, et al: Injuries of the ulnar collateral ligament of the thumb metacarpophalangeal joint. Biomechanical and prospective clinical studies on the usefulness of valgus stress testing. Clin Orthop 1993;292:165–171.
39. Smith RJ: Post-traumatic instability of the metacarpophalangeal joint of the thumb. J Bone Joint Surg Am 1977;59:14–21.
40. Durham JW, Khuri S, Kim MH: Acute and late radial collateral ligament injuries of the thumb metacarpophalangeal joint. J Hand Surg [Am] 1993;18:232–237.
41. Frank WE, Dobyns J: Surgical pathology of collateral ligamentous injuries of the thumb. Clin Orthop 1972;83:102–114.
42. Moberg E, Stener B: Injuries to the ligament of the thumb and fingers: Diagnosis, treatment, and prognosis. Acta Chir Scand 1953;106:166–186.
43. Bowers WH, Hurst LC: Gamekeeper's thumb. Evaluation by arthrography and stress roentgenography. J Bone Joint Surg Am 1977;59:519–524.
44. Stener B: Displacement of the ruptured ulnar collateral ligament of the metacarpo-phalangeal joint of the thumb. A clinical and anatomical study. J Bone Joint Surg Br 1962;44:869–879.
45. Melone CP Jr, Beldner S, Basuk RS: Thumb collateral ligament injuries. An anatomic basis for treatment. Hand Clin 2000;16:345–357.
46. Spaeth HJ, Abrams RA, Bock GW, et al: Gamekeepers thumb: Differentiation of non-displaced and displaced tears of the ulnar collateral ligament with MR imaging. Radiology 1993;188:553–556.
47. Landsman JC, Seitz WH Jr, Froimson AI, et al: Splint immobilization of gamekeeper's thumb. Orthopedics 1995;18:1161–1165.
48. Kozin SH: Treatment of thumb ulnar collateral ligament ruptures with the Mitek bone anchor. Ann Plast Surg 1995;35:1–5.
49. Lane LB: Acute grade III ulnar collateral ligament ruptures. A new surgical and rehabilitation protocol. Am J Sports Med 1991;19:234–237.
50. McCue FC, Hakala MW, Andrews JR, et al: Ulnar collateral ligament injuries of the thumb in athletes. Sport Med 1974;2:70–90.
51. Melone CP, Brodsky JW, Hendrickson RP: Primary and secondary repair of thumb metacarpophalangeal joint collateral ligament injuries. Orthop Trans 1984;8:382–383.
52. Camp RA, Weatherwax RJ, Miller EB: Chronic posttraumatic radial instability of the thumb metacarpophalangeal joint. J Hand Surg [Am] 1980;5:221–225.
53. Lamb DW, Abernethy PJ, Fragiadakis E: Injuries of the metacarpophalangeal joint of the thumb. Hand 1971;3:164–168.
54. Shah J, Patel M: Dislocation of the carpometacarpal joint of the thumb. A report of four cases. Clin Orthop 1983;175:166–169.
55. Eaton RG, Littler JW: Ligament reconstruction for the painful thumb carpometacarpal joint. J Bone Joint Surg Am 1973;55B:1655–1666.
56. Slattery PG: The dorsal plate of the proximal interphalangeal joint. J Hand Surg [Br] 1990;15:68–73.

57. Kiefhaber TR, Stern PJ, Grood ES: Lateral stability of the proximal interphalangeal joint. J Hand Surg [Am] 1986;11:661–669.

58. Green DP: Dislocations and ligamentous injuries of the hand. In Evarts CM (ed): Surgery of the Musculoskeletal System, vol 1, 2nd ed. New York, Churchill Livingstone, 1990, pp 385–448.

59. Thompson JS, Eaton RG: Volar dislocation of the proximal interphalangeal joint. J Hand Surg 1977;2:232.

60. Chabon SJ, Siegel DB: Use of the Herbert bone screw compression jig to reduce and stabilize a Bennett fracture. Orthop Rev 1993;22:97–99.

61. Duncan KH, Jupiter JB: Intraarticular osteotomy for malunion of metacarpal head fractures. J Hand Surg [Am] 1989;14:888–893.

62. Fischer MD, McElfresh EC: Physeal and periphyseal injuries of the hand. Patterns of injury and results of treatment. Hand Clin 1994;10:287–301.

63. Fitzgerald JAW, Kahn MA: The conservative management of fractures of the shafts of the phalangeal and the fingers by combined traction-splintage. J Hand Surg [Br] 1984;9:303–308.

64. Greenfield GQ: Dislocation of the interphalangeal joint of the thumb. J Trauma 1981;21:901–902.

65. McLaughlin HL: Complex "locked" dislocation of the metacarpophalangeal joint. J Trauma 1965;5:683–688.

66. Miller RJ: Dislocations and fracture dislocations of the metacarpophalangeal joint of the thumb. Hand Clin 1988;41:45–65.

67. Lane CS: Detecting occult fractures of the metacarpal head: The Brewerton view. J Hand Surg [Am] 1977;2:131–133.

68. Isani A, Melone CP: Ligamentous injuries of the hand in athletes. Clin Sports Med 1986;5:757–772.

69. Abouna JM, Brown H: The treatment of mallet finger. The results in a series of 148 consecutive cases and a review of the literature. Br J Surg 1968;55:653–667.

70. Kaplan EB: Anatomy, injuries, and treatment of the extensor apparatus of the hand and fingers. Clin Orthop 1959;13:24–41.

71. McCue FC, Wooten SL: Closed tendon injuries of the hand in athletics. Clin Sports Med 1986;5:741–755.

72. Doyle JR: Extensor tendons-acute injuries. In Green DP (ed): Operative Hand Surgery. New York, Churchill Livingstone, 1982, pp 2045–2072.

73. McFarlane RM, Hampole MK: Treatment of extensor tendon injuries of the hand. Can J Surg 1973;16:366–375.

74. Lange RH, Engber WD: Hyperextension mallet finger. Orthopedics 1983;6:1426–1431.

75. Crawford GP: The molded polyethylene splint for mallet finger deformities. J Hand Surg [Am] 1984;9:231–237.

76. Hofmeister EP, Mazurek MT, Shin AY, Bishop AT: Extension block pinning for large mallet fractures. J Hand Surg [Am] 2003;28:453–459.

77. Wehbe MA, Schneider LH: Mallet fractures. J Bone Joint Surg Am 1984;66:658–669.

78. Patel MR, Lipson LB, Desai SS: Conservative treatment of mallet thumb. J Hand Surg [Am] 1986;11:45–47.

79. Din KM, Meggitt BF: Mallet thumb. J Bone Joint Surg Br 1983;65:606–607.

80. Miura T, Nakamura R, Torii S: Conservative treatment for a ruptured extensor tendon on the dorsum of the proximal phalanges of the thumb (mallet thumb). J Hand Surg [Am] 1986;11:229–233.

81. Burton RI: Extensor tendons—Late reconstruction. In Green DP (ed): Operative Hand Surgery. New York, Churchill Livingstone, 1982, p 2073.

82. Spinner M, Choi BY: Anterior dislocation of the proximal interphalangeal joint, a cause of rupture of the central slip of the extensor mechanism. J Bone Joint Surg Am 1970;52:1329–1336.

83. Cardon LJ, Toh S, Tsubo K: Traumatic boutonniere deformity of the thumb. J Hand Surg [Br] 2000;25:505–508.

84. Elson RA: Dislocation of the extensor tendons of the hand: Report of a case. J Bone Joint Surg Br 1967;49:324–326.

85. Kettelkamp DB, Flatt AE, Moulds R: Traumatic dislocation of the long finger extensor tendon: A clinical, anatomical, and biomechanical study. J Bone Joint Surg Am 1971;53:229–240.

86. Harvey FJ, Hume KF: Spontaneous recurrent ulnar dislocation of the long extensor tendons of the fingers. J Hand Surg 1980;5:492–494.

87. Ritts GD, Wood MB, Engber WD: Nonoperative treatment of traumatic dislocations of the extensor digitorum tendons in patients without rheumatoid disorders. J Hand Surg [Am] 1985;10:714–716.

88. McCoy FJ, Winsky AJ: Lumbrical loop operation for luxation of the extensor tendons of the hand. Plast Reconstr Surg 1969;44:142–146.

89. Wheeldon FT: Recurrent dislocation of extensor tendons. J Bone Joint Surg Br 1954;36:612–617.

90. Melone CP: Hand Injuries in Boxing. Medical Aspects of Boxing. New York, CRC Press, in press.

91. McMaster PE: Tendons and muscle ruptures: Clinical and experimental studies on the causes and location of subcutaneous ruptures. J Bone Joint Surg 1933;15:705–722.

92. Leddy JP, Packer JW: Avulsion of the profundus tendon insertion in athletes. J Hand Surg 1977;2:66–69.

93. Manske PR, Lesker PA: Avulsion of the ring finger digitorum profundus tendon: An experimental study. Hand 1978;10:52–55.

94. Potenza AD: Critical evaluation of flexor tendon healing and adhesion formation without artificial digital sheaths: An experimental study. J Bone Joint Surg Am 1963;45:1217–1233.

95. Leddy JP: Flexor tendons—Acute injuries. In Green DP (ed): Operative Hand Surgery. New York, Churchill Livingstone, 1982, pp 1935–1968.

96. Stark HH, Zemel NP, Boyes TH, et al: Flexor tendon graft through intact superficial tendon. J Hand Surg 1977;2:456–461.

97. Stark HH, Jobe FW, Boyes JH, et al: Fracture of the hook of the hamate in athletes. J Hand Surg [Am] 1977;59:575–582.

98. Bishop AT, Beckenbaugh RD: Fracture of the hamate hook. J Hand Surg 1988;13:135–139.

99. Schnebel BE, Flesher D, Garcia-Moral C: Isolated traumatic avulsion of the flexor digitorum sublimes: A case report. Am J Sports Med 1989;17:692–694.

100. Bollen SR, Gunson CK: Hand injuries in competition climbers. Br J Sports Med 1990;24:16–18.

101. Rohrbough JT, Mudge MK, Schilling RC: Overuse injuries in the elite rock climber. Med Sci Sports Exerc 2000;32:1369–1372.

102. Bowers WH, Kuzma GR, Bynum DK: Closed traumatic rupture of finger flexor pulleys. J Hand Surg [Am] 1994;19:782–787.

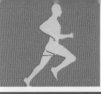

42 Hand and Wrist Rehabilitation

Constantine Charoglu

In This Chapter

INTRODUCTION

- Rehabilitation is an integral part of the treatment of hand and wrist injuries. It may be used throughout the patient's treatment course.

- Most patients with hand and wrist injuries can be treated with a general program that emphasizes splinting, edema control, range of motion, and strengthening.

- A subset of hand and wrist injuries requires specific rehabilitation protocols.

- Patients who fail to obtain adequate range of motion can be treated with dynamic and static splinting.

OVERVIEW

Rehabilitation may be used in the early, middle, and late stages of treatment of hand and wrist injuries. It will often have an impact on the patient's ultimate result. Other factors affecting outcome include the severity of the injury, the treatment of the injury, and patient-specific factors. Together these influence the physician's choice, timing, and intensity of rehabilitation protocols.

The ability of an athlete to recover from an injury depends in part on the magnitude of the trauma. Patients with high-energy injuries that involve multiple systems are likely to recover less function than those with low-energy injuries. For example, patients with extensor tendon lacerations over a fracture recover significantly less motion than those with isolated extensor tendon lacerations.

Patient-specific factors also play a role in recovery. A patient's innate ability to recover from trauma may influence the timing and nature of a rehabilitation protocol. Young patients with hypermobile joints are generally less prone to stiffness than older patients with thick brawny hands or swollen arthritic interpha-

langeal joints. Older patients with hand injuries may require early mobilization to regain a functional range of motion, whereas younger patients may tolerate longer periods of immobilization.

Most athletes with hand and wrist injuries need a simple program that emphasizes splinting, edema control, range of motion, and strengthening. A subset of injuries requires specific therapy protocols. This chapter begins with a review of the general techniques aimed at regaining motion and strength. It then describes protocols that have been developed to treat selected sports-related injuries.

GENERAL HAND AND WRIST REHABILITATION

Splinting

Static splints are often applied soon after hand and wrist injuries occur. The goal of splinting is to immobilize the hand in a position that is safe for injured tissues. When inflamed tissues are rested, a reduction in pain and inflammation follows. Splints are discontinued once the affected tissues heal and before the hand stiffens.

The safe or intrinsic plus position is recommended for most injuries, although it is not appropriate in all cases. Splints applied for tendon injuries, tendon transfers, and contracture releases often require positions that deviate from the safe position. A description of these is beyond the scope of this chapter. In addition, few injuries require immobilization beyond the minimum number of joints necessary. For example, a splint applied for a fifth metacarpal neck fracture should not preclude thumb, index, and middle finger motion.

The safe or intrinsic plus position for the hand and wrist is 20 degrees of wrist dorsiflexion, 70 degrees of metacarpophalangeal flexion, and full extension at the interphalangeal joints (Fig. 42-1). The thumb is extended and maximally abducted. Wrist extension will tend to flex the metacarpophalangeal joints by tenodesis. The metacarpophalangeal joint's collateral ligaments are placed on stretch with joint flexion, due to the anatomy of the metacarpal head. These ligaments should not be allowed to stiffen in a shortened position, as occurs with metacarpophalangeal joint extension. The interphalangeal joints are extended to prevent collateral ligament and volar plate contracture that occurs with immobilization of these joints in flexion.

Edema Control

As with splinting, edema control should be initiated as early as possible. If it is not controlled, edema leads to contractures by two mechanisms. First, significant hand edema mechanically

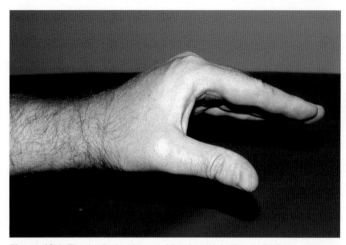

Figure 42-1 The intrinsic plus position is used when splinting to prevent contractures.

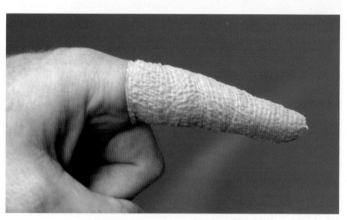

Figure 42-3 A finger wrapped in Coban.

blocks motion. Second, edematous fluid that is high in protein leads to fibroplasia and scarring (Fig. 42-2).

A number of techniques are used to decrease postinjury edema. Splints described in the previous section minimize the effects of edema on soft tissues. Elevation is extremely important in the early phases of injury. Hand elevation above the heart may be accomplished in a number of ways. A simple method available to nearly all patients is taping a pillow (or two if needed) around the forearm at night. This prevents the hand from falling to or below the level of the heart. Soft foam forearm upper extremity splints are commercially available and accomplish the same goal.

External compression also reduces edema but must be used judiciously in the early period. Patients must be monitored for compartment syndrome and capillary refill must be checked. Ace bandages provide compression while also allowing tissue expansion. They are useful in the acute phase and help prevent complications from constrictive dressings. Coban (3M, Minneapolis, MN), a self-adhesive wrap, is used in the subacute period. One-inch Coban is wrapped around digits in a retrograde fashion (Fig. 42-3). Patients are taught how to check for capil-

lary refill. The wrap is removed after 20 to 30 minutes. Larger areas of edema in the subacute period are controlled with compressive sleeves or gloves or an intermittent pneumatic compression garment.

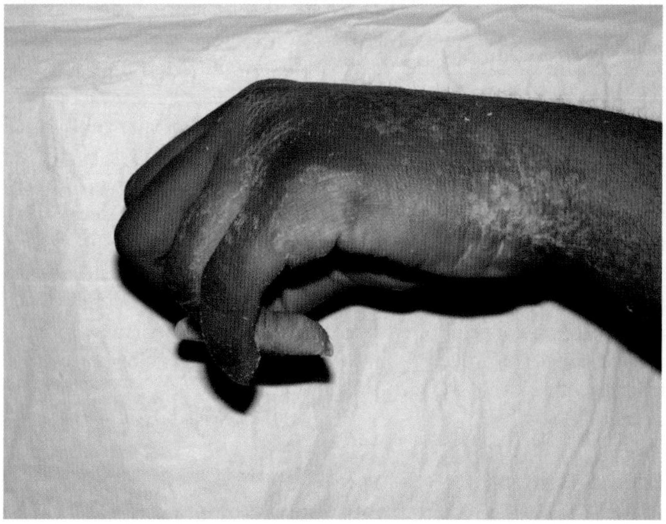

Active exercise is a very useful way of reducing edema and is used as the rehabilitation process progresses. Muscle contraction decreases hydrostatic pressure and interstitial volume. This increases lymphatic and venous return, which removes fluid from the extremity. Active motion through a full range is emphasized as limited motion will not achieve this result.

Range of Motion

Some injuries, such as tendon lacerations, ligament ruptures, and fractures require joint immobilization or specific limitations on motion in the first few weeks. Other injuries tolerate early active range of motion. The benefits of active range of motion include decreased edema, increased joint nutrition, and prevention of muscle atrophy. As a general rule, active range of motion is initiated once the injury stabilizes and is capable of withstanding forces generated by an active motion protocol.

A six-pack hand exercise program is often recommended by physicians and therapists (Fig. 42-4). When done properly, it ranges every joint in the digits and is the first set of hand exercises taught. Joint blocking techniques concentrate the patient's effort on specific joints and are used when isolated areas of digital stiffness are identified. Wrist flexion, extension, radial, and ulnar deviation exercises are also taught. Circumduction of the wrist allows patients to perform all these motions. Finally, forearm supination and pronation exercises are taught. Patients can view this motion best while holding a pen in their fist with the arm at the side and the elbow flexed 90 degrees. A hammer, or other heavy object, is used as a gentle assist if desired. Supination is often difficult to regain after distal radius fractures, and this exercise is emphasized once immobilization is discontinued.

Gentle active-assisted motion is useful when patients have difficulty regaining motion. Passive or forceful manipulation is avoided. This tears tissue and adds to the cycle of pain, edema, stiffness, and scarring. Continuous passive motion machines stretch tissue in a slow, sustained way, avoid problems with passive manipulation, and may benefit patients by preventing contractures. Unfortunately, continuous passive motion does not have the beneficial effects on edema and muscle tone that active range of motion does and is not a substitute for it.

Figure 42-2 An edematous hand after cast removal in treatment of a metacarpal fracture.

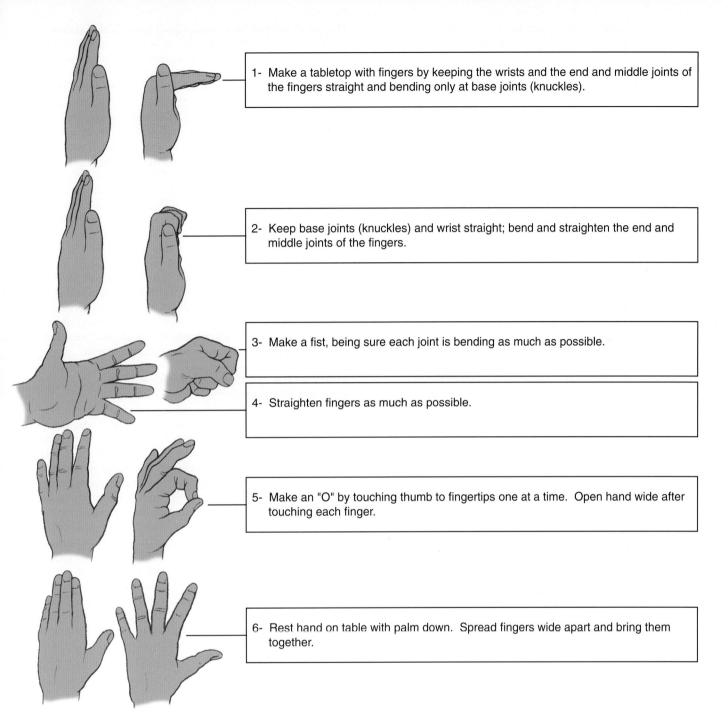

1- Make a tabletop with fingers by keeping the wrists and the end and middle joints of the fingers straight and bending only at base joints (knuckles).

2- Keep base joints (knuckles) and wrist straight; bend and straighten the end and middle joints of the fingers.

3- Make a fist, being sure each joint is bending as much as possible.

4- Straighten fingers as much as possible.

5- Make an "O" by touching thumb to fingertips one at a time. Open hand wide after touching each finger.

6- Rest hand on table with palm down. Spread fingers wide apart and bring them together.

Figure 42-4 The six-pack hand exercise program.

Strengthening

Strengthening is the final phase of hand and wrist rehabilitation and is performed once a functional range of motion is achieved and after bone, tendon, and ligament healing has occurred. A variety of exercise products are available to assist in rehabilitation of the injured athlete's hand. Rubber band grippers and Theraputty are used for strengthening grip and intrinsic and extrinsic hand musculature. Free weights, elastic tubing, Thera-Band, and weight-lifting equipment are used in training facilities, clinics, and homes to strengthen the proximal larger muscles of the wrist, elbow, and shoulder. A home exercise program with diagrams is provided to increase patient under-standing and compliance. Lower weights and higher repetitions are initially used. Patients progress to heavier weights as tolerated.

REHABILITATION FOR SPECIFIC INJURIES

While general techniques of hand and wrist rehabilitation are sufficient in most cases, some hand and wrist injuries require specific protocols. This section details rehabilitation for several common injuries seen in the athletic population. Specific rehabilitation protocols exist for many other injuries such as tendon lacerations, tendon transfers, and ligament repairs. Readers are referred to relevant chapters in this and other texts.

Finger Tip Injuries

The spectrum of finger tip injuries includes subungual hematomas, nail bed injuries, and distal finger tip amputations. The complications and rehabilitation of these injuries are similar and are treated as one entity in this section. Patients with finger tip injuries can expect some degree of cold intolerance, hypersensitivity, and stiffness. Some studies have found that cold intolerance resolves with time. Hypersensitivity and stiffness can be addressed with the specific rehabilitation protocol described.

Dressing changes are initiated 3 to 5 days after the injury. Open wounds are treated with twice-daily soaks and nonadherent dressings until they are healed. This may take as long as 4 weeks. One-inch Coban is wrapped distally to proximally for edema control. This should continue until digital edema resolves. Range-of-motion exercises are initiated after the first dressing change. Joint blocking exercises allow patients to concentrate effort at the DIP and PIP joints. Motion at the DIP joint may need to be delayed if a distal phalanx fracture is present. In this case, or if a significant soft-tissue wound is present, a protective splint over the middle and distal phalanges should be used. The splint should not impede PIP motion.

After suture removal, desensitization may be needed. The use of this technique is patient dependent. Hypersensitive patients have soft cotton balls rubbed against their finger tips four times daily for 10 minutes. Progressively more coarse substances are used as the patient's tolerance improves.

Despite the best efforts of patients, physicians, and therapists, contractures can occur. Older patients with thick brawny fingers and swollen arthritic interphalangeal joints are most likely to develop contractures. Dynamic splinting and serial casting can be used for these refractory cases.

Acute Boutonniere

Fingers with boutonniere deformities remain flexed at the PIP joint and hyperextended at the DIP joint. These deformities commonly occur after injury to the central slip. Volar subluxation of the lateral bands, contracture of the oblique retinacular ligament, and joint contractures can result if they are left untreated. Conservative management of boutonniere deformities should be attempted in almost all cases.

Acute cases without joint contractures are treated with PIP joint splinting in extension. Active and passive DIP joint flexion is encouraged. This forces the lateral bands dorsal and prevents contracture of the oblique retinacular ligament. Splint use is weaned at 6 weeks, and gradual PIP flexion is begun. If extensor lag develops, splint use can be prolonged. Extensor lags that occur late are difficult to correct. Contractures of the PIP joint with limited DIP flexion are treated with dynamic extension splinting followed by the static splinting protocol described previously.

Dorsal Proximal Interphalangeal Joint Dislocations

Dorsal PIP dislocations are the most common PIP dislocation. They occur when the middle phalanx translates dorsal to the proximal phalanx. The vast majority of these injuries can be managed with closed reduction. Dorsal PIP fracture dislocations are a different entity and are discussed in Chapter 41.

Initial management consists of closed reduction and evaluation with postreduction radiographs. These must document a reduced joint and the absence of a significant fracture. Subtle subluxation is best seen on a lateral radiograph of the finger. Stable dislocations remain reduced in extension and are treated with buddy taping and immediate motion. Unstable dislocations are immobilized in 30 degrees of flexion with a dorsal blocking splint. Radiographs must confirm a concentric reduction in this position. One-inch Coban wraps are used for edema control. Active range of motion is begun in a few days in the extension block splint. At the beginning of the fourth week, the dorsal block splint is brought out 10 degrees per week. In the sixth week, the splint is discontinued. Dynamic flexion and extension splints can be used as needed. Patients should be counseled that the PIP joint might remain swollen for up to a year. Results for simple dislocations are generally excellent, and nearly normal range of motion can be expected in most patients.

Proximal Interphalangeal Joint Collateral Ligament Injuries

PIP joint collateral ligament injuries can be simple sprains, with injured but intact ligaments. Pain, edema, and tenderness on one side of the PIP joint are present. The joint has stable endpoints with varus and valgus stress in extension and at 30 degrees. Buddy taping to an adjacent digit is the initial treatment. Tape is applied in the proximal phalanx and middle phalanx regions. It should not interfere with PIP joint motion. In cases with marked swelling and pain, splinting can be used for a short period of time. Splints are discontinued by week 3, but buddy taping is continued for 6 weeks, particularly if an early return to sports activity is anticipated.

PIP joint collateral ligaments can also rupture completely with the volar plate during a joint dislocation. Reduction usually places the ligament in its normal anatomic position. Postreduction radiographs of the finger in extension are used to evaluate stability. Stable reductions are treated with buddy taping as previously described. Dorsal subluxation is treated with the protocol for PIP dislocations.

CONCLUSIONS

Most athletic hand and wrist injuries can be treated with a standard rehabilitation protocol emphasizing splinting, edema control, range of motion, and strengthening. Patient factors and the injury itself influence the timing and intensity of these protocols. A subset of injuries may require specific rehabilitation programs.

SECTION V

Lower Back and Pelvis

43 Lumbar Spine

Robert G. Watkins

In This Chapter

Low back pain
Diagnosis
Spondylolysis and spondylolisthesis
Intervertebral disk injury
Nonoperative treatment and rehabilitation
Operative indications
Individual sports

INTRODUCTION

- Low back pain is common in all types of sports.

- The annulus and disk are excellent at resisting compressive forces, but torsional forces often lead to injury.

- An adolescent athlete with back pain that persists more than 3 weeks should undergo radiography.

- Athletes with mechanical back pain commonly have annular tears of the disk, facet joint syndrome, tears of the lumbodorsal fascia, muscle injury, or sacroiliac (SI) joint pain.

- The keys to nonoperative treatment for lumbar spine injury are controlling inflammation, restricting activity, and progressing to a spine stability rehabilitation program.

- Operative treatment is reserved for cases that are severe enough to warrant surgery, have failed conservative care, and present with an anatomic lesion that is correctable, for which a proper postoperative rehabilitation program is present.

Low back pain has been a significant factor in many different types of athletic activity. The severity and extent of back pain often determines the actual ability to compete and is a worry to all concerned from the athlete, the family, coaches and trainers to those responsible for paying the bills. Essentially, treatment of the athlete with a lumbar spine injury involves an understanding of basic anatomy and biomechanical function of the spine, the diagnosis of conditions affecting the lumbar spine, proper use of diagnostic studies, and a systematized all-inclusive history and physical examination. We must understand some factors that are important in predisposing the athlete to lumbar spine problems as well as training and therapeutic techniques to prevent lumbar spine problems in athletes. Among the predisposing factors to back pain in athletes are increased trunk length and stiff lower extremities.[1] Occulta spina bifida is found in a higher incidence of patients developing lower lumbar spondy-

lotic defects.[2] The exact relationship of exercise and back pain in athletes, when compared to the average population, does not demonstrate an increased incidence in back pain in athletes participating in organized sports as opposed to regular students. Fairbank et al[1] found that back pain was more common in students who avoided sports than those who participated. Fisk et al,[3] in 1984, found that prolonged sitting was the most important factor in the pathogenesis of Scheuermann's disease as opposed to athletes lifting weights, undergoing compressive stresses, or doing heavy lifting and part-time work. This study showed that 56% of males and 30% of females had some radiographic evidence of changes similar to Scheuermann's disease in one review of 500 students 17 and 18 years old.[3]

In an interesting review of back injuries, Keene et al[4] found that 80% of back injuries occurred during practice, 6% during competition, and 14% during preseason conditioning. The incidence was 8% in men and 6% in women, which was of no statistical significance. The nature of the injury was usually acute (59%) or overuse (12%), while aggravation of a pre-existing condition occurred in 29%.

RELEVANT ANATOMY

The vertebral column is a series of linked intervertebral joints. The joint is made up of the intervertebral disk, its two facet joints, concomitant ligaments, vessels, and nerves and is referred to as a neuromotion segment. A neuromotion segment is considered to be one of the basic units of spinal anatomy and function. The lumbar spine has a lordotic curve, which plays an important role in the biomechanics. The spine is broken down into two basic columns. The anterior column consists of the disk and vertebral bodies and the accompanying longitudinal ligaments, the anterior longitudinal ligament, and the posterior longitudinal ligament. The posterior column consists of the facet joints, lamina, spinous process, and ligamentum flavin and pars interarticularis. The disk may be described as a circular, multilaminate ligament that connects the two vertebrae together. The nucleus pulposus is the central, more gelatinous portion of the disk; the annulus is the multilayered woven basket with fibers at precise angles to resist torsional and compression forces. The annulus is firmly anchored to the end plate of the vertebrae. The annulus, nucleus, and accompanying end plates are excellent at resisting compressive forces but fare less well in resisting torsional forces. The orientation of the facet joint is different at every level of the spine. In the lumbar spine, the facet joints are oriented in a more transitional phase from parasagittal in the upper lumbar spine to a more coronal orientation in the lower lumbar spine. This parasagittal orientation allows good motion in flexion and extension and less motion in lateral flexion. The parasagittal orientation of the facet joints would naturally resist rotation, but produces victims of high torsional forces that overcome the strength of the joint, tearing the annulus and injuring the facet joints.

When considering the anatomy of the spine, one must consider the important role of the entire cylinder of the trunk and its supporting muscles. The static ligamentous structures of the spine provide considerable resistance to injury, but this resistance in itself would be insufficient to produce proper spinal strength without the additional support provided the spine through the trunk musculature and lumbodorsal fascia. Muscle control of the lumbodorsal fascia allows a much higher resistance to bending and loading stresses. The lumbodorsal fascia and the muscles attaching to it must be considered of equal importance to the more specialized function of the intervertebral disk and facet joints.

CLINICAL FEATURES AND EVALUATION

It cannot be emphasized enough that obtaining a proper diagnosis in the athlete presenting with low back pain is crucial. It is the key to initiating an appropriately aggressive diagnostic and therapeutic plan.[5,6] Particularly in the adolescent and younger athlete, a high index of suspicion must be maintained to accurately diagnose conditions such as stress fractures and spondylotic defects.[7] A great variety of pathologic conditions can be diagnosed on plain radiographs and their relationship to the athlete and his or her sport can be more specifically addressed.[8] The bone scan is a vital part of the diagnostic armamentarium of the physician caring for lumbar spine problems in athletes. An adolescent athlete with significant back pain, persisting longer than 3 weeks should have radiographs and a bone scan. Findings can range from unusual conditions such as osteoid osteoma, infection, and stress fracture of the SI joint to the more routine spondylotic defects. The incidence of spondylotic defects seen on radiography is approximately 30% to 38% and 35% of young athletes presenting with significant lumbar pain have a positive bone scan.[7,9]

In diagnosing the exact cause of lumbar spine pain in athletes, age is an important factor. Younger athletes are certainly more likely to have stress fractures and to have congenital predispositions to stress fractures. Diseases that affect growing cartilage are more common in young athletes, such as Scheuermann's disease. In the mature athlete, often the radiographic assessment involves distinguishing between age-related, asymptomatic changes and symptomatic recent trauma. Is the L5-S1 disk degeneration the symptomatic level in a 30-year-old athlete or is it an asymptomatic finding? The diagnostic plan must use an organized system of diagnosing the most common conditions as well as retain the ability to diagnose the rare conditions such as a herniation of the inferior lumbar space[10] or osteoid osteoma.

One of the most important diagnoses to make in the athlete with back and leg pain is that of peripheral nerve injury and peripheral nerve entrapment. There is a great variety of peripheral nerve problems ranging from a generalized peripheral neuropathy to carpal tunnel syndrome, pyriformis syndrome, peroneal nerve injury, femoral neuropathy, and interdigital neuroma. The chief reason for performing electromyography and a nerve conduction study of the lower extremities is to diagnose a peripheral nerve problem. The nerve conduction study combined with a careful physical examination can at least raise the distinct possibility of a peripheral nerve problem and heighten the diagnostician's skepticism concerning small, potentially asymptomatic spinal lesions in the role of the patient's extremity nerve pain.

Spondylolysis and Spondylolisthesis

Age is important in the natural history of spondylolysis and spondylolisthesis. There is a 4.4% incidence at age 6, increasing to 6% by adulthood. It is unusual for children to present with spondylolysis before the age of 5, and unusual for young children to present with severe spondylolisthesis grade III or IV. Most symptoms appear in adolescence, but fortunately the risk of progression after adolescence is low, being approximately 15%. Symptoms cannot be correlated with the degree of slip. A high degree of slip may present with deformity and very little pain. Many times, it is the pain of an injury that leads to the identification of spondylolisthesis that may not be originating in the spondylolisthetic segment.

Isthmic spondylolisthesis develops as a stress fracture. It is thought that there is a hereditary predisposition to developing the stress fracture, and there is certainly the predisposition in conditions in which the bone of the pars inarticularis is not sufficient to withstand normal stresses. Also, certain mechanical activities that expose the patient to repeated biomechanical challenge, increasing stress concentration on the pars interarticularis, have a higher incidence of spondylolisthesis. The concept of repeated microtrauma with concentration of these stresses in the pars has become increasingly recognized in adolescent athletes participating in certain sports such as gymnastics and weight lifting.

The most common site for spondylolysis and spondylolisthesis is L5-S1 (Fig. 43-1). The slippage in spondylolisthesis results from the lack of support of the posterior elements produced by the stress fracture of the pars (Fig. 43-2). The spectrum of neurologic involvement runs from rare to more common with higher degree slips. The majority of neurologic deficits are an L5 radiculopathy with an L5-S1 spondylolisthesis. Cauda equina symptoms are more likely in grade III or IV slips. Cauda equina neurologic loss is rare.

The diagnostic and therapeutic plan for spondylolisthesis begins with a high degree of diagnostic suspicion in the adolescent athlete with low back pain. As many as one third of adolescent athletes presenting with low back pain will have a

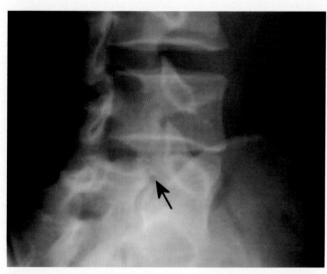

Figure 43-1 L5 spondylolysis (arrow) in a 20-year-old baseball player.

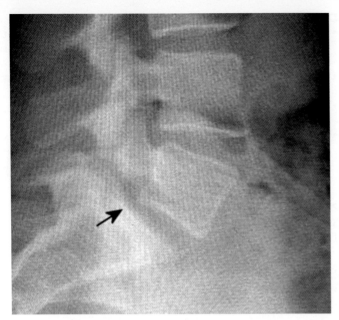

Figure 43-2 Grade I spondylolisthesis *(arrow).*

positive bone scan for a stress fracture. Certainly patients with low back pain that is not resolved within 3 weeks should have a bone scan. If the bone scan is positive, the patient should have a computed tomography scan to see whether there is a demonstrable stress fracture or whether the bone scan is positive due to impending fracture. If the bone scan is negative and the lumbosacral pain persists, magnetic resonance imaging is indicated. A combination of magnetic resonance imaging, bone scans, and computed tomography used in this manner should diagnose most significant pathologies in the lumbar spine.

The treatment plan for spondylolisthesis is basically rest or restriction of enough activity to relieve the symptoms. This may vary from simply removing the athlete from the sport until the pain has significantly improved; to immobilization in a lumbosacral corset, Boston brace, or thoracolumbosacral orthosis; to bed rest; to casting.

In summary, stop the pain through whatever amount of inactivity it takes. We routinely, with a hot bone scan, brace the patient and restrict that activity for a minimum of 3 months. Repeat the bone scan, and if it is negative, sufficient healing has taken place to allow beginning a rehabilitation program. If the bone scan is still positive and the athlete asymptomatic, it can be a very difficult decision at times whether to start the athlete back onto a rehabilitation program or continue further restriction. We usually continue restrictions another 3 months. Unilateral hot bone scans with or without fracture demonstrated have a reasonably high incidence of healing, and adolescent athletes in general should be treated with the idea of healing the defect. Bilateral stress fractures are less likely to heal despite comprehensive nonoperative therapy.

If the bone scan is cold and there is a spondylitic defect present, we should treat these patients as we would any patient with mechanical low back pain. This usually involves a progressively vigorous trunk stability rehabilitation program. We put no permanent restrictions on athletes with spondylolysis or spondylolisthesis. It should be obvious that patients with grade III to IV spondylolisthesis are less likely to be able to participate in vigorous sports activities without pain and discomfort. They

should probably avoid the heavy strength sports such as football and weight lifting.

There is a high incidence of spondylolysis and grade I and II spondylolisthesis in sports. As a long-term factor, this condition is not considered to be significant in an athlete's ability to play.

BIOMECHANICS

The understanding of the basic biomechanics of the lumbar spine begins with an understanding of the forces and stresses applied to the spine as related to the normal curvatures of the spine. Because of the lordotic shape of the spine, the results of vectorial force on the spine is usually made up of a vertical axial loading compressive force perpendicular to the surface of the disk and one horizontal to the disk, producing a shear strain. The combination of these two forces produces both tensile stresses in the annulus fibrosis and a shear force on the neural arch. The center of gravity of body weight is anterior to the spine. This weight times the distance back to the spine produces a lever arm effect of the weight of the body. This is resisted by the erector spinae muscles and the lumbodorsal fascia. When there are abnormal stresses applied to this equation, it may result in annular tears of the intervertebral disks or stress fractures of the neural arch due to this excessive resistive force. The most common place for stress fractures, of course, is the pars interarticularis.

The basic mechanism of injury produces a combined vector of force that may be difficult to analyze in a force diagram. The three basic mechanisms of injury to consider are (1) compression or weight loading to the spine; (2) torque or rotation, which may result in various shear forces in a more horizontal plane; (3) tensile stress produced through excessive motion of the spine.

The compressive type of stress is more common in sports that require high body weight and massive strengthening such as football and weight lifting. Torsional stresses occur in throwing athletes such as baseball players and golfers. Motion sports that put tremendous tensile stresses on the spine include gymnastics, ballet, dance, pole vault, and high jump.

Sprains and strains can result from direct blows. Certainly in sports like football there can be muscle contusion; muscle stretch; and tears of fascia, ligaments, and, occasionally, muscle.

Lumbar fractures can occur from direct blows to the back with fracture of the spinous process or twisting injuries that avulse the transverse process. Vertebral body end plate fracture from axial compression load on the disk is a relatively common source of compressive disk injury. While the annulus is more likely injured in rotation, the end plate is more vulnerable to compression than the annulus. Flexion rotation fracture dislocations of the cervical and lumbar spine are certainly possible. Axial loading compression injuries can result from jarring injuries in motor sports or boating. In any sport in which one athlete falls on another, the mechanism is similar to that of the coal face injury with the rock falling on the coal miner while he is on all fours. An athlete can suffer an asymmetrical loading, rotational injury to his or her thoracolumbar spine.

The intervertebral disk is injured predominantly through rotation and shear, producing circumferential and radial tears. Initially, the layers may actually separate or the inner layers break. As the inner layers weaken and are torn, there is added stress on the outer layers. This can produce a radial tear of the intervertebral disk. With the outer layers torn, the inner layers of the annulus break off and, with portions of the nucleus, are forced with axial loading to the place of least resistance, the weak area in the annulus. The outer areas of annulus are richly innervated, producing tremendous pain and reflex spasm when the annulus tears. The spasm and pain are mediated through the sinuvertebral nerve with anastomosis through the spinal nerve to the posterior primary ramus. As the herniated material extrudes and produces pain from the traversing or exiting nerve root itself, the patient may develop sciatica or radiculopathy. Intravesical infiltration of the granulation tissue adds increased potential for painful sensation in the annulus. The annulus, with time, can heal, although the healing annulus will not retain the same biomechanical function capability as the original intervertebral disk.

Biomechanical functioning of the spinal column and its relationship to the biomechanics of nerve tissue involves several basic concepts:

1. In the spine, flexion of the lumbar spine increases the size of the intervertebral canal and the intervertebral foramina.[11,12]
2. Extension decreases the size of the intervertebral canal and the intervertebral foramina.[12]
3. Flexion increases dural sac and nerve root tension.[13]
4. Extension decreases dural sac and nerve root tension.[13]
5. Front flexion, axial loading, flexion, and upright posture increase intravesical pressure.
6. With flexion, the annulus bulges anteriorly.[14]
7. With extension, the annulus bulges posteriorly.[14]
8. Nuclear shift in an injured disk is poorly documented but probably corresponds with annular bulge.[12]
9. Rotation and torsion produce annular tears and disk herniations.[15]

The conclusion of these concepts is that motion does have an effect on the nerves and the neuromotion segments of an injured area. For example, if there is a spinal obstructive problem such as spinal stenosis, extension exercises can further compress the neurologic structures and make them worse, or if there is a nerve root tension problem such as disk herniation, then flexion can produce increased tension in an already tense nerve and increase symptoms.

HISTORY AND PHYSICAL EXAMINATION

The key to a proper history and physical examination is to have a standardized plan that accomplishes the needed specific objectives.

Quantitate the Morbidity
Use a scale value of pain, function, and occupation to understand how sick the patient is. Converse in detail with the patient to hear the inflections and manner of pain description. Detail the time of disability and the time of origin of the pain.

Delineate the Psychosocial Factors
Know what psychological effect the pain has had on the patient. Know the social, economic, and legal results of the patient's disability. Understand what can be gained by his or her being sick or well. Derive an understanding of what role these factors are playing in the patient's complaints.

Eliminate the Possibility of Tumors, Infections, and Neurologic Crisis
These diseases have a certain urgency that requires immediate attention and a diagnostic and therapeutic regimen that is very different from disk disease.

Diagnose the Clinical Syndrome
- Nonmechanical back and/or leg pain: inflammatory, constant pain, minimally affected by activity, usually worse at night or early morning.
- Mechanical back and/or leg pain: made worse by activity and Valsalva maneuver and relieved by rest.
- Sciatica: predominantly radicular pain, positive stretch signs, with or without neurologic deficit.
- Neurogenic claudication: radiating leg or calf pain that is worse with ambulation, negative stretch signs that are worse with spine extension and relieved with flexion.

Pinpoint the Pathophysiology Causing the Syndrome
Three important determinations are listed:

1. What level? Which neuromotion segment?
2. Which nerve?
3. What pathology: What is the exact structure or disease process in that neuromotion segment that is causing the pain?

The history and physical examination are the first step in determining the clinical syndrome. Some key factors are the following:

- The time of day during which the pain is worse.
- A comparison of pain levels during walking, sitting, and standing.
- The effects of Valsalva maneuver, coughing, and sneezing on pain.
- The type of injury and duration of the problem.
- The percentage of back versus leg pain. We insist on getting an accurate estimate of the amount of discomfort in the back and legs. There must be two numbers that add up to 100%.

The physical examination should address the following:

- The presentation of sciatic stretch signs.
- The neurologic deficit.
- Back and lower extremity stiffness and loss of range of motion.
- The exact location of tenderness and radiation of pain or paresthesia.
- Maneuvers during the examination that reproduce the pain.

The history determines whether it is an axial (back pain) or extremity (leg pain) problem. What is the exact percentage of back versus leg pain? Is the pain made worse by the mechanical activity or is it a constant resting pain? Is the pain worsened by maneuvers that increase intradiskal or intraspinal pressure? Is there significant night pain?

Classic radiculopathy causes radicular pain radiating into a specific dermatomal pattern, with paresis, loss of sensation, and reflex loss. The radicular pattern of the pain and neurologic examination determine the nerve involved.

The classic history of radiculopathy resulting from a disk herniation is back pain that progresses to predominantly leg pain (Fig. 43-3). It is made worse by increases in intraspinal pressure such as coughing, sneezing, and sitting. Leg pain predominates over back pain and mechanical factors increase the pain. Physical examination shows positive nerve stretch signs. A dermatomal distribution of leg pain that is made worse by straight-leg raising, the sitting or supine position, leg-straight

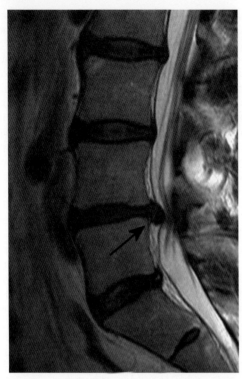

Figure 43-3 Herniated disk *(arrow)* leading to radicular symptoms in a 36-year-old golfer.

foot dorsiflexion, neck flexion, jugular compression, and direct palpation of the popliteal nerve or sciatic notch is characteristic of radiculopathy. A source of radicular pain not found in this description is that caused by spinal stenosis. Spinal stenosis usually lacks positive nerve stretch signs but has the characteristic history of neurogenic claudication (i.e., leg and calf pain produced by ambulation). Pain that does not go away immediately on stopping is made worse with spinal extension and is relieved by flexion. The pain progresses proximally to distally.

The pain drawing is a major help in accomplishing the objectives of the physical examination. Each patient completes the pain drawing using a rating system, which distinguishes organic from psychological pain fairly well. It also helps localize the symptoms for future reference with pain reproduction studies such as with diskography and postoperative evaluations.

The initial history and physical examination determine the aggressiveness of the diagnostic and therapeutic regimen. The morbidity rating and the length of time that the patient has had the problem are important parts of the history and physical examination that help determine the aggressiveness and invasiveness of the diagnostic plan. The leg pain versus back pain ratio is an important factor in determining which diagnostic tests are indicated. Leg pain leads to tests for nerve function and obstructive pathology such as electromyography/nerve conduction, myelography, contrast computed tomography, and magnetic resonance imaging. Back pain evaluation includes at times bone scan, magnetic resonance imaging, and diskography. The clinical syndrome should be divided into predominantly mechanical pain, axial pain, and leg pain. An appropriate treatment program can begin, based on the initial evaluation.

Most athletic injuries to the lumbar spine fall under the category of mechanical, axial, back, or leg pain. Within this category, a number of different syndromes exist:

1. Annular tears of the intervertebral disk, usually a loaded compressive rotatory injury to the lumbar spine producing severe, disabling back spasm and pain. The pain is usually worse in flexion with coughing, sneezing, straining, upright posture, sitting, and with any other situations that increase intradiskal pressure. There may be referred leg pain, low back pain with straight-leg raising, and anterior spinal tenderness. Annular tears can be produced with as little as 3 degrees of high torque rotation.[16] Facet joint alignment that protects the disk from rotatory forces may lead to facet joint injuries as the annulus fails in rotation.

2. Facet joint syndrome, more typically occurring in extension with rotation, reproduced with extension rotation during the examination. This may present with a pain on rising from flexion, with a lateral shift in the extension motion. Point tenderness in the paraspinous area over the facet joint occurs and may be associated with referred leg pain.

3. Tears of the lumbodorsal fascia and muscle injuries and contusions present with muscle spasm, stiffness, and many of the characteristics of facet joint syndrome in annular tears.

4. Sacroiliac joint pain and pain in the posterior superior iliac spine. The most common referred pain area for pain from the annulus in the intervertebral disk and the neuromotion segment of the spine is across the posterior surface of the ilium, which includes the posterior superior iliac spine and SI joint. Sciatic pain can hurt in the sciatic joint area as well as the sciatic notch and buttocks. While injuries can occur to the SI joint, the vast majority of syndromes presenting with SI joint pain are thought to be the result of referred pain from a neuromotion segment in the spine.

The most important thing to be done with the physical examination of the athlete is to demonstrate what types of motions reproduce the patient's pain. Where exactly is the tenderness present? What deformity is present in the spine? If there is a lateral shift, in which direction? The chief advantage that physical therapists have in the treatment of the athlete with lumbar spine pain is the hands-on approach directed specifically to motions and activities that produce and relieve the pain. Local modalities can be directed specifically to localized areas of inflammation and pain. Treatment of referred pain areas through localized treatment in the area of the referred pain plays a major role in the relief of symptoms and return to performance. Therefore, techniques of treatment of referred pain should be understood and used. This may vary from injections of local anesthetic, cortisone injection, transcutaneous electrical nerve stimulation units, ultrasound, or ice.

Another important diagnostic category in these patients is to identify areas of contracture and weakness on the physical examination. The physician and therapist can make the diagnosis by carefully examining the patient for areas of muscle atrophy and loss of range of motion. Some very sophisticated testing and dynamic electromyographic function has identified localized areas of weakness in the shoulders of pitchers as well as in the abdominal musculature of baseball pitchers.[17] There is a great deal of skill involved in the physician being able to recognize these deficiencies in the physical examination and design a rehabilitation program to correct them.

TREATMENT OPTIONS: NONOPERATIVE CARE

The nonoperative treatment plan begins with several basic rules.

1. Stop the inflammation.
2. Restore strength.
3. Restore flexibility.
4. Restore aerobic conditioning.
5. Return to full function.

To stop the inflammation of the spine in an injured athlete often requires rest and immobilization. We try to limit the rest and immobilization to the minimum. Bed rest produces stiffness and weakness, which causes the pain to persist. Stiffness and weakness are the antithesis of the body functions necessary for athletic performance. Every day of rest and immobilization may result in weeks of rehabilitation before the athlete is able to return to performance. As in motion treatment of lower extremity injuries, such as fracture bracing and postoperative continuous motion machines, rapid rehabilitation of lumbar injuries in athletes requires effective means of mobilizing the patient. Bed rest longer than 3 to 5 days is not of any benefit in the natural history of the disease. Rapid mobilization requires strong anti-inflammatory medications, ranging from epidural steroids, oral Medrol Dosepak (methylprednisolone), Indocin SR (indomethacin) to other nonsteroidal anti-inflammatories, and aspirin. Also used are lots of ice, transcutaneous electrical nerve stimulation units, and mobilization with casts, corsets, and braces. Corsets and braces are used for only limited periods of time, and strengthening techniques are started when the brace is applied in order to remove braces as soon as possible. Braces in themselves can cause a significant amount of stiffness and weakness. Exact timetables are difficult. It should be based on the individual patient's history and physical examination. As a general rule, our acute disk herniations are treated with 3 to 5 days of bed rest, then on to the physical therapist within 7 days, a corset for no longer than 10 to 14 days, and indomethacin, occasionally oral corticosteroids, and, less commonly, epidural injections. The therapist begins the neutral-position, isometric trunk strengthening program, and, depending on the response of the patient, this evolves into resistive strengthening, motion, and aerobic conditioning as tolerated.

Part of the key to being able to initiate early therapy is the understanding, based on the physical examination, of what makes the patient symptomatic. Nonoperative care should be the basis of any therapeutic approach to athletes with lumbar spine injuries. With the exception of cauda equina injuries, this should also be true in the athlete with a neurologic deficit. The key to effective nonoperative care is to have a well thought-out, balanced biomechanical approach. Common questions asked are whether to do extension exercises or flexion exercises or twisting exercises, what type of aerobic exercising should be done, when can someone lift weights, what role do Nautilus beautification exercises have in rehabilitation of the athlete, and also what type of nonoperative rehabilitation is best for the individual athlete's sport?

Everyone is concerned about the risk of increasing neurologic deficit and of producing a neurologic deficit through nonoperative care. So often, nonoperative care, in the face of a neurologic deficit, consists of no care. Bed rest is the usual initial stage for the athlete with a lumbar spine injury and neurologic deficit. It is thought that bed rest best protects the patient from increasing injury to the spine and therefore increasing neurologic deficit. Unfortunately, bed rest also produces profound weakness, loss of biomechanical function, and actually increases the risk of injury due to the weakness and stiffness that results. If the purpose of bed rest were to decrease inflammation, the logical substitute would be aggressive anti-inflammatory medication. If the objective of bed rest is to prevent motion, braces and casts can be substituted. If the objective of bed rest is to prevent abnormal motion that could injure the spine, it is with the understanding that certain mechanical functions have to take place. Patients get on and off bed pans; they get up to go to the bathroom; they roll over in bed. They cough, sneeze, and eventually have to walk. It seems logical that if we could design an exercise system that would prevent abnormal motion while restoring strength and flexibility in a biomechanically sound fashion, then the spine could be protected from the abnormal motion that produces injury and healing potentially could be enhanced. This enhancement takes place through normal biomechanical motion in the injured part through increasing strength and flexibility in the adjacent portions of the body that can absorb the stress potentially directed to the injured part and in preventing the atrophy, weakness, and stiffness caused by inactivity.

Lumbar spine injuries in athletes are a category that often demands prevention of atrophy and stiffness and restoration to maximum function as early as possible. Also, it follows that if this restoration can be achieved in athletes, it can function just as effectively in steelworkers, secretaries, weekend athletes, and housewives. The key to the program, obviously, lies in safety and effectiveness. If you could summarize an overall basis to our preferred rehabilitation program, it would lie in the concept of neutral-position isometric strengthening for the spine. This program is derived from work by Jeff Saal, MD, Arthur White, MD, and others, including Celeste Randolph, Ann Robinson, and Clive Brewster at the Kerlan Jobe Orthopedic Clinic, Inglewood, CA.

Trunk Stretching and Strengthening Program

This exercise program concentrates on trunk strength and trunk mobility, balance, coordination, and aerobic conditioning. It is a practical application of the use of trunk strengthening in back treatment, injury prevention, and improved performance in throwers.

It certainly appears that the place to begin the rehabilitation program in an injured lumbar spine, with or without neurologic deficit, should be with neutral-position isometric strengthening. The basis of the trunk stability program is to have the patient find a neutral, pain-free position, lying supine on the ground with the knees flexed and feet on the ground. This is about as atraumatic as possible a beginning to rehabilitation, but it also forms the basis of an important concept in not only athletic function, but also activities of daily living for everyone. We retrain muscles to work to support the spine while the patient is using his or her arms and legs. It is not only theoretically ideal but is practically possible. Teaching muscle control with tight, rigid contraction of the muscles, controlling the spine through the lumbodorsal fascia, with the gluteus maximus, oblique abdominals, and latissimus dorsi, not only produces protection of the lumbar spine but also improves athletic performance. The power and strength of any throwing athlete come from his or her trunk. Lifting weight requires functioning of the lumbodorsal fascia.

Trunk strength also prevents back injuries and is an important treatment method for back pain. While treatment plans for patients with symptomatic back pain may include similar exercises, each of the treatment plans should be designed to match the examination and the symptoms. Any trunk strengthening plan puts strain on the spine and can produce back pain due to overload. Therefore, it should be conducted in a controlled, progressive manner.

The key to safe strengthening is the ability to maintain the spine in a safe, neutral position during the strengthening exercises. For upper body strengthening, the spine must be well aligned with the chest-out/chin-tucked posture. Doing isometric trunk exercises and upper body exercises emphasizing this chest-out/chin-tucked posture will strengthen the support of the cervical spine, strengthen the postural muscles necessary for maintaining proper body alignment, and prevent neck pain due to athletic activity.

For the lower body, trunk control plays a vital role in the ability to rotate and transfer torque safely. Trunk strengthening exercises such as sit-ups and spine extensions produce strength. Flexibility produces a protective range of motion but often the key is providing trunk strength and control at the proper moment during the athletic activity. For example, a baseball hitter goes from flexion through rotation to extension. If his trunk musculature does not maintain rigid control, despite these changes in the axis of alignment, he may lose power or get a back injury. Therefore, one can have strong muscles but, if they do not fire in sequence at the proper time, they will not protect the athlete from injury and certainly will not enhance performance. A key to producing a safe range of motion is to begin trunk control in the safe neutral position, establish muscle control in that position, and maintain it through the necessary range of motion to perform the athletic activity.

We begin our identification of the neutral spine position with the dead-bug exercises (Fig. 43-4). Dead-bug exercises are done supine with the knees flexed and feet on the floor. With the assistance of the trainer or therapist, the player pushes his or her lumbar spine toward the mat until he or she exerts a moderate amount of force on the examiner's hand. This is not exaggerated, back flattening extreme force, but a moderate amount of painless force on the examiner's hand. The player is then taught to maintain this same amount of force through abdominal contraction while

1. Raising one foot.
2. Raising the other foot.
3. Raising one arm.
4. Raising the other arm.
5. Raising one leg.
6. Raising the other leg.
7. Doing a leg flexion and extension with one foot.
8. Doing a leg flexion and extension with the other foot.

These same exercises can be performed with weights on the arms or legs.

The next stage for torque-transfer athletes is resistance to rotation, first supine, then sitting, then standing, in which the player maintains the neutral spine control position while resisting rotation of the upper body on the lower body. The player resists the rotational activity exerted by the therapist or trainer.

In the next stage, the player maintains trunk control while actively rotating through a short range of motion against the trainer's resistance. This is done in numerous positions to teach trunk control regardless of the position of the patient.

An additional benefit can be beach ball exercises. A 4-foot diameter ball can be used to do partial sit-ups while maintaining control of the ball, with the trunk in neutral position; the sit-ups and resistive sit-ups are done on the ball.

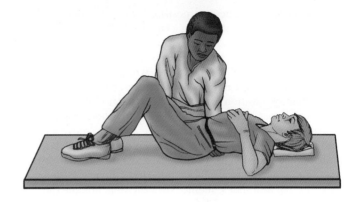
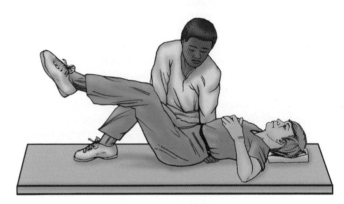
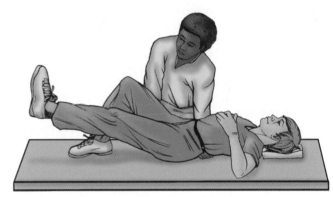

Figure 43-4 Begin identification of the neutral position with the dead-bug exercises. The dead-bug exercises are done supine, with the knees flexed and feet on the floor. With the assistance of the trainer or therapist, the patient pushes his or her lumbar spine toward the mat until he or she exerts a moderate amount of force on the examiner's hand. This is not exaggerated, extreme force, but a moderate amount of painless force on the examiner's hand. The patient is then taught to maintain this same amount of force through abdominal contraction while performing the exercises.

Lower extremity, trunk, and upper extremity strengthening must be done with concentration on maintaining the neutral trunk control position. It must be taught away from the sport, without a bat or ball, on the training table or floor. A routine is established for the player: think trunk control—neutral position—tense contractions. Trunk control is incorporated into throwing or batting. This will ultimately produce a more efficient transfer of torque from the lower to the upper extremities, that is, better bat control for a hitter and better endurance and ball control for a pitcher. An additional valuable benefit can be prevention of spinal injuries and spinal pain due to the athletic activity.

After establishing neutral position isometric control of the spine, extremity strengthening can begin. Probably the most important muscles needed to protect the spine itself are the quadriceps. The ability to return to work after a back injury has been directly related to quadriceps strength. Yet, quadriceps strengthening should not be done in the standard sitting, full knee extension position in a patient with severe lower back pain. Quadriceps strengthening should be done without irritating the lumbar spine mechanical pain. Also, the ability to move a weight from 90 degrees to zero degrees may not relate as specifically to lumbar spine function as quadriceps strength obtained through functional strengthening. Functional strengthening is done initially through wall slides, sliding down the wall, holding the position for 10 seconds, and sliding back up at varying depths. We begin this immediately postoperatively in our patients. Other activities include throwing the medicine ball in a flexed-knee position. Sports such as a Versiclimber, stationary cycle, and other techniques are used to teach quadriceps function while maintaining trunk control and during sports-related activity. Gluteal and hip extensor strengthening is important but must be done without inadvertently hyperextending the lumbar spine. Exercise bands that provide resistance to hip extension without a lot of spine extension are important as are other techniques that de-emphasize spine motion while producing isometric extensor strength. Nautilus machines can be very important in a safe, protected range of motion for extremity strengthening. The key to use of the Nautilus is good isometric trunk control in a pain-free neutral position prior to use of the machines. If you can establish trunk control first, then a safe protected range of motion is a good position for the spine. Therefore, military presses, latissimus, arm, and lower extremity leg strengthening with machines can be of benefit while protecting the spine. Spinal strength testing machines have been shown to be of benefit in predicting return to work. The ability to perform flexion extension exercises or resistance rotational exercises on a machine may not translate to functional spinal activity during athletics. We have not recommended such machines for treatment of lumbar injuries.

Stretching exercises are an important part of any rehabilitation program. The more flexible the legs, arms, and upper body are, the more likely there will be a proportional decrease in motion stress on the injured lumbar spine. If some muscle control is established first, through the strengthening program, then the spine can be held in a stable position while stretching of the extremities takes place. It is important to note that hamstring stretching too often is taken to the extent that it produces abnormal lumbar spine motion. Stretching the lower extremity past the point of pelvic motion only strains the spine and does not increase hamstring flexibility. Too often lumbar spine conditions are irritated because of excessive lumbar motion during hamstring stretching. The spine should be neutralized and held in a neutral, stable position when doing hamstring stretching exercises. Lumbar spine motion is important also, but it is not the initial stage of the rehabilitation program. Lumbar spine motion is begun with good muscle control of the spine during the motion exercises. The most common initial stage of motion is the "cat/cow" position on all fours, a position in which muscle control can be easily maintained.

The stretch exercises are a critical component of the program. Stretching increases the functional range of motion of the trunk and legs. Increasing the functional range of motion decreases the likelihood of lumbar spine injury during the strengthening program during play.

Most low back injuries occur when the player exceeds the strength of the spine and its range of motion. The stretching program provides a greater area of pain-free and injury-free function. For example, if a player who is stiff, having 10 degrees of spine extension and 20 degrees of spinal rotation, suddenly reaches for a ball producing 25 degrees of extension and 40 degrees of rotation, injury to his back can occur through tearing stiff tissue. If the mobility exercises produce a functional range of motion of 40 degrees of extension and 50 degrees of rotation, injury is less likely to occur. This is a protective range of motion.

The chief finding in our ball players with back pain is loss of spine extension, loss of rotation (usually greater in one direction), poor mechanics in rotation, and weak abdominals. Once the back pain starts, the weakness and contractions increase. However, this program is designed for performance enhancement and injury prevention, not treatment of back pain.

Aerobic Conditioning

There are numerous methods available for aerobic conditioning. Often we see athletes who prefer a specific technique such as running but have developed pain and problems directly related to running.

Cross-training is critically important in getting over aerobic exercise–induced injury. Not only does the runner with an injured back have to do the stretching and strengthening rehabilitation program, but he or she must learn cross-training for aerobic exercise. Water running, swimming, cycling, Nordic-Track, Versiclimber, and rowing machines all can produce the needed aerobic conditioning outside of the injurious sport. The benefit of swimming and water running program[18] should be obvious. The total unweighting of the spine in water removes many of the compressive loads and allows good physical activity without the tremendous pounding and straining of running. The NordicTrack builds tremendous conditioning with strong use of the arms and increases cardiac output without the pounding of running. The Versiclimber and cycling have several things in common. First, the back can be positioned in a very beneficial position for back protection while still getting good aerobic conditioning. The cycling is slightly bent forward, which, of course, helps the stenotic spine. The Versiclimber is erect, which removes as much nerve root tension as possible. Both have the same potential hazard in that the pelvis should not laterally tilt during cycling or the Versiclimber. For the Versiclimber, short steps should be taken to prevent a lot of pelvic tilting with the motion, and in cycling, the legs should not become fully extended with the effect of reaching for the peddles, as this allows the pelvis to tilt down. Keep the pelvis and spine in a firm, neutral position with good isometric control during the aerobic conditioning. Running stairs or stair-walking machines produce good leg strength and good hip extensor strength. Rowing machines obviously can injure the back, but if done properly, with rigid muscle control of the spine, in a neutral, pain-free position, the benefit from the upper extremity and lower extremity exercise can produce good aerobic conditioning without spine stress. The better aerobic condition the athlete is in, the less likely he or she will sustain injury, including lumbar spine injury. Therefore, aerobic conditioning is an important part of every spine rehabilitation program.

The summary of an effective nonoperative treatment program for lumbar spine injuries follows:

1. Stop the inflammation. We prefer anti-inflammatory medications, Indocin SR being our most standard medication.

Patients should be advised of potential complications of any anti-inflammatory medications. Medrol Dosepak may be used in more difficult clinical situations, as are epidural cortisone injections.

2. Restricted activity. This may vary from 24 to 72 hours of bed rest to immediate immobilization in a lumbosacral corset and restriction of painful activities.

3. Spinal stability rehabilitation program. We began this rehabilitation program as soon as practically possible. It may vary from in bed, in the hospital, at 24 hours to the first available outpatient appointment in physical therapy.

In reference to some of the questions asked earlier

1. Do you start flexion or extension exercises?
   The answer is you start neither. You start neutral isometric control exercises.

2. Do you use twisting exercises?
   Twisting exercises can be the most injurious exercises in any rehabilitation program, yet torsional rotation is an important part of many sports. The answer lies in producing tight, rigid trunk control that controls the spine during rotational activities with the motion occurring predominantly in the shoulders, hips, and legs, and the athlete is able to produce a parallelism between his or her shoulders and pelvis during rotation, especially during the contact portion of the rotational sport. A twisting exercise that allows loss of muscle control of the spine during exercise can be injurious and may not be of benefit. Rotational strengthening can be important but has to be started with close observation and control. We twist many times in an average day and twisting is a part of many sports. Having a pain-free rotational range of motion is important; therefore, proper, slow active stretching in rotation is important. Part of the key is not to twist, but to teach the patient to rotate the whole body.

3. What type of aerobic conditioning should be performed?
   The type that holds the spine in its most advantageous position and best unweights the spine from injurious compressive loads

4. When can someone lift weights?
   A patient can lift weights when he or she can do it safely, meaning having tight, rigid trunk control. The patient can protect the spine while strengthening the extremities. A patient can lift weights when he or she can understand the role of balance, speed, and proper mechanical advantage in weight lifting. The key to functional weight lifting for the athlete is not to lift the weight at the greatest mechanical disadvantage, but to simulate positioning used in his or her sport. Isometric trunk control and position protection are done first, then resistive weight lifting.

5. What role do weight machine exercises have?
   Weight machines can be a distinctly advantageous control situation for resistive weight lifting. All machines that strengthen the extremities require proper spinal control first. We have not used trunk strengthening machines such as the flexion, extension, and rotation machine in patients with back problems. Questions still linger as to their benefit. The key probably lies in proper use of the equipment and combining the equipment with a functional isometric control type system such as the trunk stability rehabilitation program.

6. What type of nonoperative rehabilitation is best for the individual athlete's sport?

It depends greatly on the sport and the demands as to rotational activity, compressive load, and tensile extremes of range of motion.

7. When can a professional athlete return to his or her sport after spinal surgery or a serious injury that has been treated nonoperatively?
   The athlete can return when he or she can

   - Complete level 5 of our trunk stabilization program.
   - Complete a course of sport-specific exercises for his or her sport.
   - Attain an appropriate level of aerobic conditioning for his or her sport.
   - Practice the sport fully.
   - Return slowly to the sport with some limit on the amount of time played.
   - Continue to do the level 5 stabilization exercises after the return to play.

TREATMENT OPTIONS: OPERATIVE CARE

The chief indications for spine surgery in the athlete are the same indications for spine surgery in any patient:

1. Sufficient morbidity to warrant surgery.
2. Failure of conservative care.
3. An anatomic lesion that can be corrected with a safe, effective operation.
4. A proper, fully developed postoperative rehabilitation program. A proper postoperative rehabilitation program cannot be overemphasized. The failure to do postoperative spinal rehabilitation would be similar to a failure to do postoperative knee strengthening after reconstruction of the knee. The patient wants restoration of function. The surgeon should be able to guide the patient through his or her restoration to function. The morbidity of the patient, amount of pain, loss of function, and occupation are the critical factors.

Spinal operations to enhance performance rather than relieve disabling pain are a part of managing the care of athletes, a part that requires a great deal of experience not only in spinal surgery but also in dealing with athletes.

There are numerous factors to consider. One must always keep in mind the full longevity of the patient. Young players can lay out a year after a significant spinal surgery and still return to play. Older players are less likely to return to play after a major spinal reconstructive operation.

What the player will be like after his or her career and condition of his or her spine at that time should be of major importance in decision making early in the player's career.

A major factor is calculating the risk if the operation is successful. In many sports, after a spinal fusion or a major resection of a supporting structure in a lumbar decompression, the percentage chance of return may be no greater after the operation than without the operation.

A surgeon must carefully question his or her advice concerning surgery if he or she does not have a proper alternative to the surgery and good, effective nonoperative care. Frankly, if all one knows is the surgical technique and if one does not have a proper understanding of and delivery system for a nonoperative care program, then that person should not advise surgery for the athlete. An appropriate team approach among specialists in nonoperative care and specialists in operative care can be worked out so that the decision for surgery is well founded, but the surgeon must understand and participate in that portion of the decision-making process, namely, a sufficient nonoperative treatment plan.

The anatomic lesion is critically important. A simply extruded disk herniation, of course, can be very amenable to a one-level microscopic lumbar diskectomy, but an annular tear of the intervertebral disk with mild nerve root irritation will not be made better by a decompressive laminectomy and usually will be made worse because of abnormal motion in the injured disk, segmental instability, if you will, now with a nerve root scarred to the back of the annulus. In spondylolisthesis, the obvious solution may be, as it is in the majority of the patients facing surgery for this problem, a spinal fusion. Some athletes can return to their sport after a successful spinal fusion and some may not be able to. Part of the danger is in curing the radiograph and not the patient. Another possibility is curing the patient with a successful operation and leaving the player without a job.

As with everyone, an absolute indication for surgery with lumbar disk disease is progressive cauda equina syndrome or progressive neurologic deficit. Strong, relative indications are static significant neurologic deficit, unrelenting night pain, and major loss of functional capability. Mild relative indications for surgery fall more under the category of performance enhancement and return to play. There will always be patients who could live the way they are but cannot perform the way they are. This is a relative indication for surgery but must be a frequent consideration in lumbar spine injuries in athletes.

INDIVIDUAL SPORTS

The lumbar spine is a highly vulnerable area for injury in a number of different sports. The reported incidence varies from 7% to 27%.[4,6,19] It appears that while the incidence is significant and time lost may be significant, probably the most important problems lie in fear of spinal injuries and the necessity of a therapeutic plan. Lumbar pain is a big part of many sports, but an organized diagnostic and therapeutic plan can prevent permanent injury and allow full function and maximum performance.

Gymnastics
With reference to lumbar spine injuries, gymnastics is probably the most commonly mentioned sport.[20] The motions and activities of gymnastics produce tremendous strains on the lumbar spine. The hyperlordotic position used with certain maneuvers (such as the back walkovers) exerts tremendous forces on the posterior elements and requires a great deal of flexibility. The amount of lumbar flexion/extension used during flips and vaulting dismounts requires a great deal of strength to support the spine during these extremes of flexibility. Jackson[2] pointed out that female gymnasts have an 11% incidence of spondylolysis. Spondylolysis is a fatigue fracture of the neural arch, and it is thought that the vigorous lumbar motion in hyperextension in gymnastics produces the fatigue fracture. It is also interesting to note that Jackson found spina bifida occulta in 9 of 11 gymnasts with pars interarticularis defects. It is known that there is a hereditary predisposition to spondylolysis, and the findings of occult spina bifida may point out a weakness of the dorsal arch in some of these gymnasts. But certainly the role of the sport itself plays a tremendous role in a much higher incidence of spondylolysis and a much higher incidence of back pain in

general. Garrick and Requa[21] reported a very high incidence of low back pain in female gymnasts and recommended the vigorous trunk strengthening exercises that are used today to properly prepare gymnasts for their sport.

Ballet
Many of the motions used in ballet are similar to those in gymnastics. The classic maneuver that produces back problems is the arabesque position. This position requires extension and rotation of the lumbar spine. Performing a proper arabesque maneuver is the key to preventing lumbar strain. Several points have been emphasized: keep the pelvis stable, keep the extension of the spine symmetrical over all levels, and obtain good extension through the hip joints.[22]

Ballet involves the lifting of dancers, often in awkward positions. The outstretched hand produces tremendous level arm stresses across the spine of the lifting partner. Off-balance bending and lifting is a hallmark of back problems in industrial workers and yet, ballet, while balanced, is designed often to produce some of the most difficult lifts. The male dancers follow the body weight of their female partners very closely.

Spondylolysis and spondylolisthesis are common in dancers and may often produce severe mechanical back dysfunction.

Water Sports
In addition to injuries to the wrist and cervical spine, the lumbar spine in diving is subjected to added strain not only due to rapid flexion/extension changes, but also the severe back arching after entering the water. While swimming and water exercises are a major part of any back rehabilitation program, certain kicks, such as the butterfly, produce a lot of vigorous flexion/extension of the lumbar spine, especially in young swimmers. The swimmer must develop good abdominal tone and strength in order to protect his or her back during a vigorous kicking motion. Thoracic pain and round back deformities in young female breast stroke swimmers can be a problem because of the repeated round shoulder–type stroke motion.

Pole Vaulting
Pole vaulting is another sport that involves maximum flexion/extension and muscle contraction during the sport. The range of motion of the lumbar spine has been documented with high-speed photography to change from 40 degrees of extension to 130 degrees of flexion in 0.65 seconds. One can imagine the tremendous forces generated across the spine with this functional demand.[23]

Weight Lifting
As we move from the motion sports, those sports that require tremendous amounts of flexibility (in addition to strength) and involve large degrees of changes in range of motion, we go to the heavier sports. These sports require strength, lifting, and high body weight. Of course, the most common would be weight lifting. The incidence of lower back pain and problems in weight lifters is estimated to be 40%.[24] The tremendous forces exerted on the lumbar spine by lifting weights over the head produce a tremendous lever arm effect and compressive injury to the spine. The three most important things in performing weight lifting are "technique, technique, technique." Squats and dead lifts can be done, but the technique must be perfect in order to decrease the risk of a disk injury. For example, a dead lift requires erect posture, lumbar lordosis, and balance of the weight on the heels. Most lifts are begun with the spine in tight,

rigid muscle control. Tremendous extension forces occur at the hips and knees with the spine in a rigidly stable position. Success in this portion of the lift requires the body to generate tremendous rigid immobilization of the spine in the power position of slight flexion. To do a forward bent motion with the spine out of this position can be quite dangerous, resulting in tremendous shear forces across the spine. Lifting weights with the spine flexed at 90 degrees, whether they are lighter arm weights or weights across the upper back, generates tremendous lever arm effect forces. The weight times the distance to the spine result in tremendous shear forces across the lumbar spine, especially if weight is to be moved in this position. One cannot imagine muscles that must be strengthened in this dangerous and mechanically disadvantaged position. A dangerous time for weight lifters is the shift from spinal flexion to extension that occurs with lifting the weight over the head as in the clean jerk maneuver or the "snatch." Making the transition from the flexion to extension position must be done with rigid, tight muscle control. Inexperienced lifters, especially, will have no muscle control as the spine shifts from flexion to extension. A trained lifter controls that shift with rigid muscle control of the lumbodorsal fascia. The position of holding weight over the head invariably brings increased lumbar lordosis. These tremendous extension forces of the lumbar spine naturally lead to discussion of spondylolysis and spondylolisthesis. The incidence of spondylolysis in weight lifters has been estimated at 30% and the incidence of spondylolisthesis at 37%.[25] Many newer training techniques in weight lifting emphasize the role of general body conditioning, flexibility, aerobic conditioning, speed, and cross-training in addition to the ability to lift weight.

Football

Football players lift weights. It is part of the sport. The upper body forces and leg strength necessary to play football for most of the athletes involved in the sport require tremendous strength. Some football players, of course, rely on great agility, jumping, and throwing ability and eye-hand contact, but strength is the backbone of football. Every year, every professional team needs heavier, stronger athletes, especially on the offensive line. These athletes invariably go through their period of mechanical back pain as training camp begins. It is difficult to prepare an athlete in the off-season for the tremendous, rapid back extension against weight necessary for blocking in the offensive line. Extension jamming of the spine produces facet joint pain, spondylolysis, and spondylolisthesis. It is similar to the weight-lifting position of weight over the head, except it must be generated with forward leg motion and off-balance resistance to the weight while trying to carry out specific maneuvers such as blocking a man in a specific direction. These athletes require specific training in back strengthening exercises in order to prevent lumbar spine injuries.[26,27]

Safety in weight lifting is an important part of football. To have a promising football player injured in the weight room is not an uncommon occurrence. It has been estimated that more injuries may actually occur in training rather than competition.[28] This can be avoided through proper weight-lifting techniques. In addition to these extension/lifting-type forces, football involves sudden off-balance rotation. This rotation may produce transverse process fractures, torsional disk injuries, and tears in the lumbodorsal fascia. Sudden off-balance twisting is part of the game and may be caused by tremendous loads in a loose, unloaded position. Football has the added dimension of receiving unexpected, severe blows to the lumbar spine that

may produce contusion or fracture. A helmet in the ribs produces rib fractures; a helmet in the flank can produce renal contusion, retroperitoneal hemorrhage, transverse process, and spinous process fractures. Many receivers and runners suffer spondylotic defects for the same reasons as gymnasts and ballet dancers, but the most common incidence of problems is in the weight lifting. The role of the strength coach in teaching proper weight-lifting techniques and designing training schedules that prepare the lumbar spine for what is expected with football is important in preventing lumbar spine injuries in football players.

Running

Another sport that produces stiffness is running. Distance runners must cross-train with flexibility in order to prevent injury. Running involves maintenance of a specific posture with tremendous muscle exertion over a long period of time. Low back pain as well as periscapular, shoulder, and neck pain is very commonly reported in the runner. We cure the vast majority of runners who have mechanical low back pain with stretching exercises. There is also the natural tendency in runners to develop isolated abdominal weakness. Running does not naturally involve contraction of abdominal and spinal stabilizing musculature. There frequently is a significant imbalance between flexors and extensors, not only in the legs but also in the trunk. Periscapular and back pain also results from abnormal posture during running. The key to posture is good isometric trunk strength that holds the body in an upright chest-out position. Runners with low back pain should be treated with the following:

1. Vigorous stretching program that stretches the trunk as well as lower extremities.
2. Cross-training and muscle strengthening techniques that strengthen the antagonist muscles.
3. Abdominal strengthening and isometric trunk stability exercises to enhance abdominal control.
4. Chest-out strengthening exercises. Begins with abdominal strengthening and adds upper body shoulder shrugs, arms behind the back, etc., types of exercises to emphasize chest-out posturing and tight abdominal control. The basis of treating back pain in runners is stretching exercises.
5. Proper footwear for cushioning and enhancement of foot function.

ROTATIONAL AND TORSIONAL SPORTS

Rotational and torsional sports have certain characteristics in common. Baseball, golf, and the javelin all require rotation and have distinctly different demands on the spine. The javelin requires a tremendous amount of force to be generated in going from a hyperextended to a full flexion follow-through position. You do not throw a javelin 200 feet with your arm. While shoulder and arm injuries are common in javelin throwers, the key is rigid abdominal strength that produces the torque necessary to throw the javelin. Attempting to throw with the arm only will produce arm injury and in no way can generate any type of distance. Every arm injury in a javelin thrower has to be treated with trunk exercises and trunk strengthening. A rotatory lumbar spine injury in a javelin thrower is a completely debilitating injury that requires tremendous care and correction prior to returning to the sport.

Golf

Golfers notoriously have the highest incidence of back injury of any professional athlete. Paul Callaway and Frank Jobe reviewed injuries of 300 professional golfers on the Professional Golf Association tour from 1985 to 1986. Of theses 300 golfers, 230 were injured, for an incidence of 77%: 43.8% of the total injuries were spine related and 42.4% were lumbosacral. Lumbar spine pain in golfers results from torsional stress on the lumbar spine, and the key to prevention of lumbar spine pain in golfers in to minimize the torsion stress by absorbing the rotation in the hips, knees, and shoulders and spreading the rotational stresses on the spine out over the entire spine. Maintaining rigid, tight control through the power portion of the swing is critical. Proper technique in golf begins when addressing the ball. The knee flexion of the address position tenses the abdominal musculature. This abdominal tension is initiation of the trunk control necessary for a properly placed swing. The majority of the emphasis is on maintenance of parallel shoulders and pelvis through the swing. This requires rigid abdominal control and rotation between the shoulders and hips, and loss of this rigid parallel of the shoulders and pelvis can generate rotational strain on the lumbar spine. Rotation occurs between the hips and shoulders in the back swing, and the amount of back swing is not as important to the power of the swing as the ability of the golfer to regain tight muscle control as he or she proceeds from maximum back swing down through the power portion of the swing. It is the ability to obtain tight control, parallelism, and maintain it that produces the power and protection for the lumbar spine. The first advice for any recreational golfer with back pain is to cut down the back swing and the follow-through. Concentrate on the power portion of the swing. Concentrate on tight abdominal control during the power portion and minimize the excesses of rotation with back swing and follow-through. It is important also that the golf swing be symmetrical. The same amount of extension on the back swing and follow-through is important. Lateral bending should be avoided, especially in the follow-through. There is a tendency to bend to the left side and load the spine asymmetrically, producing injury. Golf is usually restricted according to the patient's symptoms.

There is no condition of the lumbar spine for which we specifically restrict golf. Many people with spondylolisthesis, through superb conditioning and care, can play relatively pain free. Premature, symptomatic degenerative disk disease is common among golfers who play a great deal, especially among professionals who not only play, but also practice long hours. People can return to golf after decompressive lumbar surgery or spinal fusion. There are significant questions about the effect of a spinal fusion on an adult professional golfer. The effect on adjacent segments and on overall spinal function may not allow any better function. Under these circumstances, fusion should be a last resort.

Because golf is not an aerobic sport, aerobic conditioning should be included in any effective lower back rehabilitation program. Fairbank et al[1] showed that higher aerobic fitness shows a strong negative correlation with the incidence of both lower back pain and disk herniation. Exercise results in increased aerobic metabolism in the outer annulus and the central portion of the nucleus pulposus, bringing about reduction of lactate concentration.[26]

Also, aerobic conditioning plays a significant role in muscle coordination during periods of fatigue. Fatigue can produce abnormal muscle function and overcompensation and thus resultant injury. Fatigue obviously can affect performance through a lack of proper balance and coordination as a result of selectively weak muscles.

Unfortunately, some patients cannot tolerate certain types of aerobic conditioning that have high levels of loading to the spine, such as jogging. However, several types of aerobic conditioning exercises are highly effective without loading the spine (e.g., water exercises[12] and the stair climber).

As structure governs function, similarly, abnormal structure governs dysfunction.[26,28] Thus, a thorough evaluation must be undertaken before strengthening and stretching exercises are begun. The examination is completed by use of radiographs, magnetic resonance imaging, computed tomography, muscle testing, range of motion, segmental testing of vertebrae for hypomobility and hypermobility, postural evaluation, palpation, and various other methods and/or tests.

Once the dysfunction is identified, appropriate treatment techniques must be used to correct the structural abnormality. This will allow for enhanced function and therefore improve the rehabilitation process in which trunk strength, muscle coordination, and balance are stressed. Trunk strength involves the muscles of the thighs, hips, and trunk. The trunk muscles include the rectus abdominus, oblique abdominus, paraspinal musculature, latissimus dorsi, and, further up the spine, the scapular stabilizers. The muscles that insert into the lumbodorsal fascia play a key role in providing adequate balance and strength for the lumbar spine and the trunk during the golf swing. Trunk strength provides a synchrony of motion between the upper and lower extremities in that there is a controlled unwinding of the upper body relative to the trunk. The power of the golf swing is transferred from the strong leg and hip musculature through the trunk and out to the end of the club head.

Trunk fatigue produces a loss of this synchrony between the upper and lower extremities. This reduction in muscle strength prevents a proper transfer of force and leads to compensations by the body. Thus, the improvement of muscle strength, coordination, the firing sequence of muscles, and body balance underlies the entire rehabilitation process and facilitates the golfer's achieving a consistent, reproducible, effective swing.

An injury to the spine can cause pain, which produces weakness and a loss of muscle control. This loss of muscle control, which can lead to further injury because the joint is now unsupported, is similar to quadriceps weakness and its cause-and-effect relationship to a knee injury. As soon as referred pain begins, muscles in the area of referred pain become weak. Any attempt to reproduce a proper golf swing under these circumstances can be difficult and can lead to continued pain, poor swing mechanics, and subsequently poor performance. Obviously, just as in a knee injury, the solution to this problem is to first correct the structural or damaged area and then strengthen that area by use of golf-specific exercises.

Baseball

Hitters, who make up another interesting group of players, include any athlete who has to swing a bat. Hitters who take a lot of batting practice, swing with great velocity, and swing with a heavy bat are subject to lumbar spine injury. An infrequent hitter, such as a pitcher, who does not have good hitting mechanics, is also vulnerable to injury. Lumbar spine problems in hitters begin with their eyes, that is, the ability to see the ball is a critical factor in swing mechanics. Abnormal swing mechanics involve a loss of control between the hips and shoulders, essentially a loss of body synchrony. Irregular and uncoordinated motion of the upper extremity and upper torso puts undue rotational strain on the lumbar spine. Injury of the lumbar spine in someone engaging in this type of torsional activity further compounds the problem by producing stiffness, weakness, and asymmetry that add to the pain and prevent satisfactory healing. The biomechanics of hitting can be considered an ocular-muscular reflex, a reference to the fact that the triggering of the bat mechanics (the triggering of the muscles) is a split-second response to what the hitter is able to see. A hitter who is not picking up the ball well tends to open the hips too early. With the bat and upper torso lagging behind, there is a sudden torsional stress to catch the shoulders and the bat up with the rest of the body. Poor visualization of the ball produces delays in hand and arm responses.

Hitting Mechanics

To diagnose and treat lumbar spine problems in the hitter, the physician should understand that hitting mechanics require power in the legs and trunk, a rigid, solid cylinder of torque transfer, and fine muscle control of the arms and wrists.

For a more practical understanding of hitting, we turned to a hitting coach and a skilled batter.[16,29] The swing starts with the stance, which relies on balance. Every player will be a little different: open or closed, feet further apart, feet closer together. The ideal is probably placement of the feet at shoulder width, but the key is balance. The batter can fashion a hole for the back foot to use in pushing off, changing the stance slightly from closed to opposite-field open for an inside pitch. Control is based on balance in the stance and proceeds to the forward stride. As a pitcher begins the windup and approach to the plate, the hitter coils up. This coiling maneuver brings the bat to the position necessary to initiate the swing. Again, regardless of the amount of motion activity, most bats come to a relatively standard position in relation to the strike zone just before the forward stride is initiated.

The hitter assumes the correct body position: the coiled hips and head are approximately parallel to the ground and the knees are slightly bent. There is some flexion of the lumbar spine, the shoulders are level, and the head is turned as the hitter looks directly at the pitch, chin against shoulder. Hand position varies slightly according to each player. A reasonable position is 4 to 8 inches from the body, letters high to shoulder high. In the coiled position, the hitter holds the bat at approximately 45 degrees, with the elbow parallel to the ground and out from the body. Hands held too far from the body may reduce power, whereas if they are too close to the body or too low, the bat speed will be reduced. In most missed pitches, especially the fast ball, the hitter swings below the ball. Holding the hands too low reduces the bat speed and, except in exceptional cases, may reduce the contact zone. In the coiled position, the hitter begins moving with the forward arm motion of the pitcher, picking up the ball from the pitcher's hand and beginning to time his stride forward and swing.

The number one key to hitting, obviously, is vision. The hitter who does not see the ball can only guess and will not be able to make contact. Not only is visual acuity a critical factor, but eye control and eye functions are of equal importance. The hitter must have clear binocular focus to be able to visualize the ball and to predict its location. The speed of the ball makes it virtually impossible to completely follow the ball to the bat. The ideal is to follow the ball as far as possible and then make a prediction as to its line of projection. Without visualization, concentration, and focus, the hitter will fail to project the arrival

point of the ball, and inadequate ball contact is the consequence. In addition, balance and control are determined by eye focus, as in any coordinated muscle activity. If the eyes and head are locked and focused on a point, the body has a much greater chance of reproducing a coordinated, balanced motion than if the eyes are closed or poorly focused.

Thus, the key in the stance and coil position is balance, eye focus, and body readiness to start the stride. What happens before this coiling mechanism is not of great importance, but body and head position in the coiled portion of the swing should at least place the bat in a position that will facilitate the stride.

Batting coaches indicate that there are five basic aspects of the swing starting with the stride, as follows:

1. Back foot rotation, in which the heel is rotated out and the body pivots on the ball of the back foot.
2. Forward stride with the left foot.
3. Rapid hip and trunk rotation that takes the navel from a position parallel with the pitch to being perpendicular to the pitch.
4. Triangulation of the arms and extension of the arms.
5. Lateral flexion of the wrist.

Stride

Efficiency of motion is essential to the hitter.[29] The hitter must avoid needless motion. Motion must be balanced and coordinated in the forward stride. The backward motion in the coiling position precedes the forward motion. The front leg internally rotates, and the coil position will externally rotate in the stride. The stride should be directly toward the pitcher. The weight shift in a hitter is very important. With the forward stride, the weight stays back on the back foot as the forward foot strides forward lightly on the ball of the foot. The front leg now rotates externally, and the knee goes into extension. The ability to lock the knee of the front leg, providing firm rigid resistance to body motion, is important in keeping the axis of rotation of the body centered. If the knee flexes, the body weight shifts forward, and the proper axis of rotation is lost. As the foot lands evenly, it may be slightly open. The knee, of course, is initially slightly flexed as the foot lands and then locks in extension as the hips come through. This rotation around a center axis is important.

The midsection is the core of the swing action from which the hitter generates power.[29] Maintaining a center axis of motion and balance plays a critical role in maintaining head position. Too much head motion equals loss of both coordination and visualization of the ball. Locking the head to the center of axis of rotation is a key to the stride and swing positions. The bat in the coiled position is approximately at a 45-degree angle. As it comes through, there is a relative leveling of the bat, usually with less than 10 degrees of angulation. The pitch starts high because the pitcher is on the mound and throwing downward, whereas the bat comes through level. There will be a difference of a certain number of degrees of angulation between the ball and the bat. The bat comes down as the ball comes down.

Rotation

The forward stride of the legs and the rotation of the hips are reasonably standard in speed and approach. Large muscles of this type cannot be controlled quickly enough to allow the hitter to adjust to the speed at which a pitch is thrown. Therefore, the stride, at a fairly standard distance, with standard open or closed length, allows compensation. One of the important parts of batting-training technique is a rapid, sudden hip twist in which the navel goes from 90 degrees to the pitch to directly parallel to the pitch. A rapid, swift twist of the hips is what, in many ways, determines the bat speed and allows the hitter to be in a prime position to adjust to the speed and type of pitch. Therefore, stride length and hip rotation, with the navel toward the pitcher, is the same in virtually every pitch and must be a standardized, balanced, well-coordinated motion.

After this sudden hip rotation occurs, adjustments to pitches of various speed and pitch locations become crucial. As in golf, there is a ratio of derotation of the body as it leaves the coil position to the point of contact. In hitting, there is an adjustable ratio of derotation. With the power generated through hip and belly rotation, the fine control comes with the speed of (1) the upper body uncoiling, (2) elbow extension, and (3) wrist lateral flexion. Location of the pitch, of course, will vary tremendously, and the fine adjustment takes place in these latter three aspects. Therefore, the upper body trails behind the derotation of the hips. Trailing behind does not imply a helter-skelter, uncoordinated motion. Because the ratio of derotation of upper body to lower body must vary with the pitch, it requires even more muscular trunk control to allow the proper rotation to take place, depending on the pitch. Therefore, the hitter must visualize the ball and, in less than a second, determine the ratio of derotation of the upper body, as well as the position of the head, elbows, and hands for the point of contact with the ball. This requires excellent muscle control, balance, and coordination. Proper hitting depends on retraining muscles to fire and respond to changes in balance and coordination and retraining trunk muscles to maintain a tight, rigid, but mobile control between the upper and lower body. Lumbar pain that prevents proper rotation or that causes muscles to stop, to work improperly, or to work in an uncoordinated fashion can have a devastating effect on the player's ability to deliver the bat to the ball.

After hip rotation, with the upper body trailing behind slightly under maximum muscle control at a specific ratio of derotation determined by the pitch, the upper body rotates through to the point of ball contact. The head is level, going down with the pitch while the eyes focus on the ball. The chin of the right-handed batter, which is against the left shoulder in the coiling position, will end up against the right shoulder after ball contact. (The opposite, of course, is true for the left-handed hitter.) Again, head motion equals poor efficiency. At this point, with the bat coming through the strike zone, the shift is to the shoulder and upper arms, with triangulation of the arms: the chest as the base and the two arms parallel as they extend out. Locking the lead shoulder is of critical importance. Stabilization of the lead shoulder allows extension of the lead elbow and proper generation of bat speed. The bottom hand pulls and anchors the bat: the top hand pushes and guides the bat. As the arms and elbows extend, the bat is still trailing behind, with the wrists still in the cocked position.

Obviously, proper technique, including the weight shift from the back foot to the forward foot and the position of the elbows, hands, wrists, and bat, allows the hitter to delay the final commitment of bat position as long as possible. It provides longer visualization of the ball and a better prediction of the point of contact, all taking place at the same time that the body is generating tremendous torsional force. Therefore, the reproducible bat swing must generate the power and force necessary for the swing while delaying final commitment of bat position, allowing the wrists and hands to provide fine bat control and bat position at the point of contact. It is certainly possible to make contact with the ball with neither trunk rotation nor power but without

sufficient results on the field. The follow-through after ball contact is not of major consequence. Weight will be shifted to the front foot, and the left knee will be locked. Adequate control of quadriceps function of the front leg is imperative. The arms will be extended; the top hand will roll over at an appropriate time and should not be rushed.

In summary, stance, balance, control, head in proper position, stride, standardized lower body stride and position, and uncoiling of the upper body require maximum trunk control and balance to produce the correct ratio of derotation that will allow the bat to arrive at the appropriate place. The locked lead shoulder provides a rigid upper arm for proper elbow extension. Tight wrist control is obtained with proper lateral flexion of the wrist. The head rotates from the lead shoulder in the coiled position to the trailing shoulder in the follow-through.

Pitching

Some of the most difficult cases of lumbar spine problems are seen in baseball pitchers. It is extremely common in spring training to see throwers, especially baseball pitchers, having pain in the opposite side SI joint. This is due to unaccustomed torsional strain, probably in the lower facet joints, after the winter break. There is a high incidence of back stiffness in throwers as they start to regain peak mechanical functioning and begin throwing again. A common occurrence is referred diskogenic or facet joint pain in the typical pattern (through the facet joint, across the posterior superior iliac spine, SI joint, posterior ilium, and into the area of the greater trochanter). A concomitant problem is the development of secondary contractures, weakness, bursitis, tendonitis, and inflammations in the referred pain area. Often a pitcher will have greater trochanteric bursitis or SI joint pain that produces its own secondary effects.

A key aspect of a pitcher's rehabilitation is not only the resolution of the back problem; the secondary inflammatory effects of referred pain can produce the same biomechanical abnormalities in the pitching motion, thus leading to further injury. Indeed, the pain itself may prevent proper pitching and performance and thus cause additional injury. True sciatica and muscle weakness in a leg result in a critically important dysfunction in a pitcher: severe abnormalities of pitching motion that place the arm, shoulder, and elbow in jeopardy. Sciatica, especially with associated pain of increasing intradiskal and intra-abdominal pressure, can result in severe dysfunction during the throwing motion. Trunk stability is critical to a pitcher's throw, and any pain that produces weakness and stiffness can lead to a potentially catastrophic injury.

Tennis

Chard and Lachmann,[30] reporting on racquet sport injuries, separated the incidence into squash (59%), tennis (21%), and badminton (20%). Thirty-eight percent of professional tennis players have missed tournaments due to back pain. Trunk strengthening should be a major part of the tennis player's regimen.[31]

Tennis as a sport involves speed, rotation, and extremes of flexion, lateral bending, and extension. It involves the power aspects of the overhead serve, the effect of trunk strength on shoulder function, and many of the aspects brought out in the other sports. The one most consistent, important factor in protecting the spine in tennis is to bend the knees. Leg strength, quadriceps strength, the ability to play with a bent knee, and hips in a flexed positioned while protecting the back are the keys to prevention of back pain. In the serve, trunk strength in proceeding from the back extended to the follow-through position requires strong abdominal control. Gluteal, latissimus dorsi, abdominal obliques, and rectus abdominus strength controls the lumbodorsal fascia and delivers the power necessary through the legs up into the arm.

In summary, the keys to proper management of lumbar spine problems in athletes include comprehensive diagnosis, aggressive and effective nonoperative care, and pinpoint operations that do as little damage as possible to normal tissue but correct the pathologic lesion.

REFERENCES

1. Fairbank JC, Pynsent PB, Van Poortvliet JA, et al: Influence of anthropometric factors and joint laxity in the incidence of adolescent back pain. Spine 1984;9:461–464.
2. Jackson DW: Low back pain in young athletes: Evaluation of stress reaction and discogenic problems. Am J Sports Med 1979;7:364–366.
3. Fisk JW, Baigent ML, Hill PD: Scheuermann's disease: Clinical and radiological survey of 17 and 18 year olds. Am J Sports Med 1984;63:18–30.
4. Keene JS, Albert MJ, Springer SL, et al: Back injuries in college athletes. J Spinal Dis 1986;2:190–195.
5. Keene JS: Low back pain in the athlete from spondylogenic injury during recreation or competition. Postgrad Med 1983;74:209–217.
6. Spencer CW, Jackson DW: Back injuries in the athlete. Clin Sports Med 1983;2:191–215.
7. Micheli LJ: Back injuries in gymnastics. Clin Sports Med 1985;4:85–93.
8. Cacayorin ED, Hochhauser L, Petro GR: Lumbar thoracic spine pain in the athlete: Radiographic evaluation. Clin Sports Med 1987;6:767–783.
9. Papanicolaou N, Wilkinson RH, Emans JB, et al: Bone scintigraphy and radiography in young athletes with low back pain. AJR Am J Roentgenol 1985;145:1039–1044.
10. Light HG: Hernia of the inferior lumbar space. A cause of back pain. Arch Surg 1983;118:1077–1080.
11. Farfan HF: The biomechanical advantage of lordosis and hip extension for upright activity. Spine 1978;3:336–342.
12. Schnebel BE, Simmons JW, Chowning J, et al: A digitizing technique for the study of movement of intradiscal dye in response to flexion and extension of the lumbar spine. Spine 1988;12:309–312.
13. Schnebel BE, Watkins RG, Willin WH: The role of spinal flexion and extension in changing nerve root compression in disc herniations. Spine 1989;14:835–837.
14. White AA, Panjabi MM: Clinical Biomechanics of the Spine. Philadelphia, Lippincott, 1978.
15. Farfan HF: Mechanical Disorders of the Low Back. Philadelphia, Lea & Febiger, 1973.
16. Farfan HF: Muscular mechanism of the lumbar spine and the position of power and efficiency. Orthop Clin North Am 1975;6:135–144.
17. Watkins RG, Dennis S, Dillin WH, et al: Dynamic EMG analysis of torque transfer in professional baseball pitchers. Spine 1989;14:404–408.
18. Watkins RG, Buhler B, Loverock P: The Water Workout Recovery Program. Chicago, Contemporary Books, 1988.
19. Semon RL, Spengler D: The significance of lumbar spondylolysis in college football players. Spine 1981;6:172–174.
20. Schnook GA: Injuries in women's gymnastics: A five year study. Am J Sports Med 1979;7:242–244.
21. Garrick JG, Requa RK: Epidemiology of women's gymnastics injuries. Am J Sports Med 1980;8:261–264.
22. Howse AJG: Orthopedist's aid ballet. Clin Orthop 1972;89:52–63.
23. Gainor BJ, Hagen RJ, Allen WC: Biomechanics of the spine in the polevaulter as related to spondylolisthesis. Am J Sports Med 1983;11:53–57.
24. Aggrawal ND, Kaur R, Kumar S, et al: A study of changes in weight lifters and other athletes. Br J Sports Med 1979;13:58–61.
25. Kotani PT, Ichikawa MD, Wakabayashi MD, et al: Studies of spondylolisthesis found among weight lifters. Br J Sports Med 1981;9:4–8.
26. Cantu RC: Lumbar spine injuries. In Cantu RC (ed): The Exercising Adult. Lexington, MA, Collamore Press, 1980.
27. Ferguson RJ, McMaster JH, Stanitski CL: Low back pain in college football linemen. J Sports Med 1974;2:63–69.
28. Davies JE: The spine in sports injuries, prevention and treatment. Br J Sports Med 1980;14:18–20.
29. Keene JS, Drummond DS: Mechanical back in the athlete. Comp Ther 1985;11:7–14.
30. Chard MD, Lachmann SM: Racquet sports—Patterns of injury presenting to a sports injury clinic. Br J Sports Med 1987;21:150–153.
31. Marks MR, Haas SS, Weisel SW: Low back pain in the competitive tennis player. Clin Sports Med 1988;7:277–287.

44 Abdomen and Pelvis

Steve A. Mora, Bert R. Mandelbaum, and William C. Meyers

In This Chapter

Pelvis and hip stress fractures
Osteitis pubis
Apophyseal avulsion injuries
Athletic pubalgia

INTRODUCTION

- Abdominal and groin pain in the athlete can present a diagnostic dilemma.

- Many potential disorders are possible, and a careful history and physical examination are more likely than magnetic resonance imaging (MRI) to find the source of pain.

- A high index of suspicion is necessary with regard to femoral neck stress fractures, as delay in diagnosis can become highly problematic if a displaced fracture results.

- Osteitis pubis symptoms generally resolve with nonoperative treatment, but frequently last 6 to 9 months.

- Most pelvic avulsion fractures can be treated nonoperatively.

- Surgery for athletic pubalgia must be preceded by an understanding of the direct and compensatory parts of the injury.

Abdominal, groin, and pelvis pain in the athlete can be difficult to manage. Part of the reason may have been due to our shortage of good evaluation tools, interest level, and diagnostic tests. In addition, the increased popularity of soccer in North America has brought with it an increase in groin injuries and as a consequence has led to increased awareness and published reports. It is imperative that orthopedic surgeons who take care of kicking sport athletes have a thorough understanding of problems affecting the pelvic and groin areas.

Athletes presenting with groin and hip complaints pose a difficult challenge due to the long and usually unfamiliar list of diagnostic possibilities. The differential list is far reaching and not only includes orthopedic disorders but also general medical, urologic, neurologic, and gynecologic disorders. Some of the known orthopedic conditions include intra-articular hip joint disorders, acute and chronic adductor tears, pubic symphysis disorders, snapping hip syndrome, peripheral nerve entrapment,

bursitis, tumors, fractures and abdominal wall tears (Table 44-1). Usually the most sensitive tool for evaluating these difficult problems is not the "high tech" imaging study but rather the clinical history and a detailed palpation examination. It is challenging and rewarding for the clinician to gather salient clinical information, formulate a well-defined list of differentials, and plan a strategy to further define and treat the specific disorder.

Before getting into athletic pubalgia and other musculoskeletal causes of such debilitating pain in athletes, let us consider the myriad of other problems that can mimic the "pubic joint"[1] problems. We only mention, with some editorial commentary, problems that have actually been seen[2,3] rather than simply list the whole potential differential diagnosis. On the other hand, knowing the comprehensive differential is very important since other problems definitely overlap with respect to their afferent pain patterns.

We start with inguinal hernia. The issue here is particularly important since we believe strongly that the term *sports hernia* is a misnomer, leading good general surgeons to believe that they can repair the athletic problems like hernias. Inguinal hernia is different. The pain of a direct or indirect hernia is usually lateral to the pain found in most athletes. The pain relates to parietal peritoneum poking through a defect in the abdominal wall near the internal ring, either medial or lateral to the inferior epigastric vessels. The pain of a true hernia is usually associated with a distinct, palpable bulge.

With little evidence, the claim has been made that occult inguinal hernias frequently cause abdominal and pelvic pain in athletes. It is possible, rarely, that one may not detect a small hernia on physical examination. When we have seen this, the pain was well lateral to the edge of the rectus muscle. For a number of years, we have been looking for evidence of occult hernias in athletes but have seen little such evidence. We have difficulty believing reports to the contrary.

We have picked up a number of incidental hernias either on physical examination or at the time of surgery, but those hernias did not seem to account for the patterns of pain in those athletes. In each case, the pain was medial to the hernia and associated with some degree of adductor pain in the thigh.

We have also had three cases of inguinal hernias that occurred after pelvic floor repairs and may have indeed been complications of the pelvic floor repairs. We believe that pelvic floor repairs can occasionally create a small abdominal wall defect near the internal ring. In two of our cases, the patients with postoperative hernia had no pain. Those two patients presented with a bulge more than a year after the repairs. In one case, the patient presented with crampy abdominal pain and had a small bowel obstruction related to a defect that we believed that we

Table 44-1 Differential Diagnosis of Groin and Anterior Pelvis Pain
Abdominal wall strain or tear, also known as athletic pubalgia (new terminology) or a sports hernia (old terminology)
Hip muscle strain or tear (adductors, iliopsoas, and pectineus) and bursitis
Intra-articular hip joint pathology; common pathology: labral tears, cartilage defects, and ligament teres tears
Pelvis and hip fractures: stress fractures, stress reactions, and adolescent apophyseal fractures
Athletic osteitis pubis: with or without anterior pelvic ring instability (>2 mm of abnormal symphysis)
Neurologic: Referred pain from lumbar spine, peripheral nerve entrapment (obturator nerve entrapment, and ilioinguinal nerve)
Nonmusculoskeletal conditions: gynecologic disease (endometriosis, ovarian cysts, tumors), true hernias, rectal cancer, and urologic disease (cystitis, ureteral stones)

caused by our folding the lateral edge of the rectus muscle down to support the pubic joint. We identified and repaired the latter problem via laparoscopy. Exertional pain was not a factor in any of these three cases.

On the other hand, there is nothing about being an athlete that should prevent the occurrence of standard direct or inguinal hernias. We have taken care of a number of such athletes and repaired the hernias by either laparoscopic (pre- or intraperitoneal) or open techniques. The general incidence of hernia development does not seem to be particularly increased compared with nonathletes, nor does it seem to be associated with much exertional pain. Therefore, inguinal hernias do need to be considered in the differential diagnosis of most of these athletes, but rarely remain considerations after a good history and physical examination.

We now turn to some other problems that we have seen. Interestingly, in both males and females, one of the most common considerations with respect to exertional pain in this area of the body in athletes is inflammatory bowel disease. Usually, a careful history detects this possibility. The patient elicits that he or she has either had years of gastrointestinal problems or a recent change in bowel habits. In most of the cases that we have seen, there has been at least one thickened bowel loop within the pelvis. Therefore, it seems likely that the exertion caused this loop to irritate the pelvic parietal peritoneum. Sometimes the pain can go down into the thigh. Psoas signs of inflammation may also accompany the irritation.

A wide variety of other gastrointestinal problems can also mimic the musculoskeletal problems of athletes. We have now seen two patients with rectal cancer. One had resectable disease and is a long-term survivor. The other had locally metastatic disease at the time of presentation and did not do well in the long term. We have also seen one case of chronic perforated appendicitis.

Beyond a doubt, in females, there are many gynecologic problems that can mimic the athletic pubalgia pain patterns. The most common problem is endometriosis. An endometriosis implant can also occur directly within the round ligament. We suspect that several successes after pelvic floor repair in young women in our series were related to our routinely dividing the round ligament. Several of the latter patients had pelvic endometriosis and no grossly detectable round ligament implant. In one case, active endometriosis was identified histologically within the round ligament specimen. In our experience, nonendometriosis ovarian cystic disease is the second most common gynecologic problem mimicking athletic pubalgia.

We have also seen a wide variety of genitourinary problems mimicking the pain in both males and females. Overall, the most common urologic problem has been bladder or ureteral stones. It is particularly important to mention that we have also seen several testicular and other tumors. One interesting tumor resided within a seminal vesicle. In that case, the patient's pain occurred with ejaculation.

Still, a wide variety of other problems have caused enough lower abdominal, pelvic, or inguinal pain in athletes to be referred to us. Some of the more interesting other problems that we have seen associated with exertional pain include herpes disease, true spigelian hernias, pelvic inflammatory disease, and arterial insufficiency. We have also seen a chronically perforated hepatoma, a bile leak after laparoscopic cholecystectomy, and an incarcerated femoral hernia.

PELVIS AND HIP FRACTURES

General

Fractures of the pelvis and sacrum are usually pathologic due to stress or fatigue. Those fractures due to falls or high-velocity impact are uncommon and are not the focus of this section. Many stress fractures of the pelvis go undiagnosed because the prudent patient may end up self-treating with self-imposed rest until the symptoms ameliorate and activity is once again possible. When they occur, stress injuries occur at the sacrum, sacroiliac joint, pubic rami, and femoral neck. Classically, a pelvis or sacral stress fracture occurs following a recent increase in mileage or intensity. For example, stress fractures of the pubic rami are the most common in the pelvis and usually occur in long-distance runners (Fig. 44-1). Although these fractures are common, in general, the most common stress fracture is in the tibia. Stress fractures may be simplified as (1) primary osseous failure—insufficiency fracture due to inherent weakness such as osteopenia or osteoporosis, and (2) a fatigue fracture from excessive overloading of normal bone. The situation, in most cases, may be a combination of these factors. The stress fracture should also be observed as part of a spectrum of disease. On one end is a stress reaction and on the other end is a frank fracture with a distinct fracture line. Stress fracture cause is also thought to be varied. The current most widely accepted theory is that of repetitive stress causing a periosteal resorption that surpasses the rate of bone remodeling, weakening the cortex and resulting in a stress fracture. The high-intensity female athlete is at risk of stress fractures as a consequence of high-intensity training, catabolic state, poor diet, and low body mass along with menstrual problems. Risk factors for multiple stress fractures include a high longitudinal arch of the foot, leg length inequality, and excessive forefoot varus, female patients with menstrual irregularities, and high weekly training mileage.[4]

The pain pattern of a stress fracture is typically described as a "crescendo" effect beginning as a tolerable dull ache that quickly transforms into an intense pain, making the lightest exercise activity not possible. The symptoms of a stress injury are worsened with any pounding-type of weight-bearing activities. The key to the diagnosis is in the history and physical examination. The point of maximal tenderness should be identified so

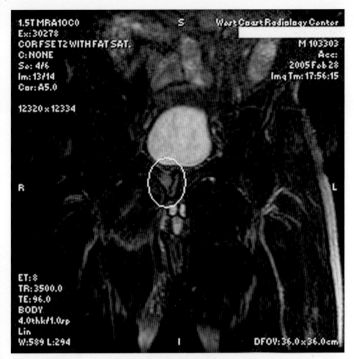

Figure 44-1 Magnetic resonance imaging of the pelvis depicts a fracture through the right parasymphyseal inferior pubic ramus in a 48-year-old sheriff reservist. The fracture occurred insidiously during endurance training. The patient presented with anterior hip flexor pain and tenderness. The plain radiographs remained negative for 4 weeks. This fracture was successfully treated with activity modification including nonimpact athletic activities and physical therapy. Despite union after 8 weeks, this patient experienced residual symptoms associated with adductor tightness.

that imaging studies may be focused to this area. Plain radiographs are usually negative because of the lack of callus formation in the early stages and sometimes when a fracture line does not form. When a fracture is thought to be occult or difficult to characterize, an MRI is considered more sensitive than a bone scan. The ideal MRI sequence for femoral neck fractures is the "fat saturation T2" (high TR and TE >60) or short tau inversion recovery (STIR) sequences, which are easier and quicker to perform than other sequences.

The treatment for pelvis stress fractures, except femoral neck, is fairly straightforward. Most resolve with 4 to 6 weeks of relative rest and progressive reintroduction of activities. When the patient is pain free, then progressive sporting activities may be initiated.

Due to their potential for major disability, femoral neck stress fractures require special consideration. This includes having increased awareness so that a timely diagnosis is made and specific treatment implemented. In general, these injuries are seen in two distinct populations: (1) young, healthy, active individuals such as runners or military recruits and (2) the elderly who have osteoporosis. In the high performance athlete, a devastating problem may occur when a seemingly simple nondisplaced femoral neck fracture becomes displaced. A delay in the correct diagnosis may be highly problematic and therefore a high index of suspicion is important.[5] The early clinical presentation of a femoral stress fracture may mimic other more common conditions. The pain is usually around the anterior groin region similar to a hip flexor strain or pull. To a lesser degree, the pain may

also be nonspecific, ill defined, or atypical around the gluteal region. Refraining from the offensive repetitive activity or excessive loading will eventually improve the symptoms and allow union.

The complication rate for femoral neck fractures is partly related to the specific type and the promptness of treatment. In an effort to efficiently guide the treatment, these fractures have been classified based on their plain radiographic and MRI appearance. The tension-type fracture involving the lateral cortex is considered more unstable and should be treated with weight-bearing protection and then expeditious surgical stabilization using a plate and screw device. The reasoning behind surgical treatment of these fractures stems from the potential for malunion and osteonecrosis if they become displaced. The compression-type fracture involving the medial side is biomechanically more stable and can usually be treated conservatively with serial radiographs, protected weight bearing, and activity modification (Fig. 44-2). In view of the fact that these fractures have potential for major disability, it behooves the clinician to order an MRI study sooner in performance athletes, especially females, to both obtain an expeditious diagnosis and avoid potential litigation. Although extremely uncommon, there have been reports of compression-type fractures also becoming displaced, and, as a consequence, some authors have recommended internal fixation if a compression type of neck fracture involves more than 50% of the cortex.[6] All patients with femoral neck fractures should be educated about potential problems with their hip joint. The surgical risks include chondrolysis, nonunion, malunion, osteonecrosis, and subtrochanteric iatrogenic fractures. An appropriate period of toe-touch weight bearing should

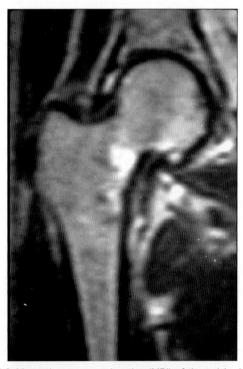

Figure 44-2 Magnetic resonance imaging (MRI) of the pelvis depicts a stable compression type of femoral neck fracture. These fractures are typically stable and can be treated with close observation, serial radiographs, protected weight bearing, and physical therapy. In an athlete with groin pain, the consideration for an early MRI should be made in order to avoid potential complications.

follow surgical fixation. Radiographic healing and signs of osteonecrosis are monitored with periodic plain radiographs. Even in cases of appropriate treatment, many patients may have persistent long-term disabling complaints. The results of surgical treatment may be influenced by the amount of fracture displacement and the quality of the fracture reduction. The incidence of osteonecrosis in nondisplaced fractures is approximately 15%.[7] Fractures that develop osteonecrosis may require a prosthetic replacement or other secondary procedure. MRI following fixation of a femoral neck fracture is usually of poor quality due to the artifactual signal from the metal screws. Routine removal of the hip fixation device is not recommended unless the hardware has failed or when a future MRI is anticipated. Hip arthroscopy after a healed femoral neck fracture has not been evaluated well in the literature. Young patients who develop symptomatic osteonecrosis may benefit from a referral to a specialist experienced in core decompression, bone grafting, and vascularized fibula transfers. Unfortunately, many patients will continue to experience differing levels of symptoms at long-term follow-up following femoral neck fractures.[8]

OSTEITIS PUBIS

Osteitis pubis in the athlete is an inflammatory condition of the pubic symphysis and surrounding structures. Due to the ubiquitous nature of this disease, it is imperative that all factors, such as infection, urologic, gynecologic, and rheumatologic issues are taken into consideration for the accurate diagnosis and treatment. The pathogenesis of this disorder remains obscure. It can occur secondary to vertical instability or as a primary condition. It may also coexist with other conditions including athletic pubalgia.

Among athletes, primary osteitis pubis is thought to be caused by repetitive microtrauma, chronic overuse injury, and muscle imbalance. The abdominal and adductor muscles have a central point of attachment on the symphysis pubis or the "pivot point," but these muscles act antagonistically to each other, predisposing the pubic symphysis to opposing forces. These forces become critical in the kicking activities associated with sports such as soccer, Australian rules football, and North American football (Fig. 44-3). When an athlete kicks, the kicking limb is hyperextended at the hip while the trunk is rotated laterally in the opposite direction. Greater than 2 mm of vertical motion is seen in cases that are associated with pubic symphysis instability.

The clinical findings include tenderness at and around the pubis symphysis area. The examination should focus on carefully defining the pathoanatomic zones. The "groin" is not sufficiently descriptive, and therefore the clinician should further define this region into the different anatomic areas including pubic, suprapubic, abdominal, anterior hip capsule, proximal thigh, inguinal ring, and perineal. A digital direct and indirect hernia examination is important to evaluate the superficial inguinal ring, spermatic cord, conjoined tendon, and deep inguinal ring. Coventry and William[9] described two provocative maneuvers: (1) the rocking cross-leg test in which examiner bears down on the crossed knee while holding down the opposite iliac crest and (2) the lateral pelvis compression test done with the patient on his or her side and the examiner pressing the presenting wing. The examiner may also glean diagnostic information by palpating the tender areas while the patient does a sit-up maneuver. Careful digital examination of the scrotum, spermatic cord, inguinal ring,

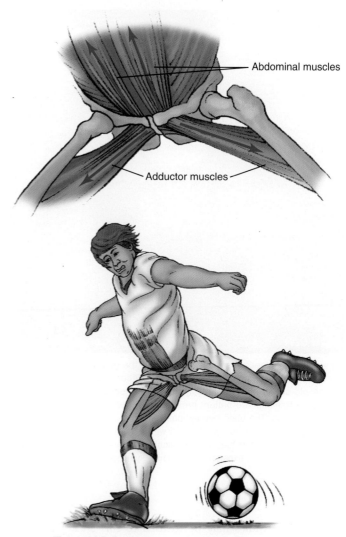

Figure 44-3 The pubis pivot point in a soccer player.

and conjoined tendon of the abdominal wall should be performed to evaluate for abdominal wall injuries (athletic pubalgia) and true hernias. If the pain is difficult to characterize or if it is of a radiating nature, the clinician should consider remote causes for the pain such as referred spinal pain or peripheral nerve entrapment. Sometimes a referral is necessary to evaluate for gynecologic, urologic, rheumatologic, or general surgery problems.

Imaging studies for osteitis pubis begins with plain radiographs as well as single-leg standing "flamingo" views to document vertical instability (abnormal if >2-mm difference in height exists). MRI may be helpful in identifying a tear of the anterior abdominal wall musculature (external oblique aponeurosis, superficial inguinal ring, conjoined tendon); however, it is frequently negative. MRI is also beneficial for nonorthopedic conditions that may be coincidentally diagnosed. A technetium 99m triple phase bone scan is useful for identifying ambiguous areas of pain caused by stress reactions or fractures.

Most of the time, nonoperative treatment will lead to resolution of symptoms. Core strengthening and flexibility, as well as an active program, are encouraged.[10–12]

The patient should be educated regarding the drawn-out clinical course and to the fact that, on average, symptoms will last

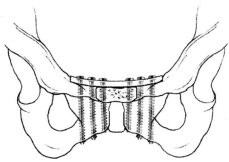

Figure 44-4 Pubic symphysis arthrodesis.

6 to 9 months. The full spectrum of conservative measures includes cessation of offending physical activity, physical therapy, ultrasonography, nonsteroidal anti-inflammatory drugs, oral glucocorticoids, radiation therapy, anticoagulation, intravenous pamidronate, and corticosteroid pubic symphysis injections. For patients who remain symptomatic, a fluoroscopically guided steroid injection may be performed in the office. If the patient does not experience immediate pain relief, then other causes, such as athletic pubalgia, need to be considered.

Rarely do patients require surgical treatment. There are a few case reports showing limited success after a proximal adductor release and drilling of the pubic bone in soccer players. Most of the literature regarding surgical management of osteitis pubis has focused exclusively on bony procedures. The procedures that have been described are either a pubic symphysis trapezoidal wedge resection or an arthrodesis with or without a compression plate (Fig. 44-4). Wedge resection of the symphysis pubis is useful as a first-line surgical procedure because of its short operative time, reliability, and low complication risk.[13] However, there is a risk of late anterior pelvis instability due to anterior pelvis disruption. Alternatively, some authors have successfully used pubic symphysis bone grafting and compression plating in athletes with documented pelvic instability.[14] There is a risk of stress fracture of the arthrodesis site if a plate is not employed. Although the surgery seems to be aggressive, there have been excellent results with low complication rates. Additionally, the issue of late instability is ameliorated.

APOPHYSEAL AVULSION INJURIES

An apophyseal avulsion fracture of the pelvis is a fracture through the physis of a secondary center of ossification. These commonly involve the anterior superior iliac spine, anterior inferior iliac spine, and ischial tuberosity apophysis. These fractures occur almost exclusively in 11- to 17-year-old patients. They are most commonly seen in soccer, track, football, and baseball. In most cases, these fractures occur during fast running, hurdling, pitching, or sprinting.[15] These injuries usually do not occur due to direct trauma. They may occur as a consequence to a hip dislocation. Fractures of the anterior superior iliac spine result from the pull of the sartorius and the tensor fascia lata muscles. Fractures through the anterior inferior iliac spine result from pull of the straight head of the rectus femoris muscle. A forceful sprint or a swing of a baseball bat will typically avulse the anterior superior iliac spine.

The injured athlete will frequently recall an associated "pop" at the moment of injury. Then acute lower extremity, hip, and groin pain with restricted range of motion and inability to bear weight will follow. Transient meralgia paresthetica may be seen due to the swelling around the lateral femoral cutaneous nerve. A displaced apophysis is usually apparent on plain radiographs, but if the clinician is not keen to the injury, a subtle opacity may be missed. An astute clinician may make the presumptive diagnosis despite "negative" radiographs. In cases of anterior inferior iliac spine avulsions, an oblique plain radiograph projection may be necessary to appreciate a subtle displacement. Despite the occasional delay in diagnosis, there is usually no major problem from wrongly receiving acute treatment for a strain instead of a fracture. On the other hand, a robust formation of callus may lead to inadvertent overtreatment due to the concern for Ewing's tumor or osteomyelitis.

The treatment of most avulsion fractures is nonoperative. The treatment can include rest and protected weight bearing with crutches followed by a supervised rehabilitation and a home exercise program. Most authors have reported excellent results following nonoperative treatment.[16] Without adequate protection, a symptomatic nonunion is possible; therefore, non-weight bearing or protected weight bearing for up to 3 weeks is a prudent decision. Despite the massive callus that frequently forms, an excellent result is likely. The most common complication of nonoperative treatment is a tender exostosis-like formation at the fracture site. Rarely will these exostosis-like lesions require surgical removal. Surgery may be considered in the case of a severely displaced fracture in a high-level athlete. A displaced fracture may create a shortened muscle and as a consequence a theoretical decrease in muscular power. Indications for open treatment and internal fixation are not well defined. Open treatment and internal fixation may be considered in a high-level athlete with displaced (>3 cm) fractures or in cases associated with hip dislocations. Reports on surgical fixation are few, and no improvement in outcome has been proven. When surgery is chosen, the apophysis is reduced and fixated using wiring and/or screw fixation.[17] Potential complications are the same as those associated with adult fracture treatment including cutaneous nerve injury, misguided hardware, hemorrhage, infection, and hip joint damage. Complete recovery, return to sports, and no long-term sequelae may be anticipated following most apophyseal fractures, regardless of the type of treatment chosen.

ATHLETIC PUBALGIA

We have recently written overviews of our current understanding of the anatomic and pathophysiologic bases for this set of syndromes.[1,3] Briefly, this set of syndromes accounts for most of the surgical problems that we see in athletes. Athletes create tremendous torque that occurs at the level of the pelvis. The anterior pelvis takes much of the brunt of these forces. The attachments to the anterior pelvis play the most important roles with respect to the direct and opposing forces that are involved in this torque. However, the posterior, lateral, and medial compartments are usually also involved and need to be considered in planning therapy.

From an anatomic perspective, it is important to understand fully the pelvic anatomy that is involved. Basically, one thinks of the pubic symphysis as the fulcrum around which the forces occur. Then one thinks of the injuries as a combination of acute or chronic weakening and compensatory overuse of various insertions or attachments. In many of these injuries, one thinks in terms of an "unstable pubic joint."

Pathophysiologically, one then can think in terms of which attachments to the joint are involved either directly in the injury or conversely as compensatory mechanisms. In addition to the attachments, one may also think in terms of there being a variety of "strap muscles" or "compensatory compartments." An example of a strap muscle might be the psoas tendon, which does not insert directly into the pubis. Nonetheless, the psoas muscle and tendon do provide considerable pubic joint stability. While the anterior compartment is the most common one involved in injury, the other compartments may also be directly involved, in which case the nondirectly involved compartments become "compensatory."

One must figure out the mechanisms of the primary injuries and then determine the method of repair. The most common injury is a weakening of the rectus abdominis muscle as it inserts on the pubis, associated with compensatory overuse of the other side, the adductor longus, adductor brevis, and/or pectineus. In total, we have described more than 18 syndromes that occur relatively commonly. One should also remember that there are other parts of these muscles or attachments that can be injured in different locations. For example, the rectus abdominis muscles can fray anywhere within the anterior abdominal wall or can also cause a subluxation syndrome of the lowermost ribs or cartilages. We have seen the latter syndromes in fighters, rowers, women tennis players, and bull riders.

We classify the pathology seen at surgery associated with the preceding syndromes as grade 1, single or multiple small tears; grade 2, partial avulsion or avulsions; and grade 3, complete avulsion or avulsions or a complete avulsion associated with another partial avulsion.

There are some other "confusors." As suggested by the previous discussion, proper diagnosis of these injuries can be tricky. At this point, we just mention some of the considerations that can be confusing.

Four of the confusors are (1) identification of patients who need surgery, (2) the type of surgery, (3) the timing of surgery, and (4) the duration of rehabilitation. Briefly, surgery is indicated when joint instability is clearly demonstrated after the acute effects of injury, for example, hematoma, have resolved and physical therapy does not seem appropriate. Surgery involves a combination of tightening, loosening, or other procedures that focus on preventing persistence of pain. The specific surgery depends greatly on understanding precisely the direct and compensatory parts of the injury as well as the principal causes of the pain. Timing of surgery depends on various medical, social, and business factors such as the proper identification of the specific injury, the degree of debility that the injury causes, the possible negative consequences of playing with the injury, and the relative risks in relation to such things as the importance of upcoming games, the player's contract, the team's interests in the player, and confidence that performance will not hurt the player's overall value. Duration of rehabilitation is a particularly tricky consideration. We get most players back within 6 weeks of the injury, depending, of course, on the type of injury. There is evidence that we could get the players back even earlier, but long-term success possibly could be negatively associated with returning too quickly.

Finally, we mention two more confusors. One is that the psoas "snapping hip" syndrome can be, but does not have to be, associated with athletic pubalgia or a labral tear. Because the iliopsoas tendon glides by the hip joint so closely, one has to consider that the patient can have one, two, or three syndromes at the same time. To make things even more confusing, one can at the same time demonstrate a clear labral tear by MRI or arthroscopy, but the tear still may be totally asymptomatic.

A second confusor is the consideration of osteitis pubis. It is important that we realize that most athlete patients with this radiographic diagnosis have a secondary type of osteitis that responds favorably to treatment of the underlying joint instability. However, there still is a "primary" type of osteitis pubis that can affect athletes. The primary form of this problem involves continuous and debilitating pain that may be aggravated or ameliorated by exertion. The pain and tenderness often involve multiple bony sites in the pelvis. The primary type of osteitis pubis is difficult to treat. Fortunately, from an athletic standpoint, the primary osteitis pubis occurs much more in nonathletes. The problem is nonetheless, of course, very unfortunate for the patients involved because it is so difficult to treat. On the other hand, the syndrome does seem usually to be time limited.

SUMMARY

Abdomen and pelvis injuries due to sports are usually a consequence of repetitive trauma and instability. These problems can become chronic problems and possibly negatively affect the athlete's performance. Due to the rising popularity of kicking sports, these types of problems are more common and are becoming better understood.

REFERENCES

1. Meyers WC, Greenleaf R, Saad A: Anatomic basis for evaluation of abdominal and groin pain in athletes. Op Tech Sports Med 2005;13:55–61.
2. Meyers WC, Foley DP, Garrett WE: Management of severe lower abdominal or inguinal pain in high-performance athletes. Am J Sports Med 2000;28:2–8.
3. Meyers WC et al: Am J Sports Med in press.
4. Korpelainen R, Orava S, et al: Risk factors for recurrent stress fractures in athletes. Am J Sports Med 2001;29:304–310.
5. Johansson C, Ekenman I, et al: Stress fractures of the femoral neck in athletes. Am J Sports Med 1990;18:524–528.
6. Shin AY, Morin WD, Gorman JD, et al: The superiority of magnetic resonance imaging in differentiating the cause of hip pain in endurance athletes. Am J Sports Med 1996;24:168–176.
7. Haidukewych GJ, Rothwell WS, et al: Operative treatment of femoral neck fractures in patients between the ages of fifteen and fifty years. J Bone Joint Dis Am 2004;86:1711–1716.
8. Weistroffer JK, Muldoon MP, Duncan DD, et al: Femoral neck stress fractures: Outcome analysis at minimum five-year follow-up. J Orthop Trauma 2003;17:34–37.
9. Coventry MB, William MC: Osteitis pubis: Observations based on a study of 45 patients. JAMA 1961;178:898–905.
10. Fricker P, Taunton J, Ammann W: Osteitis pubis in athletes: Infection, inflammatory or injury. Sports Med 1991;12:266–279.
11. Holt MA, Keene JS, Graf BK, Helwig DC: Treatment of osteitis pubis in athletes. Results of corticosteroid injections. Am J Sports Med 1995;23:601–606.
12. Harris NH, Murray RG: Lesions of the symphysis pubis in athletes. In

Proceedings of the British Orthopaedic Association. J Bone Joint Surg Br 1974;56:563–564.

13. Grace JN, Sim FH, Shives TC, Coventry MB: Wedge resection of the symphysis pubis for the treatment of osteitis pubis. J Bone Joint Surg Am 1989;71:358–364.

14. Williams PR, Thomas DP, Downes EM: Osteitis pubis and instability of the pubic symphysis. When nonoperative measures fail. Am J Sports Med 2000;28:350–255.

15. Metzmaker J, Pappas A: Avulsion fractures of the pelvis. Am J Sports Med 1985;13:349–358.

16. Sundar M, Carty H: Avulsion fractures of the pelvis in children: A report of 32 fractures and their outcome. Skeletal Radiol 1994;23:85–90.

17. Meyer NJ, Orton D: Traumatic unilateral avulsion of the anterior superior and inferior iliac spines with anterior dislocation of the hip: A case report. J Orthop Trauma 2001;15:137–140.

Hip Joint

J.W. Thomas Byrd

In This Chapter

INTRODUCTION

- Sports-related injuries to the hip joint have received relatively little attention.

- This trend is changing, but, until recently, there have been few publications in peer-reviewed journals and the topic has rarely been presented at scientific meetings. This is due to three reasons.

  - First, perhaps hip injuries are less common than in other joints.

  - Second, investigative skills, including clinical assessment and imaging studies, for the hip have been less sophisticated.

  - Third, there have been few interventional methods, including surgical techniques and conservative modalities, available to treat the hip and thus there has been little impetus to delve into this unrecognized area.

- Arthroscopy has revealed a plethora of intra-articular disorders that previously went undiagnosed and largely untreated. Uncovering the existence of these disorders has led to improved clinical assessment skills and improved imaging technology. Thus, more forms of pathology are being recognized and there are now more methods available to treat these injuries.

The indications for hip arthroscopy fall into two broad categories. In one, arthroscopy offers an alternative to traditional open techniques previously employed for recognized forms of hip pathology such as loose bodies or impinging osteophytes. In the other, arthroscopy offers a method of treatment for disorders that previously went unrecognized including labral tears, chondral injuries, and disruption of the ligamentum teres. Most athletic injuries fall into this latter category. In the past, athletes were simply resigned to living within the constraints of their symptoms, often ending their competitive careers, being diagnosed as having a chronic groin injury. Based on the results of arthroscopy among athletes, it is likely that many of these careers could have been rejuvenated with arthroscopic intervention.[1]

In a study of athletes undergoing arthroscopy, in 60% of the cases, the hip was not recognized as the source of symptoms at the time of initial treatment, and these patients were managed for an average of 7 months before the hip was considered as a potential contributing source.[1] The most common preliminary diagnoses were various types of musculotendinous strains. Thus, it is prudent to consider the possibility of intra-articular pathology in the differential diagnosis when managing a strain around the hip joint. However, the incidence of intra-articular pathology is probably quite small relative to other extra-articular injuries, and thus it is best to temper the interest in an extensive intra-articular workup for every hip flexor or adductor strain. What is important is thoughtful follow-up and reassessment of injuries, especially when they do not seem to be responding as expected.

CLINICAL FEATURES AND EVALUATION

The evaluation of a patient with hip pain focuses on whether the source of symptoms is intra-articular and thus potentially amenable to arthroscopy.[2] Characteristic features of hip joint pathology are summarized in Table 45-1. In general, a history of a specific traumatic event is a better prognostic indicator than a patient who simply develops insidious onset of hip pain. Onset of symptoms in the absence of injury implies a degenerative process or predisposition to damage that is less likely to be corrected by arthroscopic intervention. Mechanical symptoms such as sharp stabbing pain, locking, or catching are also better prognostic indicators of a potentially correctable problem.

Common examination findings are summarized in Table 45-2. Although the hip receives innervation from branches of L2 to S1 of the lumbosacral plexus, its principal innervation is the L3 nerve root. This explains why irritation of the joint may result in anterior groin and radiating medial thigh pain that follows the L3 dermatome. Posterior pain is rarely indicative of an intra-articular process but, if clinically suspected, can be confirmed with a fluoroscopically guided intra-articular injection of anesthetic, which should provide temporary alleviation of the pain.

The C sign is very characteristic of hip joint pathology. The patient cups the hand above the greater trochanter with the thumb over the posterior aspect and gripping the fingers into the groin. It may appear as if the patient is describing a lateral

Table 45-1 Characteristic Features of Hip Joint Pathology

Straight plane activity relatively well tolerated
Torsional/twisting activities problematic
Prolonged hip flexion (sitting) uncomfortable
Pain/catching going from flexion to extension (rising from seated position)
Inclines/stairs more difficult than level surfaces

problem such as the iliotibial band or trochanteric bursitis, but this maneuver is actually performed to describe deep interior joint pain.

The log roll test is the most specific test for intra-articular pathology. Gently rolling the thigh internally and externally rotates only the femoral head in relation to the acetabulum and capsule, not stressing any of the surrounding extra-articular structures. More sensitive maneuvers include forced flexion combined with internal rotation (also referred to as the impingement test) and abduction combined with external rotation. These maneuvers normally cause some discomfort and must be compared to the unaffected hip. However, more important is whether the maneuver recreates the type of pain that the patient experiences with activities. An accompanying click or pop may be elicited, but this can occur for various reasons, and, again, most important is whether it recreates the patient's symptoms.

Intra-articular lesions are usually easily differentiated from extra-articular causes of a snapping hip. Snapping of the iliopsoas tendon is a common condition that may need to be differentiated from an intra-articular problem. The tendon snaps across the anterior joint and pectineal eminence as the hip is brought from a flexed abducted externally rotated position into extension with internal rotation.[3] Iliopsoas bursography and ultrasonography are helpful in substantiating this condition.

Radiographs are an integral part of the assessment but are unreliable at detecting most lesions amenable to arthroscopy. Careful attention should be given to early signs of degenerative arthritis, which is a poorer prognostic indicator of arthroscopic outcomes.

High-resolution magnetic resonance imaging is showing more promise at detecting intra-articular pathology but requires a 1.5-T magnet and surface coil with small field of view images of the involved hip.[4] The most reliable indicators are often indirect

Table 45-2 Examination Findings

Groin, anterior, and medial thigh pain
C-sign characteristic of interior hip pain: hand gripped above greater trochanter
Log rolling of leg back and forth: most specific indicator of intra-articular pathology
Forced flexion/internal rotation or abduction/external rotation: more sensitive measure of hip joint pain; reproduces symptoms that patient experiences with activities

findings including effusion, paralabral cysts, and subchondral cysts.

Gadolinium arthrography combined with magnetic resonance imaging (magnetic resonance angiography) demonstrates superior sensitivity at detecting numerous intra-articular lesions, but the specificity is less certain with some reports of increased false-positive interpretation. In general, these studies are best for showing labral pathology and poor for demonstrating lesions of the articular surface. The intra-articular contrast injection should include long-acting anesthetic (bupivacaine) as part of the diluent. Whether the patient's symptoms are temporarily alleviated by the intra-articular anesthetic is the most reliable indicator of the joint being the source of their problem. Following the injection, it is important that the patient be instructed to perform activities that normally create symptoms in order to assess their response.

TECHNICAL OVERVIEW

The hip joint has an intra-articular and peripheral compartment. Most hip pathology is found within the intra-articular region, and distraction is necessary to achieve arthroscopic access. The patient can be placed in the supine or lateral decubitus position for performing the procedure.[5,6] Both techniques are equally effective, and the choice is simply dependent on the surgeon's preference. An advantage of the supine approach is its simplicity in patient positioning while the lateral approach may be preferable for severely obese patients.

Performing hip arthroscopy without traction has not been popular because it does not allow access to the intra-articular region. However, it is now recognized that this method can be a useful adjunct to the traction technique.[7,8] Hip flexion relaxes the capsule and allows access to the peripheral compartment, which is intracapsular but extra-articular. Numerous lesions are encountered in this area that are overlooked with traction alone. Synovial disease often covers the capsular surface, and free-floating loose bodies can hide in the peripheral recesses. This also allows generous access to the capsule for capsulorrhaphy and is essential for addressing impingement lesions of the proximal femur.

SURGERY: HIP ARTHROSCOPY

The technique illustrated is with the patient in the supine position. The important principles for performing safe, effective, reproducible arthroscopy are the same whether the patient is in the lateral decubitus or supine orientation. Portal placements, relationship of the extra-articular structures, and arthroscopic anatomy are all the same regardless of positioning.

Equipment

A standard fracture table or custom distraction device is needed to achieve effective joint space separation. A tensiometer can be helpful to monitor the traction forces intraoperatively. The C arm is important for precise placement of the instrumentation within the joint. Extra-length arthroscopy instruments are also available to accommodate the dense surrounding soft tissue.

Anesthesia

The procedure is commonly performed under general anesthesia. It can be performed under epidural anesthesia but requires an adequate motor block to ensure optimal distractibility of the joint.

Intra-articular (Central) Compartment

Setup

The perineal post is heavily padded and lateralized against the medial thigh of the operative hip (Fig. 45-1). This aids in achieving the optimal traction vector (Fig. 45-2) and reduces pressure directly on the perineum, lessening the risk of neurapraxia of the pudendal nerve. Neutral rotation achieves a constant relationship between the topographic landmarks and the joint. Slight flexion may relax the capsule, but excessive flexion should be avoided as this places undue tension on the sciatic nerve and may block access for the anterior portal. Typically, about 50 pounds of force is needed to distract the joint. In general, the goal is to use the minimal force necessary to achieve adequate distraction and keep traction time as brief as possible. Two hours is usually recognized as a reasonable limit for traction.

Portals

Three standard portals are used for this portion of the procedure (Figs. 45-3 and 45-4). Two of these (anterolateral and posterolateral) are placed laterally over the superior margin of the greater trochanter at its anterior and posterior borders. The anterior portal is placed at the site of intersection of a sagittal line drawn distally from the anterior superior iliac spine and a transverse line across the tip of the greater trochanter. With careful orientation to the landmarks in relation to the joint, these portals are a safe distance from the surrounding major neurovascular structures (Figs. 45-5 to 45-7; Table 45-3).[9]

Diagnostic Procedure

After applying traction, a spinal needle is placed from the anterolateral position and the joint is distended with fluid. The anterolateral portal is then established under fluoroscopic control for introduction of the arthroscope (Fig. 45-8). Careful

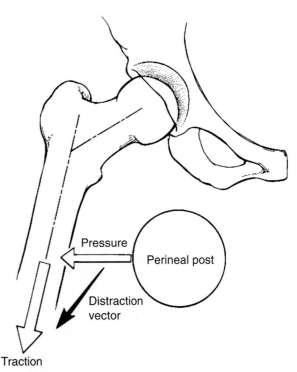

Figure 45-2 The optimal vector for distraction is oblique relative to the axis of the body and more closely coincides with the axis of the femoral neck than the femoral shaft. This oblique vector is partially created by abduction of the hip and partially accentuated by a small transverse component to the vector created by lateralizing the perineal post. (Courtesy of Smith & Nephew Endoscopy, Andover, MA.)

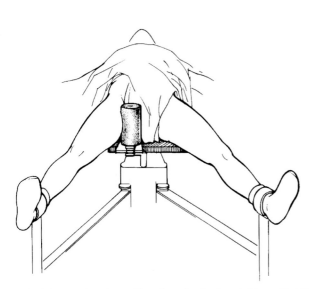

Figure 45-1 The patient is positioned on the fracture table so that the perineal post is placed as far laterally as possible toward the operative hip resting against the medial thigh. (Courtesy of Smith & Nephew Endoscopy, Andover, MA.)

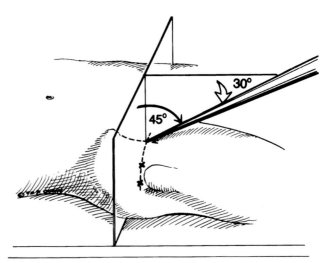

Figure 45-3 The site of the anterior portal coincides with the intersection of a sagittal line drawn distally from the anterior superior iliac spine and a transverse line across the superior margin of the greater trochanter. The direction of this portal courses approximately 45 degrees cephalad and 30 degrees toward the midline. The anterolateral and posterolateral portals are positioned directly over the superior aspect of the trochanter at its anterior and posterior borders. (From Byrd JWT: Hip arthroscopy utilizing the supine position. Arthroscopy 1994;10:275–280.)

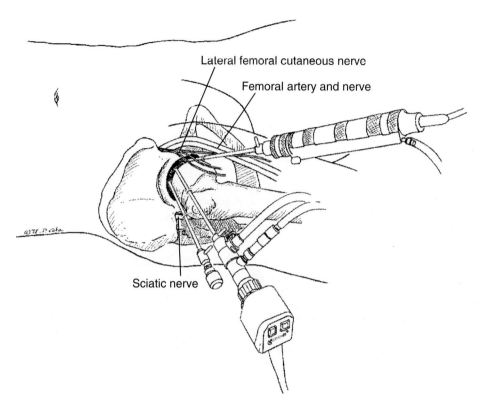

Lateral femoral cutaneous nerve

Femoral artery and nerve

Sciatic nerve

Figure 45-4 The relationship of the major neurovascular structures to the three standard portals is demonstrated. The femoral artery and nerve lie well medial to the anterior portal. The sciatic nerve lies posterior to the posterolateral portal. Small branches of the lateral femoral cutaneous nerve lie close to the anterior portal. Injury to these is avoided by using proper technique in portal placement. The anterolateral portal is established first since it lies most centrally in the safe zone for arthroscopy. (Courtesy of J.W. Thomas Byrd, MD, Nashville, TN.)

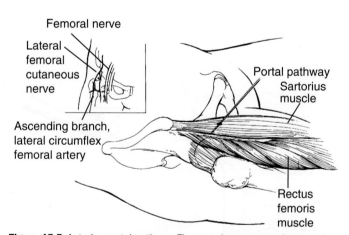

Femoral nerve

Lateral femoral cutaneous nerve

Ascending branch, lateral circumflex femoral artery

Portal pathway Sartorius muscle

Rectus femoris muscle

Figure 45-5 Anterior portal pathway. The portal penetrates the sartorius and rectus femoris before entering the anterior capsule. Its course is almost tangential to the axis of the femoral nerve, lying only slightly closer at the level of the capsule. (Courtesy of Smith & Nephew Endoscopy, Andover, MA.)

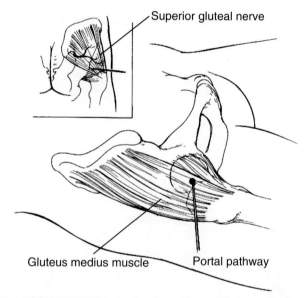

Superior gluteal nerve

Gluteus medius muscle

Portal pathway

Figure 45-6 Anterolateral portal pathway. The portal penetrates the gluteus medius, entering the lateral capsule at its anterior margin. The superior gluteal nerve lies well cephalad to this site. (Courtesy of Smith & Nephew Endoscopy, Andover, MA.)

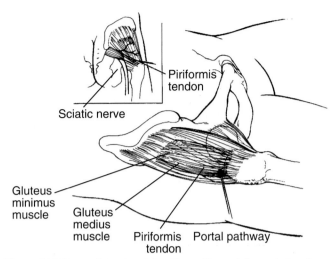

Piriformis
tendon

Sciatic nerve

Gluteus
minimus
muscle

Gluteus
medius
muscle

Piriformis
tendon

Portal pathway

Figure 45-7 Posterolateral portal pathway. The portal penetrates the gluteus and minimus, entering the lateral capsule at its posterior margin. Its course is superior and anterior to the piriformis tendon and is closest to the sciatic nerve at the level of the capsule. (Courtesy of Smith & Nephew Endoscopy, Andover, MA.)

Table 45-3 Distance from Portal to Anatomic Structures Based on an Anatomic Dissection of Portal Placements in Eight Fresh Cadaver Specimens

Portals	Anatomic Structure	Average (cm)	Range (cm)
Anterior	Anterior superior iliac spine	6.3	6.0–7.0
	Lateral femoral cutaneous nerve*	0.3	0.2–1.0
	Femoral nerve		
	Level of Sartorius†	4.3	3.8–5.0
	Level of rectus femoris	3.8	2.7–5.0
	Level of capsule	3.7	2.9–5.0
	Ascending branch of lateral circumflex femoral artery	3.7	1.0–6.0
	Terminal branch†	0.3	0.2–0.4
Anterolateral	Superior gluteal nerve	4.4	3.2–5.5
Posterolateral	Sciatic nerve	2.9	2.0–4.3

*Nerve had divided into three or more branches, and measurement was made to the closest branch.
†Measurement made at superficial branch of Sartorius, rectus femoris, and capsule.
†Small terminal branch of ascending branch of lateral circumflex femoral artery identified in three specimens.
From Byrd JWT, Pappas JN, Pedley MJ: Hip arthroscopy: An anatomic study of portal placement and relationship to the extraarticular structures. Arthroscopy 1995;11:418–423.

attention is necessary to avoid perforating the labrum or scuffing the articular surface.[10] Using the 70-degree scope, the anterior and posterolateral portals are then placed under direct arthroscopic view as well as fluoroscopy for precise entry into the joint. Diagnostic and operative arthroscopy is then achieved by interchanging the arthroscope and instruments between the three established portals. Use of both the 70- and 30-degree scopes provides optimal viewing despite limitations of maneuverability within the joint (Figs. 45-9 to 45-12).

Peripheral Compartment
Positioning
After completing arthroscopy of the intra-articular compartment, the instruments are removed, the traction released, and the hip flexed approximately 45 degrees (Fig. 45-13).

This relaxes the capsule, providing access to the peripheral compartment.

Portal Placement
Two portals are routinely used to access the peripheral compartment. These include the anterolateral portal and an ancillary portal established 4 to 5 cm distally.

Diagnostic Procedure
The anterolateral portal is redirected onto the anterior neck of the femur (Fig. 45-14). The ancillary portal is then established distally under direct arthroscopic and fluoroscopic guidance (Fig. 45-15). The arthroscope and instruments are interchanged, also using the 30- and 70-degree scopes for inspection (Figs. 45-16 and 45-17).

Figure 45-8 The arthroscope cannula is passed over a guidewire that was inserted through a pre-positioned spinal needle. Fluoroscopy aids in avoiding contact with the femoral head or perforating the acetabular labrum. (Courtesy of Smith & Nephew Endoscopy, Andover, MA.)

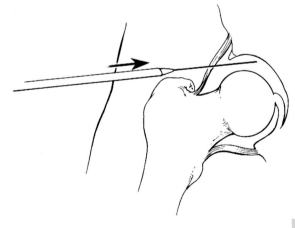

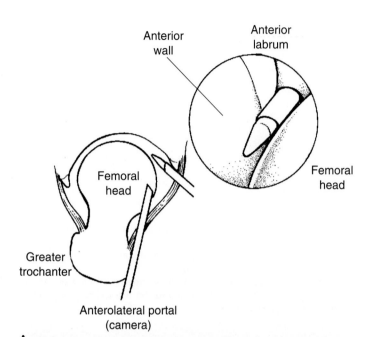

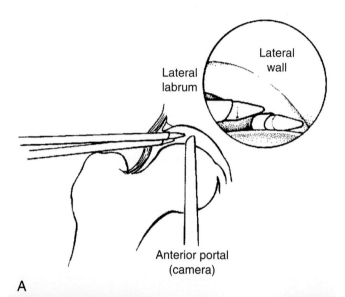

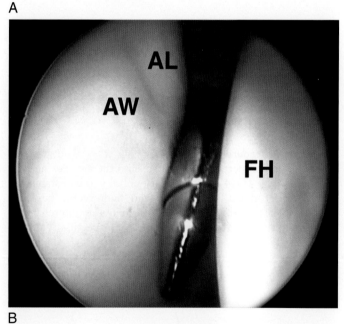

B

Figure 45-9 A, Arthroscopic view of a right hip from the anterolateral portal. (Courtesy of Smith & Nephew Endoscopy, Andover, MA.)
B, Demonstrated are the anterior acetabular wall (AW) and the anterior labrum (AL). The anterior cannula is seen entering underneath the labrum and the femoral head (FH) is on the right. (Courtesy of J.W. Thomas Byrd, MD, Nashville, TN.)

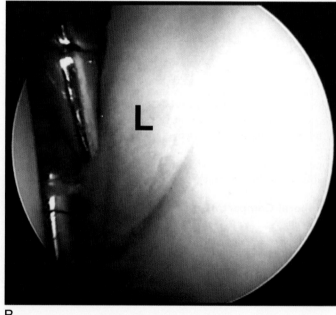

B

Figure 45-10 A, Arthroscopic view from the anterior portal.
B, Demonstrated are the lateral aspect of the labrum (L) and its relationship to the lateral two portals. (**A,** Courtesy of Smith & Nephew Endoscopy, Andover, MA.)

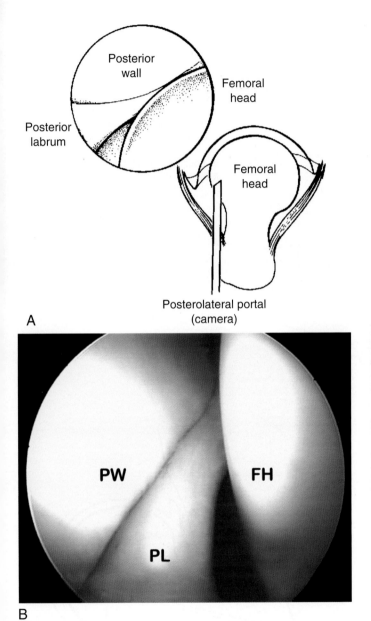

Figure 45-11 A, Arthroscopic view from the posterolateral portal. **B,** Demonstrated are the posterior acetabular wall (PW), posterior labrum (PL), and the femoral head (FH). (**A,** Courtesy of Smith & Nephew Endoscopy, Andover, MA. **B,** Courtesy of J.W. Thomas Byrd, MD, Nashville, TN.)

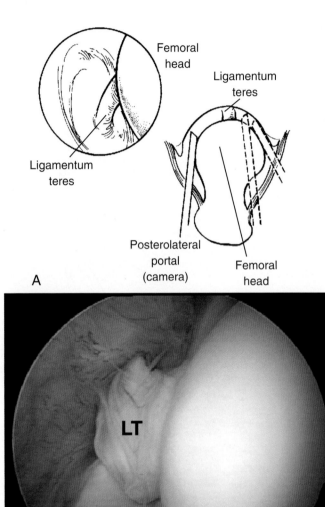

Figure 45-12 A, The acetabular fossa can be inspected from all three portals. **B,** The ligamentum teres (LT), with its accompanying vessels, has a serpentine course from its acetabular to its femoral attachment. (**A,** Courtesy of Smith & Nephew Endoscopy, Andover, MA. **B,** Courtesy of J.W. Thomas Byrd, MD, Nashville, TN.)

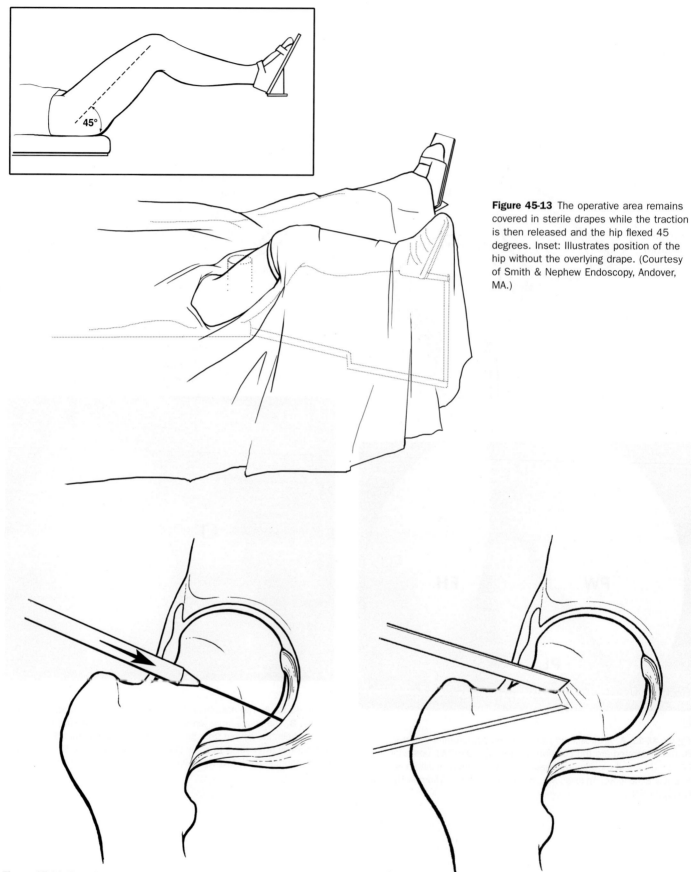

Figure 45-13 The operative area remains covered in sterile drapes while the traction is then released and the hip flexed 45 degrees. Inset: Illustrates position of the hip without the overlying drape. (Courtesy of Smith & Nephew Endoscopy, Andover, MA.)

Figure 45-14 From the anterolateral entry site, the arthroscope cannula is redirected over the guidewire through the anterior capsule, onto the neck of the femur. (Courtesy of Smith & Nephew Endoscopy, Andover, MA.)

Figure 45-15 With the arthroscope in place, prepositioning is performed with a spinal needle for placement of an ancillary portal distally. (Courtesy of Smith & Nephew Endoscopy, Andover, MA.)

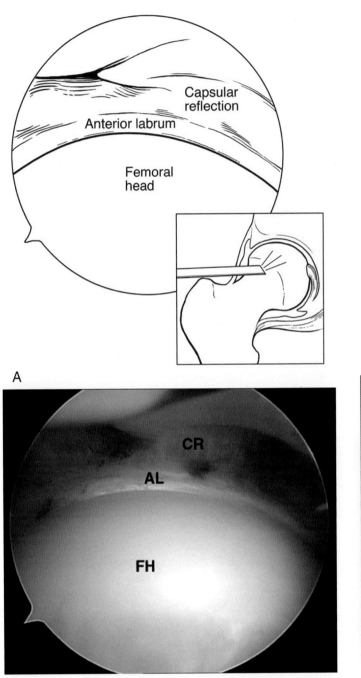

Figure 45-16 A, Peripheral compartment viewing superiorly. **B,** Demonstrated is the anterior portion of the joint including the articular surface of the femoral head (FH), anterior labrum (AL), and the capsular reflection (CR). (**A,** Courtesy of Smith & Nephew Endoscopy, Andover, MA. **B,** Courtesy of J.W. Thomas Byrd, MD, Nashville, TN.)

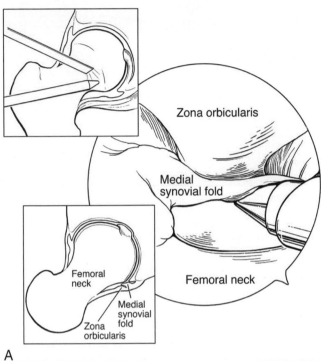

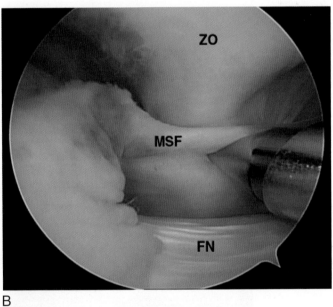

Figure 45-17 A, Peripheral compartment viewing medially. **B,** Demonstrated are the femoral neck (FN), medial synovial fold (MSF), and the zona orbicularis (ZO). (**A,** Courtesy of Smith & Nephew Endoscopy, Andover, MA. **B,** Courtesy of J.W. Thomas Byrd, MD, Nashville, TN.)

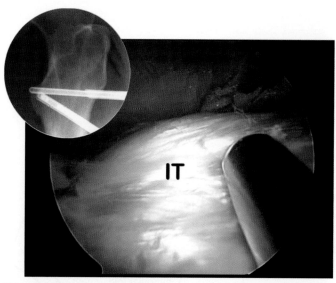

Figure 45-18 The arthroscope and shaver are positioned within the iliopsoas bursa directly over the lesser trochanter, identifying the fibers of the iliopsoas tendon (IT) at its insertion site. (Courtesy of J.W. Thomas Byrd, MD, Nashville, TN.)

Iliopsoas Bursoscopy
Positioning
Flexion is slightly less (15 to 20 degrees) than that used to view the peripheral compartment. The hip is also externally rotated, which moves the lesser trochanter more anterior and accessible to the portals.

Portals
Two portals are needed for viewing and instrumentation within the bursa (Fig. 45-18). These portals are distal to those used for the peripheral compartment and require fluoroscopy for precise positioning. These portals may be slightly more anterior to completely access the area of the lesser trochanter.

Loose Bodies
Removal of symptomatic loose bodies is not the most common indication for hip arthroscopy, but it is the clearest indication. Loose bodies can be extracted and arthroscopy offers an excellent alternative to arthrotomy, previously indicated for this condition (Fig. 45-19).[11–13] Most problematic loose bodies reside in the intra-articular compartment and are addressed with standard arthroscopic methods. However, many may remain hidden in the peripheral compartment and later become troublesome.

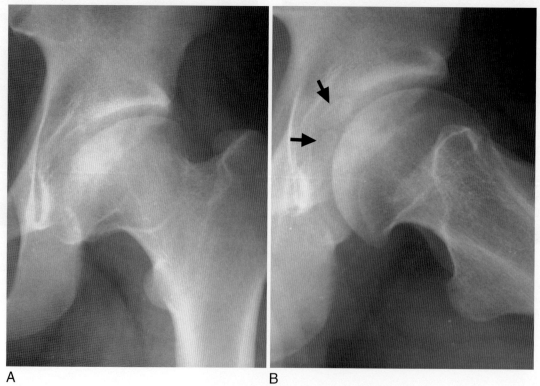

A   B

Figure 45-19 A 20-year-old male with a 3-month history of acute left hip pain. **A,** Anteroposterior radiograph demonstrates findings consistent with old Legg-Calvé-Perthes disease. **B,** Lateral view defines the presence of intra-articular loose bodies (arrows).

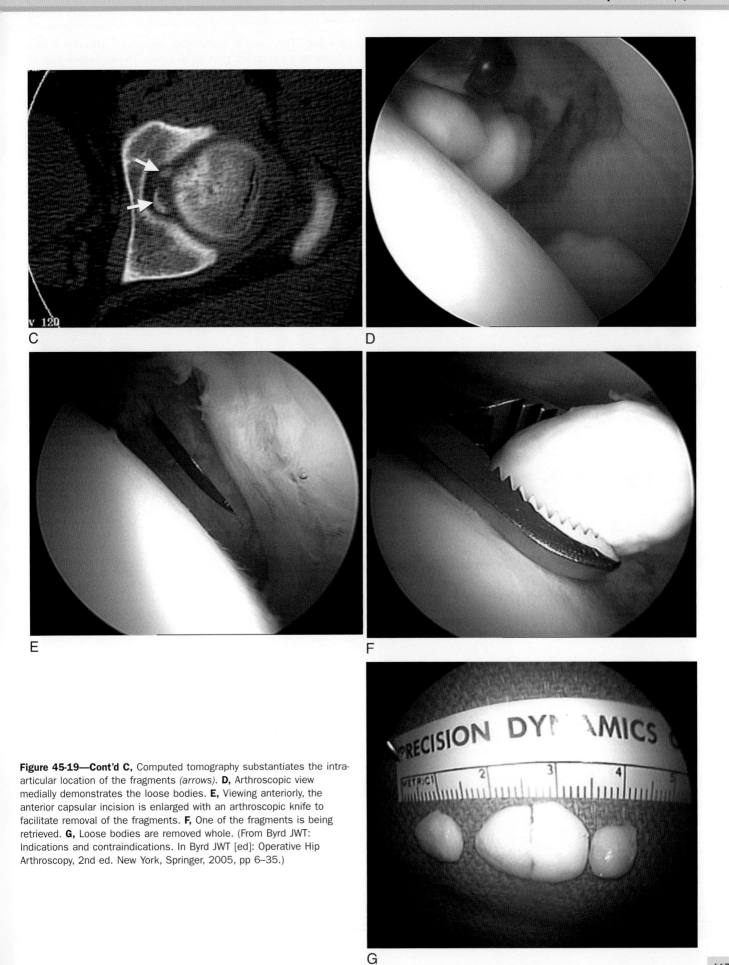

Figure 45-19—Cont'd C, Computed tomography substantiates the intra-articular location of the fragments *(arrows).* **D,** Arthroscopic view medially demonstrates the loose bodies. **E,** Viewing anteriorly, the anterior capsular incision is enlarged with an arthroscopic knife to facilitate removal of the fragments. **F,** One of the fragments is being retrieved. **G,** Loose bodies are removed whole. (From Byrd JWT: Indications and contraindications. In Byrd JWT [ed]: Operative Hip Arthroscopy, 2nd ed. New York, Springer, 2005, pp 6–35.)

Thus, arthroscopy to address symptomatic fragments must include both the intra-articular and peripheral joint.[7,8] Many can be débrided with shavers or flushed through large-diameter cannulas. Large ones can sometimes be morselized and removed piecemeal. However, often fragments may be too large to be removed through a cannula system and must be removed free hand with sturdy graspers. Once a portal tract has been developed, these larger graspers can be passed along the remaining tract into the joint in a free-hand fashion. Make sure to enlarge the capsular incision with an arthroscopic knife and the skin incision so that as the fragment is retrieved, it will not be lost in the tissues, either at the capsule or subcutaneous level.

Labral Tears

Labral lesions represent the most common indication for hip arthroscopy among athletes. Magnetic resonance imaging and magnetic resonance angiography are best at detecting labral pathology, but poor at identifying associated articular damage present in a significant portion of cases. These studies may also overinterpret pathology with lesions reported among asymptomatic volunteers, and among elite athletes, some damage may accrue simply as a consequence of the cumulative effect of their sport (Fig. 45-20). Traumatic labral tears may respond remarkably well to arthroscopic débridement (Fig. 45-21).[14-18] However, at arthroscopy, be especially cognizant of any underlying degeneration that may have predisposed to the acute tear. There will often be accompanying articular damage, and the extent of this may be a significant determinant on the eventual response to débridement (Fig. 45-22). Also, with the evolving understanding of femoroacetabular impingement and its role in the development of labral and chondral damage, it is important to make a careful radiographic assessment of accompanying bony lesions of the anterior acetabulum or femoral head that may require reshaping (Fig. 45-23).[19]

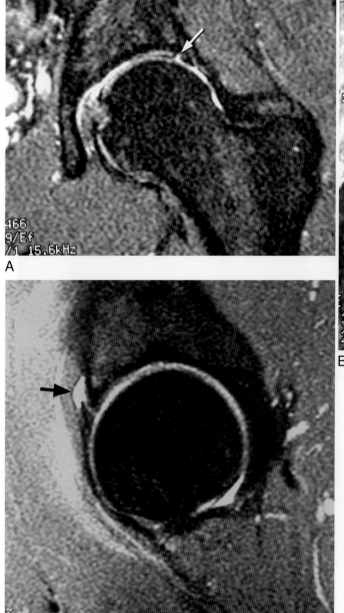

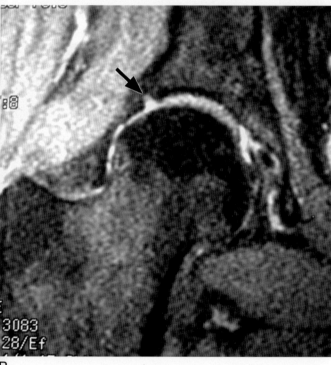

Figure 45-20 Three National Hockey League players were referred, each with a 2-week history of hip pain following an injury on the ice. Each case demonstrated evidence on magnetic resonance imaging of labral pathology *(arrows)*. These cases were treated with 2 weeks of rest followed by a 2-week period of gradually resuming activities. Each of these athletes was able to return to competition and have continued to play for several seasons without needing surgery. **A,** Coronal image of a left hip demonstrates a lateral labral tear *(arrow)*. **B,** Coronal image of a right hip demonstrates a lateral labral tear *(arrow)*. **C,** Sagittal image of a left hip demonstrates an anterior labral tear with associated paralabral cyst *(arrow)*. (Courtesy of J.W. Thomas Byrd, MD, Nashville, TN.)

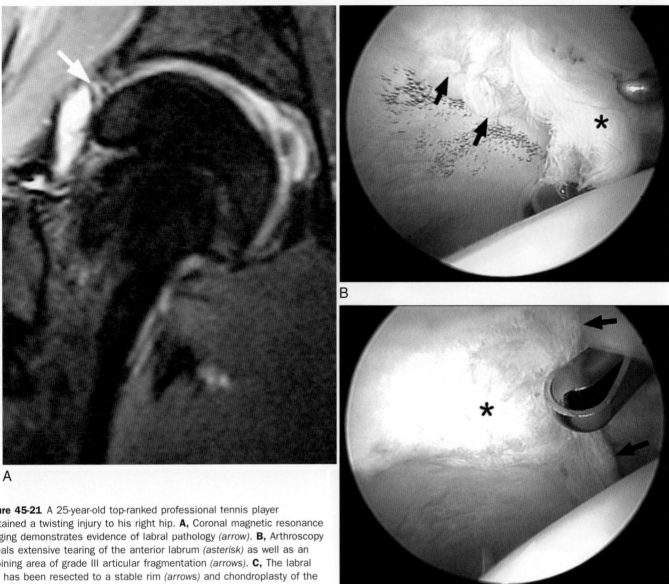

Figure 45-21 A 25-year-old top-ranked professional tennis player sustained a twisting injury to his right hip. **A,** Coronal magnetic resonance imaging demonstrates evidence of labral pathology *(arrow)*. **B,** Arthroscopy reveals extensive tearing of the anterior labrum *(asterisk)* as well as an adjoining area of grade III articular fragmentation *(arrows)*. **C,** The labral tear has been resected to a stable rim *(arrows)* and chondroplasty of the grade III articular damage *(asterisk)* is being performed. (Courtesy of J.W. Thomas Byrd, MD, Nashville, TN.)

Labral tears can be adequately accessed through the three standard portals. Similar to a meniscus in the knee, the task is to remove unstable and diseased labrum, creating a stable transition to retained healthy tissue. The most difficult aspect is creating the stable transition zone. Thermal devices have been quite useful at ablating unstable tissue adjacent to the healthy portion of the labrum. Caution is necessary because of the concerns regarding depth of heat penetration, but with judicious use, these devices have been exceptionally useful for precise labral débridement despite the constraints created by the architecture of the joint.

The natural evolution in arthroscopic management of labral pathology is from débridement to repair. Current methods of acetabular labral repair are in their infancy. A few have been attempted with mixed results. Reliable techniques remain to be developed but are probably not far off. In addition to technical advancements, there is much that remains regarding our understanding of labral morphology and pathophysiology. There is considerable variation in the normal appearance of the labrum including a labral cleft at the articular labral junction that can

be quite large.[14] It is important to distinguish this from a traumatic detachment, which can also occur. Additionally, many labral tears, even in the presence of a significant history of injury, seem to occur due to some underlying predisposition or degeneration. Under these circumstances, even with reliable techniques, repair of a degenerated or morphologically vulnerable labrum would unlikely be successful.

Articular Cartilage Injury

A propensity for acute articular injury has been identified among athletes associated with a direct blow to the trochanter (Fig. 45-24).[20] Chondroplasty can be effectively performed for lesions of both the acetabular and femoral surfaces. Curved shaver blades are helpful for negotiating the constraints created by the convex surface of the femoral head. Due to limitations of maneuverability, thermal devices have again been especially helpful in ablating unstable fragments. However, cautious and judicious use around articular surface is even more important because of potential injury to surviving chondrocytes.

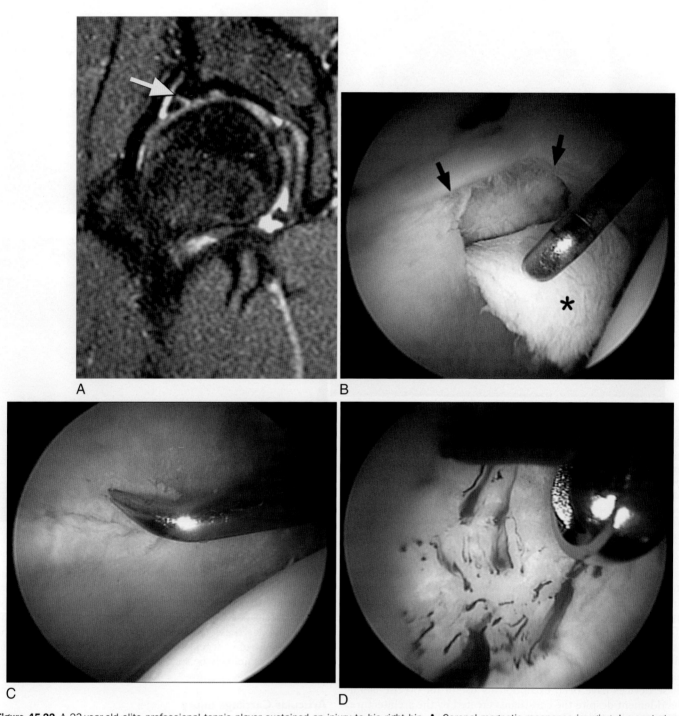

Figure 45-22 A 23-year-old elite professional tennis player sustained an injury to his right hip. **A,** Coronal magnetic resonance imaging demonstrates evidence of labral pathology *(arrow)*. **B,** Arthroscopy reveals the labral tear *(arrows)*, but also an area of adjoining grade IV articular loss *(asterisk)*. **C,** Microfracture of the exposed subchondral bone is performed. **D,** Occluding the inflow of fluid confirms vascular access through the areas of perforation. The athlete was maintained on a protected weight-bearing status emphasizing range of motion for 10 weeks with return to competition at $3\frac{1}{2}$ months. (Courtesy of J.W. Thomas Byrd, MD, Nashville, TN.)

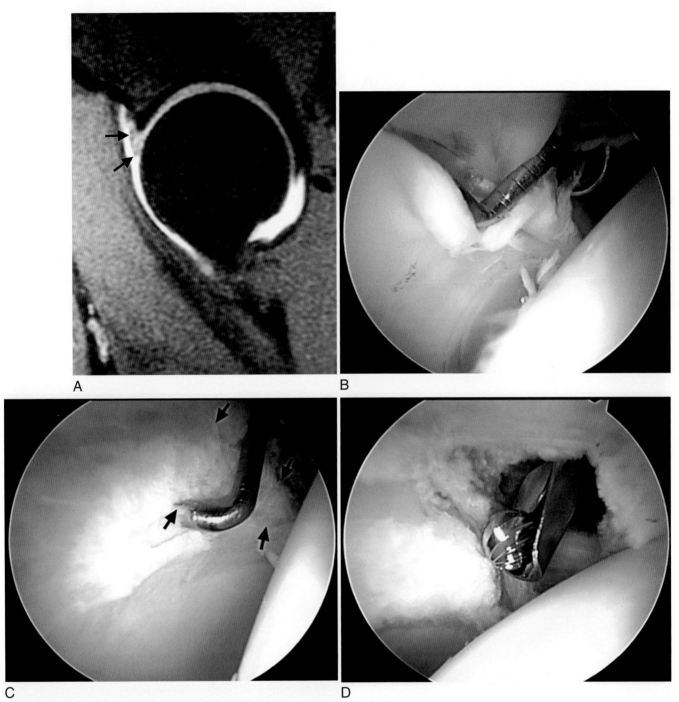

A

B

C

D

Figure 45-23 A 16-year-old high school football player develops acute onset of right hip pain doing squats. **A,** Sagittal view magnetic resonance arthrogram demonstrates a macerated anterior labrum *(arrows)*. **B,** Viewing from the anterolateral portal, a macerated tear of the anterior labrum is probed along with articular delamination at its junction with the labrum. **C,** The damaged anterior labrum has been excised, revealing an overhanging lip *(arrows)* of impinging bone from the anterior acetabulum. **D,** Excision of the impinging portion of the acetabulum (acetabuloplasty) is performed with a bur. (Courtesy of J.W. Thomas Byrd, MD, Nashville, TN.)

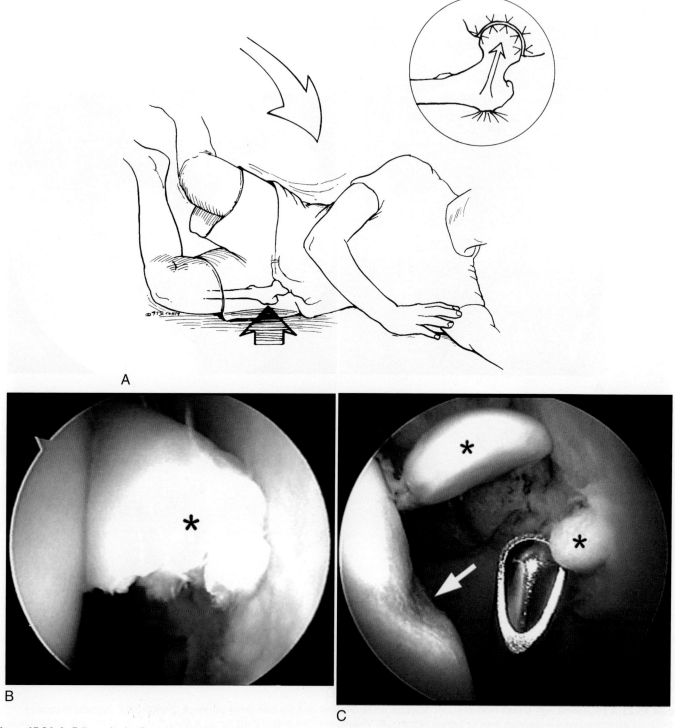

A

B

C

Figure 45-24 A, Fall results in direct blow to the greater trochanter, and, in absence of fracture, the force generated is transferred unchecked to the hip joint. **B,** Arthroscopic view of the left hip of a 20-year-old collegiate basketball player demonstrates an acute grade IV articular injury *(asterisk)* to the medial aspect of the femoral head. **C,** Arthroscopic view of the left hip of a 19-year-old male who sustained a direct lateral blow to the hip, subsequently developing osteocartilaginous fragments *(asterisks)* within the superomedial aspect of the acetabulum. (From Byrd JWT: Lateral impact injury: A source of occult hip pathology. Clin Sports Med 2001;20:801–816.)

Microfracture of select grade IV articular lesions has been beneficial (see Fig. 45-22).[18] As with other joints, it is best indicated for focal lesions with healthy surrounding articular surface. The lesion most amenable to this process is encountered in the lateral aspect of the acetabulum. This is followed by 8 to 10 weeks of protected weight bearing to neutralize the forces across the hip joint while emphasizing range of motion. Using this protocol, among a cohort of 24 patients, 86% demonstrated a successful outcome at 2- to 5-year follow-up.[21]

Ligamentum Teres Injury

Injury to the ligamentum teres is increasingly recognized as a source of hip pain in athletes (Fig. 45-25).[1] The disrupted fibers catch within the joint and can be quite symptomatic. This disruption may be the result of trauma, degeneration, or a combination of both.[22] The tear may be partial or complete with the goal of treatment being to débride the entrapping, disrupted fibers. Our recent report documented excellent success in the arthroscopic management of traumatic lesions of the ligamentum teres. The average improvement was 47 points (100-point modified Harris hip score system), with 93% showing marked (>20 points) improvement.[23]

The acetabular attachment of the ligamentum teres is situated posteriorly at the inferior margin of the acetabular fossa and attaches on the femoral head at the fovea capitis. The disrupted portion of the ligament is avascular, but the fat pad and synovium contained in the superior portion of the fossa can be quite vascular. Débridement is facilitated by a complement of curved shaver blades and a thermal device. The disrupted portion of the ligament is unstable and delivered by suction into the shaver. A thermal device can also ablate tissue while maintaining hemostasis within the vascular pulvinar.

Access to this inferomedial portion of the joint is best accomplished from the anterior portal. External rotation of the hip also helps in delivering the ligament to the shaver brought in anteriorly. The most posterior portion of the fossa and the acetabular attachment of the ligament may be best accessed from the posterolateral portal. Indiscriminate débridement of the ligamentum teres should be avoided because of its potential contribution to the vascularity of the femoral head.

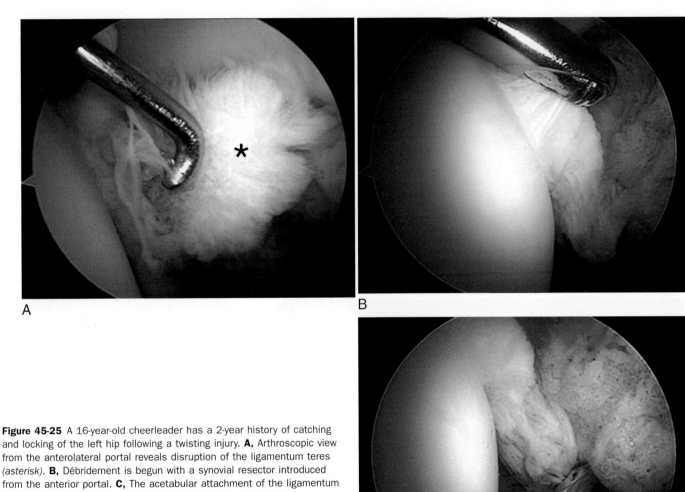

Figure 45-25 A 16-year-old cheerleader has a 2-year history of catching and locking of the left hip following a twisting injury. **A,** Arthroscopic view from the anterolateral portal reveals disruption of the ligamentum teres *(asterisk)*. **B,** Débridement is begun with a synovial resector introduced from the anterior portal. **C,** The acetabular attachment of the ligamentum teres in the posterior aspect of the fossa is addressed from the posterolateral portal. (Courtesy of J.W. Thomas Byrd, MD, Nashville, TN.)

Synovial Disease

Primary synovial disease may be encountered in athletes, but more often synovial proliferation occurs in response to other intra-articular pathology. Synovitis may be diffuse, encompassing the lining of the joint capsule, or focal, emanating from the pulvinar of the acetabular fossa. Focal lesions within the fossa may be dense and fibrotic or exhibit proliferative villous characteristics. Presumably, because of entrapment within the joint, these lesions can be quite painful and respond remarkably well to simple débridement. While a complete synovectomy cannot be performed, a generous subtotal synovectomy can be carried out. Enlarging the capsular incisions with an arthroscopic knife improves maneuverability within the intra-articular portion of the joint. For most synovial disease, arthroscopy of the peripheral compartment is necessary in order to adequately resect the diseased tissue.[7,8,19]

In the presence of arthritis, there will be arthroscopic evidence of various pathology including free fragments, labral tearing, articular damage, and synovial disease. With a meticulous systematic approach, each component can be addressed arthroscopically. Ultimately, with a well-performed procedure, the response to treatment will be mostly dictated by the extent of pathology, much of which cannot be reversed.[24-27]

Impinging Osteophytes

Post-traumatic impinging bone fragments, occasionally encountered in an active athletic population, may respond well to arthroscopic excision.[28,29] Degenerative osteophytes rarely benefit from arthroscopic excision as the symptoms are usually more associated with the extent of joint deterioration and not simply the radiographically evident osteophytes that secondarily form. However, the post-traumatic type may impinge on the joint, causing pain and blocking motion. These fragments are often extracapsular and require a capsulotomy, extending the dissection outside the joint for excision (Fig. 45-26). This necessitates thorough knowledge and careful orientation of the extra-articular anatomy and excellent visualization at all times during the procedure. In general, the dissection should stay directly on the bone fragments and avoid straying into the surrounding soft tissues. Various techniques aid in maintaining optimal visualiza-

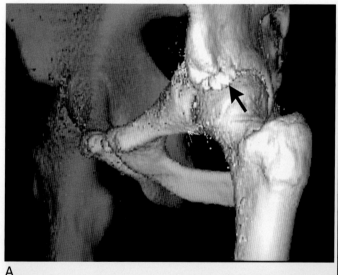

A

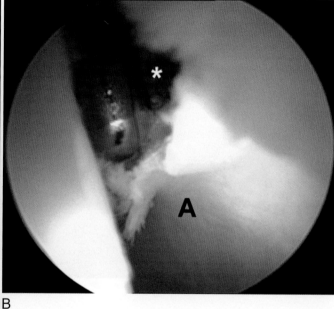

B

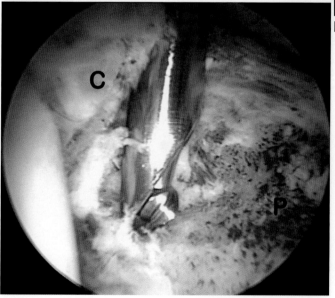

C

Figure 45-26 An 18-year-old high school football player sustained an avulsion fracture of the left anterior inferior iliac spine. **A,** Three-dimensional computed tomography illustrates the avulsed fragment *(arrow)*, which ossified, creating an impinging painful block to flexion and internal rotation. **B,** Viewing from the anterolateral portal, a capsular window is created, exposing the osteophyte *(asterisk)* anterior to the acetabulum (A). **C,** The anterior capsule (C) has been completely released allowing resection of the fragment along the anterior column of the pelvis (P). Postoperatively, the patient regained full range of motion with resolution of his pain. (From Byrd JWT: Arthroscopy of select hip lesions. In Byrd JWT [ed]: Operative Hip Arthroscopy. New York, Thieme, 1998, pp 153–170.)

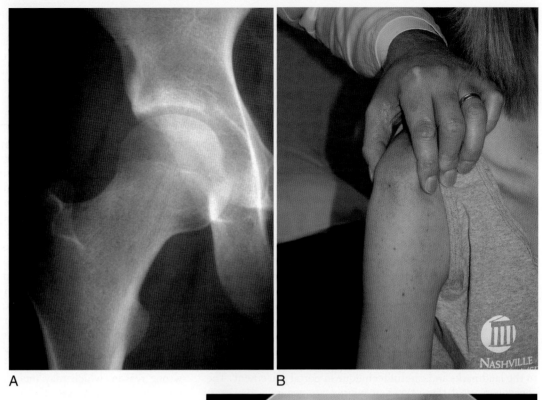

A

B

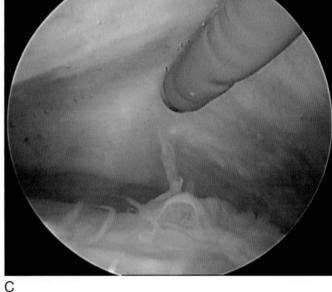

C

Figure 45-27 A 19-year-old female had undergone two previous arthroscopic procedures on her right hip for reported lesions of the ligamentum teres. Following each procedure, she developed recurrent symptoms of "giving way." **A,** Radiographs revealed normal joint geometry. **B,** She was noted to have severe diffuse physiologic laxity best characterized by a markedly positive sulcus sign. **C,** With objective evidence of laxity and subjective symptoms of instability, an arthroscopic thermal capsulorrhaphy was performed, accessing the redundant anterior capsule from the peripheral compartment. Modulation of the capsular response was controlled by a hip spica brace for 8 weeks postoperatively with a successful outcome. (Courtesy of J.W. Thomas Byrd, MD, Nashville, TN.)

tion. A high-flow pump is especially helpful, maintaining a high flow rate without excessive pressure, which would worsen extravasation. Hypotensive anesthesia, placing epinephrine in the arthroscopic fluid, and electrocautery or other thermal device for hemostasis all aid in visualization for effectively performing the excision.

Instability

Hip instability can occur but is much less common than seen in the shoulder. There are several reasons, but, most principally, it is due to the inherent stability provided by the constrained ball-and-socket bony architecture of the joint. Also, the labrum is not as critical to stability of the hip as it is in the shoulder as there is no true capsulolabral complex. On the acetabular side,

the capsule attaches directly to the bone, separate from the acetabular labrum.[30] An entrapped labrum has been reported as a cause of an irreducible posterior dislocation and a Bankart type detachment of the posterior labrum has been identified as the cause of recurrent posterior instability.[31,32] These circumstances have only rarely been reported but may be recognized with increasing frequency as our understanding of and intervention in hip injuries evolves.

Instability may occur simply due to an incompetent capsule. This is seen in hyperlaxity states and less often encountered in athletics. The most common cause is a collagen vascular disorder such as Ehlers-Danlos syndrome. With normal joint geometry, thermal capsular shrinkage has continued to meet with successful results (Fig. 45-27). If subluxation or symptomatic instability is due to a dysplastic joint, it is likely that bony correction for containment is necessary to achieve stability.

Based on this author's observations, posterior instability has been found to be associated with macrotrauma. This is due to the characteristic mechanisms of injury, including dashboard injuries and axial loading of the flexed hip encountered in collision sports. Atraumatic instability or instability due to repetitive microtrauma is anterior and develops when the normally occurring anterior translation of the femoral head exceeds the physiologic threshold and becomes pathologic. Symptoms may be due to primary instability, secondary intra-articular damage, or a combination of both.

COMPLICATIONS

The reported complication rate associated with large hip arthroscopy series ranges from 1.3% to 6.4%.[33-35] Most of these are minor or transient, but a few major complications have been reported. Traction neuropraxia is usually associated with prolonged procedures and excessive traction but can occur even when staying within established guidelines. With normal precautions, it is expected that the condition should be transient and recovery complete. Direct trauma to the major neurovascular structures should be avoidable with thoughtful orientation to the landmarks and careful technique in portal placement. The consequences of these types of injuries are generally devastating. Small branches of the lateral femoral cutaneous nerve invariably lie around the anterior portal. Even with careful technique, there is a 0.5% chance of incurring a small patch of reduced sensation in the lateral thigh due to instrumentation around one of these branches.

Potentially life-threatening intra-abdominal extravasation of fluid has been reported.[36] This is generally attributed to fresh acetabular fractures, extra-articular procedures, and prolonged operating times.[34] It is imperative that the surgeon be cognizant of the balance of ingress and egress of fluid throughout the operative procedure.

It is likely that the most common complication, which goes largely unreported, is iatrogenic intra-articular damage. Even with careful attention to the details of the procedure, this cannot be entirely avoided. However, it can be minimized and emphasizes the importance of meticulous technique in performing the procedure.

CONCLUSIONS

Hip joint injuries in athletes may go unrecognized for a protracted period of time, most commonly diagnosed as a strain. With an increase in awareness of intra-articular disorders, these problems are now being diagnosed earlier. However, much remains to be understood regarding the pathogenesis and natural history of many of these lesions that may influence the results of both surgical and conservative management. Nonetheless, arthroscopy has defined numerous sources of intra-articular hip pathology. In many cases, operative arthroscopy has met with significant success. For some, arthroscopy offers a distinct advantage over traditional open techniques, but for many, arthroscopy offers a method of treatment where none existed before. With this procedure, there are three important principles that must be thoroughly considered. First, a successful outcome is dependent on proper patient selection. A technically well-performed procedure will fail when performed for the wrong reason, which may include failure of the procedure to meet the patient's expectations. Second, the patient must be properly positioned for the procedure to go well. Poor positioning will ensure a difficult procedure. Third, simply gaining access to the hip joint is not an outstanding technical accomplishment. The paramount issue is that the joint must be accessed in as atraumatic a fashion as possible. Because of its constrained architecture and dense soft-tissue envelope, the potential for inadvertent iatrogenic scope trauma is significant and, perhaps to some extent, unavoidable. Thus, every reasonable step should be taken to keep this concern to a minimum by performing the procedure as carefully as possible and being certain that it is performed for the right reasons.

REFERENCES

1. Byrd JWT, Jones KS: Hip arthroscopy in athletes. Clin Sports Med 2001;20:749–762.
2. Byrd JWT: Physical examination. In Byrd JWT (ed): Operative Hip Arthroscopy, 2nd ed. New York, Springer, 2005, pp 36–50.
3. Allen WC, Cope R: Coxa saltans: The snapping hip revisited. J Am Acad Orthop Surg 1995;3:303–308.
4. Byrd JWT, Jones KS: Diagnostic accuracy of clinical assessment, MRI, gadolinium MRI, and intraarticular injection in hip arthroscopy patients. Am J Sports Med 2004;32:1668–1674.
5. Byrd JWT: The supine approach. In Byrd JWT (ed): Operative Hip Arthroscopy, 2nd ed. New York, Springer, 2005, pp 145–169.
6. Sampson TG: The lateral approach. In Byrd JWT (ed): Operative Hip Arthroscopy, 2nd ed. New York, Springer, 2005, pp 129–144.
7. Dienst M, Godde S, Seil R, et al: Hip arthroscopy without traction: In vivo anatomy of the peripheral hip joint cavity. Arthroscopy 2001;17:924–931.
8. Dienst M: Hip arthroscopy without traction. In Byrd JWT (ed): Operative Hip Arthroscopy, 2nd ed. New York, Springer, 2005, pp 170–188.
9. Byrd JWT, Pappas JN, Pedley MJ: Hip arthroscopy: An anatomic study of portal placement and relationship to the extraarticular structures. Arthroscopy 1995;11:418–423.
10. Byrd JWT: Avoiding the labrum in hip arthroscopy. Arthroscopy 2000;16:770–773.
11. Byrd JWT: Hip arthroscopy for post-traumatic loose fragments in the young active adult: Three case reports. Clin J Sport Med 1996;6:129–134.
12. McCarthy JC, Bono JV, Wardell S: Is there a treatment for synovial chondromatosis of the hip joint? Arthroscopy 1997;13:409–410.
13. Medlock V, Rathjen KE, Montgomery JB: Hip arthroscopy for late sequelae of Perthes disease. Arthroscopy 1999;15:552–553.
14. Byrd JWT: Labral lesions: An elusive source of hip pain: Case reports and review of the literature. Arthroscopy 1996;12:603–612.
15. Lage LA, Patel JV, Villar RN: The acetabular labral tear; an arthroscopic classification. Arthroscopy 1996;12:269–272.
16. Farjo LA, Glick JM, Sampson TG: Hip arthroscopy for acetabular labrum tears. Arthroscopy 1997;13:409–410.
17. Santori N, Villar RN: Acetabular labral tears: Result of arthroscopic partial limbectomy. Arthroscopy 2000;16:11–15.
18. Byrd JWT, Jones KS: Inverted acetabular labrum and secondary osteoarthritis: Radiographic diagnosis and arthroscopic treatment. Arthroscopy 2000;16:417.
19. Byrd JWT: Hip arthroscopy: Evolving frontiers. Op Tech Sports Med 2004;14:58–67.
20. Byrd JWT: Lateral impact injury: A source of occult hip pathology. Clin Sports Med 2001;20:801–816.

21. Byrd JWT, Jones KS: Microfracture for grade IV chondral lesions of the hip. Arthroscopy 2004;20(SS-89):41.

22. Gray AJR, Villar RN: The ligamentum teres of the hip: An arthroscopic classification of its pathology. Arthroscopy 1997;13:575–578.

23. Byrd JWT, Jones KS: Traumatic rupture of the ligamentum teres as a source of hip pain. Arthroscopy 2004;20:385–391.

24. Farjo LA, Glick JM, Sampson TG: Hip arthroscopy for degenerative joint disease. Arthroscopy 1998;14:435.

25. Villar RN: Arthroscopic debridement of the hip: A minimally invasive approach to osteoarthritis. J Bone Joint Surg Br 1991;73(Suppl II):170–171.

26. Santori N, Villar RN: Arthroscopic findings in the initial stages of hip osteoarthritis. Orthopedics 1999;22:405–409.

27. Byrd JWT, Jones KS: Prospective analysis of hip arthroscopy with five year follow up. Paper presented at the AAOS 69th Annual Meeting, February 14, 2002, Dallas, TX.

28. Byrd JWT: Indications and contraindications. In Byrd JWT (ed): Operative Hip Arthroscopy, 2nd ed. New York, Springer, 2005, pp 6–35.

29. Byrd JWT: Arthroscopy of select hip lesions. In Byrd JWT (ed): Operative Hip Arthroscopy. New York, Thieme, 1998, pp 153–170.

30. Seldes RM, Tan V, Hunt J, et al: Anatomy, histologic features, and vascularity of the adult acetabular labrum. Clin Orthop 2001;382:32–40.

31. Paterson I: The torn acetabular labrum: A block to reduction of a dislocated hip. J Bone Joint Surg Br 1957;39:306–309.

32. Dameron TB: Bucket-handle tear of acetabular labrum accompanying posterior dislocation of the hip. J Bone Joint Surg Am 1959;41:131–134.

33. Clarke MT, Arora A, Villar RN: Hip arthroscopy: Complications in 1054 cases. Clin Orthop 2003;406:84–88.

34. Sampson TG: Complications of hip arthroscopy. Clin Sports Med 2001;20;831–835.

35. Byrd JWT: Complications associated with hip arthroscopy. In Byrd JWT (ed): Operative Hip Arthroscopy, 2nd ed. New York, Springer, 2005, pp 229–235.

36. Bartlett CS, DiFelice GS, Buly RL, et al: Cardiac arrest as a result of intraabdominal extravasation of fluid during arthroscopic removal of a loose body from the hip joint of a patient with an acetabular fracture. J Orthop Trauma 1998;12:294–300.

Knee

Timothy C. Wilson

In This Chapter

Examination of specific ligaments
Patellofemoral exam
Meniscus exam
Multiligamentous knee injuries

INTRODUCTION

- The physical examination of the knee has been described as an art and a science.[1]

- The purpose of the examination is to arrive at the correct diagnosis.

- A complete patient history must be combined with a thorough physical examination in order to direct treatment.

- Additional tests such as radiographs, magnetic resonance imaging, bone scans, and angiography are sometimes used to provide information in the evaluation of a knee injury.

HISTORY

The clinical examination of the knee begins with a thorough history that focuses on the presenting symptoms and mechanism of injury. Questions should be asked regarding the onset and duration of symptoms. The location and quality of pain should be ascertained as well as the presence of any previous injuries or history of surgery. It is important to document the presence of swelling, mechanical symptoms, and instability. Mechanical symptoms may include locking and catching. Giving way may be the patient's description of instability. Many patients who experience a "pop" in their knee at the time of injury will have an anterior cruciate ligament (ACL) tear. In many cases, the history itself will direct the examiner toward the correct diagnosis.

The mechanism of injury provides useful information with regards to the direction and degree of injury. Ligament injuries are the result of forces from the opposite direction. For example, an anterior blow to the knee may cause a posterior knee dislocation. This injury pattern is commonly seen in "dashboard knee." Anterior dislocations commonly occur from extreme knee hyperextension. This happens when an anterior force occurs to the tibia against a fixed foot, and the femur is forced posterior to the tibia. Medial and lateral ligament injuries are most likely to occur from valgus and varus forces, respectively.[2] Knowledge of each patient's mechanism of injury will be useful in determining which structures may be injured and the potential risk of associated injuries. In summary, the history can lead the examiner to a specific area to inspect and improve the ability to correctly diagnose.

PHYSICAL EXAMINATION

A thorough examination of the knee involves a systematic approach. Having the patient relax is of utmost importance. The best physical examination can sometimes be obtained immediately after the injury before significant swelling and pain preclude a relaxed examination. It is helpful to examine the uninjured knee first not only to serve as a baseline, but also to gain the confidence of the patient. The least painful tests should be performed before progressing to the more painful examination techniques.

The patient's gait pattern should be inspected. An antalgic gait is demonstrated by a shortened stance phase and will confirm the involved extremity. During the stance phase the presence of a varus thrust should be noted if present. A short leg gait may be observed, and this can be noted by measuring for a leg length discrepancy. The clinical alignment of the limb should be observed for genu varus or valgus. This is measured by placing a goniometer on the patella and measuring the angular alignment of the femur in relation to the tibia. This measurement differs from the radiographic measurement of the mechanical axis.

The physical examination of the knee includes an inspection for any soft-tissue swelling or joint effusion (Fig. 46-1). It is important to distinguish between these two types of fluid accumulation. Fluid that is intra-articular signifies an injury to the joint itself. Common causes of an effusion include an ACL tear, patellar dislocation, or osteochondral injury. The finding of a ballotable patella is a sign of an effusion. Another sign of an effusion is the loss of the normal skin dimple that is visible just distal to the vastus medialis obliquus insertion on the patella. Prepatella swelling may be from a bursitis. Other soft-tissue swelling may be associated with extra-articular ligament tears and sprains. For example, a medial collateral ligament sprain may present with medial soft-tissue swelling. The ability to distinguish an effusion from soft-tissue swelling is an important aspect of the physical examination.

The range of motion of the knee should be measured. A goniometer can be used to measure the amount of knee flexion and extension. The knee should be evaluated for hyperextension as well. Both knees should always be measured as asymmetry may be a sign of injury. A locked knee is a knee with the inability to fully extend because of a mechanical block such as from a bucket handle meniscus tear or a loose body.

Measurements should be taken of the girth of the quadriceps muscle. Quadriceps atrophy is commonly seen after surgery or

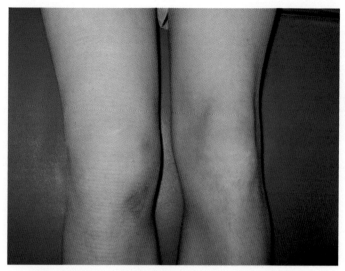

Figure 46-1 Right knee effusion after a patellar dislocation.

a chronic injury. The measurement is taken at a set distance from either the patella or joint line and the two knees are compared to one another. Subsequent measurements can be made to follow a patient's progress with rehabilitation.

Palpation is an essential part of all examinations. The bony landmarks should be assessed for tenderness. Joint line tenderness is sensitive for the diagnosis of a meniscus tear. Sometimes a meniscal cyst may be visible and palpable in the joint line. A medial patellofemoral plica can be palpable medially, just above the joint line, and is sometimes tender as it is compressed between the examiner's fingers and the medial femoral condyle. The inferior pole of the patella, patellar tendon, and tibia tubercle are common areas of tenderness in athletes with anterior knee pain. Lateral patellofemoral compression may be associated with tenderness of the lateral patellar facet. Other common areas of tenderness include the iliotibial band, pes anserine bursa, and quadriceps. Crepitation of the knee joint as it goes through a range of motion is a common sign of patellofemoral chondromalacia. The knee should be assessed for warmth. A normal knee should always feel cooler to the touch than the surrounding musculature. The back of the examiner's hand may be used to detect subtle temperature differences. Synovitis is a common cause of a subtle increase in temperature of the knee.

EXAMINATION OF SPECIFIC LIGAMENTS

In the acute setting, swelling and pain often prevent a detailed ligament examination. However, the best possible assessment should be obtained. Gross instability to varus or valgus testing in extension suggests injury to one or both cruciate ligaments, the joint capsule, and the associated collateral ligament. If the joint capsule has been disrupted, there may not be an effusion. Flexion is often not possible because of pain. This precludes anterior and posterior drawer testing. The information obtained from the physical examination should be correlated with the history and mechanism of injury.

The four main ligamentous structures include the ACL, posterior cruciate ligament (PCL), medial collateral ligament (MCL) with the posteromedial capsule, and the posterolateral corner (PLC). The PLC is composed of the lateral collateral ligament, popliteus tendon, popliteofibular ligament, arcuate ligament, fabellofibular ligament, and the posterolateral joint

capsule. It is important to specifically examine each of the four elements carefully. Magnetic resonance imaging should not be extensively relied on because the accuracy of that test is diminished without clinical correlation.

Anterior Cruciate Ligament

The ACL serves as the primary restraint to anterior translation of the tibia in relation to the femur. It provides 86% of the resistance to anterior translation.[3] The ACL also serves as a secondary stabilizer to varus, valgus, and rotational stresses about the knee.[4] The most reliable and sensitive test for assessing ACL deficiency is the Lachman test (Fig. 46-2). To perform the test, the examiner stabilizes the femur with one hand and performs an anterior drawer with the other hand on the tibia. The knee is held in 20 to 30 degrees of flexion with neutral rotation. The Lachman test measures laxity, and the examiner should appreciate the quality of an endpoint. Any increased translation is a positive result and is graded I, II, and III. A grade I is 0 to 5 mm of translation. A grade II is 6 to 10 mm, and a grade III is greater than 10 mm and lacks a firm endpoint. In multiple-ligament injured knees, this test is more difficult to perform. For example, PCL-deficient knees can mislead the examiner because of the abnormal translation. Also, a complete MCL disruption can give a false-positive result on the Lachman test if care is not taken to perform the test in neutral rotation. This results from the anteromedial rotational instability secondary to MCL disruption.

The ACL does more than just prevent anterior translation of the tibia on the femur. It also serves as the principal restraint to anterolateral rotatory instability. Tests that are designed to examine this elicit the pivot-shift phenomenon. These tests include Slocum's anterior rotatory drawer test, the Hughston-Losee jerk test, and the MacIntosh lateral pivot shift test. All these tests are performed with a valgus force during flexion and extension of the knee to elicit subluxation or reduction of the tibia on the femur. In an ACL-deficient knee, as the knee goes from flexion to extension, the iliotibial band is anterior to the center of rotation of the knee and subluxates the tibia anteriorly. The tibia is reduced as the knee goes back into flexion. These tests are difficult to perform in the acute setting because of pain and guarding.

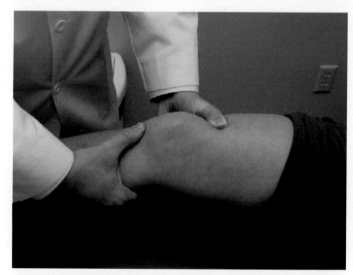

Figure 46-2 Lachman test for anterior cruciate ligament laxity. The left hand stabilizes the femur with the knee in 30 degrees of flexion. The left hand applies an anterior load and the amount of anterior translation of the tibia in relation to the femur is assessed.

The flexion rotation test combines elements of the Lachman and the pivot-shift tests. The patient is supine with the knee in neutral rotation. The leg is lifted up and the tibia subluxates anteriorly with the femur posteriorly and externally rotated. The knee is then flexed with a valgus stress and anterior force on the proximal tibia. This results in the tibia moving posteriorly as the femur internally rotates, which reduces the tibia.[5] The examiner should become proficient in the Lachman test and at least one of the pivot-shift tests.

Posterior Cruciate Ligament

Injuries to the PCL are sometimes subtle, and careful attention should be paid to a complete knee ligament examination. The PCL serves as the primary restraint to posterior translation of the tibia.[3] The physical examination of the PCL includes the posterior drawer test, posterior sag sign, and quadriceps active test. The most sensitive test is the posterior drawer test (Fig. 46-3). The posterior drawer test is performed with the knee in 90 degrees of flexion. The examiner's thumbs are placed on the joint line and a posterior drawer is applied. The anterior tibiofemoral step-off is important to note when performing this test. Normal step-off is 8 to 10 mm (tibia anterior to the femur with the knee flexed 90 degrees). This test is graded according to the amount of translation with a posteriorly directed force. A positive test has increased translation. With a grade I, the tibia remains anterior to the femoral condyles. A grade II results in the tibia being equal to the femoral condyles, and with a grade III, the tibia can be subluxated posterior to the femoral condyles and lacks a firm endpoint. Grade III laxity on the posterior drawer test is suggestive of a clinically significant injury and usually involves injury to the secondary restraints as well.

Medial Collateral Ligament

The MCL is the primary restraint to a valgus knee stress at 20 to 30 degrees of flexion. It is also a secondary restraint to ante-

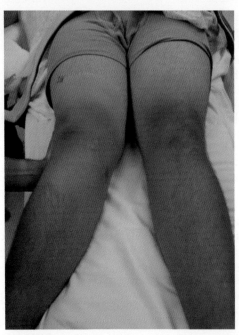

Figure 46-4 Valgus stress to right knee in full extension. The knee opened up in full extension, which signifies significant injury to the medial collateral ligament and posteromedial capsule.

rior translation. Testing is performed by applying a valgus stress at 20 to 30 degrees flexion. This test is graded according to the amount of joint line opening in millimeters and the presence of an endpoint. Grade I is less than 5 mm of opening, grade II is 6 to 10 mm, and a grade III is greater than 10 mm. The knee is also tested in full extension. Opening to valgus testing in full extension implies damage to the posteromedial capsule in addition to the superficial medial collateral ligament[6] (Fig. 46-4). The posteromedial capsule is part of the deep MCL and may need to be repaired or reconstructed in some cases.

For patients with medial collateral ligament injuries, it is important to document the precise location of the tenderness. This can help differentiate the location and severity of the injury. Although most medial collateral ligaments may do well with nonoperative treatment, a subset of MCL injuries with complete disruption off the tibia may have an indication for a direct anatomic repair. Patients with a complete disruption of the MCL off the tibia have been shown to have tenderness over the tibia as opposed to the femoral side of the MCL.[7]

Posterolateral Corner

The posterolateral corner resists varus and rotational forces to the knee. The anatomic structures of the PLC can be divided into three layers. Layer 1 is composed of the iliotibial band and the biceps femoris tendon. Layer 2 consists of the lateral retinaculum and lateral patellofemoral ligaments. Layer 3 is the deepest and contains the lateral collateral ligament or fibular collateral ligament, the fabellofibular ligament, the popliteus, the arcuate complex, and the important popliteofibular ligament. Testing of the PLC consists of varus stress to the knee at 0 and 30 degrees. Increased external rotation of the tibia at 30 and 90 degrees is tested and compared to the contralateral knee. Increased external rotation at 30 degrees that decreases at 90 degrees suggests an isolated injury of the posterolateral corner. If the external rotation does not decrease at 90 degrees, then

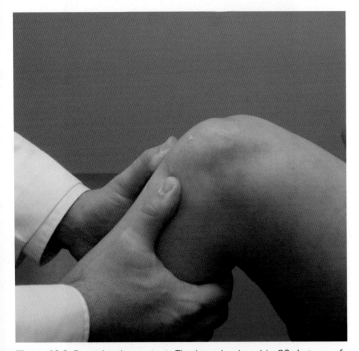

Figure 46-3 Posterior drawer test. The knee is placed in 90 degrees of flexion. A posterior force is applied to the femur. The amount of posterior displacement is assessed.

there may also be an injury to the PCL. Other tests include the posterolateral drawer test, external rotation drawer test (dial test), and reverse pivot-shift test. The posterolateral drawer test is performed with an anterior drawer at 90 degrees of knee flexion. If the posterolateral structures are torn, then the knee will have increased translation with internal rotation as compared to neutral rotation. The dial test is performed with the hips and knees flexed. Both lower extremities are evaluated by externally rotating the feet of the patient. Increased external rotation signifies injury of the posterolateral complex. A variant of this test is the external rotation recurvatum test. In this test, the examiner holds both feet by the toes and if the relaxed knee falls into recurvatum, it is a positive test result. The reverse pivot-shift test begins with the knee flexed and the tibia externally rotated. The knee is then passively extended, and when posterolateral laxity is present, a sudden shift will occur at 20 to 30 degrees of flexion as the posteriorly subluxated lateral side of the tibia abruptly reduces.

Increased opening to varus stress at 30 degrees without opening at 0 degrees or other signs of a PLC injury suggests an isolated tear of the fibular collateral ligament.[8] Failure to diagnose and treat an injury of the posterolateral corner of the knee in a patient who has a tear of the ACL or PCL can result in failure of the reconstructed ligament.

PATELLOFEMORAL EXAMINATION

The patellofemoral joint has many examination tests specific to evaluate for patellofemoral disorders. The tracking of the patella as the knee goes from a flexed to an extended position may take the form of an upside down letter J. The positive J sign suggests a tight lateral retinaculum. As previously described, the quadriceps angle or Q angle should be measured along with the lower extremity alignment. The examiner should also assess for crepitus, patellar apprehension, and specific areas of tenderness. A maneuver has been described that can detect patella instability, with the knee flexed 30 degrees and applying a distal lateral force. Increased patellar translation with a softer endpoint compared with a normal contralateral knee may suggest disruption of the medial patellofemoral ligament.[9]

MENISCUS EXAMINATION

There are many different tests used to assess for meniscus tears. The most sensitive test is joint line tenderness.[10] Other tests attempt to produce the symptoms of a torn meniscus such as McMurray's test, Apley's grind test, and others. McMurray's test is performed with passive motion from flexion to extension with internal and external rotation. A palpable click on the joint line is a positive test. Apley's grind test is performed with the patient prone and the knee flexed 90 degrees. Compression of the tibiofemoral joint will elicit pain, whereas distraction of the joint will cause diminished pain in a positive result of the Apley test. A bucket handle tear that is displaced may present with true locking of the knee. True locking of the knee is the inability of the patient to be able to fully extend the knee because of a mechanical block.

EXAMINATION OF MULTILIGAMENTOUS KNEE INJURIES

The initial diagnosis of a knee dislocation or multiple-ligament knee injury is an orthopedic emergency. Although some knee dislocations present with obvious deformity, most multiple-ligament knee injuries spontaneously reduce. One must have a high index of suspicion for these injuries. The patient's history provides essential information regarding the mechanism of injury and potential associated injuries. The direction of the force to the knee and the position of the leg are important variables. Contact versus noncontact injury is worth documenting. A high-energy motor vehicle accident is important to differentiate from a sports-related dislocation because of the greater incidence of severe soft-tissue injury and associated injuries.[11,12]

Vascular injuries, open dislocations, irreducible dislocations, and compartment syndromes require prompt diagnosis and immediate treatment. Open dislocations must be reduced with subsequent irrigation and débridement in the operating room and be treated with intravenous antibiotics for 48 hours. Soft-tissue wounds should be evaluated for problems with closure because plastic surgery consultation is sometimes necessary. Posterolateral knee dislocations may present as an irreducible dislocation (Fig. 46-5). The medial femoral condyle may become buttonholed through the medial retinaculum and present with the dimple sign.[13] This particular type of dislocation may require open reduction. Prolonged dislocation in this position has been associated with skin necrosis. Compartment syndrome must always be ruled out and emergent fasciotomies are required when this condition exists or is impending. A detailed neurovascular examination follows the visual inspection.

The initial assessment of a multiligamentous knee injury must include a thorough and expedient physical examination with particular attention directed to the vascularity of the extremity. Vascular injuries should be ruled out immediately. Vascular injuries can occur with all types of dislocations. The risk of arte-

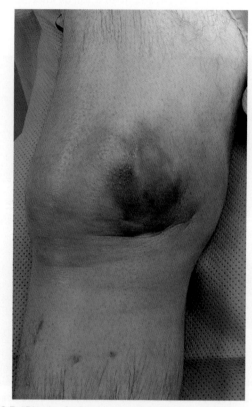

Figure 46-5 "Dimple sign" on the medial side of a right knee with an irreducible posterolateral knee dislocation.

rial injury with a knee dislocation is between 10% and 64%.[14] Green and Allen[15] reported rupture of the artery to be as high as 44% with posterior dislocations. Anterior dislocations are associated with arterial injury in as many as 39%, and the incidence with medial is reported at 25% and lateral at 6%.

The dorsalis pedis and posterior tibialis pulses should both be palpated. Never assume that a decreased pulse is normal and the result of spasm. Ankle brachial indices are assessed and a decrease of 0.15 or greater indicates a significant vascular injury.[16] The importance of early recognition of vascular injury cannot be overstated because a missed or delayed diagnosis may result in a below-knee amputation if the leg is not reperfused within 6 to 8 hours.

All patients with a normal vascular examination must have serial pulse examinations or undergo arteriography because intimal tears may be present. Intimal tears of the artery may present in a delayed fashion and are more difficult to diagnose. The initial physical examination may be completely normal in a knee with an intimal tear. Intimal tears can lead to a gradual thrombosis, which may propagate to complete arterial occlusion.

NERVE INJURIES

The neurologic examination, particularly of the peroneal nerve, should be documented. The patient is asked to actively dorsiflex the foot and to activate the extensor hallucis longus tendon. These specific tests assess the peroneal nerve function. Sensation in all the nerve distributions, as well as motor function of the tibial nerve should be examined. The incidence of nerve injury with knee dislocation is between 16% and 40%.[17-19] The peroneal nerve is most commonly injured, but injuries to the tibial nerve have occurred.[20] Injuries to the lateral corner and PLC of the knee place the peroneal nerve at increased risk because of its superficial location as it curves around the fibular head. Posterior dislocations have a high incidence of nerve injuries. The prognosis of peroneal nerve injuries is poor. Complete nerve injuries only recover about 50% of the time. Nerve injuries are generally followed conservatively for 3 months. Of these injuries, about one third will recover, one third will have minor deficits, and one third will have a complete palsy.[19]

A detailed examination of the knee ligaments is performed on the ACL, PCL, MCL, and posterolateral anatomic structures. Initial and postreduction radiographs require thorough evaluation to assess for periarticular fractures, direction of dislocation, and adequacy of reduction. Magnetic resonance imaging will provide detailed information about the ligaments, bone or subchondral bone, menisci, and articular cartilage.[21] The physical examination must be correlated with the magnetic resonance imaging findings for preoperative planning.

CONCLUSIONS

The purpose of the physical examination is to obtain the correct diagnosis. A complete patient history must be combined with a thorough physical examination in order to direct treatment of the knee injury. Additional tests such as radiographs, magnetic resonance imaging, bone scans, and angiography are sometimes used to provide information in the evaluation of a knee injury. The initial diagnosis of a knee dislocation or multiple-ligament knee injury is an orthopedic emergency. A vascular injury must be assumed until it can be ruled out. After the vascular status has been addressed, radiographs followed by a magnetic resonance imaging scan should be obtained. A complete ligament examination will help correlate the magnetic resonance imaging findings, and a preoperative plan can be established (Boxes 46-1 and 46-2).

Box 46-1 Pearls

1. In most cases, the history itself will lead the examiner to the correct diagnosis.
2. Always examine the uninjured knee for a comparison.
3. The Lachman test should be performed in neutral rotation. External rotation may cause a false-positive result in a knee with a medial collateral ligament injury.
4. Laxity of the knee joint with varus or valgus stress in full extension is a sign of a multiligamentous injury.

Box 46-2 Pitfalls

1. Failure to examine the hip and spine in conjunction with the knee can result in a misdiagnosis (e.g., knee pain in a young adolescent can be the result of a slipped capital femoral epiphysis at the hip).
2. Do not assume that all knee swelling is an effusion.
3. A missed posterolateral corner injury is a common cause of anterior cruciate ligament reconstruction failure.

REFERENCES

1. Feagin JA: Physical examination of the knee. In Garrett WE, Speer KP, Kirkendall DT (eds): Principles and Practice of Orthopaedic Sports Medicine. New York, Lippincott Williams & Wilkins, 2000, pp 613–622.
2. Kennedy J: Complete dislocation of the knee joint. J Bone Joint Surg Am 1963;45:889–904.
3. Butler DL, Noyes FR, Grood ES: Ligamentous restraints to anterior-posterior drawer in the human knee: A biomechanical study. J Bone Joint Surg (Am) 1980;62:259–270.
4. Wilson SA, Vigorta VJ, Scott WN: Anatomy. In Scott WN (ed): The Knee. St. Louis, Mosby, 1994, pp 15–54.
5. Fanelli GC, Maish DR: Knee ligament injuries: Epidemiology, mechanism, diagnosis, and natural history. In Fitzgerald RH, Kaufer H, Malkani AL (eds): Orthopaedics. St. Louis, Mosby, 2002, pp 619–636.
6. Tria AJ: Clinical examination of the knee. In Insall JN (ed): Surgery of the Knee. New York, Churchill Livingstone, 2001, pp 161–174.
7. Wilson TC, Satterfield WH, Johnson DL: Medial collateral ligament "tibial" injuries: Indication for acute repair. Orthopedics 2004;27:389–393.
8. Covey DC: Injuries of the posterolateral corner of the knee. J Bone Joint Surg Am 2001;83:106–118.
9. Tanner SM, Garth WP, Soileau R, Lemons JE: A modified test for patellar instability: The biomechanical basis. Clin J Sport Med 2003;13:327–338.
10. Eren OT: The accuracy of joint line tenderness by physical examination in the diagnosis of meniscus tears. Arthroscopy 2003;19:850–854.

11. Wascher DC: High-velocity knee dislocation with vascular injury treatment principles. Clin Sports Med 2000;19:457–477.

12. Shelbourne KD, Porter DA, Clingman JA, et al: Low velocity knee dislocation. Orthop Rev 1991;20:995–1004.

13. Quinlan A: Irreducible posterolateral dislocation of the knee with button-holing of the medial femoral condyle. J Bone Joint Surg Am 1966;48:1619–1621.

14. Cole BJ, Harner CD: The multi-ligament injured knee. Clin Sports Med 1999;18:241–262.

15. Green NE, Allen BL: Vascular injuries associated with dislocation of the knee. J Bone Joint Surg Am 1977;59:236–239.

16. Kendall RW, Taylor DC, Salvain AJ, et al: The role of arteriography in assessing vascular injuries associated with dislocations of the knee. J Trauma 1993;35:875–878.

17. Kennedy J: Complete dislocation of the knee joint. J Bone Joint Surg (Am) 1963;45:889–904.

18. Taft TW, Almenkinders LC: The dislocated knee. In Fu F (ed): Knee Surgery. Baltimore, Williams and Wilkins, 1994, pp 837–857.

19. Borden PS, Johnson DL: Initial assessment of the acute and chronic multiple-ligament injured knee. Sports Med Arthrosc Rev 2001;9:178–184.

20. Welling R, Kakkasseril J, Cranley J: Complete dislocations of the knee with popliteal vascular injury. J Trauma 1981;21:450–453.

21. Wilson TC, Johnson DL: Initial evaluation of the multiple-ligament injured knee. Oper Tech Sports Med 2003;11:187–192.

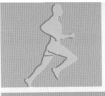

47 Principles of Knee Arthroscopy

William P. Urban

INTRODUCTION

- Knee arthroscopy is the most common procedure in orthopedic surgery.

- Originally developed as a diagnostic tool, the ability to directly visualize anatomic structures within the knee joint allows surgeons to perform intra-articular surgery through minimal incisions.

- While improvements in modern-day magnetic resonance imaging has decreased its usefulness as a diagnostic tool, advances in arthroscopic equipment and techniques have led to an increase in the number and complexity of arthroscopic procedures (Table 47-1).

- Current indications include the treatment of meniscal pathology, articular lesions, loose or foreign bodies, cruciate ligament reconstruction, patella malalignment, and intra-articular fractures. More than 600,000 knee arthroscopies are performed annually.[1]

EQUIPMENT

Knee arthroscopy requires the use of basic instrumentation for all procedures. The arthroscope is a small telescopic device that is used to visualize structures within the knee joint. While a 30-degree arthroscope is typical, a 70-degree scope is sometimes used. The remainder of the video capture equipment includes a light source, camera head, and video system. Pictures can be saved as video or computer files or printed to paper depending on the equipment. A motorized shaver system and handheld instruments are the basic implements for performing surgery, although a wide array of equipment has been developed for specific procedures. Electrothermal devices or lasers should be considered an adjunct to the basic shaver and handheld instruments.

Knee arthroscopy is performed in a fluid environment using saline. A fluid management system or infusion pump is used to maintain fluid in the joint, distend the capsule, and lavage blood or other fluids that may obscure visualization. Current systems allow the surgeon to maintain a selected intra-articular pressure and flow rate.

ANESTHESIA

Arthroscopic surgery can be performed under local, regional, or general anesthesia. Factors to be considered include the length of the procedure, tourniquet use, and postoperative pain control as well as patient and surgeon preference. Local anesthesia has become more popular with the increasing use of ambulatory surgery centers. Local anesthesia is typically used for simple cases with limited operative time. Local anesthesia is a poor choice for cases requiring additional portals or incisions. Since local anesthesia will be inadequate in 1% to 15% of cases,[2] monitored anesthesia care can be used to provide supplemental sedation in order to increase patient acceptance. An intra-articular anesthetic with epinephrine should be injected 20 minutes before surgery[3] to maximize analgesia and decrease bleeding. The skin and portals are injected prior to the incision. The use of a long-lasting anesthetic should be considered for postoperative pain control.

When additional portals or incisions are used, and hemostasis using a tourniquet is desired, regional anesthesia should be considered. Regional anesthesia, such as spinal or epidural blocks using a combination of analgesics and fentanyl, also allows manipulation and stressing of the knee to improve visualization and access to intra-articular structures. Spinal and epidural regional blocks can also be used for postoperative pain control through the use of a long-acting anesthetic or patient-controlled analgesia. Peripheral nerve blocks can be used to increase analgesia in conjunction with local anesthesia, to decrease anesthesia requirements with general anesthetics, or as a method of postoperative pain control.

General anesthesia is typically reserved for cases in which regional or local anesthesia would be inappropriate or contraindicated. Examples include long, complicated cases that require complete relaxation, cases involving infection or coagulopathy, and cases in which the patient is unable or unwilling to remain awake during surgery.

SURGICAL TECHNIQUE

Preparation

The surgical sight should be marked by the surgeon before leaving the holding area in compliance with current patient safety protocols.[4] Patients are given preoperative antibiotics 20 minutes before surgery using a broad-spectrum antibiotic covering *Staphylococcus* and *Streptococcus* organisms. This protocol can be modified when specific antibiotic coverage is needed for a known or suspected organism. Before positioning, an examination under anesthesia is performed. This examination, when the patient is pain free and relaxed (if under general anesthesia), is used to corroborate preoperative planning, the office examination, and radiographic studies. The repetitive performance of an examination under anesthesia before all surgical cases to deduce subtle findings is also an important technique for the

Table 47-1 Arthroscopic Procedure
Lavage
Removal of loose/foreign body
Plica resection/débridement
Synovectomy
Chondroplasty
Microfracture/abrasion arthroplasty
Lysis of adhesions
Lateral release/capsular imbrication
Meniscectomy
Meniscal repair
Cruciate ligament reconstruction
Arthroscopically assisted fracture open reduction/internal fixation
Osteochondral autograft transplantation

beginning arthroscopist to hone his or her physical examination skills.

Positioning

The patient is placed supine on a standard operating table with a tourniquet placed around the thigh. A wide, well-padded tourniquet should be used to decrease neurologic complications. The tourniquet should be kept as proximal as possible on the thigh to avoid the possibility of encroaching on the operative site. The decision to use a tourniquet is based on the operative procedure and surgeon's preference. New fluid management systems and high-flow cannulas, which control knee pressure and flow, make the performance of basic arthroscopic procedures without a tourniquet possible. Studies have shown that the use of a tourniquet increases postoperative quadriceps inhibition,[5] and the surgeon should weigh this against the benefits of using a tourniquet, primarily decreased bleeding, and faster operative time. Procedures requiring additional incisions and bony work should entail the use of a tourniquet. Regardless, a tourniquet is applied in case its unexpected use is necessitated.

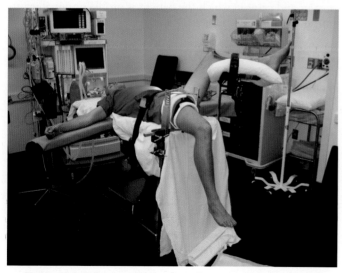

Figure 47-1 Patient positioning for arthroscopy of the right knee.

The foot of the table is dropped, and the operative leg is typically placed in an arthroscopic leg holder (Fig. 47-1). A leg holder allows the knee joint to be stressed and manipulated in order to help visualize the intra-articular compartments. Alternatively, a lateral post can be used to provide a valgus stress and the leg can be brought into a figure-four position to provide a varus stress. The nonoperative leg is placed in a leg holder to move it out of the way, allowing adequate access to the surgical extremity. With the increasing complexity of modern arthroscopic procedures resulting in increasing operative times, ensuring that the well-leg holder is appropriately padded to avoid abnormal pressure that could result in compartment syndrome or neurologic injury is critical.

Landmarks

Anatomic landmarks and incision sights should be clearly marked out before starting the case (Fig. 47-2). The use of standard landmarks that can be used consistently for most arthroscopic knee cases improves efficiency and prevents the need for determining new landmarks during unforeseen circumstances, after the knee has been distended and the anatomy altered. Standard landmarks should include the inferior pole of the patella, the medial and lateral edges of the patellar tendon, and the tibial tubercle. The medial and lateral joint line should also be marked in case posterior portals are required.

The anterolateral and anteromedial portals are then marked. The anterolateral portal is created just below the level of the inferior pole of the patella, approximately 1 cm above the joint line. The incision is placed just lateral to the patellar tendon. While the center of the "soft spot" more laterally has been advocated, this position makes accessing the posterior notch and the posterior compartment difficult in patients with a large Q angle.

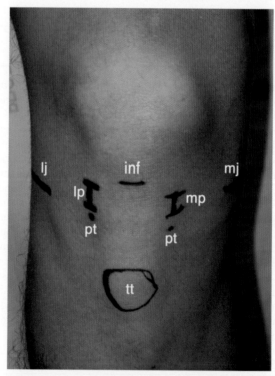

Figure 47-2 Standard landmarks include the inferior pole of the patella (inf), lateral joint line (lj), lateral portal (lp), medial joint line (mj), medial portal (mp), edges of the patella tendon (pt), and tibial tubercle (tt).

The anteromedial portal is considered the working portal for arthroscopic surgery. This portal is approximately 5 mm lower than the lateral portal or 5 mm superior to the joint line. Again, the placement of this portal close to the patellar tendon allows access to the back of the notch and posterior compartments.

Some fluid management systems require the use of a superomedial or superolateral portal. These portals are also used to remove loose/foreign bodies from the retinacular gutters or to provide direct access to the opposite side of the patellofemoral joint when a lateral release, capsular plication, or patellar microfracture is performed. The superolateral and superomedial patella portals are best created intraoperatively under direct visualization using a spinal needle for localization. Similarly, when access to the posterior compartment is required, the posterior portals are created intraoperatively using the previously marked joint lines and transillumination with the arthroscope.

A transpatellar portal through the patella tendon has also been described, but because of concerns involving the violation of the extensor mechanism, it is rarely used. During the case, new portals can be easily created along the previously marked-out joint line if specific structures need to be accessed. Using transillumination, the joint line is confirmed and then palpated under arthroscopic visualization. Once the best position is determined, a spinal needle is simply placed through the skin. If the surgeon is satisfied with the position, a small stab incision is created using a no. 11 blade. The use of additional portals is preferable to struggling with poor access during the surgery or causing iatrogenic injury by forcing the instruments.

Incision

After the patient is positioned and prepped, the anterolateral portal is established. Using a no. 11 blade, a vertical incision directed into the notch is made through the skin large enough to accommodate the arthroscope. The incision is then carried down through the capsular tissue with the blade facing up to avoid accidentally cutting the meniscus. The capsule and underlying fat pad should be cut by dropping the hand, lowering the handle, and raising the cutting edge of the blade. This results in a funnel-shaped portal, wider in the joint than superficially. This geometry allows the scope to be more easily passed around the joint than with a simple stab incision (Fig. 47-3). The stab incision results in a tunnel shaped incision in which the fat pad and retinacular tissue can hinder movement of the scope or, if wide enough, allows fluid to leak out around the arthroscope. Care should be taken not to overextend the skin incision as this will lead to flow from the portal during the procedure. If this does occur, a surgical sponge is simply hung around the scope at the level of the incision to redirect the leaking fluid into the arthroscopy bag.

Using a blunt obturator, the arthroscopic cannula is then inserted directly into the notch with the knee hanging in a flexed position. The scope should enter easily, and if resistance is encountered, the cannula should be removed and the capsular incision lengthened. The cannula is then passed behind the patellar tendon into the space anterior to the medial meniscus to ensure that it has completely passed through the fat pad and ligamentum mucosa, which attaches the fat pad to the intercondylar notch (Fig. 47-4). The knee is then brought into full extension, and the scope is directed under the patella into the suprapatellar pouch. The cannula should slip easily into the patellofemoral joint. If difficulty is encountered directing the scope superiorly, the capsular incision should be extended. The obturator is then removed, and the knee is copiously irrigated until clear in order to avoid delays caused by poor visualization. Only then is a 30-degree arthroscope inserted through the cannula. With the arthroscope inserted at a medial angle into the joint through the lateral portal, the lens should be directed laterally. The combined vectors result in a view, which is approximately straightforward (Fig. 47-5). This should be considered the standard arthroscopic position. Manipulation of the arthroscope around the joint requires smooth, mildly arcing motions because of the angle of the lens. Beginning arthroscopists mistakenly push or pull the scope straight back or forward when intending to move anteriorly or posteriorly in the knee joint.

Patellofemoral Compartment

Once in the suprapatellar pouch, the patella and trochlea should be inspected for any changes. The location and degree of any articular cartilage damage should be consistently graded should the operative report need to be reviewed without access to the intraoperative pictures. The knee should be flexed 45 degrees

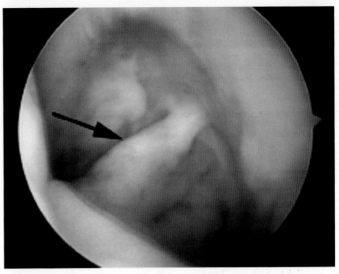
Figure 47-4 The ligamentum mucosum (arrow), viewed from above, obscures the cruciate ligaments.

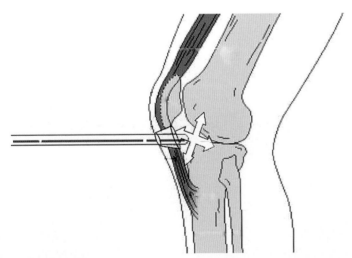
Figure 47-3 A generous capsular incision facilitates manipulation of the arthroscope with the joint.

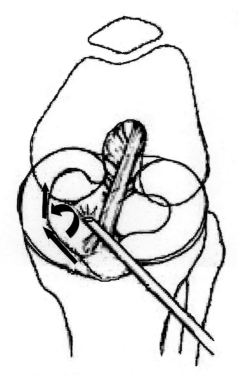

Figure 47-5 Standard arthroscopic position with the 30-degree arthroscope in the lateral portal and the lens rotated laterally.

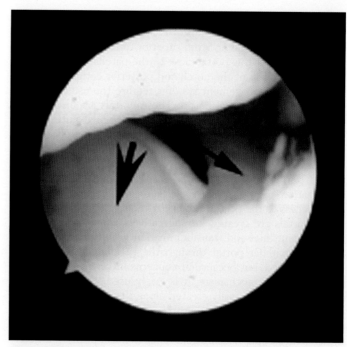

Figure 47-7 A thick fibrous plica *(thin arrow)* and wear of the femoral condyle *(arrowhead)*.

to visualize the capture of the patella into the trochlear grove (Fig. 47-6). Subluxation and tilt of the patella should be noted. While the importance of a patella that is not anatomically situated in the groove at 45 degrees of flexion during arthroscopy has been debated,[6] the technique provides general information that should be considered in conjunction with the physical examination, radiographic studies, and clinical history.

With the knee extended, the arthroscope should be directed superiorly and laterally into the lateral gutter, which is inspected for loose bodies or synovial plica. The lens should be rotated downward to visualize the gutter. The arthroscope is then directed medially into the medial gutter to visualize any loose

bodies. As the knee is brought into flexion, the lens is rotated medially and inferiorly to check for plica and any resulting damage to the femoral condyle (Fig. 47-7). As the scope continues around the curve of the condyle, the meniscocapsular junction will come into view. At this point, a valgus stress is applied to open up the medial compartment, and the arthroscope is directed into the medial compartment.

Medial Compartment

With the arthroscope in the standard position, the medial compartment is assessed for chondral and meniscal pathology (Fig. 47-8). The posterior horn should be visible, and the lens is then rotated downward to view the anterior horn as it runs off the

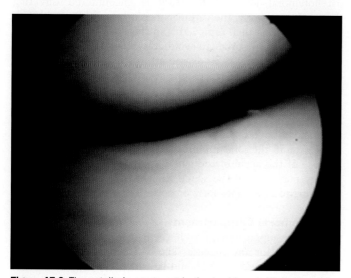

Figure 47-6 The patella is congruent in the trochlea at 45 degrees of flexion.

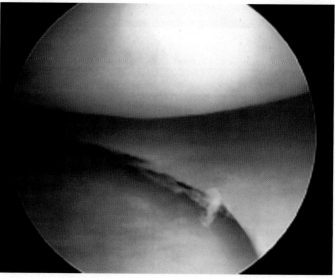

Figure 47-8 View of the medial compartment.

anterior tibial plateau. With the lens again facing laterally, the arthroscope is directed into the intercondylar notch.

Intercondylar Notch

Unless obscured by the ligamentum mucosum, the anterior cruciate ligament should be visible. If the ligamentum mucosum prevents the scope from being directed laterally, the tip of the arthroscope should be brought superiorly, tracing the outline of the notch. The scope is then directed downward along the lateral margin, posterior to the fat pad, to visualize the cruciate ligaments. If the ligamentum remains a hindrance, a medial portal should be established and the ligamentum resected with a shaver. A no. 11 blade is used to create a stab incision at the previously marked location. The blade can be visualized with the arthroscope as it is directed into the notch. The blade is removed, and the blunt obturator is inserted through the portal into the notch.

After the anterior cruciate ligament is visualized, a probe should be inserted into the medial portal (Fig. 47-9). The tension on the anterior cruciate ligament should be assessed with a probe, and it should be visualized as an anterior drawer is performed. The posterior cruciate ligament in most knees will not be visualized, but its synovial covering is apparent. The arthroscope is then brought to the anterior medial corner of the lateral plateau with the knee in flexion. With the arthroscope held in this location, a varus stress is created by bringing the leg into a figure-four position. As the compartment is distracted, the arthroscope is directed into the lateral compartment.

Lateral Compartment

The articular cartilage and the meniscus are assessed and noted (Fig. 47-10). The lens should be rotated in order to give a complete view of the meniscus starting with the posterior horn. As the meniscus is examined, the popliteus tendon should be visible as it travels through the hiatus in the posterior horn of the lateral meniscus. As the lens is rotated downward and then medially around the anterior periphery, the anterior horn is visualized anterior to the lateral tibial spine, which separates it from the posterior horn.

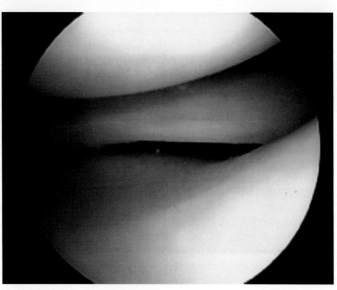

Figure 47-10 A view of the lateral compartment as the arthroscope is inserted.

Posterior Compartment

Occasionally, the posterior compartment must be inspected. In order to visualize the posterior compartment, the scope is brought anteriorly along the joint line of the medial compartment with the knee in flexion. The camera is removed and replaced with the blunt obturator. The cannula is swept laterally across the anterior joint line by moving the base of the scope medially. The tip of the cannula remains in contact with the joint line until it falls into the notch. Remaining in contact with the lateral aspect of the medial condyle, the arthroscope is advanced posteromedially. As it is directed between the anterior cruciate ligament and the lateral aspect of the medial femoral condyle, tension will be felt as it passes the posterior cruciate ligament. As this occurs, the handle of the cannula is raised and it is advanced posteriorly and inferiorly. A sudden release in tension is felt as the obturator passes the posterior cruciate ligament and enters the compartment. The obturator is then removed and the 30-degree scope is reinserted. In order to visualize the posterior aspect of the posterior horn of the medial meniscus and the posterior joint line, a 70-degree arthroscope should be introduced. The wedging of the arthroscope between the wall of the notch and the cruciate ligaments makes moving the arthroscope difficult. The compartment is visualized by rotating the 70-degree lens. The reverse techniques can be used to reposition the scope into the lateral notch, viewing the posterior aspect of the lateral joint.

In certain cases, such as posterior cruciate ligament reconstruction, a posterior working portal is necessary. The posteromedial portal places the saphenous nerve at risk, while the posterolateral portal places the peroneal nerve at risk. To avoid possible neurovascular complications, the arthroscope in the posterior compartment is used to transilluminate the posterior joint line. Palpation is used to verify the placement, and a spinal needle is inserted into the joint under arthroscopic visualization. A superficial skin incision is then created, and the tissues are bluntly dissected down to the capsule using a clamp. The capsule is then incised, and a cannula is placed into the joint to avoid having to reestablish the portal every time an instrument is removed.

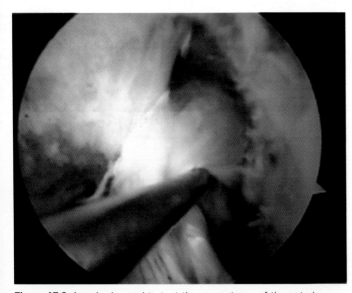

Figure 47-9 A probe is used to test the competency of the anterior cruciate ligament.

Treatment

During diagnostic arthroscopy, a probe should be used through the medial portal to test the stability and consistency of any abnormal structures. As pathology is encountered, it should be addressed using instruments through the working portals. Inserting an appropriate arthroscopic grasper through the medial portal can be used to perform the simple removal of loose or foreign bodies. If there is difficulty holding the fragment, a spinal needle inserted into the knee joint through the capsule can pin the fragment in place to allow the surgeon to grasp it without the fragment slipping away. Objects located in the gutters, suprapatellar pouch, or posterior compartment may require the use of the superior patellar or posterior portals.

Soft-tissue pathology requiring resection can usually be accomplished using an arthroscopic biter or the motorized shaver. Shavers are usually available in 3.5-, 4.5-, or 5.5-mm diameters. Care should be taken to avoid using a large shaver in a small space where it will damage normal structures. The shaver blade rotates forward or reverse or oscillates based on the settings. The speed can also be controlled, with higher speeds being used to resect bone.

Typically, for plica resection or arthroscopic meniscectomy, a full radius shaver is used. Other shavers can be used based on the surgeon's preference and experience. Soft-tissue resection should be performed with the shaver on *oscillate*. Suction is used to draw the tissue into the shaver. Bony resection is commonly performed with the shaver on *forward* or *reverse* rather than *oscillate*. While a full-radius shaver can be used, depending on the size of the resection and bone quality, burrs and specialized bone shavers are sometimes utilized.

CLOSURE

After the procedure is completed, the knee should be irrigated and drained of fluid. The skin portals may be closed with subcutaneous or simple sutures, although some surgeons opt to use Steri-Strips or leave the portals open. For basic arthroscopy, a sterile dressing should be applied that will not interfere with motion of the knee. If cryotherapy is used for postoperative pain control, the thickness of the dressing should be kept to a minimum. Cryotherapy can decrease pain, improve patient satisfaction, and decrease narcotic requirements.[7] Postoperative pain control can also be improved using a combination of analgesics or narcotics as an intra-articular injection.[8] The use of peripheral nerve blocks has also been advocated.

REHABILITATION

Postoperative pain management using a multimodal approach with opioids and nonsteroidal anti-inflammatory drugs in conjunction with local anesthetics or analgesics will facilitate rehabilitation after knee arthroscopy. Early rehabilitation after basic arthroscopy should focus on decreasing the patient's postoperative effusion, reversing quadriceps inhibition, and preventing stiffness. Typical postoperative rehabilitation regimens include quadriceps exercises, range of motion, local modalities, and cryotherapy. As inflammation and pain decrease, therapy should advance to incorporate strengthening regimens, endurance exercises, and proprioceptive training followed by functional rehabilitation programs and plyometrics.

COMPLICATIONS

Due to the use of limited incisions, short operative times, and the relative lack of neurovascular structures in proximity to the standard portals, surgical complications are uncommon,[9] especially after basic arthroscopic procedures. The unexpected nature of these complications makes their occurrence more problematic (Table 47-2). Since complications are rare, their presence may be overlooked and a diagnosis may not be made in an expeditious fashion. It is important to remain vigilant after all cases, especially after complex arthroscopic procedures where the use of additional incisions and increased operative time makes them more common.

Intraoperatively, iatrogenic cartilaginous and soft-tissue injuries can arise from trying to maneuver instruments in tight spaces. Appropriately sized instruments should always be used, especially in tight spaces, and constant visualization of the instruments is critical.

Neurovascular injuries are uncommon but have been reported even after simple arthroscopy. While the incidence of neurovascular injuries would be expected to increase as the complexity of the case increases and posterior portals are used, popliteal artery occlusion and pseudoaneurysm have been described after arthroscopic meniscectomy.[10] During meniscal repairs or simple cruciate ligament reconstructions in which instruments are used to pass sutures or wires posteriorly, visualization is more difficult, and neurovascular structures in closer proximity are more dangerous. Using a methodologic approach throughout the procedure, having a thorough understanding of the anatomy, and using direct visualization whenever possible will decrease these complications.

Compressive neurologic injuries caused by positioning, the leg holder, and tourniquet have also been reported.[11] Neurovascular injury to the nonoperative leg is possible during prolonged surgical times associated with advanced arthroscopic cases. Care should be taken to ensure that areas in contact with superficial neurovascular structures are padded. A neurovascular examination should be performed immediately postoperatively after all cases and any indication that a problem exists should be immediately investigated.

Postoperative complications after arthroscopic surgery include deep vein thrombosis, compartment syndrome, and infection. The short operative time, small incisions, and use of lavage fluid make infection after arthroscopic surgery extremely uncommon. Hemarthrosis after soft-tissue procedures (e.g., lateral release, synovectomy) and drilling bone (e.g., in anterior

Table 47-2 Complications
Intraoperative
Anesthesia Neurovascular injury Iatrogenic cartilage or ligament injury Compartment syndrome Hardware/equipment failure
Postoperative
Deep venous thrombosis Pulmonary embolus Infection Hemarthrosis

cruciate ligament reconstruction) can lead to increased pain and swelling, inhibiting postoperative rehabilitation.

The ambulatory nature of most arthroscopic procedures should decrease the rate of deep vein thrombosis, but it is important for the surgeon to have a high level of suspicion, as the incidence of deep vein thrombosis may be higher than expected.[12] When the postoperative course is complicated by unexpected swelling and pain, deep vein thrombosis should be suspected and a vascular study should be performed.

Compartment syndromes can occur in the operative or non-operative leg. Compartment syndrome of the operative leg can be caused by overdistending the joint with the infusion pump.[13] The risk is greater during arthroscopically assisted treatment of fractures, where the integrity of the joint has been disrupted, or after a knee dislocation in which the posterior capsule is torn and fluid escapes into the leg. Diagnosis can be complicated by the use of regional anesthesia. Care should be taken to ensure that the proper pressure and flow are maintained in the knee. Compartment syndrome of the nonoperative leg is a devastating complication if undiagnosed. Recognition of this complication and treatment with emergent fasciotomies are essential.

CONCLUSIONS

Arthroscopic surgery is a well-established, well-excepted method of addressing intra-articular pathologic conditions of the knee. The use of arthroscopic surgery to perform increasingly more complex procedures has been a natural progression as our techniques and equipment have improved. The use of arthroscopic techniques has led to improved visualization of pathologic structures, decreased postoperative pain, decreased soft-tissue trauma, decreased complications, faster rehabilitation, and decreased hospital costs.

REFERENCES

1. Rutkow IM: Surgical operations in the United States. Then (1983) and now (1994). Arch Surg 1997;132:983–990.
2. Horlocker TT, Hebl JR: Anesthesia for outpatient knee arthroscopy: Is there an optimal technique? Regional Anesth Pain Med 2003;28:58–63.
3. Hultin J, Hamberg P, Stenstrom A: Knee arthroscopy using local anesthesia. Arthroscopy 1992;8:239–241.
4. Wong DA: Surgical site marking comes of age. AAOS Bull 2004;52:30.
5. Saunders KC, Louis DL, Weingarden SI, et al: Effect of tourniquet time on postoperative quadriceps function. Clin Orthop 1979;143:194–199.
6. Sojbjerg JO, Lauritzen J, Hvid I, et al: Arthroscopic determination of patellofemoral malalignment. Clin Orthop 1987;215:243–247.
7. Lessard LA, Scudds RA, Amendola A, et al: The efficacy of cryotherapy following arthroscopic knee surgery. J Orthop Sports Phys Ther 1997;26:14–22.
8. Goodwin RC, Amjadi F, Parker RD: Short-term analgesic effects of intra-articular injections after knee arthroscopy. Arthroscopy 2005;21:307–312.
9. Small NC: Complications in arthroscopic surgery of the knee and shoulder. Orthopedics 1993;16:985–988.
10. Kiss H, Drekonja T, Grethen C, et al: Postoperative aneurysm of the popliteal artery after arthroscopic meniscectomy. Arthroscopy 2001;17:203–205.
11. Kieser C: A review of the complications of arthroscopic knee surgery. Arthroscopy 1992;8:79–83.
12. Michot M, Conen D, Holtz D, et al: Prevention of deep-vein thrombosis in ambulatory arthroscopic knee surgery: A randomized trial of prophylaxis with low–molecular weight heparin. Arthroscopy 2002;18:257–263.
13. Bomberg BC, Hurley PE, Clark CA, et al: Complications associated with the use of an infusion pump during knee arthroscopy. Arthroscopy 1992;8:224–228.

In This Chapter

INTRODUCTION

- The mechanisms of meniscal damage are myriad and include twisting and rotational noncontact injuries, often associated with ligament injuries.

- Medial meniscus injury is more common than lateral.

- Meniscal injuries may be difficult to diagnose since symptoms and physical findings are often nonspecific.

- Nonoperative treatment is often appropriate for less active patients and for those patients with minor symptoms.

- The tenet of surgical treatment is to preserve as much functioning meniscal tissue as possible through repair or minimal meniscectomy.

CLINICAL FEATURES AND EVALUATION

Meniscal injuries are a common source of knee pain, disability, limitation of function, and interference with athletic and recreational pursuits.[1] The most frequent mechanism is a noncontact injury resulting from deceleration or acceleration coupled with the athlete changing direction; they also may occur from a contact stress or, in the older athlete, from a degenerative process with little or no trauma. In running/cutting sports, such as soccer and football, meniscal tears can occur with cutting maneuvers. In sports involving jumping, such as basketball and volleyball, the angular momentum coupled with femoral tibial rotation that occurs with landing can cause a meniscal tear. Meniscal injuries also can result from events with a violent varus, valgus, or hyperextension force coupled with femoral tibial rotation. One of the more common events leading to meniscal tearing is an anterior cruciate ligament (ACL) tear or a buckling event from ACL insufficiency

The most frequent symptoms of a meniscal tear are pain, swelling, giving way, and locking.[1] The onset of pain is often immediate and localized to either the medial or lateral side of the knee. Because of concomitant collateral ligament sprains, the pain may not be confined to the joint line. With degenerative tears, the onset of pain and swelling may be gradual and is frequently delayed until the next day. Patients with traumatic tears usually can ambulate after an acute injury and frequently may be able to continue to participate in athletics. In some cases, large unstable fragments of meniscal tissue can become incarcerated in the intercondylar notch, leading to a "locked knee" (Fig. 48-1). More commonly, the symptoms are localized pain, with swelling and mechanical symptoms: catching, clicking, or buckling. It is theorized that displaced or nondisplaced tears alter meniscal mobility with resultant traction on the richly innervated capsule and synovium, resulting in knee pain; this pain is localized to the medial or lateral joint line, particularly with twisting or squatting activities. A torn meniscus also can alter the instant center of rotation of the knee, changing the contact area, to cause mechanical symptoms; this may lead to secondary articular cartilage lesions.[2]

The extent and timing of the effusion relating to a meniscal tear are variable. Young patients who have traumatic tears that disrupt the peripheral blood supply typically present with an early, large effusion or hemarthrosis. In degenerative tears or tears that involve the avascular central body of the meniscus, effusions are typically delayed in onset following the tear and exceedingly variable in size. Sometimes motion is limited by the feeling of tightness in the knee secondary to the effusion. Soft-tissue swelling should be distinguished from a true effusion of the knee by the finding of either a fluid wave or ballottable patella. Effusions that occur within hours of the injury are due to bleeding within the joint and often indicate rupture of the ACL or an osteochondral fracture. Although the typical effusion following the meniscal lesion develops gradually over 12 to 24 hours or more, a tear at the vascular periphery of the meniscus may cause an acute hemarthrosis.

Degenerative meniscal tears are being encountered with increasing frequency as more people over 40 years old are becoming or staying active in sports activities. Older patients with a degenerative tear may have a history of minimal or no trauma, but the diagnosis should be suspected in an older individual with a history of pain, effusions, or mechanical knee symptoms. In this older population, it is difficult to separate the symptoms of meniscal injury from articular surface damage. Meniscal tears in young patients are most commonly longitudinal (vertical) tears that result from acute flexion or rotational injury. By contrast, degenerative tears are frequently complex, showing both radial and horizontal cleavage components (Fig. 48-2).

The diagnosis of a meniscal tear can be made by history, physical examination, and appropriate diagnostic tests. The most common finding on physical examination is tenderness over the

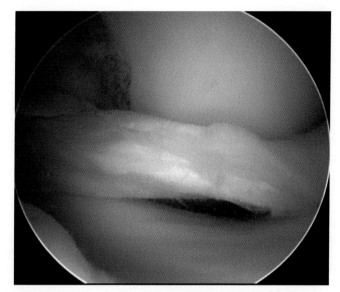

Figure 48-1 Medial meniscus bucket-handle tear locked in the notch of this right knee.

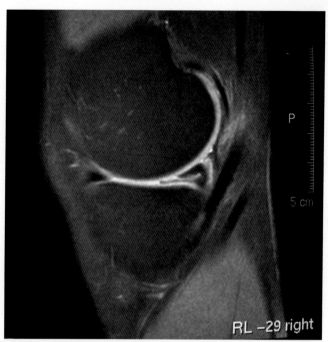

Figure 48-3 Magnetic resonance imaging demonstrating a horizontal tear of the posterior horn of the medial meniscus.

medial or lateral joint line. Knee motion may be limited secondary to pain or an effusion. More than 20 meniscal tests have been described to diagnose meniscal tears; joint line tenderness and McMurray and Apley tests are the most commonly used.[1] During provocative testing, forced flexion and circumduction (internal and external rotation of the foot) frequently elicit pain on the side of the knee with the meniscal tear. Putting together a thorough history and physical examination with plain radiographs, the overall clinical evaluation had sensitivity of 95%, specificity of 72%, and positive predictive value of 85% for the medial meniscus tears and sensitivity of 88%, specificity of 92%, and positive predictive value of 58% for lateral meniscus tears.[3] Plain radiographs should include posteroanterior weight-bearing views at 45 degrees of flexion with the x-ray beam angled 10 degrees caudad, so-called Rosenberg views, to evaluate not only

potential bony pathology, but also to assess the tibiofemoral joint spaces.[4] Magnetic resonance imaging is the best noninvasive diagnostic tool to assess the menisci, having the potential of analysis in multiple planes and the capacity to evaluate other structures in the knee. The accuracy of magnetic resonance imaging in assessing the menisci is now believed to be 95% or better (Fig. 48-3).[5] Its limitations are the relatively high cost and the potential of misinterpretation because of technical inadequacies of the study or variability in interpretation.

Relevant Anatomy

Sutton[6] first described the meniscus as "the functionless remnants of intra-articular leg muscles." Clearly, this is not borne out by the significant long-term degenerative issues that result from meniscectomy. The menisci are semilunar-shaped fibrocartilaginous structures located at the periphery of the knee joint between the tibia and femoral surfaces. The anterior and posterior horns are directly attached to bone, and the periphery of the meniscus is attached to the adjacent capsule via the coronary ligaments, also called the meniscofemoral and meniscotibial ligaments. The medial meniscus is more C shaped and has a wider diameter than the lateral meniscus, which is more circular. In addition, the lateral meniscus is free of capsular attachment at the popliteal hiatus.

The blood supply to the meniscus is via vessels from the perimeniscal capsular and synovial tissues; penetration into the meniscus is 10% to 30% of the width of the medial meniscus and 10% to 25% of the width of the lateral meniscus.[7,8] The inner 66% to 75% of the meniscus is essentially avascular and receives nutrition through diffusion and mechanical pumping.

Meniscal lesions are often classified by the location of the tear relative to the blood supply of the meniscus. The so-called "red-red" tear has a functional blood supply on both the capsular and meniscal side of the lesion and therefore has the best potential for healing. The "red-white" tear has an active peripheral blood supply, whereas the central surface of the lesion is devoid of

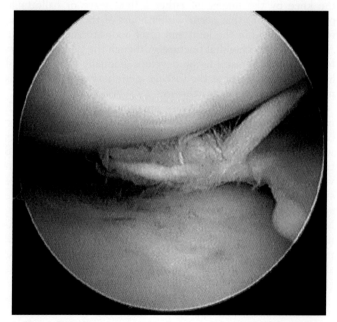

Figure 48-2 Complex degenerative tear of the medial meniscus.

vessels. These lesions should have sufficient vascularity to heal by fibrovascular proliferation. The "white-white" tears, located centrally in the meniscus, are without blood supply and have a limited healing potential.

Treatment Options

The appropriate treatment of meniscal injuries depends on understanding the basic science, the normal anatomy, and vascularity in order to determine the appropriateness of resection versus repair or nontreatment. Meniscal tears occur in virtually all age groups, and the nonoperative or operative approach to the problem must take into consideration factors such as patient age, activity level, associated injury of the knee, potential for soft tissue healing, and judicious and expeditious return to work, sports, and other recreational pursuits.

Patients involved in athletics or work endeavors that place high demands on the knee will almost always require surgery to treat a significant meniscal tear; therefore nonsurgical treatment is rarely indicated in this population. For those patients with less strenuous lifestyles, meniscal tears may be treated symptomatically. Following acute injury, protected weight bearing, ice, nonsteroidal anti-inflammatory drugs, and activity modifications are used. The athlete should avoid athletic stresses temporarily and begin a comprehensive progressive resistance exercise program until the strength deficit is within 20% to 30% of the contralateral side.[9] Resolution of the signs and symptoms suggestive of meniscal tear suggests a favorable response, and gradual resumption of preinjury activity is begun. Further evaluation is considered and offered if the patient remains symptomatic despite these nonoperative measures.

SURGERY

Historically, the surgical treatment of meniscal tears has evolved from open total meniscectomy to arthroscopic partial meniscectomy and subsequently to meniscal repair via open, arthroscopically assisted, and finally all arthroscopic means. This evolution has taken place secondary to a better understanding of the function, vascularity, and healing potential of the menisci as well as clinical studies documenting the adverse effects of removing meniscal tissue.[10–15] Arthroscopic treatment of meniscal injuries has become one of the most common orthopedic surgical procedures in the United States; in many centers, it constitutes 10% to 20% of all surgeries.[1]

Rarely is immediate surgical intervention necessary for the treatment of an isolated meniscal tear. A patient who presents with a locked knee should be operated on acutely to restore knee motion. In this situation, a displaced bucket-handle tear is usually present and should be addressed with early surgery, since a delay may result in secondary damage to the meniscus or the articular surface. When the history and examination of a young athlete suggest a meniscal tear, immediate surgery may be indicated. This is especially true if transient locking has occurred. In this situation, it is possible that recurrent catching or transient locking may cause further damage to the torn meniscus, rendering it more difficult or even impossible to repair. In addition, a delay of more than 8 weeks from the time of injury to repair may diminish the eventual healing rate.[16,17] Magnetic resonance imaging has become the diagnostic modality of choice to confirm the presence of a meniscal tear and can be very helpful in assessing the potential for repair versus resection as the treatment of choice.[5] In spite of our goal to retain meniscal tissue

through repair, more often than not partial meniscectomy is the most appropriate treatment.[18,19]

Partial Meniscectomy

Arthroscopic partial meniscectomy is currently considered state of the art in most cases of meniscal tearing not suitable for repair. The principle is to remove the torn and unstable portions of the meniscus and to retain as much functioning meniscus as possible, while leaving a well-contoured, stable meniscal remnant.[20] Metcalf et al[21] have provided general guidelines that apply for arthroscopic meniscectomy (Table 48-1). Following these guidelines for most tears not amenable to repair will preserve functioning meniscal tissue and have a low probability of residual symptoms from the retained meniscal remnant. The meniscal tear should be defined and the extent of the tear palpated with a probe. Certain tears do not require treatment; these include partial-thickness tears, relatively asymptomatic degenerative tears, and stable tears, defined clinically as those tears with less than 3 to 5 mm of movement on arthroscopic probing and those longitudinal tears less than 1 cm in length.[18] Horizontal tears less than 7 mm and radial tears less than 5 mm also do not require resection.[20,22,23] In order to provide more detail, several types of tear configuration are used here to provide examples of the steps in arthroscopic meniscectomy.

Vertical Longitudinal Tear

This is commonly seen with chronic ACL injuries and certainly may be encountered in a stable knee. In general, a longitudinal tear needs to extend for at least two thirds the circumference of the meniscus in order to produce an unstable fragment that can lock into the joint. Bucket-handle tears are three times more common in the medial than in the lateral meniscus. In most instances, displaced tears should first be reduced with the probe prior to resection. Determination as to optimal treatment is made based on proximity to the vascular supply, quality of the unstable segment, and concomitant procedures (e.g., ACL reconstruction, which improves healing rates) prior to proceeding with partial meniscectomy (Fig. 48-4). The classic cut-and-avulse technique begins with a nearly complete cut at the posterior axilla of the tear, leaving a small tissue bridge to serve as tether.[18,24] This keeps the fragment from floating free and obscuring the view of the anterior cut. The anterior axilla of the tear is then identified and cut. This can be best performed with the cutting instrument in the ipsilateral portal for those tears that end in the posterior 60% of the meniscus. Bringing the

Table 48-1 General Guidelines for Arthroscopic Partial Meniscectomy[21]
1. Remove all mobile fragments of meniscus.
2. There should be no sudden changes in the contour of the rim of meniscus.
3. It is not necessary to obtain a perfectly smooth rim following partial meniscectomy.
4. Use a probe often.
5. Protect the meniscocapsular junction.
6. Use hand and motorized instruments alternatively.
7. Whenever unsure, leave more meniscus than less.

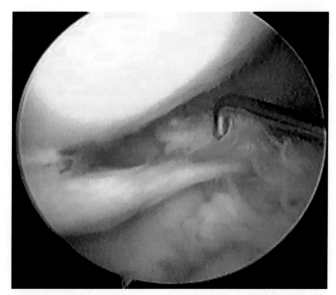

Figure 48-4 Medial meniscal tear, illustrating the most appropriate site to cut for removal.

cutting instrument in from the contralateral portal and visualizing from the ipsilateral site will facilitate balancing the remnant if the anterior axilla is in the anterior 40% of the meniscus. The free anterior edge is then grasped and the fragment is removed, avulsing the small posterior tether. Twisting of the grasper in a circular motion several times helps detach the remaining portion of the posterior horn. By this technique, the torn fragment is removed without leaving significant remnants behind. Loose edges can be smoothed with the motorized shaver.[20]

Radial Tear

These tears are most commonly located in the mid one third of the lateral meniscus, although they are also not uncommon in the posterior horn of the medial meniscus. If longer than 5 mm, then removal of the potentially unstable meniscal tissue anterior and posterior to the radial component is best achieved with the use of a manual instrument from the contralateral portal for lateral tears. Tissue anterior and posterior to the radial tear is removed so that a smooth transition to the depth of the tear is achieved without abrupt changes in the meniscal contour. The partial meniscectomy should remove the anterior and posterior lips of the tears only as deeply as the apex tear extends. Then, the remnant should be contoured as previously described. For posterior medial tears, resection is best accomplished with ipsilateral instrumentation. A radial tear of less than 5 mm in length in the mid-portion of the lateral meniscus is often an incidental finding and typically does not cause symptoms. A tear of this size and configuration may judiciously be left untreated.

Radial tears of the lateral meniscus in the mid and anterior thirds of the meniscus may lead to the formation of a parameniscal cyst, often times called cystic lateral meniscus. The cyst results from extrusion of joint fluid through the meniscus.

Horizontal Cleavage Tear

The usual cleavage plane is central or slightly inferior, leaving two distinct leaves of tissue. Often the superior and inferior surfaces of the meniscus are relatively well preserved, and the cleavage plane extends a variable distance into the meniscus. The extension of this plane determines how much meniscal

tissue should be resected. It is not essential to remove all the meniscus involved in the cleavage tear; only the unstable tissue should be resected; any hypermobile portion off superior or inferior leaflets is trimmed. Oftentimes partial resection of the inner margin of the inferior leaflet back to the end of the horizontal cleavage is the easiest and most appropriate treatment. If the tissue is of good quality, the remaining leaflet may be left in place to provide a continuous meniscal rim; in this situation, care must be taken by probing of the intact side, looking for a dimpling effect when probe pressure is applied, indicating inadequate durability of the remnant, an indication for additional resection. If the meniscus requires a partial resection of the more intact leaf to prevent recurrent tearing and the cleavage plane is deep, then a partial resection of both the superior and inferior leaves should be performed, with removal of any unstable segments, while a small cleavage between them may be left (Fig. 48-5).

Meniscal Repair

Although many specific techniques for meniscal repair have been developed over the past two decades and new techniques continue to evolve, they can be classified into four types: three arthroscopic techniques, including inside-out, outside-in, and all-inside methods and open repair. One should regard a symptomatic, potentially reparable meniscal tear as the soft-tissue equivalent of an atrophic nonunion in bone. For any surgical treatment to be successful, the intervening soft tissue with limited biologic potential should be removed by rasping both the body of the meniscus and the peripheral rim. Additionally, improved healing can be induced by thoroughly rasping the parameniscal synovium on the meniscofemoral and meniscotibial regions to stimulate both the formation of a local clot and neovascularization or potentially considering the addition of an exogenous clot.[16,25] No single study offers direct comparison of the four different techniques. In general, most authors have concluded that all techniques achieve comparable results.[17,25-28]

When considering meniscal repair, the surgeon must weigh the many factors that may affect its result[29] (Table 48-2). These include the extent, type, chronicity, and location of the tear; the

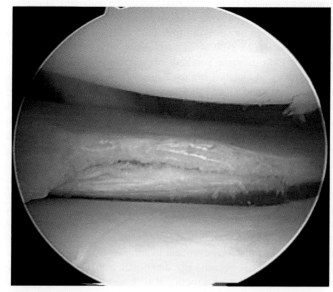

Figure 48-5 Lateral meniscus following minimal partial meniscectomy, retaining torn but stable posterior horn.

Table 48-2 Indications for Meniscal Repair
Peripheral tear
Longitudinal in orientation
Young patient
Within the red-red or red-white zone
Stable or stabilizable knee

age of the patient; and the presence of associated injuries such as an ACL tear undergoing concomitant treatment. It is known that the success of a meniscal repair depends on adequate stability and coaptation of the tear site as well as the biologic healing capacity of the meniscus. The addition of an autologous clot to the repair site, when the repair is done without ACL reconstruction, also improves healing rates. This can be done by the traditional removal of venous blood and reinsertion of the clot to the repair site or potentially through microfracture in the intercondylar notch. The indications for meniscal repair are based on an understanding of meniscal function and biology based on both basic science and clinical research. Optimally, a reparable tear would be recent and traumatic, in a young patient, localized near the capsular margin, preferably a single longitudinal tear, and in a stable or to be stabilized knee. Relative contraindications to repair include tears with significant meniscal degeneration, localized in the middle or inner third of the meniscus; oblique, radial or complex tears; or a noncompliant patient.

Outside-In Technique

This technique is considered the most simple. The instrumentation used includes 18-gauge spinal needles, a probe, and a loop curet, which is beneficial for placing countertraction on the meniscus for needle penetration. The meniscus is visualized and palpated to determine the suitability for repairs on the basis of the previous criteria. The mobility of the tear is the assessed and the segments reduced; the potential for approximation is observed. Both sides of the tear are débrided. Special care must be taken if using the rasp for abrasion to avoid injury to the articular surface. The external entry site for the needle is located on the outside of the joint by finger palpation while visualizing inside the joint. The pressure of the surgeon's finger will indent the capsule, which will be seen with the arthroscope and progressively moved to the anticipated site of insertion. Using this technique, the preferred site for needle placement is selected and the meniscus is impaled (Fig. 48-6). The needle should easily enter the joint and be visualized. A small skin incision is then made adjacent to the first needle and connecting with this needle. The needle must be free in the incision; this is confirmed by moving the hub of the needle to see that it is free of the skin. Next a hemostat is used to spread the small incision down to the capsule. This provides an opening for placement of the second needle; subsequent ligature can then be tied over the capsule and not the subcutaneous fat. This maneuver also moves small veins, cutaneous nerves, and tendons to the side of the portal. The second needle is passed through the skin opening and into the joint in such a position that subsequently inserted sutures will secure the meniscus (Fig. 48-7). Proper placement of both needles creates the route of suture placement through the tissues. This can be vertical, horizontal, or oblique. There are several techniques to accomplish transfer of the suture inside

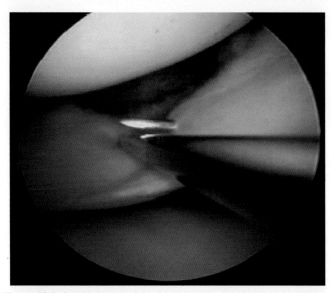

Figure 48-6 Outside-in technique for repair of posterior horn, stabilizing the body with a ring curet.

the joint. In one, a loop of wire cable is passed through the needle from the outside to the inside. The wire loop is compressed during passage through the needle and is constructed to expand upon emergence into the joint; a free 2-0 monofilament nonabsorbable suture is placed through the second needle, passage of the suture through the loop is confirmed while watching inside the joint (Fig. 48-8), and the loop is pulled out of the joint, thereby completing the loop of suture through the tear. The needles are removed, and the suture is tied outside the capsule, while watching the repair via the arthroscope. Sequential tying of the sutures helps maintain the meniscus properly reduced for subsequent needle passage. These steps are repeated at approximately 4-mm intervals until the entire tear is stabilized as confirmed both by visualization and by probing. On the basis of this inspection, sutures are removed, replaced, or added. The repair should be mechanically stable and externally secured to the joint capsule.

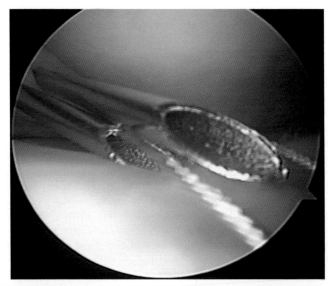

Figure 48-7 Side-by-side spinal needle passage for outside-in technique.

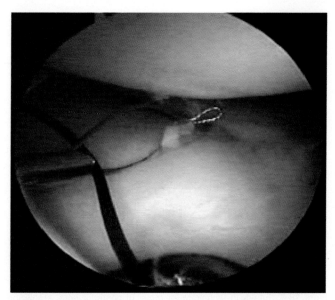

Figure 48-8 Retrieval of passed suture in outside-in technique.

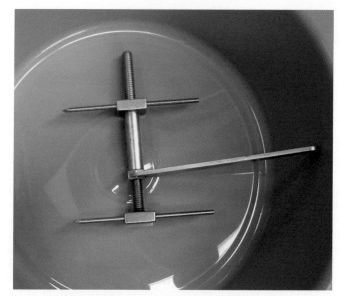

Figure 48-9 Joint distractor for meniscal repair.

Inside-Out Technique

The medial meniscus is repaired with the knee in relative extension (20 to 30 degrees of flexion), approximating the capsular tissues and meniscus to facilitate repair and avoid posterior capsular plication. The lateral meniscus, in contrast, should be repaired with the knee flexed at 50 to 70 degrees, allowing the peroneal nerve to drop back posteriorly.

Posteromedial or posterolateral extracapsular exposure should be obtained to facilitate retrieval of needles as they pass through the capsule, while protecting the neurovascular structures.[30]

Medially a 3-cm incision is made posterior to the medial collateral ligament, centered at the joint line. The sartorius fascia and sartorial branch of the saphenous nerve are retracted posteriorly along with the gracilis and semitendinous tendons. The exposure is completed by placing a spoon-type retractor anterior to the medial gastrocnemius tendon. The lateral incision is made behind the posterior margin of the lateral collateral ligament, extending from the back of the iliotibial band to the biceps tendon. The dissection is done between the anterior border of the biceps and the posterior margin of the iliotibial band. Blunt dissection is completed between the arcuate complex and capsule anteriorly and the lateral gastrocnemius muscle posteriorly, and a protective retractor is placed between the muscle belly of the gastrocnemius and the capsule. It is important to remember that the peroneal nerve lies medial to the biceps and is not protected by retraction of the biceps alone. Rather, it is the gastrocnemius muscle and the retractor that protect the peroneal nerve. We often employ a joint distractor when the involved compartment is tight, and it is difficult to obtain adequate exposure to protect the articular surfaces through manual traction alone[25] (Fig. 48-9). This is applied by inserting threaded pins 3 to 4 cm above and below the joint line into the femur and tibia through small stab incisions, as one would do in applying an external fixator. The distractor is progressively opened to take advantage of the stress relaxation of the collateral ligament (Fig. 48-10).

Various single- and double-lumen cannula systems are available to pass the sutures arthroscopically across the tear from the inside out. The number and configuration of the sutures depend on the type of tear and the clinical judgment of the surgeon. Typically, we recommend use of vertical mattress sutures due to improved coaptation and holding strength, placed at 3- to 4-mm intervals. Horizontal mattress sutures, although easier to place, have less holding strength. Sutures should be sequentially placed from both the upper and lower surfaces of the meniscus to oppose both margins of the tear. The sutures should be placed 3 to 4 mm from the margin of the tear to avoid cutting out of the sutures while also avoiding excess puckering of the meniscus. Care should be taken to avoid short tissue bridges between the arms of the mattress sutures.

Posterior horn tears are repaired via the ipsilateral portal, while mid-third tears are often most easily performed from the contralateral portal while viewing from the portal ipsilateral to the tear. For far anterior tears (extending into the anterior third

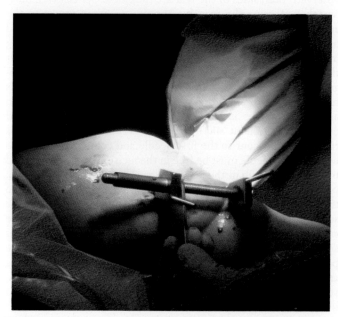

Figure 48-10 Application of a joint distractor facilitates exposure for meniscal repairs in tight joints.

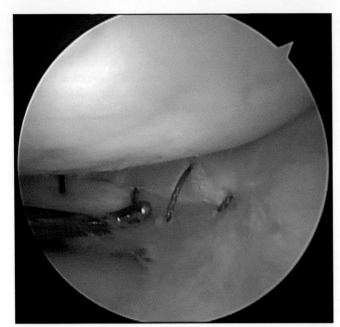

Figure 48-11 Multiple vertical mattress sutures in a lateral meniscal tear.

of the meniscus), we revert to an outside-in technique for suture passage. Using the appropriate cannula, the flexible needle of a double-arm suture is advanced. The needle-cannula unit is then advanced to "harpoon" and subsequently reduce the unstable portion of the meniscus. The needle is then advanced across the tear into the stable rim. Posteriorly, the tip of the cannula should be directed away from the midline neurovascular structures. The needle is advanced 1 to 1.5 cm, until the assistant, viewing through the posterior exposure, visualizes and grasps the needle with a needle holder. The needle, with attached suture is then delivered out of the incision. The companion needle is then passed, repeating these steps in either a vertical, horizontal, or oblique configuration (Fig. 48-11). It is our preference to tie the sutures when retrieved to simplify suture management. Soft tissue should be cleared from the suture loops, which are then tied with the knee in the position noted previously for medial or lateral tears. Securing the sutures when retrieved also facilitates the alternating passage of sutures above and below the meniscus, since a suture on the superior surface, when tied, tends to lift the meniscus and improve exposure of the inferior surface. It is important to probe the meniscus after securing each suture to assess the stability and approximation of the repair.

All-Inside Techniques

The basic principle of these techniques is avoiding the need for another incision and is the most recently developed of the four methods. This was first reported by Morgan[31] in 1991 and required a specialized set up, including the placement of a 70-degree arthroscope through the notch into the posteromedial or posterolateral compartment of the knee, the creation of posteromedial or posterolateral working portals, and the use of curved cannulated suture-passing hooks as well as arthroscopic knot-tying techniques. This technique is technically demanding and has never seen widespread use. As biomaterial technology has improved, meniscal fixation devices have been developed that eliminate the need for additional incisions, leading to a simpler, safer procedure, with reduced risk of neurovascular

injury. In the United States, the U.S. Food and Drug Administration approved the use of the BionX meniscal arrow in 1996. Since then, many companies have been quick to follow the arrow with a series of new fixators. All fixators are not the same; these devices can be divided into headless or headed, cannulated or noncannulated, and rigid or suture based, often referred to as second-generation fixators. They are made of different materials with different properties including strength, stiffness, and degradation times. Pull-out strength of these devices has been studied in cadaveric bovine and human menisci; the strength of the fixators is less than that of the gold-standard vertical mattress suture.[32-36] Most of the experience with these fixators has been with the first-generation implants, some headed and some headless. Experience has raised concerns about the increased potential with headed fixators to contact and damage the overlying femoral articular cartilage. For the all-inside techniques, we have moved to the exclusive use of suture-based implants like the Rapid Loc (DePuyMitek, Raynham, MA) and the FasT-Fix (Smith & Nephew, Andover, MA). This latest generation of meniscal repair devices has the advantage of the earlier all-inside implants, including easy intra-articular handling and short operating time, with superior biomechanical properties and the flexibility of suture material.

The FasT-Fix device consists of two 5-mm polymer suture anchors connected via a nonabsorbable braided polyester suture with a pretied, sliding, self-locking knot. After the first anchor is inserted through the meniscal body and rim to be deployed outside the capsule, the insertion needle is removed from the meniscus, the second anchor is advanced, and the meniscus is again impaled a few millimeters away. The second anchor is then deployed and the inserter removed from the joint. The sliding, self-locking knot is then pushed down, fixing the meniscus in a reduced position (Fig. 48-12). As with traditional suturing methods, different sutures should be placed with 3 to 4 mm of separation. The Rapid Loc device consists of a polyactic acid (PLA) or PDS "backstop" soft-tissue anchor, a connecting suture (absorbable Panacryl or permanent Ethibond), and a PLA or poly-

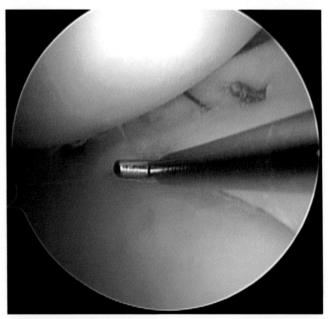

Figure 48-12 Hybrid meniscal repair, with classic inside-out sutures posteriorly, with FasT-Fix (Smith & Nephew, Andover, MA) in the foreground.

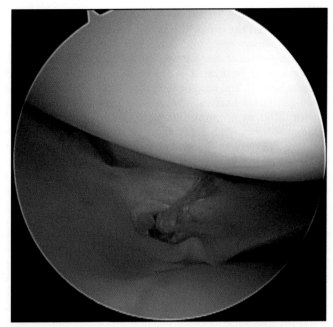

Figure 48-13 Lateral meniscal tear stabilized with a Rapid Loc (DePuyMitek, Raynham, MA) implant.

diaxone monofilament suture "top hat" with a pretied sliding-locking knot for meniscal apposition. After the soft-tissue anchor is deployed outside the capsule, the top hat is advanced along with the pretied knot to maintain reduction of the tear (Fig. 48-13). Care must be maintained to be sure that the entry site of the needle inserter is far enough from the free border of the meniscus (and hence close to the tear) to ensure adequate thickness of the meniscus to protect from having the top hat be proud and injure the femoral articular cartilage. This should be about 3 to 4 mm from the tear in most cases.

POSTOPERATIVE REHABILITATION

For arthroscopic partial meniscectomy, weight bearing is allowed as tolerated, after any intra-articular local anesthesia has worn off. We encourage protected weight bearing with crutches until the patient can ambulate without a limp. Compression and cold therapy can be employed to minimize postoperative swelling. Range-of-motion and isometric quadriceps exercises can be started immediately. Within the first week isotonic, closed kinetic chain exercises are begun. Usually, the patient regains a full range of motion within the first 2 weeks. Once adequate strength is regained and there is little pain and swelling, the athlete may resume full activities. This is usually by 3 to 4 weeks after surgery for medial tears and 1 or 2 weeks longer for lateral tears.

There is significant controversy on the postoperative rehabilitation following meniscal repair; the major controversies are in weight bearing, immobilization, and range of motion. Specific timing in the maturation of the meniscal healing process remains unclear. However, it is widely accepted that it is necessary to protect the meniscal repair during the early healing phase (4 to 6 weeks). It is our preference to limit flexion to 90 degrees and to only allow weight bearing in a brace locked in extension for the first 4 weeks after meniscal repair. The knee is protected from vigorous activity for 4 months to allow for maturation of

the healing collagen prior to cutting, jumping, or twisting sports. If an ACL reconstruction has been performed simultaneously, the basic ACL rehabilitation protocol is then followed with the additional restrictions noted previously. In isolated meniscal repairs isometric quadriceps and hamstring exercises are begun immediately. Progression varies with the individual, but once adequate strength is obtained along with full range of motion without pain or effusion, the athlete may begin jogging and half-speed running, cycling, and swimming; this occurs at about 3 months. By 4 to 6 months, the athlete is usually ready to return to full activities.

CRITERIA FOR RETURN TO SPORTS

There is no consensus on when an athlete is ready to return to competition following meniscal repair, but the ability to single-leg hop, demonstration of 80% strength of the contralateral quadriceps, and return to full, painless range of motion with no effusion are useful guidelines. The use of a brace is controversial; its main role is to aid in proprioception and comfort. Therefore, a neoprene or elastic knee sleeve provides adequate bracing.

RESULTS AND OUTCOMES

Results of arthroscopic meniscal resection tend to deteriorate over time.[10,12] In 1995, Jaureguito et al[13] compared early and long-term follow-up of 47 patients who had undergone arthroscopic lateral partial meniscectomy for isolated tears. They noted that although 92% of patients had good to excellent results at the time of maximal improvement according to the Lysholm II score, only 62% of patients had good to excellent results at an average of 8 years; 85% were able to return to their preinjury level, but only 42% had maintained that activity level at the most recent follow-up. It appears that the results are somewhat dependent on the amount of meniscal tissue resected.[11,37] Clinically, results are better after partial meniscectomy than total meniscectomy.[10] The advantage of arthroscopic meniscectomy is the ability to identify specific tear patterns, which permits greater precision on resection of meniscal tissue compared with open techniques. Because neither open nor arthroscopic techniques leave normal meniscus, the results of both methods appear to deteriorate over time[38]; however, follow-up is longer for the open technique. Apart from the amount of meniscal tissue resection, other factors that influence the outcomes of meniscal resection are listed in Table 48-3. Probably most

Table 48-3 Factors Influencing Results of Meniscal Resection
Articular degenerative changes
Malalignment
Type of meniscal tears
Lateral versus medial meniscal tear
Instability
Age
Gender

significant are the degree of arthritic change, type of meniscal tear, limb alignment, ligament instability and lateral versus medial meniscectomy; less significant are patient age and gender.[14]

The long-term success (more than 2 years follow-up) of meniscal repair reported in the literature varies between 67% and 92%,[16,19] depending on the type or location of the tear and the means of outcome measurement. Factors that have been documented to significantly influence success rates include rim width, ACL laxity and concomitant ACL reconstruction, tear length, whether the tear is acute or chronic, and whether the medial or lateral meniscus is involved. Cannon and Morgan[30] documented a 90% success rate for tears with rim widths of less than 2 mm; this success rate decreased to 74% for tears with rim widths of 2 to 3.9 mm and to 50% for tears with rim widths of 4 to 5 mm. Concomitant ACL laxity is also an important factor in meniscal healing; DeHaven[16] documented a 46% of failure rate for meniscal repairs in ACL-deficient knees; the success rate of meniscal repair has also been found higher when ACL reconstruction is performed at the same time. Other factors that were found to influence meniscal healing favorably were time from injury to surgery of less than 8 weeks, tear length less than 2.5 cm, and tear of the lateral meniscus.

Factors that do not seem to affect the healing rates include age and repair technique. The ability of successfully healed menisci to remain healed over time can be judged by the results in long-term clinical studies; Eggli et al[39] reported a 73% survival rate at 7.5-year follow-up of isolated repairs in ACL stable knees. DeHaven reported a 79% survival rate with a minimum of 10 years after repair.[2,16,17] In the future, long-term studies are needed to fully evaluate these new all-inside implants in order to confirm better results of the meniscal repair.

COMPLICATIONS

Complications in arthroscopic meniscectomy can be categorized into either errors of judgment or technique. Errors of judgment are poor clinical decisions that can affect the short- and long-term outcome. Technical errors are violations of standard operative procedures and include retained meniscal tissue, articular surface iatrogenic damage, and broken instruments. For the different meniscal repair techniques, the complications are divided into two groups: one group consists of general complications such as infection, deep venous thrombosis, arthrofibrosis, and complex regional pain syndrome and the other group is related to the specific technique or implant used for the repair such as nerve injuries, popliteal vessel injuries, synovitis, articular cartilage damage, implant migration, and extra-articular cyst formation.[26,40-50]

CONCLUSIONS

- The goal of partial meniscectomy is to retain as much functional meniscal tissue as possible.
- Meniscal tears with 3 mm or less of rim width can be repaired with a high success rate.
- When a meniscal tear is treated in association with an ACL reconstruction, one should stretch the indications for repair due to improved healing rates and the documented adverse outcomes of meniscectomy in this population.
- Lateral repairs do better than medial repairs. Lateral meniscectomies fare worse than medial.

REFERENCES

1. Greis PE, Bardana DD, Holmstrom MC, Burks RT: Meniscal injury: I. Basic science and evaluation. J Am Acad Orthop Surg 2002;10:168–176.
2. DeHaven KE, Bronstein RD: Arthroscopic medial meniscal repair in the athlete. Clin Sports Med 1997;16:69–86.
3. Terry GC, Tagert BE, Young MJ: Reliability of the clinical assessment in predicting the cause of internal derangements of the knee. Arthroscopy 1995;11:568–576.
4. Rosenberg TD, Paulos LE, Parker RD, et al: The 45° posteroanterior flexion weight-bearing radiograph of the knee. J Bone Joint Surg Am 1988;70:1479–1483.
5. Muellner T, Weinstabl R, Schabus R, et al: The diagnosis of meniscal tears in athletes: A comparison of clinical and magnetic resonance imaging investigations. Am J Sports Med 1997;25:7–12.
6. Sutton JB (ed): Ligaments, Their Nature and Morphology. London, HK Lewis, 1897.
7. Arnoczky SP, Warren RF: Microvasculature of the human meniscus. Am J Sports Med 1982;10:90–95.
8. Renstrom P, Johnson RJ: Anatomy and biomechanics of the menisci. Clin Sports Med 1990;9:523–538.
9. Shelbourne KD, Patel DV, Adsit WS, Porter DA: Rehabilitation after meniscal repair. Clin Sports Med 1996;15:595–612.
10. Andersson-Molina H, Karlsson H, Rockborn P: Arthroscopic partial and total meniscectomy: A long-term follow-up study with matched controls. Arthroscopy 2002;18:183–189.
11. Bonneux I, Vandekerckhove B: Arthroscopic partial lateral meniscectomy long-term results in athletes. Acta Orthop Belg 2002;68:356–361.
12. Fairbanks T: Knee joint changes after meniscectomy. J Bone Joint Surg Br 1948;30:164–170.
13. Jaureguito J, Elliot J, Lietner T, et al: The effects of arthroscopic partial lateral meniscectomy in an otherwise normal knee: A retrospective review of functional, clinical and radiographic results. Arthroscopy 1995;11:29–36.
14. Rangger C, Klestil T, Gloetzer W, et al: Osteoarthritis after arthroscopic partial meniscectomy. Am J Sports Med 1995;23:240–244.
15. Wu WH, Hackett T, Richmond JC: Effects of meniscal and articular surface status on knee stability, function, and symptoms after anterior cruciate ligament reconstruction: A long-term prospective study. Am J Sports Med 2002;30:845–850.
16. DeHaven KE: Current concepts: Meniscus repair. Am J Sports Med 1999;27:242–250.
17. DeHaven KE, Sebastianelli WJ: Open meniscus repair. Indications, technique, and results. Clin Sports Med 1990;9:577–587.
18. Klimkiewicz JJ, Shaffer B: Meniscal surgery 2002 update: Indications and techniques for resection, repair, regeneration, and replacement. Arthroscopy 2002;18(9 Suppl 2):14–25.
19. Rath E, Richmond JC: The menisci: Basic science and advances in treatment. Br J Sports Med 2000;34:252–257.
20. Rosenberg TD, Metcalf RW, Gurley WD: Arthroscopic meniscectomy. Instr Course Lect 1988;37:203–208.
21. Metcalf RW, Burks RT, Metcalf RS: Arthroscopic meniscectomy. In McGuinty JB, Jackson RW (eds): Operative Arthroscopy. Philadelphia, Lippincott-Raven, 1996, pp 263–297.
22. Lysholm J, Gillquist J: Arthroscopic meniscectomy in athletes. Am J Sports Med 1983;11:436–438.
23. Northmore-Ball MD, Dandy DJ, Jackson RW: Arthroscopic, open partial, and total meniscectomy. A comparative study. J Bone Joint Surg Br 1983;65:400–404.
24. Easley ME, Cushner FD, Scott WN: Arthroscopic meniscal resection. In Insall JN, Scott WN (eds): Surgery of the Knee. Philadelphia, Churchill Livingstone, 2001, pp 473–520.

25. Henning CE, Lynch MA, Yearout KM, et al: Arthroscopic meniscal repair using an exogenous fibrin clot. Clin Orthop 1990;252:64–72.

26. Al-Othman AA: Biodegradable arrows for arthroscopic repair of meniscal tears. Int Orthop 2002;26:247–249.

27. Shelbourne KD, Porter DA: Meniscal repair. Description of a surgical technique. Am J Sports Med 1993;21:870–873.

28. Warren RF: Meniscectomy and repair in the anterior cruciate ligament-deficient patient. Clin Orthop 1990;252:55–63.

29. Rispoli DM, Miller MD: Options in meniscal repair. Clin Sports Med 1999;18:77–91.

30. Cannon WD Jr, Morgan CD: Meniscal repair: Arthroscopic repair techniques. Instr Course Lect 1994;43:77–96.

31. Morgan CD: The "all-inside" meniscus repair. Arthroscopy 1991;7:120.

32. Barber FA, Herbert MA, Richards DP: Load to failure testing of new meniscal repair devices. Arthroscopy 2004;20:45–50.

33. Farng E, Sherman O: Meniscal repair devices: A clinical and biomechanical literature review. Arthroscopy 2004;20:273–286.

34. McDermott D, Richards W, Hallam P, et al: A biomechanical study of four different meniscal repair systems, comparing pull-out strengths and gapping under cyclic loading. Knee Surg Sports Traumatol Arthrosc 2003;11:23–29.

35. Miller MD, Kline AJ, Jepsen KG: "All-inside" meniscal repair devices: An experimental study in the goat model. Am J Sports Med 2004;32:858–862.

36. Rankin CC, Lintner DM, Noble PC, et al: A biomechanical analysis of meniscal repair techniques. Am J Sports Med 2002;30:492–497.

37. Schimmer RC, Brulhart KB, Duff C, Glinz W: Arthroscopic partial meniscectomy: A 12-year follow-up and two-step evaluation of the long-term course. Arthroscopy 1998;14:136–142.

38. Rockborn P, Messner K: Long-term results of meniscus repair and meniscectomy: A 13-year functional and radiographic follow-up study. Knee Surg Sports Traumatol Arthrosc 2000;8:2–10.

39. Eggli S, Wegmuller H, Kosina J: Long-term results of arthroscopic meniscal repair. An analysis of isolated tears. Am J Sports Med 1995;23:715–720.

40. Anderson K, Marx RG, Hannafin J, Warren RF: Chondral injury following meniscal repair with a biodegradable implant. Arthroscopy 2000;16:749–753.

41. Calder SJ, Myers PT: Broken arrow: A complication of meniscal repair. Arthroscopy 1999;15:651–652.

42. Ganko A, Engebretsen L: Subcutaneous migration of meniscal arrows after failed meniscus repair. A report of two cases. Am J Sports Med 2000;28:252–253.

43. Hartley RC, Leung YL: Meniscal arrow migration into the popliteal fossa following attempted meniscal repair: A report of two cases. Knee 2002;9:69–71.

44. Kumar A, Malhan K, Roberts SN: Chondral injury from bioabsorbable screws after meniscal repair. Arthroscopy 2001;17:34.

45. Lombardo S, Eberly V: Meniscal cyst formation after all-inside meniscal repair. Am J Sports Med 1999;27:666–667.

46. Menche DS, Phillips GI, Pitman MI, Steiner GC: Inflammatory foreign-body reaction to an arthroscopic bioabsorbable meniscal arrow repair. Arthroscopy 1999;15:770–772.

47. Menetrey J, Seil R, Rupp S, Fritschy D: Chondral damage after meniscal repair with the use of a bioabsorbable implant. Am J Sports Med 2002;30:896–899.

48. Otte S, Klinger HM, Beyer J, Baums MH: Complications after meniscal repair with bioabsorbable arrows: Two cases and analysis of literature. Knee Surg Sports Traumatol Arthrosc 2002;10:250–253.

49. Ross G, Grabill J, McDevitt E: Chondral injury after meniscal repair with bioabsorbable arrows. Arthroscopy 2000;16:754–756.

50. Song EK, Lee KB, Yoon TR: Aseptic synovitis after meniscal repair using the biodegradable meniscus arrow. Arthroscopy 2001;17:77–80.

Kyle R. Flik, Paul Lewis, Richard W. Kang, and Brian J. Cole

INTRODUCTION

- Cartilage injuries are increasingly recognized due to dramatic increases in sports participation at all ages and improvements in musculoskeletal imaging.

- Pain and symptoms from articular cartilage lesions are variable. Similar-appearing articular cartilage lesions in the knee may be asymptomatic or may cause disabling pain, swelling, or mechanical symptoms.

- The decision of how to treat articular cartilage lesions is dependent on lesion characteristics such as location, size, and depth coupled with patient factors such as symptom intensity, age, activity level, and the presence of concomitant pathology.

- A variety of methods are available to treat articular cartilage lesions, including microfracture, autologous osteochondral transplant, allograft osteochondral transplant, and ACI.

- The success following surgery for a focal chondral or osteochondral defect is dependent on concomitant treatment of additional knee pathology and equally dependent on patient commitment to and diligence in the postoperative physical therapy regimen.

CLINICAL FEATURES AND EVALUATION

Complete evaluation of the patient with an articular cartilage injury of the knee includes a thorough history, physical examination, specific radiographs, and review of previous surgical notes or arthroscopic images.

The initial step in the workup is the history. This should include mechanism of injury, time course and quality of symptoms, and review of previous treatments and the effects of those treatments. Patients will often report pain and swelling with weight bearing and increased activity. Direct communication with previous surgeons may be required to have a more complete understanding of the surgical history and pathoanatomy within the patient's knee.

The mechanism of injury, if determined, is a valuable source of information and should be noted. Damage to articular cartilage can be caused by an acute injury yielding a focal chondral or osteochondral defect, can be the result of a chronic development such as osteochondritis dissecans (typically in younger patients), or simply present insidiously due to focal or diffuse degeneration related to mechanical (e.g., malalignment or instability) or genetic factors.

During the physical examination, the surgeon should be careful not to assume that the articular cartilage lesion is responsible for all symptoms. Often concomitant pathology exists and can play a role in the symptoms that the patient may be experiencing. It is important to also assess gait and alignment carefully as well as range of motion and patellofemoral tracking. Evaluation for effusion, ligamentous integrity, and areas of point tenderness or crepitus are additionally valuable in considering concomitant pathologies of the knee.

Required radiographs include standing anteroposterior, lateral, patellar skyline (or Merchant), a 45-degree flexion posteroanterior weight-bearing view, and full-length alignment film. The posteroanterior flexion view is crucial for adequate assessment of the posterior femoral condyles where significant wear may not be recognized on a standard weight-bearing anteroposterior view. Full-length alignment films should be obtained to assess the mechanical axis. No cartilage restoration procedure should be performed in the setting of malalignment; therefore, if the mechanical axis bisects the affected compartment, a corrective osteotomy should be strongly considered as a concomitant or staged procedure.

Other important information can come from imaging of the knee with magnetic resonance imaging. The quality of magnetic resonance imaging technology continues to improve dramatically. In fact, magnetic resonance has established a niche in evaluating articular cartilage irregularities and the degree of cartilage pathology, while also providing information regarding ligament injury. With high-resolution fast spin echo sequencing techniques in the sagittal, coronal, and axial planes, articular cartilage surfaces can be well imaged.[1,2] Computed tomography scanning may be necessary to assess the subchondral bone for anatomic considerations including defect geometry and depth in the presence of osteochondral defects that may require bone grafting in addition to an articular cartilage restorative procedure.

An examination under anesthesia is required to better assess the knee for instability. This is performed routinely prior to every knee arthroscopy. The first operation after the diagnosis of an articular cartilage defect is often not the definitive procedure. At times, arthroscopy is performed initially as a diagnostic tool to assess the lesion, the surrounding articular surfaces in the uninvolved compartments, and the state of the menisci and to determine the presence or absence of additional pathology. If one is considering definitive treatment with ACI, a biopsy should be performed at this time. Similarly, if a significant subchondral defect exists, primary bone grafting can be performed at the index operation. Finally, in the setting of mechanical axis malalignment, preoperative discussions might include performing an osteotomy at the index procedure, especially in slightly older patients who might have articular disease patterns considered more marginal for cartilage restoration. Most importantly, however, the initial arthroscopy should be used to define the lesion fully in terms of its location, geography, surface area, and depth. Careful attention to alternative sources of pain and the condition of opposing surfaces is also important.

Lesions are most often graded based on direct visualization using the system of Outerbridge[3] or the International Cartilage Repair Society, which established a grading system to help surgeons communicate clearly about cartilage lesions.[4] The two systems are nearly identical and grade the degree of cartilage damage on a scale from 0 to 4, with a 0 indicating normal cartilage and a 4 indicating injury that penetrates the subchondral bone. A grade of 2 indicates nearly normal cartilage with minor softening or superficial fissures. Grade 3 reflects fissuring to the level of, but not violating, the subchondral bone. Regardless of the system used, always classify lesions with a written and diagrammatic description including the delineation of how the defect contacts opposing surfaces in varying degrees of flexion. In establishing a surgical plan at the time of initial arthroscopy, consider the status of the menisci for the possible inclusion of a meniscal transplant as well as the standing mechanical axis for consideration of a concomitant osteotomy.

RELEVANT ANATOMY AND BASIC SCIENCE

Chondrocytes of mesenchymal origin are responsible for the production and maintenance of the extracellular matrix of collagen. This matrix is composed mainly of type II collagen but also includes types V, VI, IX, X, XI, XII, and XIV to a lesser degree. The combination of this collagen network and water affords the viscoelastic properties that resist compressive and shear forces experienced between the articulating surfaces. Articular cartilage provides a smooth, nearly frictionless surface that protects the subchondral bone through shock absorption and wear resistance.

While highly specialized and multifunctional, this tissue ironically maintains itself with little contribution from systemic sources and is in fact avascular. As a consequence, hyaline cartilage has trouble repairing itself when damaged. Should the defect penetrate the subchondral bone (i.e., full thickness), the defect may fill with fibrocartilage repair tissue. This replacement may be sufficient in some instances to render patients less symptomatic but is typically inferior in ultrastructure and function compared to native hyaline cartilage. At this juncture, healthy articular cartilage has properties that are unmatched by any man-made substance.

TREATMENT OPTIONS

The spectrum of articular cartilage injury is broad and varies principally in terms of location, size, and depth. A diligent evaluation of these characteristics as well as considerations for patient age, activity level, concomitant pathology, and symptomatology is crucial to making appropriate treatment decisions.

It is important to recognize that not all chondral lesions cause symptoms. Conversely, not all symptoms are related to the chondral or osteochondral defect. The first step in management of articular cartilage lesions is usually conservative, nonsurgical treatment. Common methods include weight loss, shoe modification, bracing, cane use, and various pharmacologic interventions. Physical therapy may also play a role by improving strength and flexibility; however, this and the previously mentioned treatment are often ineffective in reducing the symptoms associated with an articular cartilage lesion. Medications and nutritional supplements that should be considered are nonsteroidal anti-inflammatory drugs, acetaminophen, or glucosamine and chondroitin sulfate. Intra-articular injections of corticosteroid and hyaluronic acid can be helpful for symptom control but are generally reserved for the older population.

If the preceding conservative treatments prove ineffective, both the patient and clinician need to consider surgical options. The specific surgical technique, or techniques, chosen will depend first on the general state of the knee with regard to mechanical alignment, meniscus status, and compartment involvement. Any clinically significant malalignment must be corrected before or concurrently with the cartilage restoration procedure or the restoration will likely fail because the affected compartment will continue to suffer unnecessarily high loads. In a demand-match approach, the senior author (B.J.C.) routinely performs a medial opening wedge high tibial osteotomy for the patient with a medial compartment lesion and varus alignment, a distal femoral osteotomy for the knee with valgus alignment and a lateral compartment lesion, or an anteromedialization of the tibial tubercle for most patellofemoral defects. Given this generality, it is important to note the medial shift in patellofemoral pressures as a result of anteromedialization.[5] For example, in cases of superomedial patellar disease, no anteromedialization is performed because the procedure would overload the repaired defect.

In addition to mechanical malalignment, any untreated ligament insufficiency or significant meniscus deficiency is a contraindication to articular cartilage restoration alone. While most comorbidities can be corrected simultaneously with cartilage restoration; staging of procedures is an acceptable alternative. For all surgical candidates, it is necessary that a comprehensive plan be formed and this plan be discussed with each patient so he or she understands the procedure and complies with postoperative instructions. Whenever possible, the initial treatment of an articular cartilage lesion should allow for further treatment if unsuccessful.

Despite the availability of several techniques, judicial use of each remains challenging. There are relatively few convincing data on the superiority of one technique over another for some lesions. In fact, every articular cartilage lesion is different and requires its own, unique evaluation. Part of the difficulty in treatment decision making is the fact that the natural history of asymptomatic lesions is unclear and unpredictable. However, it is widely believed that if left untreated, a symptomatic cartilage lesion is likely to persist or worsen.[6,7] The risk of a lesion being symptomatic likely depends on its location, size, depth, patient activity level, and any associated knee pathology. Pre-existing instability, meniscal damage, or malalignment provides an inhospitable environment for any articular cartilage lesion and predisposes it to progressive degeneration.

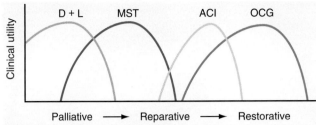

Figure 49-1 Treatment options for articular cartilage lesions overlap and range from palliative to reparative to restorative procedures. Maximal clinical utility for each should be recognized within its range. ACI, autologous chondrocyte implantation; D + L, dèbridement and lavage; MST, marrow stimulation techniques; OCG, osteochondral grafting.

Surgery

There are essentially four distinct surgical procedures used to treat chondral or osteochondral lesions in the knee. These include microfracture, osteochondral autograft, osteochondral allograft, and ACI. We conceptualize the treatment possibilities in categories depending on the clinical scenario. The categories range from palliative (dèbridement/lavage), intended to reduce mechanical irritation and inflammatory mediators, to reparative (microfracture, a marrow stimulation technique), designed to release pluripotential cells from the bone marrow that proliferate as fibrocartilage repair cells in the defect, to restorative (osteochondral grafting, either autograft or allograft), which replaces the articular cartilage and its subchondral bone. ACI bridges the boundary between a reparative technique and a restorative one (Fig. 49-1). The common goal to each of these procedures is to provide the patient with symptom reduction and a return to a high level of function while postponing, if not eliminating, the need for arthroplasty. Each recommended procedure should theoretically allow additional opportunity for cartilage restoration should the initial treatment fail.

Treatment Algorithm

Surgical treatment of a focal chondral defect is based on the characteristics of the lesion, local comorbidities, and the age and activity level of the patient. Important characteristics of the lesion include its size and depth, degree of containment, and location. For patellofemoral lesions, an anteromedialization osteotomy of the tibial tubercle is generally recommended to unload the repaired defect. For femoral condyle lesions, an intact meniscus and a mechanical axis that does not pass through the affected compartment will provide the ideal environment for healing and the greatest chance for symptom relief.

Typically, arthroscopic dèbridement with marrow stimulation is a reasonable first-line treatment, especially if performed during the initial evaluation of a defect. The intention is to reduce symptoms and provide long-term relief without eliminating options for further restorative or reparative procedures if needed. Secondary treatment for smaller lesions (i.e., 2 to 4 cm^2) includes revision with osteochondral autograft transplantation. Larger lesions may be amenable to ACI as ACI is best used in younger patients with contained shallow lesions that are 2 to 10 cm^2. Deeper lesions that are larger may be best treated with fresh osteochondral allograft transplantation. Figure 49-2 illustrates a typical treatment algorithm that considers lesion location, size, and the patient's level of physical demand.[8]

Surgical Techniques
Microfracture

Microfracture is a marrow-stimulating technique designed to allow fibrocartilage reparative tissue to form in a contained articular chondral lesion. This technique, performed arthroscopically,

Figure 49-2 Treatment algorithm for focal chondral defects of the femoral condyle or patellofemoral joint. For femoral condyle lesions, assessment must first be made regarding malalignment, meniscus status, and ligamentous stability as these comorbidities must be corrected. For trochlear and patellar lesions, patellofemoral alignment must be assessed and anteromedialization considered. High-demand individuals are more likely to require a secondary line of treatment. ACI, autologous chondrocyte implantation; AMZ, anteromedialization; OC, osteochondral.

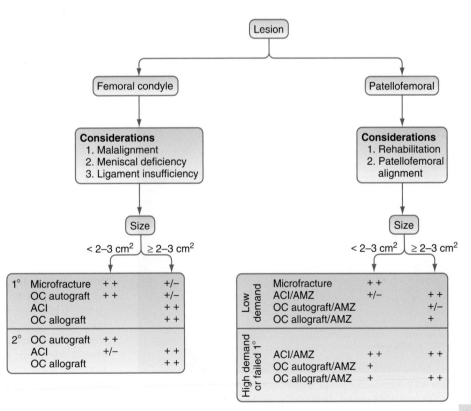

involves the creation of perforations through the subchondral bone that allow the release of blood and mesenchymal cells that form a clot in the lesion and proliferate and differentiate into a fibrocartilage repair tissue.[9]

The optimal patient for microfracture is the young, compliant patient with a focal grade III or IV articular cartilage lesion surrounded by normal cartilage without bone loss. Contraindications include significant bone loss, malalignment, or an opposing "kissing" lesion. The main advantages of this procedure are its low cost and relatively low technical difficulty. In addition, it is a procedure that does not "burn bridges" for future treatment options (i.e., it does not preclude subsequent restorative techniques if necessary). The major drawback of the procedure is that the repair tissue that forms is composed primarily of type I collagen, which is a fibrocartilage that has inferior biomechanical properties to normal hyaline cartilage and may not withstand prolonged high levels of activity with excessive biomechanical forces across a surface with reparative tissue.

The first step in microfracture is to prepare the lesion by removing all damaged cartilage, leaving a perpendicular edge of healthy articular cartilage that results in a "well-shouldered" lesion to contain the clot and reduce shear and compression of the lesion. The calcified layer of bone should then be removed with a curet. An awl is used to create holes in the lesion 2 to 3 mm apart and approximately 2 to 4 mm deep.[10] Begin by placing holes in the periphery of the lesion and work centrally until the entire surface of the lesion has been uniformly covered (Fig. 49-3). It is important to avoid subchondral bone collapse that can result from the creation of converging holes or holes placed too close together. The final step is to clamp the arthroscopy fluid inflow and confirm that blood and fat droplets emerge from each hole (Fig. 49-4). This ensures that the microfracture awl penetrated the underlying cancellous bone and that a clot is likely to form in the defect.

Osteochondral Autograft

During an osteochondral autograft procedure, a healthy intact osteochondral plug is transferred from a low weight-bearing area to the damaged lesion that is removed as a plug of matching size. Mosaicplasty is the term for this technique when multiple small plugs are used to fill a larger area. Osteochondral autograft refers

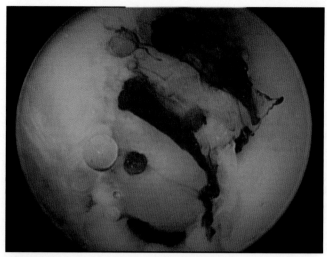

Figure 49-4 Arthroscopy image depicting adequate penetration into bleeding subchondral bone.

to the osteochondral articular transfer system devised and marketed by Arthrex Inc. (Naples, FL). This technique is limited by the amount of donor tissue that can be used.

The ideal lesion for this technique is a symptomatic distal femoral condyle defect in a knee with intact menisci and normal alignment. The senior author has the best success with lesions that are 1 to 2 cm in diameter, although larger lesions can also be treated. One disadvantage of the technique is the donor site morbidity, which increases as the size of the lesion treated increases. The major advantage of this procedure over osteochondral allograft is that the donor plug is the patient's own, so there is no infectious or immunologic risk from the transplant.

The entire procedure can be performed arthroscopically or through a small arthrotomy, depending on the size and location of the defect. The senior author uses the osteochondral autograft system (Arthrex Inc.); however, there are many commercially available systems. The first step is to use a sizer to determine the number and size of grafts that will be required to fill the area of the lesion. The graft harvester of appropriate size is then introduced perpendicular to the donor site typically through a small parapatellar arthrotomy. The typical donor sites include the femoral intercondylar notch and the periphery of the lateral femur just proximal to the sulcus terminalis (Fig. 49-5). The harvester is then tapped into the bone to a depth of 12 to 15 mm, twisted sharply 90 degrees clockwise and counterclockwise, and removed with a parallel pull. The donor plug is removed from the harvester with a plunger that will push the donor plug into the recipient hole once this has been prepared.

The recipient hole is prepared to an equal depth and extracted in an identical manner. A constant knee flexion angle is required during this portion of the procedure, so that the donor plug can be placed at the same angle. The donor harvester with plug is placed over the recipient site and advanced into the defect while maintaining perpendicular orientation and a constant angle. The donor harvester has a tendency to "back off" the articular surface and should be held securely as the donor plug is advanced. Once the donor plug has been fully released from the harvester, the plug will typically rest a few millimeters proud. The final seating of the plug is performed with an oversized tamp using a gentle tapping technique to minimize damage

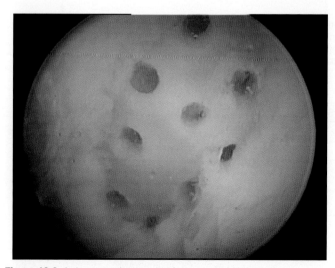

Figure 49-3 Arthroscopy image showing prepared lesion with microfracture holes placed uniformly throughout lesion 3 to 4 mm apart.

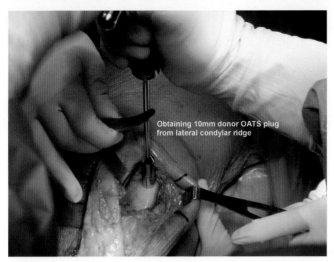

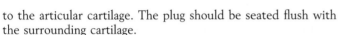

Figure 49-5 Typical harvest site for osteochondral autografts (OATS).

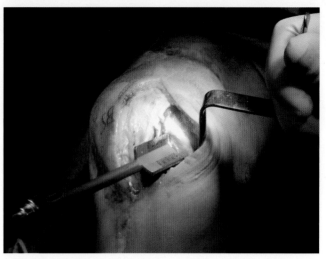

Figure 49-6 Boring the defect to create cylinder recipient site for osteochondral allograft.

to the articular cartilage. The plug should be seated flush with the surrounding cartilage.

If a mosaicplasty technique is being performed, all plugs (size and depth) should be carefully planned before placing the first one. The difficulty in using multiple smaller plugs is in creating a convexity to match the surrounding articular surface. In addition, the senior author has seen a number of patients whose smaller plugs have delaminated over relatively short periods of time postoperatively and therefore chooses to use the smallest number of larger diameter plugs possible (i.e., 10-mm diameter).

Osteochondral Allograft

This technique is employed to treat larger lesions or lesions with significant bone loss. As a salvage restorative technique, osteochondral allografts have the advantage of providing fully formed articular cartilage without limitation on size and without donor harvest morbidity. Unfortunately, a small but not negligible risk still remains with allograft tissue with respect to disease transmission and immunogenicity. In addition, the problem of cell viability at the time of implantation remains. Currently, most osteochondral allografts are transplanted as prolonged-fresh grafts stored at 4°C for between 14 and 28 days to maximally preserve cell viability, which directly correlates with the success of implantation.[11]

A parapatellar mini-arthrotomy is performed on the side of the lesion. The lesion is carefully evaluated to determine the graft shape required to best fit the defect. We use an instrumentation system (Arthrex Inc.) to size and harvest a cylindrical plug from the allograft. After matching the defect diameter to the sizing cylinder that best covers the defect, the osteochondral allograft plug is obtained. The sizing cylinder is placed perpendicular to the defect and a guide pin is drilled in the center of the lesion to a depth of 20 to 30 mm. The appropriately sized cannulated counter bore is drilled over the pin to create a cylindrical defect to a depth of 8 to 10 mm (Fig. 49-6). A small drill or Kirschner wire is then used to make multiple small perforations in the bottom of the prepared defect in order to create vascular access channels. The depth of 6 to 8 mm is a compromise between having sufficient bone to achieve a press fit and minimizing the amount of immunogenic bone implanted. The 12-o'clock position of the defect is marked with a sterile

marking pen to help with orientation of the donor plug. Each of the quadrants in the defect is measured with a depth gauge and used to tailor the exact depth of final cut of the donor allograft plug.

Attention is then turned to the allograft preparation. A flat surface must be cut first in the allograft, which makes securing the graft in the workstation easier (Fig. 49-7). The bushing on the workstation is then secured over the allograft so that the harvested plug will have a contour that best matches the defect site. With smaller defects (<2 cm²), nearly any portion of a hemicondyle allograft will closely match the defect curvature. The 12-o'clock position on the allograft is marked so that it can be easily lined up with the same position previously marked at the defect. The donor graft is then drilled through its entire depth with a harvester, and the graft is removed (Fig. 49-8). The depth of each of the four quadrants previously measured at the donor site is marked on the allograft plug, and a final cut is made with an oscillating saw (Fig. 49-9). The edge of the allograft can be slightly beveled to facilitate insertion. Prior to insertion, the bony portion of the allograft should be irrigated with a pulse lavage to remove any residual bone marrow elements that may initiate an immune response.

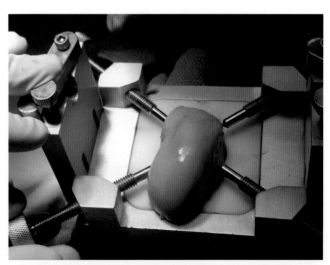

Figure 49-7 Allograft hemicondyle secured in a workstation.

509

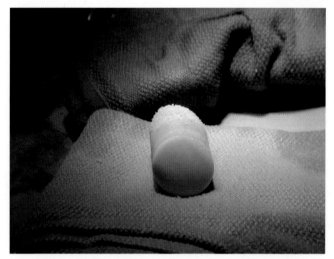

Figure 49-8 Initial allograft cylinder cut from hemicondyle.

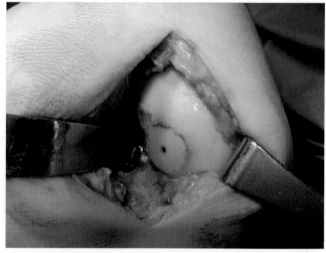

Figure 49-10 Completed osteochondral allograft.

The recipient socket is then dilated an additional 0.5 mm with a calibrated dilator and the graft is press fit into the socket by hand with the four quadrants in proper orientation. The graft can be gently impacted with an oversized tamp to ensure a flush fit, although we prefer to cycle the knee and load the ipsilateral compartment to terminally and atraumatically seat the graft. Fixation with bioabsorbable pins or a headless screw with differential thread pitch may be used to augment the press fit if needed for larger grafts (Fig. 49-10).

Autologous Chondrocyte Implantation

ACI is usually chosen to treat a defect after more traditional first-line treatments have failed. It involves the use of harvested and laboratory-grown autologous chondrocytes that are reimplanted in a defect under a watertight periosteal patch. Ideally, the patient has a symptomatic, unipolar, well-contained chondral defect in an otherwise normal knee. The defect size that can be treated with ACI ranges from 2 to 10 cm^2, although the senior author has experience in treating significantly larger lesions. The indications for use of ACI have expanded, and success has been reported with use in joints other than the knee.

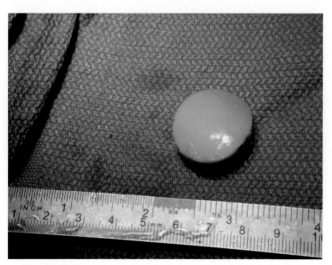

Figure 49-9 Final allograft plug to be placed in recipient bed.

In addition, patellar and tibial lesions have been treated in addition to the classic femoral condyle or trochlea. As previously discussed, contraindications include untreated malalignment and ligament or meniscus insufficiency. While a relative contraindication, in selected cases, bipolar lesions can be treated effectively with ACI.

The ACI technique requires a minimum of two operations. The first involves arthroscopy to evaluate the lesion and to obtain a biopsy of articular cartilage. The lesion should be carefully measured and assessed for containment and depth. The site from which the senior author prefers to obtain the biopsy sample is the lateral edge of the intercondylar notch. A curved bone graft harvesting gouge is used to obtain approximately 200 to 300 mg or three "Tic Tac-sized" fragments of articular cartilage. The biopsy is placed in the collection vial and into a shipping container to be mailed for processing and cell growth.

After the requisite minimum of 6 weeks of cell growth, the second stage of implantation can be performed. This is an open procedure with exposure dependent on the location of the lesion. A femoral condyle lesion is exposed through a limited parapatellar arthrotomy on the side of the lesion. For medial femoral condyle lesions, we typically expose via a limited subvastus medialis approach, and for lateral condyle lesions, we perform a limited lateral retinacular release. Patellofemoral lesions are approached through a midline incision, which allows a tibial tubercle osteotomy to be performed simultaneously, followed by a lateral retinacular release without complete eversion of the patella (Fig. 49-11). The tibial tubercle osteotomy allows increased patellar mobility and easier access to the defect; however, we avoid complete elevation and eversion of the tubercle, which are disruptive to the fat pad and patellar tendon and a potential cause of postoperative stiffness. The incision is extended distally to harvest periosteum, or if a distal realignment is not performed, an additional incision located below the pes anserine tendons is required for the periosteal patch harvest on the anteromedial tibia.

Once adequate exposure is obtained, the defect is prepared. This involves removal of any fibrocartilage or loose cartilage flaps surrounding the lesion followed by the creation of stable vertical walls of healthy cartilage around the periphery of the lesion. A no. 15 scalpel is helpful to sharply incise the defect's border. Sharp-ring curets are also used to clear tissue from the lesion

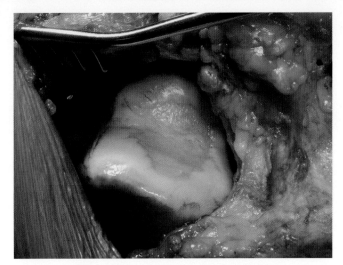

Figure 49-11 Large shallow trochlear lesion.

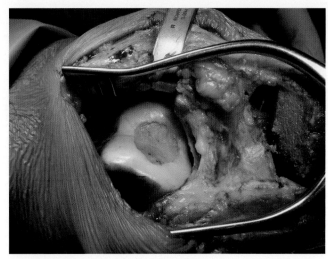

Figure 49-13 Final prepared trochlear lesion ready to be measured prior to periosteal harvest.

without penetrating the subchondral bone (Fig. 49-12). Finally, the tourniquet is deflated and neuropatties soaked in dilute 1:1000 epinephrine solution are held in the defect to achieve hemostasis. The final defect should be measured or traced so that an adequate patch of periosteum can be obtained (Fig. 49-13).

The next step is to obtain the periosteal patch through an additional incision over the anteromedial tibia 4 to 6 cm below the insertion of the hamstring tendons. Additional periosteum sites include the distal femur or contralateral tibia. Harvesting can be performed through a 3-cm longitudinal incision. Superficial subcutaneous fat and blood vessels should be carefully removed from the periosteum. This is more difficult in smokers who have more fragile periosteum and in the obese population who have greater amounts of overlying adipose tissue. Score the periosteum with a no. 15 scalpel, being sure to overestimate the required size by a few millimeters. The periosteum is elevated with a sharp, curved periosteal elevator while holding the leading edge with fine forceps (Fig. 49-14). Mark the outer surface with a sterile marking pen to distinguish it from the inner cambium layer.

The patch is then sewn onto the cartilage with the cambium layer facing down creating a taut surface. Absorbable 6-0 Vicryl sutures (Ethicon Inc, Johnson & Johnson, Somerville, NJ) on a P-1 cutting needle are used to sew the patch using sterile mineral oil so the suture passes with ease. The suture is passed first through the periosteum and then through the articular cartilage (Fig. 49-15). The knot is tied on the periosteum side, not over the healthy cartilage on the perimeter of the lesion. A small gap is left open in the patch superiorly to allow a test of water-tightness and to implant the chondrocytes with an angiocatheter.

The patch is then tested for watertightness by using a saline-filled tuberculin syringe and an 18-gauge catheter. Additional sutures are placed as necessary after removal of all the water. The edges of the patch are then sealed with fibrin glue (Tisseel, Baxter Healthcare Corp., Glendale, CA) and a second water test is performed (Fig. 49-16).

Extraction of the chondrocytes from the vials is performed under sterile technique with an 18-gauge angiocatheter on a tuberculin syringe. The angiocatheter is placed in the vial (which should always remain vertical) so that the tip is submerged in the fluid above the pellet of cells at the bottom. Repetitive

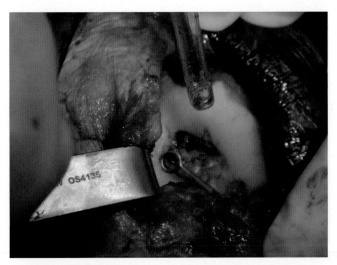

Figure 49-12 Preparing a trochlear lesion with a ring curet.

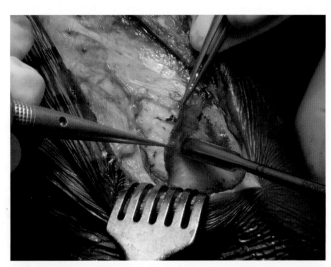

Figure 49-14 Harvesting the periosteum from the proximal medial tibia, below the medial collateral ligament insertion and Sartorius insertion.

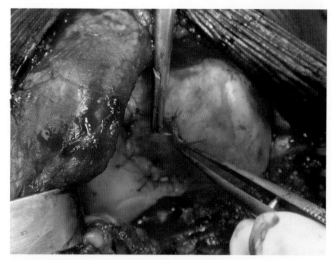

Figure 49-15 Sewing the periosteal patch in place with 6-0 colored Vicryl suture.

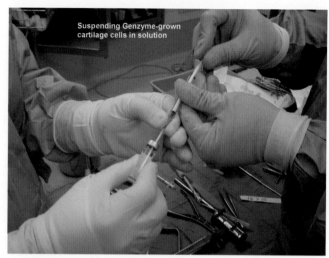

Figure 49-17 Extracting the chondrocytes for implantation.

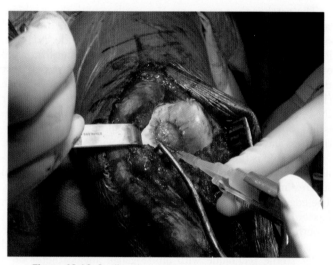

Figure 49-16 Sealing the periosteal patch with fibrin glue.

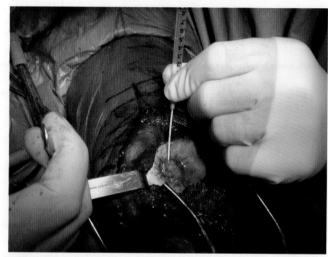

Figure 49-18 Implanting chondrocytes under the watertight periosteal patch.

gentle aspirations are the used to suspend the cells in solution. The entire volume is then aspirated and drawn into the syringe (Fig. 49-17).

To implant the cells under the periosteal patch, a new sterile angiocatheter should be placed through the opening at the top of the periosteal patch and advanced to the bottom of the defect. While injecting the cells, the surgeon slowly withdraws the angiocatheter tip to ensure even delivery of cells throughout the defect (Fig. 49-18). The remaining opening in the patch is then securely closed with additional sutures and fibrin glue (Fig. 49-19).

POSTOPERATIVE REHABILITATION

The success of all cartilage restoration techniques is highly dependent on the compliance and diligence of the patient during the rehabilitation process.

Microfracture

Following microfracture to lesions of the weight-bearing surfaces of the femoral condyle or tibial plateau, the patient is braced

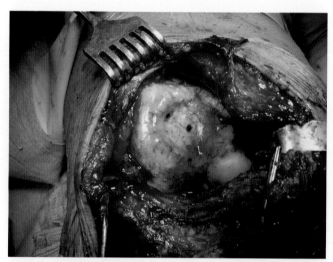

Figure 49-19 Final appearance of completed autologous chondrocyte implantation.

and remains non-weight bearing for 4 to 6 weeks with gradual advancement to full weight bearing for an additional 2 weeks. For lesions of the patellofemoral joint, the patient is braced with a flexion stop at 30 to 40 degrees in order to limit patellofemoral contact pressures but may bear weight in full extension. The brace is removed only for range-of-motion and strengthening exercises. Early passive motion is initiated, usually with a continual passive motion device immediately postoperatively used for a total of 6 hours each day for as long as 6 weeks. An alternative to continual passive motion device use is to perform 500 repetitions of knee flexion and extension three times daily.

Osteochondral Autograft

Similarly, both passive and active ranges of motion are encouraged after osteochondral autografting. Weight bearing is protected for up to 6 weeks. Once radiographic evidence of bone healing is noted at 6 to 8 weeks, the patient is advanced to full weight bearing as tolerated. Closed-chain strengthening exercises are begun after 3 months, running is usually possible at 6 months, and athletic activity involving higher shear forces can resume at 9 months.

Osteochondral Allograft

After osteochondral allografting, restricted weight bearing in a hinged knee brace is recommended for at least 8 weeks to protect the articular cartilage and to allow thorough incorporation via creeping substitution. The continual passive motion device is used for 6 to 8 hours per day at one cycle per minute for the first 4 to 6 weeks. Usually 4 to 6 months are required before return to light sporting activity. We recommend abstaining from high-impact activities after this procedure because of concern for graft collapse or deterioration of the chondral surface.

Autologous Chondrocyte Implantation

The rehabilitation following ACI involves early passive motion for 6 to 8 hours daily with the continual passive motion device. This is crucial as motion assists cellular orientation and prevents adhesions from developing. The graft is protected from overload by maintaining restricted weight bearing for 4 to 6 weeks in a hinged knee brace. Gradually impact-loading activities are phased in with increased strengthening. Full recovery and involvement in light sporting activity occurs between 4 and 6 months.

CRITERIA FOR RETURN TO SPORTS

Following all the procedures previously outlined, the general criteria for return to any sports activity include a normal gait pattern, a pain-free knee with normal or near-normal range of motion and strength, and no recurrent effusions. For patients who have undergone a microfracture, return to any sports activity is generally permitted after 16 weeks provided the preceding criteria are met. For osteochondral allograft procedures, there is the additional criterion of radiographic bony integration of the plug(s). Usually, return to lower impact sporting activities is permitted between 4 and 6 months. For autografts, return to sports involving high shear forces on the knee is delayed until approximately 6 months postoperatively. We advise our allograft patients against participating in high-impact cutting sports following an osteochondral graft procedure. Following ACI, return to light sporting activities such as jogging can usually resume by

6 to 9 months; however, high-impact activity resumes by 12 to 18 months.

RESULTS AND OUTCOMES

It is difficult to compare results for the various procedures described here. The patient population with articular cartilage defects is generally heterogeneous. Often, procedures are not performed in isolation but rather with the concomitant treatment of other comorbidities within the same knee.

Microfracture appears to have better outcomes in younger patients with smaller lesions, perhaps because the pluripotential cell count decreases with increasing age. One recent review demonstrated that 80% of patients reported themselves as improved, with patients younger than 35 showing the best outcomes.[5]

Overall, autologous osteochondral grafts perform better in isolated femoral condyle lesions (92% good or excellent) compared to tibial plateau lesions (87% good or excellent) or patellofemoral defects (79% good or excellent).[12]

Results following osteochondral allografting appear best (86% success at 7.5 years) if the lesion is the result of a purely traumatic event.[13] Bugbee[14] reported success rates of 93% for femoral lesions, 76% for patellofemoral grafts, and 65% for tibiofemoral bipolar defects at 4 years. In all studies, uncorrected mechanical limb malalignment or ligamentous instability was associated with worse outcomes.

Following ACI, results have been most favorable for femoral lesions and less favorable for patellar lesions. Peterson et al[15] reported 89% good to excellent results for femur lesions compared to 65% for the patella. As greater attention was paid to performing anteromedialization of the tibial tubercle, results after treating patellar lesions appear more promising and quite similar to femoral condyle lesions treated with ACI. We have presented 103 defects treated with ACI in 83 patients, with complete satisfaction reported in 79.3% of patients.[16]

In an attempt to compare microfracture with ACI in a similar patient population, Knutsen et al[17] randomized 80 patients with isolated focal chondral defects in stable knees with a normal mechanical axis to receive either ACI or microfracture as a first-line treatment. Both groups improved significantly; however, the microfracture group had statistically significantly greater improvement than the ACI group at 2 years.[17] Similarly, Horas et al[18] compared ACI to osteochondral autograft transplantation and noted improved symptoms in both groups but greater subjective improvement in the osteochondral autograft group.

COMPLICATIONS

Failure to recognize concomitant knee pathology is an avoidable cause of poor outcome with any cartilage restoration procedure. It is essential to have a clear understanding of the status of the knee in terms of its alignment, ligamentous integrity, and meniscal function prior to formulating a comprehensive surgical plan.

With complex or multiple procedures, stiffness is the most common complication, usually treated by arthroscopic releases and manipulation. With microfracture, overaggressive use of the awl by placing holes that are too deep or close together can lead to subchondral bone collapse. With osteochondral grafting, placement of plugs excessively proud may result in high shear forces and failure of the plug. Excessive impaction of osteochondral grafts may cause chondrocyte death. With ACI, graft overgrowth is the most common complication, which can usually be resolved with arthroscopic débridement of the hypertrophic tissue.

CONCLUSIONS

The successful management of articular cartilage lesions is challenging for both the surgeon and patient. Surgeons are faced with complex decision making in addressing the defect as well as coexisting pathology of the knee. Additionally, each patient is unique and must be evaluated individually to determine the best course of treatment. Patients are charged with the responsibility of committing to a strict postoperative regimen on which the success of the operation depends. As further advances are made in this exciting area of orthopedics, promising new methods will evolve to improve the treatment of articular cartilage lesions and narrow the use of total joint arthroplasty.

REFERENCES

1. Brown WE, Potter HG, Marx RG, et al: Magnetic resonance imaging appearance of cartilage repair in the knee. Clin Orthop 2004;422:214–223.
2. Potter HG, Linklater JM, Allen AA, et al: Magnetic resonance imaging of articular cartilage in the knee. An evaluation with use of fast-spin-echo imaging. J Bone Joint Surg Am 1998;80:1276–1284.
3. Outerbridge RE: The etiology of chondromalacia patellae. J Bone Joint Surg Br 1961;43:752–757.
4. Brittberg M, Winalski CS: Evaluation of cartilage injuries and repair. J Bone Joint Surg Am 2003;85(Suppl 2):58–69.
5. Steadman JR, Briggs KK, Rodrigo JJ, et al: Outcomes of microfracture for traumatic chondral defects of the knee: Average 11-year follow-up. Arthroscopy 2003;19:477–484.
6. Messner K, Maletius W: The long-term prognosis for severe damage to weight-bearing cartilage in the knee: A 14-year clinical and radiographic follow-up in 28 young athletes. Acta Orthop Scand 1996;67:165–168.
7. Shelbourne KD, Jari S, Gray T: Outcome of untreated traumatic articular cartilage defects of the knee: A natural history study. J Bone Joint Surg Am 2003;85(Suppl 2):8–16.
8. Cole BJ, Malek MM: Articular Cartilage Lesions: A Practical Guide to Assessment and Treatment. New York, Springer, 2004, pp 35–46.
9. Freedman KB, Nho SJ, Cole BJ: Marrow stimulating technique to augment meniscus repair. Arthroscopy 2003;19:794–798.
10. Steadman JR, Rodkey WG, Briggs KK: Microfracture to treat full-thickness chondral defects: Surgical technique, rehabilitation, and outcomes. J Knee Surg 2002;15:170–176.
11. Williams RJ 3rd, Dreese JC, Chen CT: Chondrocyte survival and material properties of hypothermically stored cartilage: An evaluation of tissue used for osteochondral allograft transplantation. Am J Sports Med 2004;32:132–139.
12. Hangody L, Fules P: Autologous osteochondral mosaicplasty for the treatment of full-thickness defects of weight-bearing joints: Ten years of experimental and clinical experience. J Bone Joint Surg Am 2003;85(Suppl 2):25–32.
13. Chu CR, Convery FR, Akeson WH, et al: Articular cartilage transplantation. Clinical results in the knee. Clin Orthop 1999;360:159–168.
14. Bugbee WD: Fresh osteochondral allografts. J Knee Surg 2002;15:191–195.
15. Peterson L, Minas T, Brittberg M, et al: Two- to 9-year outcome after autologous chondrocyte transplantation of the knee. Clin Orthop 2000;374:212–234.
16. Cole BJ, Fox J, Nho S, et al: Prospective evaluation of autologous chondrocyte implantation. Paper presented at the Annual Meeting of the American Academy of Orthopaedic Surgeons, 2003.
17. Knutsen G, Engebretsen L, Ludvigsen TC, et al: Autologous chondrocyte implantation compared with microfracture in the knee. A randomized trial. J Bone Joint Surg Am 2004;86:455–464.
18. Horas U, Pelinkovic D, Herr G, et al: Autologous chondrocyte implantation and osteochondral cylinder transplantation in cartilage repair of the knee joint. A prospective, comparative trial. J Bone Joint Surg Am 2003;85:185–192.

Graft Choices in Ligament Surgery

Andrew D. Pearle and Answorth A. Allen

In This Chapter

INTRODUCTION

- Graft choice in knee ligament surgery remains a notoriously controversial topic among sports medicine orthopedists.

- Numerous graft choices are available and studies are available to support a high rate of "good" to "excellent" results with each graft type.

- The perfect graft would have no donor site morbidity, reproduce the mechanical properties of the native ligament, provide biologic insertional incorporation, and supply neuromuscular control.

- While the perfect graft does not exist, the available choices each have pros and cons that can be tailored to the specific patient needs.

Different patient characteristics dictate certain grafts. These include lifestyle (such as job and religion), sports activity, age, and pre-existing comorbidities such as previous hamstring injuries as well as patellofemoral issues such as chondrosis/arthrosis, instability, previous trauma, and Osgood-Schlatter disease. In addition, surgeon comfort level with specific grafts and techniques affects decision making.

The purpose of this chapter is to introduce the biology, biomechanics, fixation strategies, risks, pitfalls, and outcomes of the common graft choices in ligament surgery. Basic understanding of these issues helps guide appropriate matching of graft to patient.

BASIC BIOLOGY AND BIOMECHANICS OF GRAFTS IN LIGAMENT SURGERY

Current rehabilitation protocols for knee ligament reconstruction stress immediate range of motion, return of neuromuscular function, proprioception, and early weight bearing up the kinetic chain. It is therefore essential to understand the biology and time course of graft remodeling and incorporation into the bone.

The biology of healing of the ligament replacement graft is grossly the same for all biologic graft materials. Tendon grafts go through biologic stages during the process of "ligamentization." First, the graft undergoes inflammation and necrosis. Early inflammation and neovascular proliferation is seen within the first couple of weeks after graft reconstruction. The graft then undergoes revascularization and repopulation with fibroblasts over the ensuing 4 to 8 weeks. During this stage, all the donor fibroblasts undergo cell death, but the collagen structure of the tendon serves as a scaffold for extrinsic fibroblast ingrowth. This complete repopulation of the graft with host fibroblasts is thought to occur both in autografts and allografts. The final stage involves a gradual remodeling of the graft and the collagenous structure. The rate and predictability of ligamentization vary among autograft and allograft tissues and are discussed later in the chapter.

The initial strength, stiffness, and cross-sectional areas of various ligament grafts is well characterized and summarized in Table 50-1. While these initial biomechanical properties are important determinants of graft suitability, grafts undergo a long evolution of incorporation and their structural properties are dramatically altered over time. All biologic grafts lose their initial strength during the early healing period,[1-3] and in animal models, only 10% to 50% of native anterior cruciate ligament (ACL) stiffness and strength is restored at 3 years after graft reconstruction.[4,5]

Grafts are thought to weaken during the ligamentization process because the repopulation of biologic grafts with intrinsic fibroblasts is accompanied by partial breakdown of the extracellular matrix of the graft and replacement with scarlike tissue.[6] Animal studies have demonstrated that the graft is at its weakest 3 months after surgery. This evolutionary process of graft remodeling must be understood in coordinating postoperative rehabilitation strategies.

In the early postoperative period, the main factor affecting the structural strength of the graft is not the tensile strength of the graft tissue, but the fixation of the graft to the bone.[7] Graft fixation is the "weak link" in this period as no graft fixation devices have achieved the ultimate failure strength or stiffness comparable to the native ACL. The best fixation constructs achieve pull-out strength that is almost 50% of the initial tensile strength of the graft.[8-10] The tensile load to failure of various fixation devices is shown in Table 50-2. This weak link of the graft fixation persists for up to 4 to 12 weeks; at that point, attachments to the bone are probably no longer the weakest part of the complex.

Current fixation techniques include aperture fixation strategies in which the soft tissue or bone of the graft is fixed within the bone tunnel and suspensory or periosteal fixation in which

Table 50-1 Initial Biomechanical Properties of Various Autograft Choices

Graft	Ultimate Strength (N)	Stiffness (N/mm)	Cross-sectional Area (mm²)
Intact ACL	2160	242	44
BPTB (10 mm)	2977	620	50
Quadruple hamstring	4590	861	53
Quadriceps tendon (10 mm)	2352	463	62

ACL, Anterior cruciate ligament; BPTB, bone-patellar tendon-bone.
Fu FH, Bennett CH, Lattermann C, et al: Current trends in anterior cruciate ligament reconstruction. Part 1: Biology and biomechanics of reconstruction. Am J Sports Med 1999;27:821–830.

the graft is fixed away from the joint surface (Fig. 50-1). Different fixation techniques have different biologic consequences. While no current fixation device reliably promotes complete recapitulation of the normal biology of the transition zones at the insertion of the ACL or posterior cruciate ligament (PCL), certain principles of fixation are generally recognized. There is increased knee stability with interference aperture fixation placed close to the joint. Periosteal fixation, especially with the use of indirect tendon fixation devices that rely on linkage material such as suture to connect the graft to the fixation device, are associated with the "bungee effect." This longitudinal graft micromotion along the axis of the osseous tunnel is thought to contribute to tunnel widening. Indirect fixation devices may also allow the graft to move anteriorly and posteriorly within the osseous tunnel during flexion and extension. This sagittal graft motion is termed the "windshield wiper effect." Fixation tech-

Table 50-2 Ultimate Tensile Load of Various Fixation Devices

Type of Fixation Device	Ultimate Tensile Load (N)
Indirect	
Single polyester tape loop	375
Double polyester tape loop	612–651
Single loop 5 Ethibond	238
Double loop 5 Ethibond	463
Direct Soft Tissue	
Metal interference screw (7 mm)	242
Bioabsorbable screw (7 mm)	341
Cross-pin technique (animal)	725–1600
Suture-post (animal)	374
Direct Bone	
Metal interference screw (7 mm)	640
Metal interference screw (9 mm)	276–436

Experiments performed on human cadavers, unless otherwise specified.
Fu FH, Bennett CH, Lattermann C, et al: Current trends in anterior cruciate ligament reconstruction. Part 1: Biology and biomechanics of reconstruction. Am J Sports Med 1999;27:821–830.

niques continue to evolve but are beholden on the type of graft used.

A summary of the essential criteria for comparisons of different grafts is listed in Table 50-3. Specific characteristics of the biology and biomechanical properties as well as other criteria essential for appropriate graft decision making, are explored for common types of knee ligament grafts in the remainder of the chapter.

AUTOGRAFTS

Bone-Patellar Tendon-Bone Autografts

The central third bone-patellar tendon-bone autograft has been the gold standard graft choice since it was popularized in the 1980s. Graft harvest is performed with the knee held in 90 degrees of flexion; the patella and tendon are exposed by subcutaneous dissection. A straight midline incision is made through the peritenon, which is then carefully preserved and dissected off the tendon both medially and laterally. Though the width of the graft is customized to the individual patient, typically a 10 mm wide graft from the central third of the patella tendon is used. The longitudinal strip of the central patella is harvested along with 20- to 25-mm bone plugs from the tibial tubercle and patella (Fig. 50-2).

The BPTB autograft has high tensile strength and stiffness as well as strong bony insertion points. A 10-mm patellar tendon graft has been shown to have an initial ultimate tensile load and stiffness that is higher than that of the native ACL (2977 N versus 2160 N and 455 N/mm versus 242 N/mm, respectively).[11] As mentioned, this strength and stiffness of the graft tissue is a dynamic property that undergoes predictable changes during ligamentization. While the initial soft-tissue characteristics are favorable compared to native tissue, the ultimate load to failure of the patellar tendon autograft has been shown to decrease over time and stabilizes at approximately 80% of its initial strength at 12 months.[12]

Apart from its favorable initial biomechanical properties, the most compelling advantage of BPTB autograft is the presence of the bone plug on each end of the tendon (Fig. 50-3). The native bone-tendon interface is harvested in its entirety. This obviates the issue of soft-tissue tendon-to-bone healing, which is problematic in other graft choices. In the BPTB autograft, the bone plug of the graft is fixed directly to the bone in the tunnel, ensuring bone-to-bone healing. This healing is thought to be more rapid than soft tissue-to-bone healing as appositional integration of the graft bone into the host has been demonstrated at 3 to 4 weeks after surgery in a dog model.[13]

Fixation of bone plugs is traditionally the most reliable and predictable type of graft fixation. The bone plugs themselves can provide an interference fit within the tunnel. Mechanical locking of the bone plugs with an interference screw provides rigid fixation that allows for early, aggressive rehabilitation. The ability to achieve aperture fixation with bone-to-bone healing is thought to prevent longitudinal graft motion in the tunnel.

A significant disadvantage of the BPTB autograft is donor site morbidity. Meticulous surgical technique is required to prevent intraoperative complications at the donor site such as patellar fracture and damage to the infrapatellar branch of the saphenous nerve. Major postoperative complications such as patellar tendon rupture and delayed patellar fracture are rare, but do occur.

Although major intraoperative or postoperative complications at the donor site are uncommon, there is ongoing concern about

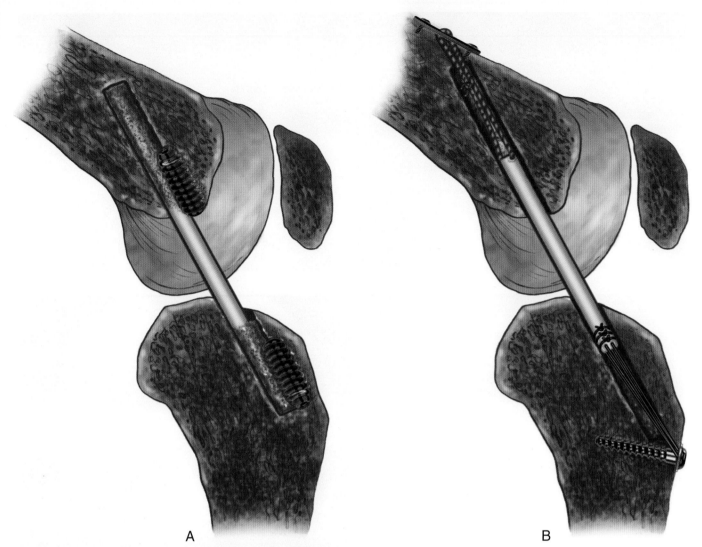

A

B

Figure 50-1 A, Aperture fixation with interference screws is the most common fixation strategy for grafts that incorporate bone plugs. Aperture fixation minimizes micromotion of the graft within the tunnel. **B,** Periosteal or suspensory fixation involves fixing the graft to posts or buttons outside the tunnel. With indirect periosteal fixation, as pictured here, linkage material such as suture is used to connect the graft to the fixation device. These types of fixation devices are often used in soft-tissue grafts without bone plugs and are thought to allow longitudinal micromotion in the tunnel (the "bungee effect").

			Table 50-3 Criteria to Compare Graft Choices		
Graft	Initial Biomechanical Properties	Incorporation	Fixation	Donor Site	Ease of Harvest
Autograft bone-patellar tendon-bone	See Table 50-1	Bone healing (approx 4 wk)	Rigid (interference screw)	Large incision	Debatable
Autograft quadruple hamstring		Soft tissue-bone (8–12 wk)	Variable	Smaller incision, less postoperative pain	Debatable
Autograft quadriceps tendon		Bone- and soft tissue-to-bone healing	Variable	Less postoperative pain than bone-patellar tendon-bone	Debatable
Achilles allograft		Bone- and soft tissue-to-bone healing, slower incorporation than autograft	Variable	None	No incision

Harner CD: Anterior Cruciate Ligament Graft Selection in 2005. Paper presented at the American Academy of Orthopaedic Surgeons 72nd Annual Meeting, 2005, Washington, DC.

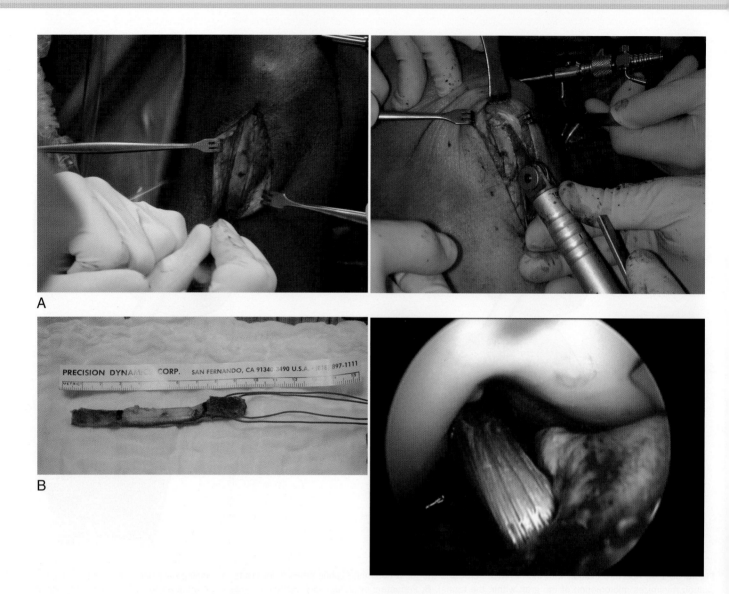

Figure 50-2 A, Bone-patellar tendon-bone (BPTB) harvest: The central third of the patellar tendon is harvested with bone plugs from the patella and tibia. **B,** Bone-patellar tendon-bone graft prepared for an anterior cruciate ligament (ACL) procedure *(left)* and arthroscopic picture after BPTB ACL reconstruction *(right).*

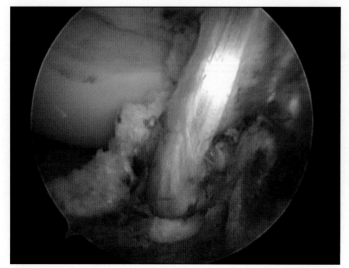

Figure 50-3 Arthroscopic picture after hamstring graft anterior cruciate ligament reconstruction.

permanent changes to the extensor mechanism resulting in altered patellofemoral biomechanics. Common long-term sequelae that have been reported after BPTB harvest include loss of quadriceps strength, patellofemoral crepitation, anterior knee pain, loss of flexion, and pain when kneeling.[14-16] Many of these reported sequelae are based on retrospective studies that lack comparison groups. For example, while anterior knee pain has been reported to occur in 10% to 40% of patients after BPTB autograft harvest, it is increasingly clear that anterior knee pain may occur after ACL reconstruction regardless of graft choice.[17] Bynum et al[18] showed that up to 40% of patients with ACL rupture will have anterior knee pain prior to their operation, suggesting that the etiology of anterior knee pain associated with ACL injury and reconstruction is multifactorial. Many reports of quadriceps atrophy after BPTB autograft harvest predate the accelerated rehabilitation programs used currently; therefore, implicating the graft type as the primary etiology of the quadriceps weakness is problematic.

Pain with kneeling, on the other hand, is supported by consistent data from randomized, controlled studies comparing

BPTB grafts to hamstring grafts.[17] This pain is usually mild and its affect on patient-relevant outcomes is unknown. For patients who are required to kneel for prolonged periods, BPTB autografts are probably not a good graft choice.

Multiple studies have demonstrated long-term stability after BPTB ACL reconstruction approaching 95%.[14–16,19,20] Proponents of this graft point to its rigid fixation constructs, predictable bone-to-bone healing, robust initial graft strength, and reliable and durable stability. It remains the most common graft used in professional athletes. Relative contraindications to BPTB autograft include patellofemoral arthritis, advanced age, and previous patellar tendon graft harvest.

Hamstring Tendon

There is a long history of successful clinical outcomes following knee ligament reconstruction using hamstring grafts.[21–25] However, concerns remain regarding the recurrence of atraumatic knee laxity, gender differences, fixation strategies, bone tunnel widening, residual hamstring weakness, and the suitability of hamstring grafts for certain athletic activities. Hamstring graft constructs continue to evolve, and it is difficult to compare results of historic studies due to variations in the reported surgical techniques. While initial hamstring grafts consisted of a single- or double-strand hamstring graft, at present, the most common type of hamstring graft is the quadrupled semitendinosus and gracilis graft.[22,26,27] This graft is a semitendinosus tendon and gracilis tendon doubled, or folded over, to produce four strands in the final construct.

Hamstring grafts are harvested through a small incision performed at the level of the pes anserinus. Dissection is taken down to the level of the sartorius fascia, which is incised. The semitendinosus and gracilis tendons are identified, freed from fascial attachments, and harvested using a tendon stripper. Meticulous care is used to free the tendon of all attachments so as to prevent transection of the tendon with the stripper. Once harvested, residual muscle is carefully dissected off the tendons and they are folded over one of a myriad of fixation devices to produce a quadruple-strand graft.

The quadruple hamstring graft has the highest initial ultimate strength and stiffness of any of the commonly used grafts.[28] However, this value is from in vitro data after equal tensioning of all strands. Clinically, this uniform tensioning may be difficult to achieve, reducing the initial biomechanical properties of the graft. In addition to its high initial strength, the dimensionality of the quadruple hamstring is more akin to the native ACL as it is round and has a larger cross-sectional area than the BPTB autograft. This provides improved "fill" of the bone tunnels with graft material. Proponents of this graft also suggest that the multiple strands of the quadruple graft construct may recapitulate the distinct functional units of the two-band ACL structure.

In general, hamstring graft harvest results in less immediate postoperative pain and morbidity than are present after a BPTB autograft. Because the incision is away from the patella, patients rarely complain of discomfort while kneeling. In skeletally immature patients, hamstring grafts offer the advantage of soft-tissue apposition to the growth plate. Bone plugs at the end of BPTB autografts could theoretically bridge the physis leading to premature closure resulting in angular deformities or limb length discrepancies; hamstring ACL reconstruction in this patient population has been shown to have a low risk of growth disturbance.[29]

While these properties of hamstring grafts are compelling, there are distinct disadvantages of hamstring grafts compared

to BPTB grafts. Fixation strategies for hamstring tendon graft have been problematic. In the past, fixation of hamstring tendons was performed by suturing the ends of the graft and fixing the sutures around posts placed outside the bone tunnels. Because of the elasticity of the sutures and the long length created by the entire graft and suture unit, there was concern about the "bungee effect" with micromotion of the graft in the tunnels. This is thought to interfere with healing of the graft soft tissue to the bone as well as resulting in graft tunnel widening.

Recently, new methods of hamstring graft fixation have evolved that provide aperture fixation and provide pull-out strength comparable with that of interference screw fixation for bone-tendon constructs. For example, soft-tissue interference screws, designed with blunt threads designed not to cut the hamstring tendons, provide aperture fixation of the tendon to the bone. These interference screws are available in bioresorbable formulations and are available impregnated with hydroxyapatite with the theoretical advantage of improved bone ingrowth.

Regardless of the fixation strategy, hamstring grafts rely on soft tissue-to-bone healing, which is thought to be slower than bone-to-bone healing. In a rhesus monkey study, the bone-bone plug interface was histologically incorporated at 8 weeks after surgery, which was the first time point at which the histology was examined.[30] In a dog model of soft tissue-to-bone healing, the soft-tissue tendon graft pulled out of the bone tunnel until 12 weeks postoperatively, indicating that incorporation of the soft tissue-to-bone interface was incomplete for as long as 3 months postoperatively.[7] However, other animal studies have suggested more rapid soft tissue-to-bone healing.[31]

Clinically, hamstring grafts have a high incidence of tunnel widening, which is sometimes seen as early as 3 months after hamstring graft ACL reconstruction. The biology behind tunnel widening is unknown but may involve an inflammatory reaction at the soft tissue-bone interface indicative of areas of incomplete incorporation. There is concern that micromotion of the soft tissue within the bone tunnel may promote this process. Williams et al[32] demonstrated that tunnel expansion was noted radiographically in all patients ($n = 85$) after hamstring ACL reconstruction using suspensory fixation for the femoral tunnel and periosteal fixation for the tibial tunnel. The clinical significance of tunnel widening is unclear as there is no direct correlation between tunnel widening and laxity.

Other disadvantages of hamstring grafts include unpredictable hamstring size, concerns about recurrent knee laxity, and hamstring weakness. While residual hamstring weakness is not drastic, it typically measures about 10% loss after recovery. This could be problematic for athletes who play a hamstring-specific sport such as running backward (e.g., a defensive back).

Comparison of Hamstring versus Bone-Patellar Tendon-Bone Autografts

A large number of studies have been published comparing hamstring and BPTB autografts expressing a myriad of different opinions. The majority of these studies are case series reporting on the use of a single graft, without an appropriate comparison group. In addition, with the evolution of graft preparation and fixation, particularly with hamstring grafts, it is difficult to use the studies to supervise graft choice decisions. In a recent meta-analysis of 34 studies involving 1976 patients, Freedman et al[33] reported a graft failure rate of 4.9% in hamstring grafts and 1.9% in bone-patellar bone grafts. Significant laxity and presence of a pivot shift was slightly higher in the hamstring groups. Anterior knee pain was present in 17.4% of BPTB patients as compared to 11.5% of hamstring patients.

Spindler et al[17] recently presented a systematic review of the nine randomized, controlled trials that compared patellar tendon and hamstring tendon autografts. A slight increased laxity (approximately 1 mm) on arthrometer testing was found in the hamstring population in three of seven studies. Knee pain with kneeling was greater for the patellar tendon population in four of four studies, but only one of nine studies demonstrated increased anterior knee pain in the patellar tendon group. There were no differences in subjective outcome, return to activity, or failure rates identified by the randomized studies. This review suggests that graft type is not the major determinant of successful outcome in ACL reconstruction when using either hamstring or patellar tendon autograft.[17]

Quadriceps Tendon

Quadriceps tendon autografts have gained attention for primary and revision knee ligament surgery.[34–36] This graft is harvested by removing a strip of the distal portion of the quadriceps along with a block of bone from the proximal patella. This results in a graft that consists of a bone plug on one end for bone-on-bone fixation and tendon of the other end for soft tissue-to-bone fixation.

Quadriceps tendon grafts have a thicker cross-sectional area than patellar tendon grafts and roughly the same tensile strength.[37] Proponents of this method suggest that postoperative pain with quadriceps tendon grafts is not as intense as with BPTB harvesting. Patients with quadriceps tendon grafts usually do not have symptoms of patellar tendonitis upon return to sports and often have minimal or no difficulty kneeling. In addition to its use in the primary setting, this graft is useful in the revision setting and can be harvested even after a previous BPTB graft.

Disadvantages of this graft include the same intraoperative and postoperative risks of patellar fracture as are seen with BPTB and a decrease of up to 20% of quadriceps strength.[38] Because quadriceps tendon harvest is not widely used and unfamiliar to many surgeons, the harvesting technique, with its subtle anatomic nuances, remains a challenge when using this graft. For example, the proximal patella has a curved surface with dense cortical bone that closely adheres to the suprapatellar pouch. When harvesting the graft, there is significant risk of entering the suprapatellar pouch and losing knee distention during ACL reconstruction.[34]

ALLOGRAFTS

Harvested from cadaveric sources, bone and soft-tissue allografts have been used successfully for a variety of conditions. Advantages of allograft ligament reconstruction include the avoidance of donor site morbidity and additional scars, decreased operative time, ease in performing multiple ligament reconstruction, and the use of a larger possible graft (Fig. 50-4). Certain scenarios are particularly attractive for allograft use. These include primary ACL reconstruction in the older patient; revision ACL reconstruction when previous autogenic sources have been used; PCL reconstruction, particularly in the setting of double bundle procedures; posterolateral corner reconstruction; multiple ligament reconstruction (ACL, PCL, lateral collateral ligament) and cases of patient preference (cosmesis, decreased postoperative pain). The most common types of allo-

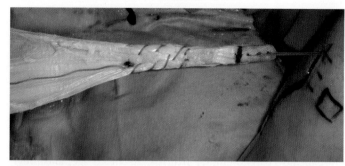

Figure 50-4 Achilles tendon allograft fashioned for anterior cruciate ligament reconstruction. The calcaneal bone plug has been contoured to fit within a 25 × 10-mm femoral tunnel. The tendinous end will be secured in the tibial tunnel.

grafts used as knee grafts include Achilles tendon, BPTB, and quadruple hamstring tendon.

Allografts are procured from donor cadavers after a detailed medical, social, and sexual history questionnaire is completed by the next of kin or life partner. Any history of exposure to communicable diseases, reports of unprotected sexual contacts, drug use, neurologic diseases, autoimmune disease, collagen disorders, or metabolic diseases is recorded, and positive findings disqualify the donor. Blood and laboratory tests are used to rule out bacterial and viral infection.

Allografts are processed using a variety of methods. Unfortunately, most methods that ensure complete sterility are unsuitable for human tissue. High doses of gamma irradiation (>3.0 mrad) are effective for sterilizing the tissue but cause structural weakening of the collagen. Lower dose irradiation does not reliably kill viruses. Chemical sterilization agents such as ethylene oxide leave behind a residue that can cause chronic synovitis.

Allografts are commonly preserved by deep freezing, cryopreservation, or freeze-drying. Deep freezing is the most common method of storage and involves an antibiotic soak prior to packaging without solution and freezing to −80°C. It can then be stored for 3 to 5 years. This process destroys all the cells in the tissue and is thought to decrease the host immune response. Cryopreservation involves controlled-rate freezing with extraction of cellular water in an effort to preserve cellular viability. Freeze-drying involves a lyophilization process to ensure residual moisture of less than 5%; the graft can then be stored at room temperature for 3 to 5 years. The freeze-dried graft requires rehydration for 30 minutes prior to implantation. Freeze-drying destroys cells in the tissue and reduces the immunogenicity of the tissue, but the strength of the graft is altered by the process. The preferred processing method for knee ligament allograft surgery remains deep freezing.

A primary concern with the use of allograft is the risk of viral and bacterial disease transmission. Hepatitis and human immunodeficiency virus can be transmitted through these tissues and bacterial infections are also a possibility; Buck et al[39] calculated the risk of human immunodeficiency virus transmission in properly screened and tested donors to be 1 : 1,600,000. A full review of the risk of disease transmission in allograft tissue is presented in Chapter 12, entitled "Safety Issues for Musculoskeletal Allografts."

Unlike organ transplants, allografts are at minimal risk of tissue rejection by the host due to the minimal protein antigen in the processed allografts. Collagen, the major constituent of the grafts, has minimal antigenicity, and frank rejection of an allograft ligament is rare. However, a low-grade immune response may occur; Harner et al[40] demonstrated a mild humoral response to allograft ligament transplantation in a majority of patients at 6 months after surgery. The clinical significance of this type of immune response is unknown.

Like autografts, allografts are thought to function as a biologic scaffold and undergo cellular repopulation, revascularization, and collagen remodeling. Initial repopulation may proceed quickly, as replacement of the graft by host cells has been evident at 4 weeks postoperatively.[41] However, the overall ligamentization process is thought to proceed more slowly for allografts compared to autografts, presumably due to a prolonged remodeling phase. Animal studies have investigated the biomechanical properties of allografts versus autografts after ligament reconstruction. In a goat model, Jackson et al[42] demonstrated that allograft patellar tendon ACL reconstruction resulted in increased anteroposterior laxity, decreased ultimate tensile load, and diminished biologic incorporation compared to autograft at 6 months after surgery. However, Nikolaou et al[43] demonstrated nearly identical ligament strength between ACL allograft and autograft reconstructions in a dog model at 9 months after surgery. It has been estimated that allograft incorporation takes up to 1.5 times as long as the incorporation of autograft tissue. Though the remodeling phase may be prolonged with allografts, once it is complete, allograft ligament tissue appears histologically and functionally similar to autograft tissue.

Comparative studies of allograft and autograft ACL reconstruction have failed to demonstrate consistent differences in objective or subjective outcomes.[44–47] There remains some concern about long-term allograft function; however, there has been no clinical difference between allograft and autograft function at 3- and 5-year follow-up.[44,45]

SYNTHETIC GRAFTS

Synthetic grafts remain an appealing alternative to biologic grafts but have a long history of failure. The ideal synthetic graft would mimic the characteristics of a normal ACL graft in terms of strength, compliance, elasticity, and durability without side effects.

In the 1990s, Gore-Tex grafts (Gore and Co., Flagstaff, AZ) were used but failed dramatically. These grafts were knitted cable with eyelets on each end that allowed for fixation to the bone outside the tunnels. Repeated cycling led to fragmentation of the grafts with shedding of particulate debris that led to persistent effusions and graft failure. Dacron and carbon fiber grafts had a similar history of failure.

More recently, the Kennedy Ligament Augmentation Device (3M, St. Paul, MN) was used to supplement ACL grafts. The purpose of this device was to protect the graft reconstruction until healing occurred. Unfortunately, the ligament augmentation device was too stiff and shielded the graft from normal stresses, delaying maturation of the graft. These devices are no longer used for ACL reconstruction. Currently, there are no prosthetic ligaments in the United States approved by the U.S. Food and Drug Administration, although several are currently being used in Europe.

CONCLUSIONS

Graft selection in knee ligament surgery remains a contentious topic among orthopedic surgeons. No single graft has been shown to be clearly superior in terms of overall patient outcome. In choosing the appropriate graft for the individual patient, surgeons must be versed in each graft's biomechanical characteristics, fixation and incorporation properties, donor site morbidities, and contraindications. In addition, graft selection is mitigated by the surgeon's comfort level with the surgical techniques required for use of the grafts.

At our institution, BPTB grafts are routinely used for ACL reconstruction in young, competitive athletes. Hamstrings grafts are commonly used in patients with pre-existing patellofemoral abnormalities such as chondrosis or arthrosis and in patients whose job requires kneeling such as firefighters or wrestlers. Achilles tendon allografts are commonly used for revision ACL surgery, primary PCL reconstruction, and multiligament knee reconstruction. Increasingly, we are using Achilles tendon allografts for primary ACL reconstruction, particularly in patients older than 30 and in recreational athletes. We have found that matching individual patients with grafts that are tailored to their needs has resulted in more targeted and appropriate graft selection.

REFERENCES

1. Butler DL: Anterior cruciate ligament: Its normal response and replacement. J Orthop Res 1989;7:910–921.
2. Fu FH, Jackson DW, Jamison J, et al: Allograft reconstruction of the anterior cruciate ligament. In Jackson DW, Arnoczky SP, Woo SL-Y, et al (eds): Anterior Cruciate Ligament. Current and Future Concepts. New York, Raven Press, 1993, pp 325–338.
3. McFarland EG, Morrey BF, An KN, et al: The relationship of vascularity and water content to tensile strength in a patellar tendon replacement of the anterior cruciate in dogs. Am J Sports Med 1986;14:436–448.
4. Ballock RT, Woo SL, Lyon RM, et al: Use of patellar tendon autograft for anterior cruciate ligament reconstruction in the rabbit: A long-term histologic and biomechanical study. J Orthop Res 1989;7:474–485.
5. Ng GY, Oakes BW, Deacon OW, et al: Biomechanics of patellar tendon autograft for reconstruction of the anterior cruciate ligament in the goat: Three-year study. J Orthop Res 1995;13:602–608.
6. Oakes BW: Collagen ultrastructure in the normal ACL and in ACL graft. In Jackson DW, Arnoczky SP, Woo SL, et al (eds): Anterior Cruciate Ligament. Current and Future Concepts, New York, Raven Press, 1993, pp 209–217.
7. Rodeo SA, Arnoczky SP, Torzilli PA, et al: Tendon-healing in a bone tunnel. A biomechanical and histological study in the dog. J Bone Joint Surg Am 1993;75:1795–1803.
8. Jomha NM, Raso VJ, Leung P: Effect of varying angles on the pullout strength of interference screw fixation. Arthroscopy 1993;9:580–583.
9. Kohn D, Rose C: Primary stability of interference screw fixation. Influence of screw diameter and insertion torque. Am J Sports Med 1994;22:334–338.
10. Matthews LS, Lawrence SJ, Yahiro MA, et al: Fixation strengths of patellar tendon-bone grafts. Arthroscopy 1993;9:76–81.
11. Cooper DE, Deng XH, Burstein AL, et al: The strength of the central third patellar tendon graft. A biomechanical study. Am J Sports Med 1993;21:818–824.
12. Johnson DL, Isbell WM, Atay OA: Grafts. In Miller MD, Cole BJ (eds): Textbook of Arthroscopy. Philadelphia, Saunders, 2004, pp 39–45.

13. Yoshiya S, Nagano M, Kurosaka M, et al: Graft healing in the bone tunnel in anterior cruciate ligament reconstruction. Clin Orthop 2000;376:278–286.

14. Bach BR Jr, Levy ME, Bojchuk J, et al: Single-incision endoscopic anterior cruciate ligament reconstruction using patellar tendon autograft. Minimum two-year follow-up evaluation. Am J Sports Med 1998;26:30–40.

15. Bach BR Jr, Tradonsky S, Bojchuk J, et al: Arthroscopically assisted anterior cruciate ligament reconstruction using patellar tendon autograft. Five- to nine-year follow-up evaluation. Am J Sports Med 1998;26:20–29.

16. O'Brien SJ, Warren RF, Pavlov H, et al: Reconstruction of the chronically insufficient anterior cruciate ligament with the central third of the patellar ligament. J Bone Joint Surg Am 1991;73:278–286.

17. Spindler KP, Kuhn JE, Freedman KB, et al: Anterior cruciate ligament reconstruction autograft choice: Bone-tendon-bone versus hamstring: does it really matter? A systematic review. Am J Sports Med 2004;32:1986–1995.

18. Bynum EB, Barrack RL, Alexander AH: Open versus closed chain kinetic exercises after anterior cruciate ligament reconstruction. A prospective randomized study. Am J Sports Med 1995;23:401–406.

19. Buss DD, Warren RF, Wickiewicz TL, et al: Arthroscopically assisted reconstruction of the anterior cruciate ligament with use of autogenous patellar-ligament grafts. Results after twenty-four to forty-two months. J Bone Joint Surg Am 1993;75:1346–1355.

20. Shelbourne KD, Gray T: Anterior cruciate ligament reconstruction with autogenous patellar tendon graft followed by accelerated rehabilitation. A two- to nine-year followup. Am J Sports Med 1997;25:786–795.

21. Aglietti P, Buzzi R, Menchetti PM, et al: Arthroscopically assisted semitendinosus and gracilis tendon graft in reconstruction for acute anterior cruciate ligament injuries in athletes. Am J Sports Med 1996;24:726–731.

22. Aglietti P, Buzzi R, Zaccherotti G, et al: Patellar tendon versus doubled semitendinosus and gracilis tendons for anterior cruciate ligament reconstruction. Am J Sports Med 1994;22:211–218.

23. Aglietti P, Giron F, Buzzi R, et al: Anterior cruciate ligament reconstruction: Bone-patellar tendon-bone compared with double semitendinosus and gracilis tendon grafts. A prospective, randomized clinical trial. J Bone Joint Surg Am 2004;86:2143–2155.

24. Barber FA: Tripled semitendinosus-cancellous bone anterior cruciate ligament reconstruction with bioscrew fixation. Arthroscopy 1999;15:360–367.

25. Giron F, Aglietti P, Cuomo P, et al: Anterior cruciate ligament reconstruction with double-looped semitendinosus and gracilis tendon graft directly fixed to cortical bone: 5-year results. Knee Surg Sports Traumatol Arthrosc 2005;13:81–91.

26. Maeda A, Shino K, Horibe S, et al: Anterior cruciate ligament reconstruction with multistranded autogenous semitendinosus tendon. Am J Sports Med 1996;24:504–509.

27. Wallace MP, Howell SM, Hull ML: In vivo tensile behavior of a four-bundle hamstring graft as a replacement for the anterior cruciate ligament. J Orthop Res 1997;15:539–545.

28. Hamner DL, Brown CH Jr, Steiner ME, et al: Hamstring tendon grafts for reconstruction of the anterior cruciate ligament: biomechanical evaluation of the use of multiple strands and tensioning techniques. J Bone Joint Surg Am 1999;81:549–557.

29. Marder RA, Raskind JR, Carroll M: Prospective evaluation of arthroscopically assisted anterior cruciate ligament reconstruction. Patellar tendon versus semitendinosus and gracilis tendons. Am J Sports Med 1991;19:478–484.

30. Clancy WG Jr, Narechania RG, Rosenberg TD, et al: Anterior and posterior cruciate ligament reconstruction in rhesus monkeys. J Bone Joint Surg Am 1981;63:1270–1284.

31. Grana WA, Egle DM, Mahnken R, et al: An analysis of autograft fixation after anterior cruciate ligament reconstruction in a rabbit model. Am J Sports Med 1994;22:344–351.

32. Williams RJ 3rd, Hyman J, Petrigliano F, et al: Anterior cruciate ligament reconstruction with a four-strand hamstring tendon autograft. J Bone Joint Surg Am 2004;86:225–232.

33. Freedman KB, D'Amato MJ, Nedeff DD, et al: Arthroscopic anterior cruciate ligament reconstruction: A metaanalysis comparing patellar tendon and hamstring tendon autografts. Am J Sports Med 2003;31:2–11.

34. Fulkerson JP, Langeland R: An alternative cruciate reconstruction graft: The central quadriceps tendon. Arthroscopy 1995;11:252–254.

35. Lee S, Seong SC, Jo H, et al: Outcome of anterior cruciate ligament reconstruction using quadriceps tendon autograft. Arthroscopy 2004;20:795–802.

36. Theut PC, Fulkerson JP, Armour EF, et al: Anterior cruciate ligament reconstruction utilizing central quadriceps free tendon. Orthop Clin North Am 2003;34:31–39.

37. Staubli HU, Schatzmann L, Brunner P, et al: Quadriceps tendon and patellar ligament: Cryosectional anatomy and structural properties in young adults. Knee Surg Sports Traumatol Arthrosc 1996;4:100–110.

38. Chen CH, Chen WJ, Shih CH: Arthroscopic anterior cruciate ligament reconstruction with quadriceps tendon-patellar bone autograft. J Trauma 1999;46:678–682.

39. Buck BE, Malinin TI, Brown MD: Bone transplantation and human immunodeficiency virus. An estimate of risk of acquired immunodeficiency syndrome (AIDS). Clin Orthop 1989;240:129–136.

40. Harner CD, Thompson W, Jamison J, et al: The immunologic response of fresh frozen patellar tendon allograft ACL reconstruction. Paper presented at American Academy of Orthopaedic Surgeons, 1995, New Orleans, LA.

41. Jackson DW, Simon TM, Kurzweil PR, et al: Survival of cells after intra-articular transplantation of fresh allografts of the patellar and anterior cruciate ligaments. DNA-probe analysis in a goat model. J Bone Joint Surg Am 1992;74:112–118.

42. Jackson DW, Grood ES, Goldstein JD, et al: A comparison of patellar tendon autograft and allograft used for anterior cruciate ligament reconstruction in the goat model. Am J Sports Med 1993;21:176–185.

43. Nikolaou PK, Seaber AV, Glisson RR, et al: Anterior cruciate ligament allograft transplantation. Long-term function, histology, revascularization, and operative technique. Am J Sports Med 1986;14:348–360.

44. Harner CD, Olson E, Irrgang JJ, et al: Allograft versus autograft anterior cruciate ligament reconstruction: 3- to 5-year outcome. Clin Orthop 1996;324:134–144.

45. Peterson RK, Shelton WR, Bomboy AL: Allograft versus autograft patellar tendon anterior cruciate ligament reconstruction: A 5-year follow-up. Arthroscopy 2001;17:9–13.

46. Shelton WR, Papendick L, Dukes AD: Autograft versus allograft anterior cruciate ligament reconstruction. Arthroscopy 1997;13:446–449.

47. Shino K, Nakata K, Horibe S, et al: Quantitative evaluation after arthroscopic anterior cruciate ligament reconstruction. Allograft versus autograft. Am J Sports Med 1993;21:609–616.

Anterior Cruciate Ligament

Armando F. Vidal and Freddie H. Fu

In This Chapter

Nonoperative management
Surgery—anterior cruciate ligament (ACL) reconstruction
  Graft harvest
  Tunnel preparation

INTRODUCTION

- ACL injuries are common, occurring in approximately one in 3000 people in the United States annually.

- ACL injuries are most commonly the result of a noncontact athletic injury; however. they can result from various forms of trauma.

- The diagnosis of an ACL tear can typically be made from a thorough history and physical examination. Imaging studies, specifically magnetic resonance imaging (MRI), can be a valuable aid in making the diagnosis and identifying associated injuries.

- Nonoperative management of ACL tears in young, active patients often fails, resulting in persistent instability, and meniscal damage. However, nonoperative management in older, more sedentary patients has been associated with good outcomes.

- Arthroscopic ACL reconstruction has been a generally successful operation at restoring knee stability and returning patients to a high level of sporting activity.

- Reconstruction can be performed with a variety of graft choices and fixation options. Overall outcomes, regardless of graft choice, have been favorable.

CLINICAL FEATURES AND EVALUATION

Isolated ACL injuries account for up to half of all ligamentous injuries to the knee and have been reported to occur in an estimated one in 3000 people in the general population.[1,2] The incidence of knee ligament injuries, overall, has increased in the past few decades secondary to the escalating activity level of the population in general. ACL ruptures are most often the result of athletic injuries, but may occur from various different types of trauma. A noncontact mechanism is the most common cause; however, they can also occur from direct contact. Contact injuries are commonly created by a direct lateral blow to the knee, imparting a valgus force. This often produces combined

ACL/medial cruciate ligament injuries. Alternatively, a direct anterior force may cause a hyperextension moment to the knee also resulting in an injury to the ACL. Noncontact injuries typically occur from acute deceleration or change-of-direction maneuvers. Patients often describe a mechanism in which they "pivot" on a fixed, planted foot. They will often report a sensation of buckling and will very commonly describe a "pop" or "tearing" sensation in the knee. Most athletes will be unable to continue with the athletic endeavor secondary to pain and giving way. A large hemarthrosis will usually develop within hours of the injury producing the characteristically large effusion that follows acute ACL injury. The presence of any acute hemarthrosis in a patient with a knee injury should raise considerable suspicion for an ACL disruption. However, hemarthrosis can be seen with meniscal tears, osteochondral fractures, and patellar dislocations as well.[3,4]

PHYSICAL EXAMINATION

A thorough physical examination of the knee, as described in Chapter 46, is the cornerstone of diagnosing an ACL injury. On first inspection, the presence of a sizable effusion can typically be detected in acute injuries. The absence of a large effusion, however, does not preclude the diagnosis of an acute ACL tear and is typical in chronically ACL-deficient knees. Palpation of the periarticular structures such as the collateral ligaments and the medial and lateral joint lines is a critical part of the examination and provides important information regarding potential injury to other intra-/periarticular structures.

Range of motion is often limited in the acute setting secondary to pain and effusion. Limited motion, however, should raise suspicion of a mechanical block resulting from displaced bucket-handle meniscal tears, displaced ACL stump remnants, or osteochondral fragments.

Stability testing of the knee should include a thorough ligamentous examination which includes anterior/posterior, varus/valgus and rotational stability testing. Acute ACL injuries often occur with other combined ligamentous injuries and these should be identified by physical examination. Unidentified associated ligamentous instability is a common cause of failure following reconstruction, and this should be detected prior to surgical planning.[5]

There are three components of the physical examination that are specific to the diagnosis of an ACL injury: the Lachman, pivot-shift, and anterior drawer tests. The Lachman test is the most sensitive of the three maneuvers[6] (Fig. 51-1). It is performed with the knee in neutral rotation at 20 to 30 degrees of flexion. An anterior translation force is imparted to the tibia with one hand while stabilizing the femur with the other hand.

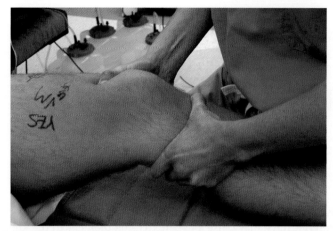

Figure 51-1 The Lachman test. With the knee in 20 to 30 degrees of flexion, the examiner stabilizes the femur with one hand while imparting an anterior force to the tibia with the other hand. Assessment of translation and endpoint is recorded. Translation is recorded as follows: I = 0 to 5 mm, II = 6 to 10 mm, III = >10 mm; A = firm endpoint, B = soft endpoint.

Degree of translation and presence or absence of an endpoint is assessed. The degree of laxity is graded as a comparison with the contralateral, uninvolved knee. The absence of a firm endpoint is indicative of ACL deficiency. Muscle splinting, effusion,

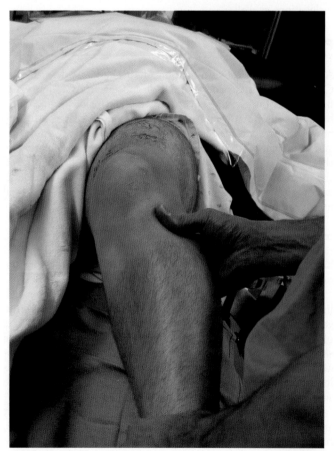

Figure 51-2 The pivot-shift is performed with the hip in slight abduction and with a valgus force applied to the extended knee. The knee is brought into flexion (from full extension) and the tibia reduces. The severity of the reduction (spin, jump, locked out) is graded.

and rotation of the leg may interfere with accurate Lachman testing. The anterior drawer is performed with the knee in neutral rotation and flexed to 90 degrees. The foot is stabilized with the examiner's thigh and an anterior stress is applied to the tibia. This test is not considered as sensitive for ACL deficiency as the Lachman.[6] Last, the pivot-shift is used to determine the rotational competency of the ACL. A positive pivot-shift is considered pathognomonic of ACL deficiency. In the ACL-deficient knee, the tibia sits in an anteriorly subluxed and internally rotated position. An axial load and a valgus torque is applied to the knee as it is brought into flexion. When the knee reaches a position of 15 to 20 degrees of flexion, the tibia reduces, thus producing the pivot shift. This phenomenon is graded as a grade 1 (spin), grade 2 (jump), and grade 3 (transient lock) based on the degree of the reduction. The sensitivity of this maneuver is poor in the awake patient, but it is very sensitive and specific when performed in a patient under anesthesia[6,7] (Fig. 51-2).

In addition to a thorough ligamentous and meniscal evaluation as described in Chapter 46, attention should also be paid to the patella. A patient with an acute patellar dislocation may present in a similar fashion and with a painful, swollen knee with a large hemarthrosis. This diagnosis must be considered when evaluating a patient with an injury suspected of being an ACL tear.

Plain radiographs are the first-line imaging modality for any acutely injured knee and should be obtained if there is any suspicion of an ACL injury. Standard posteroanterior flexion, lateral, and Merchant views should be obtained. Radiographs should be assessed for possible fractures. Occasionally, a small lateral capsular avulsion fracture of the tibial plateau can be visualized on plain films. This finding is termed a Segond fracture and has been said to be pathognomonic of an ACL injury (Fig. 51-3). Additionally, tibial spine avulsion fractures may be seen in skeletally immature and middle-aged patients with clinical examinations that are suspicious for ACL injury. In the chronic setting, intercondylar notch osteophytes, blunting of the intercondylar eminence, and accentuation of the sulcus terminalis may be observed. This accentuation of the sulcus terminalis has been termed the lateral notch sign (Fig. 51-4). Plain radiographs are also useful for assessment of overall limb alignment and degree of degenerative changes, if present.

MRI remains the gold-standard imaging modality for ACL injury. The reported sensitivity of MRI for detecting ACL injury is in excess of 90% to 95%.[8,9] Fiber discontinuity, ligament edema, and hemorrhage can be readily detected by MRI and are characteristic of an acute ACL tear (Fig. 51-5). In addition, the MRI scan often demonstrates a characteristic bone bruise pattern in the posterolateral tibial plateau and anterolateral femoral condyle with acute ACL injury. These bruises have been reported in approximately 80% of acute injuries.[10,11] The significance and long-term prognostic implications of these "bone bruises" on the natural history of the ACL-deficient knee are unknown at this time[11] (Fig. 51-6). MRI is also very useful for detecting associated meniscal, chondral, and ligamentous injuries, which are important to surgical planning.

RELEVANT ANATOMY AND BIOMECHANICS

Understanding ACL anatomy is important for interpreting imaging studies and planning surgical reconstruction. The ACL is approximately 31 to 38 mm in total length and has a midsubstance cross-sectional area of 44 mm[2].[12,13] It courses from the

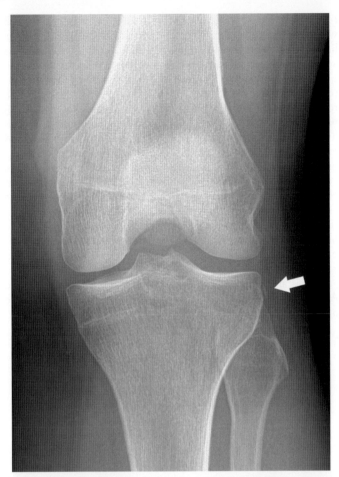

Figure 51-3 Posteroanterior flexion radiograph of an acutely injured knee revealing a classic lateral capsular avulsion *(arrow)*, termed a Segond fracture. This patient underwent magnetic resonance imaging, which confirmed an anterior cruciate ligament tear, and underwent reconstruction.

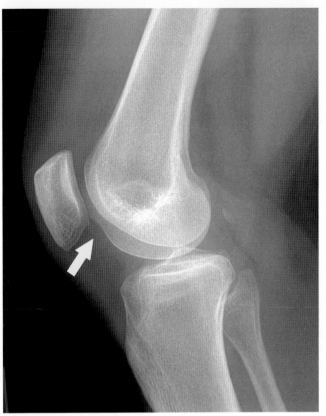

Figure 51-4 Lateral radiograph in a chronically anterior cruciate ligament–deficient patient demonstrating accentuation of the sulcus terminalis *(arrow)* termed the lateral notch sign.

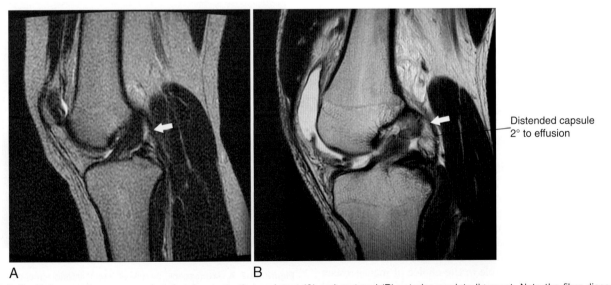

Distended capsule 2° to effusion

Figure 51-5 Sagittal magnetic resonance imaging demonstrating an intact (**A**) and ruptured (**B**) anterior cruciate ligament. Note the fiber discontinuity, hemorrhage, and sizable effusion present in the injured knee. Arrows indicated normal (**A**) and abnormal (**B**) joint capsule position.

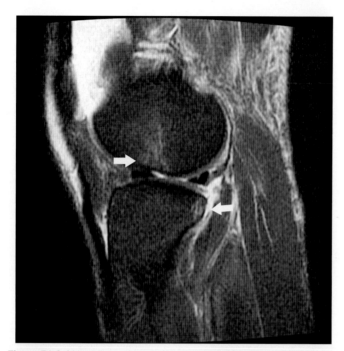

Figure 51-6 Magnetic resonance imaging demonstrating typical bone bruise pattern encountered with acute anterior cruciate ligament injury: posterolateral tibial plateau and anterolateral femoral condyle. Arrows indicate increased signal on MRI in areas of bone bruise on femoral condyle and tibial plateau.

posteromedial surface of the lateral femoral condyle in the inter-condylar notch to its tibial attachment approximately 15 mm behind the anterior border of the tibial articular surface, just medial to the anterior horn of the lateral meniscus. At both insertion sites, the ligament attaches over a broad, flattened area that is more than three times the cross-sectional area of the mid-substance ligament.[14] Additionally, the ACL has been described as being composed of two distinct anatomic and functional structures: the anteromedial and posterolateral bundles. Each bundle contributes to approximately half of the overall size of the ACL[14] (Fig. 51-7).

The ligament has an ultimate tensile load of 2160 N and a stiffness of 242 N/mm and can tolerate a strain of 20% prior to failure. The forces in the intact ACL range from 100 N during passive knee extension to about 400 N with walking, and up to 1700 N with cutting and acceleration-deceleration activities.[15,16] The individual bundles have been reported to have different bio-mechanical characteristics and tensioning patterns. Tension in the anteromedial bundle increases with flexion angles greater than 30 degrees, whereas the posterolateral bundle is more taut in extension.[17] Additionally, the role of the posterolateral bundle in resisting coupled rotatory loads is being investigated.[18]

TREATMENT OPTIONS

The natural history of ACL deficiency is not completely under-stood, and comparison of operative and nonoperative manage-ment in the literature is often difficult.[19] Numerous variables influence the decision-making process for nonsurgical or surgi-cal management of these injuries. Patient age, activity level, and associated injuries all play a role in the choice of management.

The activity level of the patient, as described by Daniel et al[4] is probably the most predictive factor regarding the need for

reconstruction. Most patients with isolated ACL injury do well with activities of daily living. They typically can participate in limited sporting activities, but will have difficulty with vigorous activity. Daniel et al[4] divided various sports and occupations into tiered levels based on the intensity of the activity. Sports that require jumping, pivoting, and hard cutting such as basketball, football, and soccer are considered level I sports. Sports such as baseball, racket sports, and skiing require lateral motion but less jumping and hard cutting than level I sports and are considered level II. Sporting activities that do not require cutting, pivoting or lateral motion such as jogging, running, and swimming are considered level III. Additionally, Daniel et al[4] expanded this classification to include occupations that similarly require cutting and pivoting type maneuvers. The challenge to the surgeon is to decide which patients will benefit from operative or nonoperative management. Generally, patients who partici-pate heavily in level I or II sports/occupations are considered candidates for reconstruction.

Age is an important consideration in the management of the ACL-injured knee. Patient age and activity level, however, are often coupled. Noyes et al[20] reviewed the results of nonopera-

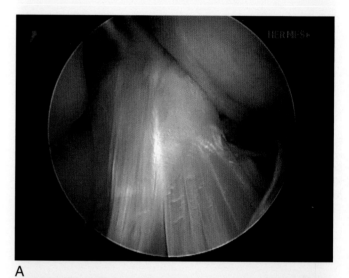

A

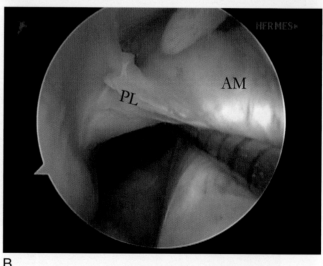

B

Figure 51-7 A, Arthroscopic picture of intact anterior cruciate ligament (ACL) demonstrating wide tibial footprint. **B,** Anteromedial (AM) bundle of the ACL is retracted, exposing the posterolateral (PL) bundle.

tive management of ACL deficiency in a group of 103 patients, with an average age of 26. In their study, a significant number of their patients progressed to have persistent instability, further meniscal damage, and ultimately joint arthroses. Only a small subset could return to turning- or twisting-type activities. Similarly, Hawkins et al[21] demonstrated that the results of nonoperative management in an active group of young patients with an average age of 22 were poor. In their cohort, 86% of the patients experienced persistent giving way, and overall 87.5% of these patients rated their knee as fair or poor. Conversely, Ciccotti et al[22] reviewed the results of nonoperative management in middle-aged patients between the ages of 40 and 60. They observed that over 80% of patients in this age group did well with nonoperative management consisting of a supervised physical therapy protocol. Patients in this age group who participated in a guided rehabilitation program and modified their activities had a satisfactory outcome without surgery. However, patients who wished to resume competitive sports requiring level I activities (e.g., pivoting) were dissatisfied with nonoperative management and required reconstruction. Overall, ACL reconstructions in the older population are less common. However, in older patients who wish to continue with vigorous or high-level activities, ACL reconstruction has been shown to be a successful option with results similar to those in younger patients.[23,24] In individuals who are older and relatively sedentary, nonoperative management of ACL has been shown to yield satisfactory results, provided the patients are willing to accept a modest amount of instability and a slight risk of meniscal injury.[25]

Nonoperative Management

The goal of nonoperative management of ACL injury is to return functional stability to the knee and prevent further injury and degeneration. Activity modification and physical therapy are the cornerstones of nonoperative management. Physical therapy initially is centered on regaining pain-free motion. Once motion is regained, rehabilitation should focus on closed-chain strengthening of both the quadriceps and hamstrings. Once sporting activities are resumed, they need to be modified to avoid high-risk, level I type behaviors. Additionally, functional bracing should be considered. The role of bracing, overall, is controversial. Its use may be helpful in managing subluxation episodes during activities that have infrequent high-risk maneuvers. However, the prevention of further subluxation episodes and injury to the articular cartilage or menisci cannot be ensured.[25,26]

Operative Management

Surgical management of ACL injury has been the subject of intense scrutiny for the past 30 years. Techniques have evolved from repair and extra-articular reconstructions to minimally invasive arthroscopic techniques with various graft choices, sophisticated fixation options, and advanced rehabilitation protocols. There are various issues surrounding ACL surgery that are critical to the success of the reconstruction. Proper surgical technique and graft placement are paramount. However, the timing of surgery, the choice of graft and fixation device, and postoperative rehabilitation also play very important roles.

ACL reconstruction in the acute period immediately following injury has been associated with an increased incidence of arthrofibrosis and knee stiffness.[27,28] Surgery should be deferred until the acute inflammatory period has passed, range of motion has returned, and strong quadriceps activation is present. This process requires preoperative rehabilitation and modalities such

Graft choice considerations

Graft choice	Advantages	Disadvantages
Patellar tendon autograft	Ease of harvest; rigid initial fixation, bone-bone healing. Excellent clinical outcomes and widespread surgeon experience	Anterior knee pain and kneeling pain (upwards of 20%). Potential donor site complications (patella fx, baja)
Hamstring autograft	Ease of harvest, Numerous fixation options, Excellent clinical outcomes	Anterior knee pain (≤ BPTB), Deep knee flexion weakness.
Allograft	No donor site morbidity, Decreased operative time, Widespread availability	Slower graft incorporation; potential bacterial contamination; possible disease transmission

Figure 51-8 Comparison of advantages and disadvantages for commonly used anterior cruciate ligament graft material.

as cryotherapy, compression, and anti-inflammatory medications. Although some authors have recommended a waiting period of 3 to 4 weeks prior to surgery, there is no true time frame and the overall condition of the knee with regard to motion and quadriceps activation should be the guide.

Numerous graft choices and fixation options have been advocated for ACL reconstruction over the years. The selection of a graft is based on various patient factors as well as surgeon philosophy and training. Current alternatives include various autograft and allograft options. At present, the most common autograft choices include autogenous hamstring and patellar tendon grafts. Allografts have gained significant popularity recently, especially in the older patient population, and include Achilles tendon, patellar tendon, and tibialis anterior/posterior tendon.

Many factors including patient age, activity level, comorbidities, and surgeon preference play a role in graft selection. Each graft choice has advantages and disadvantages (Fig. 51-8). The biomechanical properties of the graft, ease of harvest, fixation strength, donor site morbidity, and return-to-play guidelines differ with each graft choice and should be considered for each individual patient. Overall, recent prospective controlled studies and meta-analyses have failed to demonstrate a significant difference in clinical outcome between hamstring and patellar tendon autograft reconstructions.[29,30] Additionally, the overall clinical success rates of primary allograft reconstruction have been comparable to those of autograft.[31,32] An informed discussion between the surgeon and patient of the advantages and disadvantages of each graft should guide the ultimate decision.

Surgery

Prior to surgical reconstruction of the ACL, a thorough examination under anesthesia should be performed by the operating surgeon. Depending on the certainty of the diagnosis and surgeon preference, one may either proceed directly to graft harvest or diagnostic arthroscopy. In the case of allograft reconstruction, graft preparation may be performed prior to the initiation of surgery (Fig. 51-9).

Graft Harvest: Patellar Tendon

An 8 cm long incision is made just medial to the midline centered over the patellar tendon and carried down to just below the tibial tubercle. The incision is carried down to layer 1 of the knee, and full-thickness flaps are developed to expose the patel-

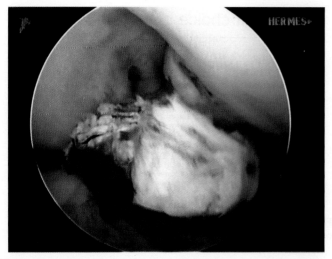

Figure 51-9 Diagnostic arthroscopy depicting acute complete anterior cruciate ligament disruption.

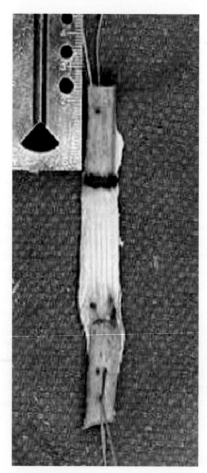

Figure 51-10 Completed bone-patellar tendon-bone graft with drill holes and sutures for graft passage.

lar tendon in its entirety. The medial and lateral borders of the patellar tendon are identified and the width of the tendon is measured. The central 10 mm of tendon (which generally corresponds with the central one third) is marked out using a sterile marking pen. The tendon is then incised along these lines longitudinally. These incisions are extended along the periosteum of the patella and tibial tubercle for an additional 2.5 cm in each direction. This serves as the guide for osteotomizing the bone plugs.

An oscillating saw is used to create the bone plugs. A trapezoidal bone plug is harvested from the tibial tubercle and a triangular bone plug is harvested from the patella. The bone plugs are then measured and contoured, and drill holes and sutures are passed through the plugs for graft passage (Fig. 51-10).

Graft Harvest: Hamstring Tendon

A 3- to 4-cm incision is made longitudinally along the anteromedial tibial crest, centered over the pes anserine tendons (Fig. 51-11A). Alternatively, transverse and oblique incisions have been described. This incision is typically approximately three finger breadths below the joint line at the level of the apex of the tibial tubercle and centered equally between the tubercle and the posteromedial aspect of the tibia. The sartorius fascia is identified, and the gracilis and semitendinosis tendon are easily palpable. If visualized, any branches of the infrapatellar branch of the saphenous nerve are preserved. At our institution, we prefer to release the tendons off their insertion on the tibia and use a closed tendon stripper for harvesting. Alternatively, the insertion site can be initially preserved and an open stripper used (Fig. 51-11B).

Once the tendons are identified, an incision is made in the sartorial fascia between the two tendons. The tendons are dissected down to the periosteum of the tibia and then reflected as one sleeve, maximizing length. Each tendon is then identified and tagged with a no. 2 nonabsorbable suture. The gracilis is harvested first. All fascial slips are released and the tendon is harvested with the closed tendon stripper. In a similar fashion, the semitendinosis is harvested. The semitendinosis often has multiple fascial connections to the medial gastrocnemius, and these must be released prior to using the tendon stripper in order to avoid premature graft amputation.[33]

Muscle remnants on the tendon grafts are removed. Final graft preparation is dependent on the fixation device. Typically, a no. 2 nonabsorbable suture whipstitch is placed in each free end and each graft is doubled over to produce a quadruplestrand construct (Fig. 51-12). Numerous fixation devices exist for both femoral and tibial fixation and are a matter of surgeon preference.

Tunnel Preparation

Diagnostic arthroscopy is performed and any intra-articular pathology is addressed. The ACL stump is debrided with a combination of a motorized shaver and electrocautery device. We leave the tibial footprint of the ACL intact for its proprioceptive and vascular contributions. The intercondylar notch is then prepared with the use of a motorized bur or shaver. We prefer to perform a limited notchplasty, taking just enough bone to expose the "over-the-top" position.

The tibial tunnel is prepared first. Tunnel placement is based on the anatomy of the intact ACL. The tibial attachment is adjacent to the anterior horn of the lateral meniscus. Numerous commercially available guide systems can be used. The tip of the guide is placed in the center of the ACL footprint on the tibia and angled about 30 degrees off the midline. The incision used for harvest of either the patellar tendon autograft or hamstring autograft can be used for the tunnel. If an allograft is used, a separate incision is made centered over the anteromedial aspect of the tibia similar to the incision described for the hamstring

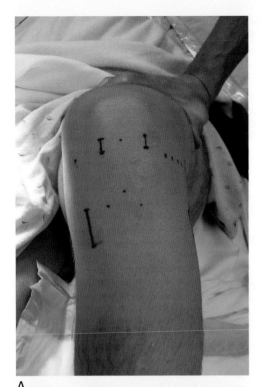

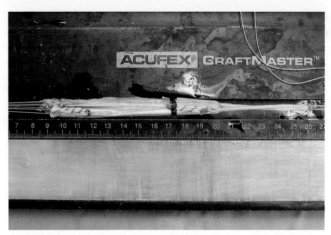

Figure 51-12 Quadruple hamstring graft being prepared for EndoButton (Smith & Nephew, Andover, MA) CL fixation.

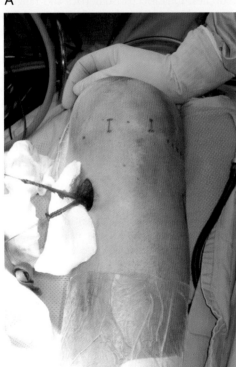

B

Figure 51-11 A, Incision site for harvest of autogenous hamstring graft. **B,** Isolation of gracilis and semitendinosis tendons. A closed tendon stripper is then used to complete the individual tendon harvest.

harvest. A provisional pin is advanced into the ACL footprint using the guide. The aiming guide is then removed and the pin is overreamed with a cannulated reamer of appropriate size (Fig. 51-13A).

Any remaining bone fragments are then removed with the use of a motorized shaver. The femoral tunnel can then be

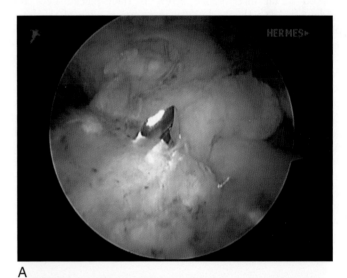

A

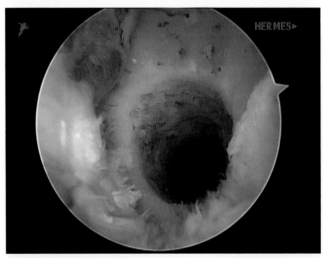

B

Figure 51-13 A, Tibial guide pin positioned in the center of the anterior cruciate ligament footprint. **B,** Femoral tunnel in 2-o'clock position with approximately 1 to 2 mm of remaining posterior wall.

addressed. The femoral tunnel can be drilled with the use of commercially available offset guides through a transtibial technique. Alternatively, a medial portal technique can be used, in which the femoral tunnel is drilled from the medial portal.[34] An offset aimer guide, typically either 6 or 7 mm, is placed in the "over-the-top" position oriented toward the 10- to 11-o'clock (right knee) or 1- to 2-o'clock (left knee) position with the knee in 90 degrees of flexion. A guide pin is then advanced approximately 3 cm and overreamed with an acorn reamer of appropriate size to a depth of about 35 mm. A 1- to 2-mm cortical wall should remain posterior to the tunnel (Fig. 51-13B).

Femoral fixation is dependent on graft choice and surgeon preference. We generally use metal interference screw fixation for bone plugs and EndoButton (Smith & Nephew, Andover, MA) fixation for soft-tissue grafts. For bone plug fixation, a Beeth pin is advanced using a transtibial technique through the femoral tunnel and out the lateral aspect of the femur. It is retrieved laterally and used to pull the sutures on the graft through the femoral tunnel. The bone-patellar tendon-bone graft is then advanced through the tibial tunnel and into the femoral tunnel. A guide pin for the interference screw is then placed between the bone plug and the tunnel. A 7 × 25-mm cannulated metal interference screw is then placed over the guidewire. With this technique, the cortical edge of the bone plug is placed posteriorly and the cancellous surface faces anteriorly.

In the case of soft-tissue grafts, after the femoral tunnel is drilled, the far cortex is breached with a 4.5-mm EndoButton drill and the depth gauge is used to assess the distance to the far cortex. Similarly, a Beeth pin is advanced through the EndoButton drill hole using a transtibial technique. It is retrieved laterally and used to pull the graft through the femoral tunnel. An appropriate length EndoButton loop is selected. Ideally between 30 and 35 mm of graft should ultimately reside within the tunnel. When EndoButton fixation is desired, the tunnel depth needs to be deep enough to accommodate the intended graft length plus an additional 8 mm for flipping the button. The quadruple-strand graft is placed in the closed loop EndoButton and sutured together using a no. 2-0 bioabsorbable stitch. Pulling sutures (using no. 2 nonabsorbable braided suture) are placed in the peripheral holes of the EndoButton, and these are advanced into the femoral tunnel using the Beeth pin. The graft is passed in a routine fashion, and the EndoButton loop is flipped to establish femoral fixation.

Once femoral fixation is achieved, the knee is cycled through a full range of motion and graft impingement is assessed. Tension is applied to the graft, and tibial fixation is performed in approximately 10 to 20 degrees of knee flexion. Bone-patellar tendon-bone grafts are secured with metal interference screw, whereas soft-tissue grafts can be secured with numerous fixation implants. Currently, we use interference fixation with a bioabsorbable screw or an Intrafix (Mitek, Innovasive Devices, Mitek, Westwood, MA) device on the tibial side for soft-tissue grafts (Fig. 51-14).

POSTOPERATIVE REHABILITATION

The goal after surgical reconstruction is to return the patient to his or her preinjury level of function without injuring the graft. In the early postoperative period, the patient is placed in a hinged knee brace locked in extension. Intermittent quadriceps sets, straight leg raises, heel slides, and continuous passive motion is encouraged during this period. The patient is allowed to be weight bearing as tolerated during this period.

For the first 6 weeks, the patient is maintained in a brace and with two crutches. Quadriceps isometrics and range-of-motion exercises are emphasized. At about 6 to 8 weeks, when the inflammation has subsided and the patient exhibits full extension, at least 90 degrees of flexion, and an adequate quadriceps set, he or she can advance to a stationary bike, closed-chain terminal extension exercises, and hamstring strengthening. Crutches and the brace can be discontinued when the patient has full extension, can perform a straight leg raise without an extension lag, and exhibits a nonantalgic gait pattern. Progressive strength, flexibility, and proprioception exercises are advanced over the course of 6 months. Functional activities and sport-specific drills are initiated between 6 and 9 months.

CRITERIA FOR RETURN TO SPORT

Multiple criteria including functional testing, clinical evaluation, and subjective assessment should be used to determine the eligibility of a patient to return to full athletic activity. A full range of motion and satisfactory return of muscle strength and endurance are necessary before return to sport is allowed. In general, a minimum of 5 to 6 months after surgery is required to attain these goals. On average, 6 to 9 months is considered a reasonable time frame for return to sport. There is considerable controversy and individual preference in regards to the timing of return to sport.[35]

Additionally, the use of a functional brace is recommended by some authors for the first 1 to 2 years after surgery. We generally recommend functional bracing for the first postoperative year and allow the patient to make a decision regarding future brace wear.

RESULTS AND OUTCOMES

Arthroscopic ACL reconstruction has proven to be a successful and reliable technique for restoring knee stability and function. Recent reports analyzing the results of patellar tendon and hamstring autograft reconstruction have demonstrated that patient

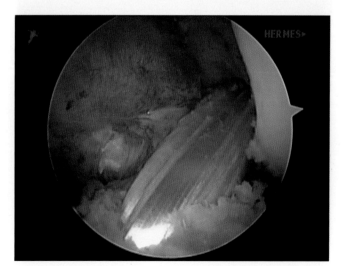

Figure 51-14 Final appearance of autogenous hamstring anterior cruciate ligament reconstruction.

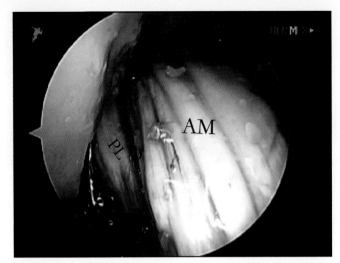

Figure 51-15 Arthroscopic image of a double-bundle anterior cruciate ligament reconstruction using tibialis anterior allograft. This reconstructive construct is a relatively new, experimental concept that attempts to improve on knee kinematics following reconstruction. AM, anteromedial; PL, posterolateral.

satisfaction following ACL reconstruction has been very high. Approximately 90% to 95% of patients are satisfied with their knee following ACL reconstruction and would have the procedure performed on their contralateral knee if it were injured. Objectively, approximately 75% to 90% of patients will have restoration of knee stability as assessed by pivot-shift testing and KT-1000 measurements. Additionally, approximately 65% of patients undergoing reconstruction return to their previous level of performance.[30,36]

Although, these numbers are encouraging, there still remains room for improvement. Innovations in surgical techniques, such as double-bundle reconstruction, and the introduction of improved fixation alternatives and biologics may ultimately improve on these already excellent results[37] (Fig. 51-15).

COMPLICATIONS

Complications following ACL reconstruction are rare. Graft failure is uncommon and occurs in approximately 2% to 5% of patients. Postoperative stiffness and arthrofibrosis can be a very disabling complication and is reported to occur in 2% to 10% of patients undergoing ACL reconstruction. However, significant, persistent motion loss greater than 5 degrees of the contralateral side is rare and is estimated at between 1% and 2%. Infection is rare, occurring in approximately 0.5% of patients undergoing reconstruction. By far, the most common complication is the presence of anterior knee pain, which occurs in approximately 10% to 20% of patients. This complication can occur in both patients undergoing bone-patellar tendon-bone and hamstring ACL reconstruction, but appears to be more common in patients undergoing bone-patellar tendon-bone reconstruction.[38]

CONCLUSIONS

Injuries to the ACL are very common and often result in symptomatic knee instability and dysfunction. Both nonoperative and operative management of ACL insufficiency can be successful in appropriately selected patients. Techniques of ACL reconstruction have advanced significantly in recent years, allowing a majority of patients to return to high-level athletics without pain and instability. Attention to surgical technique and adherence to postoperative rehabilitation protocols are the cornerstones of a successful outcome. Continued advances and improved surgical techniques and implants can be expected in the future.

REFERENCES

1. Miyasaka K, Daniel D, Stone M: The incidence of knee ligament injuries in the general population. Am J Knee Surg 1991;4:3–8.
2. Fu FH, Bennett CH, Lattermann C, et al: Current trends in anterior cruciate ligament reconstruction. Part 1: Biology and biomechanics of reconstruction. Am J Sports Med 1999;27:6 821–830.
3. Butler JC, Andrews JR: The role of arthroscopic surgery in the evaluation of acute traumatic hemarthrosis of the knee. Clin Orthop 1988;228:150–152.
4. Daniel DM, Stone ML, Dobson BE, et al: Fate of the ACL-injured patient. A prospective outcome study. Am J Sports Med 1994;22: 632–644.
5. Carson EW, Anisko EM, Restrepo C, et al: Revision anterior cruciate ligament reconstruction: Etiology of failures and clinical results. J Knee Surg 2004;17:127–132.
6. Malanga GA, Andrus S, Nadler SF, et al: Physical examination of the knee: A review of the original test description and scientific validity of common orthopedic tests. Arch Phys Med Rehabil 2003;84:592–603.
7. Bach BR Jr, Warren RF, Wickiewicz TL: The pivot shift phenomenon: Results and description of a modified clinical test for anterior cruciate ligament insufficiency. Am J Sports Med 1988;16:571–576.
8. Larson RL, Tailon M: Anterior cruciate ligament insufficiency: Principles of treatment. J Am Acad Orthop Surg 1994;2:26–35.
9. Munshi M, Davidson M, MacDonald PB, et al: The efficacy of magnetic resonance imaging in acute knee injuries. Clin J Sport Med 2000; 10:34–49.
10. Speer KP, Spritzer CE, Bassett FH 3rd, et al: Osseous injury associated with acute tears of the anterior cruciate ligament. Am J Sports Med 1992;20:382–389.
11. Faber KJ, Dill JR, Amendola A, et al: Occult osteochondral lesions after anterior cruciate ligament rupture. Six-year magnetic resonance imaging follow-up study. Am J Sports Med 1999;27:489–494.
12. Arnoczky SP: Anatomy of the anterior cruciate ligament. Clin Orthop 1983;172:19–25.
13. Girgis FG, Marshall JL, Monajem A: The cruciate ligaments of the knee joint. Anatomical, functional and experimental analysis. Clin Orthop 1975;106 216–231.
14. Harner CD, Baek GH, Vogrin TM, et al: Quantitative analysis of human cruciate ligament insertions. Arthroscopy 1999;15:741–749.
15. Markolf KL, Burchfield DM, Shapiro MM, et al: Biomechanical consequences of replacement of the anterior cruciate ligament with a patellar ligament allograft. Part II: Forces in the graft compared with forces in the intact ligament. J Bone Joint Surg Am 1996;78:1728–1734.
16. Woo SL, Hollis JM, Adams DJ, et al: Tensile properties of the human femur-anterior cruciate ligament-tibia complex. The effects of specimen age and orientation. Am J Sports Med 1991;19:217–225.

17. Sakane M, Fox RJ, Woo SL, et al: In situ forces in the anterior cruciate ligament and its bundles in response to anterior tibial loads. J Orthop Res 1997;15:285–293.

18. Gabriel MT, Wong EK, Woo SL, et al: Distribution of in situ forces in the anterior cruciate ligament in response to rotatory loads. J Orthop Res 2004;22:85–89.

19. Fithian DC, Paxton LW, Goltz DH: Fate of the anterior cruciate ligament-injured knee. Orthop Clin North Am 2002;33:621–636.

20. Noyes FR, Mooar PA, Matthews DS, et al: The symptomatic anterior cruciate-deficient knee. Part I: The long-term functional disability in athletically active individuals. J Bone Joint Surg Am 1983;65:154–162.

21. Hawkins RJ, Misamore GW, Merritt TR: Followup of the acute nonoperated isolated anterior cruciate ligament tear. Am J Sports Med 1986;14:205–210.

22. Ciccotti MG, Lombardo SJ, Nonweiler B, et al: Non-operative treatment of ruptures of the anterior cruciate ligament in middle-aged patients. Results after long-term follow-up. J Bone Joint Surg Am 1994;76:1315–1321.

23. Barber FA, Elrod BF, McGuire DA, et al: Is an anterior cruciate ligament reconstruction outcome age dependent? Arthroscopy 1996;12:720–725.

24. Plancher KD, Steadman JR, Briggs KK, et al: Reconstruction of the anterior cruciate ligament in patients who are at least forty years old. A long-term follow-up and outcome study. J Bone Joint Surg Am 1998;80:184–197.

25. Buss DD, Min R, Skyhar M, et al: Nonoperative treatment of acute anterior cruciate ligament injuries in a selected group of patients. Am J Sports Med 1995;23:160–165.

26. Fithian DC, Paxton EW, Stone ML, et al: Prospective trial of a treatment algorithm for the management of the anterior cruciate ligament-injured knee. Am J Sports Med 2005;33:335–346.

27. Harner CD, Irrgang JJ, Paul J, et al: Loss of motion after anterior cruciate ligament reconstruction. Am J Sports Med 1992;20:499–506.

28. Shelbourne KD, Foulk DA: Timing of surgery in acute anterior cruciate ligament tears on the return of quadriceps muscle strength after reconstruction using an autogenous patellar tendon graft. Am J Sports Med 1995;23:686–689.

29. Jansson KA, Linko E, Sandelin J, et al: A prospective randomized study of patellar versus hamstring tendon autografts for anterior cruciate ligament reconstruction. Am J Sports Med 2003;31:12–18.

30. Freedman KB, D'Amato MJ, Nedeff DD, et al: Arthroscopic anterior cruciate ligament reconstruction: A metaanalysis comparing patellar tendon and hamstring tendon autografts. Am J Sports Med 2003;31:2–11.

31. Harner CD, Olson E, Irrgang JJ, et al: Allograft versus autograft anterior cruciate ligament reconstruction: 3- to 5-year outcome. Clin Orthop 1996;324:134–144.

32. Strickland SM, MacGillivray JD, Warren RF: Anterior cruciate ligament reconstruction with allograft tendons. Orthop Clin North Am 2003;34:41–47.

33. Pagnani MJ, Warner JJ, O'Brien SJ, et al: Anatomic considerations in harvesting the semitendinosus and gracilis tendons and a technique of harvest. Am J Sports Med 1993;21:565–571.

34. Cha PS, Chabra A, Harner CD: Single-bundle anterior cruciate ligament reconstruction using the medial portal technique. Oper Tech Orthop 2005;15:89–95.

35. Cascio BM, Culp L, Cosgarea AJ: Return to play after anterior cruciate ligament reconstruction. Clin Sports Med 2004;23:395–408.

36. Spindler KP, Kuhn JE, Freedman KB, et al: Anterior cruciate ligament reconstruction autograft choice: Bone-tendon-bone versus hamstring: Does it really matter? A systematic review. Am J Sports Med 2004;32:1986–1995.

37. Vidal AF, Brucker PU, Fu FH: Anatomic double-bundle anterior cruciate ligament reconstruction using tibialis anterior tendon allografts. Oper Tech Orthop 2005;15:140–145.

38. Phillips BB, Haynes DE: Complications of anterior cruciate ligament reconstruction. Instr Course Lect 2002;51:329–333.

Complex Issues in Anterior Cruciate Ligament Reconstruction

L. Pearce McCarty III and Bernard R. Bach, Jr.

In This Chapter

Revision anterior cruciate ligament (ACL) reconstruction
Arthritis and ACL insufficiency
Skeletal immaturity

INTRODUCTION

- ACL injury occurs with an estimated incidence of one in 3000 among the general United States population.[1] In the majority of these cases, ACL reconstruction has proven to be a reliable and durable procedure for restoring stability, and more than 100,000 of these procedures are performed annually.[2]

- Good to excellent results in terms of patient satisfaction, stability, and return to play are observed in between 75% and 90% of these cases.[3] Clinical failure, however, remains a problem, with rates as high as 10% to 15% at short- and intermediate-term follow-up.[4]

- Despite improvements in graft fixation and a better understanding of ACL anatomy and biomechanics, this failure rate seems to be holding relatively constant, resulting in higher absolute numbers of clinical failure as the number of reconstructions performed annually continues to rise.[5]

- There are a number of complex scenarios surrounding ACL injury that require special consideration and can contribute to suboptimal clinical outcomes. Among these are revision of a failed reconstruction, ligament injury in the skeletally immature, treatment of ACL injury in the context of concomitant chondral injury, and treatment of the chronically ACL-deficient arthritic knee.

REVISION ANTERIOR CRUCIATE LIGAMENT RECONSTRUCTION

Clinical failure following ACL reconstruction can be defined as recurrent knee instability, pain, stiffness, or any combination thereof that prevents a patient from undertaking a desired set of activities.[6] Depending on the age and particular demands of the patient, these activities may range from high-level athletic competition to simple tasks of daily living. There is, therefore, a significant subjective element in the definition of clinical failure, and the treating surgeon must remain attuned to the individual needs of each patient. Once the diagnosis of clinical failure has been made, one must develop a thorough under-

standing of the etiology behind the failure such that the appropriate corrective measures can be taken.

CAUSE OF FAILURE

Failure following ACL reconstruction typically falls into one or more of four broad categories: (1) graft failure (recurrent or persistent instability), (2) secondary degenerative joint disease, (3) loss of motion, and (4) dysfunction of the extensor mechanism (Fig. 52-1).[3] These categories are not mutually exclusive, but rather the variables in each category are often interdependent. Graft failure and loss of motion are the most commonly encountered causes and most often necessitate revision of the index reconstruction.

Graft Failure

Failure of the intra-articular portion of the graft most often presents as recurrent or persistent instability. Technical errors during primary reconstruction most commonly cause graft failure, and it is estimated that malpositioned tunnels are responsible for 70% to 80% of these cases.[3,4] The most common mistake in tunnel placement has traditionally been thought to be anteriorization of the femoral tunnel, which results in loss of knee flexion, excessive tension on the graft, and early failure through cyclic loading (Fig. 52-2). This sequence of events is easily understood if one considers two anatomic and procedural factors: one, the shape of the distal femur causes the knee joint to function as a cam and two, the graft is first fixed on the femoral side and subsequently tensioned in varying degrees of extension. As the femoral tunnel is anteriorized and the knee brought into extension, the intra-articular portion of the graft progressively shortens. Tensioning and tibial-side fixation of the graft in extension then secure this shortened intra-articular graft, effectively "capturing" the knee in extension (Fig. 52-3).[1] Knee flexion then puts excessive force across the graft and potentiates graft attenuation and failure.

There also appears to be a trend toward more vertical placement of the femoral tunnel. A centralized graft may control pure anterior translation of the tibia on the femur, thereby eliminating the patient's Lachman test, but will fail to control tibial rotation resulting in a postoperative pivot-shift and persistent instability.[4] Tibial tunnel anteriorization can also result in significant dysfunction, with both loss of extension through notch impingement and loss of flexion via a mechanism analogous to that of an anteriorized femoral tunnel. However, with current endoscopic techniques, posteriorized tibial tunnels are encountered more commonly than anteriorized tibial tunnels and can cause loss of flexion through impingement against the posterior cruciate ligament (PCL). Although these may be the most com-

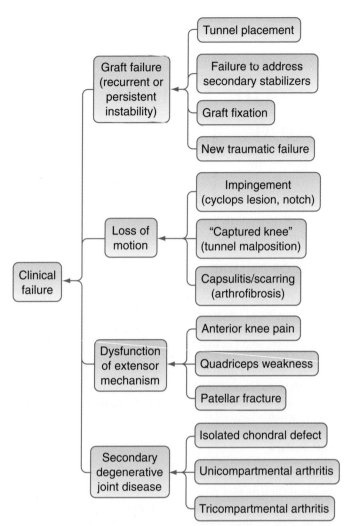

Figure 52-1 Flowchart summarizing potential causes of clinical failure following anterior cruciate ligament reconstruction.

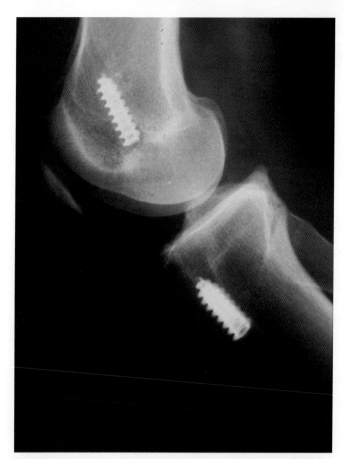

Figure 52-2 Lateral radiograph demonstrating anterior malposition of the femoral tunnel.

monly encountered types of tunnel malposition, any combination of tibial and femoral tunnel may be observed. Types of tunnel malposition and their effects on knee motion are summarized in Table 52-1.

Failure to recognize and treat combined instability patterns represents another significant cause of graft failure, thought to account for as many as 15% of cases.[7] Injury to secondary stabilizers of the knee such as the medial collateral ligament, posterolateral corner, and the posterior horn of the medial meniscus can occur during the initial trauma or can become damaged over time, placing additional stress on the graft and potentiating early failure. Posterolateral instability has been reported to accompany as many as 15% of chronic ACL injuries.[3] Unrecognized angular malalignment conditions, such as the double varus and triple varus knee (explained later in this chapter) can also lead to excessive graft strain and early failure.[8]

Catastrophic failure of graft fixation is uncommon but has been reported.[9] Certain technical errors are known to contribute to failure of fixation, including interference screw divergence and graft-tunnel mismatch.[4,10] In cases of screw divergence, the path taken by the interference screw diverges with that of the graft, decreasing contact area between the screw and the graft and weakening fixation strength.[4] This is more problematic with the dual-incision technique than the endoscopic technique,

although more common with the endoscopic technique. On the femoral side, with the endoscopic technique, screw divergence may still provide a "wedge" or "doorstop," despite suboptimal contact between the interference screw and bone block. This is not the case with femoral-side fixation using the dual-incision technique, as a result of placement of the interference screw from outside-in.

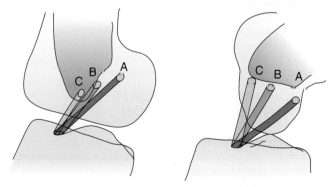

Figure 52-3 The shape of the distal femur results in a cam mechanism that puts excessive tension on grafts whose femoral point of fixation has been anteriorized. Graft A has a femoral tunnel in the desired posterior position and approximates isometry during flexion. Grafts B and C have progressively anteriorized femoral points of fixation and experience excessive strain with knee flexion as the posterior condyles engage.

Table 52-1 Tunnel Position

	Anatomic Position	Tunnel Malposition	Cause	Effect on Graft	Patient Complaint
Femur	Sagittal: 1–2mm anterior to posterior femoral cortex in notch	Anterior	Failure to identify true posterior margin of notch; "resident's ridge"	Excessive tension in flexion	Loss of flexion; recurrent instability with graft attenuation
	Coronal: 1 o'clock (left knee) or 11 o'clock (right knee) position	Central (vertical)	Placement of graft centrally in the notch	Inability to control rotatory forces	Persistent rotatory instability without elimination of pivot shift
		Posterior	Nonanatomic technique with graft fixation in "over-the-top" position	Excessive tension in extension	Loss of extension; recurrent instability with graft attenuation
Tibia	Sagittal: at point of intersection between posterior aspect of anterior horn of lateral meniscus and medial tibial spine; 1–2mm anterior to leading edge of PCL	Anterior	Excessively large angle on tibial guide/tunnel; failure to adequately débride ACL stump and identify tibial landmarks	Excessive tension in flexion; notch impingement in extension	Loss of flexion; loss of extension with notch impingement; morning stiffness; recurrent instability with graft attenuation
	Coronal: midpoint of upslope of medial tibial spine	Posterior	Excessively small angle on tibial guide/tunnel	Impingement on PCL in flexion	Loss of extension; loss of flexion; recurrent instability with graft attenuation
		Lateral	Failure to identify tibial footprint of ACL	Impingement on lateral femoral condyle in flexion	Loss of flexion; catching sensation
		Medial	Failure to identify tibial footprint of ACL	Impingement on PCL in flexion	Loss of flexion

ACL, Anterior cruciate ligament; PCL, posterior cruciate ligament.

If the length of a bone-tendon-bone graft does not match the composite length of the recipient tibial tunnel + intra-articular + femoral tunnel lengths, then a graft-tunnel mismatch exists. The surface area of bone block in the tibial tunnel for interference screw fixation is therefore reduced, again weakening fixation strength.[11] This may lead to micromotion and graft attenuation in the early postoperative period. Several strategies have been advocated for graft tunnel mismatches, including conversion to a dual-incision technique if recognized prior to femoral tunnel creation, recessing the femoral bone plug, rotating the graft 540 degrees to shorten the construct, or removing the bone block to create a free bone block modification. Traumatic tear of a well-functioning reconstruction is also a possible mode of failure, particularly within a population of high-level athletes.

Loss of Motion

Loss of motion can arise from multiple causes. Specific causes include presence of a cyclops lesion and notch impingement secondary to inadequate notchplasty or tunnel malposition. A cyclops lesion refers to the presence of a mass of scar tissue lying anterior to the tibial tunnel that impinges against the notch as the knee comes into extension. Patients typically present several months into the postoperative period with complaints ranging from a subtle click to a painless mechanical "clunk" as the knee extends. Inadequate débridement of the ACL stump is thought to be one source of this lesion, which is reported to occur in between 2% and 4% of ACL reconstructions.

More general causes of motion loss include scarring of the capsule, scarring of the patellar tendon (patella infera), and contracture of a variety of other soft-tissue structures leading to a condition known as arthrofibrosis and producing a stiff knee following an otherwise sound reconstruction procedure. Factors associated with the development of arthrofibrosis include poor preoperative range of motion, inability to achieve full extension early in the postoperative period, tunnel malpositioning, inappropriate graft tensioning, concomitant meniscal repair or medial cruciate ligament reconstruction, and male gender.[3]

CLINICAL FEATURES AND EVALUATION

History

Complaints of pain versus those of instability should be clearly delineated. A patient with a chief complaint of pain following ACL reconstruction may be treated in a markedly different fashion than one whose chief complaint is recurrent or persistent instability. ACL revision is much more successful in addressing an unstable knee in which pain is not a significant component than those in which pain is the chief complaint. Additionally, infection and complex regional pain syndrome should be considered in those patients complaining primarily of disproportional pain.

The degree to which a patient was able to return to normal activity, that is, whether the patient feels stability was ever restored to their knee, should be assessed. Persistent instability suggests failure to identify and treat a complex instability pattern in which secondary knee stabilizers have been injured. Early, abrupt, recurrent instability can be caused by failure of graft fixation. Early, gradual, recurrent instability may result from graft attenuation via tunnel malposition. Late recurrent instability following a period of return to normal activity most often results from traumatic retear.

Previous operative reports should be obtained to facilitate understanding what was done during the index procedure and to identify the manufacturer of the fixation device so that the appropriate tools for hardware removal can be made available.

Physical Examination

Skin condition and configuration of previous incisions should be inspected. Presence or absence of an effusion should be noted. Clinical varus or valgus alignment should be evaluated. Range of motion should be carefully documented and the presence and degree of flexion contracture recorded. Prone heel heights in flexion and extension can be used to assess knee flexion and extension contractures. Varus and valgus laxity should be tested at 0 and 30 degrees of flexion to evaluate collateral ligament integrity. Anterior drawer, Lachman, and pivot-shift testing should be performed and results compared to those of the contralateral, normal knee to identify the degree of instability present. Posterior drawer testing should be conducted to rule out concomitant posterior cruciate ligament injury, and the dial test should be performed at 30 and 90 degrees of flexion to rule out injury to the posterolateral corner. Patellar mobility and the presence of patellofemoral crepitation should be assessed. Finally, the patient's gait should be observed carefully.

Imaging

A standard series of plain radiographs consisting of a standing anteroposterior, Rosenberg (weight bearing posteroanterior in 45 degrees of flexion), and Merchant views of both knees, as well as a lateral of the affected side should be examined for tunnel position, tunnel enlargement, and failure of fixation (see Fig. 52-3). Clinical evidence of angular malalignment should be further evaluated with standing, long-cassette views of both lower extremities. The presence of significant tunnel enlargement

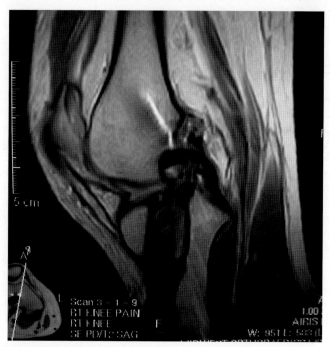

Figure 52-4 Magnetic resonance imaging of a failed anterior cruciate ligament reconstruction using Achilles tendon allograft reveals marked enlargement of the tibial tunnel that required staged treatment with tunnel débridement and grafting followed by reconstruction.

on a plain radiograph may require evaluation with computed tomography or magnetic resonance imaging (MRI) to determine whether a single or staged procedure should be undertaken (Fig. 52-4).[12] Furthermore, MRI can be useful in identifying intra-articular pathology that may require attention at the time of a revision procedure, such as chondral defects, meniscal tears, and presence of a cyclops lesion. Because instability can exist in the presence of a radiographically intact graft, however, MRI should be relied on to confirm or rule out graft failure. Failure is a clinical, not radiographic, diagnosis.

SURGERY

Preoperative Planning

Once a diagnosis of failed reconstruction has been made, a plan should be formulated to address the identified mode of failure. Not all scenarios mandate ACL graft revision. For example, presence of an isolated cyclops lesion generating loss of motion in an otherwise stable knee without tunnel malposition can be treated effectively with arthroscopic débridement. The majority of clinical failures, however, do involve index graft revision. Although a trial of functional bracing may be considered for those patients willing to make significant lifestyle modifications and accept the possibility of meniscal injury with its incumbent risk of accelerated arthrosis, most cases necessitate operative treatment. The patient should be counseled that the results of revision reconstruction are not equivalent to those of index procedures.[13] Nevertheless, proper planning and execution should result in a stable construct, and if patient expectations are appropriate, the chance of overall success remains high.

Following careful clinical evaluation as previously outlined, a preoperative checklist (Table 52-2) of key variables can be formulated to help with planning. Graft selection for revision reconstruction remains a controversial issue, and success has been reported with a variety of different allograft and autograft constructs. Consensus does exist, however, that synthetic graft materials are not recommended for either primary or revision ACL reconstruction. The most commonly reported grafts selected for revision reconstruction are bone-patellar tendon-bone (BPTB) autograft, and fresh-frozen BPTB allograft.[4] Autograft offers more rapid graft tunnel incorporation and avoids risk of disease transmission but may not be available in a revision setting and carries with it the risk of donor site morbidity. Use of allograft, on the other hand, eliminates donor site morbidity. An additional advantage of allograft use is that accompanying bone blocks are often large, a useful feature when attempting to achieve rigid fixation in the context of tunnel dilatation (Fig. 52-5). Some patients, however, may be unwilling to accept the small, but finite risk of disease transmission with the use of allografts. Commercial tissue banks often use doses of gamma irradiation between 1.5 and 2.5 mrad to treat harvested tissue. While doses in this range are considered to be bactericidal, Smith et al[14] showed that active viral replication of human immunodeficiency virus type 1 persisted in culture after doses as high as 5.0 mrad. Such high doses of gamma irradiation, however, may render allograft tissue mechanically unfit for implantation. Fideler et al[15] clearly demonstrated a dose-dependent decrease in the biomechanical properties of BPTB allograft following gamma irradiation. With use of 2.0 mrad of gamma irradiation, they observed a 15% reduction in initial biomechanical strength when compared to nonirradiated fresh-frozen controls. This reduction increased to as high as 46% when

Table 52-2 Anterior Cruciate Ligament Revision Preoperative Checklist

Preoperative Checklist	Comments
Mode of failure of index procedure	
Type of hardware used in index procedure	A selection of screwdrivers and other extraction devices when indicated should be available for hardware removal
Presence of tunnel enlargement	Marked enlargement (>15 mm) may require a staged procedure
Presence of concomitant intra-articular pathology	Meniscal tears or focal chondral defects should be addressed at the time of the revision procedure
Presence of angular malalignment	Significant angular malalignment can contribute to index graft failure and should be addressed at the time of the revision procedure
Integrity of secondary stabilizers	Posterolateral corner reconstruction may be required at the time of revision
Revision graft selection	Allograft vs. autograft; irradiated vs. nonirradiated; availability must be confirmed
Revision graft fixation	At least two means (primary and back up) of secure fixation should be available and the surgeon should be facile with each (e.g., interference screw, EndoButton)
Revision tunnel placement	The means of establishing anatomic tunnel position should be decided (e.g., overlapping tunnels, diverging tunnels, two-incision technique)

grafts were exposed to a 4-mrad dose. Use of irradiated versus nonirradiated allograft remains controversial, as does the optimal dose of gamma irradiation in the case of irradiated tissue. Current molecular screening tests, such as reverse-transcriptase polymerase chain reaction and other techniques are highly sensitive, and the surgeon and patient must make a joint, informed decision when it comes to autograft versus allograft and irradiated versus nonirradiated.

Another consideration when using allografts for revision work is the amount of tissue that will be necessary given the size of the patient. When ordering a BPTB allograft, inclusion of the patient's height may help avoid mismatch between the size of graft received and the amount of tissue needed for reconstruction. Finally, quadruple hamstring and quadriceps tendon grafts (allo- and auto-) are also possibilities for revision reconstruction, but experience with these graft selections in the setting of revision surgery is less extensive than that with BPTB grafts.

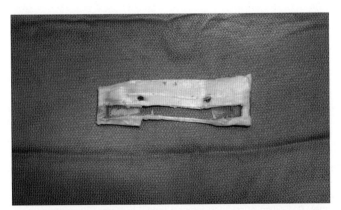

Figure 52-5 Intraoperative image of a standard bone-patellar tendon-bone allograft after the portion to be used for the reconstruction has been harvested. Ample bone stock remains in the allograft, permitting femoral and tibial bone blocks to be fashioned larger as needed and providing substrate for grafting of bony defects.

Surgical Technique with Bone-Patellar Tendon-Bone Allograft

Examination of the patient under anesthesia should confirm preoperative diagnosis of graft failure and rule out the presence of a complex instability pattern. The sequence of operative steps is in general the same as that used for primary ACL reconstruction: diagnostic arthroscopy and débridement of failed graft, tibial followed by femoral tunnel preparation, allograft preparation (alternatively, depending on anticipated needs, graft preparation can take place as the initial step or simultaneous to other steps), passage, cycling, and fixation of the graft. Most revision reconstructions can be accomplished via an endoscopic, single-incision technique.

The patient is placed in a supine position with the operative extremity held in standard ring-type leg holder. The nonoperative leg is flexed at both the knee and hip and secured in a padded gynecologic leg holder. The waist of the table is flexed and the foot is dropped, permitting easy access to both medial and lateral aspects of the knee. If the need for extensive bone grafting of widened tunnels is anticipated, then the ipsilateral iliac crest can be prepped and draped into the field. Standard arthroscopic portals are established, and a general diagnostic arthroscopy is performed. Status of the medial, lateral, and patellofemoral compartment articular cartilage as well as the menisci is evaluated and recorded. Residual ACL tissue is débrided, taking particular care to débride the tibial ACL footprint such that the medial tibial spine, the leading edge of the posterior cruciate ligament, and the posterior aspect of the anterior horn of the lateral meniscus can be identified as landmarks for accurate tibial tunnel placement. The exit point of the previous tibial tunnel and the entry point of the previous femoral tunnel are defined carefully with a shaver and arthroscopic electrocautery, and a final plan is formulated for revision tunnel preparation.

Removal of previously placed interference screws can be challenging and, if not done carefully, can lead to cortical violation of the tibia and/or femur, including posterior wall blowout. Although not routinely necessary, use of intraoperative image intensification can facilitate removal and permits evaluation of cortical integrity. A number of strategies can aid in the safe removal of a femoral interference screw. A spinal needle should be used to triangulate and establish the proper angle for removal, and at times the screw can be accessed via the tibial tunnel.

Tunnels in acceptable position are redrilled and cleared of all fibrous tissue, and the bone blocks of the allograft sized appropriately to fill the tunnels. Passage of the arthroscope through the tibial and/or femoral tunnel permits confirmation of the adequacy of débridement and maintenance of osseous integrity.

Old tunnels that are malpositioned by more than one diameter can be bypassed, as the new tunnels can be placed in anatomic position without overlap (Fig. 52-6) and may not require hardware removal. However, for cases in which preexisting hardware interferes with new tunnel placement, hardware removal and, where indicated, bone grafting of a subsequent defect should be done prior to drilling the new tibial or femoral tunnel. A clear arthroscopic cannula placed through the standard or an accessory inferomedial portal can be useful for packing allograft chips into the femoral tunnel. A solid block of allograft bone fashioned from the excess that accompanies a standard BPTB allograft can be also be used to fill bony defects in either the femoral or tibial tunnels (Fig. 52-7).

The degree of tunnel enlargement present at the time of reconstruction may require special attention. Tunnel enlargement that compromises attempts at revision graft fixation must be staged. In the first stage, the failed graft is excised, tunnels are débrided of all soft tissue, and allograft chips, autograft (e.g., iliac crest), or a mixture of both is used to fill all bony defects (Fig. 52-8). The patient is then treated with protected weight bearing for 8 to 12 weeks until bone graft incorporation is complete and new tunnels can be prepared through restored bone

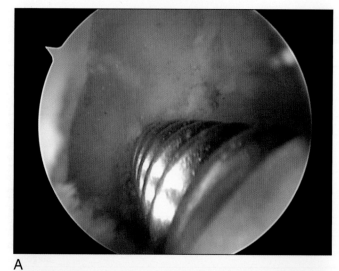

A

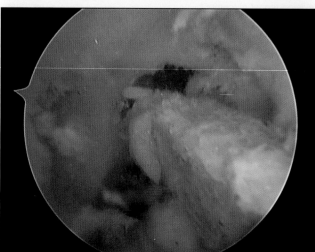

B

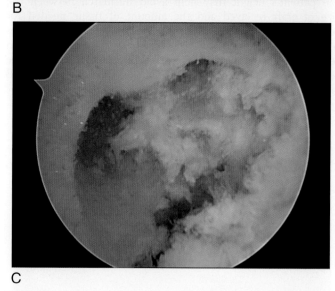

C

Figure 52-7 Series of intraoperative arthroscopic photos demonstrating revision of a malpositioned femoral tunnel. **A,** Removal of interference screw from original reconstruction. **B,** Bone grafting of original femoral tunnel. **C,** Drilling of revision femoral tunnel in isometric position.

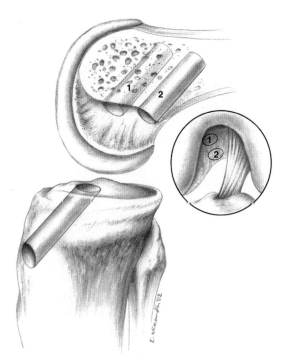

Figure 52-6 Drawing illustrating nonoverlapping tunnels. The anterior position of the existing femoral tunnel (1) allows drilling of the revision tunnel posteriorly (2) as in a primary case. (From Bach BR Jr, Mazzocca A, Fox JA: Revision anterior cruciate ligament surgery. In Grana WA [ed]: Orthopaedic Knowledge Online. Rosemont, IL, American Academy of Orthopaedic Surgeons, 2003.)

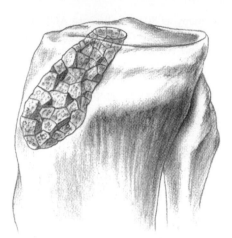

Figure 52-8 Drawing illustrating bone grafting of an enlarged tibial tunnel. (From Bach BR Jr, Mazzocca A, Fox JA: Revision anterior cruciate ligament surgery. In Grana WA [ed]: Orthopaedic Knowledge Online. Rosemont, IL, American Academy of Orthopaedic Surgeons, 2003.)

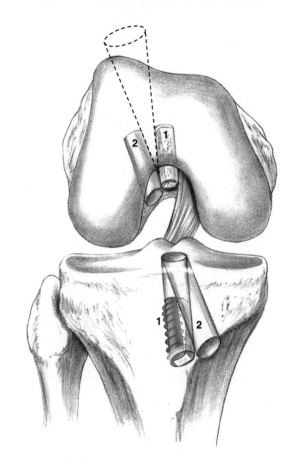

Figure 52-9 Illustration of the "divergent tunnel" concept, in this case demonstrating a revision femoral tunnel (2) drilled from outside in using a two-incision technique. (From Bach BR Jr, Mazzocca A, Fox JA: Revision anterior cruciate ligament surgery. In Grana WA [ed]: Orthopaedic Knowledge Online. Rosemont, IL, American Academy of Orthopaedic Surgeons, 2003.)

stock. For cases of mild tunnel enlargement in which a single interference screw is judged to be inadequate, techniques such as using large bone blocks on the allograft, bone grafting at the time of the reconstruction, or stacking interference screws in which a second screw is placed parallel to and alongside the first screw can enhance fixation strength.

As in index reconstruction, the tibial tunnel is prepared first. An elbow-type aiming guide is typically recommended. The tendinous portion of the graft is measured and the "n + 10" rule used to determine the appropriate guide setting. It can be helpful to leave the tibial-side bone block intentionally long to compensate for possible graft-tunnel mismatch. Excess bone block can later be trimmed as needed.

In some instances, the posterior wall of the femoral tunnel is found to be "blown out" or is violated during attempts to bypass an old anterior femoral tunnel at the time of revision surgery. Interference screw fixation is compromised in these situations because an intact osseous tube is required for interference fit. Cases of posterior wall blow out can be approached using the "divergent tunnel" concept, which refers to the fact that both the femoral and tibial tunnels can have a variety of different orientations without changing the intra-articular orientation of the graft. Arthroscopic two-incision technique permits rigid interference screw fixation through outside-in screw placement in cases in which the posterior cortex is blown out (Fig. 52-9). Alternatively, an EndoButton (Smith & Nephew, Andover, MA) technique can be used, eliminating the need for posterior wall integrity.

Following placement of new tunnels and bone grafting where needed, the graft is passed in standard fashion. Femoral-side fixation is achieved as described; and the graft is cycled in order to pre-tension the graft and evaluate isometry. The graft should translate no more than 1 to 2 mm in the tibial tunnel as the knee comes into full extension if tunnel placement is correct. Tibial-side fixation is then achieved with the knee in full extension and axially loaded. Some surgeons prefer to achieve tibial-side fixation with the knee held in a reverse Lachman position, but this maneuver raises concern about overconstraining the knee. Interference screw fixation can be reinforced using a screw and washer construct or staples if bone is deficient or osteopenic or if fixation is simply judged to be inadequate. Restoration of

stability is assessed with Lachman and pivot-shift testing intraoperatively.

POSTOPERATIVE REHABILITATION

Expectations regarding return to play and knee "normalcy" following revision ACL reconstruction should be tempered by the reality that reported results are less encouraging than those following primary reconstruction.[13] Fox et al observed a 28% failure rate (defined as presence of a pivot-shift or KT-1000 manual maximal side-to-side difference greater than 5 mm) in their series of 32 ACL revision reconstructions using nonirradiated, fresh-frozen BPTB allograft in which a standard, accelerated rehabilitation protocol was implemented. The exact effect of the rehabilitation variable in this series is unknown, but it is possible that a less aggressive protocol could have led to less graft attenuation. Nevertheless, the goals of postoperative rehabilitation following revision ACL reconstruction are in general the same as those following an index procedure, and it should be noted that in the Fox et al series no cases of arthrofibrosis were encountered.

The patient is protected in a hinged rehabilitation brace postoperatively and is permitted immediate range of motion as tolerated. Typically, weight bearing is also permitted as tolerated in the immediate postoperative period as long as the brace is locked in full extension. Weight-bearing restrictions may be indicated, however, if bone grafting was required.

Phases of rehabilitation proceed in standard fashion. Focus is initially on regaining quadriceps control and obtaining full active extension. Gait is protected with crutch use during this period. Once quadriceps control and full extension have been regained, typically at 4 to 6 weeks postoperatively, crutch and brace use is discontinued and focus shifts to obtaining full flexion and strengthening with closed-chain exercises. Once full range of motion and appropriate strength have been regained, typically at 3 months postoperatively, jogging straight ahead without cutting or pivoting is initiated. As strength and flexibility return, cutting, pivoting, plyometric, and sport-specific drills are gradually introduced. By 6 months postoperatively, the patient is generally allowed return to unrestricted activity with use of a custom ACL orthosis from 6 months to 1 year postoperatively.

ARTHRITIS AND ANTERIOR CRUCIATE LIGAMENT DEFICIENCY

Although acute meniscal and chondral injuries can occur at the time of ACL rupture, injury to articular cartilage commonly presents in the context of chronic ACL deficiency. It is well accepted that the natural history of ACL deficiency in the knee of an active individual is one of repeated episodes of instability, recurrent trauma to the menisci and articular cartilage, and accelerated arthrosis. Wear patterns in the chronically ACL-deficient knee tend to be predominantly posteromedial, with a higher relative frequency of medial meniscus and medial femoral condyle articular cartilage injury than lateral.[16-18]

Articular Cartilage Injury at Time of Anterior Cruciate Ligament Rupture

The forces that result in a tear of the ACL produce high tibiofemoral shear forces that can cause focal injury to articular cartilage.[19] Evidence of the energy transmitted to articular cartilage when the ACL is torn are the "bone bruises" of the lateral femoral condyle and posterolateral tibial plateau, recognized to

accompany as many as 80% of all acute ACL tears. The majority of bone bruises, termed reticular in nature, are seen on MRI as hemorrhage and edema in medullary bone without involvement of the subchondral plate and typically resolve by 6 to 12 months without known long-term sequelae. A minority of bone bruises, however, termed geographic, demonstrate on MRI signal change contiguous with subchondral bone and have a high likelihood of resulting in osteochondral sequelae.[19]

At the time of reconstruction, arthroscopic evaluation of the joint may reveal a focal, full-thickness chondral defect, requiring one of a variety of strategies to salvage the articular surface. If the defect involves an osteochondral fragment, the surgeon may attempt reduction and fixation using a variety of techniques. Well-defined, geographic lesions may be amenable to marrow stimulation techniques such as microfracture or osteochondral autograft transfer (Fig. 52-10). Larger lesions may demand osteochondral allograft transfer or autologous chondrocyte implantation. In addition to adding complexity to the ACL reconstruction, cartilage repair procedures require alterations in postoperative rehabilitation protocols, often with restrictions on the patient's weight-bearing status.

Chronically Anterior Cruciate Ligament–Deficient Knee

When addressing concomitant injury to articular cartilage in the context of the chronically ACL deficient knee, several very important points must be weighed: (1) the extent of damage to articular cartilage, (2) the status of the menisci, and (3) evidence of angular malalignment. Accurate determination of extent of articular involvement in the painful, unstable knee is perhaps of paramount importance. Significant involvement of two or more compartments may preclude attempts at joint salvage. Unicompartmental arthritis in the ACL-deficient knee, however, can be approached with ACL reconstruction and unloading osteotomy and/or meniscal transplantation where indicated.[20]

In select ACL-deficient patients without angular malalignment, isolated ACL reconstruction can be considered. Shelbourne et al[18] reported significant and durable pain relief (5.5 years mean follow-up) in a group of 58 patients with a chroni-

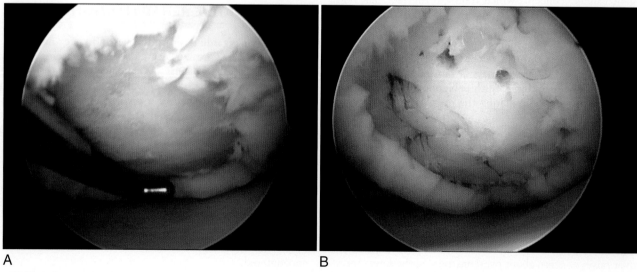

A   B

Figure 52-10 Arthroscopic images depicting microfracture of a large, full-thickness, focal, chondral lesion in a patient undergoing anterior cruciate ligament reconstruction. **A,** The lesion has been debrided down to a clean base without violation of the subchondral plate. **B,** Microfracture has been performed to stimulate fibrocartilage formation.

cally ACL-deficient knee (mean time from injury to surgery, 8.2 years) in whom an isolated ACL reconstruction was performed with BPTB autograft. Interestingly, all patients in this series had obtained temporary relief from both pain and instability with preoperative bracing using an off-the-shelf functional brace designed for ACL insufficiency.

The biomechanical importance of the meniscus is well known, and interest in meniscal transplantation has increased in recent years (Fig. 52-11). In the context of the ACL-deficient knee, the medial meniscus in particular has an important function. In addition to its role in minimizing point contact pressures via a hoop stress mechanism, the posterior horn of the medial meniscus functions as a secondary stabilizer against anterior translation of the tibia on the femur.[21] The status of the menisci at the time of reconstruction can be an important factor in determining the success of ACL reconstruction. Shelbourne et al[17] showed a significant difference in both subjective and objective measures (KT-1000 maximal manual difference) between patients who underwent ACL reconstruction with intact menisci and those status post complete or subtotal medial or medial and lateral meniscectomies. Meniscal transplantation in combination with both primary and revision ACL reconstruction has been shown to be successful in terms of both subjective measures and objective measures of stability.[22] Although not compared prospectively against a nontransplanted cohort, Sekiya et al[22] reported impressive results in a population of patients (average age, 35 years) having undergone meniscal transplantation along with either primary or revision ACL reconstruction. In their study, 96% of patients did not have pain with activities of daily living, and 71% of patients participated in moderate or strenuous sports without discomfort. Their indications for combined meniscal transplantation and ACL reconstruction included history of meniscectomy, ACL injury with symptomatic instability, joint line pain and no more than 2 mm of joint space narrowing on a weight-bearing in 45 degrees of flexion posteroanterior radiograph. Evidence of extensive grade III or IV chondrosis discovered at the time of arthroscopy precluded meniscal transplantation. Additionally, all patients were evaluated for mechanical malalignment, and two patients in their series underwent lateral closing wedge osteotomy as an added procedure. In a select group of patients with meniscal deficiency and ACL injury, meniscal transplantation at the time of ACL reconstruction should be considered as a viable option for optimizing outcome.

Mechanical alignment is also an extremely important consideration. Noyes et al[8] have described a mechanical progression that can be seen in individuals with chronic ACL deficiency and baseline varus alignment. This group of patients progress from what the authors term "single" varus to "double" varus, and finally to "triple" varus if the process is not identified and corrected. The single varus knee is one in which the tibiofemoral articulation falls into varus alignment secondary to baseline osseous geometry and degeneration of the medial meniscus and medial compartment articular surfaces. The lateral structures in this case, however, continue to tether against further varus collapse. Once the lateral structures attenuate and the knee falls further into varus, developing a lateral condylar lift off or thrust with activity, the knee is said to have developed double varus. Finally, as the posterolateral structures fail, the tibia falls into external rotation and the knee into recurvatum, resulting in the triple varus knee (Fig. 52-12). Correction of this process can require ACL reconstruction, osteotomy, and meniscal transplant where indicated.

ANTERIOR CRUCIATE LIGAMENT INJURY IN THE SKELETALLY IMMATURE

ACL injury in the skeletally immature patient represents another set of complex issues in ACL reconstruction. Intrasubstance tears of the ACL have been reported with increasing frequency as more children participate in high-level athletic activities.[23] As many as 65% of acute pediatric knee injuries (children ages 13 to 18 years) accompanied by hemarthrosis involve injury to the ACL.[24] The predicament presented by pediatric ACL injury is a difficult one. On the one hand, neglect of a complete tear of the ACL can, as in adults, lead to repeated episodes of instability, meniscal injury, and accelerated arthrosis.[25-27] On the other hand, ACL reconstruction carries the theoretical risk of limb shortening or angular deformity resulting either from direct mechanical disruption of the physis or according to the Hueter-Volkmann principle from increased mechanical loads across the physis.[28,29] With the distal femoral and proximal tibial physes together accounting for approximately

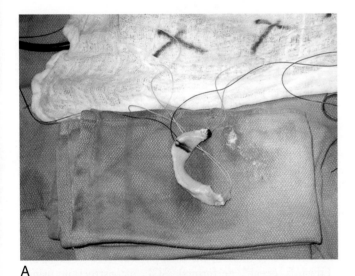

A

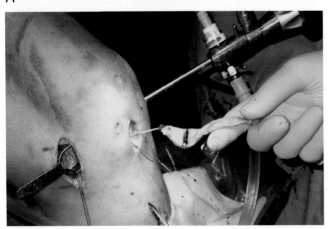

B

Figure 52-11 A, Medial meniscal allograft prepared for transplantation using double bone plug technique. **B,** Passage of medial meniscal allograft into medial compartment. A Henning retractor has been placed adjacent to the posteromedial joint capsule through a standard posteromedial approach for retrieval of inside-out meniscal sutures.

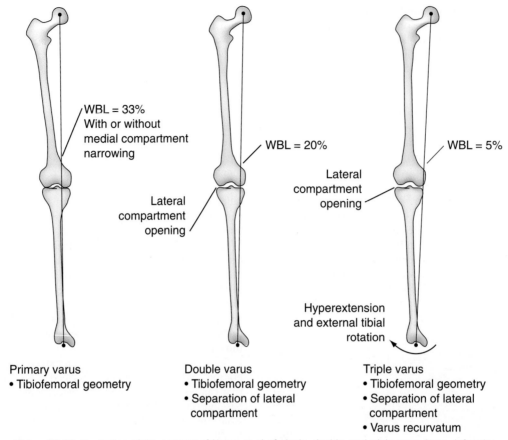

WBL = 33%
With or without
medial compartment
narrowing

WBL = 20%

WBL = 5%

Lateral
compartment
opening

Lateral
compartment
opening

Lateral
compartment
opening

Hyperextension
and external tibial
rotation

Primary varus
• Tibiofemoral geometry

Double varus
• Tibiofemoral geometry
• Separation of lateral
compartment

Triple varus
• Tibiofemoral geometry
• Separation of lateral
compartment
• Varus recurvatum

Figure 52-12 Illustration of the concept of Noyes et al of single, double, and triple varus knee deformity.

65% of total leg length, there exists the potential for significant deformity.

This scenario plays itself out most commonly in an adolescent population. Retrospective reviews of large numbers of pediatric patients suggest that intrasubstance tears of the ACL are extremely rare in young children (younger than 12 years old).[30,31] More than 80% of ligament injuries involve tibial spine avulsion rather than intrasubstance tear in children younger than 12 years of age.[30] Tibial spine avulsions invoke an algorithm different than that of intrasubstance tears, with consensus dictating that displaced fractures should be reduced and fixed anatomically. Complete tear of the ACL without concomitant meniscal or chondral injury in a slightly older, adolescent population represents perhaps the most difficult scenario with respect to decision making. These patients are often 24 to 36 months away from skeletal maturity, at which time definitive, transphyseal reconstruction of the ACL could be performed without concern for iatrogenic injury to the growth plate. This also, however, tends to be a very active population that may not easily accept the necessity of stringent activity modification for these 2 to 3 years, followed by another 3 to 6 months of postoperative rehabilitation prior to returning to preinjury level of competition.

Pathophysiology

Several animal studies have looked at growth disturbance as a function of physeal drilling, bridging with soft-tissue grafts and application of tensile force. Stadelmaier et al[32] reported that four of four canines who underwent simple transphyseal drilling without soft-tissue graft interposition went on to at least partial epiphysiodesis, where as canines with soft-tissue graft interposition following drilling did not. Of note, the grafts placed in this study were not tensioned.

Makela et al[33] drilled transphyseal tunnels in a rabbit model and observed no disturbance when the cross-sectional area of the defect was less than 3% of the total physeal area. Osseous bridging was, however, demonstrated when the size of the defect was 7% or more of the total physeal cross-sectional area.

Edwards et al[34] performed ACL reconstruction using a transphyseal, tensioned soft-tissue graft with extraphyseal fixation in a canine model. They found significant femoral valgus deformity and significant tibial varus deformity without physeal bar formation. A single degree of graft tensioning was used for all subject animals. It is somewhat difficult to interpret how this might translate to ACL reconstruction in the skeletally immature human. Furthermore, without an extraphyseal, tensioned graft control group, it is difficult to sort out the effects of transphyseal drilling versus graft tensioning on the growth disturbance observed.

Behr et al[35] conducted an anatomic study to determine the relationship between the "over-the-top" position and the distal femoral physis. They found that the femoral attachment of the ACL was at an average of 3 mm from the level of the physis and that the "over-the-top" position was at the level of the physis.

All these studies have technical ramifications when contemplating ACL reconstruction in a skeletally immature population. The findings of Stadelmaier et al suggest that soft-tissue grafts such as quadruple hamstring autograft are relatively safe from the standpoint of generating physeal disturbance. The study of Makela et al indicates that more vertically oriented transphyseal tunnels, which disturb a smaller cross-sectional area of the physis, are preferred. The relationship between the "over-the-top" position and the distal femoral physis of Behr et al cautions against reconstructive techniques that involve dissection or fixation at or near the "over-the-top" position. Finally, the findings of Edwards et al recommend against overtensioning of the graft, although it is difficult to quantify this recommendation.

Clinical Features and Evaluation

Physical examination of the pediatric knee follows the same general guidelines as that of the adult. Observation should document any skin injury and should record the presence and relative size of an effusion. Active and passive range of motion should be recorded. Stability should be evaluated with anterior and posterior drawer, Lachman, pivot-shift, and dial tests and varus/valgus stress at 0 and 30 degrees. A complete neurovascular examination should be performed.

Imaging studies should include a plain radiographic series to identify the occasional tibial spine fracture presenting as an intrasubstance ACL injury. Varus or valgus stress radiographs may be useful, as femoral physeal fractures can mimic ligamentous injuries to the knee. MRI has been criticized for high false-positive and false-negative rates in pediatric populations, but with modern techniques, MRI can be valuable in confirming a clinical diagnosis of ACL rupture, identifying osteochondral injury, and diagnosing concomitant meniscal pathology.[23,36]

The most important part of the pediatric workup is determination of skeletal maturity. Multiple methods can be used, including Tanner staging, radiographic bone age using the radiographic atlas of Greulich and Pyle, and determination peak height velocity.[29,37,38] Additionally, onset of menses is an important historical component when treating adolescent females, as it heralds an end to skeletal growth. As no single method is 100% accurate, it may be best prudent to use more than one technique prior to making establishing a definitive treatment plan.

Nonoperative Treatment

Nonoperative treatment in the context of a complete ACL tear should be reserved only for those patients willing to accept the significant degree of activity modification necessary to avoid the further meniscal and chondral injury that can lead to accelerated arthrosis. Woods and O'Connor[12] reported on a small group of adolescents with complete ACL tears managed successfully with activity modification when compared to a group who underwent early reconstruction. Their study, however, may have been underpowered to detect any real differences between the groups, making it difficult to draw any firm conclusions from their data.

Kocher et al[39] reported a 31% rate of ACL reconstruction resulting from recurrent instability and reinjury in a group of predominantly skeletally immature patients with incomplete tears of the ACL treated nonoperatively. Following a course of limited weight bearing, progressive mobilization in a hinged knee brace, and supervised physical therapy, return to sports was permitted at 3 months after injury in all cases. All episodes of instability and reinjury occurred during athletic activity. Multivariate analysis identified partial tears of the posterolateral bundle of the ACL and tears measuring more than 50% of the ligament diameter (judged arthroscopically) to be independent predictors of subsequent reconstruction.

Millet et al[26] found a statistically significant correlation between time to reconstruction following complete tear of the ACL and occurrence of medial meniscus injury in a skeletally immature population. This retrospective study did not, as did that of Woods and O'Connor, include a group treated with a specific nonoperative strategy of patient education and activity modification. These studies underscore the absolute necessity of education and strict activity modification if nonoperative treatment of complete tears of the ACL in skeletally immature patients is to be successful.

Surgery
Primary Repair
Isolated primary repair of complete intrasubstance ACL tears has not been successful in reestablishing stability to the knee and is not recommended.

Extraphyseal and Partial Transphyseal Reconstruction
Extraphyseal reconstruction, in which either the femoral- or tibial-side attachments of the graft, or both, are routed around rather than through the physis is reserved only for those patients having a significant amount of growth remaining. These reconstructions are nonanatomic and nonisometric and tend to be less durable than standard transphyseal reconstructions, possibly necessitating revision at a later age. Multiple techniques have been reported with varying results. Andrews et al[40] described a partial transphyseal technique in which a soft-tissue graft is routed through a 6- to 7-mm central, transphyseal tibial tunnel and subsequently into the "over-the-top" position on the femur. Both the femoral and tibial sides of the graft are secured in an extraphyseal fashion with posts. The authors reported on the use of this technique in a group of eight patients, ages 10 to 15 years, whom they followed through skeletal maturity with scanograms to identify any leg length discrepancy. No significant discrepancy or angular deformity was detected. All patients returned to athletic activity and KT-1000 arthrometer readings at the time of final follow-up were less than 3-mm displacement in four patients and less than 5 mm in the remaining four.

Transphyseal Reconstruction
Reconstruction with hamstring autograft is the procedure of choice for most skeletally immature patients undergoing ACL reconstruction.[41] By minimizing tunnel diameter and orienting the tunnels vertically through the physes, one reduces the cross-sectional area of physis disrupted by tunnel placement. The EndoButton (Smith and Nephew) or other extraphyseal means of fixation is used for the femoral side, and a standard post is used for tibial-side fixation. Additionally, one should avoid subperiosteal dissection around the femoral metaphysis, as this can lead to cortical bridging across the physis. The graft is tensioned with the knee in full extension.

Use of hamstring autograft versus BPTB autograft avoids the disruption of the tibial tubercle apophysis that occurs with harvest of the latter and also avoids placement of bone blocks across the physis. Nevertheless, Shelbourne et al[42] reported excellent results, without gross growth disturbance, following BPTB autograft reconstruction of Tanner stage 3 or 4 patients with "clearly" open physes. In this study, the authors altered standard BPTB technique, using a shortened tibial bone block and drilling the femoral tunnel such that the graft seated in a more proximal position than normal, resulting in both the femoral and tibial bone blocks resting proximal to their respec-

Table 52-3 Recommended Method of Anterior Cruciate Ligament Reconstruction by Skeletal Age

Skeletal Age	Gender	Graft	Femoral	Tibial
12	Male/female	HS	OTT	Transepiphyseal
13	Male/female	HS	OTT	Transphyseal tunnel with extraphyseal fixation
14	Male	HS	OTT	Transphyseal tunnel with extraphyseal fixation
	Female	HS/BTB	FT	Transphyseal tunnel
15	Male	HS	OTT/FT	Transphyseal tunnel with extraphyseal fixation
	Female	HS/BTB	FT	Transphyseal tunnel
16	Male/female	HS/BTB	FT	Transphyseal tunnel

BTB, Bone-tendon bone; FT, femoral tunnel; HS, hamstring; OTT, over the top.

From Pavlovich R, Goldberg SH, Bach BR: Adolescent ACL injury. J Knee Surg 2004;17:79–93.

tive physes. This technique requires meticulous attention to graft and tunnel lengths to avoid crossing the physis with a bony block. An algorithm of recommended reconstructive procedures based on skeletal age is presented in Table 52-3.

CONCLUSIONS

In the vast majority of cases, ligament reconstruction following complete tear of the ACL predictably restores stability to the injured knee and permits return to activity. Nevertheless, a number of difficult scenarios can complicate reconstruction, producing suboptimal results. Revision of a failed ACL reconstruction requires diligent preoperative planning, including clear identification of the mode of failure, as well as the technical ability to correct tunnel malposition and achieve secure graft fixation using multiple strategies. Chondral injury in the context of ACL injury, whether acute or in the context of the chronically ACL-deficient knee, presents a particularly challenging problem. In addition to ligament reconstruction, the surgeon may need to perform a corrective osteotomy or one of several biologic resurfacing procedures either at the time of ACL reconstruction or in a staged fashion. Finally, treatment of ACL injury in the skeletally immature requires careful evaluation of the patient's remaining growth potential and demands a shared decision-making process that involves the patient and patient's parents. The surgeon and family must weigh the risk of further intra-articular injury incumbent with nonoperative treatment versus reconstruction and the possibility of iatrogenic physeal injury with resultant length or angular deformity.

REFERENCES

1. Bealle D, Johnson DL: Technical pitfalls of anterior cruciate ligament surgery. Clin Sports Med 1999;18:831–845.
2. Brown CH Jr, Carson EW: Revision anterior cruciate ligament surgery. Clin Sports Med 1999;18:109–171.
3. Allen CR, Giffin JR, Harner CD: Revision anterior cruciate ligament reconstruction. Orthop Clin North Am 2003;34:79–98.
4. Bach BR Jr: Revision anterior cruciate ligament surgery. Arthroscopy 2003;19(Suppl 1):14–29.
5. Uribe JW, Hectman KS, Zuijac JE, et al: Revision anterior cruciate ligament surgery: Experience from Miami. Clin Orthop 1996;325:91–99.
6. Johnson DL, Fu FH: Anterior cruciate ligament reconstruction: Why do failures occur? Instr Course Lect 1995;44:391–406.
7. Getelman MH, Friedman MJ: Revision anterior cruciate ligament reconstruction surgery. J Am Acad Orthop Surg 1999;7:189–198.
8. Noyes FR, Barber-Westin SD, Hewett TE: High tibial osteotomy and ligament reconstruction for varus angulated anterior cruciate ligament-deficient knees. Am J Sports Med 2000;28:282–296.
9. Bush-Joseph CA, Bach BR Jr: Migration of femoral interference screw after anterior cruciate ligament reconstruction. Am J Knee Surg 1998;11:32–34.
10. Dworsky BD, Jewell BF, Bach BR Jr: Interference screw divergence in endoscopic anterior cruciate ligament reconstruction. Arthroscopy 1996;12:45–49.
11. Novak PJ, Wexler GM, Williams JS Jr., et al: Comparison of screw post fixation and free bone block interference fixation for anterior cruciate ligament soft tissue grafts: Biomechanical considerations. Arthroscopy 1996;12:470–473.
12. Woods GW, O'Connor PD: Delayed anterior cruciate ligament reconstruction in adolescents with open physes. Am J Sports Med 2004;32:201–210.
13. Fox JA, Pierce M, Bojchuk J, et al: Revision anterior cruciate ligament reconstruction with nonirradiated fresh-frozen patellar tendon allograft. Arthroscopy 2004;20:787–794.
14. Smith RA, Ingels J, Lochemes JJ, et al: Gamma irradiation of HIV-1. J Orthop Res 2001;19:815–819.
15. Fideler BM, Vangsness CT Jr., Lu B, et al: Gamma irradiation: Effects on biomechanical properties of human bone-patellar tendon-bone allografts. Am J Sports Med 1995;23:643–646.
16. Murrell GA, Maddali S, Horovitz L, et al: The effects of time course after anterior cruciate ligament injury in correlation with meniscal and cartilage loss. Am J Sports Med 2001;29:9–14.
17. Shelbourne KD, Gray T: Results of anterior cruciate ligament reconstruction based on meniscus and articular cartilage status at the time of surgery. Five- to fifteen-year evaluations. Am J Sports Med 2000;28:446–452.
18. Shelbourne KD, Stube KC: Anterior cruciate ligament (ACL)-deficient knee with degenerative arthrosis: Treatment with an isolated autogenous patellar tendon ACL reconstruction. Knee Surg Sports Traumatol Arthrosc 1997;5:150–156.
19. Levy AS, Meier SW: Approach to cartilage injury in the anterior cruciate ligament deficient knee. Orthop Clin North Am 2003;34:149–167.
20. Williams RJ 3rd, Wickiewicz TL, Warren RF: Management of unicompartmental arthritis in the anterior cruciate ligament-deficient knee. Am J Sports Med 2000;28:749–760.
21. Cole BJ, Carter TR, Rodeo SA: Allograft meniscal transplantation: Background, techniques, and results. Instr Course Lect 2003;52:383–396.
22. Sekiya JK, Giffin JR, Irrgang JJ, et al: Clinical outcomes after combined meniscal allograft transplantation and anterior cruciate ligament reconstruction. Am J Sports Med 2003;31:896–906.
23. Dorizas JA, Stanitski CL: Anterior cruciate ligament injury in the skeletally immature. Orthop Clin North Am 2003;34:355–363.
24. Stanitski CL, Harvell JC, Fu F: Observations on acute knee hemarthrosis in children and adolescents. J Pediatr Orthop 1993;13:506–510.
25. Kannus P, Jarvinen M: Knee ligament injuries in adolescents. Eight year follow-up of conservative management. J Bone Joint Surg Br 1988;70:772–776.

26. Millett PJ, Willis AA, Warren RF: Associated injuries in pediatric and adolescent anterior cruciate ligament tears: Does a delay in treatment increase the risk of meniscal tear? Arthroscopy 2002;18:955–959.

27. Mizuta H, Kubota K, Shiraishi M, et al: The conservative treatment of complete tears of the anterior cruciate ligament in skeletally immature patients. J Bone Joint Surg Br 1995;77:890–894.

28. Koman JD, Sanders JO: Valgus deformity after reconstruction of the anterior cruciate ligament in a skeletally immature patient. A case report. J Bone Joint Surg Am 1999;81:711–715.

29. Paletta GA Jr: Special considerations. Anterior cruciate ligament reconstruction in the skeletally immature. Orthop Clin North Am 2003;34:65–77.

30. Kellenberger R. von Laer L: Nonosseous lesions of the anterior cruciate ligaments in childhood and adolescence. Prog Pediatr Surg 1990;25:123–131.

31. Wessel LM, Scholz S, Rusch M, et al: Hemarthrosis after trauma to the pediatric knee joint: What is the value of magnetic resonance imaging in the diagnostic algorithm? J Pediatr Orthop 2001;21:338–342.

32. Stadelmaier DM, Arnoczky SP, Dodds J, Ross H: The effect of drilling and soft tissue grafting across open growth plates. A histologic study. Am J Sports Med 1995;23:431–435.

33. Makela EA, Vainionpaa S, Vihtonen K, et al: The effect of trauma to the lower femoral epiphyseal plate. An experimental study in rabbits. J Bone Joint Surg Br 1988;70:187–191.

34. Edwards TB, Greene CC, Baratta RV, et al: The effect of placing a tensioned graft across open growth plates. A gross and histologic analysis. J Bone Joint Surg Am 2001;83:725–734.

35. Behr CT, Potter HG, Paletta GA Jr: The relationship of the femoral origin of the anterior cruciate ligament and the distal femoral physeal plate in the skeletally immature knee. An anatomic study. Am J Sports Med 2001;29:781–787.

36. Lee K, Siegel MJ, Lau DM, et al: Anterior cruciate ligament tears: MR imaging-based diagnosis in a pediatric population. Radiology 1999;213:697–704.

37. Greulich WW, Pyle SI: Radiographic Atlas of Skeletal Development of the Hand and Wrist. Stanford, CA, Stanford University Press, 1950.

38. Guzzanti V, Falciglia F, Stanitski CL: Preoperative evaluation and anterior cruciate ligament reconstruction technique for skeletally immature patients in Tanner stages 2 and 3. Am J Sports Med 2003;31:941–948.

39. Kocher MS, Micheli LJ, Zurakowski D, Luke A: Partial tears of the anterior cruciate ligament in children and adolescents. Am J Sports Med 2002;30:697–703.

40. Andrews M, Noyes FR, Barber-Westin SD: Anterior cruciate ligament allograft reconstruction in the skeletally immature athlete. Am J Sports Med 1994;22:48–54.

41. Larson RV, Ulmer T: Ligament injuries in children. Instr Course Lect 2003;52:677–681.

42. Shelbourne KD, Gray T, Wiley BV: Results of transphyseal anterior cruciate ligament reconstruction using patellar tendon autograft in tanner stage 3 or 4 adolescents with clearly open growth plates. Am J Sports Med 2004;32:1218–1222.

CHAPTER

53 Posterior Cruciate Ligament

Todd C. Battaglia, Kevin J. Mulhall, and Mark D. Miller

In This Chapter

INTRODUCTION

- PCL injury is less common than injury to the anterior cruciate ligament (ACL).

- Information concerning PCL anatomy and biomechanics as well as the natural history of PCL deficiency and outcomes of surgical reconstruction is rapidly increasing.

- PCL injuries usually occur in athletic or high-energy trauma situations as a result of a posteriorly applied force to the anterior tibia.

- Most isolated, low-grade injuries are managed nonoperatively through an aggressive rehabilitation program. High-grade injuries, avulsions, and those combined with other ligamentous injuries are often treated with surgical reconstruction. Numerous surgical techniques have been described.

- Although most isolated PCL injuries are treated conservatively, some studies suggest that chronic PCL deficiency may lead to progressive joint degeneration and arthritis.

RELEVANT ANATOMY

The PCL originates in an irregular, elliptical attachment on the posterolateral border of the medial femoral condyle where the roof of the notch joins the wall, 2 to 3 mm from the articular surface[1-3] (Fig. 53-1). It extends posteriorly, inferiorly, and slightly laterally to insert in a depression between the medial and lateral tibial plateaus termed the PCL facet or fovea. This depression is located 1 to 1.5 cm below the posterior tibial rim and joint line[3] (Fig. 53-2). The PCL is an intra-articular but extracapsular (and therefore extrasynovial) structure, and reflected synovium from the posterior capsule surrounds the medial, lateral, and anterior borders of the ligament.[4-6] The ligament is in close proximity to the posterior neurovascular bundle throughout its length.[1]

The PCL is composed primarily of type I collagen, although the mean fibril diameter varies with location and decreases proximally to distally.[6] The major blood supply is via the middle geniculate artery. The average ligament length is 30 to 38 mm, and the width averages 13 mm.[1,5,6] The cross-sectional area is approximately 30 mm^2 at mid-substance; this is 1.5 times that of ACL.[5] The insertion sites are even larger, with cross-sectional areas three times larger than that in the midsubstance.[2,5] Overall, the PCL is the strongest ligament crossing the knee and may be as much as twice as strong as the ACL.

Multiple models have been used to describe intrinsic PCL anatomy, including models containing three and four bundle divisions as well as a continuum of fiber orientation. In a simplified model, however, there are three main components to the PCL complex: the anterolateral (AL) bundle, the posteromedial (PM) bundle, and meniscofemoral ligaments. The PCL proper is composed of the AL and PM bundles, of which the former is the larger and stronger. These distinctions are more functional than anatomic, as the AL and PM portions are difficult to separate macroscopically or microscopically.[7] Although the insertion sites of the two bundles are relatively equal in size, the AL bundle has approximately two to three times the cross section of the PM and may be as much as five times stronger than the PM bundle.[2-4,8]

The AL bundle begins more anteriorly on the intercondylar surface of the medial femoral condyle, runs laterally, and inserts posteriorly on the lateral aspect of the tibial fovea. The PL bundle begins more posteriorly on the intercondylar femoral surface and inserts on the medial aspect of the fovea.[7] Very few fibers of the PCL are truly isometric during the knee flexion arc.[4,5] The AL band is tighter and thus more important in knee flexion, while the PM band tightens in extension (Fig. 53-3). During a knee flexion cycle, tension in the bundles appears to develop in a reciprocal fashion.[1,9]

The PCL is considered the primary restraint to posterior tibial translation, especially when the knee is flexed more than 30 degrees. In PCL-deficient knees, translation is minimal when the knee is in full extension and maximal at 90 degrees.[9] The ligament is also a secondary restraint to varus and valgus force and to external tibial rotation, aiding the posterolateral corner complex (PLCC).[3] Since it lies near the central axis of the knee, however, the PCL has a relatively small moment arm about the knee axis of rotation.[7,8] Biomechanically, the PCL has an ultimate load of approximately 1600 N and a stiffness of 200 N/mm. Forces in response to given anterior tibial load increase as much as fourfold as the knee moves from full extension to 90 degrees of flexion.[2]

Two variable meniscofemoral ligaments originate from posterior horn of the lateral meniscus and run alongside and contribute fibers to the PCL. The ligament of Humphry passes anterior to the PCL and attaches distally, while the ligament of Wrisberg passes posteriorly and attaches proximally (Fig. 53-4).

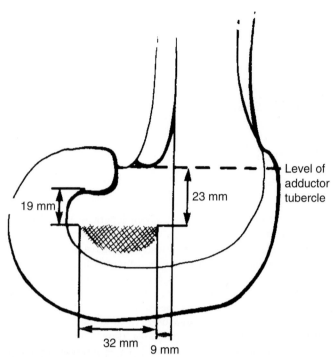

Figure 53-1 The origin of the posterior cruciate ligament forms an ellipse on the posterior portion of the medial femoral condyle. (From Giffin JR, Annunziata CC, Harner CD: Posterior cruciate ligament injuries in the adult. In DeLee JC, Drez D Jr, Miller MD [eds]: Orthopaedic Sports Medicine, 2nd ed. Philadelphia, WB Saunders, 2003, pp 2083–2106.)

At least one ligament is present in more than 90% of specimens and both are found more commonly in younger patients, suggesting that they may degenerate with age.[8,10] These meniscofemoral ligaments are believed to provide significant anatomic and biomechanical stability to the lateral meniscus, although their precise role is not currently well defined.[9] The ligament of

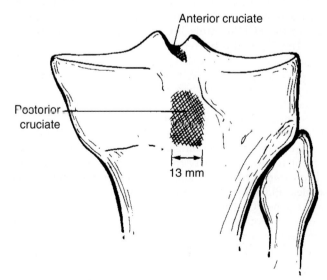

Figure 53-2 The posterior cruciate ligament inserts in a central depression called the tibial fovea located 1 to 1.5 cm below the tibial joint line. (From Giffin JR, Annunziata CC, Harner CD: Posterior cruciate ligament injuries in the adult. In DeLee JC, Drez D Jr, Miller MD [eds]: Orthopaedic Sports Medicine, 2nd ed. Philadelphia, WB Saunders, 2003, pp 2083–2106.)

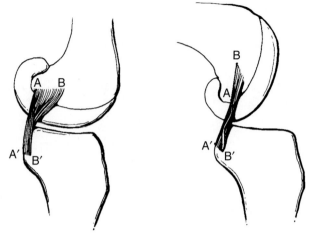

Figure 53-3 The posteromedial bundle of the posterior cruciate ligament (A-A′) is taut in extension and lax in flexion, while the anterolateral bundle (B-B′) is reciprocally tight in flexion and lax in extension. (From Giffin JR, Annunziata CC, Harner CD: Posterior cruciate ligament injuries in the adult. In DeLee JC, Drez D Jr, Miller MD [eds]: Orthopaedic Sports Medicine, 2nd ed. Philadelphia, WB Saunders, 2003, pp 2083–2106.)

Humphry is usually smaller than the ligament of Wrisberg, but the strength of each is comparable to that of each other and to that of the PM band of the PCL.[8] These ligaments may act as secondary restraints to posterior tibial translation, especially when the knee is flexed. Meniscofemoral ligaments may sometimes be preserved in the PCL-injured knee, making posterior laxity less dramatic.[2]

Other ligaments about the knee, the lateral collateral ligament, medial collateral ligament (MCL), and especially the PLCC, are secondary stabilizers to posterior tibial translation, playing a minimal role if the PCL is intact but become important if the PCL is deficient.[1] In cadaveric studies, if only the PCL is sectioned, an average posterior tibial translation of 11 to 15 mm results; however, if the PLCC is also disrupted, posterior translation approaches 30 mm.[1,2] Muscle forces about the knee also affect in situ forces on the PCL. Specifically, popliteus and quadriceps contraction can reduce PCL load, whereas hamstring and gastrocnemius contraction increase it.[9]

ETIOLOGY OF INJURY

Historically, PCL injuries have been underdiagnosed. Recent studies describe PCL tears as accounting for 3% to 20% or more of all knee ligament tears, although still occurring less frequently than injuries of the ACL, MCL, and lateral collateral ligament.[1,7,11-13] It is reported that dedicated arthroscopists and orthopedic sports physicians may perform only one tenth the number of PCL reconstructions as ACL reconstructions annually.[14]

The average age for PCL injury is approximately 30 years old. Athletic injuries account for as many as two thirds of all injuries, with high-energy trauma, especially motor vehicle accidents, accounting for much of the remainder.[14] The most common sports in which PCL injury occurs involve high-contact forces, such as rugby and football. Injury occurs less frequently in the cutting and pivoting activities classically associated with ACL injury, such as basketball and soccer. Sporting injuries more fre-

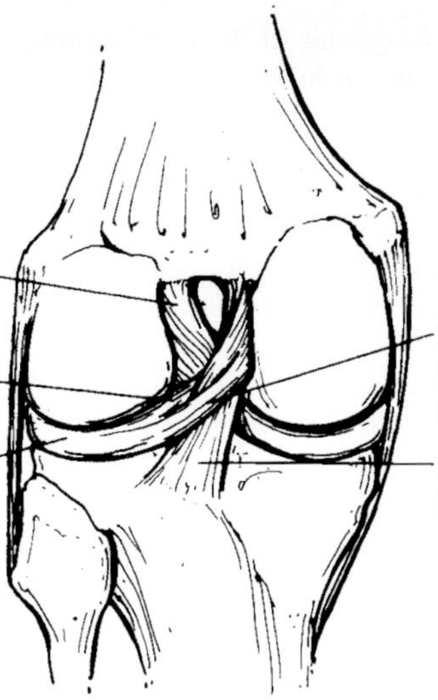

Figure 53-4 The meniscofemoral ligaments arise from the lateral meniscus and run alongside of the posterior cruciate ligament. (From Giffin JR, Annunziata CC, Harner CD: Posterior cruciate ligament injuries in the adult. In DeLee JC, Drez D Jr, Miller MD [eds]: Orthopaedic Sports Medicine, 2nd ed. Philadelphia, WB Saunders, 2003, pp 2083–2106.)

Anterior cruciate ligament

Anterior meniscofemoral ligament (ligament of Humphry)

Posterior horn of lateral meniscus

Posterior meniscofemoral ligament (ligament of Wrisberg)

Posterior cruciate ligament

quently involve isolated PCL tears, while some authors report that as many as 90% of emergency department trauma patients with PCL disruptions have combined ligamentous injuries. Typically, these arc higher grade PCL disruptions and are associated with injury involving the PLCC structures.[3,5]

Regardless of the circumstances, the most common mechanism of injury involves a posteriorly directed force to the proximal tibia of a flexed knee (Fig. 53-5). This may occur in contact sports when a tackle causes a direct blow to the anterior tibia but also may occur when a player falls forward onto the knee, especially if the foot is in plantar flexion, which allows the ground force vector to intersect the proximal tibia. When the foot is dorsiflexed, the ground force vector contacts the patella and distal femur, avoiding undue stress across the knee ligaments. In motor vehicle trauma, the classic mechanism involves a dashboard injury in which the knee and proximal tibia of a front seat rider strikes the dashboard.[1] Forced hyperflexion with or without tibial load is a less common but well-reported mechanism of injury. Indirect methods of injury include twisting and hyperextension and often lead to combined ligament injuries.[1,7] Significant varus or valgus force usually only disrupts the PCL after rupture of the appropriate collateral ligament.[13]

CLINICAL FEATURES AND EVALUATION

The first step in determining appropriate management is accurate diagnosis. Isolated PCL tears are commonly overlooked during the initial evaluation, as history is often vague and physical examination findings are subtle. Partial, or even complete, isolated tears usually present with relatively benign symptoms.[1] A thorough history should be obtained with special emphasis on the mechanism of injury, as this may give important information regarding injury severity and possible associated injuries.

Unfortunately, awareness of ligamentous injury at the moment of PCL disruption is infrequent and many patients are unable to describe precisely how the injury occurred. Some patients may describe a "pop" or tearing sensation at the moment of injury but be unable to describe the exact biomechanical forces that occurred. Location and timing of pain, sensation of instability, and performance-related impairment are important complaints to elicit. During the acute phase of injury, patients may complain of a mild or moderate effusion and posterior knee pain or pain with kneeling. Instability in isolated PCL injury is an infrequent complaint and should lead the physician to suspect associated injuries. In subacute or chronic PCL injury, complaints may include vague anterior knee pain or pain with deceleration or stair descent. Commonly in chronic injury, patients may describe dull, aching pain localized to the patellofemoral and medial compartments.[5]

On physical examination, observe the patient's gait and static weight-bearing alignment of the extremity. Varus thrust, where the knee shifts into varus during foot strike, is common in chronic posterolateral deficiency.[1,2] In acute injury, the skin

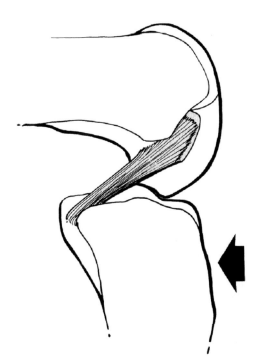

Figure 53-5 The most common mechanism of posterior cruciate ligament injury involves a direct force to the front of a flexed knee. (From Giffin JR, Annunziata CC, Harner CD: Posterior cruciate ligament injuries in the adult. In DeLee JC, Drez D Jr, Miller MD [eds]: Orthopaedic Sports Medicine, 2nd ed. Philadelphia, WB Saunders, 2003, pp 2083–2106.)

should be observed for any signs of trauma, especially over proximal tibia, and bruising may be found in the popliteal fossa from posterior capsular rupture.

There are a number of specific maneuvers described to evaluate the PCL and its associated structures. Of these, the posterior drawer test is considered the most accurate (Box 53-1).

Posterior Drawer Test

In this maneuver, the patient is supine with the feet on the table, the hip flexed 45 degrees and the knee flexed 80 to 90 degrees. Because the posterior drawer test is based on the relationship between the medial femoral condyle and the medial tibial plateau, comparison to the contralateral side is important in interpretation. First, the examiner must evaluate the tibial starting point. Normally, the tibial plateau step-off is approximately 1 cm anterior to the femoral condyle (Fig. 53-6). If a normal step-off is not palpated, PCL injury should be suspected. Next, a posteriorly directed force is applied to the anterior tibia. In a grade I injury, a palpable but diminished step-off is present, in which the tibial plateau remains anterior to the medial condyle (0- to 5-mm tibial displacement). In grade II injury, the plateau is palpated flush (5- to 10-mm displacement) but cannot be displaced behind the medial femoral condyle, and grade III refers

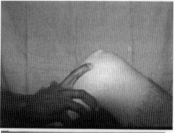

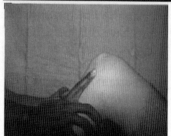

Figure 53-6 Tibial step-off is assessed during the posterior drawer test. The examiner's finger is used to palpate the relationship of the medial tibial plateau to the medial femoral condyle. (From Allen CR, Rihn JA, Harner CD: Posterior cruciate ligament: Diagnosis and decision making. In Miller MD, Cole BJ [eds]: Textbook of Arthroscopy. Philadelphia, WB Saunders, 2004, pp 687–702.)

to cases in which the plateau can be displaced posterior to the condyle (10- to 15-mm displacement)[15] (Fig. 53-7). One should also assess the endpoint when performing the posterior drawer test. Most acute injuries have an altered endpoint, although this may return to normal in chronic injuries in as quickly as a few weeks.[4]

If the tibia displaces more than 10mm (grade III laxity), a combined injury, most commonly involving the PLCC, should be suspected. Careful examination of the ACL, collateral ligaments, and PLCC is crucial. PCL injury typically allows maximal posterior translation at 90 degrees of knee flexion, which is why the posterior drawer test is performed in this position. Maximal translation at 30 degrees, which decreases at 90 degrees, may indicate isolated PLCC injury.[13] It is also critical to recognize that PCL incompetence may cause the tibia to rest in a posteriorly subluxed position, causing a false-positive Lachman test. In fact, it has been reported that 15% of patients surgically treated for isolated PCL injuries have previously undergone unnecessary ACL reconstruction as result of misdiagnosis (Box 53-2).[5]

Posterior Sag (Godfrey) Test

Here, the patient is also supine with the knee flexed 90 degrees. The examiner looks for abnormal contour or sag at the proximal tibia compared to the contralateral side. This subluxation may be accentuated by passive elevation of the heels.[1,6]

Quadriceps Active Test

Again, the patient is supine with the knee flexed 60 to 90 degrees and the foot secured on the table. In an intact knee, voluntary quadriceps activation will result in slight posterior tibial translation. In PCL injury, however, with resisted knee extension and quadriceps contraction, the posteriorly subluxated tibia reduces anteriorly. This test may be useful in assessing relative anterior and posterior instability in patients with combined ACL and PCL deficiency.[2] (Fig. 53-8).

Dynamic Posterior Shift

With the hip and knee flexed 90 degrees, the knee is slowly extended. As the knee reaches full extension, the subluxed tibia reduces, often occurring with a palpable clunk.[2]

Reverse Pivot Shift

With the patient supine and the knee flexed 90 degrees, the foot is externally rotated and the knee extended with an applied

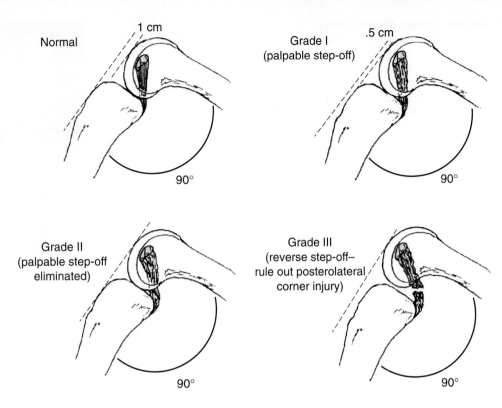

Figure 53-7 Classification of posterior cruciate ligament injury, as assessed with the posterior drawer test. In a normal knee, the anterior edge of the medial tibial plateau is palpated 1 to 1.5 cm anterior to the medial femoral condyle. In grade I injury, 0 to 5 mm of posterior tibial displacement is possible. In grade II injury, the tibia can be displaced flush with the femur (5 to 10 mm of displacement), and in grade III injury (>10 mm), the tibia can be displaced posterior to the condyle. (From Petrie RS, Harner CD: Evaluation and management of the posterior cruciate injured knee. Oper Tech Sports Med 1999;7:93–103.)

valgus stress. A positive test occurs with palpable reduction of the displaced tibia at 20 to 30 degrees of knee flexion. It is important to examine the opposite knee, as a positive reverse pivot can be a normal variant in some patients.[1]

Dial (Tibia External Rotation) Test

This is considered the most important test for posterolateral instability and is most easily performed with the patient prone.

The tibiae are externally rotated, and the thigh-foot angle measured and compared between sides. A pathologic examination is indicated by more than 10 to 15 degrees of asymmetry. The test should be performed with the knees at both 30 and 90 degrees of flexion. If asymmetry exists only at 30 degrees, this most likely indicates an isolated PLCC injury, but if asymmetry exists at both 30 and 90 degrees, combined PLCC and PCL injury should be suspected.

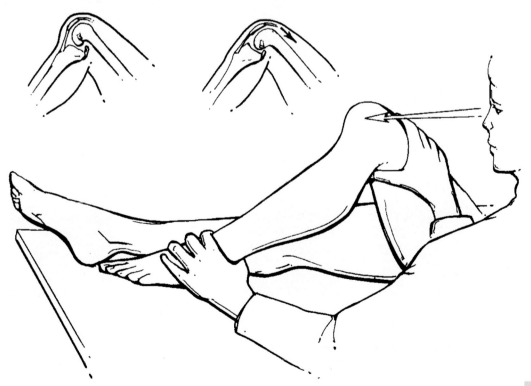

Figure 53-8 In the quadriceps active test, quadriceps contraction will reduce the posteriorly displaced tibia. (From Giffin JR, Annunziata CC, Harner CD: Posterior cruciate ligament injuries in the adult. In DeLee JC, Drez D Jr, Miller MD [eds]: Orthopaedic Sports Medicine, 2nd ed. Philadelphia, WB Saunders, 2003, pp 2083–2106.)

Whipple (Prone Drawer) Test

With the patient prone, the knee is flexed to 70 degrees. PCL insufficiency is tested by grasping the lower leg with one hand and posteriorly displacing the tibia with the other by pushing on the tibial tubercle. Although similar to the posterior drawer test, the prone position theoretically avoids quadriceps contraction, which could interfere with the examination.[5,6]

Radiography

Any knee trauma should have a complete radiographic evaluation, including anteroposterior, lateral, sunrise, and tunnel views. Avulsion injuries (of the PCL, Gerdy's tubercle, or fibular head), Segond fractures, posterior tibial sag, and lateral joint space widening should be noted (Fig. 53-9). Oblique radiographs may be necessary to evaluate for tibial plateau fractures. Flexion weight-bearing views are useful in chronic cases to assess limb alignment and medial compartment degeneration. Stress radiographs and contralateral comparison views may be useful in difficult cases; a lateral film with posterior tibial force will allow direct measure of posterior translation. A modified Laurin radiograph with or without weights (a sunrise view taken with the knee flexed 70 degrees) may demonstrate increased distance between the anterior femoral condyles and the anterior tibial edge, indicative of posterior tibial subluxation.[6]

With appropriate techniques and criteria, the sensitivity and specificity of magnetic resonance imaging in the diagnosis of complete PCL tears are thought to approach 100%. On magnetic resonance imaging, the normal PCL appears as a uniform band of low signal intensity. On sagittal images with the knee extended, the PCL is usually seen on one to two contiguous slices with an arcuate shape, whereas on coronal images, it appears as a vertically oblique band (Fig. 53-10). The meniscofemoral ligaments are seen on only 60% of magnetic resonance

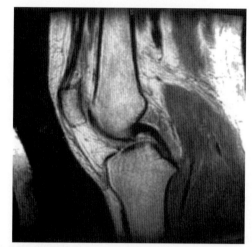

Figure 53-10 Sagittal magnetic resonance image of a normal posterior cruciate ligament. (From Allen CR, Rihn JA, Harner CD: Posterior cruciate ligament: Diagnosis and decision making. In Miller MD, Cole BJ [eds]: Textbook of Arthroscopy. Philadelphia, WB Saunders, 2004, pp 687–702.)

imaging studies, running in an oblique course adjacent to the anterior and posterior margins of the PCL.[3]

On magnetic resonance imaging, PCL injury typically appears as tearing of a portion, or the entire bulk, of PCL fibers; this is best evaluated on T2-weighted images with fat saturation (Fig. 53-11). Partial intrasubstance tears will be seen as thickening of the ligament with edema and hemorrhage causing fiber separation and associated increases in signal intensity.[1,3] Isolated tears most frequently involve the midsubstance or anterior genu and

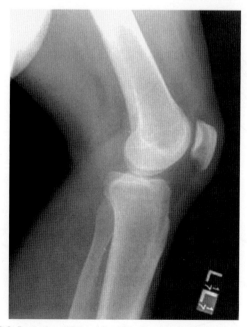

Figure 53-9 Posterior tibial subluxation in a posterior cruciate ligament–deficient knee. (From Allen CR, Rihn JA, Harner CD: Posterior cruciate ligament: Diagnosis and decision making. In Miller MD, Cole BJ [eds]: Textbook of Arthroscopy. Philadelphia, WB Saunders, 2004, pp 687–702.)

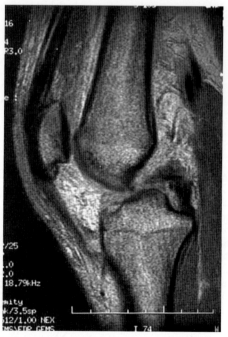

Figure 53-11 Magnetic resonance image of a complete posterior cruciate ligament tear. (From Allen CR, Rihn JA, Harner CD: Posterior cruciate ligament: Diagnosis and decision making. In Miller MD, Cole BJ [eds]: Textbook of Arthroscopy. Philadelphia, WB Saunders, 2004, pp 687–702.)

less commonly the ligament attachments, although insertions are frequently disrupted in cases of knee dislocation or combined ligament injuries. Because there is some evidence that PCL tears can heal in an elongated fashion, chronic tears (especially grades I and II) may look normal on magnetic resonance imaging. If healed with fibrosis, the ligament may demonstrate abnormal low signal along its length.[1,3]

Meniscal tears and bone bruises are less commonly associated with isolated PCL tears than with ACL tears. In injuries due to posterior tibial displacement in a flexed knee, any associated bone bruising typically occurs along the anterior tibial articular surfaces and posterolateral femoral condyles. In acute hyperextension injuries, bone bruising may be seen at the anterior tibia and anterior femoral condyles.[3,4] Finally, posterior tibial sag may create an illusion of ACL laxity and lead to false diagnoses of ACL injury.[1]

Diagnostic Arthroscopy

Although the diagnosis should be clear before surgery, anesthesia will allow full examination of all structures, and numerous arthroscopic signs of PCL injury have been described. These include partial or complete disruption of fibers, insertion site avulsions, hemorrhage, and decreased ligament tension. Indirect evidence includes ACL pseudolaxity resulting from posterior tibial displacement, altered contact points between the tibia and femur, and degenerative patellofemoral and medial compartment changes.[2,6] The PCL can usually be seen in its entirety using a 70-degree scope placed through the notch; if the tibial insertion is not visualized, a posteromedial portal will allow access. Because the PCL lies extrasynovially, it may appear normal unless the synovium is débrided.

NATURAL HISTORY

It is widely agreed that when PCL injury occurs in combination with other major knee ligament injuries or when it occurs via bony avulsion, outcomes with nonoperative treatment are much poorer than with surgical intervention. The management of isolated PCL injuries is more controversial, however, because the natural history of isolated PCL injuries continues to be debated. Most series that report the results of nonoperative treatment of PCL tears include patients with mixed injury patterns and severities.

While many authors believe that the PCL has some potential for intrinsic healing, this healing phenomena does not necessarily restore normal functional status.[1,11,16] Regardless, in some studies, as many as 80% of patients with isolated PCL injuries managed nonoperatively with quadriceps and hamstring strengthening were satisfied with their outcome, and most returned to preinjury levels of activity.[17] Furthermore, many high-caliber athletes may function well with PCL-deficient knees because as many as 2% of high-caliber college football players have been found to have a chronic PCL-deficient knee. The outcome of nonoperative treatment may depend on the patient's ability to maintain quadriceps strength, as patients with better functional results appear to be those with greater quadriceps strength in the affected extremity.[17] Many of these individuals have residual translation on posterior drawer testing, but this laxity does not appear to increase over time.[12]

Conversely, other authors suggest that even after isolated PCL injuries, many patients have frequent pain and occasional instability and giving way.[1] In one study, although 88% of com-

petitive rugby players with isolated PCL injuries were able to return to preinjury levels of play, some patients took as long as 7 months to recover and nearly all reported subjective sensations of impaired ability, most commonly manifesting in high-speed running (slower acceleration and delayed response) and while turning.[18] Long-term follow-ups have found that as many as 90% of patients with isolated PCL injuries may have persistent pain while walking, 45% report episodic instability, 65% report limitations of activity, and more than 50% demonstrate evidence of degenerative changes.[4,7] Increasing literature points to a significant incidence of knee pain, patellofemoral symptoms, and medial compartment degeneration in the PCL-deficient knee. This is likely due to altered knee kinematics, with increased quadriceps activity, altered articular contact pressures (especially patellofemoral) and abnormal tibial translation and rotation noted under complex muscle loads in the PCL-deficient knee.[19]

Overall, although there currently exists a lack of conclusive scientific and clinical information, nonoperative management of isolated PCL tears is probably not as benign as previously believed. Whereas the outcome of conservative treatment of isolated mild injuries is likely acceptable, conservative treatment of more severe isolated injuries or of combined injuries leads to a worse outcome.[15] Whether the PCL-deficient knee is at great risk of the development of significant degenerative changes is not clear, although it appears that progressive changes may occur in some affected knees.

TREATMENT OPTIONS AND RECOMMENDATIONS

Traditionally, nonoperative treatment of isolated PCL injuries has been favored, especially with lower grade injuries. This is based on both the capacity of the ligament to heal and some outcome studies demonstrating excellent results in these patients. It appears that individuals are often able to compensate for PCL insufficiency via agonist muscle function developed through a well-designed therapy program.

Nonoperative management is currently recommended for isolated, asymptomatic PCL injuries with minimal or mild laxity.[6,10] If posterior translation is less than 10 mm (i.e., grade I or II injuries), as it is in majority of isolated injuries, aggressive rehabilitation is instituted. This may also be used in cases with small tibial avulsion fractures and translation less than 5 to 10 mm. Rehabilitation for these injuries usually consists of 2 to 4 weeks of immobilization with the knee in full extension, often with protected weight bearing. This results in tibial reduction and prevents any posterior sag. Quadriceps strengthening is encouraged, while hamstring loading is prohibited to prevent posterior tibial subluxation. After 4 weeks, active-assisted range of motion and progressive weight bearing are begun.[9] Patients can usually be expected to return to sports 1 to 3 months after injury.[5] Rehabilitation focuses on closed-chain exercises, with the goal to regain 90% of quadriceps and hamstring strength (compared with the contralateral side). PCL braces have not been found helpful in low-grade chronic injuries. It is recommended that patients treated conservatively be followed yearly for any symptoms or signs of progressive instability or degenerative joint changes.[5,14]

Treatment of acute grade III injuries (displacement greater than 10 to 15 mm) is more controversial. Historically, these injuries have been treated similarly to lower grade tears, but most authors now recommend surgical intervention for all acute injuries resulting in severe tibial subluxation and for combined multiligamentous injuries.[1,6,10] Surgery is also recommended for avulsion injuries with translation greater than 10 mm. If the fragments are small, the PCL should be reconstructed, but if the fragments are sufficiently large, internal fixation may be attempted. Combined injuries are best treated within 2 weeks, after which capsular scarring develops and direct repair of collateral and posterolateral corner structures is usually not possible.[9] ACL reconstruction may be delayed, however, in order to regain knee motion and allow capsular healing. Multiple surgical options exist for ligament reconstruction, including choice of graft, single- versus double-bundle techniques, and tibial tunnel versus tibial inlay techniques. These are discussed in more detail in the next section.

The treatment of chronic instability should be based on the degree of instability, presence or absence of degenerative changes, and response of symptoms to nonoperative management. Nonoperative treatment, including physical therapy and activity modification, is successful for the majority of patients with chronic PCL instability. Surgery may be recommended if posterior displacement is greater than 10 mm and nonoperative modalities have failed to relieve symptoms. In addition, progressively increasing activity on bone scan, indicative of increased metabolic activity due to altered knee biomechanics and progressive degeneration, may be a useful evaluative factor. In the presence of medial compartment wear, valgus osteotomy with or without PCL reconstruction may be considered. One should rarely, if ever, attempt to reconstruct the PCL in patients with a fixed (irreducible) posterior drawer, and direct repair instead of reconstruction of a chronic PCL injury is also strongly discouraged.

SURGERY

Several techniques of reconstruction have been developed (Box 53-3). Current literature does not clearly indicate which is superior. Primary repair is attempted only with bony avulsions, in which fragments are fixed with a screw and washer if large enough or suture if the fragment is small. Primary repair of interstitial ligament tears has not been successful. The goals of surgery are to reproduce the normal anterior tibial step-off and restore the native restraint to posterior tibial displacement. Regardless of the chosen technique, a diagnostic arthroscopy is performed in nearly all cases, and any meniscal or osteochondral injuries are addressed. Débridement of the torn PCL, requiring complete visualization of the tibial insertion, may require a 70-degree arthroscope placed through the anterolateral portal and notch. A posteromedial portal may then be opened under direct visualization.

Single-Bundle versus Double-Bundle Techniques

The femoral side is almost always addressed arthroscopically, although two major techniques, the single bundle and the double bundle, are possible. Early reconstructive techniques, which focused on placing a single femoral tunnel in the "isometric" region of the native PCL, were found to produce abnormal knee kinematics, especially when the knee flexed more than 45 degrees.[20] Only 5% to 15% of the femoral footprint is truly isometric, and therefore current single-bundle methods have been modified to place the femoral tunnel in the anterior aspect of the footprint to reproduce only the structurally superior anterolateral bundle.

With the patient supine, a 2-cm incision over the anterior knee is necessary and should be placed just medial to the articular edge of the trochlear groove and distal to the vastus medialis obliquus. The retinaculum is incised in line with the skin incision. The proximal portion of the femoral tunnel guide is positioned midway between the patella and medial epicondyle, at least 1 cm from the patellofemoral articular edge to ensure that the joint is not violated. The tip of the drill guide is placed through the medial portal onto the anterior half of the femoral PCL footprint, 8 to 9 mm above the articular surface. The guide pin should be driven with the knee in 70 to 90 degrees of flexion and exit high in the notch at the 11- or 1-o'clock position (for left or right knees, respectively) within the anterior half of the anatomic footprint.[10,16] The tunnel is then created by drilling over the wire. Most authors drill the femoral tunnel outside-in in this manner, although an inside-out technique has also been described using an accessory anterolateral portal. It is suggested that this latter method may lead to a more acute, and therefore less favorable, angle between the intra-articular graft and bony tunnel, resulting in fraying and graft wear if the tunnel entrance is not carefully chamfered[21] (Fig. 53-12).

Because the PCL exhibits a very small zone of isometric fibers, only anatomic reconstructions can accurately restore native function.[21] Reconstruction of only the AL bundle may over time allow graft elongation secondary to nonuniform distribution of forces across the graft. To improve the success of reconstruction, some surgeons have added a second bundle to better replicate the native PCL orientation and provide a more uniform load distribution.[20] Theoretically, a two-bundle technique offers a biomechanical advantage and is superior to single-

---

Box 53-3 Principles of Posterior Cruciate Ligament Reconstruction[2]

- Identification and treatment of all pathology
- Protection of neurovascular structures
- Accurate tunnel placement
- Recreation of anatomic insertion sites
- Appropriate graft tension and fixation
- Structured postoperative rehabilitation

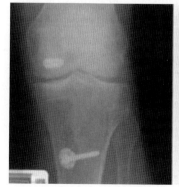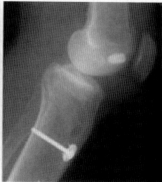

Figure 53-12 Postoperative radiographs of a single-bundle posterior cruciate ligament reconstruction. (From Allen CR, Rihn JA, Harner CD: Posterior cruciate ligament: Diagnosis and decision making. In Miller MD, Cole BJ [eds]: Textbook of Arthroscopy. Philadelphia, WB Saunders, 2004, pp 687–702.)

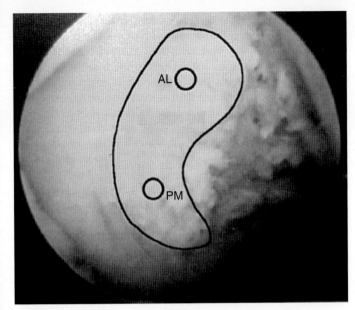

Figure 53-13 Anatomic position of femoral tunnels for single-bundle (anterolateral [AL] only) or double-bundle (AL and posteromedial [PM]) posterior cruciate ligament reconstruction. (From Allen CR, Rihn JA, Harner CD: Posterior cruciate ligament: Diagnosis and decision making. In Miller MD, Cole BJ [eds]: Textbook of Arthroscopy. Philadelphia, WB Saunders, 2004, pp 687–702.)

tubercle through a longitudinal 2- to 3-cm incision. This results in a trajectory of 50 to 60 degrees to the long axis of the tibia, creating a graft orientation at the posterior tibia of approximately 45 degrees. This reduces the effects of the "killer turn," a term referring to the sudden bend that the graft must take as it passes from the tunnel into the knee joint.[10] The anterior skin incision can also be placed lateral to the tubercle, which may further reduce graft angulation.[21] It has been recommended that one make a 2-cm safety incision posteromedially, which will allow access for the surgeon's finger to directly protect the neurovascular structures and monitor any instruments placed in posterior knee[10] (Fig. 53-14). A guidewire is drilled under arthroscopic visualization, and a 10- to 12-mm tunnel then drilled over the wire, taking care to protect the neurovascular structures at all times because, even with the knee flexed 90 degrees, the distance between the popliteal artery and posterior tibia is less than 1 cm. (Because of this, the inlay technique should be avoided in patients who have had recent or remote vascular repairs, which causes increased scarring and altered anatomy in the posterior knee.) The posteromedial portal and fluoroscopy may be used for direct observation during this step. The final drilling of the posterior cortex should also be completed by hand. The edge of the tibial tunnel must be chamfered to avoid excessive graft wear at the turn (Fig. 53-15).

bundle methods because it replaces both major portions of the native PCL. As each bundle is tensioned at the appropriate degree of flexion, this technique may decrease posterior laxity and better restore normal knee biomechanics through a greater range of knee motion.[14,22] Proper placement of this second bundle is critical, however, as position greatly affects the tension of the AL bundle. A middle or distal second bundle allows cooperative load sharing and decreases anterior bundle tension, but proximal placement of the second bundle may not alter peak anterior bundle tension.[20] Clinical studies have not yet consistently demonstrated improved resistance to posterior translation or improved in vivo joint kinematics between the two techniques.[5,14]

Although technically more challenging, the two-bundle method is similar to the single tunnel except for the fact that two femoral tunnels are drilled, one for the AL bundle in the anterior half of the femoral footprint and a smaller tunnel posteriorly (Fig. 53-13). Both grafts are routed through same tibial tunnel or can originate from the same tibial bone block. Again, the tunnel for the AL band is centered at the 1-o'clock position (for right knee), 2 to 3 mm behind the condylar articular margin, while the tunnel for the PM band is centered on the footprint at about 3:30-o'clock position.

Transtibial versus Tibial Inlay Techniques

Two disparate methods for tibial fixation also exist. In the transtibial technique, the tibial tunnel and fixation are performed completely arthroscopically. With the patient supine, the tibial tunnel is drilled from front to back. First, any posterior adhesions are lysed and the posterior capsule separated from the tibial ridge. A PCL drill guide is passed through the intercondylar notch and positioned slightly lateral and distal to the anatomic tibial footprint.[7] The anterior portion of the drill guide is placed on the anteromedial tibia 1 to 2 cm below the tibial

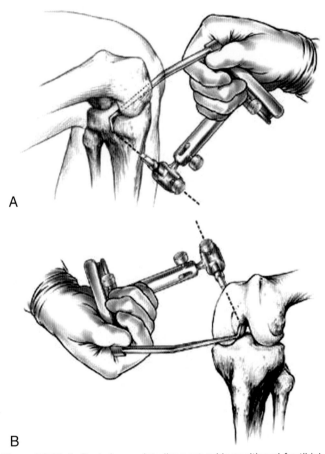

Figure 53-14 A, Posterior cruciate ligament guide positioned for tibial tunnel guidewire placement. **B,** Position for femoral tunnel guidewire placement. (From Johnson DH, Fanelli GC, Miller MD: PCL 2002: Indications, double-bundle versus inlay technique and revision surgery. Arthroscopy 2002;18:40–52.)

It is sometimes difficult to pass a graft around the sharp angle at the back of tibial tunnel, and this bend poses several potential long-term disadvantages: tibial tunnel erosion may occur, excessive bending may increase graft strain and wear, and the abrasive ridge may lead to elongation, fraying, or failure.[23] Drilling of the tibial tunnel also risks neurovascular injury. Furthermore, the tibial tunnel technique requires a longer graft (usually at least 40 mm), which may be a problem, especially when using bone-patellar tendon-bone grafts. The tibial inlay method is an alternate technique that uses direct exposure and visualization for tibial fixation, eliminating the acute turn because the graft is fixed directly to a trough on the posterior tibia via a bone block. This is theoretically more secure, allows use of a bone-tendon or bone-tendon-bone allograft with bone-to-bone healing and may improve isometry. However, patient positioning is more difficult, as is hardware removal if necessary, and revision is more challenging and dangerous due to scarring in posterior knee. Recent studies have debated whether any differences exist in the outcome between inlay and tunnel techniques, and some authors reserve inlay methods for revision or osteopenic bone.[5,21]

For inlay procedures, the patient is placed in the lateral decubitus position, from which the hip can be externally rotated for arthroscopy. After arthroscopic débridement and preparation of the femoral tunnel(s), a horizontal incision is made in the knee flexion crease, exposing the interval between the semimembranosus and the medial head of the gastrocnemius. A hockey stick incision may also be used, with the inferior arm overlying the medial gastrocnemius. This muscle is then retracted laterally along with the neurovascular structures, allowing the posterior capsule to be incised vertically and the PCL insertion to be visu-

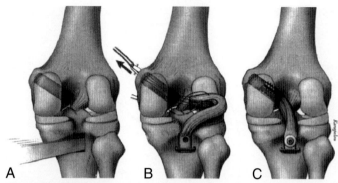

Figure 53-16 Posterior cruciate ligament reconstruction using the tibial inlay technique. After creation of the posterior tibial trough (**A**), the graft is secured with staple or screw (**B**), and passed through the femoral tunnel (**C**). (From Miller MD, Gordon WT: Posterior cruciate ligament reconstruction: Tibial inlay techniques—principles and procedures. Oper Tech Sports Med 1999;7:127–133.)

alized. Pins or sharp-tipped 90-degree retractors can be placed in the posterior tibial cortex to assist with exposure. The hamstrings, if required for a multiligament reconstruction, can also be harvested through this approach.

The posterior tibial plateau is exposed and prepared by fashioning a unicortical window to fit the bone block of the graft. A vertically oriented rectangular trough is made in the tibia with an osteotome. This should match the dimensions of the graft bone plug. The upper end of the slot should lie within the tibial anatomic footprint, above the transverse ridge where the posterior capsule inserts. After the graft is impacted into the slot, graft fixation is completed with screws and washers (Fig. 53-16).

Graft Passage and Tensioning

Graft passage and tensioning will depend on the exact techniques chosen on the tibial and femoral sides. If using tibial and single femoral tunnels, a looped 18-gauge wire or tunnel smoother is passed through tibial tunnel, grasped under arthroscopic visualization, redirected through femoral tunnel, and delivered externally. The graft is then pulled anterograde through the femoral tunnel and into tibial tunnel. The tibial tunnel may be oversized by 1 mm to assist with graft passage around the killer turn. The femoral side is usually secured first with an interference screw, and the graft then tensioned with the knee in 70 to 90 degrees of flexion with an anterior drawer force performed to eliminate any posterior sag. Any tension beyond that needed to reestablish normal step-off is excessive. It is critical to tension with the knee in flexion, after which the tibial side may be secured with an interference screw or with a screw and spiked washer. Many authors prefer double fixation on both sides.[10]

If using a tibial inlay technique, the graft will typically first be fixed to the tibial trough, passed retrograde through the femoral tunnel, and tensioned and fixed as just described. If using a double-bundle technique, the graft limbs will also be passed retrograde (if using a single bone block on the tibial side) or may be passed anterograde if using two separate grafts. Regardless, to reproduce the normal PCL biomechanics, the AL bundle should be tensioned and fixed with the knee flexed 90 degrees, and the PM bundle tensioned and fixed at or near full extension.

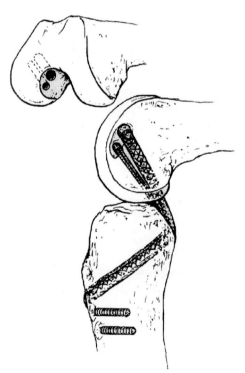

Figure 53-15 Posterior cruciate ligament reconstruction using a transtibial tunnel and a double-bundle femoral technique. (From Petrie RS, Harner CD: Double bundle posterior cruciate ligament reconstruction technique: University of Pittsburgh approach. Oper Tech Sports Med 1999;7:118–126.)

Box 53-4 Considerations for Posterior Cruciate Ligament Reconstruction

- Arthroscopic versus open
- Tibial tunnel or tibial inlay
- Single bundle or double bundle
- Graft choice
- Graft fixation technique
- Postoperative rehabilitation/weight bearing

Graft Selection

Although the perfect PCL graft does not exist, graft selection is an essential part of surgery. Ideally, a graft would have structural properties similar to those of the intact PCL, with minimal harvest site morbidity, easy passage, secure fixation, and fast incorporation.[24] One must also consider requirements for additional graft materials, if there are multiple injured ligaments. Autograft options include bone-patellar bone-bone, quadriceps tendon, and hamstring. Bone-patellar bone-bone usually consists of a 10- to 12-mm strip of patellar tendon with 20- to 25-mm bone blocks at each end. Incorporation through bone-to-bone healing is believed to occur within 4 to 6 weeks. Quadriceps grafts consist of a 10- to 12-mm strip of quadriceps tendon with a distal patellar bone block. Quadriceps is typically thicker than patellar tendon, although this does not translate to greater strength. The bone block can be used on the tibial or femoral side, while the other end of the graft requires tendon-to-bone healing. Quadriceps grafts may also be used as split grafts for double-bundle techniques. Hamstrings are usually used as quadruple-stranded grafts or as two double strands for a two-tunnel technique. Hamstrings are associated with less graft site morbidity, but fixation appears inferior to that of bone-patellar bone-bone, as it requires tendon-to-bone healing on both ends. All these grafts appear to possess in vitro strength and stiffness greater than those of the native PCL, with quadrupled hamstring having the greatest stiffness and strength and quadriceps tendon the least.[24]

Allograft choices include all the previously cited tissues in cadaveric form, as well as allograft Achilles, tibialis anterior, and tibialis posterior tendons. Allografts may especially be necessary if multiple ligaments are being reconstructed. Advantages of allografts include the absence of donor site morbidity and reduced operative time. Some allografts (e.g., Achilles tendon) also provide thicker tendons and larger amounts of collagen, which can completely fill larger tunnels.[9] Availability, price, risk of disease transmission, tissue quality, and graft incorporation are concerns. Synthetic grafts are not recommended because of high complication rates, including generation of wear debris, cystic changes in bone tunnels, and graft failures (Box 53-4).[6]

POSTOPERATIVE REHABILITATION

Rehabilitation after surgical reconstruction focuses on restoring knee range of motion while simultaneously avoiding excessive graft stress until healing has occurred. Specific protocols are highly variable depending on the authors consulted. Most surgeons brace the knee in full extension from a few weeks to 2 months, and most allow early partial or full weight bearing using crutches with the knee in full extension. Range-of-motion (often

using a continuous passive motion device) and quadriceps exercises are begun within the first 1 to 4 weeks.[1,13,14] In this period, efforts are concentrated on unweighted knee extension exercises and straight leg raises. At 4 to 6 weeks after surgery, the brace is unlocked and closed-chain exercises including biking and leg presses are started, followed by treadmill walking or pool jogging at 3 months. Running is allowed at 5 to 6 months and agility drills at 6 to 7 months. A return to regular sporting activities is anticipated at about 9 months, although some patients may take significantly longer. Return to sports is allowed only after the recovery of normal (90% of contralateral side) quadriceps strength is achieved. Loss of motion may be a problem, and some authors report that as many as 20% of patients require a manipulation under anesthesia 6 to 8 weeks after reconstruction to regain full flexion.[9]

SURGICAL COMPLICATIONS AND OUTCOMES

Successful PCL reconstruction is technically more difficult than ACL reconstruction. Factors contributing to this include the fact that the PCL has a complex fiber pattern that is impossible to duplicate precisely, as its broad femoral footprint causes wider variation of fiber tension during knee motion than that of the ACL. In addition, PCL reconstruction is more commonly performed in the setting of combined ligamentous injuries.

The most common intraoperative complications concern neurovascular injury, particularly involving the popliteal artery. Techniques to reduce this are discussed in the preceding section and are especially important during procedures using a transtibial approach. Hematoma formation and drainage from a posterior arthrotomy may occur as a result of gravity drainage or bleeding from inferior geniculate vessels. Because of this, some authors recommend routine ligation of the inferior medial geniculate vessels.[16] Postoperatively, residual laxity, loss of motion or arthrofibrosis, infection, painful hardware, and anterior knee pain are the most common complications. Reconstructed PCL knees may be slow to regain full flexion; this may be worsened by poor tunnel placement.[6] As importantly, patient age, severity of trauma, and ability to actively rehabilitate are important factors often beyond the surgeon's control.

Results comparing different reconstruction techniques are somewhat inconsistent. Choice of autograft versus allograft has not been proven to play a significant role in outcome.[16] Theoretically, use of a transtibial approach may decrease accuracy of tunnel placement, and the acute posterior turn of the graft may lead to tunnel erosion, higher graft stresses, and graft elongation. Some authors believe that tibial inlay techniques allow greater initial stability due to avoidance of the killer turn, and, indeed, some recent evidence indicates that tibial inlay techniques may result in less graft laxity. In addition, two-bundle techniques may afford improved stability in both flexion and extension when compared to single-bundle reconstructions.[2,3] To date, however, there is no consensus regarding the superiority of one technique over another. Overall, good to excellent results can be expected regardless of the specific operative technique used, with normal or near-normal posterior drawer test results found in more than 95% of postoperative patients. Most knees with grade III laxity before surgery are reduced to grade I, and nearly all are reduced to at least grade II.[4-6] In addition, statistically significant improvements in posterior tibial displacement on stress radiographs and KT-1000 testing have been documented after multiple reconstructive techniques.[10]

Box 53-5 Causes of Failed Primary Posterior Cruciate Ligament Surgery[16]

- Biologic
  Poor graft incorporation or remodeling, tunnel erosion, tunnel expansion
- Technical
  Failure of fixation (bone plug breakage, loss of interference fixation, graft creep or slippage)
  High internal graft stress (nonisometric placement of anterolateral bundle, internal stress at tunnel edges)
- Surgical decision making
  Failure to treat associated injuries, primary repair versus delayed reconstruction
- Inappropriate rehabilitation
  Early aggressive range-of-motion or hamstring resistance exercises, early weight bearing in combined injuries

---

It is important to note, however, that PCL reconstruction may not consistently correct abnormal patellofemoral contact pressures or altered knee kinematics.[19] This may be related, at least in part, to difficulties with anatomic tunnel placement. To date, there have been no long-term studies providing conclusive proof that operative intervention decreases the risks of long-term degenerative changes. With identification of the PCL reconstruction that most accurately restores knee kinematics and joint contact pressures, one might expect to demonstrate decreases in late-onset arthritis (Box 53-5).

SPECIAL CONSIDERATIONS

Pediatric PCL injuries are uncommon. The usual injury pattern described in children involves periosteal stripping of the femoral attachment or a bony avulsion from the tibia. For the former, a suture technique used to reattach the ligament through drill holes in the femur is recommended, while for the latter, bony reattachment similar to that performed in adults is the treatment of choice.[25]

Revision PCL cases are also fairly uncommon, comprising only 10% or fewer of all PCL reconstructions.[14] When evaluating potential surgical failures, it is important to remember that the reference position of the anterior tibial plateau with respect to medial femoral condyle can be significantly altered after PCL reconstruction. This can, therefore, markedly affect subsequent evaluation and interpretation of posterior tibial translation.[15] If clinical and radiographic examination leads to the diagnosis of surgical failure, special consideration must be given to prior surgical scarring, potential loss of bone stock from tunnel enlargement, interference from previous tunnel positions, and location of hardware. As a rule, final stability in revision cases is usually worse that that obtained in primary procedures.[10]

Finally, although covered in detail in another chapter, multiligament injuries have relatively poor outcomes if treated nonoperatively. Most commonly, these occur as grade III PCL injury combined with posterolateral corner insufficiency, resulting in additive laxity in the posterior and external rotation vectors. For acute injuries, attempts to repair all damaged structures are warranted. The posterolateral corner especially will scar and obliterate normal anatomy if not addressed within 2 to 3 weeks of injury. Combined ACL and PCL injuries often represent an unrecognized knee dislocation. Some authors recommend acute repair or reconstruction, while others initiate early range-of-motion exercises and delay surgery for fear of arthrofibrosis.[1] Treatment of combined PCL and MCL injuries may depend on the degree of MCL laxity. Low-grade MCL tears may heal with bracing and protection, while high-grade MCL injuries will have marked valgus instability and typically require acute repair.

CONCLUSION

PCL injuries, although less common than ACL injuries, may be seen in variety of clinical settings. These can usually be diagnosed by the skilled physician through a thorough physical examination and confirmatory radiographic studies. Low-grade, isolated PCL injuries are usually treated nonoperatively with acceptable outcomes. Recent studies, however, suggest that chronic PCL deficiency may lead to progressive joint degeneration and arthritis. Multiple surgical options exist for reconstruction of the PCL, although there is little evidence to date demonstrating that PCL reconstruction significantly alters this natural history. Further research is needed to evaluate surgical techniques and treatment controversies.

REFERENCES

1. Cosgarea AJ, Jay PR: Posterior cruciate ligament injuries: Evaluation and management. J Am Acad Orthop Surg 2001;9:297–307.
2. Miller MD, Cooper DE, Fanelli GC, et al: Posterior cruciate ligament: Current concepts. Instr Course Lect 2002;51:347–351.
3. White LM, Miniaci A: Cruciate and posterolateral corner injuries in the athlete: Clinical and magnetic resonance imaging features. Semin Musculoskelet Radiol 2004;8:111–131.
4. Dowd GSE: Reconstruction of the posterior cruciate ligament: Indications and results. J Bone Joint Surg Br 2004;86:480–491.
5. Margheritini F, Rihn J, Musahl A, et al: Posterior cruciate ligament injuries in the athlete: An anatomical, biomechanical and clinical review. Sports Med 2002;32:393–408.
6. St. Pierre P, Miller MD: Posterior cruciate ligament injuries. Clin Sports Med 1999;18:199–221.
7. Schulte KR, Chu ET, Fu FH: Arthroscopic posterior cruciate ligament reconstruction. Clin Sports Med 1997;16:145–156.
8. Amis AA, Bull AMJ, Gupte CM, et al: Biomechanics of the PCL and related structures: Posterolateral, posteromedial and meniscofemoral ligaments. Knee Surg Sports Traumatol Arthrosc 2003;11:271–281.
9. Harner CD, Honer J: Evaluation and treatment of posterior cruciate ligament injuries. Am J Sports Med 1998;26:471–482.
10. Johnson DH, Fanelli GC, Miller MD: PCL 2002: Indications, double-bundle versus inlay technique and revision surgery. Arthroscopy 2002;18:40–52.
11. Shelbourne KD, Carr DR: Combined anterior and posterior cruciate and medial collateral ligament injury: Nonsurgical and delayed surgical treatment. Instr Course Lect 2003;52:413–418.
12. Shelbourne KD, Gray T: Natural history of acute posterior cruciate ligament tears. J Knee Surg 2002;15:103–107.
13. Veltri DM, Warren RF: Isolated and combined posterior cruciate ligament injuries. J Am Acad Orthop Surg 1993;1:67–75.

14. Harner CD, Fu FH, Irrgang JJ, et al: Anterior and posterior cruciate ligament reconstruction in the new millennium: A global perspective. Knee Surg Sports Traumatol Arthrosc 2001;9:330–336.

15. Ma CB, Kanamori A, Vogrin TM, et al: Measurement of posterior tibial translation in the posterior cruciate ligament-reconstructed knee. Am J Sports Med 2003;31:843–848.

16. Cooper DE, Stewart D: Posterior cruciate ligament reconstruction using single-bundle patella tendon graft with tibial inlay fixation. Am J Sports Med 2004;32:346–360.

17. Parolie JM, Bergfeld JA: Long-term results of nonoperative treatment of isolated posterior cruciate ligament injuries in the athlete. Am J Sports Med 1986;14:35–38.

18. Toritsuka Y, Horibe S, Hiro-oka A, et al: Conservative treatment for rugby football players with acute isolated posterior cruciate ligament injury. Knee Surg Sports Traumatol Arthrosc 2004;12:110–114.

19. Gill TJ, DeFrate LE, Wang C, et al: The effect of posterior cruciate ligament reconstruction on patellofemoral contact pressures in the knee joint under simulated muscle loads. Am J Sports Med 2004;32:109–115.

20. Shearn JT, Grood ES, Noyes FR, et al: Two-bundle posterior cruciate ligament reconstruction: How bundle tension depends on femoral placement. J Bone Joint Surg Am 2004;86:1262–1270.

21. Christel P: Basic principles for surgical reconstruction of the PCL in chronic posterior knee instability. Knee Surg Sports Traumatol Arthrosc 2003;11:289–296.

22. Giffin JR, Haemmerle MJ, Vogrin TM, et al: Single- versus double-bundle PCL reconstruction: A biomechanical analysis. J Knee Surg 2002;15:114–120.

23. Margheritini F, Mauro CS, Rihn JA, et al: Biomechanical comparison of tibial inlay versus transtibial techniques for posterior cruciate ligament reconstruction: Analysis of knee kinematics and graft in situ forces. Am J Sports Med 2004;32:587–593.

24. Hoher J, Scheffler S, Weiler A: Graft choices and graft fixation in PCL reconstruction. Knee Surg Sports Traumatol Arthrosc 2003;11: 297–306.

25. Larson RV, Ulmer T: Ligament injuries in children. Instr Course Lect 2003;52:677–680.

54 Medial Collateral Ligament

Matthew Alan Rappé and Peter Indelicato

In This Chapter

INTRODUCTION

- The management of MCL injuries has evolved over the past 30 years.

- Whereas most isolated anterior cruciate ligament (ACL) injuries are treated surgically, there remains a place for non-operative management of isolated MCL injuries.

- In combined lesions with other ligaments, surgical repair/reconstruction of the MCL may be indicated.

- Whereas the knee has little tolerance for ACL laxity, as an isolated entity, it copes much better with residual MCL laxity even in athletes who perform high-level sports.

CLINICAL FEATURES AND EVALUATION

The management of MCL tears continues to evolve as our understanding of the functional anatomy, biomechanics, and physiologic healing of this important extracapsular structure increases. The majority of patients who injure their MCL do so via a twisting or external rotation injury to the knee (during activities such as snow skiing). Another common mechanism in athletics involves a valgus blow to the lower thigh or upper leg (Fig. 54-1). Isolated MCL injuries, irrespective of the mechanism of injury, are not necessarily very painful. In fact, the more severe isolated tears are generally less painful than other injuries that occur about the knee.

The key to a successful knee examination is relaxation of the thigh. We have found that gentle stress is more revealing than forceful stress. In order to isolate the superficial MCL and test its integrity, the knee must be flexed to 30 degrees and a valgus stress applied (Fig. 54-2).[1,2] The amount of medial opening detected with the knee in 30 degrees of flexion compared with the uninjured knee is a direct reflection of the damage to the MCL. Just like in performing the Lachman test for suspected ACL damage, the quality of the endpoint must also be considered. When a complete MCL injury is present, an absent endpoint is discovered where one is expected. Further valgus load will eventually elicit one and that endpoint may, in fact, be the intact ACL.

To evaluate for associated ligamentous injuries, a valgus stress to the knee while in extension is performed. Asymmetrical medial joint space opening to a valgus stress occurring in full extension is strongly suggestive of combined MCL and posterior oblique ligament (POL) damage and should caution the examiner to suspect associated ACL and/or posterior cruciate ligament involvement.

In addition, one should illicit tenderness along the course of the MCL. If the patient is seen acutely, the location is generally related to the mechanism of injury. Twisting, noncontact injuries usually demonstrate proximal tenderness. Valgus contact injuries usually demonstrate distal tenderness. Any asymmetry of opening greater than 4 mm compared to opposite side, especially coupled with a "soft" endpoint, is strongly indicative of a complete disruption of the superficial MCL and underlying medial capsular ligament.[1]

The gold standard for radiographic evaluation of an MCL injury is magnetic resonance imaging. Magnetic resonance imaging is highly sensitive in identifying injury or detachment of the MCL as well as other associated ligamentous or meniscal injuries about the knee[3] (Figs. 54-3 and 54-4).

For skeletally immature patients with suspected MCL injuries, it is of paramount importance to perform stress radiographs to rule out the possibility of physeal plate injury (Fig. 54-5). Diagnostic arthroscopy is rarely helpful in deciding to what extent the medial supporting structures of the knee joint have been damaged.

RELEVANT ANATOMY

It is important to understand knee anatomy in order to fully comprehend the principles of both nonoperative and operative treatment of MCL injuries. The MCL is composed of both a superficial and deep portion. The MCL's position about the medial knee is best described by Warren and Marshall[4] who introduced the three-layer description of this anatomy. These authors defined layer 1 as that which involves the sartorius and sartorius fascia. Layer 2 includes the superficial MCL, POL, and the semimembranosus. Layer 3 includes the deep MCL and the posteromedial capsule. Layers 1 and 2 blend anteriorly, while layers 2 and 3 blend posteriorly.

The proximal attachment site of the superficial MCL is somewhat circular and located on the medial femoral epicondyle. Its distal attachment is much larger and located 4 or 5 cm below the joint on the medial metaphyseal area of the tibia. It is divided from the deep MCL by a bursa. The deep MCL inserts directly into the edge of the tibial plateau and medial meniscus

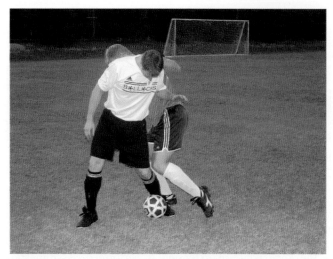

Figure 54-1 Valgus contact resulting in medial collateral ligament tear.

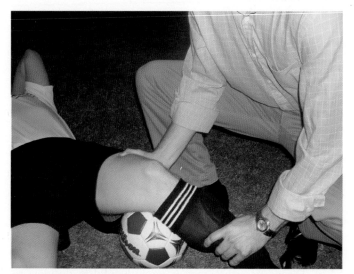

Figure 54-2 Valgus stress in 30 degrees of flexion isolating the superficial medial collateral ligament.

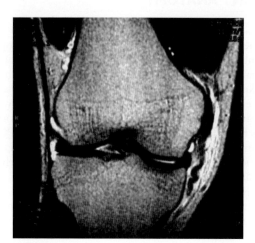

Figure 54-3 Magnetic resonance imaging of the knee demonstrating a distal tear of the medial collateral ligament.

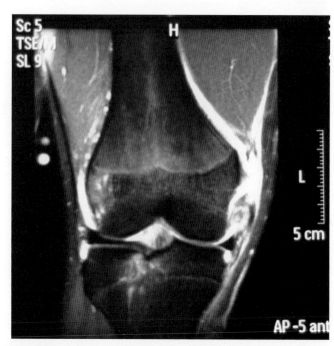

Figure 54-4 Magnetic resonance imaging of the knee demonstrating a proximal tear of the medial collateral ligament.

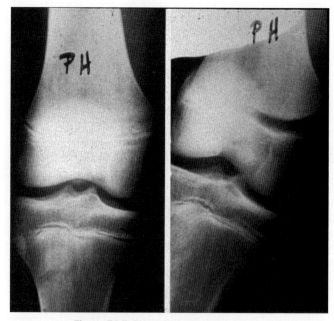

Figure 54-5 Distal femoral physeal injury.

via its two divisions: the meniscotibial and meniscofemoral attachments.

Biomechanical studies have shown that the MCL is the prime medial stabilizer of the knee, which resists valgus loading.[1,2] Due to the parallel arrangement of the collagen that composes the MCL, only a relatively small increase of laxity (approximately 5 to 8 mm) is indicative of a complete failure of the ligament. Another point to remember is that the deep capsular ligament (layer 3) is an important anchoring location for the medial meniscus. Therefore, although damage to this layer can extend into the substance of the meniscus, true substance tears of the medial meniscus are seldom seen in conjunction with complete disruption of the MCL.

The location of the proximal attachment site of the MCL places it near the knee's center of rotation. An intact MCL is fan shaped, and, as a result, some aspect of its structure is always under tension during knee flexion. As the knee goes into flexion, the anterior fibers of the MCL remain tight, whereas the posterior fibers slacken. The POL blends in with the posterior edge of the MCL and helps prevent medial opening with valgus loading with the knee in full extension. In a flexed position, the anterior aspect of the POL actually lies underneath the MCL. The bursa that separates the superficial from the deep MCL allows for the 1- to 2-cm anteroposterior excursion that must occur to the MCL during flexion/extension of the knee. While surgically repairing damage to the area, this relationship must be kept in mind. Suturing the anterior aspect of the POL to the posterior fibers of the MCL with the knee in more than 30 degrees of flexion could limit the necessary excursion of the MCL and lead to a significant flexion contracture postoperatively.

The complexity of the medial structures of the knee have led some authors to focus on the specific structures injured as opposed to grouping them as simply an injury to the MCL. Specifically in the work of Hughston and Eilers,[5] Hughston,[6] and Muller,[7] the importance of the posteromedial corner of the knee as a dynamic and static stabilizer has been emphasized. These anatomic structures include the posterior horn of the medial meniscus, the POL, semimembranosus, meniscotibial attachments, and oblique popliteal ligament and serve as a restraint to anteromedial rotatory instability.[7,8] In a series of 93 knees treated operatively for medial-side knee injuries by Sims and Jacobson[8] of the Hughston Clinic and Tulane, 99% of the knees were found to have injury of the POL ligament and 70% had semimembranosus capsular attachment injuries.

TREATMENT

The treatment of the MCL continues to evolve. Historically, predictably good or excellent results were achieved with primary repair of the torn MCL and POL.[5,9–13] In O'Donoghue's series[14] from 1950, he strongly advocated suture repair immediately after injury. Furthermore, Hughston and Barrett[15] supported immediate primary repair of MCL and posterior oblique tears. In their series, they emphasized anterior advancement of the POL in order to restore medial stability.

The nonoperative approach to management of complete tears of the MCL was first advocated by Ellsasser et al.[16] Fetto and Marshall[17] also reported excellent results following complete isolated MCL tears, irrespective of whether they were treated with an open or closed surgical technique. In 1983, the senior author published the results of a series of isolated MCL tears of the knee treated nonoperatively.[18] He found no advantage

to direct suture repair when compared with a nonoperative approach that involved a structured rehabilitation program. In a subsequent article, the senior author and colleagues[19] showed that this conservative approach was successful, even for the highly competitive athlete who returned to contact sports. In 1993, Reider et al[20] reported excellent results in 35 athletes who had undergone conservative management of MCL tears with functional rehabilitation and been monitored for more than 5 years.

In patients with combined MCL and ACL injuries, many authors favor nonoperative management of the MCL after reconstruction of the ACL. Shelbourne and Porter[21] claim that excellent subjective and objective results can be achieved with proper reconstruction of the ACL and nonoperative management of the MCL, even in the elite athlete. In most cases of combined injuries, Noyes and Barber-Westin[22] also favor nonoperative management of the MCL. They state that after reconstruction of the ACL, high-demand athletes with extensive medial joint space laxity may require operative repair of the medial structures.[22]

More recent work at other centers continues to support nonoperative management of concomitant ACL and MCL injuries. Millett et al[23] showed patients with 19 combined ACL tears and minimum grade II MCL tears. These patients underwent early reconstruction of the ACL and nonoperative treatment of the MCL. Serial clinical examinations demonstrated good functional outcomes, range of motion, and strength. No patient experienced ACL graft failure or valgus instability or required subsequent surgery for chondral or meniscal damage at 2 years.[23]

Acute Medial Collateral Ligament Tear Management

For the treatment of incomplete tears, we recommend minimal immobilization for 1 to 3 weeks followed by physical therapy focusing on quadriceps- and hamstring-strengthening exercises.

The senior author's management of grade III acute MCL injuries has evolved over the past 20 years. His initial recommendations were to immobilize all knees with MCL tears in a cast brace in 30 degrees of flexion for 2 weeks, which limited range of motion from 30 to 90 degrees of flexion as well as weight bearing for 6 weeks.[18]

Now, for complete proximal isolated tears of the MCL, the senior author prefers to place the knee in a commercially available splint in full extension for 2 weeks. A concern with these lesions is the possibility of excessive stiffness developing in the knee early in the healing process; therefore, immobilization should be minimized in any degree of flexion. For distal-based tears of the MCL, we immobilize the knee (splint versus cylinder cast) for 2 weeks in 30 degrees of flexion. Irrespective of the location of the tear, after 2 weeks of immobilization has passed, we begin to mobilize the knee throughout a comfortable range of motion without any set limitations. Weight bearing as tolerated is encouraged. We focus on quadriceps- and hamstring-strengthening exercises similar to those used in an incomplete MCL tear rehabilitation program.

Once isokinetic studies show that the extremity has recovered at least 80% of its strength, power, and endurance, then an on-the-field agility program is begun. For contact sports, we recommend a double upright knee orthosis for the first season. After that, the use of an orthosis is left to the patient's discretion. Since writing the original article in 1983, the senior author does not know of any patient who has developed functional laxity as a result of being treated in this fashion.

Indications for Primary Repair

Indications for primary repair both for isolated and combined ligament injuries of the knee remain somewhat controversial. Most surgeons still choose not to operate on isolated complete tears, especially those that demonstrate no laxity to valgus stress in full extension. When asymmetrical laxity occurs in full extension, some surgeons may choose to perform primary repair of the MCL and posterior capsule. Wilson et al[24] reported that in their series distal tears healed less reliably, leading to the need for late reconstructions. This led them to advocate acute surgical repair for distal tears in athletic populations.[24]

At our institution, we seldom perform acute MCL repair when there is a concomitant anterior and/or posterior cruciate ligament tear(s). In this clinical situation, we immobilize the knee for 3 to 4 weeks to allow early primary healing of the MCL. Following this, patients are started on a rehabilitation program in order to recover most of their motion. This may take up to 6 to 8 weeks, especially if the lesion is proximal. Once most motion and quadriceps control of the leg has been recovered, an ACL reconstruction is performed. Intraoperatively, following the ACL reconstruction, the knee is reexamined for medial laxity, both in 30 degrees of flexion and in full extension. Using this approach, the senior author seldom has needed to perform an MCL repair and/or reconstruction. If the knee remains grossly unstable, particularly in full extension, a small posteromedial incision is made and the POL is tightened by advancing it as advocated by Hughston.[5,6] Care is taken to avoid significant anterior advancement or reefing of this ligament because of the risk of developing a flexion contracture, as discussed earlier.

Surgical Technique

If an acute MCL repair is deemed necessary, it is performed using a straight medial incision extending from the medial epicondyle to 5 cm distal to the medial joint line. The sartorius fascia is divided and the sartorius retracted distally. Flexing the knee further retracts the sartorius and the pes anserinus components, giving visualization of the superficial MCL. If the MCL is torn distally, it is important to reflect it proximally, exposing the deep meniscocapsular ligaments. If these are torn, and they frequently are, they are repaired with simple interrupted suture. The sequence of repair thus proceeds from deep to superficial. If the posterior capsule is torn mid-substance, it is approximated with interrupted sutures. If the posterior capsule is torn from the femoral or tibial attachment, it is advanced and reattached to either the femur or the tibia, respectively, with suture anchors. Once this is accomplished, repair of the superficial MCL is addressed. Reapproximation of mid-substance tears is performed using Bunnell-Kessler suture configuration. Proximal or distal tears are advanced and reattached with anchors or over a post depending on tissue quality. If tissues are deemed inadequate, we commonly will augment this repair with Achilles tendon allograft secured via interference screws. Irrespective of open or closed treatment of a complete MCL tear, normal medial tightness is almost never completely achieved. Despite this fact, the senior author rarely has seen this result in a functionally unstable knee unless there was coexisting laxity in other structures (Figs. 54-6 through 54-10).

Rehabilitation for Primary Repair

Following surgery, the knee is immobilized in full extension for the first 3 weeks. The focus of the early rehabilitation program

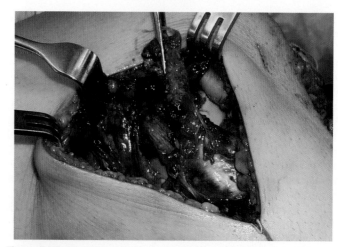

Figure 54-6 Surgical approach for repair of acute proximal medial collateral ligament tear.

is quadriceps-strengthening exercises in order to minimize muscle atrophy. It is critical to avoid any loss of full extension, particularly if the MCL lesion is more proximal. Hip and ankle exercises also should be included throughout the entire program.

Chronic Medial Collateral Ligament Reconstruction

In cases in which the patient is first seen 3 weeks or more after the injury, it is probably too late to treat grade III MCL injuries successfully with either open primary repair or closed conservative management. In reviewing the literature, there are multiple ways to attempt to reconstruct the MCL. This usually means that there is no one procedure available that is always successful. In past years, the senior author reconstructed the MCL mainly by detaching its proximal end and either advancing it or countersinking it in an attempt to "retension" the

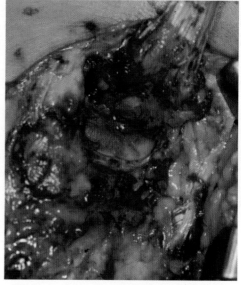

Figure 54-7 Higher magnification demonstrating a torn posterior capsule.

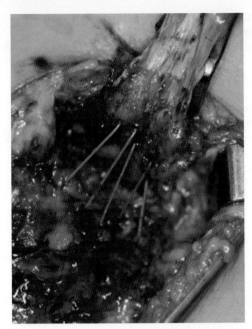

Figure 54-8 Surgical repair of the posterior capsule with interrupted suture.

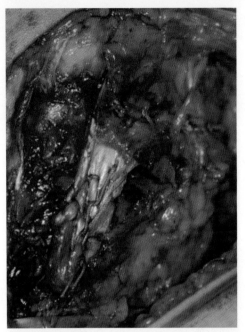

Figure 54-10 Repair of medial collateral ligament using Bunnell-Kessler suture configuration.

ligament. In addition, he would advance the posteromedial capsule anteriorly in an attempt to reestablish stability in full extension.

Recently, the senior author has used Achilles tendon allograft to reconstruct the MCL (Fig. 54-11). The allograft dimensions are similar to the MCL with the ACL length being greater. The femoral attachment site receives the calcaneal bone (10- to 12-mm plug) with interference screw. The tibial attachment site is sutured over a post and/or biodegradable interference screws are used to achieve fixation via a transtibial tunnel (Fig. 54-12). In addition, a posteromedial capsular advancement is performed, but care is taken following each suture to ensure the ability to achieve full extension, thus preventing a situation in which the advancement "captures" the knee.

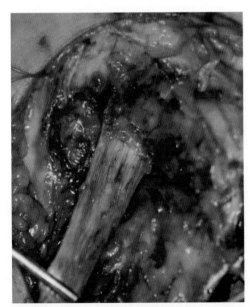

Figure 54-9 Higher magnification demonstrating torn medial collateral ligament.

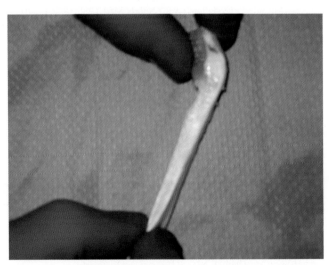

Figure 54-11 Achilles tendon allograft.

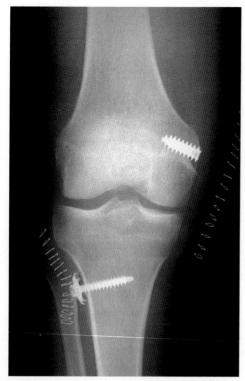

Figure 54-12 Postoperative radiograph demonstrating femoral and tibial fixation of Achilles tendon allograft used for reconstruction of a chronic medial collateral ligament–deficient knee.

Medial Collateral Ligament Reconstruction Rehabilitation

Just as in primary repair, we immobilize the knee for the first 3 weeks in full extension. Following that time, the rehabilitation program is identical to that for ACL reconstruction.

Combined Medial and Posterior Collateral Ligament Injury

Associated posterior collateral ligament (PCL) and MCL damage usually implies posterior capsule involvement, and the knee, therefore, will demonstrate some laxity in full extension to valgus stress. As a result, the senior author routinely performs either a primary repair (acutely) or a reconstruction (chronically) of the MCL in this situation. In mild to moderate PCL laxity, the senior author awaits any functional deficit that may develop prior to performing a PCL reconstruction. In severe PCL laxity, he performs a combined PCL and MCL repair/reconstruction at the same time.

CONCLUSIONS

The management of MCL injuries continues to evolve. When injuries are isolated to the MCL, most orthopedic surgeons prefer conservative management. In combined lesions of the MCL and ACL, surgical repair of the ACL may be all that is necessary for treatment. If the knee continues to demonstrate medial laxity, repair or reconstruction of the MCL is indicated.

REFERENCES

1. Grood E, Noyes F, Butler D, Suntay W: Ligamentous and capsular restraints preventing straight medial and lateral laxity in intact human cadaveric knees. J Bone Joint Surg Am 1981;63:1257–1269.
2. Warren L, Marshall J, Girgis F: The prime stabilizer of the medial side of the knee. J Bone Joint Surg Am 1974;56:665–674.
3. Mandelbaum B, Finerman G, Reicher M, et al: Magnetic resonance imaging as a tool for evaluation of traumatic knee injuries: Anatomic and pathoanatomical correlations. Am J Sports Med 1986;14:361–370.
4. Warren F, Marshall J: The supporting structures and layers on the medial side of the knee: An anatomical analysis. J Bone Joint Surg Am 1979;61:56–62.
5. Hughston J, Eilers A: The role of the posterior oblique ligament in tears of acute medial (collateral) ligament tears of the knee. J Bone Joint Surg Am 1973;55:923–940.
6. Hughston J: The importance of the posterior oblique ligament in repairs of acute tears of the medial ligaments in knees with and without an associated rupture of the anterior cruciate ligament. J Bone Joint Surg Am 1994;76:1328–1344.
7. Muller W: The Knee: Form, Function, and Ligament Reconstruction. Berlin, Springer-Verlag, 1983.
8. Sims F, Jacobson K: The posteromedial corner of the knee: Medial-sided injury patterns revisited. Am J Sports Med 2004;32:337–345.
9. Hughston J, Andrews J, Cross M, Moschi A: Classification of knee ligament instabilities. Part I. The medial compartment and cruciate ligaments. J Bone Joint Surg Am 1976;58:159–172.
10. Abbott L, Saunders J: Injuries to the ligaments of the knee joint. J Bone Joint Surg Am 1944;26:503–521.
11. England R: Repair of the ligaments about the knee. Orthop Clin North Am 1976;7:195–205.
12. Marshall J, Fetto J, Botero P: Knee ligament injuries. A standardized evaluation method. Clin Orthop 1977;123:115–129.
13. Quigley T: The treatment of avulsion of the collateral ligaments of the knee. Am J Surg 1949;78:574–581.
14. O'Donoghue D: Surgical treatment of fresh injuries to the major ligaments of the knee. J Bone Joint Surg Am 1950;32:721–738.
15. Hughston J, Barrett G: Acute anteromedial rotatory instability. Long-term results of surgical repair. J Bone Joint Surg Am 1983;65:145–153.
16. Ellsasser J, Reynolds F, Omohundro J: The non-operative treatment of collateral ligament injuries of the knee in professional football players: An analysis of seventy-four injuries treated non-operatively and twenty-four injuries treated surgically. J Bone Joint Surg Am 1974;56:1185–1190.
17. Fetto J, Marshall J: Medial collateral ligament injuries of the knee: A rationale for treatment. Clin Orthop 1978;132:206–218.
18. Indelicato P: Non-operative treatment of complete tears of the medial collateral ligament of the knee. J Bone Joint Surg Am 1983;65:323–329.
19. Indelicato P, Hermansdorfer J, Huegel M: Nonoperative management of complete tears of the medial collateral ligament of the knee in intercollegiate football players. Clin Orthop 1990;256:174–177.
20. Reider B, Sathy M, Talkington J, et al: Treatment of isolated medial collateral ligament injuries in athletes with early functional rehabilitation. A five-year follow-up study. Am J Sports Med 1994;22:470–477.
21. Shelbourne K, Porter D: Anterior cruciate ligament-medial collateral ligament injury: Nonoperative management of medial collateral ligament tears with anterior cruciate ligament reconstruction: A preliminary report. Am J Sports Med 1992;20:283–286.
22. Noyes F, Barber-Westin S: The treatment of acute combined ruptures of the anterior cruciate and medial ligaments of the knee. Am J Sports Med 1995;23:380–389.
23. Millett P, Pennock A, Sterett W, Steadman J: Early ACL reconstruction in combined ACL-MCL injuries. J Knee Surg 2004;17:94–98.
24. Wilson T, Satterfield W, Johnson D: Medial collateral ligament "tibial" injuries: Indication for acute repair. Orthopedics 2004;27:389–393.

55 Posterolateral Corner

Amir R. Moinfar, Daniel S. Lorenz, and Claude T. Moorman III

In This Chapter

INTRODUCTION

- The posterolateral corner (PLC) of the knee has been misunderstood and poorly described. In fact, it has been termed the "dark side" of the knee.[1] It was defined as a clinical entity as recently as 1976, and there continues to be considerable debate over the proper nomenclature for this region of the knee.

- To illustrate, Covey[2] reported that the popliteofibular ligament has been termed the short external lateral ligament, popliteofibular fascicles, fibular origin of the popliteus, and the popliteofibular fiber.

- There has been no clear algorithm or surgical technique that has been established as a gold standard for either acute or chronic instability.[3]

- Examination findings have been poorly described and confusing. Complicating this even more, structures in the PLC oftentimes are not well visualized by magnetic resonance imaging, making certain diagnoses challenging.[4]

- The PLC has received attention in recent years due to its role in the stabilization of the knee joint, especially in the success or failure of concomitant cruciate ligament repair.[5]

RELEVANT ANATOMY

The PLC of the knee has classically been described to include the lateral collateral ligament (LCL), popliteofibular ligament, popliteus tendon, and the arcuate ligament complex. Some authors have included the iliotibial band[2,5] and the fabellofibular ligament[5,6] in this group. Seebacher et al[7] divided the lateral aspect of the knee into three layers: (1) lateral fascia, iliotibial tract, and biceps femoris tendon; (2) patellar retinaculum and patellofemoral ligament; and (3) joint capsule, LCL, arcuate ligament, fabellofibular ligament, and popliteus tendon. It is this third layer that is the focus of this discussion.

The LCL arises from the lateral femoral condyle and attaches on the fibular head. It begins 2 cm above the joint line,[5] slightly proximal and posterior to the lateral epicondyle, and then proceeds distally and posteriorly to the posterior aspect of the fibular head.[5] The functions of each ligamentous structure in the knee are highlighted in Table 55-1.

The popliteus muscle originates on the anterior aspect of the lateral condyle of the femur, courses inferomedially, and inserts on the posterior tibia, proximal to the soleal line.[8] It also has attachments to the posterior and middle segments of the lateral meniscus (popliteomeniscal fascicle) and the apex of the fibula (popliteofibular fascicle).[5] The popliteus tendon itself lies in the lateral one third of the popliteal fossa, and it is anterior to the LCL femoral attachment.[9]

The arcuate ligament complex is intimately associated with the popliteus. The arcuate ligament is a Y-shaped ligament arising from the posterior part of the joint capsule. It tapers down to the insertion of the posterior aspect of the fibular head, running over the popliteus muscle.[5] The lateral limb of the arcuate ligament blends with the lateral gastrocnemius near its condylar insertion and the oblique popliteal ligament joins the semimembranosus tendon.[4] Because of its association with the arcuate ligament complex, the popliteus muscle is both intra-articular and extra-articular. The popliteus tendon passes under the LCL in the popliteal hiatus and then goes under the arcuate ligament before becoming extra-articular and joining the muscle belly of the popliteus.[4] Despite its connection with the popliteus, the arcuate ligament complex is often not included in the PLC literature because it is not consistently present in all knees. Researchers have found it to be present in 24%[10] to 80%[7] of knees.

The popliteofibular ligament is the ligamentous scaffolding attaching the popliteus tendon and the fibular head. Researchers[9] have shown that it has an anterior division and a posterior division. The anterior division attaches proximal to the musculotendinous junction of the popliteus muscle and distally to the anteromedial fibula, while the posterior division attaches to the posteromedial fibula. Much like the arcuate ligament, there is some debate over the prevalence of the popliteofibular ligament. Maynard et al[3] reported it in 100% of cadaver specimens, while Watanabe et al[11] reported it in 93% of knees and Sudasna and Harnsiriwattanagit[10] in 98% of knees.

The fabellofibular ligament is often not referred to in the PLC literature because the fabella is not present in all knees. The fabella is a sesamoid bone in the lateral head of the gastrocnemius at its proximal attachment to the femur. The fabellofibular ligament runs parallel to the LCL from the fabella to the fibula, inserting posterior to the insertion of the biceps tendon on the fibular head.[5] The fabellofibular ligament is found to be tight in extension and lax with increasing flexion.[12]

Table 55-1 Function of Knee Ligaments

	Posterior Cruciate Ligament	Lateral Collateral Ligament	Anterior Cruciate Ligament	Posterolateral Corner
Primary restraint	Posterior translation of tibia, IR of tibia	Varus at 30 degrees of knee flexion and 0 degrees of knee extension	Anterior translation of tibia, IR of tibia	ER of tibia
Secondary restraint	Valgus and varus forces	ER of tibia	Valgus and varus forces	Varus at 0 degrees and 30 degrees of knee extension

ER, External rotation; IR, internal rotation.

The iliotibial band, while often not discussed as being part of the PLC, is worth noting as it is important in preventing varus opening of the knee.[12] It inserts on Gerdy's tubercle on the anterolateral aspect of the tibial eminence. Through its origin on the gluteus maximus, it functionally helps to decelerate internal rotation of the tibia during gait.

More recent terminology has simplified the posterolateral anatomy into two surgically important structures: the LCL and the popliteus/popliteofibular ligament. Current reconstruction techniques thus focus on restoring stability to these two structures.

Blood Supply and Innervation

The popliteal artery and its genicular branches supply blood to the PLC.[2] The popliteal artery is a continuation of the femoral artery as it passes through the adductor hiatus. Innervation to the PLC is from multiple sources. The common peroneal nerve arises from the tibial nerve, just distal to the adductor hiatus, and courses inferolaterally posterior to the fibular head. The posterior tibial nerve, which is the distal continuation of the tibial nerve, and branches of the obturator nerve innervate the posterolateral capsule and lateral meniscus. A branch of the common peroneal nerve provides nervous fibers to the inferior/lateral capsule and the LCL. The popliteus is innervated by the tibial nerve, L4-S1.[8]

BIOMECHANICS

Much like the anatomy of the PLC, the biomechanics of this region and its resulting clinical implications are becoming better understood. The PLC helps to prevent posterior tibial translation, varus, and external rotation of the tibia.[3] Isolated PLC injury is uncommon and is often associated with concomitant cruciate ligament injury. DeLee et al[13] reported that in 735 knees treated for knee injury, only 12 (1.6%) had acute isolated PLC injury.

Prior to exploring the complex nature of the biomechanics, it is noteworthy that there are coupled motions that occur in the knee joint. With the foot fixed on the ground and the knee fully extended, as a person begins to flex the knee (as in sitting on a chair), the femur rolls posteriorly on the tibia, but glides anteriorly. The initial 10 degrees of knee flexion actually involves a medial rotation of the tibia to "unlock" the knee. Likewise, as the knee is extended with a closed kinetic chain, the femur rolls forward, glides posteriorly, and the tibia externally rotates for the last 10 degrees of extension. The last 10 degrees of external rotation is known as the screw home mechanism. The posterior cruciate ligament (PCL) helps to resist the posterior translation of the tibia, and the PLC resists the rotational forces. When an anterior force is applied to an intact knee, the tibia

rotates internally. Likewise, with a posterior force, the tibia rotates externally.[14] Therefore, it is apparent that the PLC and the cruciates are intimately related in the function of the knee. Brunnstrom[15] noted that the popliteus complements the PCL by preventing forward slide of the condyles in flexed knees, while also unlocking the lateral aspect of the knee in flexion.

The roles of the various parts of the ligamentous and capsular components have been elucidated in studies whereby each structure was selectively sectioned and the resulting biomechanical implications were analyzed. Davies et al[5] recently have summarized what is currently known from the literature (Box 55-1; Table 55-2).

Collectively, these studies show that sectioning of the posterolateral structures resulted in increased primary posterior translation, primary varus rotation, primary external rotation, and coupled external rotation. LaPrade et al measured forces on anterior cruciate ligament[16] and PCL grafts[17] following sectioning of posterolateral structures. In both grafts, forces on these grafts increased with varus load at 0 and 30 degrees of knee flexion and was even greater with coupled varus and external rotation than with an intact PLC. In the anterior cruciate ligament graft, coupled varus and internal rotation at 0 and 30 degrees increased graft force beyond that with varus alone. In PCL grafts[17], force on the graft was higher with the posterolateral structures transected during varus load at 30, 60, and 90

Box 55-1 Biomechanics of Posterolateral Rotary Instability

- If the lateral collateral ligament or posterolateral corner is cut individually, there is no change in the posterior translation at all angles of knee flexion. Lateral collateral ligament sectioning resulted in greater varus angulation than with posterolateral corner sectioning.
- If the lateral collateral ligament and posterolateral corner are cut together, there is increased posterior translation at all angles of knee flexion, and an increase in coupled external rotation and posterior forces. Additionally, there was increased varus, maximal at 30 degrees of knee flexion. Combined lateral collateral ligament/posterolateral corner sectioning revealed increased varus, greater than if the lateral collateral ligament alone is cut.
- If the posterior cruciate ligament alone is sectioned, there is increased posterior translation at all angles of flexion, increasing as the knee flexes from 0 to 90 degrees. Also, there is a cessation of coupled external rotation with posterior force.
- If the posterior cruciate ligament, lateral collateral ligament, and posterolateral corner complex are all cut, there is much greater posterior translation at all angles of flexion, increased varus rotation in response to varus forces, which is maximal at 60 degrees of flexion. Finally, there is an increase in primary external rotation.

Table 55-2 Motions Restricted by Ligamentous Structures in the Knee

	Posterior Cruciate Ligament	Lateral Collateral Ligament	Anterior Cruciate Ligament	Posterolateral Corner
ER of tibia	At 90 degrees of flexion		√	√
Varus at 30 degrees of flexion		√	Possibly	√
Posterior translation	All angles of flexion			
Anterior translation			√	
ER and posterior translation		√		√
Varus, ER, posterior translation	√	√		√
Varus at 0 degrees of extension	Possibly	√	Possibly	√
IR of tibia			√	√

ER, External rotation; IR, internal rotation.

degrees of knee flexion than with the posterolateral structures intact. In addition, coupled external rotation with a posterior force increased graft force at 30, 60, and 90 degrees compared to that with the posterolateral structures intact.

Veltri et al[14] studied the rotational contributions of the LCL, popliteofibular ligament, and popliteus tendon attachments. The popliteofibular ligament and the popliteus tendon were found to be crucial in the resisting of posterior translation, varus, external rotation, and coupled external rotation. In addition, they found that isolated sectioning of the anterior cruciate ligament and PCL resulted in increased primary anterior and posterior translation, respectively, and increased coupled external rotation and posterior force, increased varus, and increased primary internal rotation. Finally, at all angles of knee flexion, PCL and PLC sectioning resulted in increased primary posterior translation, increased primary external rotation, and increased varus. These increases were greater at 90 degrees of knee flexion compared to isolated posterior cruciate sectioning. Maynard et al[3] demonstrated that after simulation of a varus load, the LCL fails first, followed by the popliteofibular ligament, then the muscle belly of the popliteus.

From these studies, one can conclude that in order to differentiate posterior cruciate from PLC involvement, external rotation must be evaluated at both 30 and at 90 degrees of knee flexion. If there is greater external rotation at 30 degrees of flexion but not at 90 degrees of flexion, isolated PLC pathology is likely.

CLINICAL FEATURES AND EVALUATION

Posterolateral corner injuries occur from a blow to the anteromedial aspect of the knee, contact and noncontact hyperextension injuries, and varus contact of a flexed knee. There has been some speculation as to certain predisposing factors such as genu varum, pre-existing excess external tibial rotation, ligamentous laxity, recurvatum, and epiphyseal dysplasia. Patients having suffered an acute injury of the PLC describe a traumatic event and report pain over the posterolateral aspect of the knee. Patients may also complain of lower extremity weakness or numbness secondary to peroneal nerve injury. Patients also may report gait difficulties and instability, particularly complaining of hyperextension during toe off.

Physical examination that specifically isolates the structures of the posterolateral aspect of the knee is critical. Hughston and Norwood[18] described two tests, the posterolateral drawer test

and the external rotational recurvatum test, as key in detecting posterolateral rotatory instability. The posterolateral drawer test is performed to assess posterolateral rotation with the knee at 90 degrees of flexion. The foot is placed in 15 degrees of external rotation, and knee rotation is assessed while a posterolateral force is applied. An increase in rotation compared to the contralateral side typically reflects injury to the popliteus complex.[12] The external rotation recurvatum examination is performed by lifting both lower extremities by the hallux with the patient in the supine position. A positive test refers to increased hyperextension and resultant external rotation.[19] The reverse pivot shift is performed by slowly extending the knee from 45 degrees of flexion while applying a valgus and external rotational force to the knee. Reduction of the subluxated knee with extension connotes a positive result. Varus testing should be performed at both 0 and 30 degrees of flexion. Varus opening at 0 degrees is likely indicative of severe combined ligamentous injury, while opening at 30 degrees reflects incompetence of the LCL and possibly of other posterolateral structures.[18] The posterolateral rotation test, also referred to as the dial test, is performed at both 30 and 90 degrees of knee flexion. Although the test may be performed in the supine or prone position, the senior author prefers the prone position with the knees held tightly together to help eliminate hip rotation. A greater than 15-degree increase in external rotation compared to the contralateral side only with the knee at 30 degrees of flexion suggests an isolated PLC injury. A greater than 15-degree increase at 90 degrees of flexion reflects a concomitant PLC and PCL injury.[20] The knee should also be carefully evaluated for anterior and posterior cruciate ligamentous incompetence, in addition to medial-side knee injury. A thorough neurovascular examination is also necessary.

The gait status of an individual with suspected PLC insult will also help confirm clinical findings. Because of the role the PLC has in stabilizing varus forces, patients will typically present with a varus thrust or hyperextension at midstance, due to external rotation of the tibia at full extension.[5] Some patients may also walk with a flexed knee[2,5,21] to avoid pain and instability experienced with hyperextension. DeLeo et al[22] reported in a case study a patient with pain in terminal stance and push-off. In this phase of gait, the knee is flexing rapidly from full extension. Stresses to the lateral structures of the knee are increased here, resulting in decreased stance time on the involved limb.

Radiographic examination should consist of standard standing bilateral posteroanterior, lateral, and Merchant knee views.

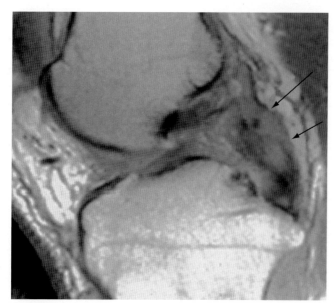

Figure 55-1 Posterolateral corner injury. Sagittal spin-echo intermediate-weighted magnetic resonance image (2000/20) through the intercondylar notch shows a thickened posterior cruciate ligament *(arrows)* with intermediate signal intensity throughout, indicative of a torn posterior cruciate ligament. (From Helms CA: The impact of MR imaging in sports medicine. Radiology 2002;224:631–635.)

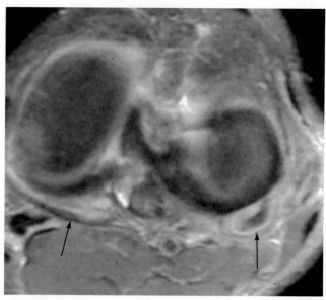

Figure 55-3 Transverse fast spin-echo T2-weighted fat suppressed magnetic resonance image (3000/70) at the level of the joint shows the posterior capsule *(left arrow)* of the medial side of the joint, which is not evident on the lateral side. This indicates a torn arcuate ligament (which should be seen as a thickening of the lateral capsule at the joint line). In addition, the popliteus tendon *(right arrow)* has high signal intensity within and a distended tendon sheath. (From Helms CA: The impact of MR imaging in sports medicine. Radiology 2002;224:631–635.)

Plain radiographs may reveal an avulsion fracture of the proximal fibula (arcuate sign), an avulsion of Gerdy's tubercle, or a Segond fracture (although more common with an anterior cruciate ligament injury). Stress radiographs may show lateral joint space widening. Chronic instability often reveals changes consistent with post-traumatic degenerative joint disease. If malalignment is also suspected, long-cassette hip-to-ankle films should be taken as they may serve beneficial in the planning of a possible osteotomy as an adjunct to ligament repair or recon-

struction. Magnetic resonance imaging is key in the evaluation of the specific individual components of the PLC of the knee. A high-powered magnet of at least 1.5 T is recommended in order to adequately assess the iliotibial band, long and short heads of the biceps femoris, LCL, popliteus, and the popliteofibular and fabellofibular ligaments (Figs. 55-1 through 55-4). A bone contusion of the anteromedial femoral condyle is also a common finding.

TREATMENT OPTIONS

Injuries of the PLC are rarely isolated injuries and are most often the result of significant trauma, with approximately 40% being athletic injuries.[14] Although the natural history of posterolateral instability is poorly understood, this injury is associated with the potential for significant morbidity. There is also increased disability when posterolateral instability is part of a combined ligament injury pattern. Unrecognized or inappropriately treated PLC injury has commonly been identified as a leading cause of anterior cruciate ligament reconstruction failure. Nonoperative management is reserved for mild instability without significant functional limitation.[23] These patients typically have no varus instability and are free from other associated ligamentous injury. Patients with a negative posterolateral rotation test are also often best suited by nonoperative management. Treatment entails 2 to 4 weeks of immobilization with protected weight bearing for the initial 2 weeks.

SURGERY

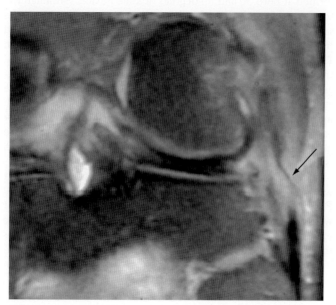

Figure 55-2 Coronal fast spin-echo T2-weighted fat-suppressed magnetic resonance image (3000/70) reveals a torn lateral collateral ligament *(arrow)*. (From Helms CA: The impact of MR imaging in sports medicine. Radiology 2002;224:631–635.)

If possible, primary surgical repair should be performed within 6 weeks from injury. A concern with isolated repair or recon-

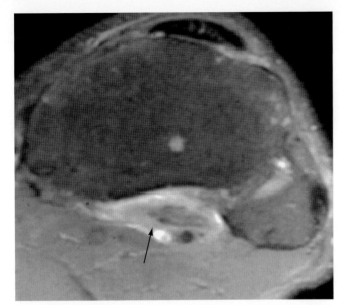

Figure 55-4 Transverse fast spin-echo T2-weighted magnetic resonance image (3000/70) several centimeters distal to the joint shows high signal intensity surrounding the popliteus muscle *(arrow)*, indicative of injury. At surgery, the popliteus muscle was torn at the musculotendinous junction, and the posterior cruciate, medial collateral, and arcuate ligaments were torn. (From Helms CA: The impact of MR imaging in sports medicine. Radiology 2002;224:631–635.)

struction is varus knee alignment. Varus deformity places increased tensile forces on the repair or reconstruction and may subsequently lead to incompetence and failure of the structures. A high tibial osteotomy may be recommended prior to, or concomitant with, posterolateral repair of reconstruction in this setting. In the case of chronic posterolateral rotary instability (PLRI) in the varus knee, the osteotomy is generally the first stage of a two-stage procedure with ligament reconstruction performed at a later setting.

SURGICAL TECHNIQUE

The patient is placed supine on the operating room table, with both the injured and uninjured legs in the extended position. A lateral valgus bar is placed next to the injured thigh. A thorough examination under anesthesia is carried out prior to proceeding with the definitive procedure. A bump of towels is placed under the injured knee. We have found arthroscopic evaluation of the knee with both acute and chronic posterolateral rotatory instability as a valuable adjunct to the open procedure. Noyes et al described the amount of lateral joint line opening under a varus load during arthroscopy. Incompetence of the PLC resulted in at least 12, 10, and 8 of opening at the periphery, mid-portion, and innermost medial edge of the lateral tibiofemoral compartment, respectively.[24] In addition, concomitant ligamentous, meniscal, and chondral injuries can be diagnosed and treated during arthroscopy. Open or arthroscopic cruciate reconstruction is at the surgeon's discretion. Acute PLC repair can be successful in the first 6 weeks following injury, assuming adequate tissue quality without severe injury. Successful surgical repair is aided by early intervention, prior to profound scar formation, in order to allow identification of anatomic structures.

At the conclusion of the arthroscopic portion of the procedure, the limb is exsanguinated, and a tourniquet is inflated to

300 to 350 mm Hg. A no. 10 blade is used to dissect a full-thickness skin flap through a laterally based hockey-stick incision that starts 8 cm proximal to the lateral joint line, immediately posterior to the lateral epicondyle, and courses approximately 7 cm distally between Gerdy's tubercle and the fibular head (Fig. 55-5). Care is taken to preserve at least a 7-cm skin bridge from other incisions, particularly from an anterior-based incision from open cruciate reconstruction (Fig. 55-6). The interval between the iliotibial band and biceps femoris tendon is developed, which allows exposure of the lateral head of the gastrocnemius and the posterior capsule (Fig. 55-7). The LCL and the popliteus tendon can be evaluated proximally by incising the iliotibial band at the level of the epicondyle. As the peroneal nerve runs posterior to the biceps femoris tendon, it must be carefully protected throughout the procedure (Fig. 55-8). Knee flexion and biceps femoris retraction helps to protect the peroneal nerve. LCL or popliteus avulsion from the femoral origin typically occurs concomitantly and can be repaired with direct sutures to bone, suture anchors, or soft-tissue screws with washers. Popliteus avulsion from the tibia can also be repaired in similar fashion. Disruption of the popliteofibular ligament can be treated by tenodesis of the popliteus to the posterior fibular head, reinforcing it with the fabellofibular ligament if present. Distal LCL avulsion accompanied by a large amount of bone can be repaired with screw or suture fixation. Most primary repairs benefit from tissue augmentation, which helps to allow more expeditious mobilization and rehabilitation.[25]

When repair is not a feasible option, numerous alternative techniques have been described to address the insufficient PLC. Hughston and Jacobsen[26] described advancement of the entire

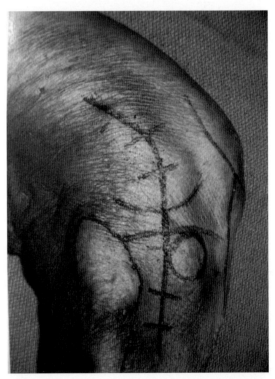

Figure 55-5 Position of preferred lateral incision for posterolateral corner reconstruction. (From Richards RS, Moorman CT: Open surgical treatment. In Fanelli GC [ed]: The Multiple Ligament Injured Knee. New York, Springer-Verlag, 2004, pp 143–146.)

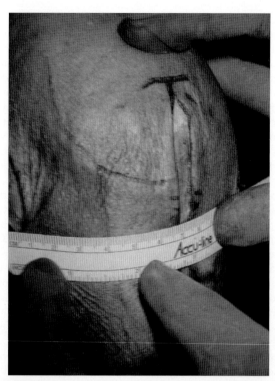

Figure 55-6 Relationship of the lateral incision to the anterior incision. (From Richards RS, Moorman CT: Open surgical treatment. In Fanelli GC [ed]: The Multiple Ligament Injured Knee. New York, Springer-Verlag, 2004, pp 143–146.)

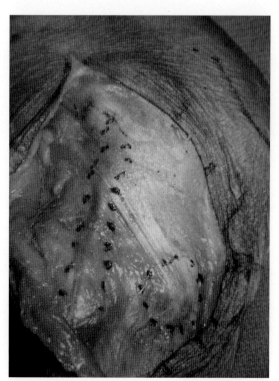

Figure 55-7 Exposure of the posterolateral corner with development of full-thickness skin flaps. Note relationship of the fibular head to Gerdy's tubercle. (From Richards RS, Moorman CT: Open surgical treatment. In Fanelli GC [ed]: The Multiple Ligament Injured Knee. New York, Springer-Verlag, 2004, pp 143–146.)

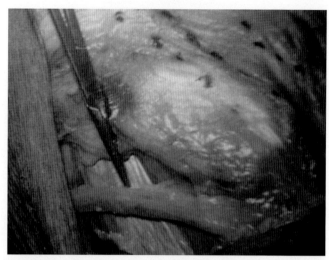

Figure 55-8 Peroneal nerve identification, dissection, and protection are critical in posterolateral corner exposure and reconstruction. (From Richards RS, Moorman CT: Open surgical treatment. In Fanelli GC [ed]: The Multiple Ligament Injured Knee. New York, Springer-Verlag, 2004, pp 143–146.)

PLC complex. Popliteal bypass procedures have been described using various tissues in order to reconstruct the popliteus muscle tendon unit. Clancy et al[27] popularized tenodesis of the biceps femoris to the anterolateral femoral epicondyle. The senior author employs a modified figure-eight fibular-based technique using double-stranded hamstring autograft. Research involving the senior author revealed that both fibular-based and combined tibiofibular-based PLC reconstruction techniques are equally effective in restoring external rotation and varus stability after simulated PLC injury.[28]

The approach to the PLC of the knee is the same as that for repair. The proximal fibula and biceps femoris tendon are isolated. The femoral fixation site for reconstruction is identified as the point between the footprint of the LCL and the insertion of the popliteus (Fig. 55-9). Next, attention is turned to the fibula. The fibula is drilled with a guide pin in an anterior-to-posterior direction, just superior to the fibular neck. Using a 7-mm acorn reamer, a tunnel is created over the guidewire (Fig. 55-10). The hamstring graft is then pulled through the fibular head, with the long limb of the graft passed posteriorly and around a 30- to 35-mm cancellous synthes screw with a washer (Fig. 55-11). The anterior limb is also passed around the washer; however, in the opposite direction. This produces a figure-eight type arrangement underneath the biceps femoris and iliotibial band. The posterior loop reproduces the popliteofibular complex, while the anterior loop reproduces the LCL (Fig. 55-12). The screw is then tightened in place, and the remaining posterior loop is placed through the fibular tunnel again in a posterior-to-anterior direction (Fig. 55-13). The two loops are then tied to one another with 2-0 Vicryl sutures. The posterolateral complex is then tensioned in 30 degrees of knee flexion, with the knee in slight valgus and internal rotation (Figs. 55-14 and 55-15). The posterolateral capsule is then fixed to the posterior aspect of the construct using no. 2 nonabsorbable sutures.

REHABILITATION

There is a paucity of literature on the rehabilitation of PLC injuries, treated both nonoperatively and operatively. No con-

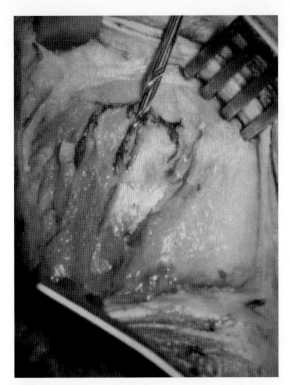

Figure 55-9 Identification of lateral femoral position for posterolateral corner reconstruction between the lateral collateral ligament and the popliteus tendon. (From Richards RS, Moorman CT: Open surgical treatment. In Fanelli GC [ed]: The Multiple Ligament Injured Knee. New York, Springer-Verlag, 2004, pp 143–146.)

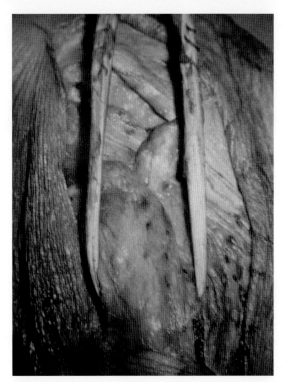

Figure 55-11 Passage of the double-hamstring autograft through the fibular head. (From Richards RS, Moorman CT: Open surgical treatment. In Fanelli GC [ed]: The Multiple Ligament Injured Knee. New York, Springer-Verlag, 2004, pp 143–146.)

trolled studies to date have been done on this region. Isolated low-grade injuries may do well with conservative treatment.[5] LaPrade and Wentorf[12] suggest that grade I to II PLC injuries can initially be treated nonoperatively in a knee immobilizer in full extension for 3 to 4 weeks non-weight bearing with no motion allowed. Patients may do quadriceps setting and straight

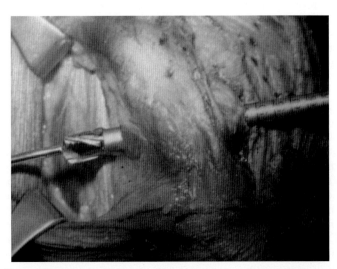

Figure 55-10 Preparation of the fibular head for passage of double-hamstring autograft. A 7-mm reamer is used in an anterior-to-posterior direction over a guidewire. (From Richards RS, Moorman CT: Open surgical treatment. In Fanelli GC [ed]: The Multiple Ligament Injured Knee. New York, Springer-Verlag, 2004, pp 143–146.)

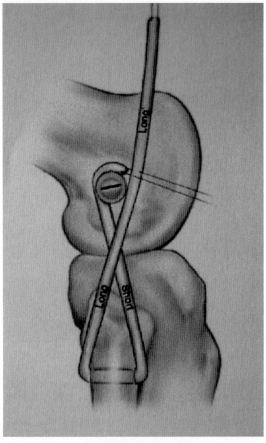

Figure 55-12 Reconstruction of the posterolateral corner.

573

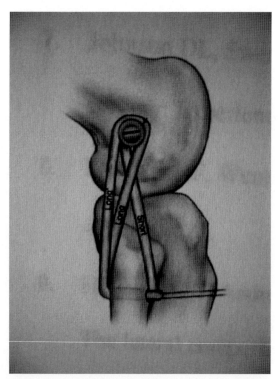

Figure 55-13 Posterolateral reconstruction. Screw and washer are placed.

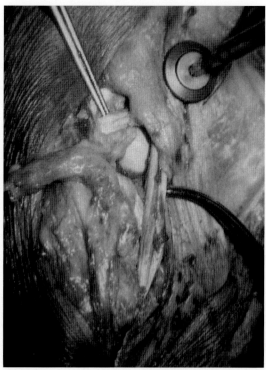

Figure 55-14 Fixation of the posterolateral corner "O" autograft. The graft is passed in a figure-of-eight fashion such that the posterior limb *(left)* serves as the popliteofibular complex and the anterior limb *(right)* serves as the reconstructed lateral collateral ligament. (From Richards RS, Moorman CT: Open surgical treatment. In Fanelli GC [ed]: The Multiple Ligament Injured Knee. New York, Springer-Verlag, 2004, pp 143–146.)

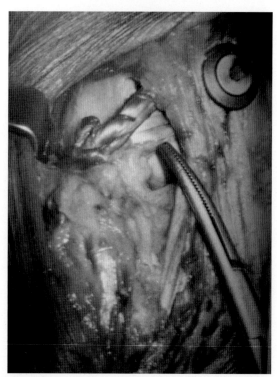

Figure 55-15 Fixation of the posterolateral corner graft often allows overlapping of the anterior and posterior limbs with extra tendon. Care is taken to ensure that the tendon is captured by the soft-tissue washer. (From Richards RS, Moorman CT: Open surgical treatment. In Fanelli GC [ed]: The Multiple Ligament Injured Knee. New York, Springer-Verlag, 2004, pp 143–146.)

leg raises. It is currently advised, however, that the leg raises be performed in a brace, with the brace locked at 20 degrees of flexion to minimize the effects of gravity causing either posterior translation or external rotation of the tibia. In this position, a straight leg raise is a misnomer. Bent leg raise is more appropriate terminology. Ultimately, weight-bearing status is at the discretion of the physician. At 4 weeks, LaPrade and Wentorf allow patients to begin range-of-motion exercises and gradual weight bearing. They also propose that closed-chain quadriceps strengthening with no active open-chain hamstring activity is done from weeks 6 to 10.

Wilk described, in the case study of DeLeo et al[22] a nonoperatively managed PLC injury, that strengthening of the hamstrings, gastrocnemius, popliteus, and hip musculature is indicated to help control varus at the knee. Also, a foot orthosis with a lateral heel wedge may be helpful to unload the lateral structures of the knee during stance phase, as well as a knee brace to offload the medial compartment. A brace may be necessary due to shifting of the axis for tibial rotation to the medial compartment with PLC sectioning.[14] The clinician must also be mindful of concomitant cruciate or collateral ligament injury. If present, it will change precautions and indications for therapy. Determining the plan of care for PLC injuries should be managed on a case-by-case basis involving all members of the health care team.

In cases of nonoperative management, goals of therapy are to protect the PLC and maintain quadriceps function. Thus, quadriceps setting and bent leg raises with the brace in 20 degrees of flexion are advocated. Achieving full active extension to 0 degrees is contraindicated for 4 weeks due to the tensile forces that will be placed on the PLC at full extension. Limiting extension ensures that proper healing of the tissues is optimized. As stated previously, weight bearing is at the discretion of the physician, but current standard of practice is for an initial period of protected weight bearing as tolerated with the brace locked at 10 to 20 degrees of flexion. Weight bearing may be indicated because a lack of articular compression deprives articular cartilage of nutrition, which may hasten degeneration of the cartilage matrix.[29] Once the patient can bear weight, balance/proprioceptive exercises should be initiated in a closed chain to encourage cocontraction of the hamstrings and quadriceps in stance. Active open-chain knee flexion against gravity is not advised until 6 to 8 weeks after the injury. Pool exercise may also be useful to help with motion and gait status.

One study elucidated the results of PLC reconstructions and rehabilitation outcomes. Noyes and Barber-Westin[21] reconstructed posterolateral complex injuries using allograft tissues in 20 patients. They reported a 76% success rate by means of stress radiographs and knee stability examinations. The day after surgery, patients did patellar mobilizations, straight (bent) leg raises, electrical muscle stimulation, and isometrics. Patients were non-weight bearing for 4 weeks, and they completed active-assisted range-of-motion exercises six to eight times per day from 10 to 90 degrees. Pool exercises commenced at the third month, and no hamstring activity was done until week 12. Patients were gradually progressed to full weight bearing by the 16th week. Bracing was used for the first 9 months postoperatively to prevent abnormal hyperextension, varus, and external rotation of the tibia. Full hyperextension was avoided until 6 months after surgery.

Key considerations in the postoperative care of PLC reconstructions are prevention of (1) varus and external rotation of the tibia, (2) active knee flexion against gravity, and (3) extension/hyperextension of the tibia to protect the grafts. Therefore, no active knee flexion against gravity is done until 12 weeks postoperatively due to the internal rotation of the tibia during the first 10 degrees of flexion and the posterior translation, which places tensile forces on the graft. Passive extension to 0 degrees with gravity eliminated and without overpressure is advocated. Additionally, full hyperextension is not emphasized until up to 3 months postoperatively. Hyperextension should be based on bilateral comparison of the uninvolved limb. Achieving extension of the involved limb should be based on the uninvolved. Contrary to isolated ACL reconstruction in which hyperextension is emphasized immediately, hyperextension after PLC reconstruction can potentially lead to graft failure,[30] but 0 degrees of extension is achieved. Not only does it help minimize scar tissue infiltration in the joint, but extension to 0 degrees also helps decrease anterior knee pain. If the knee cannot reach 0 degrees, the quadriceps must contract more forcefully to achieve terminal knee extension needed for heel strike and the midstance portions of gait.

Protected motion is also advocated with the brace unlocked, using passive or active-assisted range of motion to tolerance. Complete immobilization is not recommended due to the deleterious effects associated with it, including decreased bone mass, articular cartilage changes, synovial adhesions, muscular inhibition,[29] and increased risk of arthrofibrosis due to ligament and capsule stiffness.[30] In addition, it leads to loss of lubrication between joint surfaces.[29] The paradox is that the knee must be protected against undue forces, but also must be moved to prevent the negative effects secondary to prolonged immobilization.

Following surgical repair, gait is gradually progressed beginning at week 6. It is imperative that assistive devices not be discontinued without normal, nonantalgic gait. Often crutches are discontinued completely, and patients ambulate with a Trendelenburg gait pattern. It is advised that patients progress from bilateral axillary crutches, then to one crutch on the contralateral side, and then a standard cane if necessary. The Trendelenburg gait pattern can cause subtle malfunctions in the kinetic chain that may lead to pain or pathology in other joints, particularly the hip and low back. Careful gait observation should be made by both the physician and rehabilitation professional to ensure that proper gait has been achieved.

Because of the non-weight-bearing status, the ipsilateral hip abductors can weaken, complicating gait status once it is allowed at week 6. The gluteus medius stabilizes the ipsilateral pelvis to prevent the contralateral pelvis from dropping inferiorly at midstance. Thus, active hip abduction exercises of the involved limb, standing with a brace, are advocated early to help minimize the presence of the Trendelenburg gait pattern due to gluteus medius weakness. Hip abduction exercises with the hip in neutral and in slight external rotation are effective exercises to be included as part of physical therapy and/or the home exercise program. Resistance should be placed above the knee in order to minimize potential varus forces that would exist if the resistance were placed distal to the knee. Likewise, side-lying exercises are contraindicated initially due to the deleterious effects of varus forces on the reconstructed grafts. Repeating this exercise bilaterally once the patient can fully weight bear will help with control of the involved limb in unilateral stance.

Aquatic therapy can be very beneficial for improving range of motion and gait status. Noyes and Barber-Westin[21] proposed that this start at 12 weeks. Currently, 6 weeks should be sufficient for the patient to begin careful weight bearing and gait training in the pool. In chest deep water, the patient is approximately 75% unweighted. Buoyancy of water minimizes stress placed on the injured knee.[29] Therefore, the water can assist the patient in achieving a normal gait pattern. The patient can be progressed to shallower water, as 50% of body weight is present at waist level. As gait normalizes, this will likely transfer benefit to land-based gait training.

A protocol for postoperative rehabilitation is presented in Box 55-2. With proper communication between patient, physician, and rehabilitation professional, safe return to full activity is anticipated following reconstruction of the PLC. In addition, a systematic, graded progression of exercise while being mindful of the healing process will ensure that dynamic stability and strength returns to the involved limb.

COMPLICATIONS

Posterolateral corner injuries rarely occur in isolation, and the complex nature of this injury leads to numerous potential complications. Neurologic and vascular injuries may be sustained secondary to the traumatic incident itself. Iatrogenic complications may include neurologic injury and intraoperative fracture during the course of the reconstruction. Failure to appreciate and identify other areas of instability may lead to early failure. In addition, arthrofibrosis, infection, persistent postoperative pain, and painful hardware are also potential complications.

Box 55-2 Protocol for Postoperative Rehabilitation

Phase I: Postoperative weeks 1 to 6
Goals
1. Decrease pain and swelling
2. Maintain patellar mobility
3. Protect against varus, external rotation, and flexion forces
4. Initiate and sustain active quadriceps set
5. Maintain cardiovascular endurance via upper body ergometer

Weight-bearing status: Non-weight bearing
Brace: Physician preference; but current standard is locked at full extension, unlock for physical therapy at week 4
Exercises
1. Ankle pumps
2. Patellar mobilizations: superior/inferior, medial/lateral
3. Passive extension to 0 degrees without overpressure/with gravity eliminated
4. Quadriceps sets, adductor setting with quadriceps sets, gluteal sets, bent leg raises
5. Begin passive/active-assisted range of motion for flexion at week 4

Phase II: Weeks 6 to 10
Goals
1. Begin weight bearing with unlocked brace
2. Progress to full range of motion in gravity-eliminated position
3. Continue to protect against varus, external rotation, and flexion forces

Weight-bearing status: Weight bear as tolerated and progress to full weight bearing
Brace: Unlock brace, may discharge when gait is normalized
Exercises
1. Active knee flexion in seated position, not against gravity
2. Initiate biking, emphasizing range of motion
3. Initiate pool exercises to help increase range of motion and help with weight bearing
4. Initiate progressive resistance exercise for the quadriceps (i.e., knee extension)

5. Initiate active knee flexion against gravity at week 10 and progress to progressive resistance as tolerated

Phase III: Weeks 12 to 16
Goals
1. Full weight bearing without assistive devices and nonantalgic
2. Begin closed-chain exercises
Exercises
1. Bicycle for range of motion and endurance
2. Pool program (strengthening, swimming, walking)
3. Closed-chain exercises:
   a. Mini-squats
   b. Front lunges
   c. Ball/wall squats
   d. Leg press
   e. Step ups: forward, side
   f. Step downs
   g. Lateral lunges
   h. Multidirectional lunges
4. Continue isotonic strengthening for the knee extensors, hip abductors/adductors, and hamstrings
5. Stairmaster, elliptical trainer for endurance
6. Proprioceptive/balance exercises
   a. Progress from stable to unstable surfaces, unidirectional to multidirectional, single plane to multiple plane
   b. Eyes open, eyes closed
   c. Cervical movement to help enhance vestibular input

Phase IV: 4 to 6 months postoperatively
Goals
1. Gradually initiate pool running and agility drills in the pool
2. Continue all strengthening exercises
3. Progress to land-based agility as pool exercises are pain free
4. Gradual return to sports activities at least 6 months postoperatively following isokinetic testing, multidirectional functional and sport-specific testing

CONCLUSIONS

PLC injuries present numerous challenges to the orthopedic surgeon. Expeditious and accurate diagnosis of this condition and all other concomitant injuries is critical in achieving a successful outcome. The decision to pursue nonoperative or operative management should be carefully analyzed and based on patient expectation, level of function, and motivation and only after a comprehensive physical examination and review of pertinent radiographic studies. We believe that a fibular-based reconstruction using hamstring autograft in conjunction with a specific, carefully supervised rehabilitation protocol can successfully achieve the goal of a stable and functional knee.

REFERENCES

1. Andrews JR, Baker CL, Curl WW: Surgical repair of acute and chronic lesions of the lateral capsular ligamentous complex of the knee. In Feagin JA (ed): The Cruciate Ligaments: Diagnosis and Treatment. New York, Churchill Livingstone, 1988, pp 425–438.
2. Covey DC: Injuries to the posterolateral corner of the knee. J Bone Joint Surg Am 2001;83:106–118.
3. Maynard MJ, Deng XH, Wickiewicz TL, Warren RF: The popliteofibular ligament: Rediscovery of a key element in posterolateral stability. Am J Sports Med 1996;24:311–315.
4. Recondo JA, Salvador E, Villanua JA, et al: Lateral stabilizing structures of the knee: Functional anatomy and injuries assessed with MR imaging. Radiographics 2000;20:S91–S102.
5. Davies H, Unwin A, Aichroth P: The posterolateral corner of the knee: Anatomy, biomechanics, and management of injuries. Injury 2004;35:68–75.
6. Kim YC, Cheng IH, Yoo WK, et al: Anatomy and magnetic resonance imaging of posterolateral structures of the knee. Clin Anat 1997;10:397–404.
7. Seebacher JR, Inglis AE, Marshall JL, Warren RF: The structure of the posterolateral aspect of the knee. J Bone Joint Surg Am 1982;64:536–541.
8. Kendall FP, McCreary EK, Provance PG: Muscles: Testing and Function, 4th ed. Baltimore, Williams & Wilkins, 1993.
9. LaPrade RF, Ly TV, Wentorf FA, Engebretsen L: The posterolateral attachments of the knee: A qualitative and quantitative morphologic

analysis of the fibular collateral ligament, popliteus tendon, popliteofibular ligament, lateral gastrocnemius tendon. Am J Sports Med 2003;31:854–860.

10. Sudasna S, Harnsiriwattanagit K: The ligamentous structures of the posterolateral aspect of the knee. Bull Hosp Jt Dis Orthop Inst 1990; 50:35–40.

11. Watanabe Y, Moriya H, Takahashi K, et al: Functional anatomy of the posterolateral structures of the knee. Arthroscopy 1993;9:57–62.

12. LaPrade RF, Wentorf F: Diagnosis and treatment of posterolateral knee injuries. Clin Orthop 2002;402:110–121.

13. DeLee JC, Riley MB, Rockwood CA Jr: Acute posterolateral rotatory instability of the knee. Arthroscopy 2002;18(2 Suppl 1):1–8.

14. Veltri DM, Deng XH, Torzilli PA, et al: The role of the cruciate and posterolateral ligaments in stability of the knee: A biomechanical study. Am J Sports Med 1995;23:436–443.

15. Brunnstrom S: Clinical Kinesiology, 3rd ed. Philadelphia, FA Davis, 1983.

16. LaPrade RF, Resig S, Wentorf F, Lewis JL: The effects of grade III posterolateral complex knee injuries on ACL graft force: A biomechanical analysis. Am J Sports Med 1999;27:469–475.

17. LaPrade RF, Muench C, Wentorf F, Lewis JL: The effect of injury to the posterolateral structures of the knee on force in a PCL graft: A biomechanical study. Am J Sports Med 2002;30:233–238.

18. Hughston JC, Norwood LA Jr: The posterolateral drawer test and external rotation recurvatum test for posterolateral rotatory instability of the knee. Clin Orthop 1980;147:82–87.

19. LaPrade RF, Terry GC: Injuries to the posterolateral aspect of the knee: Association of anatomic injury patterns with clinical instability. Am J Sports Med 1997;25:433–438.

20. Grood ES, Stowers SF, Noyes FR: Limits of movement in the human knee: Effect of sectioning the posterior cruciate ligament and the posterolateral structures. J Bone Joint Surg Am 1988;70:88–97.

21. Noyes FR, Barber-Westin SD: Surgical reconstruction of severe chronic posterolateral complex injuries of the knee using allograft tissues. Am J Sports Med 1995;23:2–12.

22. DeLeo AT, Woodzell WW, Snyder-Mackler L: Resident's case problem: Diagnosis and treatment of posterolateral instability in a patient with lateral collateral ligament repair. J Orthop Sports Phys Ther 2003; 33:185–194.

23. Chen FS, Rokito AS: Acute and chronic posterolateral rotatory instability of knee. J Am Acad Orthop 2000;8:97–110.

24. Fanelli GC: Treatment of combined anterior cruciate ligament-posterior cruciate ligament-lateral side injuries of the knee. Clin Sports Med 2000;19:493–501.

25. Veltri DM, Warren RF: Anatomy, biomechanics, and physical findings in posterolateral knee instability. Clin Sports Med 1994;13:599–614.

26. Hughston JC, Jacobsen KE: Chronic posterolateral rotatory instability of the knee. J Bone Joint Surg Am 1985;67:351–359.

27. Clancy WG, Meister K, Craythome CB. Posterolateral corner collateral ligament reconstruction. In Jackson D (ed): Reconstructive Knee Surgery. New York, Raven Press, 1995, pp 143–159.

28. Moorman CT, Clancy WG: American Orthopaedic Society for Sports Medicine. Annual Meeting, July 1, 2002, Lake Buena Vista, FL.

29. Zachazewski JE, Magee DJ, Quillen WS: Athletic Injuries and Rehabilitation. Philadelphia, WB Saunders, 1996.

30. Irrgang JJ, Fitzgerald GK: Rehabilitation of the multiple ligament injured knee. Clin Sports Med 2000;19:545–571.

56 Multiligament Knee Injuries

James R. Gardiner and Darren L. Johnson

In This Chapter

Classification
Associated injuries
Initial evaluation and management
Nonoperative management
Surgery

INTRODUCTION

- A multiligament knee injury is a serious injury that presents the orthopedic surgeon with a complex treatment challenge.

- Multiligament knee injuries result from a minimal disruption of two or more of the major stabilizing ligaments of the knee and often result in multidirectional instability patterns.

- Knee dislocation may be misleading because the majority of knee dislocations present after having spontaneously reduced. Therefore, the term multiligament knee injury may be more appropriate.

- Treatment of this injury may be complicated by associated neurovascular, articular cartilage, meniscal, osseous, and soft-tissue injuries.

- Effective treatment requires the clinician to be aware of the associated injury patterns and to be proficient in the evaluation and treatment of multiligament injuries.

INCIDENCE

Acute knee dislocations are a rare event, accounting for less than 0.02% of all orthopedic injuries.[1-3] The true incidence is probably unknown because the majority of multiple-ligament-injured knees present after spontaneous reduction. In one series, the incidence of multiligament injuries in an athletically active population was 1.2% of orthopedic trauma.[4]

RELEVANT ANATOMY

A thorough understanding of the complex anatomy surrounding the knee is essential to accurate diagnosis and appropriate decision making during treatment of the multiligament-injured knee. The anatomy of the major stabilizing ligaments of the knee (anterior cruciate ligament [ACL], posterior cruciate ligament [PCL], medial cruciate ligament [MCL], lateral collateral ligament) as well as secondary stabilizers (posterolateral corner, pos-

teromedial capsule, menisci, and musculotendinous units) have been well studied and are thoroughly reviewed in other chapters.[5]

In addition to knowledge of major stabilizing ligaments, it is important to be familiar with the relevant neurovascular anatomy. The popliteal artery is the continuation of the superficial femoral artery as it passes through the tendinous hiatus of the adductor magnus. The popliteal artery is tethered proximally at the adductor hiatus and distally as it passes under the soleus arch making it susceptible to traction injuries in these areas. The skin surrounding the knee receives a rich blood supply from the superior, middle, and inferior geniculate branches of the popliteal artery. However, this anastomotic ring provides inadequate collateral circulation for lower limb perfusion in the event of disruption of popliteal flow. The sciatic nerve divides proximal to the popliteal space into posterior tibial and common peroneal divisions. The common peroneal nerve courses inferolaterally deep to the biceps femoris and passes around the fibular neck causing it to be more susceptible to injury.

CLASSIFICATION

Classification of orthopedic injuries can be useful for both effective communication between physicians and development of appropriate treatment strategies. Multiligament-injured knees can be classified based on the following parameters: (1) joint position, (2) injured structures, (3) energy level, and (4) chronicity. Classification of knee dislocations is summarized in Table 56-1.

Historically, knee dislocations like other joint dislocations, have been classified based on the position of the distal bone (tibia) in relation to the proximal bone (femur). Kennedy[2] noted five main types of dislocations: anterior (40%), posterior (33%), lateral (18%), medial (4%), and rotational (5%). This classification system is limited because the majority of dislocations present following spontaneous reduction.

Although the least common type, the posterolateral dislocation, is well described and is one of the few useful aspects of the positional classification system. The hallmark of this type of dislocation is its frequent irreducibility secondary to "button-holing" of the medial femoral condyle through the medial capsule and invagination of the MCL into the medial joint space[6] (Fig. 56-1). The posterolateral dislocation often produces a dimple sign on the medial aspect of the knee (Fig. 56-2).

The anatomic system classifies multiligament-injured knees based on functional evaluation of injured structures,[7] which is determined by a thorough clinical examination. The anatomic system clearly defines which structures are injured and can be used to guide surgical planning.

Table 56-1 Classification of Knee Dislocations

Anatomic Classification	
KDI	Cruciate intact knee dislocation
KDII	Both cruciates torn, collateral intact
KDIII	Both cruciates torn, one collateral torn
KDIIIM	MCL torn
KDIIIL	LCL torn
KDIV	All four ligaments torn
KDV	Periarticular fracture-dislocation
Joint Position	
Anterior	40%
Posterior	33%
Lateral	18%
Rotational	5%
Medial	4%
Energy Level	
High	Fractures and neurovascular injury common
Low	
Chronicity	
Acute	<3 wk
Subacute	3–12 wk
Chronic	>3 mo

Data obtained from references 2, 4, 6, 9, 11.

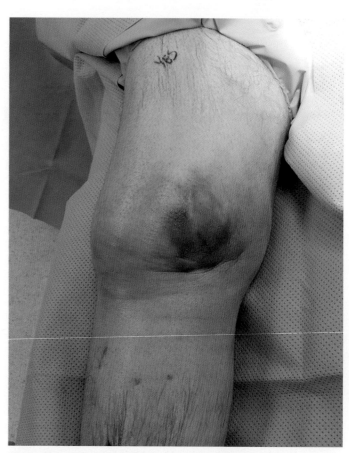

Figure 56-2 Clinical photograph of a right posterolateral knee dislocation showing dimple sign. Orientation is with the patient's head toward the top. This photograph corresponds to the magnetic resonance image shown in Figure 56-1.

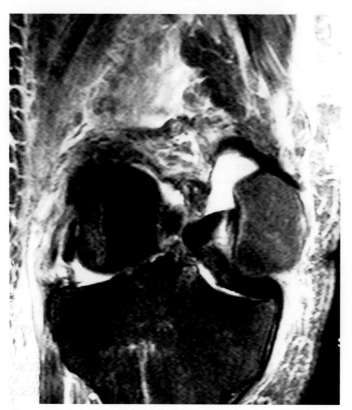

Figure 56-1 Coronal magnetic resonance image of a multiligament-injured knee showing displacement of the medial collateral ligament and medial capsule into joint space.

In addition to the anatomic classification, knee dislocations can be classified based on the energy level or chronicity of the injury. Higher energy level injuries are often associated with additional musculoskeletal or systemic injuries. Low-energy dislocations have a lower incidence of vascular, neurologic, and meniscal injuries.[8] In high-energy dislocations, the rate of popliteal artery injury ranges from 14% to 65%. Fifty percent to 60% of patients will have fractures, and 41% will have multiple fractures. Patients with these high-energy injuries often have other significant injuries to their head or chest, which precludes early aggressive treatment of their knee ligaments.[9]

The chronicity of the injury is also important with regard to associated injuries and surgical planning. Surgical treatment gives improved results in acute versus chronic cases.[10] Some structures may be repaired if treated acutely, whereas late treatment may require a reconstruction. A knee dislocation is acute if seen within 3 weeks, subacute if seen between 3 to 12 weeks, and chronic if seen after 3 months.[11]

MECHANISM OF INJURY

The mechanism of injury provides useful information regarding the direction and degree of injury. The mechanisms for the two most common patterns, anterior and posterior dislocations, are well described. Kennedy[2] was able to reproduce anterior dislocation by using a hyperextension force acting on the knee. At 30 degrees of hyperextension, the posterior capsule fails. This is followed at about 50 degrees by the ACL, PCL, and popliteal artery. Posterior dislocations can be caused by a force applied to the anterior proximal tibia in the knee flexed 90 degrees. This has been referred to as the so-called dashboard injury and may be associated with a hip fracture or dislocation.

Knee dislocations can also occur from sports-related or low-velocity mechanisms. Shelbourne and Klootwyk[8] reported that the most commonly involved sports were football (35%), wrestling (15%), and running (10%). Industrial accidents and falls are other common mechanisms.[2]

ASSOCIATED INJURIES

All anatomic structures surrounding the knee are at risk of injury following a knee dislocation. By definition, more than one of the four primary ligamentous stabilizers of the knee is disrupted following a multiligament injury. In addition, neurovascular injuries are common. Bony injuries may occur and range from simple avulsions to intra-articular fracture-dislocations. High-energy dislocations may be associated with significant injury to the surrounding soft tissue including skin and myotendinous units. Patients who sustain a high-energy knee dislocation will present with spontaneous reduction up to 50% of the time, leading to delayed or missed diagnosis.[9]

Vascular Injuries

Vascular injuries may occur with all types of knee dislocations. The presence of a multiligament-injured knee obligates the clinician to carefully evaluate the circulatory status of the injured extremity. The overall incidence of recognized popliteal vessel injury ranges from 10% to 44%.[12-14] The popliteal artery is an end artery for the leg as the genicular arteries provide inadequate collateral circulation to maintain limb perfusion. Obstruction of the popliteal vessels can lead to prolonged ischemia and eventual amputation.

Nerve Injuries

The incidence of nerve injuries with knee dislocations is 20% to 30%.[15,16] The injury can range from stretching of the nerve (neurapraxia) to transection. The peroneal nerve is most commonly injured, but injuries to the tibial nerve can occur. Injuries to the lateral and posterolateral corner of the knee place the peroneal nerve at increased risk because of its superficial location at the level of the fibular neck. The prognosis of severe peroneal nerve injuries is poor. Complete nerve injuries only recover about 50% of the time.[15,17] First-degree injuries (neurapraxia) commonly recover within 1 to 4 months.[15]

Other Injuries

Open dislocations may occur in as many as 30% of high-energy dislocations. The highest incidence is in dislocations that are in the sagittal plane. Cole and Harner[11] reported injuries to the patellar tendon or biceps in 20% of these patients (Fig. 56-3). Associated fractures of the distal femur and tibial plateau may occur in up to 30% of high-energy dislocations.[11] Patients who sustain high-energy dislocations also often have multiorgan system trauma requiring specialized evaluation and treatment. Recognition and treatment of associated injuries may take precedence and have implications upon definitive treatment of ligamentous injuries.

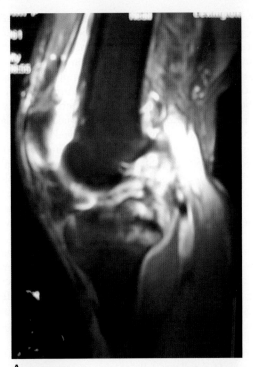

A

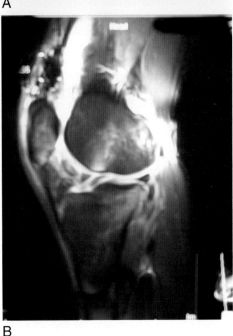

B

Figure 56-3 Sagittal magnetic resonance images of high-energy multiligament knee injury. **A,** Disruption of anterior and posterior cruciate ligaments. **B,** Partial quadriceps rupture and open anterior wound.

INITIAL EVALUATION AND MANAGEMENT

History and Physical Examination

Although some knee dislocations present with obvious deformity, most multiligament knee injuries spontaneously reduce. One must have a high index of suspicion, particularly in the polytrauma setting where these injuries may go overlooked. Important elements from the history include injury mechanism, direction of force, and position of the leg.

After obtaining a history, a thorough physical examination must be performed. Careful visual inspection should note any deformity, wound, or skin discoloration. Patients with a knee dislocation will often have a large effusion and even swelling of the entire extremity. The presence of a dimple sign or tight compartments must be assessed. A detailed neurovascular examination of both lower extremities must be performed. Evaluation of the sensory and motor functions of peroneal and tibial nerves should be well documented and followed serially. Careful assessment of the circulatory status of the limb should include observation of capillary refill, palpation of the popliteal, posterior tibial and dorsalis pedis pulses, as well as Doppler ankle brachial indices. Keep in mind that a patient with brisk capillary refill and palpable pulses may still have a vascular injury.

In the acute setting, swelling and pain often prevent a detailed ligament examination. However, the best possible assessment should be obtained. The four main ligamentous structures include the ACL, PCL, MCL with posteromedial capsule, and the lateral collateral ligament with posterolateral corner. Each of these structures must be systematically evaluated for stability. The most sensitive test for ACL rupture is the Lachman test performed with the knee held in 20 to 30 degrees of flexion.[18] The most sensitive test for detecting PCL injury is the posterior drawer test performed with the knee in 90 degrees of flexion.[19] The collateral ligaments are assessed by applying varus and valgus stress at both 30 degrees of flexion and full extension. Laxity in full extension denotes disruption of a cruciate ligament and the posteromedial or posterolateral capsule in addition to collateral injury. These patients will exhibit rotatory instability that must be identified initially and addressed at the time of surgery. Techniques for a comprehensive knee examination have been described in a previous chapter.

Imaging

Upon completion of the initial examination, anteroposterior and lateral radiographs of the affected extremity should be obtained. This should be done prior to any attempts at manipulation. Obtaining radiographs allows for diagnosis of any associated fractures and will assist in planning the appropriate reduction maneuver. Magnetic resonance imaging (MRI) is necessary to evaluate the ligamentous structures and other soft tissues (Fig. 56-4). It may help to diagnose patellar tendon or quadriceps rupture, which would require early repair. MRI may also identify meniscal injuries, articular cartilage lesions, bone bruises, and occult fractures. We recommend performing MRI in all cases in which repair or reconstruction is planned. This imaging study can be obtained in a nonemergent fashion.

Reduction

An unreduced knee dislocation represents a true orthopedic emergency. A reduction should be performed expeditiously after completion of initial evaluation and radiographs. Following administration of appropriate sedatives, reduction is performed by applying gradual longitudinal traction through the ankle with manipulation of the proximal tibia in the appropriate direction. Following reduction, with the patient still sedated, a repeat examination of the stability of the knee can be performed. Reduction should be confirmed with radiographs. It is imperative to reassess the neurovascular status of the limb following manipulation.

Keep in mind that an anteromedial dimple sign indicates a posterolateral dislocation. In this setting, closed reduction is unlikely to be successful and probably should not be attempted.

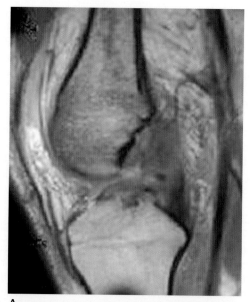

A

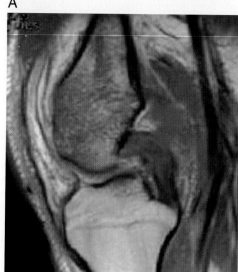

B

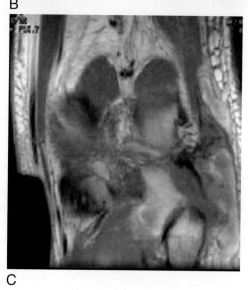

C

Figure 56-4 Sagittal magnetic resonance images of multiligament knee injury showing anterior cruciate ligament disruption (**A**), posterior cruciate ligament disruption (**B**), and fibular collateral ligament disruption (**C**).

Because of interposed soft tissue within the medial joint space, open reduction is warranted.[20]

Stabilization

Once reduction has been confirmed radiographically, the knee needs to be temporarily stabilized. Potential modes for temporary stabilization include a hinged knee brace, long-leg splint, and knee-spanning external fixation. The choice depends on the patient's body habitus, presence of concomitant musculoskeletal or systemic injuries, and overall stability of the knee. For most low-energy injuries, immobilization in full extension with a hinged knee brace or long-leg splint is appropriate. For high-energy injuries, in select polytrauma patients, and patients with significant soft-tissue injuries, external fixation may be more appropriate. Whatever mode of stabilization is selected, it is important to radiographically verify that reduction is maintained immediately after immobilization and at regular intervals thereafter.

Vascular Injuries

Popliteal artery injury is often associated with knee dislocation following blunt trauma. The risk of amputation is high if revascularization is not accomplished within a 6- to 8-hour window.[1,2,13] Patients who present with signs of vascular compromise, including diminished or absent pulses, pallor, or temperature changes clearly require emergent vascular surgery consultation. However, the most appropriate method of vascular evaluation for a patient with a knee dislocation without signs of ischemia remains controversial.

Historically, authors have advocated routine angiography on all patients with a multiligament-injured knee secondary to the relatively high incidence of popliteal vessel injury.[1,2,21,22] Routine angiography is also supported by the fact that as many as 30% of patients with popliteal artery injuries will have palpable distal pulses.[9,23] However, more recent literature has supported the role of serial physical examination, including an ankle brachial index with use of selective angiography only if abnormalities are detected on physical examination.[13,22] Additional noninvasive techniques include duplex ultrasonography.[24]

Stannard et al[22] performed a prospective cohort study evaluating the role of physical diagnosis in determining the need for angiography. They evaluated 138 consecutive patients with an acute multiligament knee injury. All patients underwent serial physical examination for 48 hours. Arteriography was obtained in patients with a decrease in pedal pulses, temperature or color changes, expanding hematoma, or documented abnormal vascular examination prior to presentation. In their cohort, physical examination had a positive predictive value of 90%, a negative predictive value of 100%, sensitivity of 100%, and specificity of 99%.

We have incorporated the use of serial physical examination and selective angiography in our algorithm for initial evaluation and management of multiligament knee injuries. This is based on advocacy of selective arteriography in more recent literature as well as the associated cost and risk of routine arteriography. Table 56-2 provides an algorithm for the initial evaluation and management of multiligament knee injuries.

Table 56-2 Algorithm for Initial Evaluation and Management of Multiligament Knee Injuries

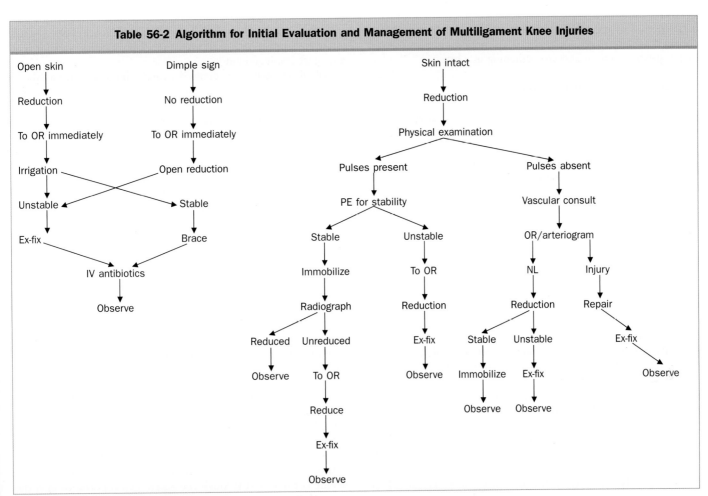

Ex-fix, External fixation; OR, operating room; PE, physical examination.
From Wilson TC, Johnson DL: Initial evaluation and management of the acute multiple-ligament-injured knee. Op Tech Sports Med 2003;11:187–192.

TREATMENT OPTIONS AND RECOMMENDATIONS

Definitive management of multiligament knee injuries has not been well studied using prospective, randomized techniques. Interpretation of current literature is made difficult because of the varied combinations of ligamentous, meniscal, and osseous injuries, as well as multiple treatment approaches and outcome measures. The primary goals of treatment include achieving knee stability, maintaining knee motion, and restoring overall knee function to allow for daily activities.

Nonoperative Management

Historically, nonsurgical management of knee dislocations was standard.[25–27] Treatment typically consisted of cast immobilization for 4 to 12 weeks. Selecting duration of treatment represented a compromise between stability and motion. Knee stability generally improved while knee motion declined with longer periods of immobilization. Given the results of modern reconstruction techniques, nonoperative management should probably be reserved for those patients who are elderly or very sedentary or have significant medical comorbidities.

Nonoperative treatment consists of 6 weeks of immobilization in extension using a cast, brace, or external fixation. The form of immobilization depends on the patient's habitus, energy level of the injury, and associated soft-tissue, vascular, or systemic injuries. Typically, obese patients, high-energy injuries, and injuries requiring soft-tissue or vascular surgery are best served by treatment in an across-knee external fixator. During the initial period of immobilization, regular radiographs should be obtained to confirm reduction. Initial immobilization is followed by progressive motion and strengthening in a brace.

Surgical Management Principles

Most authors currently recommend surgical treatment of acute multiligament knee injuries.[3,9–11,27,28] Some disagreement remains concerning surgical timing, surgical technique, graft selection, and rehabilitation protocols. Generally, addressing cruciate ligament injuries as well as all grade III collateral instabilities will allow for the greatest restoration of overall knee function. Careful preoperative planning must include review of MRI, radiographs, initial physical examination, and availability of all equipment and graft sources. Careful examination under anesthesia is performed to confirm the presence of pathologic laxity. Diagnostic arthroscopy should be carried out to confirm ligament injuries and identify any chondral or meniscal injury. Reconstructions should be performed with accurate tunnel placement, strong graft material, and secure fixation. Repairs should be anatomic and secure.

Surgical Timing

Absolute surgical indications include irreducibility, vascular injury, open injury, compartment syndrome, and inability to maintain reduction with nonoperative methods. When there are no indications for emergent surgical intervention, reduction, immobilization, and MRI can be performed followed by delayed surgical intervention.

Delaying surgery for 7 to 14 days will allow for appropriate vascular monitoring and reduction of swelling. This period will also allow for some capsular healing, which allows the use of arthroscopically assisted techniques with less risk of fluid extravasation. In cases in which collateral ligaments repair is indicated, surgery should not be delayed beyond 3 weeks as scar-

ring will obscure tissue planes and repair of individual structures will be difficult.

Graft Selection

The physician planning surgical treatment for a multiligament-injured knee should be adept at using multiple graft sources including autograft and allograft. Most authors currently advocate reconstruction using allograft sources.[3,10,28] The advantages of allograft use in surgical management of multiligament injuries include less graft site morbidity, shorter operative time, less surgical dissection in an already traumatized knee, and the potential for less postoperative stiffness. More detailed discussion on the advantages and disadvantages of autograft and allograft tissue are discussed in Chapters 12 and 50.

Combined Cruciate Reconstruction

We use a single-stage arthroscopic combined ACL/PCL reconstruction using a bone-patellar tendon-bone allograft for the ACL and an Achilles tendon allograft via a transtibial approach for the PCL. The patient is positioned supine with the operative leg in an arthroscopic leg holder and the well leg widely abducted in the lithotomy position. A tourniquet is applied and used if visualization is impaired. A fluid pump is used judiciously with regular examination for fluid extravasation.

Diagnostic arthroscopy is performed and all meniscal and articular pathology is addressed. This is followed by the notchplasty consisting of débridement of the ACL and PCL stump and contouring of the medial and lateral walls and the intercondylar roof. Use of a radiofrequency ablater may help minimize bleeding and improve visualization. Notchplasty should allow for appropriate anatomic tunnel positioning and prevent any graft impingement.

Tibial tunnels are created using commercially available ACL and PCL guides. Preparation of the PCL tibial tunnel is always done with the use of an accessory posteromedial portal and a 70-degree arthroscope. The medial meniscal root is used as a landmark for the PCL tibial tunnel position.[29] The tip of the guide is placed just posterior to the meniscal root 1 cm off of the tibial plateau. The tunnel should start 4 cm distal to the joint and 2 cm medial to the tibial tubercle. Care must be used in passing the guidewire because of its close proximity to the posterior neurovascular bundles. The ACL tibial guide is placed in the posteromedial footprint of the ACL stump leaving a 2- to 3-cm bridge in the PCL tunnel (Fig. 56-5). Proper guidewire position can be confirmed fluoroscopically, if needed.

Femoral tunnels are created next. The ACL femoral tunnel should be positioned at the 10- or 2-o'clock position, leaving a 1- to 2-mm posterior wall. The PCL femoral tunnel is created through the anterolateral arthroscopic portal. It should be positioned in the center of the stump of the anterolateral bundle 2 mm from the articular surface. All soft tissue and sharp edges should be removed from the margins of the tunnels to facilitate graft passage and prevent graft abrasion.

PCL graft passage is performed next by passing a long looped wire antegrade through the anterolateral portal into the tibial tunnel. The wire is then used to pass the suture secured to the tendinous portion of the graft retrograde through the tunnel. A blunt trochar placed through the posteromedial portal can assist with graft passage around the corner of the tibial tunnel. A Beath needle is then used through the anterolateral portal to pass the graft into the femoral tunnel, after which it is secured with a bioabsorbable interference screw. The ACL graft is then passed

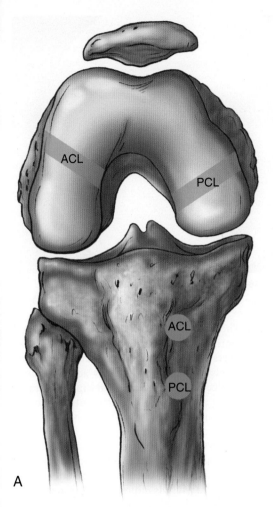

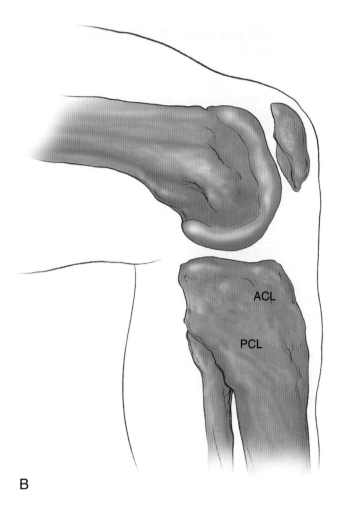

A

B

Figure 56-5 Diagram of tunnel placement in combined anterior cruciate ligament (ACL)/posterior cruciate ligament (PCL) reconstruction. (From Rihn JA, Groff YJ, Harner CD, et al: The acutely dislocated knee: Evaluation and management. J Am Acad Orthop Surg 2004;12:334–346.)

in a retrograde fashion and fixed on the femoral side with an interference screw.

If repair of collateral structures is required, it should be performed prior to fixation of the grafts on the tibial side. While visualizing the grafts arthroscopically, the knee should be taken through a range of motion to ensure there is no graft impingement (Fig. 56-6) The PCL is tensioned and fixed on the tibial side in 90 degrees of flexion. Prior to fixation, a gentle anteriorly directed force is applied to the proximal tibia to recreate the normal step-off between the tibial plateau and femoral condyle. The PCL is then secured on the tibial side with an interference screw. The ACL is tensioned with the knee in full extension and fixed on the tibial side with an interference screw. Table 56-3 summarizes the order of reconstruction.

Medial-Side Injury

Grade I or II MCL injuries alone or in combination with ACL or PCL injuries can be treated successfully nonoperatively with edema control, bracing, early motion, and functional rehabilitation.[30,31] Treatment of acute grade III MCL injuries in association with ACL/PCL injuries remains controversial. Treatment recommendations have included nonoperative treatment of the MCL and early reconstruction of the ACL/PCL, nonoperative treatment of the MCL, and delayed cruciate reconstruction, or

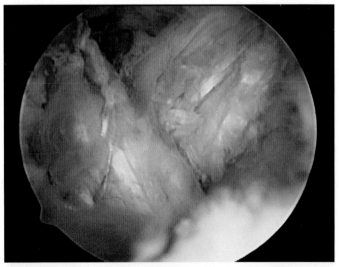

Figure 56-6 Arthroscopic view of completed anterior/posterior cruciate ligament reconstruction.

Table 56-3 Order of Bicruciate Ligament Reconstruction in the Multiligament Injured Knee

Step 1	Drill tibial tunnels	PCL, then ACL
Step 2	Drill femoral tunnels	ACL, then PCL
Step 3	Graft passage and femoral fixation	Pass PCL retrograde into femoral tunnel and fix Pass ACL retrograde and fix femoral side
Step 4	Collateral repair or reconstruction	
Step 5	PCL fixation: tibia	Fix PCL graft on tibia at 90 degrees of flexion. Re-create anteromedial step-off
Step 6	ACL fixation: tibia	Fix ACL graft on tibia in full extension

ACL, Anterior cruciate ligament; PCL, posterior cruciate ligament.
From Cole BJ, Harner CD: The multiligament injured knee. Clin Sports Med 1999;18:241–262.

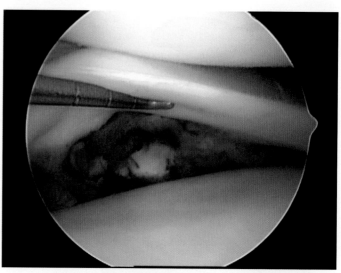

Figure 56-8 Arthroscopic picture of medial lift-off.

treatment of all acute grade III injuries.[10,31–33] Others have advocated treating grade III MCL tears based on the location of the tear, selecting nonoperative treatment for proximal or midsubstance tears, and treating more distal tears with early repair because of a propensity for poor healing.[34,35] It is important to check for involvement of the posteromedial capsule. If patients have laxity to valgus stress in full extension with associated rotatory instability, acute repair of the MCL and posteromedial capsule is warranted. Regardless of the protocol chosen, important principles to follow include accurate diagnosis of both the degree of medial instability and the location of the acute injury. All tools of diagnosis must be used including initial examination, examination under anesthesia, MRI (Fig. 56-7), and arthroscopic findings (Fig. 56-8).

Repair of acute medial instability is performed through a straight medial incision extending from the medial epicondyle to 4 cm distal to the joint line. Care must be taken to protect the saphenous nerve. This approach allows access to the superficial MCL, deep MCL, medial meniscus, and posteromedial

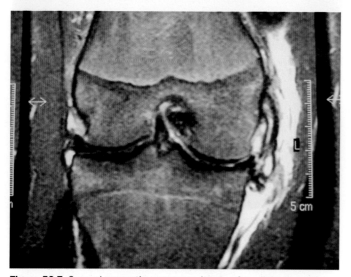

Figure 56-7 Coronal magnetic resonance image of medial collateral ligament avulsion off the tibia with proximal retraction.

capsular structures. The superficial MCL should be isolated and the zone of injury identified. The injury will usually be located either proximally or distally, allowing the ligament to be tagged with a locking whipstitch and reflected to allow access to deep structures. Tears in the deep MCL and meniscal capsular attachments are repaired using a minimum of three suture anchors placed just below the articular margin. The posteromedial capsule should be evaluated and repaired mid-substance or reattached with suture anchors if avulsed. The superficial MCL can then be repaired to its anatomic position either proximally or distally and secured with a spiked washer or suture anchors. In cases in which the superficial MCL is injured mid-substance, the repair may be augmented with either a hamstring autograft or an allograft. The medial-side repair should be completed prior to final fixation of the cruciate ligaments.

Lateral-Side Injury

Unlike medial-side injury, there is widespread agreement that grade III lateral-side injuries in association with ACL/PCL injury are best treated with acute repair.[36,37] Grade III lateral-side injuries most commonly represent avulsions from the tibia/fibula. Direct anatomic repair of all injured structures will provide the greatest chance of favorable outcome.[37]

The posterolateral corner is approached through a curvilinear incision extending from the lateral epicondyle to Gerdy's tubercle. A systematic evaluation of all structures should take place including the iliotibial band, biceps femoris, lateral collateral ligament, popliteus, popliteofibular ligament, lateral meniscus, and peroneal nerve. Repair should proceed from deep to superficial with either a direct end-to-end suture repair or suture anchors as needed. Repairs should be performed with the knee in 30 degrees of flexion.

In cases of significant mid-substance injury or poor tissue quality, direct repair may be augmented with hamstring autograft, allograft, biceps femoris, or iliotibial band tendon. Numerous techniques have been described.[38–40] These same techniques can be applied to cases of chronic laxity requiring reconstructions. We perform reconstructions of the fibular collateral ligament and popliteofibular ligament using a split Achilles tendon allograft fixed on the lateral femoral condyle with an interference screw and passed through tunnels in the proximal tibia and fibula with interference screw fixation.

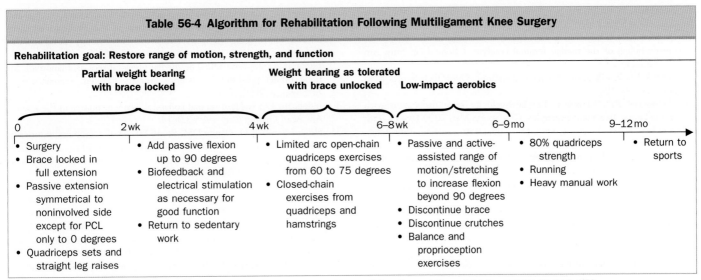

Table 56-4 Algorithm for Rehabilitation Following Multiligament Knee Surgery

Rehabilitation goal: Restore range of motion, strength, and function

Partial weight bearing with brace locked | Weight bearing as tolerated with brace unlocked | Low-impact aerobics

0 — 2 wk — 4 wk — 6–8 wk — 6–9 mo — 9–12 mo

- Surgery
- Brace locked in full extension
- Passive extension symmetrical to noninvolved side except for PCL only to 0 degrees
- Quadriceps sets and straight leg raises

- Add passive flexion up to 90 degrees
- Biofeedback and electrical stimulation as necessary for good function
- Return to sedentary work

- Limited arc open-chain quadriceps exercises from 60 to 75 degrees
- Closed-chain exercises from quadriceps and hamstrings

- Passive and active-assisted range of motion/stretching to increase flexion beyond 90 degrees
- Discontinue brace
- Discontinue crutches
- Balance and proprioception exercises

- 80% quadriceps strength
- Running
- Heavy manual work

- Return to sports

From Harner CD, Waltrip RL, Bennett CH, et al: Surgical management of knee dislocations. J Bone Joint Surg 2004;86:262–273.

POSTOPERATIVE REHABILITATION

Postoperative rehabilitation is an important element in the successful treatment of multiligament knee injuries. A comprehensive postoperative rehabilitation program following multiligament reconstructions has been well described.[41,42] A summary is provided in Table 56-4. The knee is placed in a hinged knee brace kept in full extension for the first 4 to 6 weeks. The patient is kept partially weight bearing. For the first 4 weeks, passive extension is emphasized and passive flexion is limited to 90 degrees. After 4 weeks, patients begin closed-chain quadriceps and hamstring exercises. After 6 weeks, the brace can be discontinued with good quadriceps control, and progressive open-chain strengthening and range-of-motion exercises are started. If sufficient motion and strength have been obtained, return to sports and heavy labor can be considered after 9 months.

COMPLICATIONS

Given the severity of the injury and the nature of the complex reconstructions, complications with traumatic knee dislocations do occur. Major complications include vascular injury, neurologic injury, compartment syndrome and soft-tissue trauma, and infection associated with open injuries. Other complications include loss of motion, residual laxity, painful hardware, and complex regional pain syndrome.

RESULTS AND OUTCOMES

Published results of surgical management of knee dislocations are heterogeneous, small in number, and retrospective. This makes interpreting results difficult. Harner et al[10] recently published their results in 33 patients treated with repair or reconstruction of all grade III instabilities at a minimum of 24 months of follow-up. Mean Lysholm score was 87 (range, 50 to 100), average Knee Outcome Survey Activities of Daily Living score was 89 (range, 64 to 99), and final overall International Knee Documentation Committee rating was nearly normal for 11 knees, abnormal for 12, and severely abnormal for eight. These results are similar to ones in other published reports.[26–28,43–47] Table 56-5 summarizes subjective assessments of operatively treated multiligament-injured knees.

Table 56-5 Subjective Outcome in Operatively Treated Multiligament Injuries

Study	Year	No. of Knees	Lysholm Score
Walker et al[43]	1994	13	84.6 (73–94)
Montgomery et al[45]	1995	13	80 (60–95)
Shapiro et al[47]	1995	7	74.7 (34–93)
Fanelli et al[48]	1996	20	91.3 (80–100)
Wascher et al[44]	1994	13	88 (42–100)
Yeh et al[46]	1999	25	84.1 (79–93)
Harner et al[27]	2004	33	87 (50–100)

Modified from Almekinders and Dedmond.[27]

REFERENCES

1. Green NE, Allen BL: Vascular injuries associated with dislocations of the knee. J Bone Joint Surg Am 1977;59:236–239.
2. Kennedy J: Complete dislocation of the knee joint. J Bone Joint Surg Am 1963;45:889–904.
3. Rihn JA, Groff YJ, Harner CD, et al: The acutely dislocated knee: Evaluation and management. J Am Acad Orthop Surg 2004;12:334–346.
4. Schenk R: Knee dislocations. Instruct Course Lect 1999;48:515–522.

5. Goldblatt, JP, Richmond JC: Anatomy and biomechanics of the knee. Oper Tech Sports Med 2003;11:172–185.
6. Quinlan AG: Irreducible posterolateral dislocation of the knee with button-holing of the medial femoral condyle. J Bone Joint Surg Am 1977;59:236–239.
7. Schenk R: Classification of knee dislocations. Oper Tech Sports Med 2003;11:193–198.
8. Shelbourne KD, Klootwyk TE: Low-velocity knee dislocation with sports injury. Treatment principles. Clin Sports Med 2000;19:443–456.
9. Wascher DC: High-velocity knee dislocations with vascular injury. Treatment principles. Clin Sports Med 2000;19:457–477.
10. Harner CD, Waltrip RL, Bennett CH, et al: Surgical management of knee dislocations. J Bone Joint Surg [Am] 2004;86:262–273.
11. Cole BJ, Harner CD: The multiligament injured knee. Clin Sports Med 1999;18:241–262.
12. Miranda FE, Dennis JW, Veldenz HC, et al: Confirmation of the safety and accuracy of physical examination in the evaluation of knee dislocation for injury of the popliteal artery: A prospective study. J Trauma 2002;52:247–251.
13. Armstrong PJ, Franklin DP: Treatment of vascular injuries in the multiple-ligament-injured knee. Oper Tech Sports Med 2003;11:199–207.
14. Mills WJ, Barei DP, McNair P: The value of the ankle-brachial index for diagnosing arterial injury after knee dislocation: A prospective study. J Trauma 2004;56:1261–1265.
15. Monahan TJ: Treatment of nerve injuries in the multiple-ligament-injured knee. Oper Tech Sports Med 2003;11:208–217.
16. Goitz RJ, Tomaino MM: Management of peroneal nerve injuries associated with knee dislocations. Am J Orthop 2003;32:14–16.
17. Mont MA, Dellon AL, Chen F, et al: The operative treatment of peroneal nerve palsy. J Bone Joint Surg Am 1996;78:863–869.
18. Donaldson WF, Warren RF, Wickiewicz T: A comparison of acute anterior cruciate ligament examinations. Am J Sports Med 1992;10:100–102.
19. Rubinstein RA, Shelbourne KD, McCarroll JR, et al: The accuracy of the clinical examination in the setting of posterior cruciate ligament injuries. Am J Sports Med 1994;22:550–557.
20. Wand JS: A physical sign denoting irreducibility of a dislocated knee. J Bone Joint Surg Br 1989;71:94–102.
21. McCoy GF, Hannon DG, Barr RJ, et al: Vascular injury associated with low-velocity dislocations of the knee. J Bone Joint Surg Br 1987;69:285–287.
22. Stannard JP, Sheils TM, Lopez-Ben RR, et al: Vascular injuries in knee dislocations: The role of physical examination in determining the need for arteriography. J Bone Joint Surg [Am] 2004;86:910–915.
23. McCutchan JD, Gillham NR: Injury to the popliteal artery associated with dislocation of the knee: Palpable distal pulses do not negate the requirement for arteriography. Injury 1989;20:307–310.
24. Bynoe RP, Miles WS, Bell RM, et al: Noninvasive diagnosis of vascular trauma by duplex ultrasonography. J Vasc Surg 1991;14:346–352.
25. Taylor AR, Arden GP, Rainey HA: Traumatic dislocation of the knee: A report of forty-three cases with special reference to conservative treatment. J Bone Joint Surg Br 1972;54:96–102.
26. Richter M, Bosch U, Wipperman B, et al: Comparison of surgical repair or reconstruction of the cruciate ligaments versus nonsurgical treatment in patients with traumatic knee dislocations. Am J Sports Med 2002;30:718–727.
27. Almekinders LC, Dedmond BT: Outcomes of the operatively treated knee dislocation. Clin Sports Med 2000;19:503–518.
28. Fanelli GC, Edson CJ: Arthroscopically assisted combined anterior and posterior cruciate ligament reconstruction in the multiple ligament injured knee: 2 to 10 year follow-up. Arthroscopy 2002;18:703–714.
29. Kantaras AT, Johnson DL: The medial meniscal root as a landmark for tibial tunnel position in posterior cruciate ligament reconstruction. Arthroscopy 2002;18:99–101.
30. Indelicato PA: Isolated medial collateral ligament injures in the knee. J Am Acad Orthop Surg 1995;3:9–14.
31. Hillard-Sembell D, Danile DM, Stone ML, et al: Combined injuries of the anterior cruciate and medial collateral ligaments of the knee. Effect of treatment on stability and function of the knee. J Bone Joint Surg Am 1996;78:169–176.
32. Noyes FR, Barber-Westin SD: The treatment of acute combined ruptures of the anterior cruciate and medial ligaments of the knee. Am J Sports Med 1995;23:380–391.
33. Klimkiewicz JJ, Petrie RS, Harner CD: Surgical treatment of combined injury to anterior cruciate ligament, posterior cruciate ligament, and medial structures. Clin Sports Med 2000;19:479–492.
34. Robins AJ, Newman AP, Burks RT: Postoperative return of motion in anterior cruciate ligament and medial collateral ligament injuries: The effect of medial collateral ligament location. Am J Sports Med 1993;21:20–25.
35. Wilson TC, Satterfield WH, Johnson DL: Medial collateral ligament "tibial" injuries: Indications for acute repair. Orthopedics 2004;27:89–93.
36. Covey DC: Injuries of the posterolateral corner of the knee. J Bone Joint Surg Am 2001;83:106–118.
37. Veltri DM, Warren RF: Anatomy, biomechanics and physical findings in posterolateral knee instability. Clin Sports Med 1994;13:599–614.
38. Noyes FR, Barber-Westin SD: Treatment of complex injuries involving the posterior cruciate and posterolateral ligaments of the knee. Am J Knee Surg 1996;9:200–214.
39. Veltri DM, Warren RF: Operative treatment of posterolateral instability of the knee. Clin Sports Med 1994;13:615–627.
40. Clancy WG, Sutherland TB: Combined posterior cruciate ligament injuries. Clin Sports Med 1994;13:629–647.
41. Irrgang JJ, Fitzgerald GK: Rehabilitation of the multiple-ligament-injured knee. Clin Sports Med 2000;19:545–571.
42. Edson C: Postoperative rehabilitation of the multiple-ligament reconstructed knee. Oper Tech Sports Med 2003;11:294–301.
43. Walker DN, Hardison R, Schenck RC: A baker's dozen of knee dislocations. Am J Knee Surg 1994;7:117–124.
44. Wascher DC, Becker JR, Dexter JG, et al: Reconstruction of the anterior and posterior cruciate ligaments after knee dislocation: Results using fresh-frozen nonirradiated allografts. Am J Knee Surg 1994;27:189–196.
45. Montgomery IJ, Savoie FH, White JL, et al: Orthopedic management of knee dislocations: Comparison of surgical reconstruction and immobilization. Am J Knee Surg 1995;8:97–103.
46. Yeh WL, Tu YK, Su JY, et al: Knee dislocation: Treatment of high velocity knee dislocations. J Trauma 1999;46:693–701.
47. Shapiro MS, Freedman EL: Allograft reconstruction of the anterior and posterior cruciate ligaments after traumatic knee dislocation. Am J Knee Surg 1995;23:580–587.
48. Fanelli GC, Gianotti BF, Edson CJ: Arthroscopically assisted combined anterior and posterior cruciate ligament reconstruction. Arthroscopy 1996;12:5–14.

57 Patellofemoral Instability

Kevin Charron and Anthony Schepsis

In This Chapter

- Finally, the role of proximal and distal realignment for treatment of patients with patellofemoral malalignment and/or instability is explored. The decision-making process in assessing malalignment/instability of the patellofemoral articulation, the criteria for tibial tubercle transfer in both the medial and anteromedial direction versus proximal realignment, and details of the surgical techniques are addressed.

INTRODUCTION

- Patellofemoral instability encompasses a continuum of abnormal patellofemoral joint mechanics, ranging from subluxation to dislocation, the cause of which can be either traumatic or atraumatic.

- Patellofemoral instability is defined as abnormal, clinically symptomatic, lateral, or, in rare cases, medial translation of the patella out of the trochlear groove. In cases of recurrent subluxation, there is lateral translation of the patella early in the flexion range.

- Patients may experience a sense of giving way, slipping, or abnormal motion of the patella, unless the patient has permanent lateral tracking of the patella, which is most often secondary to malalignment.

- Recurrent subluxation encompasses a spectrum from minor subtle translation of the patella that is not associated with a clinically evident relocation to episodes of major recurrent subluxation when the patella nearly dislocates in the early stages of flexion and then reduces with a clinically apparent snap or shift.

- Permanent lateral subluxation is often defined under the category of malalignment and is characterized by a persistent laterally displaced patella through the range of motion (ROM) of the knee, with little or no tendency to recenter in the trochlea. It is often associated with patellar tilt.

- The usual mechanism of traumatic patellar dislocation is external rotation of the tibia with concomitant contracture of the quadriceps.

- Relevant anatomy, history, physical examination, and imaging modalities that would aid in diagnosis are discussed.

- Conservative therapy for the treatment of the various instabilities is briefly discussed.

RELEVANT ANATOMY

The anatomy of the entire lower extremity is paramount in the discussion of patellofemoral instability. Starting proximally at the hip, femoral version (anterior or posterior) can affect patellofemoral mechanics. With femoral anteversion, the distal femoral trochlea is internally rotated with a neutral hip alignment. Conversely, with femoral retroversion, the distal femoral trochlea is externally rotated with a neutral hip alignment. Normal femoral anteversion is approximately 14 degrees. Excessive hip anteversion causes the patella to displace laterally. Varying degrees of femoral torsion may also be present, which affects the position of the trochlea. Excessive femoral anteversion with or without internal femoral torsion is usually accompanied by tibial external rotation, which has the effect of further displacing the patella laterally. Dysplasia of the medial or lateral femoral condyle also affects patellofemoral mechanics. If the lateral condyle is hypoplastic, the bony constraint to lateral subluxation is not present in flexion at 20 degrees and beyond.

The patella is a sesamoid bone contained within the extensor mechanism. It is made up of a medial and lateral facet separated by a median ridge. Usually the lateral facet is longer and more sloped to match the corresponding condyle. The rectus femoris, vastus lateralis, vastus medialis, and vastus intermedius all send fibers to the extensor mechanism at the proximal aspect of the patella and respective retinaculum. All muscles originate from the proximal femur except for the rectus femoris, which originates on the anterior inferior iliac spine (reflected head) and superior acetabulum (direct head). The orientation of the quadriceps muscle fibers is important in patellofemoral mechanics because they create varying vectors of force on the patella during contraction. The vastus medialis obliquus originates on the medial intermuscular septum and the adductor tubercle and inserts on the medial proximal third of the patella. The vastus medialis obliquus is the most obliquely oriented muscle and therefore provides a medially directed force vector to the patella during extension, which decreases lateral subluxation. All the quadriceps muscles are innervated by the femoral nerve.

At the distal aspect of the patella is the patellar tendon, which inserts on the tibial tubercle. The tendon is separated from the anterior tibia by the deep infrapatellar bursa. Further posterior to this is the infrapatellar fat pad. Other static restraints to the patella are the medial and lateral patellofemoral ligament and the medial and lateral patellotibial ligament. The MPFL has an almost 90-degree orientation to the patella and therefore is one of the main static restraints to lateral subluxation. The MPFL has been found to be the primary restraint to lateral patellar translation at 20 degrees of flexion, contributing 60% of the total restraining force.[1]

CLINICAL FEATURES AND EVALUATION

History

The events surrounding the onset of the knee instability often point to a diagnosis. If the patient's instability is a result of trauma, most often a ruptured MPFL with or without underlying malalignment may be suspected. In the acute setting, the patient may present with a large hemarthrosis and tenderness over the medial femoral epicondyle and medial border of the patella, in addition to pain or apprehension with lateral translation of the patella. If the patient's instability is indolent in nature and has occurred over years, most likely the patient has some component of malalignment. In the chronic setting, the patient may give a history of the knee "giving way" with increasing activity. These patients also may complain of an intermittent effusion and pain over the lateral retinaculum and lateral patellar facet. By history, it is important to determine whether the patient has symptomatic instability, either subluxation or dislocation, or purely patellofemoral pain secondary to chondrosis or arthrosis associated with malalignment.

Physical Examination

After an appropriate history is taken, the patient is examined standing. Overall varus or valgus alignment of the lower extremity, which can affect patellofemoral mechanics, can be evaluated. A valgus knee tends to increase the quadriceps angle (Q angle) and loading of the lateral facet of the patella. The position of the patella can also be assessed. If the patellae are facing each other when the feet are parallel there may be some degree of femoral anteversion or femoral internal torsion. This is usually accompanied by some degree of tibial external rotation, which can be assessed by palpating the tibial tubercle. The position of the plantigrade foot also can give some insight to overall alignment. With excessive external rotation of the tibia, there is usually a compensatory foot pronation with heel valgus. Leg length discrepancy may also be evaluated at this time by noting any pelvic obliquity. Finally, the patient's gait may be evaluated for any asymmetry. With proper mechanics, the hip and ankle center should line up so that the overall mechanical axis passes through the center of the knee. Any noticeable pelvic obliquity could be attributed to abductor deficiency. Last, a loaded flexion squat can be performed. Pain and crepitus referable to the patellofemoral articulation is often accentuated by this maneuver.

The sitting examination is then performed with the legs flexed 90 degrees over the examination table. Again, the orientation of the patella can be observed. Laterally facing patellae can indicate extensor mechanism malalignment. The tuberosulcus angle can also be measured while the knee is flexed to 90 degrees (Fig. 57-1). It represents the angle between a perpendicular to the transepicondylar axis and a line drawn from the

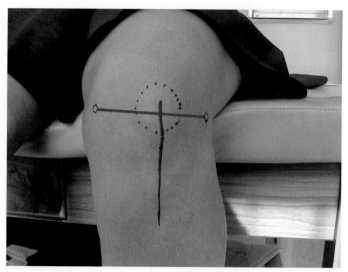

Figure 57-1 The tuberosulcus angle.

midpoint of the patella to the tuberosity. Normally this measures 0 degrees, and greater than 10 degrees is considered abnormal.[2] Tibial torsion can also be evaluated by palpating the tibial tubercle. In normal alignment, the tibial tubercle should lie lateral to the midline of the femur, although this is highly variable in the population. Vastus medialis obliquus atrophy can also be appreciated at this point. With flexion and extension of the knee, crepitus can be palpated and patellar tracking observed. The flexion arc in which the patient has pain is sometimes a tip-off as to the location of the patient's disease. Early range flexion pain and crepitus indicate a more distal lesion, a painful arc and crepitus between 30 and 70 degrees indicate a mid-patellar lesion, and a painful crepitus in greater degrees of flexion indicates a more proximal lesion on the patella. The soft tissues are responsible for stability of the patellofemoral articulation in the first 30 degrees of flexion, whereas the bony anatomy becomes more critical beyond 30 degrees of flexion. At approximately 20 degrees of flexion, the patella should seat fully in the femoral trochlea. A pathologic J sign can be observed as the patella seated in the trochlea subluxates laterally with terminal extension. ROM and muscle strength of the knee and ankle should be documented.

From the sitting position, the patient is then placed supine. With the extensor mechanism relaxed, any effusion can be noted and the entire knee should be palpated to include the medial and lateral facets, retinaculum, common extensor tendon, tibial tubercle, and patella tendon. Next the patella should be compressed against the trochlea and moved medially and laterally. Pain during this maneuver implicates the patellofemoral articulation. Lateral glide of more than 50% of the width of the patella is considered abnormal unless there is symmetrical patellar hypermobility associated with generalized ligamentous laxity. A patellar apprehension sign may be encountered when the patient has a sense of dislocation or subluxation with a laterally directed force. Several measurements can now be taken. Leg length can be measured by taking the distance from the anterior superior iliac spine to the tip of the medial malleolus. The Q angle can also be measured (Fig. 57-2). This is measured from the anterior superior iliac spine to the center of the patella to the tibial tubercle. Normal values are up to 15 degrees in the male and up to 18 degrees in the female. The larger Q angles in females are due to the wider pelvis and increase in genu valgum as com-

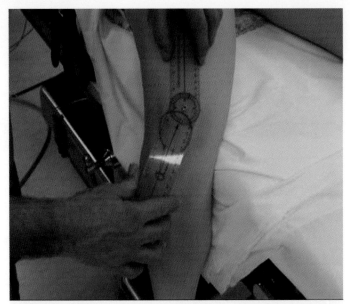

Figure 57-2 Measuring the quadriceps (Q) angle. A line is drawn from the anterior superior iliac spine to the center of the patella to the center of the tibial tubercle. The angle between the two is the Q angle.

pared to males. The author believes that the most accurate Q-angle measurement is made at 30 degrees of flexion because the patella should be well centered in the trochlear groove by 20 to 25 degrees of flexion. If the Q angle is measured in extension, an inaccurate low value may be obtained since the patella lies laterally in terminal extension from lack of bony constraint. Excessive femoral anteversion, internal femoral torsion, genu valgum, and external tibial torsion all increase the Q angle. A thorough examination would not be complete without a ligamentous examination. Last hamstring tightness should be evaluated by measuring the popliteal angle. The angle can be measured by flexing the hip to 90 degrees, extending the knee to the maximum, and then measuring the angle between the femur and tibia. Values greater than 25 degrees indicate hamstring tightness.

From the supine position, the patient should then be placed prone. In this position, hip ROM can be assessed by internally and externally rotating the flexed knees. With the knees flexed in this position, femoral and tibial lengths can be assessed. Finally, quadriceps tightness can be assessed by flexing the knees. With the pelvis level, the heel should come toward the buttocks in a symmetrical level and increased tightness in the anterior thigh, as compared to the contralateral side, could be an indication of quadriceps tightness.

Imaging Modalities

Evaluation of patellofemoral pain starts with a standard bilateral standing anteroposterior view of the knees. This probably has the least amount of information as it pertains to patellofemoral disease but may give insight into degenerative joint disease and accessory ossification centers of the patella as possible sources of pain. A modification of this radiograph is a flexed knee anteroposterior view called the tunnel view. This gives insight into disease of the femoral condyles and can diagnose an osteochondral defect.

With the lateral view of the knee, patella alta (high) or patella baja (low) can be evaluated. The Insall Salvati technique[3] measures the ratio of the length of the patellar tendon to the largest diagonal measurement of the patella on the lateral projection. Normal ratios are 0.8 to 1.2. Ratios less than 0.8 indicate patella baja and ratios greater then 1.2 indicate patella alta. Another similar method is that of Blackburn and Peel,[4] who measure the distance from the tibial plateau to the inferior articular surface of the patella as compared to the length of the patella articular surface. A ratio from between 0.54 to 1.06 is normal. Values greater than 1.06 indicate patella alta. This measurement has been found to be more accurate in the evaluation of patella alta and baja. The lateral view can also give an indication to the amount of patellofemoral arthritis by the amount of joint space that is present.

The last view obtained is the axial view (Fig. 57-3). Traditional sunrise views are taken with the knee in various degrees of flexion depending on institutional guidelines. Typically they are taken at greater degrees of flexion (i.e., greater than 45 degrees). At these degrees of flexion, almost all patellae are well seated in the trochlea and mild patellofemoral malalignment may be missed. Two standardized views are typically used. The Merchant view[5] is taken with the knee flexed to 45 degrees. The x-ray source is placed proximal to the knee with the plate distal to the knee. The congruence angle, described by Merchant, can be measured from this radiograph. On the axial view, the angle between the medial and lateral condyle is bisected. Then a line is drawn from the femoral trochlea to the lowest point on the median ridge of the patella. The angle between these two lines represents the congruence angle. If the line falls medial to the bisector, it is a negative value and if it falls to the lateral side, it is a positive value. Merchant found the average congruence angle in 100 normal subjects was −6 degrees with a standard deviation of 11 degrees. In a normal knee, the median ridge of the patella lies on the medial condyle. The Laurin view[6] is another axial view, taken at 20 to 30 degrees of knee flexion. The x-ray tube is placed between the ankles and the x-ray plate is held proximal to the knees. On this view, the lateral patellofemoral angle can be measured. This angle is measured from a line drawn across the most anterior portions of the medial and lateral femoral condyles in the axial view to a line that follows the slope of the lateral patella facet. Normally this angle should increase laterally. In patients with patellar tilt or lateral patellar subluxation, the angle is parallel or increased medially.

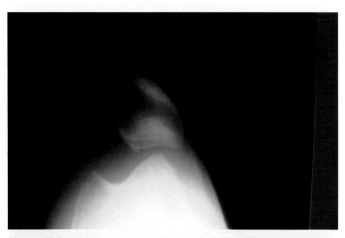

Figure 57-3 Axial view demonstrating marked tilt, subluxation, and arthrosis of the lateral facet.

Standing mechanical axis view can be taken to assess lower extremity limb alignment. Normally the mechanical axis, a line from the femoral head to the middle of the tibial plafond, should fall just medial to the center of the knee joint. The Q angle, as described before, can also be measured on the radiograph. Varus or valgus angulation at the knees can be measured and an appreciation of femoral anteversion/torsion and tibial torsion can be visualized.

A computed tomography (CT) of the knee at various angles of flexion can give insight to the patellofemoral dynamics (Fig. 57-4). Axial images through the midpoint of the patella are taken at 10-degree increments from 0 to 60 degrees of flexion. Congruence angle and lateral patellofemoral angle can be measured from these images at varying degrees of flexion.

Another use of CT is the measurement of the anterior tibial tubercle to trochlear groove distance (Fig. 57-5).[7] Axial images are taken from the proximal trochlea through the tibial tubercle on the same sequence, with the extremity fixed in extension. It is thought that more than a 2-cm distance is highly abnormal, representing excessive lateralization of the tibial tubercle with a high valgus vector on the knee. Although one study suggests that the normal range is 2 to 9 mm and greater than 10 mm is abnormal,[7,8] the exact cutoff between "normal" and "abnormal" would be very difficult to ascertain because of the very wide range of anatomic variations.

A final use of CT is in the evaluation of the rotational alignment of the lower extremity. Femoral anteversion/torsion can be evaluated by measuring the angle between the line bisecting the femoral neck and a line drawn across the posterior condyles of the femur on subsequent cuts. In the same way, tibial torsion can be evaluated by measuring the angle between the line across the posterior tibial plateau superimposed on the transmalleolar axis. If excessive femoral anteversion results in patellofemoral malalignment, a femoral derotational osteotomy may be in order.

Magnetic resonance imaging can also be helpful in diagnosis. Although CT is better for visualization of bone detail, magnetic

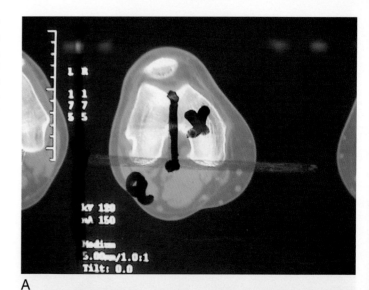

A

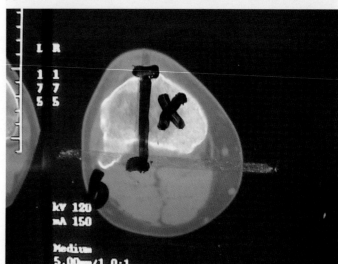

B

Figure 57-5 The anterior tibial tubercle to trochlear groove distance. A computed tomography measurement of the distance between the center of the trochlear groove and the attachment of the patella tendon to the anterior tibial tubercle. Axial images are taken from the proximal trochlea through the tibial tubercle on the same sequence with the extremity fixed in extension. **A,** A line is drawn along the posterior femoral condyles on the cut through the deepest portion of the trochlear groove. A perpendicular (x) is drawn from the center of the groove to this line and measured. The distance (a) is measured from this intersection to a fixed point; in this case, the edge of the frame. **B,** The same parallel line is transposed with a parallel rule to the cut through the midportion of the tendon attachment on the tubercle at the same perpendicular distance (x). The distance (b) is measured to the same fixed point. The anterior tibial tubercle to trochlear groove distance is a − b. In this instance, it was 5 mm, well within normal range.

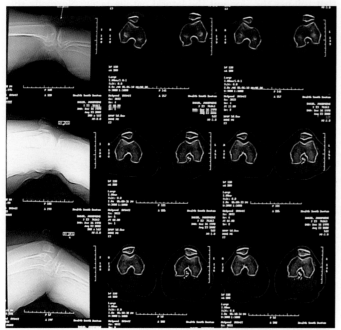

Figure 57-4 Patellofemoral computed tomography tracking study.

resonance imaging is more sensitive for osteochondral, ligament, and meniscal injuries that may be caused by a traumatic patellar dislocation. These findings include disruption of the MPFL and osteochondral bone bruises or fractures involving the inferomedial patella and lateral femoral condyle.[9-11]

Last, in some cases, a bone scan may be useful. With patellar instability, the biomechanical and metabolic processes that maintain homeostasis of the cartilage and soft-tissue structures are affected. The loss of this homeostasis is typically undetectable with radiographs or magnetic resonance imaging. The bone scan, on the other hand, can demonstrate a persistently abnormal technetium scintigram of the involved area prior to the development and progression of irreversible degenerative changes that would be evident on radiograph or magnetic resonance imaging.[12] In the arena of patellar instability, an area of uptake on the lateral patella facet could mean abnormal articular loading in the face of other normal imaging modalities.

TREATMENT OPTIONS

Conservative Treatment

Nonsurgical treatment of patellofemoral instability is the cornerstone of treatment. Henry[13] reported an approximately 80% success rate in the literature for the conservative treatment of patellofemoral instability. The mainstay of treatment involves the selective strengthening of the vastus medialis obliquus with de-emphasis on strengthening the vastus lateralis. This focus has changed from general quadriceps strengthening that was previously prescribed for patellofemoral pain. McConnell[14] has developed a treatment plan for patellofemoral pain that has a reported success rate of 96%. Her method consists of muscle re-education focusing on the vastus medialis obliquus and taping of the patella to modify tilt or subluxation. The use of a patella-stabilizing brace is another treatment modality that may have some benefit. Closed-chain exercises, stationary bike, elliptical runner, and other core strengthening exercises help strengthen and stabilize the knee joint without excessive loading of the joint. Prone quadriceps stretching, iliotibial band stretching, and lateral retinacular stretching are paramount. Lower extremity strengthening, patellar stabilization, lower extremity flexibility, and proprioception are important treatment modalities. Correction of excessive foot pronation or supination with orthotics can have a positive effect on alignment in that this limits compensatory external and internal rotation of the tibia, respectively. Nonsteroidal anti-inflammatory drugs may be used as an adjunct to treatment, and a level of activity modification to limit loading of the patellofemoral joint can be beneficial.

In the realm of patella dislocations, there are numerous retrospective studies in the literature that detail the success of nonoperative and operative treatment of first-time patella dislocators. Consensus between the studies is problematic due to the varying sample sizes, differing follow-up, varied surgical techniques, and heterogeneity between populations. One prospective, randomized study demonstrated equivalent results between operative and nonoperative treatment for first-time patella dislocation.[15] Conservative treatment, which includes immobilization of the knee in extension for 2 to 3 weeks, followed by strength and ROM exercises, has therefore become the author's treatment of first-time dislocators. The author's only indications for acute surgical intervention for first-time dislocators include unstable osteochondral fractures and asymmetrical unreduced lateral subluxation of the patella.

Surgical Management

When conservative treatment fails to provide satisfactory results, surgery may be indicated. Surgical techniques can be grouped into proximal and distal realignment procedures. Proximal alignment procedures include a lateral release (open or arthroscopic), lateral release and medial plication (open or arthroscopic), and MPFL reconstruction. Distal realignment procedures include the medialization of the tibial tubercle and anteromedialization of the tibial tubercle. The Maquet technique, anteriorization of the tibial tubercle, has been used mainly to unload the patellofemoral joint in patients with patellofemoral arthritis without malalignment. The Hauser technique is a tibial tubercle osteotomy and moves the tibial tubercle medial, distal, and posterior due to the triangular cross-section of the proximal tibia. This technique has been abandoned because it increases the patellofemoral joint reactive forces, resulting in the subsequent development of patellofemoral arthritis. In this chapter, lateral retinacular release, arthroscopic proximal realignment, MPFL reconstruction, medial tibial tubercle transfer, and anteromedialization of the tibial tubercle are discussed in detail.

Lateral Retinacular Release

Abnormal patellar tilt increases loading of the lateral patella facet, causes contracture of the lateral retinaculum, and increases the incidence of patellofemoral arthritis on the lateral side. Current indications for lateral release consist of (1) patellofemoral pain with lateral tilt, (2) lateral retinacular pain with lateral tilt or lateral patella position, and (3) tight lateral retinaculum/excessive lateral pressure syndrome.[16] This operation is done for pain and is not indicated as a stand-alone procedure for instability. If lateral release is done for instability, the results deteriorate with time. Lateral release is contraindicated with a hypermobile patella. In addition, the authors do not perform lateral release as an isolated procedure for the treatment of recurrent lateral patellar dislocation. Lateral retinacular release can be performed either arthroscopically or open. During knee arthroscopy, the patellar tracking is best observed through a superomedial or superolateral portal. Selective femoral nerve stimulation can be used under general anesthesia to allow active quadriceps contraction and thus evaluate dynamic tracking. If at this point, lateral retinacular release is appropriate, the lateral retinaculum should be divided within 1 cm of the patella starting approximately 2 cm proximal to the proximal pole and extending 2 cm distal to the distal pole. Electrocautery can be used and care must be taken to cauterize the lateral superior geniculate vessels. The tendon fibers of the vastus lateralis should be avoided as this could cause relative weakness of the lateral compartment and a medial patella subluxation. The most common complication of a lateral release is hemarthrosis from laceration of the superolateral geniculate vessels. An open technique can also be employed, which entails an approximately 3-cm longitudinal incision, about 1 cm lateral to the patella. Skin and subcutaneous tissue are divided with a scalpel down to the retinaculum. A Z-plasty is then performed on the transverse fibers of the retinaculum. Once adequate correction is obtained, sutures can be used to prevent further lengthening of the lateral retinaculum. As in the arthroscopic procedure, care is taken to identify and coagulate the superolateral geniculate vessels.

Arthroscopic Proximal Realignment

Medial reefing is often indicated with a lateral release in proximal realignment. This can be done open, arthroscopically assisted (mini-open), or done all arthroscopically. The author's ideal indications for proximal realignment include traumatic onset, recurrent episodes associated with an abnormal lateral patellar glide indicating insufficiency of the MPFL and medial soft-tissue restraints, no significant arthrosis of the medial facet, and normal alignment and quadriceps angle. The author uses this arthroscopic technique only in cases of mild instability and uses a formal MPFL reconstruction for cases of moderate to severe instability.

Using a thigh holder and standard arthroscopy portals, an epidural needle is introduced through the medial retinaculum next to the proximal medial border of the patella. A no. 1 polydiaxone monofilament suture is introduced through the spinal needle into the joint and withdrawn through an accessory portal with a grasper. The spinal needle is then withdrawn from the retinaculum only, into the subcutaneous tissue, and then reinserted into the joint after moving it posterior to the first needle tract. This loop of suture is then withdrawn through the accessory portal and the process is repeated. This procedure can be repeated until the amount of medial imbrication is deemed adequate. An arthroscopic lateral release, if necessary, can then be performed as described previously. The sutures in the medial capsule can then be tied using standard arthroscopic knot-tying techniques.

Postoperative Rehabilitation Postoperatively the patient is placed in a hinged knee brace in extension for 1 week followed by ROM exercises with physical therapy. ROM is gradually increased to a maximum of 90 degrees over a 4-week period. Bracing is continued until quadriceps strength returns. The patient is weight bearing as tolerated postoperatively.

Results The all-inside technique of proximal realignment has been successful. In Halbrecht's review[17] of 5-year results, 93% of patients who underwent the procedure reported significant improvement. The average Lysholm score improved from 41.5 to 79.3 ($P < 0.05$). There were no complications or redislocations. Patients in the study reported significant improvement in pain, swelling, stair climbing, crepitus, and ability to return to sports ($P < 0.05$).

Medial Patellofemoral Ligament Reconstruction

The author prefers to use formal MPFL in cases of moderate to severe instability. His other indications include traumatic onset, recurrent episodes associated with an abnormal lateral patellar glide (indicating insufficiency of the MPFL and medial soft-tissue restraints), no significant arthrosis of the medial facet, and normal alignment and quadriceps angle.

Technique First, make an incision the length of the patella, located over the junction of the medial and middle thirds of the patella (in line with the medial border of the expansion of the patellar tendon at the distal patellar pole). If a tibial tubercle realignment procedure is indicated, this should be performed first before MPFL reconstruction. The goal of MPFL surgery is to provide a checkrein to lateral displacement of the patella; this surgery is not performed to pull the patella into the trochlea. Perform a subperiosteal dissection, extending medially deep to layers 1 and 2, exposing layer 3 (the capsular layer) at the medial border of the patella. Deeper dissection, between layers 2 and 3, is preferable to dissection superficial to layer 2 because it allows incorporation with advancement of the MPFL (layer 2) superficial to the graft during wound closure. Using a curved clamp to develop the selected tissue interval, bluntly dissect medial retinacular layers between the patella and medial femoral epicondyle.

A single-strand semitendinous allograft or autograft approximately 5 to 7 mm in diameter is prepared for the MPFL substitute. If the graft is small in diameter, it may be doubled to achieve the 5- to 7-mm diameter. A running baseball stitch with

no. 2 FiberWire is placed for approximately 15 mm from one end of the graft to help in seating the graft in the femoral tunnel. If the graft is doubled, it should be run from the two free ends.

The origin of the MPFL is now identified on the distal femur. The adductor tubercle and medial epicondyle should be identified. The saddle between these two structures is the femoral origin of the MPFL. A 2.4-mm drill pin is then placed in the center of the saddle. A suture is then wrapped around the drill pin and then attached to the insertion of the MPFL on the patella. The insertion of the MPFL lies on the medial proximal one half of the patella. The knee is placed in 30 degrees of flexion, and the suture is tensioned slightly. The knee is taken through a ROM to evaluate the length change of the suture. Maximum tension should be seen between 0 degrees and 30 degrees, with progressive laxity between 30 degrees and full flexion. The femoral origin point is adjusted to minimize length change of the suture with knee flexion. If lengthening occurs in flexion, replace the pin more distally toward the medial femoral epicondyle. If lengthening occurs in extension, move the pin more proximally toward the adductor tubercle. Slight lengthening will not affect the overall results. Adjustment of the femoral origin of the MPFL is complete when the isometric point is established.

Now with the MPFL femoral origin identified, the femoral tunnel can be made with the appropriately sized reamer over the guide pin to a depth of 20 mm. The graft is then fixed in the femoral pilot hole with the appropriately sized Bio-Tenodesis screw. The sutures previously placed in the end of the graft can be brought in through the cannulated Bio-Tenodesis screwdriver to facilitate seating of the graft. The screw should be placed on the medial aspect of the femoral tunnel with the graft exiting laterally. The Bio-Tenodesis screw should be advanced until it is flush with cortical bone. Security of the graft then can be evaluated.

Next, a 2.4-mm Beath pin is placed at the insertion of the MPFL on the medial patella, as previously identified. The pin is advanced transversely across the patella until it exits laterally. Isometry should be again tested by provisionally fixating the free end of the graft to the patella. The tendon should be marked at the cortical edge of the patella and cut an additional 15 mm distal to this point. After confirming correct placement of the insertion of the graft, an appropriately sized reamer is placed over the pin and a patella tunnel of 20 mm in depth is made. Usually a 6-mm reamer is used with a 5.5-mm Bio-Tenodesis screw. A no. 2 fiber wire (FiberWire; Arthrex, Naples, FL) then is run as a baseball stitch at the distal aspect of the graft for approximately 15 mm. The free ends of the suture are then placed through the eyelet of the Beath pin and pulled into the patellar tunnel to the previously marked depth and fixated with another Bio-Tenodesis screw. The Bio-Tenodesis screw is advanced over the superior portion of the graft until flush with the patellar cortex. A medial imbrication can now be performed if there is redundant medial tissue. The wound is then closed in the standard fashion.

Alternatively, a suture anchor technique can be used for patellar fixation. A cancellous bone trough is created in the medial edge of the patella, anterior to the articular surface, from the midwaist superiorly. Two Bio-Suture Taks (Arthrex, Naples, FL) are placed in this trough and the free end of the graft is fixed with suture.

Postoperative Rehabilitation Postoperatively the patient is placed in a hinged knee brace in extension for 1 week followed by ROM exercises with physical therapy. ROM is gradually increased to a maximum of 90 degrees over a 4-week period. Bracing is continued until quadriceps strength returns. The patient is weight bearing as tolerated postoperatively. Return to sports is allowed at 6 months postoperatively if there is full motion, no pain or swelling, and strength at least 80% of the unoperated side.

Results   Various techniques of anatomic reconstruction of the MPFL have been described and have met with success. At 2-year follow-up, Drez et al[18] found that 93% of their patients had good to excellent results after MPFL reconstruction. In another study by Gomes et al,[19] 94% of patients had good to excellent results at over 5 years of follow-up after MPFL reconstruction.

Medial Tibial Tubercle Transfer

The author's principal indications for medial tibial tubercle transfer are given in Box 57-1. If significant patella alta is present, tightening the proximal medial restraints will not correct the problem and will create abnormal forces. In these cases, the patellar centers into the groove in higher degrees of flexion. Some of the best results of distal realignment or medial tubercle transfers occur in patients with patella alta and lateral patellar instability. Likewise, J tracking, where the patella "jumps" out laterally in terminal extension, is an indicator of a "valgus vector" from bony malalignment, which starts at the hip from internal femoral torsion. The more practical solution would be to make the correction at the tibial tubercle, although on a theoretical basis, a femoral derotation osteotomy would correct the problem at its source.

The advantages of distal realignment are listed in Box 57-2. Numerous studies have looked at the effects of medialization

and anteromedialization on patellofemoral mechanics. The effect of anterior displacement of the tuberosity on patellofemoral contact forces is discussed in a later section. However, there are numerous publications in the literature that show that medial tubercle transfer corrects tilt as well as subluxation and transfers force at the patellofemoral joint from a lateral to a medial direction.

In a recent study by Ramappa et al[20] it was shown that increasing the Q angle increases patellofemoral contact pressures and transfers forces to the lateral facet of the patella. An increased Q angle also tilts and subluxates the patella laterally. It was further established that medialization corrects the maltracking and partially corrects the increased contact pressures in the patellofemoral articulation.

Medial tubercle transfer, however, is contraindicated in patients with a normal Q angle or no clinical or radiographic evidence of tubercle malalignment. In a cadaver study by Kuroda et al,[21] medialization in the presence of a normal Q angle increased patellofemoral contact pressures, along with increasing the contact pressures in the medial tibiofemoral compartment. These authors also concluded that overmedialization should be avoided in the varus knee, the knee with medial compartment arthrosis, and the knee with previous total or subtotal medial meniscectomy.

Distal realignment is sometimes indicated in combination with proximal realignment when there is both traumatic insufficiency of the MPFL as well as tubercle malalignment. In these cases, both abnormalities need to be corrected.

There are a number of disadvantages of distal realignment that should be recognized before performing this procedure. They are listed in Box 57-3.

Technique   Medial tubercle transfer was first described by Trillat et al[22] in 1964. It was then popularized by Cox as the Elmslie-Trillat procedure.

Arthroscopy is first performed to address any associated lesions, chondroplasty is performed if necessary, and patellar tracking assessed. At this time, a decision must be made as to whether to perform anteromedialization rather than straight medialization. In general, even in the presence of significant chondral changes at the time of arthroscopy, if the patient is not symptomatic from the chondrosis or arthrosis, straight medialization to correct patellar instability and/or malalignment would be indicated. If the patient has symptomatic arthrosis or chondrosis, the location and severity of the lesion should be noted before deciding which direction to move the tibial tubercle. Furthermore, in some patients with very severe grade IV disease in both the patella and trochlea in diffusely, no further surgery may

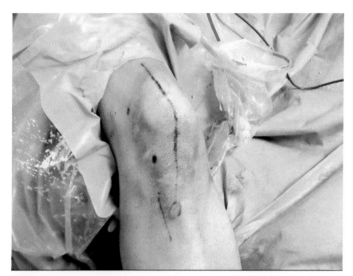

Figure 57-6 Lateral incision for tibial tubercle medialization (Elmslie-Trillat). The tibial tubercle *(circle)* and Q angle are marked.

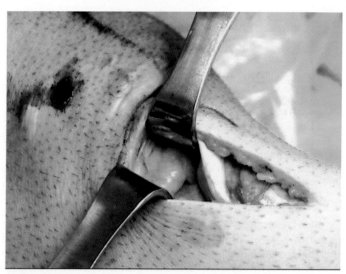

Figure 57-7 Exposing the patellar tendon. Both sides of the tendon must be freed up to prevent tethering when the tubercle is shifted.

be indicated at this time and the patient may be a better candidate for other procedures.

The decision as to whether to perform a lateral retinacular release, either arthroscopic or open, should be made next. Lateral retinacular release is performed in those cases where there is excessive tightness of the lateral retinaculum secondary to a passive patellar tilt, in patients with symptomatic arthrosis or chondrosis in the lateral compartment of the patellofemoral joint, and radiographic or CT imaging evidence of a decreased lateral patellofemoral angle. Lateral release alone, in these cases, is only indicated for excessive lateral pressure syndrome, with lateral facet pain, a tight lateral retinaculum, minimal or only grade 1 to 2 lateral facet changes, and no subluxation or clinical instability symptoms.

The medial tubercle transfer is performed through a small 3- to 4-cm longitudinal incision just lateral to the tibial tubercle (Fig. 57-6). A 1 to 1.5 cm thick, 5 to 6 cm long osteoperiosteal shingle with hand osteotomes is created. The patellar tendon is mobilized so that the undersurface of its attachment can be well visualized with retraction (Fig. 57-7). The first cut is performed from lateral to medial with a 1- to 1.5-inch wide hand osteotome 1 cm thick at the level of the tibial tubercle (Fig. 57-8). Care should be made to make this osteotomy directly in the coronal plane. However, if one is to err, err on the side of going from posterior to anterior when going from the lateral to the medial direction so that when the tubercle is transferred, it will move slightly anteriorly and never posteriorly, which would increase patellofemoral contact pressures. A mark is made on the skin distally, 5 to 6 cm distal to the tubercle, and a curved osteotome is used to aim for this point to angle quickly toward the anterior cortex. A small osteotome is used to complete the osteotomy transversely just on the proximal side of the tibial tubercle to prevent propagation into the tibial plateau. Osteoclasis is performed, leaving the distal soft tissues intact, and the tibial tubercle is gently rotated medially (Fig. 57-9). The parameters used by the author are that the patella is fully engaged and congruent by 20 degrees of flexion and that the Q angle is corrected to below 10 degrees as measured intraoperatively. Temporary fixation is achieved with a 3.2-mm drill bit to, but not through, the posterior cortex, at which time a final assessment

of tracking is made (Fig. 57-10). In general, the transfer ranges from a 1- to 1.5-cm shift. If the surgeon is satisfied with the degree of tubercle transfer and the tracking is satisfactory, fixation is performed with a fully threaded 4.5-mm bicortical screw with metal washer (Fig. 57-11). Since this osteotomy is a short, thin osteoperiosteal shingle, the author routinely uses only one bicortical screw, allowing rigid fixation and an aggressive postoperative rehabilitation program. However, if the osteotomy is on the larger side, one can consider fixation with two screws. Care must be taken when drilling through the posterior cortex of the tibia in this area. Drilling should be performed with the knee in at least 90 degrees of flexion and taking care not to plunge through the posterior cortex (Fig. 57-12). In

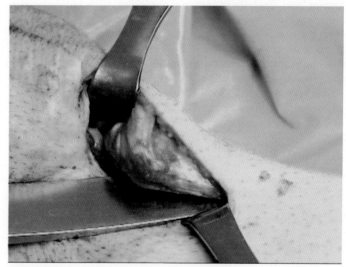

Figure 57-8 For medialization, a 1 to 1.5 cm thick, 5 to 6 cm long shingle is adequate. It is left attached by periosteum distally at the anterior cortex. The osteotomy is performed with hand osteotomes laterally to medially. The osteotomy must be made directly in the coronal plane for true medialization. Care must be taken not to angle posteriorly or else posteromedialization will occur. This could lead to overloading.

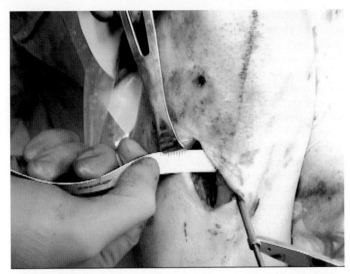

Figure 57-9 The amount of medialization is measured. A 10- to 15-mm transfer is usually adequate. The Q angle should be corrected to less than 10 degrees.

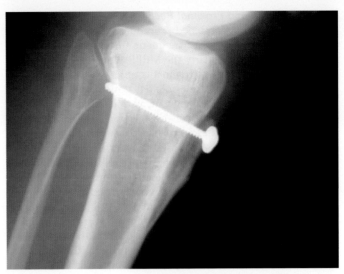

Figure 57-12 Lateral radiograph of a completed tibial tubercle medialization. The screw should be placed with the knee in flexion to avoid injury to posterior neurovascular structures.

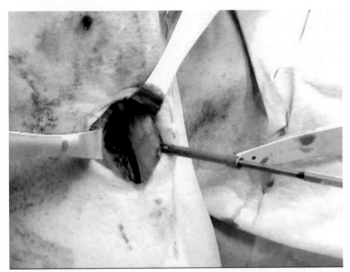

Figure 57-10 The osteotomy is temporarily fixed and patellofemoral tracking assessed.

those cases in which MPFL deficiency is a problem and instability and tracking are not fully corrected, it can be addressed, either arthroscopically or open at this time.

We use the tourniquet for the open part of this case and then release it prior to closure and achieve hemostasis. A drain is not usually necessary as it is for anteromedialization. The subcutaneous tissues and skin are closed carefully, and the patient is placed in a long-leg brace locked in extension.

Postoperative Rehabilitation The biomechanics of a flat versus oblique osteotomy have been described by Cosgarea et al.[23] In cases of straight medial tubercle transfer with a small thin flat osteotomy, weight bearing can be allowed right away, whereas in a patient with an anteromedialized tubercle, with a larger oblique osteotomy, weight bearing should be prohibited for the first 4 to 6 weeks postoperatively.

In general, full ROM is allowed immediately and usually these patients regain full ROM within a couple of weeks after surgical intervention. Protected weight bearing for the first 3 to 4 weeks with the brace locked in extension is encouraged until the patient has good quadriceps control. Since the quadriceps and extensor mechanism are not violated, early quadriceps isometrics are allowed with resisted quadriceps strengthening allowed at 6 to 8 weeks, at which point there is some early bony healing.

Results Multiple large series have reported a very high success rate with a low rate of complications.[24–26] In summary, the major conclusions of these clinical studies of medial tubercle transfer are the following:

1. It is best in young patients without evidence of severe systematic chondrosis or arthrosis.
2. Medial tubercle transfer corrects subluxation (congruence angle) as well as tilt (lateral patellofemoral angle).
3. Adequate postoperative Q-angle correction (<10 degrees) correlates with a good outcome.
4. Patella alta patients do well with this procedure.
5. Screw removal is common.

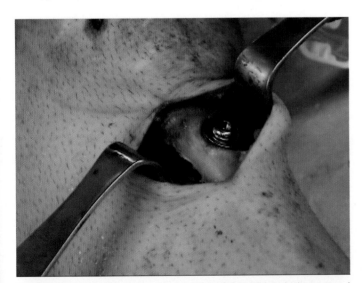

Figure 57-11 The osteotomy is fixed with a 4.5-mm bicortical screw and washer. A second screw and washer can be added if necessary.

Combined Distal and Proximal Realignment

The indications for a combined procedure are a combination of tubercle malalignment and traumatic incompetence of the medial restraints, particularly the MPFL. Usually this occurs in a patient with recurrent (traumatic onset) lateral instability leading to proximal insufficiency and a static lateral position of the patella from distal malalignment, with an increased Q angle and radiographic evidence of tilt and/or subluxation. The author's approach in these cases is to correct the tubercle malalignment first and then reassess patellar tracking. This is to eliminate the valgus vector pulling the patella laterally. In this instance, if only proximal realignment is performed, the Q angle and the valgus vector forces would be increased even more and create abnormal stresses on the patellofemoral joint. With this approach, after the tubercle malalignment correction is performed, if it is thought that patellar tracking is still not corrected and there is still lateral instability of the patella, the additional proximal realignment necessary to correct the problem is then performed. In the author's practice, an arthroscopic medial imbrication has been sufficient to correct the problem in the majority of patients. Open reconstruction of the MPFL, which is performed in cases of severe insufficiency of this ligament, has been only rarely necessary. If tibial tubercle malalignment is borderline and the patella is very lax, the author chooses to do the proximal realignment first followed by evaluation of patellar tracking and possible tubercle transfer.

Symptomatic Arthrosis and Anteromedialization

If pain is a significant component of the patient's symptom complex, in combination with malalignment, a decision must be made as to whether to move the tubercle straight medially or anteromedially. In general, if the patient has symptomatic chondrosis or arthrosis that is lateral or distal, anteriorization is considered in addition to the medialization. One must ask when is it appropriate to move the tubercle anteromedially instead of just medially and when should a tubercle transfer be avoided altogether?

When considering tibial tubercle osteotomy for patellofemoral arthrosis with malalignment, it is important to define which patients will benefit most from anteromedialization. In general, these are patients with pain secondary to symptomatic arthrosis of the patellofemoral articulation with malalignment, with or without symptoms of lateral patellar instability. The role of medialization has already been discussed. The goal in these patients is to unload and relieve the pain of symptomatic lesions as well as to realign by anteriorization of the tibial tubercle. At the same time, one must be wary of loading other areas of diseased cartilage and causing more pain by performing this procedure.

Anteriorization of the tibial tubercle dates back to 1963 with the so-called Maquet principle (which may have actually first been described by Bandi in 1962).[27-31] The Maquet principle stated that elevation of the tibial tubercle reduces patellar tendon forces and decreases the vector angle between the quadriceps and the patellar tendon force and thus reduces the resultant patellofemoral joint reaction vector force. In Maquet's initial biomechanical studies,[28-31] he concluded that 2 cm of advancement of the tibial tubercle reduced the compressive patellar forces by about 50% and also decreased the tibiofemoral forces. By his theory, the greater the elevation of the tubercle is, the greater the benefit of decreasing the patellofemoral contact forces. In the 1970s and 1980s, in both Europe and the United States, this procedure was commonly used for patients with symptomatic patellofemoral arthrosis. Unfortunately, elevation of the tibial tubercle up to 2 cm led to many complications, such as skin necrosis, wound breakdown, infection, fracture, and nonunion. Furthermore, in Maquet's biomechanical studies, he did not account properly for rotational or horizontal vectors in his calculations and he assumed that the vector force of the quadriceps pole was equal to the vector force of the patellar tendon pole, which is erroneous.

Subsequently, between the hallmark study of Ferguson et al[32] in 1979 to the present, numerous authors have studied tibial tubercle transfer extensively.[32-60] A summary of the conclusions of these biomechanical studies on anteriorization are listed in Box 57-4.

Clinical confirmation of these biomechanical findings has been further demonstrated by the excellent clinical studies by Fulkerson et al.[35,44,51,52] They demonstrated that the patients who gained the most benefit from anteromedialization of the tibial tubercle were those with chondrosis or arthrosis in the lateral or distal portion of the patella.

Anteromedialization of the tibial tubercle was first described by Fulkerson[44] in 1983 with a subsequent follow-up in 1990.[35] It is indicated for patients with patellar malalignment consisting of tilt and/or subluxation in association with arthrosis, preferably in the areas described. Fulkerson's biomechanical studies were in concert with others showing that anteriorization of 12 to 15 mm and medialization of 9 to 10 mm of the tibial tubercle results in decreased lateral facet pressures and a shifting of the contact pressures of the patella proximally and medially.[20,32-34,36,37,47,61,62]

The obliquity of the cut can be varied so that a maximal obliquity (which is limited by the lateral intermuscular septum to approximately 60 degrees) is indicated for patients with arthrosis, more pronounced than malalignment, to maximize anteriorization and minimize medialization. On the other hand, an osteotomy with less obliquity can be created for more medialization when malalignment is more of an issue than arthrosis.

Box 57-4 Conclusions of Biomechanical Studies on Anteriorization

1. Anteriorization of the tibial tubercle more than 12 to 15 mm is never necessary because further elevation has minimal biomechanical effect (it may, in fact, have a deleterious effect by loading the proximal portion of the patella) and increases the risk of complications. In particular, wound complications increase dramatically with an elevation of more than 15 mm.
2. Anteromedialization of the tibial tubercle decreases contact pressures, mostly on the distal and lateral portions of the patella, and transfers the load proximally and medially.
3. Anteriorization of the tibial tubercle rotates the patella on its horizontal axis and relieves pressure on the distal portion of the patella, but loads the proximal portion of the patella. This is particularly evident at elevations of more than 15 mm.
4. Anteromedialization of the tibial tubercle shifts contact forces from the distal lateral portion of the patella to the proximal medial portion of the patella.
5. There is an extremely variable effect of anterior or anteromedial tibial tubercle transfer from patient to patient because every tracking pattern is different and the problem is multifactorial. There is a wide range of changes and shifting of contact pressures with anteromedialization and anteriorization.[61]

In summary, most biomechanical and clinical studies suggest that the location of the arthrosis is a much more important factor than the extent of disease.

Ideal Indications: Anteromedialization

1. A patient has symptomatic arthrosis of the patellofemoral joint that is located in the lateral or distal portion of the patella associated with clinical and radiographic evidence of malalignment consisting of tilt and/or subluxation.
2. The patient has failed an extensive nonoperative rehabilitation program.
3. In combination with cartilage restoration procedures of the patella or trochlea to unload and protect the concomitant procedures unless the primary symptomatic and treated lesion is located on the proximal one-third of the patella. These patients may have undergone a microfracture, autologous chondrocyte implantation, or patellar or trochlear OATS procedure. Anteromedialization is often combined with these procedures to correct malalignment and unload the treated areas of the articular cartilage.

In most patients with symptomatic arthrosis, unless secondary to direct trauma, a degree of malalignment is frequently present. Oftentimes this is subtle and can only be identified by the CT studies described previously. Careful assessment of the tubercle alignment is mandatory.

Technique After arthroscopic evaluation and treatment, if a final decision to perform the anteromedialization has been made, this procedure is performed through a laterally based incision (Fig. 57-13), and, if necessary, a lateral retinacular release is performed (Fig. 57-14). If there are pre-existing incisions, a skin bridge of at least 5 cm is mandatory and the incision can be modified if necessary. It is important to free up the patellar tendon on both sides to allow proper transfer of shift in forces to the patella (Fig. 57-15). The tibialis anterior is carefully dissected off the lateral tibial crest, subperiosteally, back to the limit of the lateral intermuscular septum. The osteotomy should be approximately 8 cm in length, so the incision should allow adequate exposure of the tibia to this extent (Fig. 57-16).

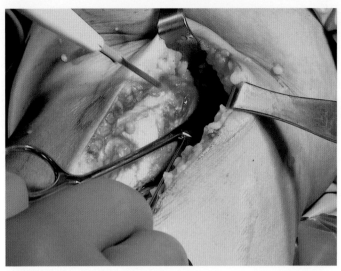

Figure 57-14 A lateral release may be necessary to decrease lateral tethering.

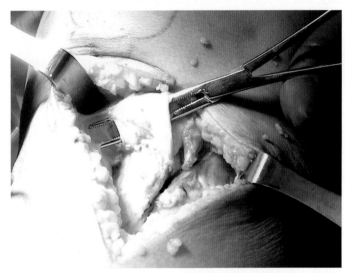

Figure 57-15 The patellar tendon is exposed and freed on both sides to allow unrestrained shift of the patella with tubercle transfer.

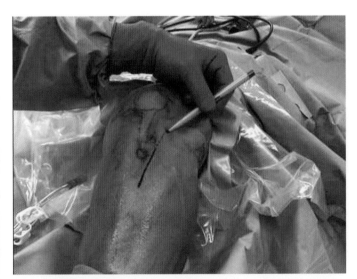

Figure 57-13 Lateral incision for anteromedialization procedure. Care must be taken to identify previous incisions or wounds that could impair skin circulation.

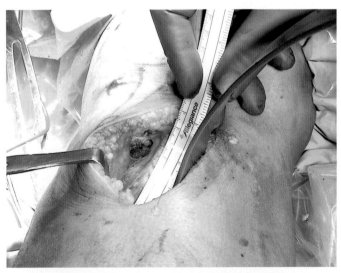

Figure 57-16 An 8-cm tubercle shingle is planned.

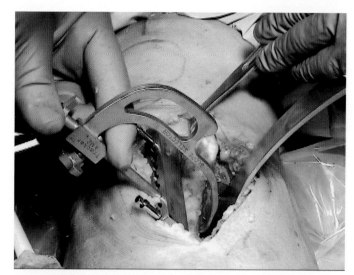

Figure 57-17 The AMZ Guide (DePuy-Mitek, Norwood, MA) in position on the medial tibial slope. A caliper is used to identify the exit point of the saw blade on the lateral side. Care must be taken to ensure that the blade exits anterior to the lateral intermuscular septum.

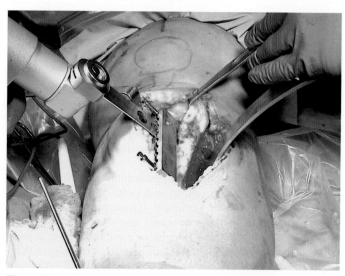

Figure 57-18 The osteotomy is initiated with an oscillating saw. A special retractor is used to protect the anterolateral musculature, which has been elevated off the lateral tibial slope subperiosteally.

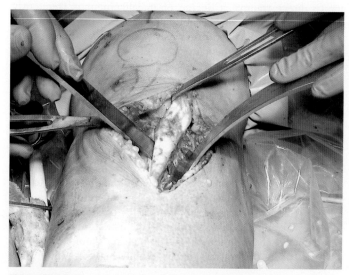

Figure 57-19 The initial cut is completed with an osteotome distally as it tapers toward the anterior cortex.

The author prefers to use an AMZ Guide (DePuy-Mitek, Norwood, MA; Fig. 57-17). This is helpful to predetermine the exact obliquity of the cut and to ensure a flat cut so that there are no incongruities in the contact areas between the two surfaces when shifting the tubercle anteriorly and medially. As an alternative, a flat pin block from a commercially available external fixation system can be used.

The AMZ Guide is placed in the proposed spot and a specially designed caliper can be placed inside the holes of the guide to determine where the osteotomy will exit on the lateral side. The more proximal part of the osteotomy will exit the tibia more posteriorly and taper more anteriorly as it courses distally. As mentioned previously, the maximum obliquity possible is approximately 60 degrees, so that the osteotomy exits just anterior to the lateral intermuscular septum. This is a tapering cut from the medial border of the patellar tendon insertion to the tibial crest approximately 8 cm distally. A specially designed retractor is used to protect the lateral soft tissues and the vital neurovascular structures posterior to the lateral intermuscular septum. A power saw is used to make the initial oblique cut, and the final cuts are performed using hand osteotomes (Figs. 57-18 and 57-19). A transverse cut is made just proximal to the patellar tendon with a 0.5-inch straight osteotome (Fig. 57-20) with a connecting cut between the transverse cut and the longitudinal osteotomy posterior to the tibial tubercle at its proximal extent to prevent propagation into the tibial plateau (Fig. 57-21).

The osteotomy is carefully completed from proximal to distal using a small hand osteotome, attempting to leave the distal soft tissues intact. Once the osteoclasis is complete, the tubercle is rotated anteriorly and medially the desired amount (Figs. 57-22 and 57-23). The two proposed screw sites are marked on the anterior tibial cortex and the osteotomy is fixed temporarily with a 3.2-mm drill bit at the planned distal screw site, going through the osteotomy and the anterior cortex of the tibia but not the posterior cortex (Fig. 57-24). At this point, the patellar tracking is assessed clinically and the amount of anteriorization and medialization is determined as well as the correction of the

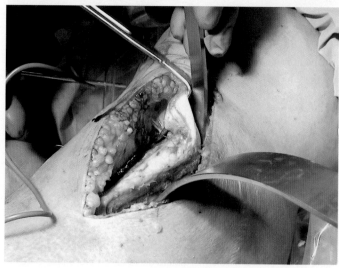

Figure 57-20 A transverse cut is made just proximal to the insertion of the patellar tendon.

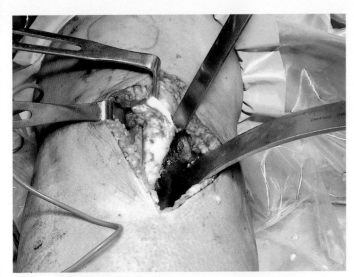

Figure 57-21 An oblique cut is made to connect the transverse and longitudinal cuts and prevent propagation of the osteotomy into the tibial plateau.

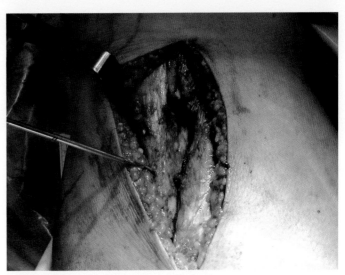

Figure 57-23 The location of two 4.5-mm bicortical screws is marked. The tubercle is temporarily fixed distally with a 3.2-mm drill bit to, but not through, the posterior cortex. With the tubercle fixed here, the knee is ranged and patellofemoral tracking inspected.

Q angle (Fig. 57-25). If the tubercle position is adequate and patellar tracking is normalized, final fixation is performed using two bicortical 4.5 cortical screws with metal washers. Leaving the distal drill bit in place, the proximal screw is inserted in a routine fashion and then the distal drill bit is advanced carefully through the posterior cortex and the second screw and washer are inserted. The knee should be flexed when placing anterior to posterior screws to avoid damage to the neurovascular structures posteriorly (Fig. 57-26). The procedure adequately corrects for patellar tilt and subluxation as shown by the preoperative and postoperative radiographs (Figs. 57-27 and 57-28).

The author usually performs the open part of the procedure under tourniquet control, and the tourniquet is deflated prior to

closure and careful hemostasis is achieved. The author believes that it is important to drain after anteromedialization because of the large area of exposed bone that can cause significant bleeding. Furthermore, release of the tourniquet is important to ensure that with closure of the wound, there is no compromise of the capillary circulation to the skin. In general, anteriorization limited to 12 to 15 mm has not been associated with skin circulatory problems. However, if the patient has pre-existing scars and incisions or vascular compromise, skin circulation should be carefully assessed. If there is any evidence that there is excessive pressure on the skin from the shift of the tubercle, the anteriorization should be decreased accordingly. This is usually not necessary. The fascia is never closed, and careful closure of the subcutaneous tissue and skin is performed. The

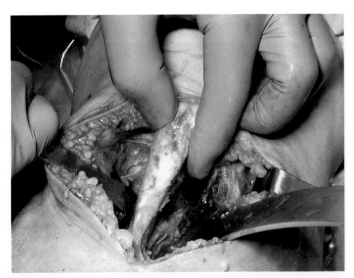

Figure 57-22 The tubercle shingle is now free to be shifted anteromedially along the oblique osteotomy plane. Note the shingle remains attached distally by periosteum and soft tissue.

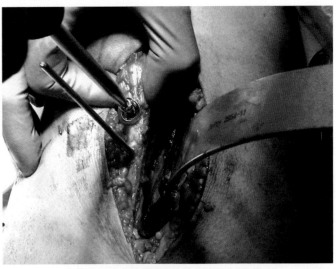

Figure 57-24 If patellofemoral tracking is deemed adequate, the tubercle is fixed with the proximal and then distal screws and metal washers. These screws are placed with the knee flexed 90 degrees to protect the posterior neurovascular structures that are at risk with posterior cortex penetration.

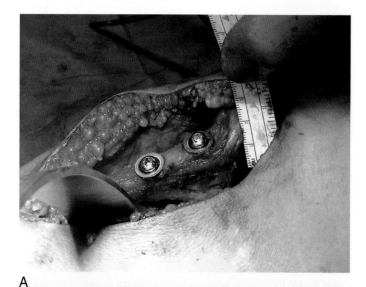

A

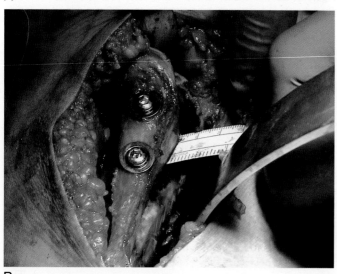

B

Figure 57-25 A, The amount of anteriorization is measured on completion of the transfer. Anteriorization is generally limited to 12 to 15 mm but must be individualized based on the patient's symptomatology and location of chondral lesions. **B,** Medialization is measured. Again, the amount of medialization must be individualized dependent on the amount of preoperative tubercle malalignment.

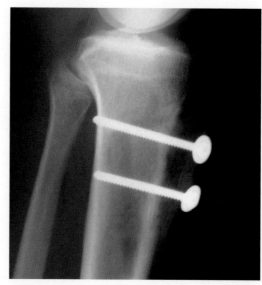

Figure 57-26 Lateral radiograph after placement of the screws.

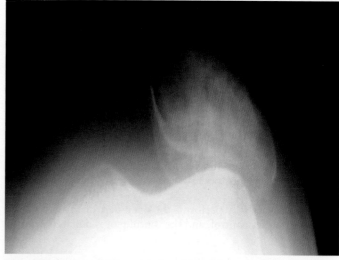

Figure 57-27 Preoperative axial view demonstrates patellar subluxation and excessive tilt.

patient is mobilized in a straight-leg locked brace position. Overnight hospitalization is necessary and the drain is removed prior to discharge. The author allows 2 to 3 days for the swelling in the soft tissues to subside and then a continuous passive motion machine is used at home for progressive ROM of the knee. Early goals with physical therapy are to regain ROM and quadriceps control.

Postoperative Rehabilitation As mentioned previously, there are high stress forces on the tibia with an oblique osteotomy and the author recommends no weight bearing for 6 weeks postoperatively. The more vertical the cut is, the higher the stress risers are, so that with a maximum oblique cut of 60 degrees, no weight bearing for 6 weeks is paramount. With lesser degrees of obliquity, weight bearing can probably be allowed a little earlier. Full ROM is allowed postoperatively. Quadriceps isometric

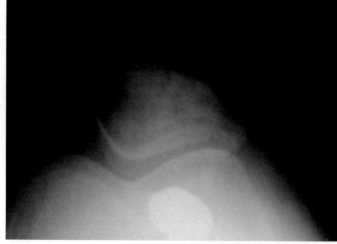

Figure 57-28 Postoperative axial view demonstrating correction of patellar tilt and subluxation after anteromedialization.

exercises are encouraged early, but no resistive exercises are allowed until approximately 2 months postoperatively to allow for osseous healing.

Results As in most procedures, the proper patient selection is critical to the success of this procedure. Fulkerson (along with others)[35,44,47,51,52] has well documented that this procedure can be very beneficial to the patient with arthrosis associated malalignment, particularly with lateral or distal disease.

CONCLUSIONS

Proximal realignment, lateral retinacular release, medial capsular reefing, and MPFL reconstruction can be used as stand-alone procedures if indicated or in conjunction with a distal realignment procedure. Tibial tubercle transfer, either in a medial, anteromedial, or anterior direction, can play a valuable role in the treatment of the patient with symptomatic patellofemoral arthrosis associated with malalignment and/or instability. Figure 57-29 demonstrates the author's treatment algorithm for the decision regarding which direction the tibial tubercle should be transferred in these cases. Patient selection is absolutely critical to the success of these procedures. With careful attention to technique and rehabilitation, in most cases, a successful outcome and a happy patient will be the final result.

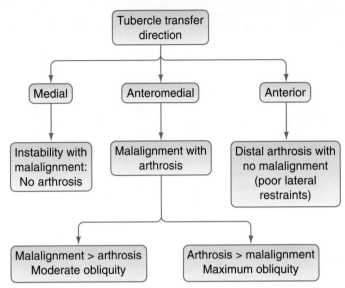

Figure 57-29 Algorithm for direction of tibial tubercle transfer when distal realignment is indicated.

REFERENCES

1. Desio S, Burks R, Kent B: Soft tissue restraints to lateral patellar translation in the human knee. Am J Sports Med 1998;26:59–65.
2. Kolowich P, Paulos L, Rosenberg T, Farnsworth S: Lateral release of the patella: Indications and contraindications. Am J Sports Med 1990;18:359–365.
3. Insall J, Goldberg V, Salvati E: Recurrent dislocation and the high-riding patella. Clin Orthop 1972;88:67–69.
4. Blackburn JS, Peel TE: A new method of measuring patellar height. J Bone Joint Surg Br 1977;59:241–242.
5. Merchant AC, Mercer RL, Jacobsen RH, Cool CR: Roentgenographic analysis of patellofemoral congruence. J Bone Joint Surg Am 1974;56:1391–1396.
6. Laurin CA, Levesque HP, Dussault R, et al: The abnormal lateral patellofemoral angle. J Bone Joint Surg Am 1978;60:55–60.
7. Muneta T, Yamamoto H, Ishibashi T, et al: Computerized tomographic analysis of tibial tubercle position in the painful female patellofemoral joint. Am J Sports Med 1994;22:67–71.
8. Beaconsfield T, Hons B, Pintore E, et al: Radiologic measurements in patellofemoral disorders: A review. Clin Orthop 1994;308:18–28.
9. Elias DA, White DM, Fithian DC: Acute lateral patellar dislocation at MR imaging: Injury patterns of medial patellar soft tissue restraints and osteochondral injuries of the inferomedial patella. Radiology 2002;225:736–743.
10. Virolainen H, Visuri T, Kuusela T: Acute dislocation of the patella: MR findings. Radiology 1993;189:243–246.
11. Kirsch M, Fitzgerald S, Friedman H, Rogers LF: Transient lateral patellar dislocation: Diagnosis with MR imaging. AJR Am J Roentgenol 1993;161:109–113.
12. Dye SF, Chew MH: The use of scintigraphy to detect increased osseous metabolic activity about the knee. J Bone Joint Surg Am 1993;75A:1388–1406.
13. Henry JH: Conservative treatment of patellofemoral subluxation. Clin Sports Med 1989;8:261–278.
14. McConnell J: The management of chondromalacia patellae: A long term solution. Aust J Physiother 1986;2:215–223.
15. Nomura E, Inoue M, Kurimura M: Chondral and osteochondral injuries associated with acute patellar dislocation. Arthroscopy 2003;19:717–721.
16. Fulkerson JP, Kalenak A, Rosenberg TD, Cox JS: Patellofemoral pain. Instruct Course Lect 1992;41:57–71.
17. Halbrecht J: Arthroscopic patella realignment: An all-inside technique. Arthroscopy. J Arthrosc Relat Surg 2001;17:940–945.
18. Drez D, Edwards T, Williams C: Results of medial patellofemoral ligament reconstruction in the treatment of patellar dislocation. Arthroscopy. J Arthrosc Relat Surg 2001;17:3:298–306.
19. Ellera Gomes JL, Stigler Marczyk LR, Cesar de Cesar P, Jungblut CF: Medial patellofemoral ligament reconstruction with semitendinous autograft for chronic patellar instability: A follow-up study. Arthroscopy 2004;20:147–151.
20. Ramappa A, Apreleva M, Harrold F, et al: The effects of medialization and anteromedialization of the tibial tubercle on patellofemoral mechanics and kinematics. AOSSM Instructional Course presented at AOSSM Annual Meeting, July 2003, San Diego, CA.
21. Kuroda R, Kambic H, Valdevit A, Andrish J: Articular contact pressures after tibial tubercle transfer. Am J Sports Med 2001;29:403–409.
22. Trillat A, Dejour H, Couette A: Diagnostic et traitement des subluxation recidivantes de la rotule. Rev Chir Orthop 1964;50:813–824.
23. Cosgarea A, Schatzke M, Seth A, Litsky A: Biomechanical analysis of flat and oblique tibial tubercle osteotomy for recurrent patellar instability. Am J Sports Med 1999;27:507–512.
24. Cox J: Evaluation of the Roux-Elmslie-Trillat procedure for knee extensor realignment. Am J Sports Med 1982;10:303–310.
25. Shelbourne K, Porter D, Rozzi W: Use of a modified Elmslie-Trillat procedure to improve abnormal patellar congruence angle. Am J Sports Med 1994;22:318–323.
26. Farr J: Distal realignment for recurrent patellar instability. Op Tech Sports Med 2001;9:176–182.
27. Bandi W: Chondromalacia patella und femo-patellare arthrose. Helv Chir Acta 1972;11:1–70.

28. Maquet P: Un traitement biomecanique: L'arthrose femore-patellaire: L'avancement du tendon rotulien. Rev Rhum Mal Osteoartic 1963;30:779–783.

29. Maquet P: Advancement of the tibial tuberosity. Clin Orthop 1976;115:225–230.

30. Maquet P: Mechanics and osteoarthritis of the patellofemoral joint. Clin Orthop 1979;144:70–73.

31. Maquet P: Biomechanics of the Knee, 2nd ed. Berlin, Springer-Verlag, 1984.

32. Ferguson A, Brown T, Fu F, Rutkowski R: Relief of patellofemoral contact stress by anterior displacement of the tibial tubercle. J Bone Joint Surg Am 1979;61:159–166.

33. Ferguson A: Elevation of the insertion of the patellar ligament for patellofemoral pain. J Bone Joint Surg Am 1982;64:766–771.

34. Ferrandez L, Usabiaga J, Yubero J, et al: An experimental study of the redistribution of patellofemoral pressures by anterior displacement of the anterior tuberosity of the tibia. Clin Orthop 1989;283:183–189.

35. Fulkerson J, Becker G, Meaney J, et al: Anteromedial tibial tubercle transfer without bone graft. Am J Sports Med 1990;18:490–496.

36. Hungerford D, Barry M: Biomechanics of the patellofemoral joint. Clin Orthop 1979;144:9–15.

37. Nakamura T: Advancement of tibial tuberosity: A biomechanical study. J Bone Joint Surg Br 1985;67:255–260.

38. Pan H, Kish V, Boyd RD, et al: The Maquet procedure: Effect of tibial shingle length on patellofemoral pressures. J Orthop Res 1993;11:199–204.

39. Radin E: The Maquet procedure: Anterior displacement of the tibial tubercle. Indications, contraindications, and precautions. Clin Orthop 1986;213:241–248.

40. Radin E: Anterior tibial tubercle elevation in the young adult. Orthop Clin North Am 1986;17:297–302.

41. Radin E, Pan H: Long-term follow-up study on the Maquet procedure with special references to the causes of failure. Clin Orthop 1993;290:253–258.

42. Bellemans J, Cauwenberghs F, Witvrouw E, et al: Anteromedial tibial tubercle transfer in patients with chronic anterior knee pain and a subluxation type patella malalignment. Am J Sports Med 1997;25:375–381.

43. Bessette G, Hunter R: The Maquet procedure. A retrospective view. Clin Orthop 1998;232:159–167.

44. Fulkerson J: Anteromedialization of the tibial tuberosity for patellofemoral malalignment. Clin Orthop 1983;177:176–181.

45. Heatley FW, Allen PR, Patrick JH: Tibial tubercle advancement for anterior knee pain. Clin Orthop 1986;208:215–224.

46. Hirsch D: Experience with Maquet anterior tibial tubercle advancement for patellofemoral arthralgia. Clin Orthop 1980;148:136–139.

47. Koshino T: Changes in patellofemoral compressive force after anterior or anteromedial displacement of tibial tuberosity for chondromalacia patella. Clin Orthop 1991;266:133–138.

48. Leach R, Radin E: Anterior displacement of the tibial tubercle for patellofemoral arthrosis. Orthop Trans 1979;3:291–294.

49. Leach R, Schepsis A: Anterior displacement of the tibial tubercle: The Maquet procedure. Contemp Orthop 1981;3:199–204.

50. Lund F, Nilsson BE: Anterior displacement of tibial tuberosity in chondromalacia patella. Acta Orthop Scand 1980;51:679–688.

51. Pidoriano A, Weinstein R, Buuck D, Fulkerson J: Correlation of patellar articular lesions with results from anteromedial tibial tubercle transfer. Am J Sports Med 1997;25:533–537.

52. Post W, Fulkerson J: Distal realignment of the patellofemoral joint. Orthop Clin North Am 1992;23:631–643.

53. Putnam M, Mears D, Fu F: Combined Maquet and proximal tibial valgus osteotomy. Clin Orthop 1985;197:217–223.

54. Rappaport LH, Browne MG, Wickiewicz TL: The Maquet osteotomy. Orthop Clin North Am 1992;23:645–656.

55. Rozbruch J: Tibial tubercle elevation: A clinical study of 31 cases. Orthop Trans 1979;3:291.

56. Schepsis A, DeSimone A, Leach R: Anterior tibial tubercle transposition for patellofemoral arthrosis: A long-term study. Am J Knee Surg 1994;7:13–20.

57. Schmidt F: The Maquet procedure in the treatment of patellofemoral osteoarthritis. Clin Orthop 1993;294:254–258.

58. Siegel M: The Maquet osteotomy: A review of risks. Orthopedics 1987;10:1073–1078.

59. Sudmann E, Salkowitsch B: Anterior displacement of tibial tuberosity in the treatment of chondromalacia patella. Acta Orthop Scand 1980;51:171–174.

60. Weisbrod, H, Treiman N: Anterior displacement of tibial tuberosity for patellofemoral disorders. Clin Orthop 1980;153:180–182.

61. Cohen Z, Henry J, McCarthy D, et al: Computer simulations of patellofemoral joint surgery: Patient-specific models for tuberosity transfer. Am J Sports Med 2003;31:87–98.

62. Benvenuti J, Rakotomanana L, Leyvraz P, et al: Displacements of the tibial tuberosity: Effects of the surgical parameters. Clin Orthop 1997;1:224–234.

58 Tendon Ruptures

Jeff C. Brand, Jr.

In This Chapter

INTRODUCTION

- Extensor mechanism disruptions include quadriceps and patellar tendon rupture.

- Bilateral atraumatic simultaneous quadriceps tendon ruptures tend to occur in patients with systemic disease.

- Diagnosis is made by clinical examination and radiographic findings in most instances.

- Surgery is necessary to restore the extensor mechanism anatomy.

- Rehabilitation is determined by the type and strength of the repair.

- Weakness, atrophy, and functional losses are common postoperative problems.

QUADRICEPS TENDON RUPTURES

Relevant Anatomy

The quadriceps tendon is the tendinous confluence, approximately 3 cm proximal to the patella, of the vastus lateralis, medialis longus and obliquus, rectus femoris, vastus intermedius, and articularis genu. The tendon is broad based and has a trilaminar depth with fat between the tendon planes. The rectus femoris is the most superficial of the three layers. The rectus direct head arises from the anterior inferior spine and indirect head is from the anterior capsule of the hip. Innervation as for all the quadriceps is from the femoral nerve. It is a two-joint muscle unique among the quadriceps muscles. Distally, fibers form the superficial layer of the quadriceps tendon that traverse over the patella and insert in the infrapatellar tendon. The trilaminar expansion of the quadriceps tendon consists of the superficial layer described, the intermediate layer of the lateralis and medialis, and the deep layer of the intermedius. The lateralis sends fibers to the lateral patellofemoral ligament as well. The vastus lateralis arises from the lateral flare of the greater trochanter along the linea aspera. The vastus intermedius arises from the mid-anterior femur. The vastus medialis originates at the ante-

rior femur just below the level of the lesser trochanter and inserts in the middle layer on the superior medial border of the patella. Its distal fibers contribute to the medial retinaculum. The articularis genu, an anatomic variant, arises deep to the intermedius and inserts on the superior capsule of the knee serving to retract it from the patella.[1]

Biomechanics

The patella acts as a moment arm for knee extension through the quadriceps mechanism and patellar tendon attachment on the tibia. Forces in the quadriceps tendon and patellar tendon vary with flexion angle but are consistently reported to be greater at 60 degrees of knee flexion. At 30 and 120 degrees, forces in both structures are roughly one half of these peak values. At 60 degrees of knee flexion, the forces in each tendon are approximately equal. The force in the patellar tendon (F_L) is approximately 30% greater than the force in the quadriceps tendon (F_Q) at 30 degrees of knee flexion. At 90 degrees of knee flexion, F_Q is 30% greater than F_L. The patellar contact area moves proximally with increased knee flexion. With the knee in 30 degrees of flexion, the patellar contact area is on the distal portion positioning the patellar tendon at a mechanical disadvantage and increasing forces within the patellar tendon compared to the quadriceps tendon. This suggests that the patella functions as more than a simple pulley that would have equal forces in each the patellar tendon and quadriceps tendon at all knee flexion angles.[2] Changing the length of the lever arm by changing the length of either the patellar tendon or the quadriceps tendon can occur with extensor mechanism tendon repair. This will change force loading in each tendon and the contact area of the patella.

Cause of Injury

An intact healthy extensor mechanism, particularly the quadriceps tendon, is unlikely to rupture. The tendon most commonly ruptures through a histologically proven degenerative area.[3] Patients with bilateral simultaneous quadriceps tendon ruptures frequently have degeneration as a result of a systemic disease. Although the spontaneous atraumatic rupture of bilateral quadriceps tendons simultaneously is a frequent subject of case reports, it is uncommon in case series.

Clinical Features and Evaluation

The patient with a quadriceps tendon rupture is commonly a male in the sixth decade of life, may have systemic disease, and suffers an indirect eccentric load to the knee with a misstep. Historically, quadriceps tendon rupture was thought to be rare in the patient younger than 40 years of age.[4] Forty-five years ago Scuderi stated, "There should be no difficulty in diagnosing a

Table 58-1 Clinical Evaluation of Patients with Extensor Tendon Disruption
Mechanism of injury
Consider systemic medical conditions
Hemarthrosis
Loss of active knee extension
Palpable defect
Patella alta (patellar tendon rupture) or baja (quadriceps tendon rupture) on plain radiographs
Magnetic resonance imaging if diagnosis is not clinically evident

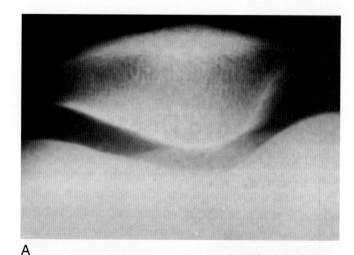

A

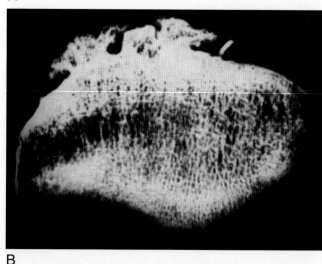

B

Figure 58-2 A, Normal patella as seen on a tangential view. **B,** A superoinferior radiograph of the specimen demonstrates the toothlike structures intimately fused with the anterior cortex of the proximal pole of the patella. (From Greenspan A, Norman A, Kia-Ming Tchang F: "Tooth" sign in Patellar degenerative disease. J Bone Joint Surg Am 1977;59:483–485.)

ruptured quadriceps tendon, but the diagnosis is all too frequently missed."[5] An inability to voluntarily extend the leg, patella baja on exam and a hemarthrosis combined are quite accurate (Table 58-1). Plain radiographs may reveal avulsion fractures and patella baja, which can be assessed with the Insall-Salvati method of measurement. Less than 0.8 suggests patella baja (Fig. 58-1). The "tooth" sign seen on the axial patellar radiographs may be an indication of quadriceps tendon degeneration at its insertion on the patella[6,7] (Fig. 58-2).

Magnetic resonance imaging, as reported in small series, shows a discontinuity in all three layers of the quadriceps tendon.[8,9] The patellar tendon, with an intact quadriceps tendon and normal tension in the extensor mechanism, displays a linear or nearly linear appearance. If the quadriceps tendon is ruptured, the patellar tendon has a corrugated or wrinkled appearance due to lack of tension in the extensor mechanism[10] (Fig. 58-3). Most authors agree that magnetic resonance imaging is not necessary in patients who have the usual findings of extensor mechanism disruption, but it may be useful when the diagnosis is in doubt.

Surgery

Acute Repair

A longitudinal incision offers an extensile approach that can be used for secondary procedures such as a total knee arthroplasty.

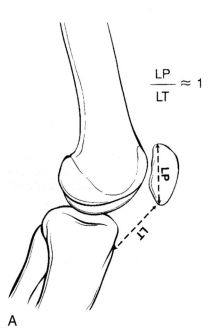

$$\frac{LP}{LT} \approx 1$$

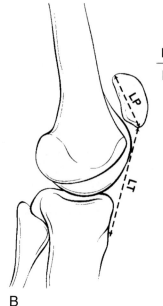

$$\frac{LP}{LT} \approx 0.50$$

Figure 58-1 The Insall-Salvati ratio in a normal knee (**A**) and in one with patella alta (**B**). LP, length of the patella; LT, length of the patellar tendon. (From Rose PS, Frassica FJ: Atraumatic bilateral patellar tendon rupture. A case report and review of the literature. J Bone Joint Surg Am 2001;83:1382–1386.)

A

B

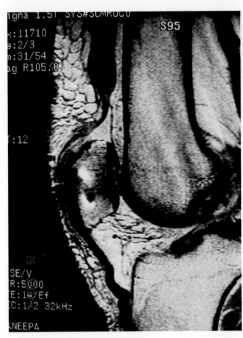

Figure 58-3 Magnetic resonance imaging of a patient 3 months after quadriceps tendon repair with suture anchors, demonstrating failure of the repair. The end of the quadriceps tendon is attenuated with signal change within the attenuated portion. The patellar tendon is wrinkled, consistent with relaxation of tension within the patellar tendon due to lengthening of the extensor mechanism.

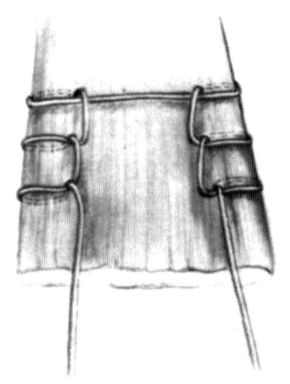

Figure 58-4 Schematic diagram of ligament fixation with the Krackow grasping suture. (From Krackow KA, Thomas SC, Jones LC: A new stitch for ligament-tendon fixation. J Bone Joint Surg Am 1986;68:764–766.)

After the incision, the hematoma is evacuated. Intra-articular structures are inspected for further injury to the degree that is possible. The margins of the quadriceps tendon and retinaculum are débrided. As the majority of these lesions occur at the insertion of the tendon onto the superior pole of the patella, the bone of the superior pole of the patella is prepared. Classic descriptions include a trough; however, soft-tissue removal from cortical bone may be adequate as is performed in rotator cuff repair preparation of the greater tuberosity.

Three longitudinal drill holes are drilled in the patella. One is drilled in the center of the patella in the coronal plane. A parallel drill hole is positioned on either side of the middle drill hole for a total of three drill holes. An anterior cruciate ligament drill guide may be used to drill the holes in a more controlled fashion.[11] Two no. 5 braided Ethibond sutures (Ethicon, Somerville, NJ) or similar suture is passed through the quadriceps tendon in a grasping configuration, such as a Krackow stitch (Fig. 58-4). The sutures are positioned to allow the central limbs of each suture to pass through the central drill hole of the patella. The opposite limb of each suture is passed with a Beath pin or suture passer (Fig. 58-5) through the drill holes along the medial and lateral sides of the patella, respectively. Opposite ends of each suture loop are knotted over the distal pole of the patella (Fig. 58-6). Alternatively, suture anchors drilled and deployed in the position where the bone tunnels would normally be drilled can provide fixation to the patella. The suture from the suture anchors is passed through the tissue in weave or grasping suture.[12] Usually there is a defect in the medial and lateral retinaculum that is repaired with no. 2 braided nonabsorbable suture in an interrupted figure-eight fashion. The natural space that is anterior to the repair and deep to the skin should be obliterated in the closure. Meticulous hemostasis and possibly a surgical drain prevent a postoperative hematoma that can become infected.

Chronic Repair

For patients who have near-normal length of the quadriceps tendon, standard repair techniques perform well. For the patients without normal length and tension in the quadriceps mechanism, the surgeon must decide between measures to add length to the tendon and those meant to substitute for the defect. Often the defect in the quadriceps tendon consists of variable amount of amorphous, nonfunctional scar tissue that should be resected.[13] Length may be restored to the quadriceps tendon mechanism through the Codivilla technique described by Scuderi[14] (Fig. 58-7). An inverted V is cut through the full thickness of the proximal segment of the quadriceps tendon with the inferior ends of the V ending 1.5 to 2 cm proximal to the rupture. The triangular flap thus fashioned is split into an anterior part of one third of its thickness and the posterior part of two thirds. The tendon ends of the rupture are then apposed with interrupted nonabsorbable sutures. The anterior one third thickness is turned distally and sutured (see Fig. 58-7). The open upper part of the V is closed with interrupted sutures. The stability of the repair is evaluated with passive range of motion (ROM).[15]

Postoperative Treatment

A hinged rehabilitative brace provides protection, controlled ROM and access to the incision. For the rare patient who may not be compliant with postoperative instruction, a cast may be more secure. Initially the brace is locked into full extension for 1 to 2 weeks to allow wound healing. This period varies depend-

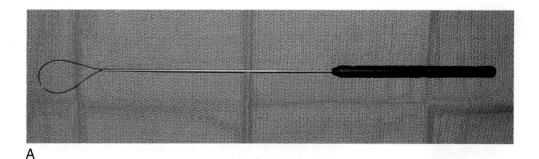

A

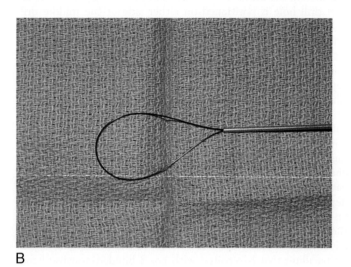

B

Figure 58-5 A, Hewson suture passer (Smith & Nephew, Memphis, TN). **B,** The tip of the suture passer.

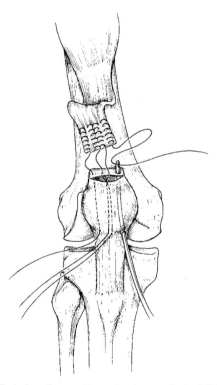

Figure 58-6 Technique for quadriceps tendon repair via drill holes in the patella. Sutures *(dashed lines)* are passed through three parallel drill holes and tied distally. The central two suture strands are passed through the same central hole and tied to the corresponding medial or lateral strand. (From Ilan DI, Tejwani N, Keschner M, Leibman M: Quadriceps tendon rupture. J Am Acad Orthop Surg 2003;11:192–200.)

ing on coexistent medical issues, immunosuppressive medications, and repair strength. After wound healing is achieved, progressive ROM starts from 0 to 30 degrees for 1 to 2 weeks, 0 to 60 degrees for the next 1 to 2 weeks, 0 to 90 degrees for the following 1 to 2 weeks. Most braces allow a 15-degree progression of ROM if the surgeon desires a slower progression of ROM. Weight bearing is full from the time of surgery with the hinges of the brace locked in full extension. Until 4 to 6 weeks postoperatively, strengthening is by isometrics, quadriceps-setting exercises, and straight leg raises in the brace with the hinges on the brace locked in full extension. At 4 to 6 weeks, the patient may start closed-chain strengthening. Proprioceptive or neuromuscular activities are an important part of the rehabilitative process as many of these injuries likely result from a misstep. At 10 to 12 weeks, plyometrics and functional activities may be added depending on the patient's demands and capabilities.

This progression of activities can be slowed for chronic repairs or reconstructions of the extensor mechanism. The quality of tissue, quality of the repair, and knee flexion obtained at the time of surgery all are important factors that influence the progression of activities.

Results

If proven surgical principles and techniques are practiced, patient results are generally good, independent of the quadriceps tendon repair method.[4,13,16] Weakness is the most common adverse outcome that may occur as often as 30% or more with isokinetic testing.[17] Extensor lag, although less common with more aggressive rehabilitation programs, still affects some patients after repair, and particularly after delayed reconstruction. Return to daily or occupational activities takes approxi-

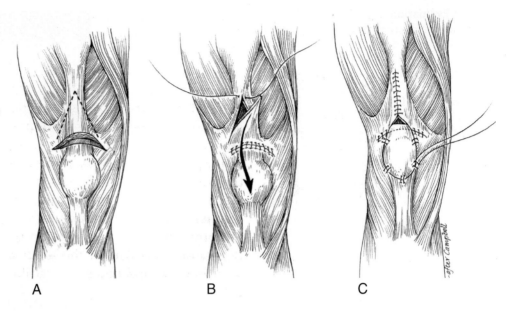

Figure 58-7 Codivilla method of quadriceps tendon lengthening and repair. **A,** Chronic quadriceps tendon tear exposed. Proximal retraction prevents direct opposition of the tear. *Dashed lines* represent inverted V cut (full thickness) to be made. **B,** The inverted V cut allows the tear to be approximated and repaired. **C,** The proximal aspect of the inverted V repaired side to side. A full- or partial-thickness flap may be used to augment the repair, as in the Scuderi technique. (From Ilan DI, Tejwani N, Keschner M, Leibman M: Quadriceps tendon rupture. J Am Acad Orthop Surg 2003;11:192–200.)

A   B   C

mately 4 months, but full recovery is longer with some patients. Most patients are able to return to vigorous occupations, but as many as 50% are unable to return to previous recreational activities.[18,19]

Scuderi stated,[5] "It is axiomatic that the earlier a ruptured quadriceps tendon is diagnosed and repaired, the better the end result will be." A delay in surgical repair results in a greater need for ambulatory aids, a decreased ability to climb stairs, and an increased incidence of an extensor lag. Return to work and recreational activities are similarly affected. Patient satisfaction scores are lower with a delayed surgical repair. Although the best results have been seen in patients who were repaired within 7 days, surgical repair for a chronic rupture is recommended.[12,15]

Patients with bilateral simultaneous quadriceps tendon rupture do not perform as well as patients with unilateral rupture. The majority of these patients are affected by chronic medical conditions (76%). In one study, results in 57% were considered favorable and 43% had a poor outcome. Older patients did not fare as well as younger patients.[20]

Complications
In a review of multiple series of quadriceps tendon repairs, the most common complication is postoperative stiffness, either extensor lag or loss of flexion. Wound-healing problems and infection are also potential complications. Rerupture of the repair can occur, although it is relatively rare. Other described complications include postoperative hemarthrosis, and deep venous thrombosis or pulmonary embolus.

PATELLAR TENDON RUPTURES

Relevant Anatomy
The patellar tendon is the distal insertion of the extensor mechanism into the proximal tibia through the tibial tubercle. It is obliquely orientated in the coronal plane with the patella lying slightly medial to the tibial tubercle. It is wider and thinner proximally at its attachment on the distal pole of the patella. The patellar tendon fibers merge to attach on the tibial tubercle. Consequently, the tibial insertion is narrower and thicker than the patellar origination. The patellar origination on the distal pole of the patella arcs a crescent in the coronal plane with

the medial and lateral fibers attaching more proximally. The patellar tendon attaches to the anterior aspect of the distal pole of the patella. The nonarticular zone is largely devoid of patellar tendon attachment.[21]

Cause of Rupture
The patellar tendon ruptures through an area of degeneration or impairment[3] (Table 58-2). Mechanical impairment may be due to harvest of the middle third of the tendon for ligament reconstruction surgery. Compared to a control group, a test group that experienced harvest of the middle third of the patella in young human cadavers (mean age 24.86 ± 7.13 years) measured a mean area of 48.67 mm^2 (49.64% less) and load of 2226.58 N (51% less), and energy level at failure of 32.58 J (45.14% less).[22]

Cortisone injections into the patellar tendon for inflammatory conditions or anterior knee pain are discussed in several reports as a cause of patellar tendon rupture.[6,23] A biochemical investigation demonstrated that dexamethasone significantly decreased cell viability, suppressed cell proliferation, and reduced collagen synthesis in cultured human tenocytes.[24]

Table 58-2 Patellar Tendon Ruptures

Causes	Mechanism
Harvest of the middle third of the patellar tendon for ligament reconstruction[22]	Mechanical
Cortisone injection[6,24,33]	Decreased cell viability, suppressed cell proliferation, and reduced collagen synthesis
Jumper's knee[6]	Degeneration
Rheumatoid arthritis[1]	Fibrosis, synovitis
Obesity[1]	Fatty degeneration
Fluoroquinolones[1]	
Osgood-Schlatter disease[6,30]	Mechanical

Clinical Evaluation

The clinical findings of patellar tendon rupture mirror those of the quadriceps tendon rupture (see Table 58-1). Patients with a patellar tendon rupture are generally younger than those with a quadriceps tendon rupture.

Biomechanics of Repairs

In an investigation of elderly cadaveric knees (mean age, 66 years), three methods of patellar tendon repair were loaded in a cyclical fashion for 250 cycles at 0.25 Hz. In the first group, the patellar tendon was sutured with no. 5 Ethibond in a Krackow stitch passed through longitudinal drill holes in the patella (mean gap across the repair site 11.3 ± 0.5 mm). The second group added a no. 5 Ethibond suture augmentation as a cerclage passed through a transverse drill hole at the mid-patella and then passed through a transverse drill hole through the tibial tubercle and tied at 90 degrees of flexion (mean gap, 4.9 ± 0.5 mm). The third group used a 2.0 Dall-Miles cable (Howmedica Inc., Rutherford, NJ) augmentation (mean gap, 3.5 ± 0.8 mm). Although this investigation was a biomechanical evaluation, the authors believed that the Dall-Miles augmentation allowed an accelerated rehabilitation consisting of full weight bearing in extension, knee ROM from 0 to 90 degrees, and isometric quadriceps/hamstring muscle strengthening.[25]

A similar method of augmentation with the semitendinosus tendon placed through drill holes allowed an accelerated rehabilitation program that obtained ROM through continual passive motion for 2 weeks combined with passive and active-assisted ROM. Low-resistance cycling started at 2 weeks postoperatively. Three of four patients were identical to the contralateral leg with Cybex dynamometer, Lysholm knee scoring scale, one-legged hop test, ROM, and radiographic evaluation.[26]

Acute Repair

A longitudinal midline approach to the patellar tendon from the vastus medialis oblique to just beyond the tibial tubercle allows other procedures at the same time or as a delayed procedure.[27] Creating thick skin flaps prevents wound-healing complications.

A 60-degree lateral radiograph of the contralateral knee preoperatively serves as a guide to patellar tendon length (Fig. 58-8) that restores normal patellar tracking in all planes. Skin incision and prepatellar bursa excision expose the ruptured patellar tendon. Mid-substance tears and the tendinous portion of the proximal and distal repairs can be sutured with a grasping suture such as the Krackow stitch. For either proximal or distal tears, an anatomic attachment to bone needs to be recreated. The bone should be débrided of soft tissue to allow restoration of the normal tendon to bone insertion. Insertion site anatomy can be restored through either bone anchors or tunnels placed through bone. Transosseous tunnels are favored by history; bone anchors are favored by ease and exposure. A braided no. 5 nonabsorbable suture has been traditionally chosen for these repairs (Fig. 58-9). Newer suture with improved biomechanical properties (Fiberwire; Arthrex, Naples, FL) is currently available.

Augmentation with wire,[28] Dall-Miles cable,[27] or biologic tissue (semitendinosus[26]) is advocated by some authors. Augmentation can allow a more rapid or accelerated rehabilitation program through improved biomechanical properties of the surgical repair site.[25,27] It is most commonly used in circumstances in which tissue quality is considered compromised or when patient compliance with a postoperative program is a concern. Shelbourne et al[27] apply the Dall-Miles device after the sutures

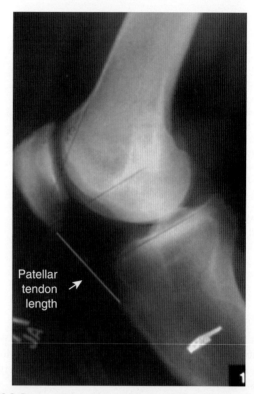

Figure 58-8 Preoperative lateral radiograph is taken of the normal knee to obtain the normal patellar tendon length. (From Shelbourne KD, Darmelio MP, Klootwyk TE: Patellar tendon rupture repair using Dall-Miles cable. Am J Knee Surg 2001;14:17–21.)

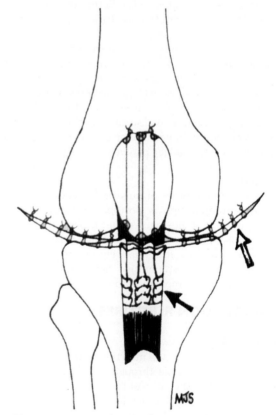

Figure 58-9 Diagram of the repair technique with tendon reattachment through vertical drill holes in the patella using nonabsorbable suture (*solid arrow*) and reapproximation of the retinaculum using interrupted absorbable sutures (*open arrow*). (From Kuechle DK, Stuart MJ: Isolated rupture of the patellar tendon in athletes. Am J Sports Med 1994;22:692–695.)

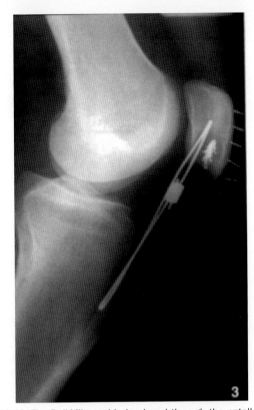

Figure 58-10 The Dall-Miles cable is placed through the patella and tibia and is clamped at the joint line. The placement of the cable allows knee flexion to approximately 120 degrees without placing undue tension on the patellar tendon repair. (From Shelbourne KD, Darmelio MP, Klootwyk TE: Patellar tendon rupture repair using Dall-Miles cable. Am J Knee Surg 2001;14:17–21.)

are positioned but before they are tied. A drill hole is placed transversely across the patella at the mid-portion. A similar transverse hole is drilled across the tibial tubercle. The Dall-Miles cable, neutralization wire, or semitendinosus can be tensioned and lateral radiograph obtained with the knee in 60 degrees of flexion that is compared to the preoperative contralateral knee radiograph. The length of Dall-Miles cable or neutralization can be adjusted until the repaired tendon length is equal to the opposite side (Fig. 58-10). Grasping sutures are tied and knee flexion is evaluated for the limits to postoperative rehabilitation. The space anterior to the repair and deep to the skin is closed with meticulous hemostasis and possibly a surgical drain to prevent a postoperative hematoma.

Chronic Repair or Reconstruction

If possible, the chronic repair should be performed using the techniques and principles detailed in the acute repair section previously discussed. This approach will not likely be possible beyond 6 weeks from the time of injury. By that time, due to the retraction of the patella alta from the quadriceps muscle, the patellar tendon has healed in an elongated position with biomechanically inferior fibrous tissue.

Allograft tissue as a reconstructive option offers ease of use, avoidance of graft site morbidity, availability, and often shorter operating times. Unfortunately, viral or bacterial disease may be transmitted by the allograft tissue. Allograft tissues add to the expense of the operation and are not available in all parts of the world. Anterior cruciate ligament reconstruction results with allograft tissue have been comparable, in some series, to those results obtained with autogenous tissue. The results of patellar tendon reconstruction are limited to either case reports or small case series.

Mills[29] published a very complete description of the reconstruction of the patellar tendon with an allograft Achilles tendon, and the reader may wish to refer to this description for further details. Five- to 10-degree flexion contractures are treated with physical therapy, dynamic splinting, and possibly serial casting. Flexion contractures greater than 10 degrees are treated surgically as the first stage of a two-stage reconstruction. The second stage is reconstruction of the patellar tendon. Extensive quadriceps retraction and scarring are treated with a quadricepsplasty. This procedure may reduce flexion after surgery, and the patient should be warned of this possibility.

A longitudinal incision from 2 cm proximal to the patella to the distal extent of the tibial tubercle is created. Thick skin flaps are made to protect the vascular supply to the skin edges. The patellar tendon scar is incised in midline providing a sleeve for the allograft. This soft tissue is subperiosteally elevated off the patella and tibial tubercle. Retropatellar and suprapatellar adhesions are resected. The patellar fat pad should be protected and retained if not diseased. A large Weber reduction clamp applies traction to restore the patella to its anatomic position after it is mobilized. If the patella cannot be restored to its anatomic position, a series of quadriceps releases are performed. First, the quadriceps is elevated through the suprapatellar pouch, dissecting between the periosteum of the anterior femur and vastus intermedius with a Cobb elevator. If this fails to restore length to the extensor mechanism, a V-lengthening of the scarred distal vastus intermedius from the undersurface of the quadriceps mass is performed. The next step is to resect the vastus intermedius, maintaining the fibers of the rectus femoris, if inadequate length of quadriceps tendon is not obtained with the measures mentioned previously.

The Achilles allograft bone plug is shaped into a rectangular block 30 mm in length, 10 mm in depth, and 10 mm wide. The tendon is divided into a two-tailed graft. The tendinous ends of the graft are tubularized to fit through 6-mm bone tunnels (Fig. 58-11A). A trough is created with a small oscillating saw on the tibial tubercle to match the bone plug on the tendon allograft. The bone plug is extracted from the tibial tubercle with a thin osteotome. A vertical proximal wall of the trough stops graft migration proximally. The bone plug is secured in the trough with two 3.5-mm small fragment cancellous screws (ASIF; Synthes, Paoli, PA).

The bone tunnels in the patella are drilled over a Beath pin. The Beath pin can be positioned with the anterior cruciate ligament tibial drill guide. The bone tunnels are parallel and about 8 mm from the midline in the coronal plane. The grafts are passed with the Beath pin. A plain lateral radiograph or fluoroscopy with the knee in 30 to 45 degrees of flexion confirms the correct length of the reconstructed patellar tendon. The allograft tendon tails are sutured with braided nonabsorbable suture material into the quadriceps expansion. The remaining tails are brought over the superficial surface of the patella and sutured to allograft tails (Fig. 58-11B). The soft-tissue envelope is sutured over the graft. Knee flexion is evaluated in order to guide postoperative knee flexion.[29]

Postoperative Treatment

The techniques and principles of rehabilitation discussed in the postoperative treatment section of the quadriceps tendon repair apply to the patellar tendon repair.

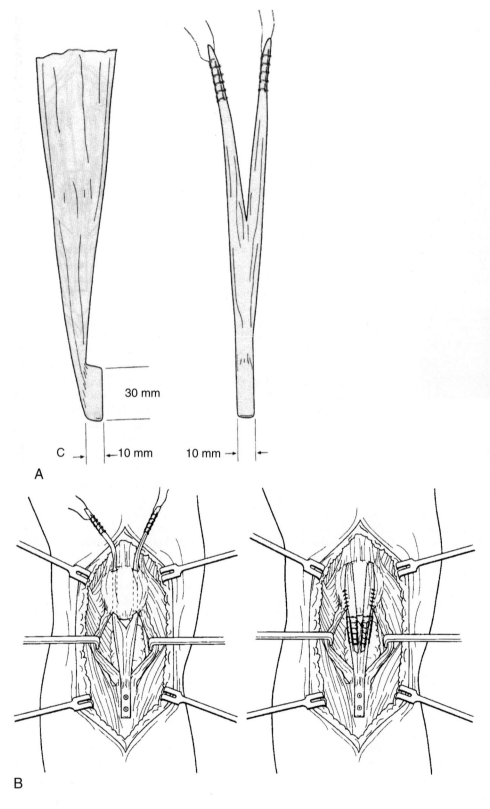

30 mm

C

←10 mm

10 mm →

←

A

B

Figure 58-11 Achilles tendon allograft preparation. Line drawings of the allograft with 30 × 10 × 10-mm bone block, before and after fashioning the two tails of the graft. **A,** Small-fragment fixation of the calcaneal bone block. Graft passage through the patellar drill holes. **B,** The limbs of the graft are sutured to the quadriceps tendon and medial and lateral retinaculum and then turned down for suture to the patellar tendon graft as well. (From Mills WJ: Reconstruction of chronic patellar tendon rupture with Achilles tendon allograft. Tech Knee Surg 2004;3:154–162.)

The patient who undergoes reconstruction of the patellar tendon with an Achilles tendon allograft follows a similar program but is carefully monitored. Knee motion is not allowed until the wound seals. For 2 weeks, 30 degrees of knee flexion is allowed in a hinged rehabilitative brace. If patellar tendon length is maintained, motion is advanced to 60 degrees of knee flexion for 2 weeks. Again, the position of the patella is con-

firmed with a plain lateral radiograph. If the position is the same as immediately postoperatively, knee flexion is advanced to 90 degrees. Assuming that patellar tendon length is maintained, unlimited motion is allowed at 6 weeks.[29] The quality of tissue, quality of the repair, and knee flexion obtained at the time of surgery determine the progression of activities after repair or reconstruction of the extensor mechanism.

Results

Weakness of the quadriceps muscle may occur in as many as 40% to 50% of patients. Extensor lag is less common in patellar tendon repair compared to those who undergo quadriceps tendon repair. Most patients regain close to full ROM, an argument against the use of augmentation devices and accelerated rehabilitation for repair of the patellar tendon.

Unfortunately, patellofemoral incongruence or osteoarthrosis is seen all too frequently on postoperative radiographs, for example, 12 of 29 patients in one series.[30] Of the 12 patients, three had unsatisfactory results. All the patients with unsatisfactory results due to pain in the series of Larsen and Lund[31] had patellar incongruence. The Insall-Salvati ratio differed more than 10% from the uninvolved knee in 16 of 29 patients in one series of repairs.[30] In a series of 10 patients with athletic patellar tendon ruptures treated with immediate suture repair to bone, two of those patients had significant patella alta (Insall-Salvati ratios of 0.55 and 0.59) that was increased in each patient from preoperatively. Those two had patellar pain postoperatively that limited their sporting activities.[5] Even though patients with patellar tendon repair are generally younger than those with quadriceps tendon rupture, return to preoperative activities is not universal for every patient.

Patients with a delayed diagnosis of patellar tendon rupture who undergo reconstruction are less likely to return to full activities. Mills[29] reported on five patients with Achilles tendon allograft reconstruction of the patellar tendon. Mean average flexion was 123 degrees. Four of five patients achieved full active terminal extension without an extensor lag. No wound complications or graft ruptures were encountered.

Complications

A second operation to remove a cerclage wire is usually necessary as painful hardware or wire breakage is common with this method of augmentation. Other complications closely parallel those described previously for quadriceps tendon repair.

CONCLUSIONS

Randomized clinical trials are uncommon involving treatment of extensor mechanism disruption. The body of science on extensor mechanism injuries consists of case series, review articles, and a large number of case reports; as such, clinical decision making relies on data with a low level of clinical evidence. Box 58-1 summarizes the general principles involved in diagnosing and treating extensor mechanism injuries.

Due to the strong biomechanical properties of the extensor mechanism, rupture occurs through damaged or degenerative tissue. Particularly in patients with disruption of the quadriceps tendon, systemic disease should be sought and addressed.

Box 58-1 General Principles

1. Recognize the diagnosis early.
2. Recognize systemic disease.
3. Restore appropriate tension to the extensor mechanism.
4. Repair with grasping suture.
5. Respect the biology of the injury.
6. Rehabilitate appropriate to the patient.

Failure to address these factors may jeopardize postoperative success.

A delay in diagnosis and treatment of extensor mechanism disruption is the single most negative impact on outcome from treatment. The clinical findings are straightforward. If the diagnosis is suspected, it is unlikely to be missed.

Extensor mechanism length restoration using the contralateral knee as a control is the first priority. Patients with incongruence or malalignment of the patellofemoral articulation after repair or reconstruction are at increased risk of pain.[6,30,31] The standard of care is primary repair of the extensor mechanism within 2 weeks of injury with a grasping suture on the tendinous portion of the repair with the suture passed through drill holes. A relatively conservative rehabilitation program focused on restoration of strength, mobility, and functional activities will likely allow the patient to return to daily activities and may allow a return to sporting activities.

Augmentation of the primary patellar tendon repair with wire, Dall-Miles cables, suture, and pull-out wire can be advised for patients undergoing an accelerated rehabilitation program. Factors that affect tissue integrity, healing response, or noncompliant patients may be considered for an augmented repair. In general, augmentation is not necessary in the absence of these factors.

Repair of the chronically ruptured extensor mechanism presents controversy. Up to 6 weeks after injury a repair may be possible; beyond that time, most authors would recommend the Codivilla V-Y plasty as described by Scuderi for the chronic ruptured quadriceps tendon. Use of allograft tissue, prosthetic devices, and soft-tissue grafts should be confined to individual situations rather than general use. Treatment of the chronic patellar tendon rupture is even more controversial. The first principle is to restore length to the extensor mechanism with the use of the normal side as a control if available. Up to 6 weeks from time of the injury, it may be possible to do a primary suture repair. Proponents of allograft tissue report the use of tendon allograft.[29] Autogenous semitendinosis and gracilis may substitute for the patellar tendon after appropriate length is restored.

REFERENCES

1. Ilan D, Tejwani N, Keschner M, et al: Quadriceps tendon rupture. J Am Acad Orthop Surg 2003;11:192–200.
2. Huberti H, Hayes W, Stone J, et al: Force ratios in the quadriceps tendon and ligamentum patellae. J Orthop Res 1984;2:49–54.
3. Kannus P, Józsa L: Histopathological changes preceding spontaneous rupture of a tendon: A controlled study of 891 patients. J Bone Joint Surg Am 1991;73:1507–1525.
4. Siwek CW, Rao JP: Ruptures of the extensor mechanism of the knee joint. J Bone Joint Surg Am 1981;63:932–937.
5. Scuderi C: Ruptures of the quadriceps tendon. Study of twenty tendon ruptures. Am J Surg 1958;95:626–634.
6. Kelly DW, Carter VS, Jobe FW, et al: Patellar and quadriceps tendon ruptures-jumper's knee. Am J Sports Med 1984;12:375–380.
7. Greenspan A, Norman A, Tchang FK-M: "Tooth" sign in patellar degenerative disease. J Bone Joint Surg Am 1977;59:483–485.
8. Zeiss J, Saddemi S, Ebraheim N: MR imaging of the quadriceps tendon: Normal layered configuration and its importance in cases of tendon rupture. Am J Roentgenol 1992;159:1031–1034.

9. Yu J, Petersilge C, Sartoris D, et al: MR imaging of injuries of the extensor mechanism of the knee. Radiographics 1994;14:541–551.

10. Berlin R, Levinsohn E, Chrisman H: The wrinkled patellar tendon: An indication of abnormality in the extensor mechanism of the knee. Skeletal Radiol 1991;20:181–185.

11. Ong BC, Sherman O: Acute patellar tendon rupture: A new surgical technique. Arthroscopy 2000;16:869–870.

12. Richards DP, Barber FA: Repair of quadriceps tendon ruptures using suture anchors. Arthroscopy 2002;18:556–559.

13. Rougraff BT, Reeck CC, Essenmacher J: Complete quadriceps tendon ruptures. Orthopaedics 1996;19:509–514.

14. Scuderi G: Quadriceps and patellar tendon disruption. In Scott W (ed): The Knee. St. Louis, Mosby, 1994, pp 469–478.

15. Yilmaz C, Binnet MS, Narman S: Tendon lengthening repair and early mobilization in treatment of neglected bilateral simultaneous traumatic rupture of the quadriceps tendon. Knee Surg Sports Traumatol Arthrosc 2001;9:163–166.

16. Wenzl M, Kirchner R, Seide K, et al: Quadriceps tendon ruptures—is there a complete functional restitution? Injury 2004;35:922–926.

17. De Baer T, Geulette B, Manche E, et al: Functional results after surgical repair of the quadriceps tendon rupture. Acta Orthop Belg 2002;68:146–149.

18. Konrath G, Chen D, Lock T, et al: Outcomes following repair of quadriceps tendon ruptures. J Orthop Trauma 1998;12:273–279.

19. Vidil A, Ouaknine M, Anract P, et al: Trauma-induced tears of the quadriceps tendon: 47 cases. Rev Chir Orthop Reparatrice Appar Mot 2004;90:40–48.

20. Shah K: Outcomes in bilateral and simultaneous quadriceps tendon rupture. Orthopaedics 2003;26:797–798.

21. Basso O, Johnson D, Amis A: The anatomy of the patellar tendon. Knee Surg Sports Traumatol Arthrosc 2001;9:2–5.

22. Lairungruang W, Kuptniratsaikul S, Itiravivong P: The remained patellar tendon strength after central on third removal: A biomechanical study. J Med Assoc Thailand 2003;86:1101–1105.

23. Kennedy JC, Willis RB: The effects of local steroid injections on tendons: A biomechanical and microscopic correlative study. Am J Sports Med 1976;4:11–21.

24. Wong M, Tang Y, Lee S, et al: Effect of dexamethasone on cultured human tenocytes and its reversibility by platelet-derived growth factor. J Bone Joint Surg Am 2003;85:1914–1920.

25. Ravelin R, Mazzocca A, Grady-Benson J, et al: Biomechanical comparison of patellar tendon repairs in a cadaver model: An evaluation of gap formation at the repair site with cyclic loading. Am J Sports Med 2002;30:469–473.

26. Larson RV, Simonian RT: Semitendinosus augmentation of acute patellar tendon repair with immediate mobilization. Am J Sports Med 1995;23:82–86.

27. Shelbourne K, Darmelio M, Klootwyk T: Patellar tendon rupture using Dall-Miles cable. Am J Knee Surg 2001;14:17–21.

28. Bhargava SP, Hynes MC, Dowell JK: Traumatic patella tendon rupture: Early mobilization following surgical repair. Injury 2004;35:76–79.

29. Mills WJ: Reconstruction of chronic patellar tendon rupture with Achilles tendon allograft. Tech Knee Surg 2004;3:154–162.

30. Kasten P, Schewe B, Maurer F, et al: Rupture of the patellar tendon: A review of 68 cases and a retrospective study of 29 ruptures comparing two methods of augmentation. Arch Orthop Trauma Surg 2001;121:578–582.

31. Larsen E, Lund PM: Ruptures of the extensor mechanism of the knee joint: Clinical results and patellofemoral articulation. Clin Orthop 1986;213:150–153.

In This Chapter

INTRODUCTION

- An aging population that desires to remain active has resulted in increased demands on medical providers to treat arthritis in athletic individuals.

- Generalized conditioning, reduction in body mass index, and strength and flexibility training have all been shown to be beneficial in improving symptoms.

- Glucosamine, chondroitin sulfate, NSAIDs, viscosupplementation, and intra-articular corticosteroids all have a role in the treatment of arthritis.

- Unloader bracing is used to improve the distribution of forces through the entire joint.

- Realignment osteotomy can provide significant symptomatic relief by redistributing load to more normal articular cartilage while preserving the patient's own joint.

One of the goals of modern medicine is to extend the quality-of-life years of the population. Advances in this direction have resulted in a population who is living longer and more active lives. Improvements in workplace productivity, personal income, and better working conditions have also created more time for leisure activities for the population. These factors, combined with the aging "baby boomer" population, who will comprise almost 20% of the United States population aged 60 or older by the year 2020, have created a significant population of "aging athletes" (Population Division of the Department of Economic and Social Affairs of the United Nations Secretariat, 1998). Sports medicine physicians are being challenged to create a treatment strategy for arthritis in the athlete.

For the purposes of this volume, we examine the occurrence and treatment of primary osteoarthritis in the adult athletic population. Figures for the United States in the year 2000 indicate that arthritis is a public health burden second only to heart disease in disability expenses, with approximately 38 million people requiring treatment at a cost of $72 billion or 2.5% of the gross national product.[1,2]

The development and progression of osteoarthritic cartilage changes are influenced by genetic, physiologic, and geometric factors. An error in the DNA sequence for type II collagen that represents an amino acid substitution of one base sequence of cysteine for arginine has been shown to be present in osteoarthritic cartilage.[3] There are changes in the load-bearing properties of articular cartilage with age, such as increased cellular death, proteoglycan loss, and a loss of the cartilage matrix. While these changes do occur with age, the symptoms of osteoarthritis are, fortunately, present in only half of the population older than 65 years. The development and progression of symptomatic osteoarthritis are potentiated by a change in the joint architecture. Nonanatomic joint geometry will lead to degeneration of the articular cartilage surface at an increased rate. It is common in the athletic population to have sustained an injury to a joint at an earlier time, such as a small meniscus tear or a low-grade ligament strain, changing the joint architecture slightly, which can later lead to a rapid progression of symptomatic arthritic change. Adults who have previously competed at high-level sports and those who remain active are keenly aware that sporting activities can take a toll on their bodies and lead to the "wear and tear arthritis" that is common in the "master athlete." They must also be made aware of the tremendous benefits that can be gained from maintaining an active lifestyle, an appropriate body mass index, and good muscle tone and encouraged to continue to participate in activities that are appropriate for their abilities.

TREATMENT OPTIONS

Physical Therapy and Conditioning

The physician treating symptomatic osteoarthritis has a number of interventions at his or her disposal. Patients with symptomatic osteoarthritis in a weight-bearing joint who have an elevated body mass index can expect an improvement in their symptomatology with a 10% reduction in mass. A dedicated physiotherapy regimen that focuses on improving the strength and flexibility of musculature surrounding an arthritic joint will improve objective pain scores in symptomatic arthritis. The athletic population with arthritis tend to be excellent candidates for a focused physical therapy and conditioning program as they often have participated in these type programs during their competition days. The role of preactivity stretching, maintaining muscle conditioning, and the use of rest, ice, compression, and elevation of the affected body part is usually well-known in the adult athlete and should always be encouraged as a first-line therapy and maintenance strategy. The opportunity for group activities such as conditioning classes with goals formed around some manner of competition, weight loss, or strength improvements can be excellent motivational tools.

Nutritional Supplements

The use of nutritional supplements is now quite common in the athletic population. Athletes who are experiencing arthritic symptoms are likely to try to treat their pain with the use of nutritional supplements in addition to other modalities. Chondroitin sulfate and glucosamine sulfate are the most commonly used supplements in this role. As substances that are classified as nutritional supplements that have an intended effect of treatment of a medical condition, they have commonly become referred to as "nutriceuticals."

In both osteoarthritis and rheumatoid arthritis, patients have an increased excretion of glucosamine in the urine. As a naturally occurring substance, it stimulates glycosaminoglycan and proteoglycan synthesis, which are involved in the formation and repair of articular cartilage. Chondroitin sulfate is a glycosaminoglycan composed of units of glucosamine with attached sugar molecules. Both chondroitin sulfate and glucosamine are derived from animal sources.[4]

As dietary supplements, nutriceuticals such as glucosamine and chondroitin sulfate are not subjected to analysis by the U.S. Food and Drug Administration prior to sale. There exists no standardization of testing, and producers regulate the content of their product according to their own guidelines. This has created a concern that substances in this category may not be exactly represented by the labeled amounts of ingredients of the package. A recent consumer monitoring group completed a study that concluded that almost half of the glucosamine/chondroitin supplements tested did not contain the labeled amounts of ingredients.[5]

To date there has been only one scientific study that has shown an improvement in symptoms with glucosamine compared to placebos. In this study, 212 patients with symptomatic knee arthrosis received either 1500 mg glucosamine daily for 3 years or placebo. A digital knee radiograph study before and after treatment showed progressive joint space narrowing in the placebo group versus no significant narrowing in the glucosamine group. WOMAC (Western Ontario and McMaster University Osteoarthritis Index) knee scores were improved in the glucosamine group and worse in the placebo group.[4] With the results of this single study, there is at present no compelling evidence from randomized, double-blind, controlled trials that shows a clear benefit of glucosamine or chondroitin sulfate as a medication for the treatment of painful osteoarthritis.

The National Institutes of Health are currently completing what is hoped to be the definitive trial (the Glucosamine/Chondroitin Arthritis Intervention Trial [GAIT]) of these nutritional supplements. The study is designed to determine whether glucosamine, chondroitin sulfate, and/or the combination of glucosamine and chondroitin sulfate are more effective than placebo and whether the combination is more effective than glucosamine or chondroitin sulfate alone in the treatment of knee pain associated with osteoarthritis of the knee.

Nonsteroidal Anti-inflammatory Drugs

Athletes may to be used to the concept of minor aches and pains associated with their sporting activity, and "playing with pain"

is often a common scenario in the athlete with arthritic symptoms. It is also very common for athletes to have taken various analgesic remedies during their competition days and the history of analgesic use should be determined for each patient. As a treating physician of an athlete with arthritic symptoms, it is important to establish the medications that an athlete has used previously for his or her condition and to determine whether the medications have been used on an appropriate dosing schedule. Often medications are taken as an occasional pain reliever on an irregular and inappropriate dosing schedule that may not be of help to the patient and may even be harmful. Our role should be to assess the patient's symptoms and to create an appropriate treatment plan that can realistically be followed.

Pharmaceutical interventions target the painful inflammation from the joint capsule, ligaments, synovium, and subchondral bone, which are responsible for the noxious nerve stimuli and pain of arthritis. Interestingly, articular cartilage does not contain nerve tissue. The transmission of painful stimuli is mediated by prostaglandin synthesis. NSAIDs decrease the production of prostaglandins by inhibiting cyclooxygenase (COX), an enzyme that catalyses the first two steps in the production of prostaglandins from arachidonic acid. Prostaglandins are also involved in the maintenance and protection of gastric mucosa, and it is the disruption of this role that can potentiate NSAID-associated gastrointestinal bleeding.

While NSAIDs remain a mainstay of treatment for management of arthritis related pain, the incidence of NSAID-associated gastrointestinal bleed complications has created a significant public health burden, where an estimated 33% of the money spent to treat arthritis each year is spent on treatment of NSAID-related gastrointestinal disorders.[1] This recognized complication rate has created a tremendous need for the development of NSAIDs that are less harmful to the gastrointestinal tract. COX has more than one form; COX-I has a role in the physiologic maintenance of all tissues, including gastric mucosa, while COX-II is the inducible form of the enzyme involved in the conversion of arachidonic acid to prostaglandins. COX-II–specific NSAIDs or COX-II inhibitors were developed to decrease prostaglandin production with less effect on the COX-I homeostasis role. COX-II inhibitors have been shown to have a lower rate of gastrointestinal complications at a rate of 0.2% of patients per year of use versus 1.7% of patients per year of use of traditional NSAIDs.

COX-II inhibitors as a class of drug include several different proprietary formulae, one of which is sulfonamides or celecoxib (Celebrex). As sulfur-containing compounds, there had been concerns that people with "sulfa allergies" would also have a hypersensitivity reaction to these sulfonamides. However, sulfonamide antimicrobials as a derivative of sulfanilamides are arylamines, while celecoxib is a nonarylamine as is hydrochlorothiazide and DiaBeta (glyburide). A meta-analysis of the North American trials of nonarylamine sulfanilamide COX-II inhibitors showed no statistical increase in hypersensitivity reactions in sulfa-allergic patients treated with celecoxib compared to placebo. There may be, however, a cross-reactivity in patients with a confirmed allergy to nonarylamine sulfanilamide compounds such as hydrochlorothiazide and celecoxib, and thus prescribing physicians need to proceed with appropriate caution.[1]

Recently, concerns regarding the possibility of increased cardiovascular events such as myocardial infarction and stroke in patients taking COX-II inhibitors prompted a voluntary removal of rofecoxib (Vioxx) from the market (Merck and Co. news release, "Merck Announces Voluntary Worldwide Withdrawal of Vioxx," September 30, 2004; available at: www.vioxx.com/), and the U.S. Food and Drug Administration requested a withdrawal of valdecoxib (Bextra) from the market ("FDA Announces Series of Changes to the Class of Marketed Nonsteroidal Anti-inflammatory Drugs [NSAIDs]," April 7, 2005) and a change in the labeling of all NSAIDs (other than aspirin) to reflect the possibility of cardiovascular and gastrointestinal risks. In 1999, researchers had reported that COX-II inhibitors had an inhibitory effect on prostacyclin, which, through its action on the endothelial cells lining blood vessels, maintains thrombosis homeostasis and vascular resistance. With the progression of clinical trials using COX-II inhibitor medications, the possibility of increased occurrence of myocardial and cerebrovascular thrombotic events has been postulated, yet not all COX-II inhibitors appear to have this association, and investigations of the safety of these medications are ongoing. While complete understanding of the clinical safety of all COX-II inhibitor–specific and non–COX-II inhibitor–specific NSAIDs remains to be determined, at present they remain a useful treatment for the inflammation-associated pain of arthritis in the appropriate patient.

Corticosteroid Injections

Corticosteroids inhibit the production of the pain mediator prostaglandin from arachidonic acid. Intra-articular steroid injections aim to deliver a higher dose of corticosteroid directly to the site of inflammation and pain in arthritis than would be achievable with oral or intravenous delivery. In addition, high-dose local delivery of corticosteroid decreases the vasodilation and permeability of inflammation and may improve the edema and pain of arthritis. Intra-articular steroid delivery has a lengthy clinical history. Recent meta-analyses reported, from the six studies reviewed, an improvement in the various outcome measures at 2 weeks in 74% of patients treated with steroid injection versus 45% of patients treated with placebo. In the three studies that included results at 16 to 24 weeks after injection, the reported improvement decreased to 33% of patients treated with steroid injection versus 16% of patients who received placebo.[6,7]

Injectable steroid preparations vary in their solubility, and insoluble steroid esters may have a longer duration. More insoluble steroids are appropriate for intra-articular delivery, while soft-tissue injections should use more soluble steroid preparations (such as Celestone [betamethasone]) to limit soft-tissue atrophy.[4] While there is no established dose or delivery frequency for the administration of intra-articular steroid in the arthritis literature, the frequency of steroid injections should not exceed one every 3 months.[8]

Viscosupplementation

Arthritis involves changes in the joint surface as well as the synovial fluid within the joint. Osteoarthritic joints have a lower than normal concentration of hyaluronic acid, and viscosupplementation delivers a preparation of hyaluronic acid within the joint with the goal of restoring a more normal joint fluid viscosity and improving the viscoelastic properties for proper joint mechanics. Viscosupplementation has been used in Europe for several years and received U.S. Food and Drug Administration approval in 1997. Hyaluronic acid preparations derived from rooster combs or those manufactured from bacterial cultures are available. Patients with severe hypersensitivity to poultry products are advised to consider the manufactured preparation. The schedule of injections for viscosupplementation delivery varies by proprietary preparation.

While the effect appears to be transient, viscosupplementation has been shown to restore rheologic homeostasis in the osteoarthritic joint with improved WOMAC pain and function scores by 10% to 15% at 12 months following delivery in 62% of patients.[9] Many athletes may have previously received intra-articular steroid injections and thus may be quite open to the concept of a trial of viscosupplementation. It is important, however, that patients understand that viscosupplementation will work gradually, does not contain analgesic agents, and requires a full course of injections to determine its effect.

The U.S. Food and Drug Administration classifies viscosupplements as a device and not a drug. Medical insurance coverage may reimburse the cost of devices and procedures that are deemed "medically necessary" as treatment for arthritis, according to the labeled uses of the "medical device" as approved by the U.S. Food and Drug Administration. At present, Medicare will provide coverage of hyaluronic acid–based products that are used to treat osteoarthritis of the knee only. Current Medicare policy requires radiographic evidence of the established diagnosis of osteoarthritis and the current approved treatment course will be paid for only if given not more than once every 6 months.

Bracing and Orthotics

Symptomatic knee arthrosis is often associated with nonanatomic joint malalignment, which results in uneven load distribution of the weight-bearing axis through the knee. The malalignment may be a result of a previous cartilage injury with cartilage volume loss (such as a meniscal injury that may have been surgically repaired) or a ligament insufficiency leading to attenuation of the remaining structures and nonanatomic joint loading, or it may be due to progressive bone deformation as part of an arthritic process in addition to a primary joint malalignment such as tibia vara. Whatever the cause of nonanatomic joint loading, the concentration of load-bearing forces through one point rather than anatomic distribution of the forces will lead to degenerative joint disease progression at an increased rate.

The role of orthotics and bracing in the treatment of osteoarthritis is to attempt to alter the joint architecture to better distribute the effective forces of the weight-bearing axis through the entire joint. Orthotics are intended to realign the foot and ankle to create a solid, stable platform for the rest of the body during the stance phase of weight bearing. Functional knee bracing may be helpful in patients with unicompartmental arthrosis and a malalignment that is correctable with a force that is attainable by the brace.[10] Typically this may be a custom-molded medial unloader brace for a correctable varus malalignment, with isolated medial compartment symptoms. Custom-molded unloader braces can also be made for valgus malalignment and used with success. Important considerations for the use of unloader bracing and orthotics are whether the implement can achieve the desired correction to relieve the symptoms and whether the patient tolerates the application of this corrective force through the contact points with the implement for the desired period of symptomatic benefit. The well-fitted functional brace will not benefit the patient if use of the brace cannot be tolerated.

Discussion of the use of bracing in a protective role for ligaments and menisci is beyond the scope of this chapter, and the reader is directed to the position statement of the American Association of Orthopaedic Surgeons on the use of knee braces for a more complete discussion. This resource also contains recommendations for some common clinical scenarios where knee bracing has been considered.

SURGICAL INTERVENTION

Arthroscopy and Arthroscopic Débridement

Arthroscopic débridement is commonly considered as an intervention for treatment of symptomatic knee arthrosis in the athletic population. There are several theories as to the possible mechanism of benefit of an arthroscopy to relieve arthritic symptoms. With arthroscopy, the irrigation of the joint may remove particulate debris and dilute and remove inflammatory mediators and degenerative enzymes, and it has been postulated that pain impulses may be interrupted by chloride ions from the irrigation solution. Arthroscopic instruments can also be used for mechanical débridement to create a smoother remaining articular surface with stable borders. With intra-articular instrumentation, it is also possible to remove painful impinging osteophytes, débride degenerative meniscal tears, and remove loose bodies. It may also be that the benefit of arthroscopy is in some way a placebo effect.[11]

The published results of the benefit of arthroscopy have varied, with no standardization of inclusion and exclusion criteria, and no standardization of the outcome measures or the surgical technique of the intervention. This lack of standardization makes prediction of the success rate of arthroscopic débridement for symptomatic knee arthrosis difficult[12]; however, a nonrigorous meta-analysis indicates that approximately 60% of appropriately selected patients reported improved symptomatology at 3 years postoperatively.[4] While many patients report an improvement in their symptoms, arthroscopic débridement does not stop the progression of arthrosis and the benefits predictably decrease with time.

Knee arthroscopy primarily involves the use of an arthroscopic shaver to mechanically débride tissue and can be used to attempt to create a smooth cartilage surface. Attempts to use radiofrequency probes to débride irregular osteoarthritic cartilage have been successful in creating débrided surfaces that may be smoother than what is achievable with standard arthroscopic shavers. Radiofrequency energy imparts high temperature on the chondrocytes, which are very temperature sensitive, and may lead to chondrocyte cell death.

For treatment of full-thickness lesions, microfracture to promote fibrocartilaginous ingrowth in the area of the lesion has been shown to have good to excellent results for focal lesions.[13] Instrumentation such as a microawl is used to penetrate down through the base of the focal lesion, through the subchondral bone, into the vascularized metaphyseal bone. It is postulated that the pluripotent stem cells in the marrow are then released into the area of the focal defect where they form a fibrin clot that can reform into fibrocartilage. Continuous passive range of motion and limited weight bearing for 6 weeks postoperatively may be beneficial to the stability of the fibrocartilage "repair." As primarily type I cartilage, fibrocartilage expectedly has less rigorous wear characteristics than type II hyaline cartilage, and attempts to encourage more extensive fibrocartilaginous ingrowth for advanced degenerative arthrosis have not been shown to be any more successful than arthroscopic débridement alone.[14]

Cartilage Transplantation

Focal articular cartilage defects are difficult to treat, and the surgical options for this entity have previously been relatively limited. In addition to the previously discussed microfracture technique that attempts to patch an articular defect with type I fibrocartilage, there are emerging technologies focusing on transplanting viable type II articular cartilage into these defects.

"Mosaicplasty" refers to the transfer of full-thickness articular cartilage with its corresponding subchondral bone plug from a non-weight-bearing area of the knee to a corresponding bone plug hole drilled into the base of the full-thickness cartilage lesion. This procedure is technically challenging but its use is increasing. While still considered an advanced surgical principle that is not universally offered, it has shown favorable bone growth and favorable cartilaginous incorporation for focal defects.[15]

Realignment Osteotomy

Knee arthrosis is frequently associated with malalignment. The load across the knee joint is a function of alignment; changes in the axial alignment of the femur or tibia in either the coronal or sagittal plane will influence the distribution of this load resulting in abnormal stresses on articular cartilage. The goal of realignment osteotomy for treatment of knee pain related to arthrosis is to transfer the effective weight-bearing axis from the arthritic cartilage to the more normal cartilage.

While the definition of "appropriate" postoperative alignment has been studied extensively, there is no clear consensus on the desired correction angle when performing an osteotomy in the younger patient with a cartilage defect.[16] In the patient with varus gonarthrosis, we prefer a weight-bearing line that intersects at a point 62% of the tibial width from the edge of the medial plateau to produce a mechanical axis of 3 to 5 degrees.[17] Traditionally, varus gonarthrosis was considered the indication for a valgus-producing osteotomy. The indications for realignment osteotomy have grown to include a correction of valgus malalignment, as an adjunct to ligament reconstruction to help protect the repair and restore joint mechanics, or as an unloading procedure in the event of a significant cartilage defect[18] (Table 59-1).

The treatment options for an active patient with isolated cartilage lesions are relatively limited, and an osteotomy can be considered as a treatment option to help unload the involved compartment, but there are limitations to the application of this procedure. While a realignment osteotomy through the knee to transfer the load-bearing axis away from the lesion may be a viable treatment, severe degeneration in the opposite tibiofemoral compartment and a gross loss of range of motion will certainly affect the outcome of an osteotomy and may be considered a relative contraindication. A valgus osteotomy should be avoided in those who have previously undergone a

Table 59-1 Indications for Knee Osteotomy			
Malalignment and arthrosis	Malalignment and instability	Malalignment and arthrosis and/or instability	Malalignment and articular cartilage procedure and/or instability

Table 59-2 Specific Indications for Individual Osteotomy Techniques

	Varus <25 deg	Varus >25 deg	Valgus <15 deg	Valgus >15 deg	Increased Tibial Slope	Decreased Tibial Slope
Medial opening HTO	X					
Lateral closing HTO	X					
Medial closing HTO			X			
Lateral opening HTO			X			
External fixation HTO		X			X	X
Anterior closing HTO					X	
Anterior opening HTO						X

HTO, High tibial osteotomy.

lateral meniscectomy. However, in the very young athlete with early signs of degenerative joint disease, a lateral meniscectomy should be considered only a relative contraindication, and in the case of severe varus alignment, a high tibial osteotomy to correct to a neutral alignment will preserve favorable joint mechanics (Table 59-2). Higher correction angles may require a change in the traditional fixation implants, but the principles remain the same.

Limb alignment is determined by the line extending from the center of the hip to the center of the ankle, that is, the mechanical axis of the limb. This line typically passes immediately medial to the center of the knee, and, by definition, malalignment occurs when this line does not lie close to the center of the knee.[19] Sagittal plane alignment should also be considered. This involves evaluation of the posterior tibial slope angle on a lateral radiograph. Tibial slope has been defined as the angle between a line perpendicular to the mid-diaphysis of the tibia and the posterior inclination of the tibial plateau. Measurements based on lateral radiographs have shown the tibial slope of the knee to average 10 ± 3 degrees.

Surgical Technique for High Tibial Osteotomy

For the treatment of varus arthrosis, common in athletes, a medial opening, high tibial osteotomy is a very useful tool for correction of alignment in the coronal and sagittal planes. The procedure is carried out through a vertical skin incision, which extends 5 cm distally from the medial joint line and is centered between the anterior tubercle and the posteromedial border of the tibia (Fig. 59-1A). The gracilis and semitendinosus tendons and the superficial medial collateral ligament are preserved and retracted medially to expose the posteromedial border of the proximal tibia (Fig. 59-1B). A guide pin is inserted obliquely along a line proximal to the tibial tubercle starting approximately 4 cm below the medial joint line in the region of the transition between metaphyseal and diaphyseal cortical bone on radiographs and extending to a point 1 cm distal to the lateral joint line.

Figure 59-2 illustrates the opening wedge technique, which is monitored throughout with a mobile, low-dose ionizing radiation fluoroscopy unit. The osteotomy is made below the guide pin using a small oscillating saw to breech the medial, anteromedial, and posteromedial cortices. This is followed by narrow, sharp, thin, flexible osteotomes to a point just 1 cm short of the lateral cortex. Frequent imaging helps prevent violation of the lateral cortex and/or misdirection of the osteotome. The osteotomy is opened gradually to the desired correction angle first with distracting osteotomes to confirm the mobility of the osteotomy and then a calibrated wedge to maintain the appropriate measured distraction. The distracted osteotomy is then fixed with a four-hole Puddu plate secured with two 6.5-mm cancellous screws proximally and two 4.5-mm cortical screws distally. Bone grafting is recommended in all opening wedge osteotomies greater than 7.5 mm. Allograft cancellous bone chips and/or tricortical blocks may be used unless there is an expressed desire by the patient for autograft bone. In our practice, osteotomies less than 7.5 mm are rarely grafted.

The pearls and pitfalls of a medial opening wedge osteotomy are presented in Table 59-3. Dissection of the most superior fibers of the patellar tendon insertion on the tibial tubercle improves exposure and protects the patellar tendon when completing the anterior extent of the corticotomy, which must be distal to the patellar tendon insertion. The use of a low-dose ionizing radiation fluoroscope throughout the procedure is critical to ensure all the following: proper guide-pin placement, prevention of lateral cortex violation, avoidance of misdirection of the osteotome, avoidance of intra-articular screw placement, and adequate setting of the bone graft and filling of the defect.

The tip of the fibular head is a helpful reference when aiming the guide pin. The correct obliquity of the osteotomy relies on proper placement of the guide pin. For larger corrections, placement should be more horizontal. Greater obliquity increases the risk of fixation failure but, on the other hand, provides increased depth, which may be appropriate for smaller corrections. The osteotomy should always be carried out parallel to the joint line in the sagittal plane and below the guide pin to help prevent intra-articular fracture. The use of thick, traditional-type osteotomes can apply a greater distraction moment when completing the osteotomy and carries an inherent risk of creating an extra- and/or intra-articular fracture. This is considerably minimized with thin, flexible osteotomes (Fig. 59-3). However, these should be advanced with frequent fluoroscopy checks to avoid misdirection.

To avoid altering the posterior tibial slope, the distraction of the osteotomy anteriorly (at the tibial tubercle) should be approximately one half its distraction posteromedially. This is facilitated by using trapezoidal distraction block Puddu plates rather than the traditional rectangular version. The plate should be positioned as far posterior as possible along the medial cortex

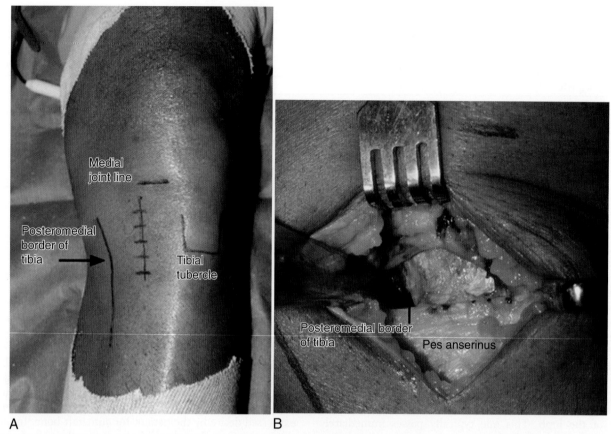

Figure 59-1 The surgical approach to medial opening wedge high tibial osteotomy. **A,** The skin incision is centered between the posteromedial border of the tibia and the tibial tubercle and extends distally from the medial joint line. **B,** The posteromedial border of the tibia is exposed with a blunt retractor placed deep to the superficial medial collateral ligament. The pes anserinus is left intact.

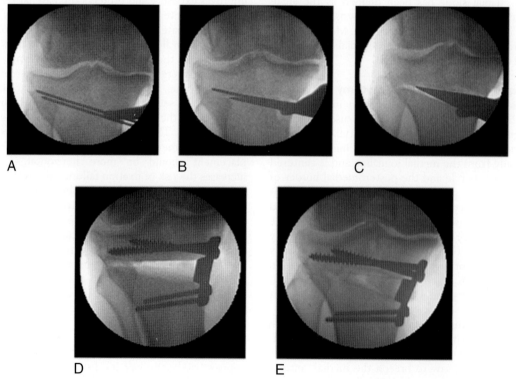

Figure 59-2 The use of intraoperative fluoroscopy during medial opening wedge high tibial osteotomy. **A,** The guide pin is directed toward the tip of the fibular head and from a point 4 cm distal to the medial joint line. Placement should be optimal before proceeding. **B,** The osteotomy is made below the guide pin. **C,** The osteotomy is gradually opened to the desired width using a calibrated wedge. **D,** Fixation is achieved with a four-hole Puddu plate. Care is taken to avoid intra-articular or intraosteotomy screw placement. **E,** Here the defect has been filled with tricortical bone graft.

Table 59-3 Pearls and Pitfalls of Corrective Osteotomy

	Pearls	Pitfalls
All osteotomies	Adequate exposure Use of intraoperative fluoroscopy and guide pins Accurate preoperative planning and radiographic evaluation	Violation of opposite cortex Making asymmetrical bone cuts in sagittal plane Opening the osteotomy before the anterior and posterior cortices are osteotomized
High tibial lateral closing	Make osteotomy 2 cm distal to lateral joint line Complete posterior cortical resection in piecemeal fashion with Kerrison rongeurs	Decreasing tibial slope inadvertently
High tibial medial opening	Use oscillating saw to breach cortex only Make osteotomy below the guidepin Pay particular attention when securing osteotomy plate	Suboptimal guidepin positioning Neglecting the posterior tibial slope when making the osteotomy

to ensure that the distraction is maximized posteromedially and minimized anteriorly. Careful attention to this detail will help decrease the risk of increasing tibial slope on distraction of the osteotomy. Tension of the medial collateral ligament should be assessed during distraction and lengthening by fenestration of the medial collateral ligament may assist in achieving larger corrections.

Finally, strict attention to detail is necessary to avoid intra-articular or intraosteotomy screw penetration during fixation of the plate and to ensure that the defect is completely obliterated with bone graft or a substitute; frequent rechecks with fluoroscopy are beneficial.

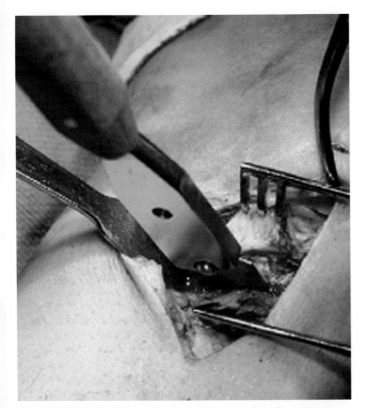

Figure 59-3 Thin flexible osteotomes used to complete the osteotomy. The osteotomy can then subsequently be opened with distracting osteotomes to the desired correction. This applies less distraction moment on the initial bone cut and thus decreases the chance of intra-articular fracture.

Rehabilitation Following an Osteotomy

The rehabilitation schedule is presented in Table 59-4. Early postoperative knee range-of-motion exercises benefit joint healing and articular cartilage nourishment as well as lower limb neuromuscular function. In addition, the return to normal weight bearing is essential for healthy bone turnover and healing. Postoperative physical therapy programs should focus on these components while respecting the desired outcomes of the realignment procedure, which include union and restoring and maintaining alignment.

Restoring full range of motion is an important factor in the long-term success of the surgical procedure, and we encourage range-of-motion exercises to begin as soon as possible. Full extension should be achieved by postoperative week 6. If progress is behind schedule, active exercises with slight volitional overpressure are recommended.

The weight-bearing progression will depend on the nature of the osteotomy and any other cartilage restoration procedure performed. After an opening wedge osteotomy, patients are restricted to touch weight bearing, equivalent to 25 to 40 pounds, for the first 6 weeks. If any osteocartilaginous procedure has been performed in combination, the opening wedge protocol takes preference. Following closing wedge osteotomy, we allow protected weight bearing for the first 6 weeks. If a cartilage restoration procedure has been performed also, a partial weight-bearing protocol should take preference.

From the 6-week mark, the progression of weight bearing is dependent on the appearance of the radiograph at this stage. It would be anticipated that any closing wedge osteotomy could progress to weight bearing as tolerated at this point, with the use of a cane or a single crutch, if consolidation and progression to union are occurring. An opening wedge osteotomy should progress to partial weight bearing for 3 weeks and then to protected weight bearing for 3 weeks if consolidation is evident on the radiograph, and there is no evidence of hardware loosening or change in position.

Neuromuscular programs aimed at the maintenance of surrounding joint strength and muscle function, as well as pain management modalities, should be employed during the initial postoperative 6 weeks. During weeks 6 to 12, a more functional program can be instituted, while methods to improve muscular endurance can be instituted after postoperative week 12. Gait retraining and returning to a fully functional state should be additional goals throughout the rehabilitation process. More directed therapy to correct additional functional impairments should also take place after week 12.

Table 59-4 Postoperative Rehabilitation Guidelines	
Timeline	Exercise
0–3 wk	Passive range of motion using slider board
	Pedal rocking on bicycle
	Isometric quadriceps setting
3–6 wk	Full-circle pedaling on bicycle, very light resistance
	Active range of motion
	Side-lying gluteus medius strengthening
	Hip abduction/adduction, flexion, and extension with resistance fixed above knee, e.g., pulley or resistance tubing
	Pool exercises, hip abduction/adduction, flexion, and extension; knee flexion and extension
	Gait pattern training with crutches focusing on proper heel strike/toe off
	Pool, deep water running or cycling
	Leg press or squat with weight off-loaded to 24–40 pounds (watch range-of-motion restriction associated with any cartilage/meniscus restoration/repair)
6–9 wk	Pool, shallow water walking as weight-bearing restrictions allow
	As a general guideline, when 60% of body is submerged, 60% of body weight is off-loaded
	Standing/seated calf raise
	Bilateral wobble board balancing as weight-bearing status allows
	Knee flexion/extension with very light resistance
Upon full weight bearing	Gait training to restore normal gait
	Step up and step down to work on alignment and eccentric control
	Elliptical trainer and bicycle for cardiovascular conditioning

Complications of an Osteotomy

The list of possible intraoperative, early postoperative, and late postoperative complications following any realignment procedure around the knee is exhaustive. The early complications of upper tibial osteotomy are those of any surgical operation on the lower extremity including compartment syndrome, infection, neurovascular injury, deep vein thrombosis, and pulmonary embolus. These, as well as some that require specific mention, should be included in any list of complications of osteotomy around the knee, namely, delayed or nonunion.

The frequency of thromboembolic disease is lower following osteotomy than total knee arthroplasty, and the proper method of prophylaxis is controversial. We currently do not use chemical prophylaxis in patients undergoing knee osteotomy. Mobilization is encouraged on postoperative day 1. Patients with specific risk factors for deep venous thromboembolism or pulmonary embolism are anticoagulated with low molecular weight heparin given subcutaneously for the perioperative period and undergo lower limb venous studies prior to discharge from the hospital. Patients with a history of deep vein thromboembolism or pulmonary embolism are anticoagulated for 6 weeks with Coumadin.

The avoidance of intraoperative complications of any osteotomy is especially important with osteotomy around the knee. Intra-articular fracture, intra-articular screw placement, and violation of the opposite cortex with resultant instability of the osteotomy are all avoidable and will all have a significant outcome on the osteotomy. Prevention of these complications by continuous fluoroscopy use is the best form of management; otherwise, early recognition and immediate management are suggested.

Intra-articular fracture should be assessed intraoperatively with fluoroscopy and a decision made whether interfragmentary screw stabilization is required. A fracture detected postoperatively may require internal fixation with or without revision of the osteotomy or a simple modification of the postoperative rehabilitation protocol with immobilization and non-weight bearing for a period and radiographic monitoring of the fracture. Violation of the opposite cortex in an opening wedge osteotomy of the tibia usually does not require any additional treatment.

Under- and overcorrection is a significant concern in tibial realignment osteotomies. Numerous authors have discussed overcorrection into valgus.[20,21] Because, cosmetically, producing a valgus deformity is less well tolerated than producing varus alignment, it is best to err on the side of "avoiding excessive valgus." Critical assessment of the alignment both intraoperatively and in the early postoperative period should take place, and if "overcorrection" or "excessive" varus or valgus correction has occurred, the osteotomy should be revised, as the primary surgical goals have not been attained.

Realignment osteotomy about the knee is a very useful tool for the treatment of arthrosis with the benefits of a capacity for correction in multiple planes, the capacity to restore anatomy to a more favorable alignment, and the benefit of maintaining the integrity of the patient's own joint with the goal of a high level of function (Fig. 59-4).

Arthroplasty in the Athlete

Joint arthroplasty has provided a tremendous tool for the relief of arthritis sufferers and is one of the most cost-effective medical interventions available to restore functional lives.[22] The goal of arthroplasty is to alleviate pain first and to maintain function. Improvement in function is not the specific intended goal. This is especially true of total knee arthroplasty. With respect to active athletes who are severely affected by arthritis pain, it is most important that this type of patient understand that a unicondylar or a total knee arthroplasty is intended for pain relief, and a modification of activities to avoid high-impact and loading activities would be advised to prolong the life span of the implant.

Because the technical challenges of early revision surgery and the morbidity associated with early implant failure are so sig-

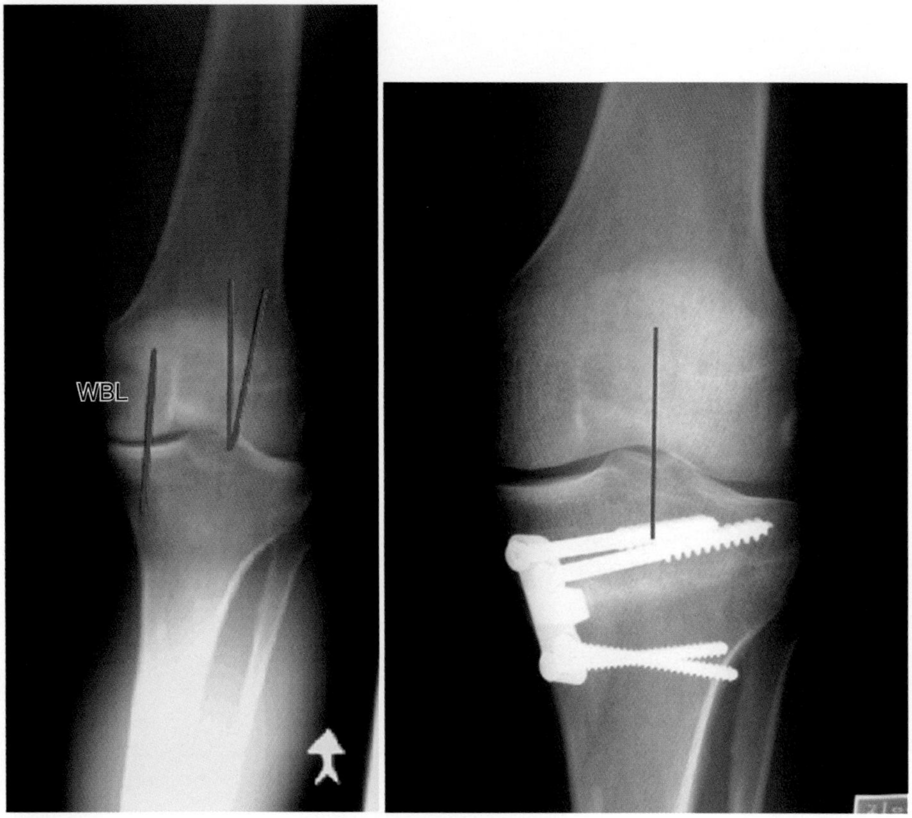

Figure 59-4 A 31-year-old man with isolated medial compartment articular cartilage disease, varus malalignment, and intact anterior and posterior cruciate ligaments. **A,** The anteroposterior view shows the weight-bearing line (WBL) through the center of the medial compartment and the predicted correction angle. **B,** Postoperatively, the mechanical axis of the limb is normalized.

nificant (autolysis, bone loss, nerve and blood vessel compromise), active and athletic patients who are considering knee arthroplasty are best served by a full understanding of the limitations of the procedure. In some cases, the procedure must be delayed until the patient reaches the point at which his or her activity level is appropriate for the limitations of the implant.

REFERENCES

1. Laine L: COX-2 selective drugs: Improving safety. Clin Dilemmas 2001;3–6.
2. Reuben S: Orthopaedic applications of COX-2 inhibitors. Orthop Today 2001;5–6.
3. Hochberg M, Brandt K: Guidelines for the medical management of DJD of the hip and knee. J R Coll Physicians Lond 1993;27:391–397.
4. Bert JM, Gasser SI: Approach to the osteoarthritic knee in the aging athlete: Debridement to osteotomy. Instructional course 306. Arthroscopy 2002;18:9107–9110.
5. American Academy of Orthopedic Surgeons: AAOS Research Committee fact sheet: Osteoarthritis, June 2001.
6. Godwin M, Dawes M: Intra-articular steroid injections for painful knees: Systematic review with meta-analysis. Can Fam Physician 2004;50:241–248.
7. Arroll B, Goodyear-Smith F: Corticosteroid injections for osteoarthritis of the knee: Meta-analysis. BMJ 2004;328:869–870.
8. Gaffney K, Ledingham J, Perry JD: Intra-articular triamcinolone hexacetonide in knee osteoarthritis: Factors influencing the clinical response. Ann Rheum Dis 1995;54:379–381.
9. Marshall KW: Intra-articular therapy in knee osteoarthritis: The role of viscosupplementation. Am J Orthop 2001;23–27.
10. Kirkley A, Webster-Bgaert S, Litchfield R, et al: The effects of bracing on varus gonarthrosis. J Bone Joint Surg Am 1999;81:539–548.
11. Moseley JB, O'Malley K, Petersen NJ, et al: A controlled trial of arthroscopic surgery for osteoarthritis of the knee. N Engl J Med 2002;347:81–88.
12. Wai EK, Kreder HJ, Williams JI: Arthroscopic debridement of the knee for osteoarthritis in patients fifty years of age and older. J Bone Joint Surg Am 2002;84:17–22.
13. Miller BS, Steadman JR, Briggs KK, et al: Patient satisfaction and outcome after microfracture of the degenerative knee. J Knee Surg 2004;17:13–17.
14. Bert JM: Role of abrasion arthroplasty and debridement in the management of osteoarthritis of the knee. Rheum Dis Clin North Am 1993;19:725–739.
15. Barber FA, Chow JC: Arthroscopic osteochondral transplantation: Histologic results. Arthroscopy 2001;17:832–835.
16. Coventry MB, Ilstrup DM, Wallrich SL: Proximal tibial osteotomy: A critical long-term study of 87 cases. J Bone Joint Surg Am 1993;75:196–201.
17. Dugdale TW, Noyes FR, Styer D: Pre-operative planning for high tibial osteotomy. Clin Orthop 1992;274:248–264.
18. Giffin JR, Vogrin TM, Zantop T, et al: Effects of increasing tibial slope on the biomechanics of the knee. Am J Sports Med 2004;32:376–382.
19. Paley D, Herzenberg JE, Tetsworth K, et al: Deformity planning for frontal and sagittal plane corrective osteotomies. Orthop Clin N Am 1994;25:425–465.
20. Insall JN, Joseph DM, Msika C: High tibial osteotomy for varus gonarthrosis. A long-term follow-up study. J Bone Joint Surg Am 1984;66:1040–1048.
21. Yasuda K, Majima T, Tsuchida T, Kaneda K: A ten- to 15-year follow-up observation of high tibial osteotomy in medial compartment osteoarthrosis. Clin Orthop 1992;186–195.
22. Hawker GA, Wright JG, Coyte PC, et al: Differences between men and women in the rate of use of hip and knee arthroplasty. N Engl J Med 2000;342:1016–1022.

60 Overuse Injuries

Stephen F. Brockmeier and John J. Klimkiewicz

In This Chapter

Patellar tendinosis
Quadriceps tendinosis
Iliotibial band friction syndrome
Popliteus tendonitis
Semimembranosus tendonitis
Prepatellar bursitis
Pes anserine bursitis
Infrapatellar fat pad syndrome

INTRODUCTION

- Overuse injuries of the knee are a common clinical entity encountered by primary care physicians, general orthopedists, physical medicine and rehabilitation physicians, and sports medicine specialists.

- Among the many diagnoses that fit in this category are tendonitis/tendinosis, bursitis, and other chronic and/or degenerative processes that result from repetitive trauma and overuse.

- While overuse syndromes occur elsewhere, the knee is the most commonly affected joint. The overall prevalence of these disorders is unknown. In some populations, such as distance runners, the incidence has been estimated to be as high as 30% each year.[1]

- Management of these disorders can be problematic due to a considerable rate of chronicity and the disability that can be encountered in active patients.

The etiology of overuse injuries can often be attributed to both intrinsic and extrinsic factors. Intrinsic causes can include limb malalignment, leg length discrepancy, muscle/tendon tightness or imbalance, foot abnormalities, and concomitant pathology or injuries about the knee such as meniscal or ligamentous injuries. Extrinsic factors are thought to play a large role in the development of many overuse injuries. The concept of Leadbetter's "Rule of Toos" in which athletes train *too* hard, *too* often, and return to sport *too* soon and *too* much after an injury often applies.[1] A recent change in the rate, duration, or intensity of activity frequently precedes the development of one of these disorders. Specific activities and training errors are often associated with specific conditions.

Overuse injuries are chronic syndromes, initiated by cyclic mechanical trauma. Repetitive trauma to the involved area leads to an initial injury. The body's physiologic response to this often subclinical injury includes inflammation about the injured tendon and eventually weakness or dysfunction of the involved muscle(s). A premature return to full activity prior to complete healing can lead to further tissue damage and ultimately chronic degeneration. Many of these syndromes have historically been referred to as tendonitis due to a proposed inflammatory nature of disease. Pathologic and histologic investigation has challenged this terminology. Microscopic evaluation of the diseased tissue has revealed changes consistent with a chronic, degenerative process. Mucoid degeneration or angiofibroblastic hyperplasia is often noted, with a remarkable lack of inflammatory cells.[2,3] For this reason, tendonopathy or tendinosis have become the more accurate terminology.

The management of these disorders often begins with a period of rest or a decrease in the frequency or intensity of activity. Conservative management, consisting of rest, ice, oral anti-inflammatories, and physical therapy aimed at stretching and strengthening of involved muscle groups, is often successful. Corticosteroid injections may have a role in some of these disorders. Surgical intervention can be indicated in recalcitrant cases after a failed period of nonsurgical management.

This chapter addresses some of the more commonly encountered overuse injuries about the knee, including patellar tendinosis, quadriceps tendinosis, iliotibial band friction syndrome, popliteus tendonitis, semimembranosus tendonitis, prepatellar bursitis, pes anserine bursitis, and infrapatellar fat pad syndrome.

PATELLAR TENDINOSIS

Also called "jumper's knee," patellar tendinosis is a common cause of anterior knee pain in athletes that participate in jumping sports or activities with repetitive knee extension, such as basketball, volleyball, and soccer. The term jumper's knee was coined by Blazina et al[4] in 1973, referring to both patellar and quadriceps tendonopathy. Today, however, the term is usually reserved for only patellar tendinosis. Repetitive eccentric contraction of the extensor that occurs with landing on one leg or kicking is thought to lead to mechanical overload in affected patients.[4] This disorder is seen most commonly in adolescents and young adults; symptoms sometimes commence during the adolescent growth spurt as the tendon does not lengthen as fast as the adjacent bone. Multiple predisposing factors have been reported. These include abnormal patellofemoral tracking, patella alta, chondromalacia patella, leg length discrepancy, limb malalignment, and Osgood-Schlatter disease. Patellar tendinosis can occasionally be confused with Sindig-Larsen-Johansson disease, which is a traction apophysitis of the distal pole of the patella. This disorder presents in a younger age group.

The most frequently affected area is the deep fibers at the tendon's insertion on the inferior pole of the patella; involvement of the distal tendon at the tibial tubercle is less frequent (one sixth as often).[5] Biomechanical evidence suggests that the process likely results from heavy cyclic loading causing a traction injury to the deep fibers of the patellar tendon at its proximal insertion. Others have postulated that repeated impingement of the inferior pole of the patella on the patellar tendon during flexion is causative.[6] Pathologically, the process is initiated by microscopic damage to the tendon fibers, leading to an initial inflammatory response and increased vascularity. These physiologic attempts at healing are impeded by repetitive injury. Pathologic changes noted on biopsy include fibroblast proliferation, neovascularization, mucoid degeneration, lipomatosis, and calcification of the tendon, with an absence of inflammatory cells.[3,7]

Patients typically present with the insidious onset of anterior knee pain and soreness localized to the inferior pole of the patella. Depending on the chronicity of the process, they may report pain after activity, during sports, or a continuous dull ache within the tendon. Ultimately, the pain interferes with the ability to compete and can be present at night, disturbing sleep. Blazina et al[4] classified patellar tendonopathy based on the patient's symptoms. Stage I is characterized by pain experienced after activity. In stage II, pain is present at the beginning of activity, only to disappear and return near the end of activity with muscle fatigue. Stage III is characterized by constant pain both with activity and at rest. Stage IV (added later by Martens et al[5]) is frank tendon rupture.

On examination, the most reproducible finding is point tenderness with palpation of the tendon at the inferior pole of the patella. The tenderness is maximal with the knee in full extension and diminishes with flexion as the tendon is placed under tension. Resisted knee extension and squatting can also be painful. Weakness, tightness, or atrophy of the quadriceps can also be noted.

While patellar tendinosis is a clinical diagnosis, imaging can be confirmatory. Plain radiographs are typically normal; however, occasionally one can note abnormalities such as calcification within the proximal tendon. Magnetic resonance imaging (MRI) and ultrasonography are the most useful modalities. MRI evaluation will often reveal an area of increased signal within the deep substance of the tendon, distal to the inferior pole of the patella (Fig. 60-1). The tendon may appear amorphous and often will be increased in thickness.[6,8] Ultrasonography can reveal the lesion as a focal area of decreased echogenicity as well as tendon enlargement. Some authors have reported abnormal tendons seen on MRI or ultrasonography in asymptomatic patients.[3]

Initial management of patellar tendonopathy is conservative. A treatment approach that includes a decrease or cessation of the inciting activity, ice, nonsteroidal anti-inflammatory drugs, and physician-directed physical therapy has been shown to be successful in more than 90% of patients. Most reports are retrospective and review variable populations. However, reported outcomes are consistent, with most patients reporting symptom-free resumption of sports within 6 months. Poorer response is seen in those with concomitant pathology or Blazina stage III disease.[9] Rehabilitation should initially focus on quadriceps stretching as well as the correction of any predisposing factors. Isometric exercises to strengthen the quadriceps can be initiated

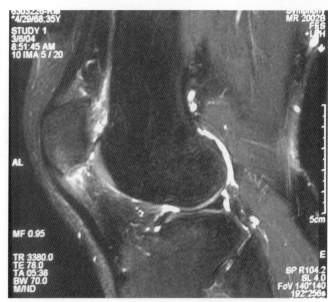

Figure 60-1 Magnetic resonance imaging (MRI) of patellar tendinosis. Characteristic MRI findings include increased signal within the deep tendon at the inferior pole of the patella and generalized tendon thickening.

early, but isotonic and isokinetic exercises should be delayed until the patient's symptoms subside. A gradual advancement to an eccentric quadriceps strengthening program is critical for a successful outcome.[1,3,9–11] Accumulating basic science evidence has pointed to a detrimental effect of corticosteroids on tendon tissue. Some authors do advocate corticosteroid injection in more severely affected patients. Complications of injection include resultant tendon rupture and subcutaneous atrophy/skin changes. We do not recommend corticosteroid injection for patellar tendinosis.

Operative intervention is generally reserved for recalcitrant patients who have not improved after 3 to 6 months of appropriate conservative management. A number of surgical procedures have been described. The recovery and rehabilitation after operative treatment can be prolonged, frequently lasting 6 to 12 months. While the majority of patients have been reported to have successful results with respect to resolution of pain, the percentage of those who return to their previous level of competition is significantly less after operative treatment.[9,12–14]

The described surgical techniques involve incision of the proximal tendon with the excision of the degenerative tissue. Often, the inferior pole of the patella is débrided, drilled, or freshened.[5,9] The remaining healthy tendon can be imbricated and the paratenon closed. For larger lesions, some authors have advocated a wide excision with reattachment of the tendon using heavy suture.

Recently, arthroscopic techniques have been described for this population of patients.[12,15] After a diagnostic arthroscopy is performed to examine the intra-articular portion of the patellar tendon and evaluate for concurrent intra-articular pathology, the pathologic tissue and overlying fat pad can be débrided from within the joint using a shaver. A recently published report found arthroscopic tenotomy to be equivalent to open tenotomy with respect to the resolution of symptoms and return to athletics.[12]

QUADRICEPS TENDINOSIS

Tendonopathy of the quadriceps is much less common than patellar tendonopathy.[4] The superior mechanical strength of the quadriceps combined with its improved vascularity provides reasonable protection from significant injury in most patients. However, a similar cascade of microinjury leading to chronic, degenerative tendinosis can occur in some active individuals. The involved portion is commonly at the quadriceps insertion on the superior pole of the patella. Predisposing risk factors can include extensor mechanism malalignment, increased frequency and intensity of activity, and hard playing surfaces.[7,10] Most affected patients report less limitation of athletic participation than those with patellar tendonopathy. However, long-standing symptoms can eventually curb performance. In some cases, chronic tendonopathy can lead to partial or frank rupture.[7]

Patients with quadriceps tendonopathy present with the insidious onset of pain and tenderness at the proximal pole of the patella. A recent increase in running, jumping, kicking, or climbing may be reported. Examination reveals point tenderness over the superior pole of the patella and pain with resisted extension. Attention should be given to the rotational alignment of the limb and to extensor mechanism tracking. As with patellar tendinosis, imaging can be confirmatory with similar findings often seen on MRI or ultrasonography.

Nonoperative management of quadriceps tendinosis is almost universally successful. Activity modification, nonsteroidal anti-inflammatory drugs, and physical therapy focusing on hamstring flexibility and quadriceps strengthening are generally effective in most patients. Strengthening exercises should build up to eccentric muscle training in order to fortify the tendon to withstand higher stresses. By 3 months, most patients have full resolution and are able to resume activities. Operative intervention is again only indicated after failure of a 3- to 6-month period of conservative treatment. Surgery consists of excision of the diseased tendon and drilling or débridement of the proximal pole of the patella to stimulate healing.[10] In the setting of a partial tendon rupture, operative repair is indicated if greater than 50% of the tendon is compromised.

ILIOTIBIAL BAND FRICTION SYNDROME

Also called "lateral runner's knee," iliotibial band (ITB) friction syndrome is the most common cause of lateral-side knee pain in long-distance runners. Also seen in cyclists, weight lifters, football and soccer players, and cross-country skiers, ITB friction syndrome is an overuse disorder caused by excessive friction between the ITB and the lateral femoral epicondyle.[16] Friction is maximal at 30 degrees of knee flexion, which is the position of greatest discomfort. This disorder was described by Renne[17] in 1975 in a cohort of marine recruits. He postulated that repeated flexion and extension of the knee during training caused the ITB to rub back and forth over the lateral epicondyle causing direct irritation of the band or periosteum and inflammation of the interposed bursa (Fig. 60-2).

The overall incidence has been reported to range from 1.6% to as high as 52% in certain populations.[17–19] It is very common in long-distance runners, especially those who run downhill. A number of intrinsic and extrinsic factors have been reported. Prominent lateral femoral epicondyle, genu varum, tightness of the ITB, limb length discrepancy, hindfoot varus, and foot prona-

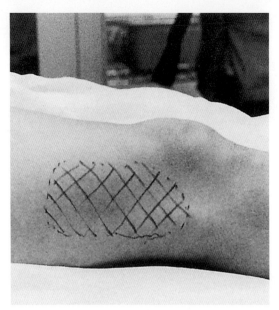

Figure 60-2 Area of pain and tenderness in iliotibial band friction syndrome. (From Safran MR, Fu FH: Uncommon causes of knee pain in the athlete. Orthop Clin North Am 1995;26:547–559.)

tion have all been implicated. An increase in the distance or frequency of running, a change in training surface, or an increase in downhill training can contribute. When running downhill, the angle of knee flexion at foot strike is decreased. This leads to increased contact between the epicondyle and the ITB. The pathogenesis is often a combination of extrinsic training factors in susceptible individuals.

Patients present clinically with lateral-side knee pain that usually begins during a long run. Pain is generally not present at rest but returns with resumption of the offending activity. The pain is often progressive, worsening to the point that the patient has to cease running. Discomfort is often increased with downhill running, and frequently patients can participate in other activities without symptoms.

Physical examination findings include point tenderness over the lateral femoral epicondyle, approximately 3 cm proximal to the joint line. Provocative testing using the "creak" test can be helpful. The patient stands with full weight on the affected extremity. A positive test is noted when the patient experiences a stinging pain over the epicondyle at 30 degrees of knee flexion.[17] Noble's test can be confirmatory (Fig. 60-3). It is performed with the patient supine and the affected knee in 90 degrees of flexion. While applying pressure over the lateral femoral epicondyle, the knee is extended and pain is elicited at approximately 30 degrees of flexion.[17] Ober's test is helpful to gauge ITB tightness (Fig. 60-4). The patient is placed in the lateral decubitus position with the affected extremity upward. The uninvolved hip and knee are flexed to correct lumbar lordosis. The affected knee is flexed to 90 degrees and the hip is gently hyperextended and abducted to catch the proximal ITB on the greater trochanter. Tightness in the ITB will prevent the affected limb from adduction below the horizontal created by the patient's torso.[16,18]

Imaging is usually not necessary unless other diagnoses are being ruled out. Radiographs are negative in ITB friction syndrome. MRI can be useful to differentiate ITB friction syndrome

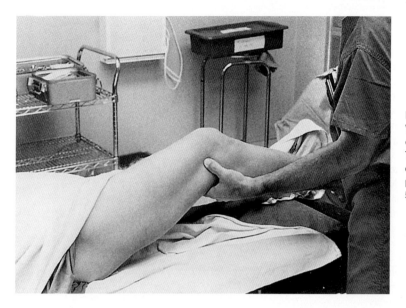

Figure 60-3 Noble's test for iliotibial band friction syndrome. With the patient supine and the affected knee flexed, the examiner applies pressure over the lateral femoral epicondyle. The knee is extended and pain is elicited at about 30 degrees of flexion. (From Safran MR, Fu FH: Uncommon causes of knee pain in the athlete. Orthop Clin North Am 1995;26: 547–559.)

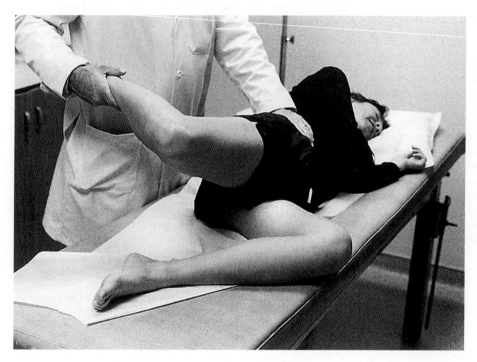

Figure 60-4 Ober's test for iliotibial band (ITB) tightness. With the patient in the lateral decubitus position, the uninvolved hip and knee are flexed to correct lumbar lordosis. The affected knee is flexed to 90 degrees, and the hip is gently hyperextended and abducted to catch the proximal ITB on the greater trochanter. Tightness in the ITB will prevent the affected limb from adduction below the horizontal created by the patient's torso. (From Safran MR, Fu FH: Uncommon causes of knee pain in the athlete. Orthop Clin North Am 1995;26:547–559.)

from other intra-articular pathology. MRI findings in ITB friction syndrome can include focal thickening of the ITB and/or fluid between the ITB and the lateral condyle.

Treatment of this disorder is usually conservative. Principles include modification of activity, control of inflammation, and correction of the contributing factors. Training modification includes a period of rest and the cessation of downhill running. Ice, nonsteroidal anti-inflammatory drugs, and phonophoresis can assist with controlling local inflammation. Local corticosteroid injection into the bursa can be helpful to reduce pain and inflammation in the acute phase.[20] Shoe modifications or orthotics can help correct foot pronation. Therapy should focus on entire limb kinetics. ITB stretching is essential as well as stretching and strengthening the tensor fascia latae, hip abductors, and hamstrings.[16]

Surgical intervention may be warranted in the atypical situation in which a patient fails an appropriate course of conservative treatment. In these recalcitrant patients, surgical release, as described by Noble,[19] of the posterior ITB with excision of a 2-cm triangular portion at the level of the lateral epicondyle has been effective. A number of small series have been reported using variations of this technique with satisfactory outcomes.[16,18]

POPLITEUS TENDONITIS

The popliteus travels from its origin on the lateral femoral condyle (tendinous portion) posterolaterally through the popliteal hiatus of the lateral meniscus (intra-articular portion) to form a broad, muscular insertion on the posterior proximal tibia. It functions to derotate the knee joint at the initiation of

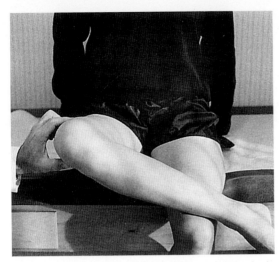

Figure 60-5 Evaluation of popliteus tendonitis by palpation in the figure-four position. (From Safran MR, Fu FH: Uncommon causes of knee pain in the athlete. Orthop Clin North Am 1995;26:547–559.)

flexion and aids the posterior cruciate ligament in preventing posterior displacement of the tibia on the femur. Injuries to this structure can occur acutely (with concomitant disruption of the anterior cruciate ligament, posterior cruciate ligament, or the posterolateral corner stabilizers) or chronically with overuse. Overuse injury to the popliteus, called popliteus tendonitis, is not uncommon in active individuals, especially in downhill runners or walkers (backpackers). Hyperpronation of the foot on the affected side due to running on banked terrain has been reported to be associated. Pronation leads to external rotation of the tibia and places chronic stress on the popliteus tendon.[16,21]

Patients usually complain of the insidious onset of lateral or posterior knee pain. There is usually no history of inciting trauma. Findings on examination include tenderness to palpation over the popliteus tendon at its origin on the lateral femoral condyle. This is best appreciated with the leg in the figure-four position[21] (Fig. 60-5). Pain with resisted external rotation can also be noted. The differential diagnosis includes ITB friction syndrome, lateral meniscal tear, and biceps femoris tendonitis. As the ITB and biceps femoris act to resist internal rotation and the popliteus prevents external rotation, pain with external rotation can aid in differentiating these entities.

Treatment of popliteus tendonitis includes rest and modification of training techniques in the form of eliminating downhill activities. Ice, ultrasound therapy, iontophoresis, nonsteroidal anti-inflammatory drugs, and physical therapy aimed at stretching can be helpful as well.[16] If the patient hyperpronates, orthotics may be beneficial. Symptoms usually resolve over 1 to 2 weeks, and a gradual return to running may be initiated. Uphill running and/or changing sides of the road during runs may help to prevent recurrence.

SEMIMEMBRANOSUS TENDONITIS

Semimembranosus tendonitis is an often neglected cause of medial-side knee pain. It occurs in endurance athletes as the result of repetitive loading and unloading and is often associated with other pathologic disorders of overuse. It can result from compensation for other knee problems in the nonathlete.[21] Patients present with pain posteromedially just below the joint line that is noted during or after activity. Tenderness is elicited with palpation of the anterior medial tendon of the semimembranosus distal to the joint line and is accentuated with knee flexion and external rotation. The differential diagnosis includes pes anserine bursitis and medial meniscal tear. Treatment is almost always conservative with rest, activity modification, nonsteroidal anti-inflammatory drugs, and physical therapy focusing on hamstring stretching. In the rare refractory patient, surgical exploration, débridement, and drilling of the semimembranosus insertion has been successful.[21]

PREPATELLAR BURSITIS

The prepatellar bursa is a potential space of synovial tissue that functions to decrease the friction between the subcutaneous tissue and the patella. Inflammation of this synovial sac can result from direct trauma, chronic activity or overuse, systemic disease (e.g., gout), or infection. It is most commonly encountered in wrestlers and in those with occupations that require frequent kneeling.[22,23] The incidence in wrestlers has been reported to be 9%.[22] The proposed mechanism involves repetitive trauma to the bursa leading to aseptic inflammation and chronic anterior knee swelling.

Patients present clinically with swelling located superficial to the patella. Knee range of motion is usually painless except at the extremes of flexion (depending on the size of the collection). There is no associated effusion. Thickening and crepitation of the tissue can be seen in more chronic cases.

Warmth, erythema, pain, and systemic symptoms signify septic bursitis. This must be confirmed by aspiration, as not all infected bursae are clinically demonstrable. A polymorphonuclear cell count of greater than 75% is the most accurate finding on synovial fluid analysis. Total white blood cell count and glucose levels are less specific.[23] Fluid should also be sent for Gram stain, culture, and crystalline analysis. The most common infecting organisms are *Staphylococcus aureus* and *Streptococcus* species.[23]

Following aspiration, treatment of aseptic prepatellar bursitis involves activity modification, compressive wrapping, and anti-inflammatory medications. Recurrence is common. Aspiration in combination with immobilization can be helpful in these situations. Surgical excision of the bursa is indicated in multiply recurrent or chronic cases. Septic bursitis is best rectified by surgical excision followed by a period of postoperative antibiotics. Both open and endoscopic techniques for excision have been described.[23] Whether treated conservatively or operatively, return to sports or work should be allowed once the inflammation has subsided, and the patient has regained normal strength and range of motion in the involved extremity.

PES ANSERINE BURSITIS

The pes anserine bursa is the synovial tissue overlying the attachment of the sartorius, gracilis, and semitendinosus tendons at the pes anserinus (goose foot). It is located approximately 5 to 6 cm below the anteromedial joint line. Inflammation of this bursa (or less commonly the neighboring Voshel's bursa, which is located just proximal to the pes anserine bursa, deep to the superficial medial collateral ligament) is a potential cause of medial knee pain in runners and athletes who participate in pivoting sports.[21]

Pes anserine bursitis can be incited by overuse or by direct trauma. Pes tendonitis, while less common, can be superimposed. Patients will present with pain, tenderness, and swelling over the pes bursa. In addition, resisted active knee flexion may be painful. This entity must be distinguished from other sources of medial-side pain, including medial meniscal pathology, saphenous nerve entrapment, proximal tibial stress fracture, and degenerative arthritis of the medial compartment.

The treatment is conservative with activity modification, ice, moist heat, anti-inflammatory drugs, and physical therapy focusing on hamstring stretching and strengthening modalities. Recalcitrant cases often respond to corticosteroid injections.[23] A premature return to activity can lead to recurrence. Surgical excision is rarely indicated.[21]

INFRAPATELLAR FAT PAD SYNDROME

Infrapatellar fat pad syndrome is a disorder associated with anterior knee pain secondary to hypertrophy and inflammation of the infrapatellar fat pad. Also known as Hoffa's disease, this syndrome is relatively rare. The cause is not fully known, but some have postulated that trauma of the infrapatellar fat pad occurs in those who participate in activities that entail repetitive maximal extension of the knee. With extension or hyperextension, the fat pad is pinched between the distal femur and the tibial spine leading to injury, hypertrophy, and inflammation.[21]

Patients present with pain below the inferior pole of the patella, which is exacerbated with activity or knee extension. On examination, tenderness with palpation of the fat pad, deep to the patellar tendon, can be noted. Swelling or an effusion can be present. The bounce test involves passive hyperextension of the knee, which reproduces the patient's pain.[21] Hoffa's disease is a diagnosis of exclusion. Reduction of symptoms with an injection of Xylocaine into the fat pad can be helpful in confirming the diagnosis.[21]

In most instances, patients respond to a conservative regimen consisting of rest, ice, and anti-inflammatory drugs. Activity modification with the prevention of hyperextension is effective. In recalcitrant patients, arthroscopic resection of the fat pad may be indicated.[21]

REFERENCES

1. James SL: Running injuries to the knee. J Am Acad Orthop Surg 1995;3:309–318.
2. Almekinders LC: Tendinitis and other chronic tendinopathies. J Am Acad Orthop Surg 1998;6:157–164.
3. Warden SJ, Brukner P: Patellar tendinopathy. Clin Sports Med 2003; 22:743–759.
4. Blazina ME, Kerlan RK, Jobe FW, et al: Jumper's knee. Orthop Clin North Am 1973;4:665–678.
5. Martens M, Wouters P, Burssens A, et al: Patellar tendinitis: Pathology and results of treatment. Acta Orthop Scand 1982;53:445–450.
6. Johnson DP, Wakeley CJ, Watt I: Magnetic resonance imaging of patellar tendonitis. J Bone Joint Surg Br 1996;78:452–457.
7. Bottoni CR, Taylor DC, Arciero RA: Knee extensor mechanism injuries in athletes. In DeLee JC, Drez DD, Miller MD (eds): DeLee and Drez's Orthopaedic Sports Medicine, 2nd ed. Philadelphia, WB Saunders, 2003, pp 1857–1867.
8. Shalaby M, Almekinders LC: Patellar tendinitis: The significance of magnetic resonance imaging findings. Am J Sports Med 1999;27:345–350.
9. Panni AS, Tartarone M, Maffulli N: Patellar tendinopathy in athletes, outcome of nonoperative and operative management. Am J Sports Med 2000;28:392–397.
10. Panni AS, Biedert RM, Maffuli N, et al: Overuse injuries of the extensor mechanism in athletes. Clin Sports Med 2002;21:483–498.
11. Teitz CC, Garrett, WE, Miniaci A, et al: Tendon problems in athletic individuals. J Bone Joint Surg Am 1997;79:138–152.
12. Coleman BD, Khan KM, Kiss ZS, et al: Open and arthroscopic patellar tenotomy for chronic patellar tendinopathy, a retrospective outcome study. Am J Sports Med 2000;28:183–190.
13. Ferretti A, Conteduca F, Camerucci E, et al: Patellar tendinosis, a follow-up study of surgical treatment. J Bone Joint Surg Am 2002; 84:2179–2185.
14. Popp JE, Yu JS, Kaeding CC: Recalcitrant patellar tendinitis, magnetic resonance imaging, histologic evaluation, and surgical treatment. Am J Sports Med 1997;25:218–222.
15. Romeo AA, Larson RV: Arthroscopic treatment of infrapatellar tendonitis. Arthroscopy 1999;15:341–345.
16. Nemeth WC, Sanders BL: The lateral recess of the knee: Anatomy and role in chronic iliotibial band friction syndrome. Arthroscopy 1996;12: 574–580.
17. Renne JW: The iliotibial band friction syndrome. J Bone Joint Surg Am 1975;57:1110–1111.
18. Kirk KL, Kuklo T, Klemme W: Iliotibial band friction syndrome. Orthopedics 2000;23:1209–1215.
19. Noble CA: Iliotibial band friction syndrome in runners. Am J Sports Med 1980;8:232–234.
20. Gunter P, Schwellnus MP: Local corticosteroid injection in iliotibial band friction syndrome in runners: A randomised controlled trial. Br J Sports Med 2004;38:269–272.
21. Safran MR, Fu FH: Uncommon causes of knee pain in the athlete. Orthop Clin North Am 1995;26:547–559.
22. Mysnyk MC, Wroble RR, Foster BT, et al: Prepatellar bursitis in wrestlers. Am J Sports Med 1986;14:46–54.
23. Neuschwander DC: Peripatellar pathology. In DeLee JC, Drez DD, Miller MD (eds): DeLee and Drez's Orthopaedic Sports Medicine, 2nd ed. Philadelphia, WB Saunders, 2003, pp 1867–1878.

The Stiff Knee

Craig S. Mauro and Christopher D. Harner

INTRODUCTION

- Loss of motion is a common and potentially debilitating problem following knee ligament injury. Depending on the ligament injured and the subsequent repair or reconstruction, loss of motion may involve loss of extension and/or loss of flexion.

- Previous studies have identified several risk factors that are associated with loss of motion. The etiology of loss of motion is multifactorial; it may be the result of diffuse joint inflammation and scarring or a mechanical block.

- Preventive strategies are the most important means of combating loss of motion. Additionally, early recognition of even a modest loss of motion may lead to an earlier intervention and improved outcome.

- Treatment options include nonoperative measures, such as range-of-motion and strengthening exercises, and arthroscopic and open surgical interventions.

- Recent studies have demonstrated improved outcomes when steps are taken to prevent, identify early, and aggressively treat loss of knee motion.

CLINICAL FEATURES AND EVALUATION

For the purposes of this chapter, the stiff knee is one that has lost some degree of flexion or extension. Throughout the literature, terms such as *arthrofibrosis*, *ankylosis*, *flexion contracture*, and *infrapatellar contracture syndrome* are used to describe knee motion loss in an attempt to characterize the etiology of the motion loss. To avoid any confusion that may be generated by such descriptions, we use the term *loss of motion* and, specifically, *loss of extension* and *loss of flexion* to describe any decrease from normal knee motion. When a specific diagnosis is discussed, we refer to that entity as it relates to loss of motion.

Most people demonstrate some degree of hyperextension in their normal knee range of motion, with men averaging 5 degrees and women averaging 6 degrees of recurvatum.[1] Loss of motion has been defined in various ways in the numerous clinical studies on the subject. Some have defined loss of extension as a loss of greater than 10 degrees relative to the zero-degree position, while others have defined it as a symptomatic lack of motion compared with the other side.[2,3] In 2000, the International Knee Documentation Committee (IKDC) revised the IKDC Knee Form, which is a knee-specific measure of symptoms, function, and sports activity.[4] One specific modification was a change in the way in which loss of extension is identified. In the original IKDC knee ligament guidelines, loss of extension was defined in terms of the difference from the zero-degree position.[5] In the 2000 IKDC Knee Examination Form, extension in the involved knee is compared to that of the normal, noninvolved knee to calculate the motion deficit. The 2000 IKDC Knee Examination Form defines passive motion deficits compared to the noninvolved knee (Table 61-1). These definitions have helped to standardize measurements and communication concerning loss of motion following knee injuries.

Loss of motion may be the result of factors specific to a knee injury or, more commonly, the treatment of this injury. Loss of motion may involve loss of flexion and/or loss of extension. Loss of extension usually results in greater functional deficits, as patients may walk with a bent knee gait, which places increased strain on the quadriceps and increases contact forces in the patellofemoral joint.[6] Consequently, patients with loss of extension may experience quadriceps weakness, patellofemoral pain, and fatigue.[7] Loss of flexion rarely causes functional difficulties unless the knee fails to flex at least 120 degrees. This degree of deficit may interfere with functional activities such as sitting, squatting, stair climbing, and running.

The true incidence of loss of motion following knee ligament injury and surgery, as defined by the IKDC classification system, is unknown and, as described previously, very much depends on the injury pattern and surgical intervention. The majority of the research concerning loss of knee motion has been focused on loss of motion following anterior cruciate ligament (ACL) injury and subsequent reconstruction. In 1984, Johnson et al[8] reported an incidence of loss of extension of 67.9% and loss of flexion of 76.5% following ACL reconstruction compared to the contralateral side. Since then, authors have reported the incidence of motion loss as between 1% and 25% following ACL reconstruction, with those studies more strictly defining loss of motion demonstrating a higher incidence.[2,3,9,10] The incidence of loss of motion is higher in the multiple ligament–injured knee, with some authors reporting an incidence between 18% and 30%.[11,12]

The risk factors associated with loss of motion have been studied most extensively following injuries to the ACL. As men-

Table 61-1 Passive Motion Deficit Compared to the Noninvolved Knee

Normal	<3 degrees extension or <5 degrees flexion
Nearly normal	3–5 degrees extension or 6–15 degrees flexion
Abnormal	6–10 degrees extension or 16–25 degrees flexion
Severely abnormal	>10 degrees extension or >25 degrees flexion

2000 International Knee Documentation Committee/Examination Form.

tioned, an injury pattern involving multiple ligaments, especially the medial collateral ligament, has a higher risk of loss of motion.[11,12] Other risk factors for loss of motion that have been identified are related to the surgery itself or postoperative rehabilitation. Several such factors have been described in the ACL reconstruction patient (Table 61-2).

Patients with knee dislocations and multiple ligament injuries are at highest risk of loss of motion because of the extensive injury sustained by the tissues during the injury and subsequent reconstruction. Injuries to, and procedures involving, the medial side of the knee may accentuate the fibrotic response of the knee joint, resulting in excessive scar formation and increased loss of motion. Interestingly, patients with multiple ligament injuries who undergo surgery within the first 3 weeks after injury tend to have better subjective functional ratings and better restoration of ligamentous stability.[12] This finding may be the result of the easier dissection and repair facilitated by the acute reconstruction prior to the initiation of the fibrous healing response. Further, the timing of surgery in the multiple ligament–injured knee may not affect motion.[12]

The timing of ACL reconstruction has been a very controversial aspect of reconstructive knee surgery. While several studies have reported that acute ACL reconstruction results in a higher incidence of loss of motion,[3,9,13] others have demonstrated no such relationship.[14–16] The time frame of an acute ACL reconstruction has traditionally been defined as within 3 weeks of the injury. The association between time from injury to surgery and loss of motion has been attributed to the healing response that begins following any injury. Fibrinogenic cytokines have been shown to promote fibroblast proliferation and extracellular matrix production. Before surgery is performed, it is important to allow the acute sequela of the injury to subside. The quiescence of this episode is manifested by a decrease in swelling, restoration of extension within 5 degrees of the non-involved side, and the ability of the patient to perform a good quadriceps contraction, such as a straight leg raise without a lag. Even those studies that endorse acute surgery suggest that

Table 61-2 Risk Factors for Loss of Motion After Anterior Cruciate Ligament Reconstruction

Acute reconstruction
Decreased preoperative motion
Graft malposition
Poor rehabilitation
Excessive immobilization

restoring the motion deficit preoperatively is an important measure to prevent postoperative loss of motion.

Preoperative motion has been demonstrated to be an important risk factor for loss of motion postoperatively in most studies. The preoperative motion may be the most important clinical marker of the inflammatory response that is seen after the initial injury. This response and the consequent risk of motion loss following surgery may be minimized by restoring motion preoperatively. The time from injury to surgery to minimize the risk of loss of extension may vary for each patient, and we believe that the best indicator of when to proceed with ACL reconstruction is restoration of preoperative extension.

ACL graft malposition is an important technical factor that may place a patient at risk of loss of motion postoperatively. An anterior tibial tunnel may cause impingement between the graft and the intercondylar notch during terminal extension. This impingement may lead to loss of extension or, ultimately, graft failure.

Patients who take part in physical therapy programs that stress early motion and weight bearing tend to have fewer problems with loss of motion.[2,9] Excessive immobilization that limits extension following surgery is associated with a higher incidence of loss of extension.[3] Achievement of full extension, which may be assisted through bracing and crutches in the early postoperative period, may engage the graft within the intercondylar notch, minimizing hemorrhage and intercondylar notch scarring.

RELEVANT ANATOMY

The etiology of loss of motion following ligament surgery is multifactorial but may be attributed to one or more of the following pathoanatomic processes. A mechanical block to flexion or extension may be caused by impingement resulting from an intra-articular block. Alternatively, diffuse inflammation or capsulitis may lead to loss of motion through the development of adhesions and intra-articular scar formation or arthrofibrosis.

Impingement

Impingement may be the result of intercondylar notch scarring, a fibrovascular proliferation from the tibial side of the reconstruction, or an anteriorly placed ACL graft. Intercondylar notch scarring may result from bleeding and regrowth of the notch. Also, failure to perform an adequate notchplasty may lead to a physical block to extension.[17]

An ACL nodule may develop following ACL rupture or reconstruction of the ACL, causing a mechanical block to extension. When the lesion develops following ACL rupture, prior to reconstruction, full extension may be not be achieved within 2 months, even with aggressive rehabilitation. It has been reported that this nodule may develop from the torn fibers of the ligament at the tibial attachment site.[18]

The ACL nodule that may develop following ACL reconstruction was first described by Jackson and Schaefer[19] in 1990, as a "cyclops lesion" because of its arthroscopic appearance. These nodules may arise from the graft and the surrounding tissue overlying the tibia, typically anterolateral to the tibial tunnel (Fig. 61-1). The nodule is composed of fibroelastic connective tissue proliferation, and it is unclear whether the lesion is the result of repetitive trauma to the graft or from hypertrophy of the remains of the native ACL. With knee extension, the cyclops lesion impinges between the graft and the intercondylar notch, preventing full extension.

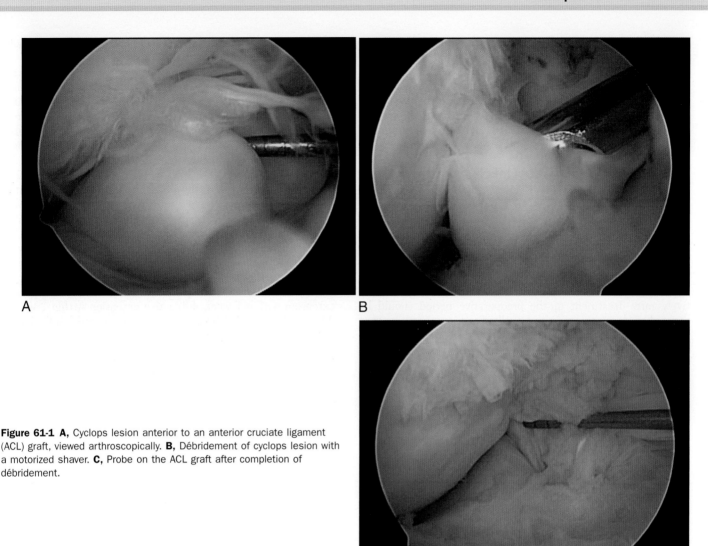

Figure 61-1 A, Cyclops lesion anterior to an anterior cruciate ligament (ACL) graft, viewed arthroscopically. **B,** Débridement of cyclops lesion with a motorized shaver. **C,** Probe on the ACL graft after completion of débridement.

The ideal position of the tibial tunnel is within the ACL footprint. Anterior placement of the graft on the tibial side may lead to impingement of the graft in the intercondylar notch when the knee approaches terminal extension. Impingement from an improperly placed tunnel may lead to graft damage and subsequent fibroproliferation within the notch.

Symptoms of impingement include stiffness in the morning that may improve with motion, anterior knee pain, and crepitus at terminal knee extension. Loss of motion with impingement is usually loss of terminal extension, with normal flexion. Usually, the knee is not diffusely inflamed, swelling is minimal, and patellar mobility is not affected.

Capsulitis/Arthrofibrosis

Loss of motion following any knee ligament surgery may be due to capsulitis. Capsulitis refers to diffuse periarticular inflammation and swelling. This inflammatory response may lead to varying degrees of arthrofibrosis, a condition of diffuse intraarticular fibrous adhesions. Capsulitis, and the subsequent arthrofibrosis, is the result of cytokine release during the inflammatory response to an injury or surgery. Cytokines stimulate fibroblasts to produce the fibrous adhesions, which leads to the arthrofibrosis.

Shelbourne et al[20] developed a classification system of arthrofibrosis based on the motion of the injured knee compared to motion in the uninjured knee. In this classification system, patients with type I arthrofibrosis have an extension loss of 10 degrees or less and normal flexion. Patients with type II arthrofibrosis have greater than 10 degrees of extension loss and normal flexion. Patients with type III arthrofibrosis have greater than 10 degrees of extension loss, greater than 25 degrees of flexion loss, and decreased patellar mobility. Patients with type IV arthrofibrosis have greater than 10 degrees of extension loss, greater than 30 degrees of flexion loss, and patella inferna with markedly decreased patellar mobility.

Inflammation in the peripatellar tissues is associated with decreased patellar mobility. Patellar baja may result from the diffuse inflammation because of fibrous hyperplasia of the anterior fat pad. In 1987, Paulos et al[21] coined the term *infrapatellar contracture syndrome* to refer to patients with patellar entrapment associated with loss of extension and flexion despite multiple corrective procedures. The cause of this entrapment is hyperplasia of the anterior fat pad, prolonged immobility, and lack of extension. When the fat pad becomes hyperplastic and adherent to the underlying tibia, the patella has limited excursion, and loss of motion may result.

Capsulitis results in diffuse constant pain and stiffness. The knee is actively inflamed with diffuse swelling and warmth. Both extension and flexion are limited as a result. Patellar mobility is usually limited and, consequently, contraction of the quadriceps fails to create enough tension to actively extend the knee completely. Arthrofibrosis is the end product of capsulitis, and the knee may demonstrate decreased flexion, extension, and patellar mobility, but the swelling and warmth usually subside.

PREVENTION AND TREATMENT OPTIONS

Prevention

Preoperative

Preoperative steps are the most important interventions to take to prevent loss of motion. Loss of motion following an injury is usually the result of pain, swelling, quadriceps inhibition, and hamstring spasm. A locked knee from a torn meniscus is relatively rare. Treatment in the preoperative period should be focused on decreasing pain and swelling and improving range of motion. Preoperatively, management consists of the use of ice to reduce pain and swelling, range-of-motion exercises, hamstring and calf stretching, and isometric quadriceps exercises. It is also important to counsel the patient about the possible complication of loss of motion and the importance of appropriate physical therapy.

Intraoperative

Some of the important intraoperative considerations to prevent loss of motion postoperatively were discussed earlier in the clinical features section. Accurate surgical technique and meticulous attention to graft placement are necessary to minimize the risk of loss of motion postoperatively. With ACL reconstruction, improper tibial tunnel placement may lead to motion problems. Most commonly, an anterior tibial tunnel may lead to impingement between the graft and the roof of the intercondylar notch with knee extension.[17] Ideally, the tibial tunnel should be drilled within the ACL footprint. For less experienced surgeons, or whenever any surgeon is unsure about tunnel location (especially in revision cases where arthroscopic anatomy is potentially distorted), intraoperative lateral radiographs with the knee in extension are critical. A notchplasty should be performed to allow adequate clearance for the graft within the intercondylar notch. As previously discussed, an inadequate notchplasty or regrowth and scarring of the notch is one of the commonly identified causes of loss of extension following ACL reconstruction.

Postoperative

An appropriate rehabilitation program that stresses early motion is the most important postoperative measure to take to avoid loss of motion in this period. The goals of the rehabilitation program are to minimize inflammation, restore motion and strength, enhance proprioception and dynamic stability, and return the patient to full function. Our ACL postoperative physical therapy program stresses early motion with passive extension, heel/wall slides, hamstring/calf stretching, and active-assisted range of motion. Straight leg raises, quadriceps sets, half squats/wall slides, standing heel raises, and lateral step-ups are important for early postoperative muscle function. It is important to see the patella glide superiorly with the quadriceps sets to prevent infrapatellar contracture syndrome. These exercises may be performed several times daily in the early postoperative period. Modalities such as cold and compression may be helpful to decrease inflammation and swelling.

Postoperative rehabilitation following ACL reconstruction must be done in such a manner that minimizes inflammation, pain, and swelling but stresses early motion to minimize adhesive scar formation. During week 1, we lock the knee brace in extension but allow range-of-motion exercises several times during the day. In most cases, we allow the patient to weight bear as tolerated. Beginning week 2, the brace is unlocked for ambulation. We stress the heel-toe gait to emphasize terminal extension. After week 4, the brace and crutches are discontinued if the patient has reached full extension and 100 degrees of flexion, has no knee extensor lag and minimal swelling, and is able to walk without a bent knee gait. Crutches are critical for successful rehabilitation in the first month postoperatively to achieve and maintain terminal extension without development of a bent knee gait.

Critical milestones for patients to achieve are full passive extension within 1 week, full active extension within 2 weeks, 90 to 100 degrees of flexion within 2 weeks, and full flexion by 6 weeks. The surgeon should recognize that patients who are not meeting these milestones may require more specific and intense treatment for loss of motion.

Treatment

Recognition of loss of motion must occur as early as possible to allow for immediate initiation of treatment. Although the preventative measures described previously are optimal, treatment of loss of motion must be initiated if these measures fail. The treatment process begins with a systematic approach to identify the cause of loss of motion. Successful treatment of loss of motion depends on early recognition of the cause. Early recognition of loss of motion and appropriate intervention should decrease long-term complications for the patient.

Some patients experience loss of motion because the affected knee continues to be diffusely swollen, painful, and inflamed in the postoperative period. This type of response may be associated with capsulitis and, if left untreated, arthrofibrosis. When identified in the period of active inflammation, the appropriate treatment for the inflamed knee is anti-inflammatory agents, rest, and ice. Patients may continue with pain-free active range-of-motion exercises and strengthening but should avoid forceful manipulation of the knee. Stretching techniques should be gentle to avoid aggravation of pain and swelling.

Efforts toward regaining motion should be focused on reducing the motion deficit in one direction at a time. We address loss of extension first because it tends to cause more functional deficits and patellofemoral pain if left untreated. Patients should be encouraged to perform quadriceps sets and straight leg raises to minimize any knee extensor lag.

A drop-out cast may be used overnight to provide a sustained stretch and prevent further loss of extension. The drop-out cast is constructed by applying a cylindrical long-leg cast with the knee at the end range of extension. Padding is incorporated into the cast anteriorly superior to the patella and posteriorly on the proximal thigh and distal calf to create a three-point pressure system to increase knee extension. After the cast has hardened, a window is cut to expose the anterior aspect of the patella and lower leg. The amount of stretch is then adjusted by incorporating a wedge between the cast and the distal aspect of the calf. The cast is left in place overnight and then removed by splitting it anteriorly over the thigh.

During the active stage of capsulitis, gentle patellar mobilization is also important. Superior excursion of the patella, which is necessary for proper functioning of the extensor mechanism, may be restored by performing quadriceps sets in terminal extension. This mobilization must not be overly aggressive and must be pain free, as further inflammation of the peripatellar tissues may lead to further delay in restoration of motion.

The surgeon, physical therapist, and the patient must have patience in the management of capsulitis. Overly aggressive stretching, manipulation, or surgical intervention during the period of active inflammation may only further inflame the knee and worsen the problem. Once the active inflammation has subsided, which may be 6 months or longer after reconstruction, surgery or manipulation may be considered if the patient has persistent loss of motion.

Manipulation under anesthesia is a more invasive means of gently flexing and extending the knee under general or regional anesthesia to loosen scar tissue in patients with arthrofibrosis not responsive to standard physical therapy techniques. Manipulation is most effective for mild arthrofibrosis leading to flexion loss, as knees with greater extension deficits have been shown to achieve significantly less final extension than knees with smaller deficits.[22] We believe that manipulation is most effective around 3 months postoperatively, after the acute response has subsided, but before the fibrotic response is complete. Manipulation under anesthesia should be performed gently to prevent chondral damage or stimulation of myositis ossificans or ossification of the medial collateral ligament.

When loss of motion appears to be caused by impingement, physical therapy to improve extension should be the focus of the initial management. Gentle stretching techniques that employ a sustained, low-amplitude force should be used. Quadriceps strengthening exercises are stressed to eliminate any quadriceps lag that may be contributing to the loss of extension. A drop-out cast may also be used in this setting to provide a sustained stretch and prevent further loss of extension.

If impingement is the suspected cause of loss of motion and extension fails to improve with physical therapy within 2 or 3 weeks, arthroscopic evaluation and débridement of the intercondylar notch (as described in the following section) may be necessary. Aggressive nonoperative manipulation should not be performed in the setting of a physical impingement. Forceful stretching may result in graft failure and will not be successful unless the physical block to motion is removed.

SURGERY

Surgical management of loss of knee motion is indicated when nonoperative interventions have failed or if a specific, correctable abnormality exists. Several techniques have been described, including open débridement, arthroscopic débridement, and combined open and arthroscopic débridement.

Arthroscopic Débridement

Arthroscopic débridement has been advocated as the first-line surgical treatment for loss of motion. It is often successful and may be performed on an outpatient basis. Loss of extension following ACL reconstruction may be particularly appropriate for arthroscopic intervention, as correction of loss of extension secondary to pathology localized to the notch or scarring may be particularly amenable to this approach.

Prior to undertaking a surgical intervention to address loss of motion, the surgeon should have an idea of the etiology of the loss of motion. Even when the surgeon has a strong suspicion preoperatively of the underlying pathology, it is important to thoroughly visualize all compartments of the knee. We use a diagnostic arthroscopic approach to evaluate the knee in the setting of loss of motion that is similar to the nine-step approach described by Millett et al.[23] We create the standard anterolateral and anteromedial portals immediately adjacent to the respective border of the patellar tendon, at previous arthroscopy portal sites if possible. We first evaluate the suprapatellar pouch, the medial gutter, and the lateral gutter, using a motorized shaver to reestablish these spaces if scarring has compromised their visualization (Fig. 61-2).

We then turn our attention to the infrapatellar fat pad, which is débrided and mobilized to reestablish the pretibial recess. Any infrapatellar adhesions between the anterior tibia and the fat pad must be débrided to allow patellar mobilization and superior patellar excursion. The medial and lateral retinaculum are then evaluated and released with a motorized shaver if tight or scarred. If the anterior aspects of the menisci are involved in the scarring, this scarring should be released to allow normal anterior-posterior meniscal translation.

Evaluation of the intercondylar notch is next. When loss of knee extension following ACL reconstruction is a result of impingement, the offending pathology may be visualized in the intercondylar notch. Proliferation of a cyclops lesion from the tibial side of the reconstruction is usually first visualized with any attempt to visualize the intercondylar notch. This nodule should be débrided, and the intercondylar notch should be evaluated for scarring.

Regardless of the presence of a cyclops lesion, intercondylar notch scarring should be débrided to allow the knee to reach as nearly normal extension as possible. Once the excess scarring is excised, the graft should lock into the notch without impinging on it during knee extension. Impingement of the graft in the intercondylar notch may result in failure of the graft to incorporate. The graft insertion should be evaluated for evidence of failure. An inadequate notchplasty may cause impingement and loss of extension following ACL reconstruction. A notchplasty should be performed if there is evidence of continued impingement despite débridement of the notch scarring. In severe cases of intercondylar notch scarring, the ACL and/or posterior cruciate ligament may need to be released. Following intercondylar notch débridement, a drop-out cast may be applied.

An anteriorly placed ACL graft may contribute to the loss of motion following ACL reconstruction. In the case of an anteriorly placed ACL graft causing impingement and loss of extension, an adequate notchplasty must be completed to provide the anterior graft the opportunity to reduce into the notch without impingement. If elimination of the impingement is not feasible through notchplasty, the ACL graft may have to be resected. If necessary, revision reconstruction is performed later as a staged procedure.

The posterior capsule should be evaluated at its tibial and femoral insertions, as tightness of the posterior capsule may contribute to loss of extension. Some authors advocate release of the posterior capsule if tightness is noted.[23] This débridement must be performed carefully, with special consideration given to the neurovascular anatomy of the posterior knee. We do not routinely perform a posterior capsule release and have found a drop-out cast in the postoperative period to be effective for relieving posterior knee tightness.

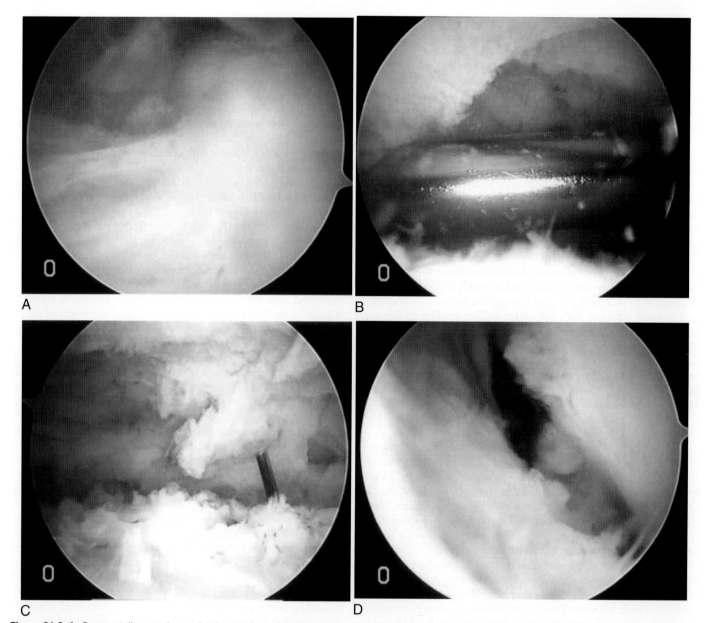

Figure 61-2 A, Suprapatellar pouch scarring in a patient with severe arthrofibrosis after a tibial plateau fracture (preoperative flexion <60 degrees). **B,** Creating a space with the shaver. **C,** Suprapatellar pouch after nearly completed excision of adhesions. **D,** Scarring in the lateral gutter in the same patient.

Open Débridement

Open débridement procedures are indicated in patients in whom nonsurgical and arthroscopic surgical procedures have been unsuccessful for resolving the motion deficit or for patients with severe motion deficits and patellar baja. Most patients respond to the less invasive means previously described. Open procedures are usually salvage interventions that involve an extended hospital stay, analgesia, and prolonged rehabilitation.

Open débridement may be indicated in patients with diffuse periarticular and intra-articular scarring who have failed arthroscopic intervention or in whom arthroscopic intervention is not feasible. Patients with arthrofibrosis and no localizable lesion may benefit from this approach. When performing an open approach, it is important to completely remove all scar tissue encountered. A systematic approach to the knee is important to ensure complete débridement. We also place all patients who undergo open débridement in a drop-out cast postoperatively.

Our technique is similar to that described by Millett et al.[24] We approach the knee through a medial parapatellar arthrotomy. The knee is inspected to identify any areas of particular involvement. A release of the medial soft tissues over the medial tibial cortex is first performed if medial scarring is identified. These areas deep to the medial collateral ligament overlying the tibial plateau and femoral condyle are particularly important to release. The infrapatellar fat pad is then débrided, and a lateral peripatellar release may be performed if additional exposure or mobilization is needed. The undersurface of the extensor mechanism is then débrided to allow full mobilization of the patella. We then address any intra-articular adhesions, paying particular attention to the intercondylar notch and the posterior capsule.

Once all identifiable impediments to motion are addressed, the knee is closed and adequate analgesia ensured.

POSTOPERATIVE REHABILITATION

The postoperative rehabilitation following surgery to address loss of motion is structured according to the intervention undertaken. Patients undergoing limited arthroscopic débridement to address impingement, such as with cyclops lesion excision, may more aggressively rehabilitate. These patients may continue with the previously described exercises for regaining extension. Following open débridement, patients may benefit from cryotherapy, early bracing in extension, and early active and active-assisted range-of-motion exercises. In patients being treated for more severe deficits with loss of flexion and extension, we focus our postoperative rehabilitation on regaining extension first, as full extension may be more difficult to achieve and lack of extension may cause more functional deficits.

CRITERIA FOR RETURN TO SPORTS

We use the same criteria for return to sports following treatment for knee loss of motion as we would following any knee injury or reconstruction. Following an ACL reconstruction, our patients begin running at an average of 4.3 months postoperatively, light sports at 5 months, moderate sports at 5.8 months, jumping at 6.5 months, and strenuous sports at 8.1 months. We use the following criteria to guide this return: absence of pain and swelling, laxity, quadriceps strength greater than 80% to 90%, hop test, and proprioception and neuromuscular control. Following treatment of loss of motion, we use these same criteria to guide the patient's return to sports. If the patient's loss of motion was due to intercondylar notch scarring that was treated with an arthroscopy, the patient may advance very quickly to meet these criteria and return to sports. However, if the patient required open débridement following loss of motion after a knee dislocation and multiligament reconstruction, the return to sports will be significantly delayed. Usually a patient will need a deficit of less than 3 degrees of extension to return to full athletic activity. Loss of flexion is more forgiving and usually does not interfere with activity unless the patient has a loss of flexion to approximately 125 degrees.

RESULTS AND OUTCOMES

Several authors have reported outcomes following treatment of the knee with loss of motion. Sprague et al[25] were the first to describe the arthroscopic treatment of patients with limited knee motion following open knee surgery. They described 24 patients whose mean total range of motion increased from 70 degrees preoperatively to 115 degrees at final follow-up. They found that the morbidity associated with the procedure was low and complications were infrequent and mild.

Shelbourne et al[20] reported the results of 72 patients who sustained loss of motion following ACL reconstruction. These patients were classified by their staging system and treated arthroscopically. They classified and recorded passive motion as a/b/c with "a" representing the degree of hyperextension, "b" representing the degree of flexion that is short of 0 degrees of extension, and "c" as the degree of flexion present. The patients underwent arthroscopic scar resection at an average of 12.5 months following the initial ACL reconstruction and were exam-

ined at a mean follow-up of 35 months. Patients with type I arthrofibrosis improved from a preoperative mean of 0/3/140 degrees to a postoperative mean of 4/0/140 degrees. Patients with type II arthrofibrosis improved from 0/11/135 degrees to 3/0/137 degrees, while patients with type III arthrofibrosis improved from 0/10/111 degrees to 3/0/139 degrees. Patients with type IV arthrofibrosis improved from 0/15/103 degrees to 3/0/130 degrees. The authors also noted a considerable improvement in mean modified Noyes knee score, stiffness score, self-evaluation score, and functional activity for patients in all groups.

Jackson and Schaefer[19] reported on a series of 13 patients who were found to have cyclops nodules anterolateral to the tibial tunnel placement of the ACL graft following reconstruction. They noted improvement in mean extension following arthroscopic excision of the nodule and knee manipulation from 16 degrees preoperatively to 3.8 degrees at final follow-up. Loss of motion secondary to a discrete cyclops nodule carries a more favorable prognosis for recovery than does recovery from diffuse arthrofibrosis.

We recently reported the results of a series of 229 patients undergoing ACL reconstruction.[10] Twenty-eight patients underwent an arthroscopic procedure to improve loss of motion. The majority of the patients (25 of 28) were found to have intercondylar notch scarring, resulting in graft impingement and a physical block to extension. Following arthroscopy and débridement, 4 patients, or 1.7% of the original series, continued to have passive motion deficits between 6 and 10 degrees, while no patients had a deficit greater than 10 degrees.

Millett et al[24] recently reported on the outcomes of eight patients who underwent open débridement for severe loss of knee motion. In this series, mean extension was 18.8 degrees and mean flexion was 81 degrees preoperatively. Following débridement, mean extension improved to 1.25 degrees and mean flexion improved to 125 degrees. They noted improvement in function, patient satisfaction, and Lysholm II scores, but a high incidence of patellofemoral arthritis and patellar tendon shortening at follow-up.

COMPLICATIONS

The complications of loss of knee motion are more obvious with loss of extension than flexion, as patients usually experience greater functional deficits. Patients with loss as little as 3 degrees of extension may walk with a bent knee gait, which places increased strain on the quadriceps and increases contact forces in the patellofemoral joint.[6] As a result, patients may experience quadriceps weakness, patellofemoral pain, and fatigue.[7] Loss of flexion rarely causes functional difficulties unless the knee fails to flex at least 120 degrees. This degree of deficit may interfere with functional activities such as sitting, squatting, stair climbing, or running.

Despite treatment of loss of motion through nonoperative or operative means, continued loss of motion may persist. This finding is the most frequent complication of attempted treatment. Other complications of treatment are less frequent. Manipulation may cause chondral damage, stimulation of myositis ossificans, ossification of the medial collateral ligament, or femoral or tibial fracture. Arthroscopic débridement places a patient at risk of all complications associated with knee arthroscopy, such as neurovascular injury, chondral damage, numbness, and deep vein thrombosis. Open débridement also carries the risk of postoperative hematoma or hemarthrosis.

CONCLUSIONS

Loss of motion is a potentially debilitating problem following knee ligament injury or knee surgery. Multiple risk factors for diffuse joint inflammation and scarring or a mechanical block leading to loss of motion have been identified. Preventive strategies and early recognition of loss of motion are the most important means of combating loss of motion. Loss of motion often may be treated with appropriate range-of-motion and strengthening exercises. Arthroscopic treatment of loss of motion is an effective and safe alternative when less invasive therapies fail.

REFERENCES

1. DeCarlo MS, Sell K: Normative data for range of motion and single leg hop in high school athletes. J Sport Rehabil 1997;6:246–255.
2. Shelbourne KD, Gray T: Anterior cruciate ligament reconstruction with autogenous patellar tendon graft followed by accelerated rehabilitation. A two- to nine-year followup. Am J Sports Med 1997;25:786–795.
3. Harner CD, Irrgang JJ, Paul J, et al: Loss of motion after anterior cruciate ligament reconstruction. Am J Sports Med 1992;20:499–506.
4. Irrgang JJ, Anderson AF, Boland AL, et al: Development and validation of the international knee documentation committee subjective knee form. Am J Sports Med 2001;29:600–613.
5. Hefti F, Muller W, Jakob RP, Staubli HU: Evaluation of knee ligament injuries with the IKDC form. Knee Surg Sports Traumatol Arthrosc 1993;1:226–234.
6. Perry J, Antonelli D, Ford W: Analysis of knee-joint forces during flexed-knee stance. J Bone Joint Surg Am 1975;57:961–967.
7. Sachs RA, Daniel DM, Stone ML, Garfein RF: Patellofemoral problems after anterior cruciate ligament reconstruction. Am J Sports Med 1989;17:760–765.
8. Johnson RJ, Eriksson E, Haggmark T, Pope MH: Five- to ten-year followup evaluation after reconstruction of the anterior cruciate ligament. Clin Orthop 1984;122–140.
9. Shelbourne KD, Wilckens JH, Mollabashy A, DeCarlo M: Arthrofibrosis in acute anterior cruciate ligament reconstruction. The effect of timing of reconstruction and rehabilitation. Am J Sports Med 1991;19:332–336.
10. Mauro CS, Herrera MF, Irrgang JJ, et al: Loss of extension following ACL reconstruction: Analysis of incidence and etiology using new IKDC criteria. Presented at the annual meeting of the American Orthopaedic Society for Sports Medicine, Quebec City, 2004.
11. Noyes FR, Barber-Westin SD: Reconstruction of the anterior and posterior cruciate ligaments after knee dislocation. Use of early protected postoperative motion to decrease arthrofibrosis. Am J Sports Med 1997;25:769–778.
12. Harner CD, Waltrip RL, Bennett CH, et al: Surgical management of knee dislocations. J Bone Joint Surg Am 2004;86:262–273.
13. Shelbourne KD, Johnson G: Evaluation of knee extension following anterior cruciate ligament reconstruction. Orthopedics 1994;17:205–206.
14. Sterett WI, Hutton KS, Briggs KK, Steadman JR: Decreased range of motion following acute versus chronic anterior cruciate ligament reconstruction. Orthopedics 2003;26:151–154.
15. Hunter RE, Mastrangelo J, Freeman JR, et al: The impact of surgical timing on postoperative motion and stability following anterior cruciate ligament reconstruction. Arthroscopy 1996;12:667–674.
16. Bach BR Jr, Jones GT, Sweet FA, Hager CA: Arthroscopy-assisted anterior cruciate ligament reconstruction using patellar tendon substitution. Two- to four-year follow-up results. Am J Sports Med 1994;22:758–767.
17. Howell SM, Barad SJ: Knee extension and its relationship to the slope of the intercondylar roof. Implications for positioning the tibial tunnel in anterior cruciate ligament reconstructions. Am J Sports Med 1995;23:288–294.
18. McMahon PJ, Dettling JR, Yocum LA, Glousman RE: The cyclops lesion: A cause of diminished knee extension after rupture of the anterior cruciate ligament. Arthroscopy 1999;15:757–761.
19. Jackson DW, Schaefer RK: Cyclops syndrome: Loss of extension following intra-articular anterior cruciate ligament reconstruction. Arthroscopy 1990;6:171–178.
20. Shelbourne KD, Patel DV, Martini DJ: Classification and management of arthrofibrosis of the knee after anterior cruciate ligament reconstruction. Am J Sports Med 1996;24:857–862.
21. Paulos LE, Rosenberg TD, Drawbert J, et al: Infrapatellar contracture syndrome. An unrecognized cause of knee stiffness with patella entrapment and patella inferna. Am J Sports Med 1987;15:331–341.
22. Dodds JA, Keene JS, Graf BK, Lange RH: Results of knee manipulations after anterior cruciate ligament reconstructions. Am J Sports Med 1991;19:283–287.
23. Millett PJ, Wickiewicz TL, Warren RF: Motion loss after ligament injuries to the knee. Part II: Prevention and treatment. Am J Sports Med 2001;29:822–828.
24. Millett PJ, Williams RJ 3rd, Wickiewicz TL: Open debridement and soft tissue release as a salvage procedure for the severely arthrofibrotic knee. Am J Sports Med 1999;27:552–561.
25. Sprague NF 3rd, O'Connor RL, Fox JM: Arthroscopic treatment of postoperative knee fibroarthrosis. Clin Orthop 1982;165–172.

62 Pediatric Knee

Nathalee S. Belser and Craig S. Roberts

In This Chapter

Osteochondritis dissecans (OCD)
Osgood-Schlatter disease (OSD)
Intercondylar eminence fractures
Salter-Harris fractures

INTRODUCTION

- There is a gamut of knee disorders in the skeletally immature knee.

- Disorders range from repetitive overuse injuries to growth plate fractures.

- This chapter covers OCD, OSD, intercondylar eminence fractures, distal femoral physeal/epiphyseal fractures, proximal tibial physeal/epiphyseal fractures, distal pole patellar sleeve fractures, and tibial tubercle fractures.

OSTEOCHONDRITIS DISSECANS

The term OCD appears to have originated with Konig, who in 1888 postulated that spontaneous necrosis of the subchondral bone and the overlying cartilage was caused by loose bodies and inflammation.[1] Fairbanks in 1933[2] suggested that OCD stemmed from a violent internal rotation of the tibia that caused impingement of the tibia spine on the femoral condyle.[3]

OCD is an epiphyseal disorder in which a localized segment of subchondral bone undergoes necrosis and demarcation from the surrounding normal bone.[4] Fracture and failure of healing can result in the bone becoming separated partially or completely from the joint surface, forming an osteocartilaginous loose body. Although OCD can also involve the medial or lateral femoral condyle or patella,[5] the lateral side of the medial femoral condyle is the most frequent site of involvement, seen in 75% of the cases.

Traditional beliefs about the causes of OCD such as trauma, ischemia, and genetics have proven to be wrong.[3] In addition, studies concerning familial incidence of OCD document an autosomal dominant pattern of heredity with a high degree of expression.[4]

Clinical Features and Evaluation

Early symptoms of OCD are vague (Box 62-1). As the fragment begins to separate, the patient experiences catching, locking and joint effusion and may limp on ambulation.[6] Patients complain of medial knee pain and partial giving way after strenuous physical activity.[7] Physical findings include local tenderness over the site of the fragment and quadriceps weakness.

The patient may present with Wilson's sign, which is based on the fact that tibial spines may impinge against the femoral condyle when the OCD is located at the classic site at the lateral side of the medial femoral condyle[6] (Box 62-2). The patient is placed in a supine position and the knee is flexed to a right angle. The leg is internally rotated and is gradually extended. The test is positive when pain is felt at 25 to 30 degrees of knee flexion and the tibia is internally rotated. Pain is relieved when the tibia is externally rotated. However, the validity of Wilson's sign has recently been questioned by Conrad and Stanitski,[8] who, in a series of 32 patients, found that Wilson's sign was of minimal clinical diagnostic value.

OCD is usually divided into three stages. Stage I is a well-demarcated prominence of the articular surface; the cartilage covers the elevation that is continuous with the rest of the cartilage surface but is a different color.[4] The prominence can be easily separated, and beneath it there is an excavation of bone and chondral portion of the articular end of the bone.

In stage II, the fragment is distinctly separated but still lies within its anatomic bed on the articular surface. In stage III, the fragment is displaced out of its anatomic bed into the joint.

Diagnostic Imaging

Imaging recommendations for OCD include anteroposterior, lateral, tunnel, and merchant views.[9] Magnetic resonance imaging (MRI) can assess lesion size and the status of cartilage and subchondral bone and subsequent healing of the lesion (Fig. 62-1).[9] Luhmann et al[10] noted that routine review of MRI scans for pediatric knee disorders such as OCD increased the diagnostic accuracy of the MRI.

Treatment Options

Treatment decisions are based mainly on the stability of the lesion (Box 62-3). Stable lesions are treated with conservative measures in skeletally immature patients. A debate exists regarding therapeutic or detrimental effects of immobilization, which centers on which tissue the treating physician considers most important in healing.[9] Advocates who focus on the subchondral bone believe that OCD should be treated like a fracture, with a cast or knee immobilizer. In contrast, those who focus on the cartilaginous component of OCD recommend early knee motion.

The conservative management protocol can be divided into three phases. First, the knee is immobilized in a long-leg cast for 6 weeks with toe touch (10 pounds) weight bearing with crutches and regular straight leg raise exercises. In the second

Box 62-1 Osteochondritis Dissecans: Signs and Symptoms

- Catching, locking, knee effusion, limping
- Quadriceps atrophy
- Presenting complaint of knee giving away while walking in a straight line or during strenuous activity
- Wilson's sign: if the knee is flexed to a right angle and the tibia is internally rotated, pain is experienced as the knee is extended. Pain is relieved by external rotation.

Box 62-2 Osteochondritis Dissecans: Anatomic Lesions

- Avascular area with overlying articular cartilage that becomes loose and detaches
- Typically occurs on lateral aspect of medial femoral condyle

Box 62-3 Osteochondritis Dissecans: Treatment Options

- If lesion is intact, a period of observation is recommended with avoidance of sports. Close follow-up with imaging such as radiographs or magnetic resonance imaging is recommended over the next year to demonstrate healing of the lesion.
- If symptoms persist or the fragment is detached, knee arthroscopy with fixation of the fragment or excision.
- Operative treatment is indicated on a semiurgent basis for detached or unstable lesions.

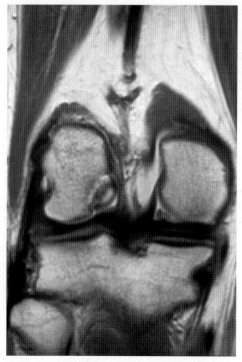

Figure 62-1 Magnetic resonance imaging of a loose osteochondritis dissecans fragment of the lateral femoral condyle, an atypical location, in a nearly skeletally mature individual.

phase (weeks 6 to 12), weight bearing is permitted without immobilization. A rehabilitation program is initiated emphasizing knee range of motion and low-impact quadriceps and hamstring strengthening exercises. If the patient remains pain free, phase three begins at 3 months after diagnosis. This phase includes running, jumping, and sports readiness activities, but high-impact and shear activities are restricted until the child has had several months of pain free, low-impact conditioning and radiographs document healing. MRI can be repeated if clinically indicated in phase three to assess healing.

Operative treatment is indicated for patients who have detached or unstable lesions, who are approaching epiphyseal closure, or when nonoperative management fails to alleviate symptoms. The goals of operative treatment include rigid internal fixation of unstable fragments and repair of osteochondral defects. Surgical options include drilling, bone grafting, internal fixation in situ, open or arthroscopic reduction with internal fixation, fragment excision, autologous osteochondral grafting, and allogenic osteochondral grafting.[11] For patients who fail nonoperative treatment but have a stable lesion and intact articular surface, arthroscopic drilling of the lesion creates channels for potential revascularization and healing. The drilling may either pass through the epiphysis without articular penetration or continue transarticularly. While drilling through the epiphysis avoids articular surface violation, it is associated with the technical challenges of maintaining drill depth and placement accuracy.

In cases of flap lesions, fibrous tissue found between fragments should be removed. Débridement of significant portions of bone from the fragment and subchondral base of the lesion should be avoided. Wright et al[12] reported that only six of 17 patients (35%) had a good result from fragment excision, an average of 8.9 years postoperatively, and recommended "aggressive attempts to preserve the articular cartilage and avoid excision of the fragments when possible." In patients who have unstable lesions with subchondral bone attached that can be anatomically reduced, fixation can be performed by a variety of arthroscopic or open methods. These options include metallic, cannulated, partially threaded small fragment screws; metallic self-compressing screws; bioabsorbable pins; and bioabsorbable screws.

Unique situations include bone and cartilage defects when osteochondral fragments cannot be saved. Newer surgical options include autologous chondrocyte implantation, which involves the transplantation of cloned cartilage cells under a periosteal cover and cylindrical osteochondral autograph transfer. Yoshizumi et al[13] treated three cases of OCD in patients with closed growth plates with a 10-mm diameter osteochondral autograph transfer with excellent clinical and radiographic results, but areas of signal intensity remained on MRI scans at short-term follow-up.

Recent reports on juvenile OCD have noted a significant number of poor results at follow-up.[3] To date, there have been no controlled prospective studies on OCD that accurately measured the effect of different treatments.[3]

Surgery

Knee arthroscopy is performed in order to evaluate the size and reducibility of the osteochondral fragment. The bony bed of the lesion is débrided, the fragment is anatomically reduced, and provisionally fixed with a percutaneously inserted guide wire. The guide wire is then overreamed with a cannulated reamer. A partially threaded, cannulated screw is inserted percutaneously; the fragment is compressed, and the guide wire is removed. The

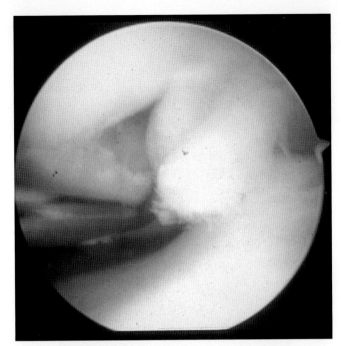

Figure 62-2 Arthroscopic view of the loose osteochondritis dissecans fragment of the lateral femoral condyle.

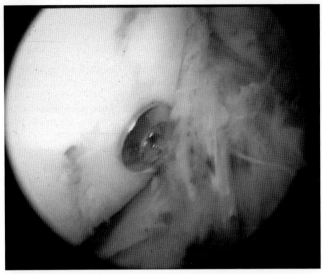

Figure 62-4 Arthroscopic view of the seated cannulated screw that has been used to fix the osteochondritis dissecans fragment.

screw is subsequently removed arthroscopically at 10 to 12 weeks after insertion in a similar manner (Figs. 62-2 through 62-5).

OSGOOD-SCHLATTER DISEASE

OSD is an overuse injury or traction apophysitis of the tibial tubercle that commonly occurs in boys 13 to 14 years of age and in girls 10 to 11 years of age. Inflammation and new bone formation at the patellar tendon insertion are characteristic. The differential diagnosis includes patellar tendonitis, Sinding-Larsen-Johansson syndrome, avulsion fracture of the tibial

tuberosity, tumor, and infection. The association of patella alta with OSD has been reported.[14,15]

The precise cause of OSD is unknown.[14] The most common theory is that repeated contractions of the quadriceps mechanism result in an extra-articular osteochondral stress fracture of the apophysis.[16] Tension forces produce fracture separation of an osteochondral fragment that includes a segment of the secondary ossification center of the tibial tubercle and the cartilage anterior to it. With healing, new bone forms in the gap between the separated osteochondral fragment and the tibial tubercle, which is deviated and prominent. OSD is usually unilateral but has been reported to occur bilaterally in 20% to 30% of cases.[14]

Ross and Villard[17] reported that subjects with a 7-year history of OSD had significantly lower scores than subjects in a control

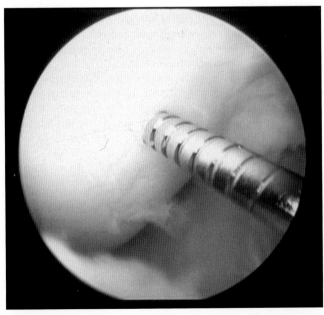

Figure 62-3 Arthroscopic view of provisional fixation after reduction of the osteochondritis dissecans fragment.

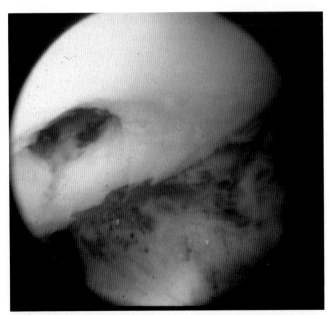

Figure 62-5 Follow-up arthroscopic view of the healed osteochondritis dissecans lesion at the time of implant removal.

group on both the Knee Outcome Activities of Daily Living Scale and Sports Activity Scale. Browner-Elhanan et al[18] noted a lack of flexibility and strength imbalance of the leg muscles associated with OSD in nine patients who were an average of 11.8 years old.

Clinical Features and Evaluation

Patients present with complaint of pain in the anterior aspect of the knee in the region of the proximal tubercle, which is swollen, prominent, and tender. The onset of symptoms is vague and intermittent.[16] Running and jumping aggravate the severity of pain, while rest relieves symptoms. Physical examination reveals swelling and localized tenderness over the tibial tubercle without other abnormalities. Boys are frequently more affected than girls, and about a half of the patients have a history of precipitating trauma. Pain is reproduced by extension against forced resistance. In addition, there may be quadriceps atrophy (Boxes 62-4 and 62-5).

Diagnostic Imaging

The lateral radiograph is the most useful view and shows soft-tissue swelling and a separate ossicle over the tubercle (Fig. 62-6).[14] In addition, there may be bilateral accessory ossification centers. MRI can be useful in detecting partial avulsion or an avulsion fracture of the apophyseal cartilage with fragmentation of the accessory centers.

Treatment Options

OSD is generally a self-limited condition.[19] Treatment of acute avulsion of the tubercle depends on the size of the fragment and the degree of displacement (Box 62-6). The condition usually resolves within 1 to 2 years, but in about 10% of patients, the formation of a discrete ossicle and bursa results in persistent pain and tenderness.

OSD is managed by modification of activities, nonsteroidal anti-inflammatory drugs, and a knee pad to control discomfort. If OSD is severe or persistent, a knee immobilizer may be effec-

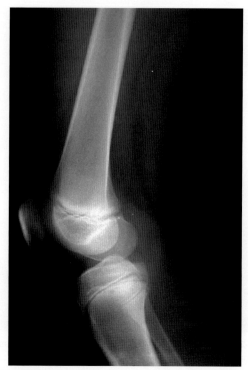

Figure 62-6 This lateral radiograph of the knee is from a mild case of Osgood-Schlatter disease with ossification over the tibial tubercle.

tive. Duri et al[14] warned, "The ossicle can be easily enucleated from the patellar tendon by way of a longitudinal fiber-splitting incision. The patient and the family should be forewarned that some residual soft tissue and bony prominence may remain." Operative treatment is reserved for nonunited ossicles and persistent symptoms after the physes have closed. Excision is performed through a short incision by splitting the distal fibers of the patellar tendon. Postoperative casting for 6 weeks may be necessary if more dissection is performed. Excellent results have been reported with surgical excision. Flowers and Bhadreshwar[20] reported that 88% of patients reported complete relief of pain an average of 13.5 months after surgical excision of the ossicle after a trial of conservative treatment failed. Overall, the prognosis for OSD is excellent as patients usually are able to return to full activity and participate in athletics.

Concerns have been raised about safety of harvesting a bone-patellar tendon-bone autograft for anterior cruciate ligament (ACL) reconstruction in patients with an ossicle associated with OSD. However, Di Gennaro et al[21] noted that an autogenous bone-patellar tendon-bone graft can be safely harvested in ath-

Box 62-7 Intercondylar Eminence Fractures: Signs and Symptoms

- Inability to bear weight
- Hemarthrosis
- Knee held in a flexed position

letes who have an ossicle associated with OSD. McCarroll et al[22] noted the importance of recognizing the OSD ossicle preoperatively, so that it is not mistaken for the tibial tubercle intraoperatively. The surgeon can safely excise the ossicle intraoperatively with a small surgical knife blade after graft harvest.

INTERCONDYLAR EMINENCE FRACTURES

Intercondylar eminence fractures are the children's equivalent of an ACL tear in the adult.[23,24] The reported mechanisms of injury in the child are similar to those in the adult and include motor vehicle accidents, falls, and sports activities.[23,25] Because the collagenous portion of the ACL is stronger than the bony attachments in the skeletally immature individual, bony avulsion occurs at the tibial ACL insertion site (the intercondylar eminences), usually as a result of an athletic, noncontact, twisting injury. Although the bony avulsion appears to be the primary pathology, interstitial tearing of the ACL also occurs in most cases.

Clinical Features and Evaluation
Patients present with knee pain and limited knee motion and are unable to bear weight. An effusion caused by the hemarthrosis is present (Boxes 62-7 and 62-8). Patients hold the knee in a fixed position, once pain is controlled. The presence of a locked knee (usually determined on examination under anesthesia) is indicative of concomitant knee pathology or that the fracture is not fully reduced due to an interposed meniscus or a transverse intermeniscal ligament. Neurovascular status should not be affected and the skin should be intact.

These injuries have traditionally been classified into three types according to the system first described by Meyers and McKeever[26] in 1959. Type I injuries are nondisplaced or minimally displaced fractures of the intercondylar eminence. Type II injuries have partial displacement of the eminence fracture proximally and anteriorly with a "beaklike" deformity on the lateral radiograph.[27] In type III injuries, the eminence is completely displaced from its tibial attachment, and in type IV injuries, a displaced, comminuted fracture is present.[28]

Diagnostic Imaging
Standard anteroposterior and lateral radiographs are obtained. The lateral radiograph is the most helpful because it can demonstrate the degree of displacement.[29] Alternatively, MRI can be used to assess for displacement, possible interposition of the meniscus, ACL injury, and other concomitant bony and soft-tissue injuries.

Treatment Options
Nonoperative treatment of type I injuries is generally accepted. Historically, conservative treatment has also been recommended for type II injuries (Box 62-9). However, authors have reported that 26% of type II injuries involve entrapment of either the anterior horn of the medial meniscus, transverse meniscal ligament, or the anterior horn of the lateral meniscus.[30] Hunter and Willis[27] reported on arthroscopic fixation of type II and III eminence fractures in a series of 17 patients who were an average of 26.6 years old. Eight of the 17 subjects were 16 years of age or younger, and these patients had better outcomes as measured by the International Knee Documentation Committee functional and overall rating scores. These authors noted the phenomenon of interposition of the meniscal ligament between the avulsed fragments in 17 patients (59%). They equated the intermeniscal ligament with the Stener lesion (interposed adductor pollicis tendon), associated with ulnar collateral ligament of the thumb tears where the lesion prevents the tendon or bony avulsion from returning to its anatomic position.[27] Kocher et al[30] reported on arthroscopic reduction and cannulated screw fixation of six patients with type III injuries and reported persistent laxity but excellent functional outcome.[30] The use of bioabsorbable fixation of the fracture has been used in a small number of patients.[31] A metallic screw shorter than 25 mm can be used to avoid the proximal tibial growth plate. Alternatively, Lubowitz et al[32] recommended repair using nonabsorbable suture fixation, citing the advantages of eliminating the risks of comminution of the fracture fragment, vascular injury, and future hardware removal. Patients and parents should be counseled that persistent laxity is normal even after the surgical treatment of intercondylar eminence fractures. Persistent laxity is nonetheless still associated with an excellent clinical outcome. Future surgical procedures will most likely be necessary for removal of implants and possible ACL reconstruction in athletically active patients or those who subsequently experience symptoms of knee instability.

Surgery
Knee arthroscopy is performed and may require the use of a pump for inflow or a tourniquet. The knee joint is inspected. Particular attention is paid to visualization of the avulsed fragment. The anterior infrapatellar fat pad may prevent adequate visualization and may require débridement. The fracture bed is inspected for possible incarceration of the anterior horn of the

Box 62-8 Intercondylar Eminence Fractures: Anatomic Lesions

- Fracture of the intercondylar eminence
- Variable amount of fracture displacement
- Possible entrapment of the meniscus
- Interstitial tearing of the anterior cruciate ligament

Box 62-9 Intercondylar Eminence Fractures: Treatment Options

- Type I injuries: nonoperative treatment (immobilization)
- Type II injuries: treatment is controversial (recent trend toward operative treatment)
- Type III and IV injuries: operative management

lateral meniscus. If present, the meniscus must be retracted and preserved and the fragment reduced. Reduction maneuvers include decreasing the amount of knee flexion and manual manipulation of the fragment with a nerve hook. The ACL should also be carefully assessed for interstitial stretching, partial tearing, and loss of function. Optimal viewing of the ACL from the anteromedial portal will usually be required. Decision making for choice of fixation of the fragment is based on the operative pathology. If the fragment is not comminuted (type II or III), then cannulated screw fixation can be used. Guide wire insertion often requires placing an arthroscopic portal somewhat higher than usual. Positioning the knee in less flexion also helps reduce the fragment. The portal location can be precisely localized using a percutaneously inserted spinal needle. Oftentimes, three anterior portals are required: one for the arthroscope, one for the nerve hook to maintain reduction, and one to insert the cannulated screw over a guide wire. Small fragment, partially threaded screws about 25 mm long are usually used. If the fragment is comminuted (type IV), options include one or two cannulated screws and washers (Figs. 62-7 and 62-8) or suture methods that pass sutures through the base of the ACL using arthroscopic suture passers. Sutures can be tied over an anterior tibial bone bridge.

FRACTURES ABOUT THE KNEE

Fractures of the growth plates around the knee occur in skeletally immature individuals. These injuries can be thought of in terms of "3s": the three major physes or growth plates (femur, tibia, and fibula), the three major epiphyses (femur, tibia, and fibula), and three traction sites (patella, tibial tubercle, and tibial intercondylar spines). Although many of these injuries occur by mechanisms that would cause a ligamentous injury in an adult, the determining factor of which injury occurs is a function of the rate and magnitude of the injuring force.[33] High-magnitude forces at a low rate of application result in physeal fractures, whereas low-magnitude forces applied at a high rate produce lig-

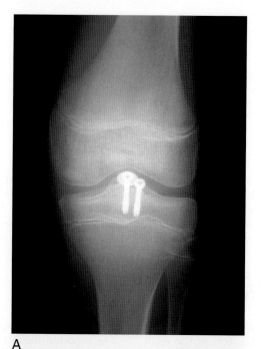

A

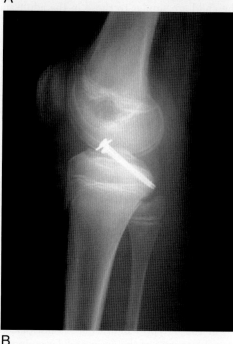

B

Figure 62-8 Postoperative anteroposterior (**A**) and lateral (**B**) radiographs after fixation of an intercondylar spine fracture.

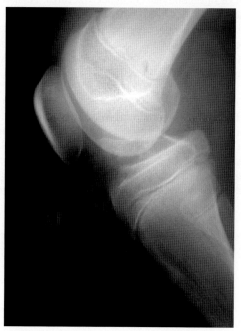

Figure 62-7 Lateral radiograph of a displaced intercondylar eminence fracture (type IV).

ament injuries. Physeal fractures are generally classified according to the Salter-Harris classification, which divides injuries into types I through V. A Salter type I injury is an epiphyseal separation.[34] A Salter type II fracture is also an epiphyseal plate injury, but after the fracture line continues a variable distance across the physis, it then extends out into the metaphysis producing the characteristic Thurston-Holland fragment. The Salter type III fracture is intra-articular and extends from the joint surface to the physis and then out perpendicularly across the physis. A Salter IV fracture is also intra-articular. The fracture line extends from the joint surface through the physis and then through the metaphysis producing a complete split. A Salter type V fracture is a rare occurrence and involves a crushing injury to the epiphysis and physis. This section includes the following fractures: distal femoral physeal fracture, proximal tibial physeal fracture, patellar sleeve fracture, and tibial tubercle avulsion fracture (Boxes 62-10 and 62-11).

The knee physes are immature tissues and vulnerable to injury. Effects on future growth from these fractures may occur. As a general rule, the femur has more remodeling capacity than the tibia. Although the prognosis of these injuries traditionally has been assumed to be favorable, these injuries can cause future problems. Careful follow-up is important.

Clinical Features and Evaluation
Distal Femoral Physeal Fractures
Although knee ligament ruptures can occur in children, most prepubescents and adolescents suffer growth plate injuries rather than ligamentous injuries. The distal femoral physis is the largest in the body. The epiphysis is the first to ossify and provides 70% of the overall growth of the femur.

Proximal Tibial Physeal Fractures
About 50% of proximal tibial fractures occur in sports. These fractures are about one fourth as common as distal femoral physeal fractures. The mechanism of injury is usually hyperextension and valgus stress. The most important part of the initial treatment of these injuries is the recognition that these injuries can be the pediatric equivalent of an adult dislocation of the knee. Associated vascular injuries, compartment syndromes, or neurologic deficits may be present and must be recognized. Arteriograms are necessary if there is any question about the vascular status. Metaphyseal injuries are more common than tibial plateau fractures (epiphyseal injuries). Proximal tibial metaphyseal injuries commonly occur between the ages of 2 and 8. Patients and parents need to be counseled about the unpredictability of possible valgus deformity from medial overgrowth after fracture or subsequent hyperextension deformity secondary to anterior growth plate arrest. Salter type II fractures are the most common tibial epiphyseal injuries.[35] Physical examination demonstrates severe tenderness and swelling over the proximal tibial physis for epiphyseal injuries.

Patella Sleeve Fractures
Patella sleeve fractures are commonly misdiagnosed and usually involve the distal rather than the proximal pole of the patella.

Clinical findings include an extensor lag and patella alta. Differential diagnosis includes Sinding-Larsen-Johansson syndrome and bipartite patella.

Tibial Tubercle Avulsion Fractures
These injuries tend to occur in the robust athlete, near skeletal maturity, usually as a result of a jump or fall.[36] There is a possible association with OSD.[36] Fractures of the tibial tuberosity are classified according to the system of Ogden et al.[37] Associated injuries are uncommon but must be ruled out. These include tears to the menisci, medial collateral ligament, lateral collateral ligament, and ACL as well as compartment syndromes and neurovascular injuries.

Diagnostic Imaging
As a general rule, nondisplaced fractures may not be visible on plain radiographs. Subtle radiographic findings such as a small fleck of bone at the periphery of the metaphysis may be the only radiographic finding of a proximal tibial epiphyseal fracture.[35] Stress views for the diagnosis of radiographically occult fractures in the skeletally immature patient were previously thought to be of value but have fallen out of vogue since the advent of MRI. The Thurston-Holland sign is a metaphyseal, wedgelike component of a physeal fracture. It is the sine qua non of a Salter type II fracture. Patella sleeve fracture radiographic findings include a small avulsion or "chip" about the distal pole of the patella.

Treatment Options
Distal Femoral Physeal Fractures
All fractures of the distal femoral physis usually require surgical stabilization[38] (Box 62-12). Surgical options include crossed Kirschner wires, wires/screws parallel to the growth plate for a Salter type II, and a transepiphyseal screw for a Salter type IV. Salter type I fractures are usually treated with smooth pins. Salter type II fractures with large metaphyseal fragments can often be treated with 4.5 or 7.3 mm screws. Salter type III or IV fractures can be treated with percutaneous screws parallel to the physis. Postoperatively, a long-leg cast is usually required.

Proximal Tibial Physeal Fractures
Fractures that cannot be reduced require an operative reduction. Fracture reduction may be blocked by soft-tissue interposition that requires removal from the fracture site.

Valgus deformity after proximal tibial metaphyseal fracture can correct spontaneously up to 3 years after injury. In the rare cases in which the deformity does not correct itself, surgical options that may be considered include proximal tibial osteotomy or proximal tibial hemiepiphysiodesis. Irreducible displaced fractures require reduction and fixation, usually with a transmetaphyseal screw.

Patellar Sleeve Fractures
Patellar sleeve fractures (Fig. 62-9) are treated operatively and usually require open reduction and internal fixation, except in exceptional cases of no or only minimal displacement.

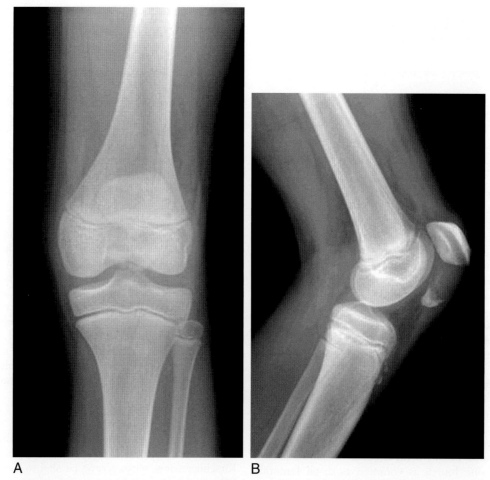

Figure 62-9 Anteroposterior (**A**) and lateral (**B**) radiographs of a displaced patellar sleeve fracture.

Treatment options include a periosteal suture, tension band (Fig. 62-10), and screw fixation.

Tibial Tubercle Avulsion Fractures

Type I tibial tubercle injuries (Fig. 62-11) are treated with cast immobilization for 3 weeks. Type II and III injuries are treated with open reduction and internal fixation, especially for the articular component of the injury. Options for internal fixation include sutures, threaded pins, and, if the fragment is large, screws (Fig 62-12). Prognosis is usually excellent, and the risk of recurvatum is minimal because the growth plate is usually almost closed.

CONCLUSIONS

There is a wide range of pediatric knee disorders. Because early symptoms and imaging findings of OCD and OSD can be non-specific, a high level of clinical suspicion ought to be maintained for the relevant clinical features. In contrast, intercondylar eminence fractures present in a similar manner to adult ACL tears and can be easily diagnosed and expeditiously treated. Fractures of the growth plates and apophyses about the knee can be radiographically occult or difficult to image and require timely treatment for the best functional outcome. Although the prognosis of injuries to growing knees is usually favorable, these injuries can cause future problems. Careful follow-up of these patients is important.

ACKNOWLEDGMENT

The authors thank David Antekeier, MD, for providing some of the radiographs and intraoperative photographs (Figs. 62-6 through 62-12) for this chapter.

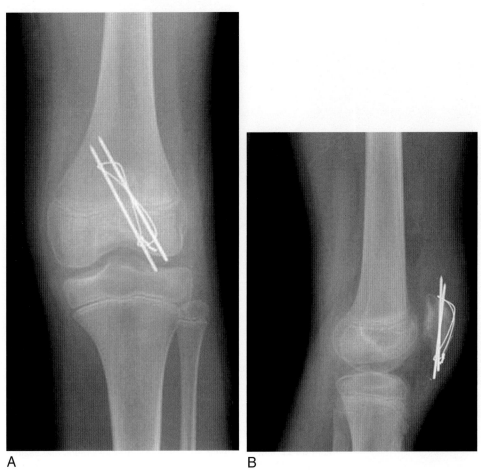

A   B

Figure 62-10 Postoperative anteroposterior (**A**) and lateral (**B**) radiographs after open reduction and internal fixation of a patellar sleeve fracture using a tension band technique.

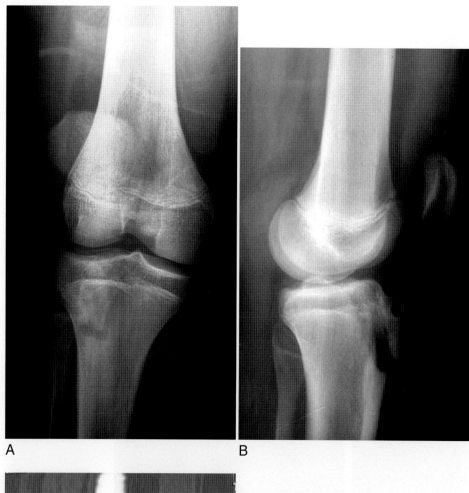

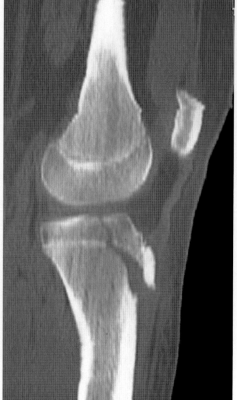

Figure 62-11 Anteroposterior (**A**) and lateral (**B**) radiographs and sagittal computed tomography scan image (**C**) of a displaced fracture of the tibial tubercle. The lateral radiograph (**B**) shows the presence of an associated Osgood-Schlatter disease lesion.

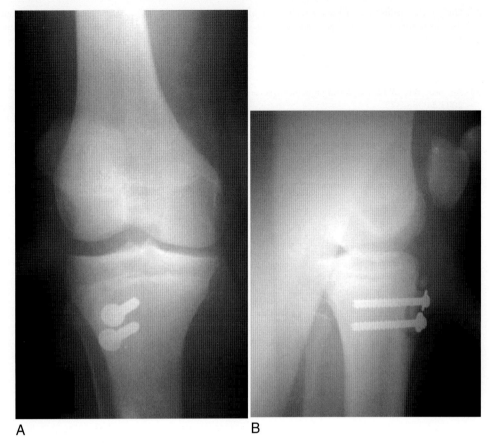

Figure 62-12 Postoperative anteroposterior (**A**) and lateral (**B**) radiographs after open reduction and internal fixation of the fracture of the tibial tubercle.

A   B

REFERENCES

1. Cain EL, Clancy WG: Treatment algorithm for osteochondral injuries of the knee. Clin Sports Med 2001;20:321–342.
2. Fairbanks H: Osteochondritis dissecans. J Bone Joint Surg Br 1933;21:67–71.
3. Wall E, Von Stein D: Juvenile osteochondritis dissecans. Orthop Clin N Am 2003;34:341–353.
4. Shapiro F: Pediatric Orthopedics Deformities. Orlando, FL, Academic Press, 2001, pp 466–469.
5. Staheli LT: Fundamentals of Pediatric Orthopedics, 3rd ed. New York, Lippincott Williams & Wilkins, 2001, p 71.
6. Benson M, Fixsen H, Macnicol M, et al: Children's Orthopaedics and Fractures. New York, Churchill Livingstone, 1994, pp 420–421.
7. Herring JA: Disorders of the knee. In: Tachdjian's Pediatric Orthopaedics, 3rd ed. Philadelphia, WB Saunders, 2002, pp 789–792.
8. Conrad JM, Stanitski CL: Osteochondritis dissecans: Wilson's sign revisited. Am J Sports Med 2003;31:777–778.
9. Pill SG, Ganley TJ, Milam RA, et al: Role of magnetic resonance imaging and clinical criteria in predicting successful nonoperative treatment of osteochondritis dissecans in children. J Pediatr Orthop 2003;23:102–108.
10. Luhmann SJ, Schootman M, Gordon JE, et al: Magnetic resonance imaging of the knee in children and adolescents. J Bone Joint Surg Am 2005;87:497–502.
11. Robertson W, Kelly BT, Green DW: Osteochondritis dissecans of the knee in children. Curr Opin Pediatr 2003;15:38–44.
12. Wright RW, McLean M, Matava MJ, et al: Osteochondritis dissecans of the knee: Long-term results of excision of the fragment. Clin Orthop 2004;424:239–243.
13. Yoshizumi Y, Sugita T, Kawamata T, et al: Cylindrical osteochondral graft for osteochondritis dissecans of the knee. Am J Sports Med 2002;30:441–445.
14. Duri ZA, Patel DV, Aichroth PM: The immature athlete. Clin Sports Med 2002;21:461–482.
15. Jakob RP, Von Gumppenberg S, Engelhardt P: Does Ogood-Schlatter's disease influence the position of the patella? J Bone Joint Surg Br 1981;63:579–582.
16. Herring JA: Disorders of the knee. In: Tachdjian's Pediatric Orthopaedics, 3rd ed. Philadelphia, WB Saunders, 2002, pp 812–813.
17. Ross MD, Villard D: Disability levels of college-aged men with a history of Osgood-Schlatter disease. J Strength Cond Res 2003;17:659–663.
18. Browner-Elhanan KJ, Small E, Coupey S, et al: Lower limb flexibility and muscle strength in Osgood-Schlatter disease. Med Sci Sports Exerc 1999;31:S359.
19. Krause BL, Williams JPR, Catterall A: Natural history of Osgood-Schlatter disease. J Pediatr Orthop 1990;10:65–68.
20. Flowers MJ, Bhadreshwar DR: Tibial tuberosity excision for symptomatic Osgood-Schlatter disease. J Pediatr Orthop 1995;15:292–297.
21. Di Gennaro S, Calvisi V, Magaletti M: Bone patellar tendon bone and ACL reconstruction in Osgood-Schlatter's disease. J Bone Joint Surg Br 2001;83(Suppl II):170.
22. McCarroll JR, Shelbourne D, Patel DV: Anterior cruciate ligament reconstruction in athletes with an ossicle associated with Osgood-Schlatter's disease. Arthroscopy 1996;12:556–560.
23. Kendall N, Hsu S, Chan K: Fracture of the tibial spine in adults and children. J Bone Joint Surg Br 1992;74:848–852.
24. Meyers M, McKeever F: Fracture of the intercondylar eminence of the tibia. J Bone Joint Surg Am 1970;52:1677–1684.
25. Gronkvist H, Hirsch G, Johansson L: Fracture of the anterior tibial spine in children. J Pediatr Orthop 1984;4:465–468.
26. Meyers M, McKeever F: Fracture of the intercondylar eminence of the tibia. J Bone Joint Surg Am 1959;41:209–222.

27. Hunter RE, Willis JA: Arthroscopic fixation of avulsion fractures of the tibial eminence: Technique and outcome. Arthroscopy 2004;20: 113–121.

28. Zaricznyj B: Avulsion fracture of the tibial eminence: Treatment by open reduction and pinning J Bone Joint Surg Am 1977;59:1111–1114.

29. Accousti WK, Willis RB: Tibial eminence fractures. Orthop Clin N Am 2003;34:365–375.

30. Kocher MS, Micheli LJ, Gerbino P, et al: Tibial eminence fractures in children: Prevalence of meniscal entrapment. Am J Sports Med 2003;31:404–407.

31. Shepley RW: Arthroscopic treatment of type III tibial spine fractures using absorbable fixation. Orthopedics 2004;27:767–769.

32. Lubowitz JH, Elson WS, Guttmann D: Part II: Arthroscopic treatment of tibial plateau fractures: Intercondylar eminence avulsion fractures. Arthroscopy 2005;21:86–92.

33. Stanitski CL: Knee trauma and epiphyseal disorders. Paper presented at the American Academy of Orthopaedic Surgeons, Review and Update for Practicing Orthopaedic Surgeons Course, November 1, 2003, Washington, DC.

34. Salter RB: Injuries involving the epiphyseal plate. J Bone Joint Surg Am 1963;45:587–622.

35. Beaty JH, Kumar A: Current concepts review. Fractures about the knee in children. J Bone Joint Surg Am 1994;76:1870–1880.

36. Stanitski CL: Physeal fractures about the knee. Paper presented at the American Academy of Orthopaedic Surgeons, Review and Update for Practicing Orthopaedic Surgeons Course, October 23, 2004, Washington, DC.

37. Ogden JA, Tross RB, Murphy MJ: Fractures of the tibial tuberosity in adults. J Bone Joint Surg Am 1980;62:205–212.

38. Reynolds R: Proximal tibia and distal femur fractures. Paper presented at the 81st AO Course, December 13, 2004, Davos, Switzerland.

CHAPTER 63

Knee Rehabilitation

Terry Malone

In This Chapter

General algorithm
Functional progression
Rehabilitation for specific conditions

INTRODUCTION

- A functional progression from lower levels of function to more demanding activities is critical.

- While protocols are helpful, flexibility is necessary according to the needs and progression of the individual patient.

- Frequent assessment drives the rehabilitation.

- Specific injuries require specialized rehabilitation, often varying by whether surgery is implemented.

- Communication with the surgeon and a consistent message to the patient are essential.

This chapter is designed to provide the reader a well-defined process of rehabilitation progression in relationship to numerous knee conditions and their corresponding interventions. Rather than attempting to go into great detail on the rehabilitation sequence for each condition outlined in previous chapters, clinical pearls or unique observations are shared regarding each major area. The term functional progression is frequently used to describe the transition of the patient from lower levels of function to higher, more demanding levels, thus enabling a return to desired activity. These progressions are provided for each condition with the unique challenges of that specific patient presentation. A key part of these progressions is that certain rules always are observed, that is, controlled actions before less controlled actions, stable before unstable, partial weight bearing before full weight bearing, thus outlining a general algorithm of progression. This concept is also a part of the required patient assessment and allows the clinician to have a linkage of assessment to rehabilitation through well-defined sequences.

One of the major advances available to clinicians today is protocol information from Web sites of universities or centers enabling a quick review of patient progressions following specific interventions. Although readily available, clinicians must be cautious in the application of these external protocols to the individual patient, not blindly accepting a time-driven approach. The best application of protocols is to use them as a general "flight plan" that may need to be altered as "weather" conditions change.

GENERAL ALGORITHM OF ASSESSMENT AND PROGRESSION

Safe progression for rehabilitation requires appropriate patient assessment to demonstrate that he or she possesses the requisite skills and is able to perform in less controlled environments or more demanding circumstances. Figure 63-1 provides an assessment algorithm that demonstrates this process.

If a patient has no major differences at the anthropomorphic level, that patient is then assessed at the strength and power level and so forth. If he or she has deficiencies (involved to uninvolved differences of greater than 10% open chain or 5% closed chain), the rehabilitation program will then be focused on this level of activities initially. This is a demonstration of how assessment and rehabilitation are linked. Patients progress in rehabilitation only after demonstrating appropriate performance through assessment.

Application of this process is seen in Figure 63-2. Functional progression in rehabilitation is an organized, sequential approach of providing incrementally increasing demands to the patient.

This type of progression attempts to mimic the multiple joint interactions and coordinated muscle activations required of skilled functional tasks. The nonathletic patient would not proceed beyond the job-related functional task level while the athlete must move onto the advanced levels to enable a safe return to the competitive environment. Importantly, the clinician selects activities for rehabilitation emphases based on the patient's performance during assessment (anthropomorphic, strength and power, or functional), which then likewise correlate with tasks within the functional progression. True progression also occurs through the clinician selecting varied cadences, intensities, and durations. Communication with a patient is facilitated by these processes as he or she can appreciate his or her inability to do an upper level task while doing relatively well on less demanding requests. Thus, assessment and rehabilitation are linked in both outcomes and applications. The remainder of this chapter provides applications of this linked process in specific entities as described in previous chapters with the adjustments required through their unique features. This includes the "special progressions" that may be required for optimal rehabilitation outcomes.

PATELLOFEMORAL CONDITIONS

While these patients are among those most common seeking orthopedic care, they are not necessarily consistently treated with the best evidence-based approaches.[1] Clinicians attempt to use a single protocol of care that often has included a focus on vastus medialis obliquus strengthening. This approach traces its

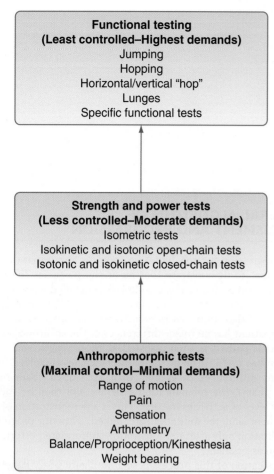

Figure 63-1 Assessment algorithm. The patient is assessed initially at the anthropomorphic level and then at more demanding levels if safe and reliable performance is observed. (Davies GD, Wilk K, Ellenbecker TS: Assessment of strength. In Malone TR, McPoil T, Nitz AJ [eds]: *Orthopaedic and Sports Physical Therapy,* 3rd ed. St. Louis, Mosby Year Book, 1997, pp 225–227.)

roots to Lieb and Perry,[2] who described the important function of the vastus medialis obliquus in patellar alignment. Unfortunately, since 1968, many patients have received terminal extension exercises to "isolate the vastus medialis obliquus" while other approaches may have been more beneficial. Recent data demonstrate that we cannot selectively train the vastus medialis obliquus but rather strengthen the quadriceps as a group.[3–5]

It is important to recognize that patellofemoral conditions are multifactorial and the assessment provides the information that allows the proper grouping of the patient into a treatment or rehabilitation protocol. Four patient groups are outlined in Figure 63-3 as a rehabilitation classification of patellofemoral patients. This process is built on assessment (allowing classification) and then the application of a specific rehabilitation protocol. The four areas are ligamentous instability, tension, friction, and compression with specific rehabilitation pearls to assist with each classification. It is important that clinicians recognize that their level of successful outcomes should be greater than 80% generally in patellofemoral patients, but not necessarily within each individual class.

The rehabilitation "protocol" for each of these classes is quite different. Tables 63-1 through 63-4 respectively outline the clinical approach for each class. This is based on the concept of what

we control as clinicians and what is affecting the patient's response to exercise. These factors are initiated through answering the question: What do we control?

The factors that we control include range of motion (ROM) of contact (patellofemoral and tibiofemoral), length of time (and) level of pressure applied to the surface, activation type,

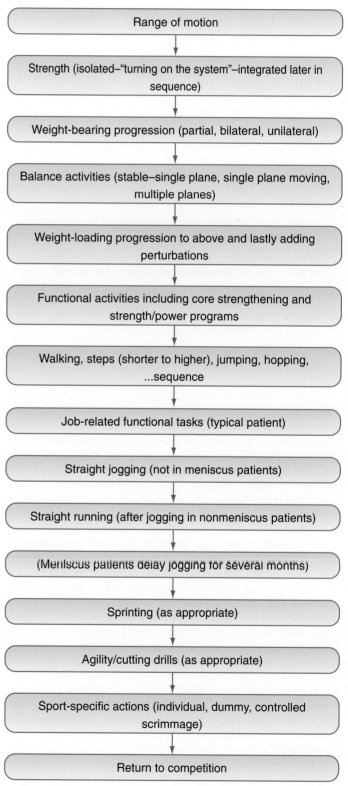

Figure 63-2 Functional progression for the lower extremity patient.

Patellofemoral patients

Assessment determines the primary factor.

Patients are then classified with:

1. Ligamentous instability (ligament incompetency/laxity)
2. Tension (inability to tolerate high loads, especially eccentric loads)
3. Friction (inability to tolerate repeated flexion/extension activities)
4. Compression (inability to tolerate compression loads, weight-bearing activities)

Figure 63-3 Patellofemoral patients.

Table 63-4 Compression Rehabilitation Pearls*

- Pain-free exercise: partial range of motion, multiple-angle isometrics
- Avoid full range of motion loaded activities that cause pain, viscolastic inserts
- Strengthen the quadriceps: open and closed chain but pain free, do not abuse the damaged surface
- High-speed isokinetics can be used (low torque and short time of loading)

*Common problems: articular defects, arthritis, abnormal muscular absorption.

Table 63-1 Ligamentous Instability Rehabilitation Pearls*

- Avoid terminal extension (patella must not laterally bias excessively)
- Exercise in the groove (lower range of motion, patella within the sulcus). Fingers, tape, brace, get the patella medial for exercise, exercise must be pain free
- Remember gluteals, adductors, and abductors
- Strengthen the quadriceps: open and closed sequences

*Common problems: patellar dislocation/subluxation, lateral instability.

Table 63-5 Articular Cartilage Rehabilitation Pearls: Nonoperative*

- Strengthen the quadriceps: open and closed chain but pain free, do not abuse the damaged surface, open lower in range of motion, closed closer to extension range of motion
- Control shear forces (use submaximal exercises, high-speed exercise, partial range-of-motion exercises, again pain free)
- Decrease maximal loads: pool programs/aquatic approach
- Walking: soft, multidensity absorbent inserts, limit fatigue, 12-minute rule
- Limit range of motion of some exercise devices (cross-country simulator and stepmachine)

*Common problem: articular abnormality.

Table 63-2 Tension Rehabilitation Pearls*

- Avoid high-speed isokinetics
- Emphasis on eccentric maximal exercise
- Use plyometrics but late in rehabilitation sequence (advance weight prior to speed)
- 10–12 week rule (it takes several weeks for eccentric program to work)

*Common problems: jumper's knee, tendonitis/tendonosis, muscle strains.

motor program/pattern selected, open/closed, shear/compression, and external modifiers (e.g., braces, tape, medications, orthotics). Each protocol is designed to optimally use these factors through an evaluation-based selection/application.

The application of this process has been described previously with a more specific listing of diagnostic classifications.[6] The categorization into four rehabilitation patterns is somewhat arbitrary and designed to illustrate the special concepts for patellofemoral patients. However, Table 63-4 (compression rehabilitation concepts) is quite reflective of the approach to patients with arthritis or articular injury. Table 63-5 presents approaches to these patients in a nonoperative situation.

ARTICULAR CARTILAGE

When surgery is performed, the rehabilitation program still is designed with the aforementioned concepts, but implementation often is dictated by the surgical impact and the patient's individual response to the intervention. Articular cartilage problems that do not respond to strengthening and the general approach outlined in Table 63-5 are extremely challenging for all concerned parties: patient, surgeon, and therapist. Surgical interventions were outlined in a previous chapter but basically include abrasion/débridement, microfracture, drilling, autograft osteochondral transplantation, allograft transplantation, autogenous chondrocyte implantation, and joint replacement. A recent

---

Table 63-3 Friction Rehabilitation Pearls*

- Avoid repetitive flexion/extension loaded patterns
- Avoid high-speed isokinetics
- Multiple-angle isometrics and partial range-of-motion exercise sequences
- Modify footwear if pronation related but remember other leg (often pronating to shorten the long leg, put heel lift under other leg)

*Common problems: plica, iliotibial band, bursal irritation.

two-part series on these topics nicely defines a treatment sequence.[7,8] Specific protocols are used with each of these, but several special pearls are provided:

1. Passive ROM can be facilitated very nicely in water and gentle assisted/active motion is easily incorporated in this medium as well.
2. It is better to protect the surface from weight-bearing loads and particularly sudden impacts longer rather than shorter time frames.
3. Patients must be able to demonstrate appropriate gait before moving from assistive devices; do not let them apply loads without muscular absorption/protection.
4. General articular surface problems may respond well to quadriceps strengthening, although the radiographic appearance is of significant involvement; we do not treat radiographs. Patients frequently will see dramatic improvements in function and pain through quadriceps strengthening while radiographs would point toward the need for surgical intervention.

MENISCAL REHABILITATION

Rehabilitation of meniscal patients includes nonoperative intervention, post partial or complete meniscectomy, and following meniscal repair. Meniscal surgery has been refined primarily with the evolution of the use of the arthroscope and the acknowledgment of the importance of the meniscus in long-term joint health. In younger patients, surgeons make every attempt to preserve as much of the meniscus as is possible when a partial meniscectomy is performed and often will use a reparative technique if success can be anticipated. These concepts are defined well in a recent publication that also includes some rehabilitation recommendations.[8]

In general terms, repair is best performed in cases in which a peripheral, longitudinal tear (such as a bucket handle) is present in the younger patient while resection is the better option in segmental nonvascularized tears. From the rehabilitation perspective, the presence of ligamentous incompetence and/or chondral injury has major implications for long-term outcome.

NONOPERATIVE TREATMENT

The traditional patient is one with joint line tenderness but no locking and exhibiting essentially a full ROM. The knee often has a small effusion and consequently a level of muscle inhibition. Weight bearing may be minimally painful, particularly near full extension.

The early rehabilitation sequence should focus on strengthening in an open kinetic chain in pain-free portions of the available range, most commonly working from 90 degrees to approximately 30 degrees, while also urging the patient to eliminate activities that result in pain. Another pearl in these patients is to use a heel lift under the involved extremity or to have the patient wear a shoe with an elevated heel (1 to 2 inch) as this minimizes the knee extension required during gait, which frequently facilitates pain-free ambulation.

PARTIAL OR COMPLETE MENISCECTOMY

When nonoperative care is unable to provide pain-free function or the knee demonstrates locking, surgical intervention is nearly

always performed using arthroscopic techniques. Following these procedures, patients should be urged to regain quadriceps control as quickly as possible. A useful treatment pearl is to initiate quadriceps contraction with the knee flexed at least 30 degrees to increase capsular volume (open pack joint position), also placing the muscle on a slight stretch to facilitate activation. The reason quadriceps activation is important relates to the ability of this muscle-tendon unit to absorb and dissipate energy during the gait cycle. Without adequate quadriceps activation, the patient may develop a chronic effusion, which makes function and continued rehabilitation difficult. With today's arthroscopic techniques, patients typically regain full motion rather easily unless they had "lived with" a limitation for a period of time prior to surgery. Patients are progressed as described in Figure 63-2 with the functional cycle being altered slightly, allowing running rather than jogging for these individuals. It has been the author's experience that running (up on the ball of the foot) helps minimize knee extension and increases the demand on the musculature to protect (absorb and dissipate loading) the joint. One of the greatest difficulties is communicating the long-term implications to these patients. Significant alterations in knee function do occur (particularly related to loading on underlying articular surfaces), thus placing them at risk of late postoperative degenerative joint disease.

Meniscal Repair

A large variety of meniscal repair techniques are available to the surgeon and are described well by Sgaglione et al.[9] Surgeons should provide the treating therapist guidelines that are based on the unique circumstances of the individual, which includes location and size of tear, method of fixation, quality of tissues, condition of articular surfaces, condition of other structures (e.g., ligamentous competence, valgus/varus orientation concerns), and concomitant surgical procedures (e.g., anterior cruciate ligament [ACL] reconstruction, articular débridement/microfracture). Although some authors have demonstrated success with early motion, weight bearing, and return to activities,[10,11] others have espoused a more controlled approach that emphasizes the individual nature of the needs of the patient and possible degenerative nature of more complex situations.[12]

Specific rules are hard to provide as all the unique features observed by the surgeon greatly affect how quickly "progression" may occur but as general rules:

1. No aggressive strengthening for 3 to 4 (or more) weeks
2. Be careful of hamstring activation tensioning the posterior medial meniscus
3. ROM is 0 to 90 degrees for 3 to 6 weeks
4. Weight bearing is in extension and protected for 3 to 4 weeks
5. Open-chain 90 to 30 degrees strengthening is often the best option for basic strength training; avoid large closed-chain loads, particularly in more flexed positions (>60 degrees)
6. Return to function when no joint line tenderness and the patient has successfully completed the Figure 63-2 progression to the required level

LIGAMENT: NONSURGICAL CONCEPTS

The most commonly used nonsurgical ligamentous approach is that devised for patients following medial collateral injury. This model of what might be termed "functional rehabilitation" for these patients emerged during the 1970s and 1980s. It is now widely accepted that the vast majority of isolated medial collateral ligament–injured patients may effectively be treated with a nonoperative approach allowing immediate controlled motion and strengthening.[13,14] It is important to note that concomitant injury to other ligaments or structures may alter the opportunity for nonoperative treatment. Typically, a phased rehabilitation approach is implemented starting with maximal protection (protected weight bearing, controlled ROM, quadriceps activation), moderate protection (normalization of gait, strengthening, full ROM), minimal protection (increase strength/power, return to work activities), and return to higher levels as in the later portions of progression as presented in Figure 63-2. Most of these patients proceed through this sequence in approximately 3 to 4 weeks with a partially torn (grade I to II) medial collateral ligament injury but take 6 or more weeks with a complete disruption (grade III). The location of the injury (femoral insertion versus tibial insertion) does affect the early phase, as some surgeons do recommend a period of immobility with grade III tibial disruptions.[15] Clinical pearls in the rehabilitation of these patients include the following:

1. When the femoral insertion is the tender site: immediate, controlled ROM and strengthening in the nonpainful portion of the ROM and protected weight bearing is the treatment of choice.
2. If the patient has posterior medial corner tenderness, have the patient wear shoes with a slight heel (1 to 2 inches) during ambulation to minimize knee extension, particularly in the early phases of rehabilitation.
3. If there are concomitant injuries, treatment may not be able to be nonoperative or of the normal progressive nature.

ANTERIOR CRUCIATE LIGAMENT REHABILITATION

Reconstructive surgery of the ACL has become one of the most common orthopedic surgical procedures performed in the United States. The surgical technique and graft sources were described in a previous chapter. The surgeon works with the patient to plan the surgery after the patient has regained his or her ROM and normalized muscular function. This may require recommending preoperative physical therapy visits if the patient appears to be having difficulty performing activities independently.

The therapist must know the type of graft and fixation used to best design the early phases of the rehabilitation program. In general terms, the normal initial progression/maximal protection phase is to achieve full extension in the immediate postoperative week, use protected weight bearing until the patient can activate the quadriceps effectively to absorb and transfer loads (1 to 3 weeks), maintain patellar mobility, regain quadriceps control, and prevent development of a chronic effusion.

The patient progresses after becoming fully weight bearing to an integrated approach of open- and closed-chain activities. Bilateral closed-chain activities progress to unilateral demands, and core strengthening is often added to be emphasized in the home exercise program. Therapists are urged to be aware of red flags such as difficulty in regaining motion, development of chronic effusion, and inability to adequately control the extremity during normal activities of daily living and functional tasks.

Readers are urged to examine the numerous protocols that are available for these procedures through university and sports medicine center Web sites. It is important to see these materials as guidelines because the unique circumstances of the patient may require adjustments, particularly if the protocol is somewhat time focused in its approach. The special clinical pearls for ACL reconstruction rehabilitation include the following:

1. Prevent problems rather than treat them whenever possible; see problems emerging and treat them early.
2. Imperative: Get extension early and in the first few days, be protective of requested function; do not "beat" a dead extremity.
3. Know which graft is used: If a hamstring graft, avoid isolated open-chain hamstrings for several weeks; if contralateral patellar tendon, implement donor site tendon program; if ipsilateral patellar tendon, get patellar mobility.
4. Quadriceps activation is facilitated by working in flexion and not attempting to activate initially in full extension.
5. Do not discard assistive device until able to activate the quadriceps effectively and demonstrate a normal gait.
6. Integrate your program; do not use just open chain or closed chain; integrate both to gain complete rehabilitation.
7. You may wish to avoid large loads in terminal extension (particularly open chain) during the initial months postoperatively.

POSTERIOR CRUCIATE LIGAMENT REHABILITATION

Although ACL injury results in significant disability and joint deterioration, posterior cruciate ligament (PCL) injury is less predictable. Some patients can function well and do not develop symptoms as they "live with" their condition, while others will develop symptoms, often after several years. ACL surgical technique has become well defined, but PCL surgery is more controversial. Nonoperative treatment of PCL disruption is still a common option as the surgical challenges have made for less predictable outcomes. Optimal surgical reconstruction of the PCL remains controversial, with tibial tunnel and inlay techniques described, along with single- and double-bundle reconstructions. Each has potential advantages, with long-term outcomes to be determined.[16,17]

Nonoperative Treatment
The normal instability seen with PCL injury is more of a straight posterior displacement that allows some compensation by the quadriceps. There is greater lateral compartment displacement that manifests as increased external tibial rotation in the PCL-deficient patient. The patients who do not do well typically develop medial compartment arthritis and patellofemoral pain. This is provided via education of the patient as the nonoperative program is instituted. A phased approach to rehabilitation is implemented with the maximal protection including: protected ROM (not greater than 0 to 60 to 70 degrees), protected weight bearing, open-chain quadriceps strengthening, no hamstring strengthening, and control of inflammation. This is followed by moderate protection including full weight bearing, full ROM, emphasis on open-chain quadriceps strengthening, pool activities (which are excellent), and avoiding large closed-chain loaded activities. A functional training program is then used after approximately 10 weeks of the foregoing programs.

Posterior Cruciate Ligament Reconstruction Rehabilitation

The special features of surgical technique make the use of the surgeon's protocol most important in these patients. The therapist and physician must be able to present the same picture to the patient to maximize outcomes. As a general rule, things are progressed more slowly than in ACL patients as the PCL grafts may have greater inherent risks of stretching or loosening, resulting in instability. The following are general guidelines for PCL reconstruction:

1. Know the surgeon and the procedure: same ideas
2. Get motion early; do not keep them in strict immobilization
3. Protected weight bearing (bilateral crutches)
4. Protected ROM, 0 to 90 degrees in first 4 to 6 weeks
5. Progression after 6 weeks in the moderate protection phase
6. Long term: avoid large loads in closed-chain exercises (e.g., leg presses, squats); always monitor for the development of arthritic change; thus, be careful with biking activities.

COMPLEX LIGAMENTOUS CONDITIONS

The patient with instability related to multiple ligament/capsule injuries is a great challenge for surgeon and therapist as outlined in a previous chapter. Certain combinations, such as ACL or PCL with posterolateral injury require surgical intervention, which make rehabilitation more difficult as the required early postoperative ROM limitations may provide a challenge to normalizing the ROM long term. Ambulatory abnormalities are often seen in these patients as they may have adopted a varus thrust gait preoperatively. A clinical pearl is to keep the knee flexed during gait by wearing a heel or heel lift under the involved extremity. In the clinic, patients may be instructed in an exaggerated form of this by walking in significant flexion (Groucho walk, as in Groucho Marx). Another activity to avoid is heavy closed-chain loading as the posterolateral corner and PCL both lead to posterior arthritic changes. Open-chain strengthening is often the modality of choice but should be limited in its ROM (typically 90 to 30 degrees) as we do not want to aggressively load the last 30 degrees of extension (thus minimizing loading to the posterolateral corner as well as minimizing possible patellofemoral reaction). Again, it is imperative for the therapist and surgeon to have strong communication and provide a unified standard of expectation. Unfortunately, some of these patients expect too much improvement and are not able to accept that there are limitations as to what level of success will be achieved following surgery and rehabilitation.

CONCLUSIONS

Rehabilitation of patients with knee conditions has greatly evolved through the past 25 years. Evidence of clinical and functional improvement is readily available, particularly as it relates to specific conditions. The use of a structured assessment integrated with a functional progression is very appropriate in most nonsurgical patients. A key to success in the more complex situations is the communication between the physician and therapist as they must be certain to provide a consistent message reinforced by each during their interactions with the patient. The functional progression approach is still used with these more challenging patients but with the recognition of special limitations and also expected outcomes following certain interventions.

REFERENCES

1. Malone T, Davies G, Walsh WM: Muscular control of the patella. Clin Sports Med 2002;21:349–362.
2. Lieb FJ, Perry J: Quadriceps function: An anatomic and mechanical study using amputated limbs. J Bone Joint Surg 1968;50:1535–1548.
3. Bolgla L, Malone T: Exercise prescription and patellofemoral pain: Evidence for rehabilitation. J Sport Rehabil 2005;14:72–88.
4. Powers CM, Landel R, Perry J: Timing and intensity of vastus muscle activity during functional activities in subjects with and without patellofemoral pain. Phys Ther 1996;76:946–955.
5. Powers CM, Ward SR, Frederickson M, et al: Patellofemoral kinematics during weight-bearing and non-weight-bearing knee extension in persons with lateral subluxation of the patella; a preliminary study. J Orthop Sports Phys Ther 2003;33:677–685.
6. Wilk KE, Davies GJ, Mangine RE, Malone TR: Patellofemoral disorders: A classification system and clinical guidelines for nonoperative rehabilitation. J Orthop Sports Phys Ther 1998;28:307–322.
7. Alford JW, Cole BJ: Cartilage restoration, part I: Basic science, historical perspective, patient evaluation, and treatment options. Am J Sports Med 2005;33:295–306.
8. Alford JW, Cole BJ: Cartilage restoration, part II: Techniques, outcomes, and future directions. Am J Sports Med 2005;33:443–460.
9. Sgaglione NA, Steadman JR, Shaffer B, et al: Current concepts in meniscus surgery: Resection to replacement. Arthroscopy 2003;19(Suppl 1):161–188.
10. Mariani P: Accelerated rehabilitation after arthroscopic meniscal repair. Arthroscopy 1997;13:731–736.
11. Barber F: Accelerated rehabilitation for meniscus repairs. Arthroscopy 1997;13:206–210.
12. Tenuta J, Arciero R: Arthroscopic evaluation of meniscal repairs: Factors that effect healing. Am J Sports Med 1994;22:797–802.
13. Vailas AC, Tipton CM, Matthes RD, et al: Physical activity and its influence on the repair process of medial collateral ligaments. Connect Tissue Res 1981;9:25–31.
14. Woo SL-Y, Orlando CA, Gomez MA, et al: Tensile properties of the medial collateral ligament as a function of age. J Orthop Res 1986;4:133–139.
15. Shelbourne KD, Patel DV: Management of combined injuries of the anterior cruciate and medial collateral ligaments. J Bone Joint Surg Am 1995;77:800–806.
16. Noyes FR, Medvecky MJ, Bhargava M: Arthroscopically assisted quadriceps double-bundle tibial inlay posterior cruciate ligament reconstruction. Arthroscopy 2003;19:894–905.
17. Dennis MG, Fox JA, Alford JW, et al: Posterior cruciate ligament reconstruction: Current trends. J Knee Surg 2004;17:133–139.

In This Chapter

INTRODUCTION

- Soft-tissue injuries of the thigh and leg, while not receiving the attention or requiring operative intervention as often as joint injuries, can still be a significant cause of morbidity and lost playing time for the athlete.

- The leg is the weight-bearing structure that is the critical column on which balancing and locomotion depend. Any kinematic or kinesiologic compromise may cause significant impact.

- We briefly address some of the more commonly seen injuries, mention some of the less prevalent syndromes, and discuss the etiology, evaluation, treatment plans, and prognosis as indicated. With the recent trend of increased sports-mindedness of those of all ages, you will likely see variations of the spectrum of these injuries.

- A working cognition of the anatomy, biomechanics, and athletic kinesiology will aid the thought process as you consider how sport-specific injuries are incurred and related.[1]

THIGH

Quadriceps Contusion

These injuries are most commonly seen in contact sports. In the United States, quadriceps contusions are typically seen in football where the helmet of a tackler hits a running back in the anterior thigh. The thigh pads are specifically designed to absorb this injury, but sometimes players do not like to wear them (against regulations) because they feel that they slow them down or they may slide off to one side. Quadriceps contusions cause immediate muscular damage,[2] intramuscular bleeding, and pain. With severe injuries, the patient may be unable to continue playing. The trainer will typically place an Ace bandage around the thigh, an ice bag, and another Ace bandage over that, trying to apply compression and ice in order to avoid the development

of a large hematoma and decrease the swelling. Depending on the position of the knee at contact and the degree of involvement, flexion (and/or extension) deficits may develop. The degree of difficulty with postinjury range of motion, most specifically regaining flexion, is a significant prognostic indicator.[3] The amount of flexion at 48 hours after injury was found by Jackson and Feagin[3] to be a predictor of and guide to rehabilitation prognosis and progression. The ice can be removed after about 20 minutes and reapplied every 2 hours. Radiographs are usually not needed immediately. They may be helpful after several weeks to evaluate for myositis ossificans. Immobilization in as much flexion as comfortable for the first 24 hours using an adjustable hinged knee brace may help maintain range of motion. Heat and ultrasound are not used in the initial phase. After the initial injury phase[2] and swelling are resolved, the range of motion is gently reestablished without undo stressing of the extensor muscle mass. This may be begun in the inflammatory stage and continued through remodeling.[4] Ice massage and soft-tissue techniques are used to try to mobilize the knee and reestablish dynamic functionality of the quadriceps musculature.

A progressive resistance exercise program may be undertaken when 90 degrees of flexion is obtained. Prognostic factors include regaining a range of motion of at least 45 degrees of flexion in the first 3 weeks.[5] The trainer or therapist needs to be careful with regard to aggressively trying to establish range of motion, as scarring and increased contracture have been noted with aggressive or manipulative attempts to regain knee flexion. Generally, the prognosis is good with return to play at 2 to 3 weeks when the athlete passes isokinetic and functional testing, although in severe cases, it may take several months.

The overall outlook for functional return is good, and the risk of myositis ossificans is proportional to the amount of bleeding and degree of the original injury.[1] If myositis ossificans becomes a significant factor, range of motion may be more difficult to obtain and the patient may develop a hard mass in that area on a long-term basis. Increased or specialized padding to protect that area for future contact may be appropriate. Excision of myositis ossificans deposits has met with limited success. Compartment syndrome after thigh contusion has been reported, and this entity is discussed later.

Myositis Ossificans

Myositis ossificans is the ossification caused by the osteogenic progenitor cells released in the periosteal soft tissue with bleeding and hematoma formation (Fig. 64-1). The mass effect it has on the quadriceps muscle after maturation is usually the only sequelae of formation.[3] It is commonly painless, unless reinjured by contusion, but may not decrease in size with time. After ath-

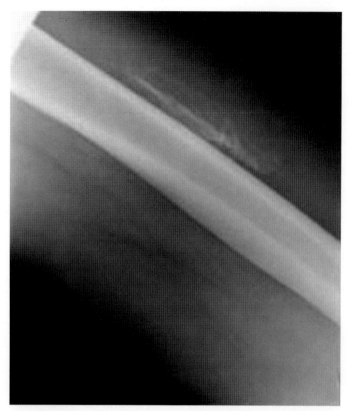

Figure 64-1 Myositis ossificans after a quadriceps contusion.

letic thigh contusion, the incidence of myositis ossificans is 9% to 20%.[5]

Radiographic maturation is usually seen at approximately 4 to 6 months. If a biopsy is performed to rule out osteosarcoma, the biopsy specimen should come from the mature periphery. Serial radiographic follow-up is usually adequate without biopsy. Rarely is the athlete symptomatic or is excision indicated. Increased or specialized padding to protect that area for future contact may be appropriate. If excision is undertaken, it must be done after the bony mass has matured or recurrence may be an issue. Prophylactic treatment with indomethacin postoperatively is recommended.

Rhabdomyolysis

Rhabdomyolysis is a disease process whereby damage sustained by the muscle fibers leads to the dissolution of the compromised structural components of the muscle fibers of the involved area. The subsequent elimination of the waste products released can be toxic to the kidneys and can lead to renal failure. Rhabdomyolysis is seen after crushing injuries and contusions but has been reported after extreme overuse episodes such as heavy or maximized weight training. It may be seen as well with compartment syndrome.

The patient usually presents with acute pain and swelling in the thigh or involved area. Urine output may decrease with darkening of the urine as the renal involvement becomes more apparent. Laboratory studies will show increased myoglobin in the blood and urine. Fluid support and alkalinization of the patient's urine is initiated to maintain output, which is monitored with a Foley catheter in a hospital setting. This syndrome usually develops over a period of several hours. The patient's condition will deteriorate unless the syndrome is recognized and the afore-

mentioned medical intervention is undertaken. Medical support is usually adequate for management with resolution of rhabdomyolysis, but, depending on the cause, appropriate compartment release or débridement may also be needed.

Compartment Syndrome of the Thigh

Compartment syndrome of the thigh can also be seen on a rare occasion after extensive workouts or contusion to the anterior thigh.[6] Symptoms are similar to those in the leg as outlined later in this chapter, which is more commonly seen. A high index of suspicion is needed when pain out of proportion to any injury is reported. Other signs include paresthesias and severe pain with passive motion or stretch of the muscles in the involved compartment. Treatment includes catheter pressure monitoring and fasciotomies as indicated. Compartment pressures[7] of more than 30 mm Hg or within 30 of the diastolic blood pressure have both been used as thresholds for considering compartment fascial releases. The thigh has anterior, posterior, and medial compartments. The anterior and posterior compartments can usually be released from a lateral incision. The medial compartment often does not need to be released, and some surgeons will do the lateral incision, release the anterior and posterior compartments, and then check the medial compartment by palpation to see if it is soft.

Muscle Strains

"Pulled" muscles are a common occurrence on the athletic field.[8,9] These strains are a physiologic failure of the musculotendinous unit to remain in complete functional continuity. Tissue tension failure can occur at the origin or insertion, muscle belly, and, most commonly, at the musculotendinous junction. Failure may be graded by the degree of involvement of the acting cross-sectional area damaged. The usual mechanism is an overwhelming extension force on an eccentrically contracting muscle.[10,11] Warm-up programs may have a preventive effect.[12] Treatment is similar to that outlined for a thigh contusion and initially includes rest, ice, compression, and elevation (RICE). Magnetic resonance imaging (MRI) may be helpful to delineate degree of damage. Healing and rehabilitation progress through the three stages of tissue injury, inflammation, and remodeling.[3] The different muscles typically involved are discussed.

Hamstring Strain

Hamstring strains are most commonly seen[13] and especially occur in those sports requiring sprinting or jumping. These muscles (long head of the biceps femoris, semimembranosus, semitendinosus) cross two joints so they are susceptible to fast, heavy loads. Strain location can be an avulsion at the origin on the ischial tuberosity. A mid-substance muscular strain is occasionally seen, but failure is most commonly at the musculotendinous junction, at the junction of the middle and distal thigh. The lateral hamstrings are more commonly involved than the medial hamstrings. Poor flexibility and fatigue have been implicated.[9] Pain, a pop, or a tearing sensation is usually acutely felt during a jumping or running activity. This most commonly occurs during eccentric contraction of the muscle. There are acute pain and swelling. The degree of strain may be classified as in Table 64-1.[14] If the tear is severe with a major portion of the substance involved, a gap or mass may be palpable. This is most easily checked with the athlete lying prone and the knee flexed to about 90 degrees with slight resistance. If the tear is contained within the fascial constraints of the belly, ecchymosis may not be appreciated. However, if the fascial sheath is vio-

Table 64-1 Hamstring Strain Classification	
Grade I	Small disruption of structural integrity at musculotendinous junction
Grade II	Partial tear, some musculotendinous fibers remain intact
Grade IIIA	Complete rupture of musculotendinous unit
Grade IIIB	Avulsion fracture at tendon's origin or insertion site

From DeLee JC, Drez D: DeLee & Drez's Orthopaedic Sports Medicine: Principles & Practice, 2nd ed. Philadelphia, WB Saunders, 2003, pp 1487–1488.

lated, blood and ecchymosis will usually appear subsequently in the dependent portion of the leg. Immediate care is icing, compression wrapping, and limitation of activities (RICE) with immobilization/crutches as needed. Rehabilitation by the trainer or therapist typically has an acute injury phase, a healing phase with stretching, and a return to activity phase with return to play in a few days to several weeks depending on the degree of strain (Table 64-2).[15] Suspected complete tears may be evaluated by MRI, and reattachment of avulsions at the ischial tuberosity has been described. Steroid injections for recalcitrant enthesopathic-type partial tears at the ischial tuberosity may give successful long-term symptomatic relief. If return to activity has been attained, it is important that the athlete continue with a regular stretching program to avoid recurrent injury. Return to play usually is determined by functional evaluation by the team trainer for sprinting and jumping.

Quadriceps Strain
Quadriceps strains are less common. The rectus femoris is usually involved. This may be because it acts across two joints. Isolation testing of the rectus femoris involves changes in the examination at varying degrees of hip extension. The quadriceps muscle typically works as an antagonist to the hamstrings. Again, injury is usually focused at the musculotendinous junction, but more proximal tears have been described.[16] Treatment algo-

Table 64-2 Hamstring Treatment Protocol[6]
Phase I
Rest, ice, compression, elevation (RICE)
Phase II
Ice, stretch, NSAIDs, electrical stimulation, isometrics ± isotonics, condition
Phase III
Ice, stretch, NSAIDs ± electrical stimulation, isotonics ± isokinetics,* condition
Phase IV
Ice, stretch, isokinetics,* running, sport-specific training
Phase V
Return to sports

NSAIDs, Nonsteroidal anti-inflammatory drugs.
*Concentric high speeds at first, proceeding to eccentric slow speeds.
From DeLee JC, Drez D: DeLee & Drez's Orthopaedic Sports Medicine: Principles & Practice, 2nd ed. Philadelphia, WB Saunders, 2003, pp 1487–1488.

rithms are similar to those for the hamstrings, but with severe injuries progress may be slower secondary to painful weight acceptance. Conservative care with rehabilitation is successful in the vast majority of patients. Bicycling is often helpful to restore endurance and eliminate fatigue, weakness, and deficits. Most athletes can return to play in 2 to 6 weeks. Neoprene sleeves or shorts may provide symptomatic support. Surgery for proximal tears of the indirect head of the rectus or acute complete tears at the musculotendinous junction[16] and chronic attritional microtears with lengthening[17] and extension lag has been described.

Adductor Strain
Adductor strains are a significant cause of lost playing time for athletes in sports that require pushing off from side to side (e.g., skating, baseball, soccer). "Groin pulls" are usually of the adductors (mainly the proximal musculotendinous area of the longus) and pectineus. Preparticipation stretching is the key to prevention. Palpation of the painful structure and increased pain with passive stretching aid in diagnosis. Inguinal hernia should be ruled out by physical examination. "Sports hernias"[18] or inflammation/enthesopathy at the insertion on the pubis may be the cause of recalcitrant cases. MRI may be helpful in cases where localization is difficult or treatment is not causing resolution as expected. Treatment is similar to that outlined for hamstring and quadriceps strains, and future preventive stretching is essential to avoid falling into a pattern of recurrent injury. Obturator nerve entrapment may mimic a groin strain but will usually have accompanying symptoms of paresthesias of the inner upper thigh. Surgery for chronic adductor tendonitis has been described.[19] Surgery is also considered for acute, complete avulsion injury. However, conservative care allows resolution and return to play in a few weeks in the vast majority of patients.

Femoral Stress Fractures: Shaft
Stress fractures of the femoral neck are more commonly seen and are described in Chapter 44. Stress fractures of the femoral shaft[20] are occasionally seen and have the typical dull, aching pain seen with other stress fractures that increases with activity and resolves with rest. Usually, a history of changes in training, intensity, or frequency can be elicited from the athlete. Stress fractures are a sign of trabecular bony compromise in the attempt to balance bone remodeling due to unusual loads. Clinical tests as simple as levering the femur over an object (fulcrum test) have been used (Fig. 64-2).[21] Bone scan or MRI is used as a diagnostic test. Rest or change of activity level or type will typically allow resolution of symptoms. Pool running can aid in maintaining conditioning with a return to activity in 2 to 4 months.

Saphenous Nerve Entrapment
Saphenous nerve entrapment is a rarely seen pain syndrome. The patient will describe paresthesias in a distribution along the saphenous nerve that can fluctuate with activities or exertion. The nerve can be entrapped in Hunter's canal or the fascial soft tissue on the medial aspect of the thigh. Using Tinel sign to locate the involved area has been helpful as well as a diagnostic (and sometimes therapeutic) injection[22] with local anesthetic and a corticosteroid. Release of the nerve from the involved area has been reported with satisfactory results. This is a syndrome that needs to be considered for nonspecific medial distal thigh pain of undetermined cause. Involvement including compression of the superficial femoral artery in the adductor canal (Hunter's)

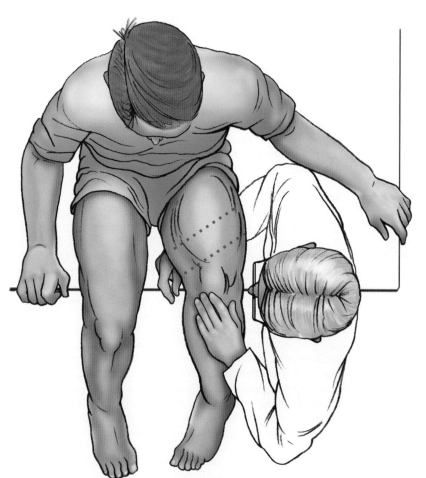

Figure 64-2 The fulcrum test with the examiner's arm (fulcrum) moved proximally under the thigh. Pain develops when the arm is placed directly under a stress fracture of the femoral shaft and gentle pressure is applied to the dorsum of the knee. (From Johnson AW, Weiss CB, Wheeler DL: Stress fractures of the femoral shaft in athletes-more common than expected. A new clinical test. Am J Sports Med 1994;22:248–256.)

has also been reported.[23] Vascular occlusion type of symptoms may be reported, and surgical release has been described.

LEG

Compartment Syndrome of the Leg
Acute

Acute compartment syndrome of the leg is usually caused by injury: bony, muscular, or vascular. This discussion deals mostly with acute compartment syndrome due to muscular contusion and hematoma or bleeding as seen in sports injuries. The pathophysiology is similar to compartment syndrome seen with high-energy bony or vascular injury as seen in a traumatic scenario. This includes increased fluid and pressure contained within the fascial envelope to such a degree that ischemia ensues. A high index of suspicion is necessary. Careful monitoring for pain with passive range of motion and checking compartment pressure measurement is appropriate. Guidelines for compartment pressure indications for fasciotomies vary significantly in the literature, anywhere from 30 mm Hg below diastolic blood pressure to any measurement above a threshold pressure of 30 mm Hg. Treatment for acute compartment syndrome includes fascial release on an emergent basis. This typically involves the anterior and lateral compartments and is done in an open fashion through longitudinal incisions on the lateral[24] and, if needed, medial aspects of the leg. There are four anatomic compartments in the leg: anterior, lateral, superficial posterior, and deep posterior (Fig. 64-3).[24] The lateral incision is used to identify the intermuscular septum and decompress the anterior and lateral compartments. The fascia is opened anterior and posterior to the

septum, with care to avoid the superficial peroneal nerve. It is important in doing the release to make certain the entire length of the compartment tightness is released as anatomy can vary and some people have tight areas at the far proximal and distal extremes. Lateral release is usually adequate depending on the area and involvement. If needed, a medial incision is used to release the posterior compartments. This incision is at the posterior aspect of the tibia to release the superficial compartment. By following the posterior aspect of the tibia to the intermuscular septum and dissecting just behind that septum, a careful release of the fascia proximally and distally is performed, thereby releasing the deep posterior compartment. Typically, this provides a visible softening of the compartments, and the wounds are then covered with gauze and later wet-to dry dressings are applied. Delayed primary closure or skin grafting is done at approximately 5 days after the initial swelling has resolved.

Chronic Exertional Compartment Syndrome

Chronic exertional compartment syndrome has symptoms similar to those of the acute entity but to a lesser degree and is a more difficult diagnosis to make. Patients typically complain of aching pain or paresthesias (and occasionally vascular complaints) after exercises that stress or challenge the leg muscles.[25] Runners complain of insidious pain that begins to limit their activity level. Symptoms originate after beginning activity, and typically resolve after 10 to 30 minutes upon completing the activity. Symptoms most commonly occur in the anterior and lateral compartments. Anterior compartment symptoms include paresthesias in the first web space. Recent studies outlining vascular flow as well as MRI findings in exertional compartment

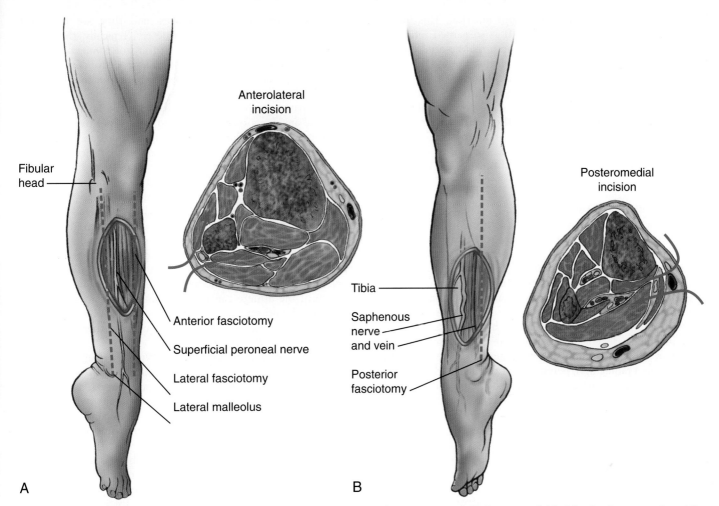

Figure 64-3 A, Anterolateral incision for decompression of the anterior and lateral compartments. **B,** Posteromedial incision for decompression of the superficial and deep posterior compartments. (From Mubarak SJ, Owen CA: Double-incision fasciotomy of the leg for decompression in compartment syndromes. J Bone Joint Surg Am 1977;59:184–187.)

syndrome have been used to noninvasively evaluate this syndrome. Pre- and postexercise MRI changes in blood flow or fluid in the involved area have been documented, but results of MRI in diagnosing this entity have been equivocal. Invasive catheter measurements for significant increases in pressure postexercise have also been used.[26] This is more invasive but currently more reliable and reproducible. After the diagnosis has been made, for symptoms that are significant and recalcitrant to conservative care, release of the involved (typically the anterolateral) compartments has been described. This can be done using a large or small open[24] approach as previously described or a percutaneous endoscopic approach.[27] This includes three small skin incisions and subcutaneous evaluation of the fascia with use of an endoscope to delineate the intermuscular septum and the fascia anteriorly and posteriorly for release (Fig. 64-4).[27] This minimizes the invasiveness with regard to the skin incisions and has been reported to have satisfactory success (approximately 90%). Return to play is typically in a few weeks.

Medial Gastrocnemius Strain (Tennis Leg)

Medial gastrocnemius strain, or tennis leg, is a syndrome in which a sudden vigorous load causes pain and often a tearing sensation in the upper calf. Pathophysiology is an eccentric

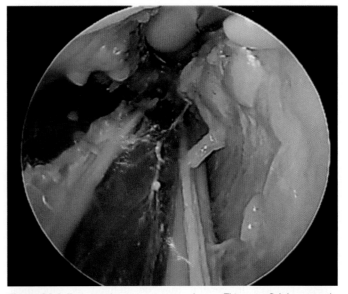

Figure 64-4 Endoscopic compartment release. The superficial peroneal nerve is seen centrally.

loading failure at the musculotendinous junction. This muscle spans both the knee and the ankle. It is so named tennis leg because it is commonly encountered in a middle-aged individual during the push-off phase while playing tennis.[28] Swelling and sometimes ecchymosis are seen. Seldom is a major defect palpated, but often there may be acute or chronic slight muscle mass loss in that area. Concomitant acute compartment syndrome has been reported.[29] As with other muscular strains, the phases of injury, inflammatory healing, and remodeling occur as a rehabilitation course is undertaken. Resolution of symptoms and no significant loss in functional performance are the typical course.

Contusion of the Anterior Tibia

Rarely, blows to the tibia may cause a fracture. Much more commonly, these contusions cause a painful soft-tissue injury. This type of injury is seen in youth soccer or sports in which direct blows to the subcutaneous border of the anterior tibia causes hematoma formation. If the hematoma is subperiosteal, it causes severe pain and may result in a significant bony prominence in that area as it consolidates. The use of shin guards for soccer serves to almost eliminate this unless the shin guards are too short, in which case, contusions above the level of the shin guard can occur. While it is impossible to definitively rule out a fracture without a radiograph, percussion of the heel and gentle torsional stressing by rotating the foot may be helpful. Palpation of the noninvolved posteromedial aspect of the tibia may be nontender, thus supporting absence of a fracture. The contusion injury resolves with conservative care, and symptoms are in large part in proportion to the amount of bleeding. Careful padding speeds return to play and any resulting osseous prominence may be permanent.

Shin Splints or Medial Tibial Stress Syndrome

Shin splints is a catch phrase for pain in the medial tibial area, usually with overuse activities. Multiple causes[30] have been proposed. Soft-tissue sources have been implicated, with tendonitis or periostitis due to overload or unbalanced tendon effects. These can be due to biomechanical sources, such as a foot or ankle malalignment. Poor balancing of the gastrocsoleus posteriorly, the posterior tibialis medially, the anterior tibialis anteriorly, or the peroneals laterally may cause symptoms. The most commonly accepted source of shin splints is a periosteal reaction due to stressing of the insertional fascial areas from the gastrocsoleus or posterior tibialis. Tenderness is elicited by palpation of a length of the involved tibia. Careful evaluation[11] of shoes, feet, ankle, tendons, lower extremity alignment, and gait as well as training history should allow changes that will bring symptomatic relief. Orthotics may help with hyperpronation. Rest until symptoms resolve, followed by pool running and bicycling, which may aid conditioning, are recommended until return to play. Surgery has been mentioned for recalcitrant symptoms.[31] Radiographs may show a periosteal reaction. A bone scan[32] may rule out a transverse osseous involvement (i.e., stress fracture) versus the linear periostitis reaction seen with shin splints.

Tibial Stress Fracture

A tibial stress fracture is another source of leg pain in the athlete. Stress fractures in general may be defined as subclinical microfractures that progress to become symptomatic and may even result in a displaced fracture when improperly treated. In the tibia, they are relatively common, representing approxi-

mately 17% of all stress fractures, and they are the most common stress fracture in the athlete.[33] Typically, they occur posteriorly in the proximal or distal third of runners and tend to heal with rest.[34] However, they may also occur in other sports and, more significantly, may occur at the anterior mid-diaphysis where healing is less predictable.[35]

Most patients present with a characteristic history. The leg pain is of insidious onset, associated with repetitive activities, and relieved by rest. Running and jumping sports are most often affected, including track, basketball, volleyball, dance, and football. While the cause is not completely clear, there is an obvious association with overuse. Thus, the athlete may describe an increase in training frequency or intensity, a change of shoes or practice surface, or another variation that could lead to excess biomechanical stresses. At the time of presentation, most often the pain has been present for weeks to months and sometimes even years. The pain may initially occur only after strenuous exercise, later becoming present even with simple walking. It may fluctuate with athletic seasons or gradually worsen with time until the athlete can no longer participate in sports. The examiner should obtain a history regarding amenorrhea in the female, thyroid disease, nutritional deficits, or other factors that may influence bone health.

On physical examination, there is typically point tenderness only at the fracture, with relatively normal surrounding soft tissues. In contrast, shin splints are tender over a larger extent of the medial tibia. Symptoms of paresthesias, weakness, or motion restriction are generally absent. Some authors describe the use of tuning forks or distant bony percussion as pain reproductive methods.

Imaging studies include radiography, bone scan, computed tomography, and MRI. Radiographs are generally normal for the first few weeks and may take months to show typical abnormalities, which include periosteal reaction, cortical lucency, sclerosis, or even a distinct fracture line. The anterior tibial stress fracture is recognized by its characteristic "dreaded black line": on a lateral radiograph, this is a thickened area of anterior cortex in the middle third of the tibia with a distinct radiolucent line extending anterior to posterior (Fig. 64-5). While both bone scan and MRI are more sensitive than radiography, a bone scan is thought to be the more sensitive of the two, especially early in the disease course. In fact, it can continue to be positive long after clinical symptoms have resolved and should therefore not be used to monitor healing. The advantages of MRI include its noninvasive nature, ability to visualize soft-tissue pathology, and higher specificity.

Treatment of tibial stress fractures depends on location. As stated previously, they most commonly occur on the compressive side of the bone (posterior), typically posteromedially, at the proximal and distal thirds of the bone. Treatment with nonsteroidal anti-inflammatory drugs, ice, physiotherapy, and activity modification generally reduces symptoms within 1 month and allows full sports participation by 3 months. Activity modification includes complete rest until pain free, cross-training, or restriction from running and jumping. Use of a long pneumatic splint has been reported to allow continued sports participation and symptom resolution within a month.[36]

Treatment of anterior tibial stress fractures is far more controversial. While most authors continue to recommend a trial of conservative treatment, it is well established that, without surgery, the healing rate of these fractures is significantly lower. In addition, the risk of progression to complete fracture is a real, albeit undefined, risk. A review of the literature revealed 15

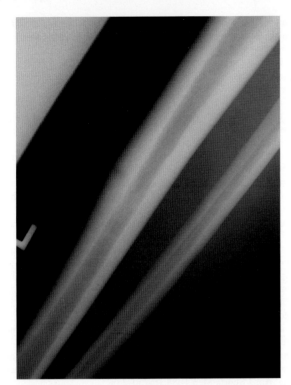

Figure 64-5 Anterior tibial stress fracture, the "dreaded black line."

documented stress fractures progressing to complete fracture.[37] Both physician and athlete alike should be aware of this possibility and its consequences should the athlete be allowed to continue play prior to documented healing. This same review noted that of 73 attempts at conservative treatment, only 20 (27%) went on to radiographic healing. Surgical treatment has varied widely, including nonunion excision and bone grafting, intramedullary nailing, and plating. Of 57 surgical interventions reported in the literature, 32 (56%) had documented healing within 6 months. Many athletes were able to return to play prior to radiographically proven healing. In general, for patients with a radiographically apparent stress fracture of the anterolateral tibia, early surgery is commonly now employed. The most common surgical treatments are reamed intramedullary nailing and compression plating.

Proximal Tibial-Fibular Joint Pain

While not common, inflammation or instability of the proximal tibia-fibula articulation is occasionally seen.[38] Symptoms along the interosseous area may be localized to the proximal tibia-fibular junction. Often instability is difficult to identify and symptoms are limited to tenderness or slight swelling in that area. Cysts around the joint may also be symptomatic.

Peroneal nerve irritation just posterior to the fibular head may be evaluated using Tinel's test. Testing the anterior and lateral muscles by resisted dorsiflexion and eversion of the foot will stress the tibial-fibular joint and sometimes elicit symptoms, including pain and popping or shifting in that area. Plain radiographs, fluoroscopy, computed tomography scan, and MRI may be useful, but are frequently normal. A diagnostic/therapeutic injection of local anesthetic and corticosteroid can also be used. Treatment is generally conservative, but surgical stabilization has been described in recalcitrant cases, when instability of the joint is present.

Nerve Entrapment

Nerve entrapments in the leg, similar to those previously described for the thigh, can include medially branches of the saphenous nerve, anterolaterally the peroneal[39] or superficial peroneal nerve,[40,41] and laterally the sural nerve. These are all described in rare cases. Localized areas of possible constriction are best identified by a positive Tinel sign along the course of the involved nerve. A diagnostic and potentially therapeutic injection of local anesthetic and corticosteroid may be helpful, especially if surgical release of constricting fascial soft tissue is considered.[41]

Vascular Entrapment

Vascular compression entities such as popliteal artery entrapment[40] and effort-induced venous thrombosis have been described. Popliteal artery entrapment reportedly causes intermittent claudication, and symptoms may be mimicked by passive dorsiflexion of the foot and checked by Doppler or radiographic studies. Effort-induced venous thrombosis may involve the upper or lower extremity. Diagnosis is confirmed by venous Doppler ultrasonography.

Muscle Herniation

In the thigh and more commonly in the leg, aching symptoms may be due to muscle herniation through a defect in the encompassing fascial sheath. These defects can be congenital, spontaneous, or post-traumatic. Herniation sometimes can be grossly seen or palpated. Appreciation may be enhanced with positioning or stressing the muscle belly. MRI or ultrasonography may also be helpful in delineating areas of involvement. The most commonly encountered area of involvement is in the anterolateral distal leg, where the superficial peroneal nerve exits the fascia. If conservative treatment is ineffective, surgery to enlarge the fascial defect (fasciotomy) is performed, eliminating the small confined defect through which the underlying muscle can herniate.

REFERENCES

1. Fu FH, Stone DA: Sports Injuries: Mechanisms, Prevention and Treatment. Baltimore, Williams & Wilkins, 1994.
2. Crisco JJ, Jokl P, Heinen GT, et al: A muscle contusion injury model: Biomechanics, physiology and histology. Am J Sports Med 1994;22:702–710.
3. Jackson DW, Feagin JA: Quadriceps contusions in young athletes: Relation of severity of injury to treatment and prognosis. J Bone Joint Surg Am 1973;55:95–105.
4. Noonan TJ, Garrett WE: Muscle strain injury: Diagnosis and treatment. J Am Acad Orthop Surg 1999;7:262–269.
5. Ryan JB, Wheeler JH, Hopkinson WJ, et al: Quadriceps contusions, West Point update. Am J Sports Med 1991;19:299–304.
6. Colosimo AJ, Ireland ML: Thigh compartment syndrome in a football athlete: A case report and review of the literature. Med Sci Sports Exerc 1992;24:958–963.
7. Whitesides TE, Haney TC, Morimoto K, et al: Tissue pressure measurements as a determinant for the need of fasciotomy. Clin Orthop 1975;113:43–51.
8. Garrett WE: Muscle strain injuries. Am J Sports Med 1996;24:S2–S8.

9. Mair SD, Seaber AV, Glisson RR, et al: The role of fatigue in susceptibility to acute muscle strain injury. Am J Sports Med 1996;24:137–143.

10. Garrett WE, Nikolaou PK, Ribbeck BM, et al: The effect of muscle architecture on the biomechanical failure properties of skeletal muscle under passive extension. Am J Sports Med 1988;16:7–12.

11. Viitasalo JT, Kvist M: Some biomechanical aspects of the foot and ankle in athletes with and without shin splints. Am J Sports Med 1983;11:125–130.

12. Styf J: Entrapment of the superficial peroneal nerve. J Bone Joint Surg Br 1989;71:131–135.

13. Clanton TO, Coupe KJ: Hamstring strains in athletes: Diagnosis and treatment. J Am Acad Orthop Surg 1998;6:237–248.

14. Zarins B, Ciullo JV: Acute muscle and tendon injuries in athletes. Clin Sports Med 1983;2:167–182.

15. DeLee JC, Drez D: DeLee and Drez's Orthopaedic Sports Medicine: Principles and Practice, 2nd ed. Philadelphia, WB Saunders, 2003, pp 1487–1488.

16. Hughes C, Hasselman CT, Best TM, et al: Incomplete, intrasubstance strain injuries of the rectus femoris muscle. Am J Sports Med 1995;23:500–506.

17. Temple HT, Kuklo TR, Sweet DE, et al: Rectus femoris muscle tear appearing as a pseudotumor. Am J Sports Med 1998;26:544–548.

18. Meyers WC, Foley DP, Garrett W, et al: Management of severe lower abdominal or inguinal pain in high-performance athletes. Am J Sports Med 2000;28:2–8.

19. Akermark C, Johansson C: Tenotomy of the adductor longus tendon in the treatment of chronic groin pain in athletes. Am J Sports Med 1992;20:640–643.

20. Hershman EB, Lombardo J, Bergfeld JA: Femoral shaft stress fracture in athletes. Clin Sports Med 1990;9:111–119.

21. Johnson AW, Weiss CB, Wheeler DL: Stress fractures of the femoral shaft in athletes: More common than expected. Am J Sports Med 1994;22:248–256.

22. Romanoff ME, Cory PC, Kalenak A, et al: Saphenous nerve entrapment at the adductor canal. Am J Sports Med 1989;17:478–481.

23. Balaji MR, DeWeese JA: Adductor canal outlet syndrome. JAMA 1981;245:167–170.

24. Mubarak SJ, Owen CA: Double-incision fasciotomy of the leg for decompression in compartment syndromes. J Bone Joint Surg Am 1977;59:184–187.

25. Fronek J, Mubarak SJ, Hargens AR, et al: Management of chronic exertional anterior compartment syndrome of the lower extremity. Clin Orthop 1987;220:217–227.

26. Pedowitz RA, Hargens AR, Mubarak SJ, et al: Modified criteria for the objective diagnosis of chronic compartment syndrome of the leg. Am J Sports Med 1990;18:35–40.

27. Ota Y, Senda M, Hashizume H, et al: Chronic compartment syndrome of the lower leg: A new diagnostic method using near-infrared spectroscopy and a new technique of endoscopic fasciotomy. Arthroscopy 1999;15:439–443.

28. Leach RE: Leg and foot injuries in racquet sports. Clin Sports Med 1988;7:359–370.

29. Straehley D, Jones WW: Acute compartment syndrome (anterior, lateral, and superficial posterior) following tear of the medial head of the gastrocnemius muscle. Am J Sports Med 1986;14:96–99.

30. James SL, Bates BT, Osternig LR: Injuries to runners. Am J Sports Med 1978;6:40–50.

31. Detmer DE: Chronic shin splints. Classification and management of medial tibial stress syndrome. Sports Med 1986;3:436–446.

32. Rupani H, Holder L, Espinola D, et al: Three-phase radionuclide bone imaging in sports medicine. Radiology 1985;156:187–196.

33. Morris JM, Blickenstaff LD: Fatigue Fractures: A Clinical Study. Springfield, IL, Charles C Thomas, 1967.

34. Devas MB: Stress fractures of the tibia in athletes or "shin soreness." J Bone Joint Surg Br 1958;40:227–239.

35. Rettig AC, Shelbourne KD, McCarroll JR, et al: The natural history and treatment of delayed union stress fractures of the anterior cortex of the tibia. Am J Sports Med 1988;16:250–255.

36. Dickson TB: Functional management of stress fractures in female athletes using a pneumatic leg brace. Am J Sports Med 1987;15:86–89.

37. Hurt JH, Mair SD: Anterior tibial stress fracture: A systematic review of the literature. 2006 (In press).

38. Ogden JA: Subluxation and dislocation of the proximal tibiofibular joint. J Bone Joint Surg Am 1974;56:145–154.

39. Leach RE, Purnell MB, Saito A: Peroneal nerve entrapment in runners. Am J Sports Med 1989;17:287–291.

40. Lysens RJ, Renson LM, Ostyn MS, et al: Intermittent claudication in young athletes: Popliteal artery entrapment syndrome. Am J Sports Med 1983;11:177–179.

41. Safran MR, Garrett WE, Seaber AV, et al: The role of warm-up in muscular injury prevention. Am J Sports Med 1988;16:123–129.

In This Chapter

Ankle
Hindfoot
Midfoot
Forefoot
Special tests

INTRODUCTION

- Accurate diagnosis of foot and ankle pathology requires a careful, systematic approach.

- Knowledge of the fundamental biomechanics of the foot is essential in making a correct diagnosis.

- This chapter describes the foot and ankle examination with regard to the athlete, making mention of relevant biomechanics when necessary.

INSPECTION

The foot and ankle physical examination begins with a thorough visual inspection. Begin by noting the athlete's training shoes if possible. The size, type, and condition of the shoe should be appropriate for the training being done. The force across the foot for each foot strike is approximately 3 times the body weight during running, occurring approximately 3000 times every mile for the average jogger.[1] Obviously, a shoe's ability to absorb force is critical for injury prevention. After 500 miles, remember that a shoe retains less than 60% of its cushion.[2] Also, note any abnormal wear patterns. Normally, the heel has a slight tendency to have more wear laterally. Excessive medial sole wear along the heel may indicate overpronation. In a similar fashion, a large degree of distal sole wear over the metatarsals can indicate an equinus contracture or may simply be secondary to the athlete's normal running style. Comparison with the other shoe is helpful, especially if complaints are unilateral and the shoe wear is not symmetric.

Next, make sure that both legs are visible from the knee down. The patient should begin standing, first facing away from and then toward the examiner. As always, throughout the examination, compare any findings with the contralateral side to check for asymmetry. Note the alignment of the hindfoot. As viewed from behind, the heel should be neutral (Fig. 65-1). In addition, provided the knees both face directly forward, the same number of toes should be visible on the lateral side. With

pes planus conditions (e.g., posterior tibialis dysfunction), an increased number of toes will be seen on the lateral side. This "too many toes" sign is usually accompanied by a valgus position of the heel. On double heel rise, the hindfoot should move into a position of relative varus (Fig. 65-2). Failure to do so is most often consistent with a posterior tibialis tendon dysfunction. Likewise, inability to perform a single heel rise (while keeping the knee in extension) may indicate the same pathology of the Achilles tendon-gastrocsoleus complex, or a bony abnormality. If a varus position of the hindfoot is noted on initial examination, a Coleman lateral block test should be performed (see later discussion).

Next, the patient should face the examiner. Note overall alignment of the hind-, mid-, and forefoot and the status of the midfoot arch. The talar head may be abnormally protruded medially with a flatfoot deformity. Crossover and hammer toes, hallux valgus, and other distal pathology are best observed in a weight-bearing position. Finally, have the patient walk while carefully watching symmetry, ability to achieve a plantigrade foot, avoidance patterns, and flow of the stance phase (heel strike to toe off).

Inspect the feet as the athlete sits on the examination table. Take note of calluses on the side and undersurface of the foot. Note areas of swelling and contusion and reinspect the arch for comparison with the weight-bearing state. An arch that remains flat even while non-weight bearing may indicate a fixed deformity such as a tarsal coalition.

EXAMINATION

Hindfoot

Palpation should begin at nontender areas to maintain a relaxed, compliant state. Progression to areas of tenderness can help lead to a provisional diagnosis (Figs. 65-3 and 65-4). In the posterior hindfoot, examine the heel cord for continuity, tenderness, and swelling. Achilles tendonitis may present with simply pain or may have associated tendon enlargement. Try to distinguish between tenderness in the tendon itself and pain located more anterior in the retrocalcaneal bursa. In addition, Haglund's or "pump-bump" deformity will present as a painful bony prominence of the posterior superior calcaneal process (Fig. 65-5). When symptomatic, it usually results in tenderness proximal and lateral to the Achilles tendon insertion. A calcaneal stress fracture may be differentiated from these latter entities by compressing the medial and lateral calcaneal surfaces between the bases of the hands, causing pain when the test is positive. In late childhood and early adolescence, Sever's disease (calcaneal apophysitis) usually presents with tenderness more distal than the Achilles tendon insertion, at the most posterior and plantar

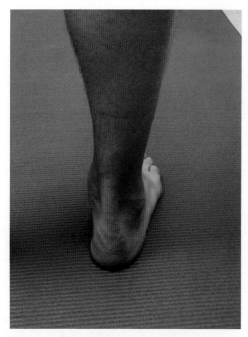

Figure 65-1 Neutral hindfoot.

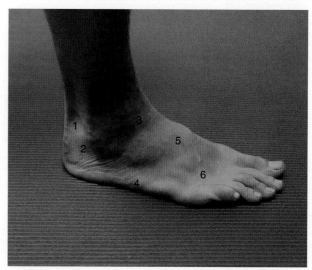

Figure 65-3 Lateral side of the foot/ankle. Areas of tenderness correspond to the following diagnoses: 1, retrocalcaneal bursitis; 2, peroneal tendonitis; 3, anterior ankle joint line synovitis; 4, fifth metatarsal base fracture; 5, navicular stress fracture; 6, Morton's neuroma.

aspect of the calcaneus. On both the lateral and medial hindfoot, tendon sheaths may be identified and then palpated along their course. For instance, instruct the patient to evert the foot in order to tense the peroneal tendons for identification. Pain with resisted eversion as well as localized peroneal tendon tenderness helps to diagnose peroneal tendonitis. This method of examination may be repeated for all tendons in the foot, including the flexor hallucis longus, flexor digitorum longus, and posterior tibialis tendons on the medial hindfoot. Furthermore, in the case of the peroneal tendons, specific signs of tendon subluxation may be sought as indicated. Test by palpating the

tendons as they pass posterior to the lateral malleolus and have the patient actively move the foot from a position of inversion to eversion. When the test is positive, the examiner will feel the tendons snap over the bone. Occasionally, resisted eversion will be necessary to elicit tendon subluxation.

Ankle

Next inspect the ankle joint proper. The medial and lateral malleoli, anterior tibiotalar joint line, and the regions of the deltoid, anterior talofibular (ATFL), and calcaneofibular (CFL) ligaments are all readily available to direct palpation, thus facil-

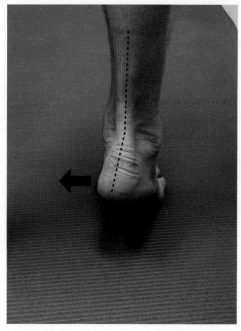

Figure 65-2 Single heel rise with hindfoot inversion.

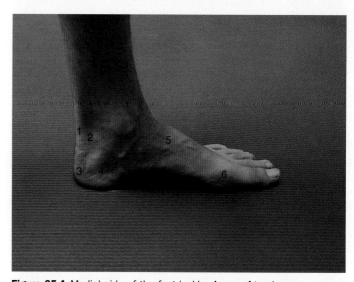

Figure 65-4 Medial side of the foot/ankle. Areas of tenderness correspond to the following diagnoses: 1, Achilles tendonitis; 2, retrocalcaneal bursitis; 3, calcaneal apophysitis; 4, calcaneal stress fracture; 5, tibialis posterior tendonitis/symptomatic accessory navicular; 6, bunion.

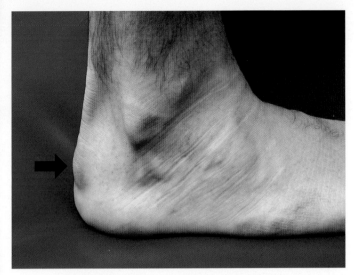

Figure 65-5 Haglund's deformity (pump bump).

itating diagnosis. For instance, tenderness to touch over only the ATFL and not the lateral malleolus helps differentiate an ankle sprain from a fracture. Care must also be taken to distinguish tenderness over the ATFL from a painful sinus tarsi, as can occur with sinus tarsi syndrome. When an isolated syndesmotic injury (i.e., high ankle sprain) is suspected, perform the squeeze test by compressing the tibia and fibula at the junction of the middle and distal thirds to reproduce the pain, or, alternatively, dorsiflex and externally rotate the foot while stabilizing the leg at the knee. The resulting torque on the lateral malleolus will cause pain if the syndesmosis is injured.

The tibiotalar joint itself should be examined along the anterior joint line where painful spurs can develop, by plantar flexing the ankle and directly palpating the talar dome (to evaluate for osteochondral injury), and by differentiating soft-tissue edema from effusion. Check for an ankle effusion by simultaneously compressing the anteromedial (medial to the tibialis anterior tendon) and anterolateral clear spaces (lateral to the extensor digitorum longus tendon). A distinct fluid wave will be felt when an effusion is present. In addition, the foot is generally held in a slightly plantar-flexed position to relieve intra-articular pressure. Last, painful plantarflexion-dorsiflexion or inversion-eversion of the hindfoot will help differentiate tibiotalar versus subtalar joint pathology, respectively.

Midfoot

The midfoot joints should be manipulated to check for inflammation. Simply stabilize the hindfoot with one hand and move the forefoot in a circular motion. Follow this up with joint specific palpation including the talonavicular, calcaneocuboid, naviculocuneiform, and tarsometatarsal joints. On the medial side, specifically examine for tenderness over the navicular bone itself (to rule out a stress fracture) as well as at its medial border. This is where both the posterior tibialis tendon inserts and a symptomatic accessory navicular is located. On the lateral midfoot, be sure to check for tenderness over the insertion of the peroneus brevis at the proximal fifth metatarsal. Pain here could be indicative of avulsion fracture, tendonitis, or a symptomatic os peroneum. This should be differentiated from a fifth metatarsal stress fracture (e.g., Jones fracture), which will typically be tender just distal to the metaphysis.

Forefoot

In the forefoot, palpate the metatarsal heads and necks for excessive tenderness to diagnose lesser metatarsal overload (as may occur after bunion surgery) or metatarsal stress fractures, respectively. The pain from an interdigital neuroma (i.e., Morton's neuroma) is similar in location but localized specifically between metatarsal heads, most often the third interspace. Mediolateral compression of the metatarsal heads may produce a click (Mulder's click) and generally reproduces the pain of a Morton neuroma, sometimes requiring 20 to 30 seconds of constant pressure. Special attention should be paid to the first metatarsophalangeal (MTP) joint. Hallux rigidus often presents with painful first MTP motion (especially dorsiflexion) and a tender, prominent dorsal spur. Likewise, an obvious hallux valgus deformity (i.e., bunion) will typically be quite tender over the prominent medial first MTP joint line. If there is concern for hallux rigidus, perform the grind test, which entails simultaneous compression and circumduction of the first MTP. Reproduced pain and crepitus is a positive indicator of first MTP osteoarthritis. Lesser MTP synovitis may be diagnosed by direct superior-inferior joint line compression. This condition may also have painful hyperlaxity in the superior-inferior plane. Grasp the proximal phalanx and the corresponding metatarsal head and reciprocally translate up and down; excessive motion combined with pain will often be present.

The toes should be separated to visualize painful corns and calluses, and ingrown toenails should be easily distinguished from other sources of discomfort. Common toe deformities include hammer, mallet, and claw toes. A hammer toe entails a neutral or extended MTP joint, a flexed proximal interphalangeal (PIP) joint, and an extended distal interphalangeal (DIP) joint. Often, a painful callous is present on the dorsal skin of the PIP. The second toe is most often affected (due to its longer length), and it is uncommon to find multiple hammer toes on the same foot. A mallet toe presents as a neutral MTP joint, a neutral or extended PIP joint, and a flexed DIP joint. Finally, a claw toe has a flexion deformity at both the PIP and DIP joints. A tender callus generally occurs at the dorsal PIP, similar to a hammer toe. Multiple claw toes are most commonly due to long-term use of shoes that are too constrictive, although other etiologies such as Charcot-Marie-Tooth or MTP inflammatory disease should be considered.

Plantar Surface

The plantar surface of the foot should likewise be specifically palpated. In the hindfoot, a painful heel pad should be differentiated from plantar fasciitis. The latter typically has tenderness at the anteromedial border of the calcaneus, whereas the former is more painful in the center of the fat pad. Warts may be distinguished from calluses by their punctate bleeding when shaved, greater tenderness with side-to-side (versus direct) compression, and the absence of skin wrinkles passing through their substance. On the plantar surface of the first MTP, the sesamoids should be examined for point tenderness as may occur with sesamoiditis or fracture. The plantar surface of the first MTP will similarly be tender after turf toe in which the plantar capsule has been injured or disrupted.

Functional Range of Motion

Normal values for joint range of motion can be found in Table 65-1. Start by evaluating the heel cord and gastrocsoleus complex (GSC) for excessive tightness. Passively dorsiflex the foot while the knee is flexed and note the motion. Then pas-

Table 65-1 Normal Joint Range of Motion[5]

Ankle	20 degrees of dorsiflexion	50 degrees of plantarflexion
Subtalar	20 degrees of inversion	10 degrees of eversion
First MTP	70 degrees of dorsiflexion	45 degrees of plantarflexion

MTP, metatarsophalangeal.

sively extend the knee while holding the foot dorsiflexed. Because the GSC crosses the knee and ankle joints, when tight, it will force the foot into relative plantarflexion as the knee extends (Figs. 65-6 and 65-7). A supple GSC is essential for prevention of multiple foot injuries including bunions, forefoot overload, and tendonitis. At least 10 degrees of ankle dorsiflexion is required during the support phase of running.[3]

The tibiotalar joint should then be checked for range of motion while the knee is flexed (to eliminate the GSC contribution). To evaluate the subtalar joint, first place the ankle in a plantigrade position, locking the talus in the ankle mortise. Then passively invert and evert the hindfoot. It is normal to have twice as much inversion. The subtalar joint is critical for accommodating uneven surfaces, and lack of motion here may indicate a tarsal coalition or fibrosed joint as may occur in late stages of posterior tibialis dysfunction. In the midfoot, examination for excessive plantar-dorsal motion (more than approximately 1 cm) of the first tarsometatarsal joint is useful in making treatment decisions for bunions.[4] Similarly, the first MTP should be checked to ensure motion, particularly full, painless dorsiflexion that may be limited by hallux rigidus or turf toe.

Neurovascular Examination

In most athletes, the neurovascular examination will be relatively normal. However, it is still important to verify, particularly with an established diagnosis of diabetes.

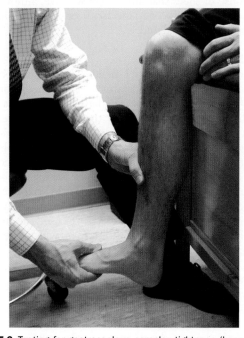

Figure 65-6 Testing for gastrocsoleus complex tightness (knee flexed).

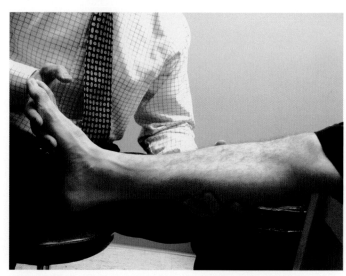

Figure 65-7 Testing for gastrocsoleus complex tightness (knee extended). Note relative plantarflexion of the foot indicating a tight gastrocsoleus complex.

Neurologic Examination

Knowledge of the foot and ankle neuroanatomy is helpful in combining physical examination findings to make a diagnosis. Initial evaluation begins with testing patients for sensation to light touch. If further investigation is indicated, a 5.07 Semmes-Weinstein monofilament should be used to test sensation.[6] Diabetics and others with distal neuropathies unable to feel this monofilament are thought to be below the threshold for protective sensation and at high risk of neuropathic ulceration. Occasionally, an isolated decrease in sensation may be present in the plantar aspect of toe web spaces with corresponding interdigital neuromas. This finding is highly specific when present.[4] To distinguish diffuse distal neuropathy from a superficial peroneal nerve palsy, note that in the latter, the foot dorsum will be numb except for first web space sparing (innervated by branches of the deep peroneal nerve). In patients with previous foot surgery, signs of peripheral nerve injury should be sought. These include point tenderness over a possible neuroma, percussion-induced paresthesias, and anesthesia distal to the suspected injury.

All motor units should be checked for strength with standard 0 through 5 grading. Most of the muscle units may be checked with simple manual resistance. For instance, to check the posterior tibialis and accessory foot invertors, have the patient actively invert the foot and then resist that force with the examiner's hand. Compare with the contralateral side if normal. Not only will this help determine strength and neurologic function, but pain reproduced only with resisted active motion (i.e., not with passive motion) is indicative of pathology in the musculotendinous unit being tested. Two special circumstances should be noted. First, testing of the peroneus longus is not intuitive. To check strength for this tendon, have the patient perform resisted plantar flexion of the first ray (the primary function of the peroneus longus). Second, the GSC is generally too strong to be tested by hand. Even a deficient GSC can typically overcome manual resistance without detection of weakness. Instead, have the patient perform multiple single-limb heel rises and compare with the contralateral side to identify deficits. If any part of the neurologic examination is abnormal, a thorough neurologic assessment should be performed to check for possible etiologies in the proximal leg or the CNS.

Vascular Examination

This generally involves palpation of the dorsalis pedis pulse (just proximal and lateral to the first metatarsal base) and the posterior tibial pulse (approximately 1 cm posterior to the medial malleolus). If pulses are absent or diminished, a full vascular assessment including Doppler pulse pressure measurements is indicated.

SPECIAL TESTS

Thompson Test

The Thompson test is designed to diagnose an Achilles tendon rupture. Have the patient lie prone on the examining bed with the feet dangling off the end. Start with the normal side by squeezing the calf musculature and noting the normal, brisk plantarflexion of the foot. Next, perform the same maneuver on the leg in question. The test is positive for a rupture if absent (or significantly diminished) plantarflexion is noted. In this case, a palpable defect is usually present in the Achilles tendon (Fig. 65-8).

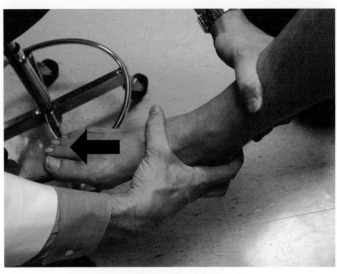

Figure 65-9 Anterior drawer test.

Coleman Lateral Block Test

During examination, if a hindfoot varus deformity is found (as can occur with Charcot-Marie-Tooth disease), it is important to determine whether it is fixed or flexible. The Coleman lateral block test, designed to answer this question, is performed by having the patient stand on a block (approximately 1 inch high) with support under only the heel and lateral metatarsals. Specifically, the first metatarsal is permitted to plantarflex freely. If the deformity is flexible, the hindfoot will correct from a position of varus to neutral. If it is fixed, it will remain in varus, significantly influencing treatment options.

Anterior Drawer Test

After an ankle sprain, the anterior drawer test is used to evaluate the integrity of the ATFL and, to a lesser extent, the CFL. It is most useful in cases of suspected chronic ankle instability. Brostrom[7] showed that this test's sensitivity was relatively low in the acute setting secondary to guarding. First, have the patient relax the affected extremity with the knee flexed. Then, stabi-

lize the leg with one hand while grasping the heel with the other hand and applying an anterior force to affect anterior talar translation. Perform in both plantarflexion (tests ATFL) and dorsiflexion (tests CFL). A few millimeters of movement is normal, and variation among different individuals can be significant. Comparison to the contralateral side is thus essential (Fig. 65-9).

Talar Tilt Test

Similar to the anterior drawer test, the talar tilt test is used in cases of suspected chronic ankle instability. However, it differs from the drawer test by examining primarily the CFL instead of the ATFL. Again, with the patient relaxed and the knee flexed, stabilize the leg with one hand and grasp the heel with the other. Then, with the foot first dorsiflexed (for CFL examination) and then plantarflexed (for ATFL examination), invert the hindfoot. Excessive motion may indicate instability of the tibiotalar joint, subtalar joint, or both (Fig. 65-10).

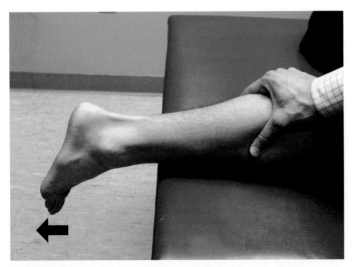

Figure 65-8 Thompson test. Absent or diminished plantarflexion indicates Achilles tendon rupture.

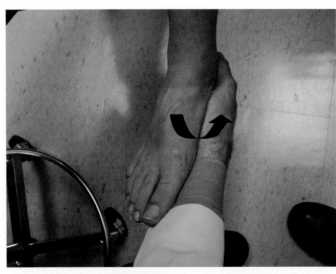

Figure 65-10 Talar tilt test.

REFERENCES

1. Southmayd W, Hoffman M: Sports Health: The Complete Book of Athletic Injuries. Quick Fox, 1981.
2. Barber FA, Sutker AN: Iliotibial band syndrome. Sports Med 1992;14:144–148.
3. James SL: Running injuries to the knee. J AAOS 1995;3:309–318.
4. Alexander IJ: The Foot: Examination and Diagnosis. New York, Churchill Livingstone, 1997.
5. Sammarco GS: Foot and Ankle Manual. Baltimore, Williams & Wilkins, 1998.
6. Brodsky W: Outpatient diagnosis and care of the diabetic foot. Instruct Course Lect 1993;42:121–139.
7. Brostrom L: Sprained ankles: III Clinical observations in recent ligament ruptures. Acta Chir Scand 1965;130:560–569.

Ankle Ligament Injury and Instability

Jeffrey D. Willers and Robert B. Anderson

In This Chapter

INTRODUCTION

- Ankle sprains are among the most common athletic injuries.

- The majority of ankle sprains involve the lateral ligament complex.

- Chronic instability is a relatively common sequelae.

- Associated injuries are common with acute lateral ligament injury and should be considered when symptoms persist.

- Rehabilitation generally allows return to sport.

- In chronic cases, surgical reconstruction of the lateral ligaments is considered.

Ankle sprains are the most common sports-related and recreational injury, representing an estimated 40% of all athletic injuries.[1] Ankle sprains comprise an especially significant percentage of injuries in selective sports: 45% to 53% of all basketball injuries, 21% to 31% of soccer injuries, and 10% to 15% of football injuries that result in time lost.[2,3] Jackson et al[4] likely reported the truest incidence of ankle injuries in an athletic population in a study of U.S. Military Academy cadets. This study found that approximately one third of all cadets will sustain an ankle injury requiring medical treatment during their 4-year term at the Academy.

The vast majority (approximately 75%) of ankle sprains involve injury to the lateral ligament complex. The medial ligaments, however, are infrequently injured with eversion injuries. These medial injuries are rarely isolated injuries but instead usually occur in conjunction with lateral ankle injury or fracture.[5] The anterior portion of the deltoid ligament is most frequently injured. An in-depth discussion of medial ligament injury and instability is beyond the scope of this chapter; thus, we focus on lateral ligament injury and instability.

Although most ankle sprains do heal with conservative treatment, it has been estimated in multiple studies that long-term sequelae do occur in a significant percentage of patients (up to 50%).[6–9] Chronic instability has been reported to occur in 20% to 42% of patients with acute ankle sprains.[10,11]

RELEVANT ANATOMY

Lateral ankle stability is provided by both static and dynamic restraints. Both the lateral ligaments and the bony configuration of the ankle afford static restraint. The peroneal tendons supply the ankle's primary dynamic restraint. The bony configuration of the talus contributes approximately 30% of the resistance to rotational forces about the ankle, whereas soft tissues provide the remaining 70%.[12]

The talus has a flare in its anterior half, which provides significant bony restraint to lateral motion when the talus is engaged in the mortise with the ankle in dorsiflexion. As the talus plantarflexes, the narrower surface of the talus moves into the mortise, resulting in a marked reduction of bony stability and increased susceptibility of the ankle to inversion injury.

The lateral ligaments of the ankle are comprised of three main bands (Fig. 66-1): the anterior talofibular ligament (ATFL), the calcaneofibular ligament (CFL), and the posterior talofibular ligament (PTFL). The ATFL is a thickening of the anterior capsule that courses anteromedially from its origin on the distal anterior tip of the lateral malleolus to insert on the talar body just anterior to the lateral articular surface of the talus. The ATFL is the weakest of the lateral ankle ligaments.[13] The CFL is a round (6 to 8 mm in diameter) ligament that originates from the lower anterior border of the lateral malleolus and courses obliquely in a posteromedial direction across both the tibiotalar and subtalar joints to insert on the lateral surface of the calcaneus.[14] The CFL imparts stability to both the tibiotalar and subtalar joints. The CFL acts as the floor of the peroneal sheath; thus, injury to the CFL is frequently associated with disruption of the peroneal sheath and infrequently with a tear of the peroneal tendons. Last, the PTFL runs horizontally from its origin on the posterior margin to the lateral malleolus to the posterolateral tubercle of the talus.

The lateral ligament complex functions as a unit during ankle motion to provide stability. In the neutral position the ATFL is relaxed, but its strain increases significantly as the ankle moves into plantarflexion. The CFL is relaxed in the neutral position and under significantly increased strain as the ankle is dorsiflexed.

The tibiotalar joint is inherently stabilized with stance (loading) due to the configuration of the mortise and the normally valgus positioned hindfoot. Subtalar joint stability is not enhanced by loading but instead relies completely on the ligamentous complex. It is for this reason and the fact that the CFL

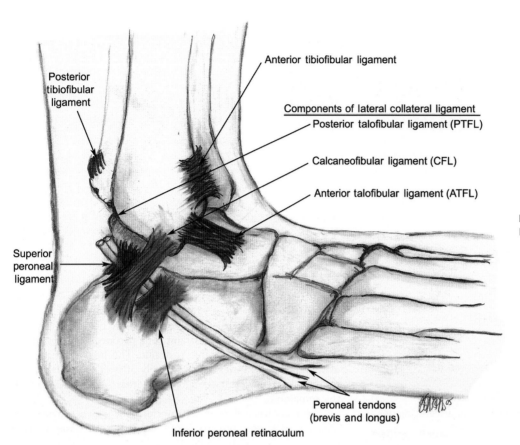

Anterior tibiofibular ligament

Posterior tibiofibular ligament

Components of lateral collateral ligament
Posterior talofibular ligament (PTFL)

Calcaneofibular ligament (CFL)

Anterior talofibular ligament (ATFL)

Superior peroneal ligament

Peroneal tendons (brevis and longus)

Inferior peroneal retinaculum

Figure 66-1 Essential anatomy of the lateral ligament complex of the ankle.

imparts stability across both joints that we often consider the presence of combined instability patterns.

ACUTE LATERAL ANKLE INJURY

Clinical Features and Evaluation
An acute injury to the ankle ligaments is generally apparent from the patient's history. The patient typically complains of lateral ankle pain and swelling following a forced plantarflexion and inversion injury. Frequently, the history will include a "pop" or "snap" during the traumatic event, but this does not appear to correlate with severity or with long-term sequelae.[15]

Proper examination should include evaluation of range of motion, swelling, tenderness, and stability. The area of maximal swelling and tenderness is usually indicative of the area of ligament injury; the ATFL is most frequently injured at its fibular origin and the CFL at its calcaneal insertion.

Additionally, lateral ligament injuries are commonly categorized by severity into three grades (Table 66-1).[16]

Many associated injuries can be found in patients with acute lateral ankle injury (Table 66-2).[17] These should all be considered when evaluating the patient and thorough examination performed to rule out occult injury.

Diagnostic Studies
Although radiographs are frequently obtained in the evaluation of ankle pain, they are often not necessary for the evaluation of ankle sprains. The Ottawa Ankle Rules was developed to establish criteria for performing radiographs.[18] According to the Ottawa Ankle Rules, radiographs are necessary only with (1) bony tenderness at the posterior edge or tip of either malleolus,

(2) inability to bear weight immediately following the injury and for four steps in the emergency department, or (3) bony tenderness at the base of the fifth metatarsal. These criteria reduce the number of unnecessary radiographs without reducing the sensitivity for diagnosing fractures (remains at nearly 100%).[18] If indicated, standard radiographs should include three views of the ankle (anteroposterior, lateral, and mortise).

The role of stress radiographs of the ankle remains controversial. While numerous articles cite parameters of "significant" instability, the anterior drawer and talar tilt stress radiographs have not been shown to be reliable in diagnosing instability and we have not found them helpful in our decision making process.

Magnetic resonance imaging also has a role in the evaluation of select acute ankle injuries. This sensitive test can be benefi-

Table 66-1 Acute Lateral Ankle Injury Grading

Grade	Ligament Involvement	Physical Examination
I	Ligament stretch, no tear	Minimal swelling, mild tenderness, no instability, can weight bear
II	Torn ATFL, intact CFL	Moderate swelling and tenderness, difficulty with weight bearing
III	Complete tear of both ATFL and CFL	Marked swelling, diffuse tenderness, inability to bear weight

ATFL, anterior talofibular ligament; CFL, calcaneofibular ligament.

Table 66-2 Potential Associated Injuries with Acute Lateral Ankle Ligament Injury

Ligamentous Injuries
Hindfoot sprain
Midfoot sprain (Lisfranc)
Bony Injuries/Fractures
Malleoli (medial, lateral, or posterior)
Anterior process of calcaneus
Base of fifth metatarsal
Lateral posterior talar process
Proximal fibula
Midtarsal
Osteochondral Lesions
Talus (usually posterolateral or anteromedial)
Distal tibia
Tendon Injuries
Peroneal brevis
Peroneal longus
Peroneal instability/retinacular tear
Os peroneum syndrome
Neurapraxic Injuries
Superficial peroneal nerve
Sural nerve

cial if the clinician suspects associated injuries or, more subacutely, if the recovery is not following the typical course of recovery.

Treatment Options

Patients with grade I or II ankle injuries respond well to conservative treatment.[10,19] A functional treatment protocol is initiated that consists of several phases (Table 66-3). Treatment immediately following the injury consists of RICE (rest, ice, compression, and elevation) with the goal to reduce swelling, hemorrhage, and pain.

During the 1- to 3-week period (proliferation phase), protection in the form of taping or bracing should be used. Weight bearing should be initiated as soon as it is tolerated as it is considered beneficial to the healing process.

Table 66-3 Functional Rehabilitation Program

Stage		Time After Injury	Treatment
1	Acute injury phase	Immediate	RICE (rest, ice, compression, elevation)
2	Proliferation phase	1–3 wk	Protection with tape or brace
3	Maturation	3–6 wk	Controlled stretching and range of motion
4	Remodeling	6–8 wk until 6–12 mo	Continued motion and strengthening with goal of full return to activity

At approximately 3 weeks following injury, ankle mobilization is initiated through gentle range-of-motion and controlled stretching. When pain-free range of motion and weight bearing have been established, strengthening and proprioception training can begin; timing of this varies depending on severity of the injury.

Multiple studies have compared functional treatment/early protected mobilization with both cast immobilization and acute surgical repair (including a large meta-analysis by Kannus and Renstrom[20]). Functional treatment results in a more rapid recovery of ankle mobility and an earlier return to work or physical activity without sacrificing mechanical stability.[21,22] Additionally, if a patient does fail initial nonoperative treatment, delayed reconstruction can be performed even several years following the injury with comparable results to primary repair.

CHRONIC LATERAL ANKLE INSTABILITY

Clinical Features and Evaluation

Patients with isolated chronic lateral ankle instability typically presents with complaints of periodic "giving way" and a history of several previous severe ankle sprains. Although these intermittent episodes are typically associated with a brief period of pain and dysfunction, most patients with isolated instability are essentially pain free between episodes and do not experience mechanical symptoms. If pain is present between episodes of giving way, secondary diagnoses must be considered (Table 66-4).[23]

Table 66-4 Lesions to Consider in Patients with Persistent Symptoms and Chronic Lateral Ankle Instability

Bone
Anterior process of calcaneus fracture
Lateral/posterior talar process fracture
Malleolar fracture
Base of fifth metatarsal fracture
Anterior ankle bony impingement
Tarsal coalition (osseous or fibrous)
Ligament
Subtalar instability
Syndesmosis injury
Medial ankle instability
Tendon
Peroneus longus or brevis tear
Peroneal instability/superior peroneal retinacular injury
Painful os peroneum syndrome (POPS)
Cartilage
Osteochondral lesions of talus or tibia
Neural
Neurapraxia of sural or superficial peroneal nerve
Soft Tissue
Anterolateral ankle soft-tissue impingement
Sinus tarsi syndrome

A complete physical examination of the ankle should include assessing the joint above (knee) and below (subtalar). Lower extremity alignment should also be assessed; hindfoot varus predisposes the ankle to inversion injury. Hindfoot/midfoot mobility should also be evaluated, as it is not uncommon for tarsal coalition to present as recurrent ankle sprain.

The peroneal tendons should also always be assessed as they can also be injured. Peroneal examination should involve an assessment of eversion strength, stability of the tendons in the fibular groove, and tenderness and swelling along the course of the tendons.

The anterior drawer test evaluates the integrity of the ATFL by assessing the amount of anterior translation of the talus with respect to the tibia. This test is properly performed with the patient sitting, the knee flexed 90 degrees, and the ankle positioned in 10 degrees of plantar flexion. The tibia is stabilized while an attempt is made to draw the talus forward. A positive drawer is defined as greater than 5 mm more than the contralateral side or absolute value of 10 mm of translation.[24-26] The quality of the endpoint is also noted. A positive test is only significant if it correlates with the history; Brostrom and Sundelin[7] found that only one half of those with a positive anterior drawer had symptomatic instability.

The talar tilt test is another common test performed. This test, first described by Faber in 1932, is performed by grasping the calcaneus and talus in one hand while stabilizing the distal tibia in the other. The calcaneus and talus are then inverted. Increased talar tilt, when compared with the contralateral side, indicates rupture of both the CFL and ATFL. Debate remains on what constitutes physiologic tilt; Cox[27] reports the normal range of tilt values between 5 and 23 degrees.

Nonoperative Treatment Options

As with treatment of acute lateral ankle injuries, functional treatment remains the mainstay of initial treatment for chronic lateral instability. Functional treatment protocols emphasize stretching, muscle strengthening (particularly peroneal), and proprioception.[28] Prior to considering surgery, most agree that a trial of a minimum of 6 weeks of aggressive physical therapy should be attempted.

Shoe wear modifications or orthotic devices can be used for flexible foot and ankle malalignment and instability. Most patients with lateral ankle instability, particularly those with dynamic supination, will benefit from an external lateral heel wedge.

External stabilization of the ankle by taping or braces is also employed. Taping demonstrates excellent initial support, but the amount of support decreases substantially with time, with a 50% reduction at 10 minutes[29,30] and no support after 1 hour of exercise.[31] A wide variety of commercially available ankle braces exists. These braces consist of rigid or flexible materials in combination with special systems of straps.

Surgical Treatment Options

If symptomatic instability persists despite an adequate functional rehabilitation program and bracing, lateral ligament reconstruction is indicated. More than 80 surgical procedures have been described to reconstruct the lateral ankle ligaments. These procedures can be grouped into either anatomic repair or nonanatomic repair. Anatomic repair is preferred as it preserves the natural biomechanics of the ankle. Nonanatomic biotenodesis techniques are used in select cases: obesity, poor soft tissue (revision procedures or connective tissue disorder/generalized

ligamentous laxity), or high-demand patients at risk of repetitive external varus stresses (e.g., football linemen).[23]

In patients with osteochondral or impingement lesions, arthroscopy is performed as the primary procedure followed immediately by open lateral ligament reconstruction. In 2000, DiGiovanni et al[32] published a retrospective review of associated injuries found during primary lateral ankle ligament reconstruction. They found significant intra-articular pathology: anterolateral impingement lesions (67%), ankle synovitis (49%), loose bodies (26%), and talar osteochondral lesions (23%). Similarly, Komenda and Ferkel[33] found a 25% prevalence of chondral injuries in 55 unstable ankles. Others have reported cartilage damage in up to 95% of chronically unstable ankles.[34] Due to the high percentage of associated intra-articular pathology in patients with chronic lateral ankle instability, some advocate arthroscopy as the initial diagnostic step during reconstruction of ankle ligaments.

Modified Brostrom Anatomic Lateral Ligament Reconstruction

In 1966, Brostrom[14] first reported on 60 patients who underwent delayed direct repair of the ATFL and CFL by shortening of the torn ends and midsubstance suturing (Fig. 66-2). Gould et al[35] modified this procedure in 1980 by adding an advancement of the extensor retinaculum over the Brostrom repair. The Gould modification reinforces the repair, limits inversion, and helps to correct the subtalar component of instability.

Two surgical approaches are commonly used for this procedure: (1) an anterior incision along the distal and anterior border of the fibula (if no extra-articular pathology is suspected) or (2) a curvilinear posterior incision along the posterior border of the fibula (if peroneal tendon or retinacular pathology is suspected). An anterolateral arthrotomy is performed with caution to identify and protect branches of the sural and superficial peroneal nerves. The ATFL and CFL are divided in midsubstance and shortened/imbricated in standard vest-over-pants technique with 2-0 nonabsorbable braided suture. With the ankle in slight plantarflexion and eversion, the CFL sutures are secured first. The posterior heel is suspended and the ATFL sutures are then tied with caution to avoid anterior subluxation of the talus. Last, the repair is reinforced with the Gould modification as the extensor retinaculum is advanced and secured to the distal fibula.

Modified Brostrom–Split Evans Procedure

In 1953, Evans[36] described a biotenodesis procedure in which the peroneus brevis tendon is released at the musculotendinous junction, rerouted through the fibula, and then reattached to its proximal stump. This procedure was later modified by suturing the tendon back to itself instead of reattaching it to the proximal stump.[37] In 1999, Girard et al[38] reported on their results of the modified Brostrom-Evans procedure, a procedure that augments the Brostrom reconstruction with the addition of the anterior third of the peroneus brevis (Figs. 66-3 and 66-4). This procedure adds static restraint without a significant sacrifice of dynamic peroneal restraint. The authors believe that the modified Brostrom–split Evans has a role in revision surgery, obese individuals, heavy athletes (e.g., football lineman), laborers, and in patients with generalized ligamentous laxity. It is also our procedure of choice in patients with suspected combined instability patterns. Girard et al[38] reported results in 21 patients at an average follow-up of approximately 2.5 years, finding that when compared to the uninjured contralateral side, there was no

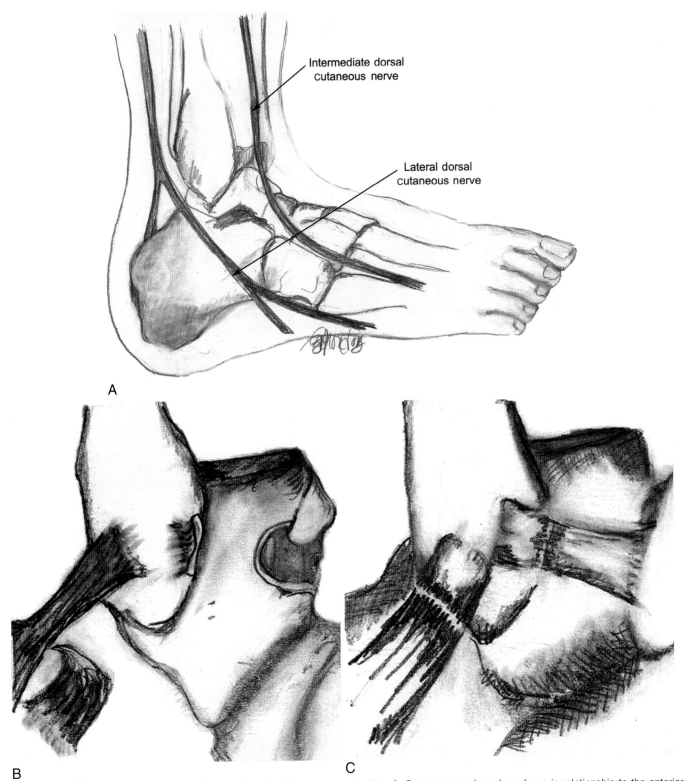

Figure 66-2 Modified Brostrom-Gould anatomic lateral ankle ligament reconstruction. **A,** Sensory nerve branches shown in relationship to the anterior incision. **B,** Midsubstance tears of the anterior talofibular ligament (ATFL) and calcaneofibular ligament (CFL). **C,** Modified Brostrom repair with imbrication of the ATFL and CFL.

Continued

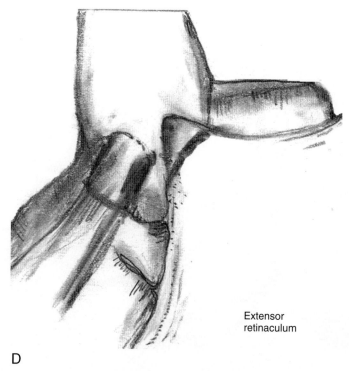

Extensor
retinaculum

D

Figure 66-2—Cont'd D, Gould modification with interior extensor retinaculum–reinforcing repair.

significant difference in ankle plantarflexion or dorsiflexion and no significant loss of peroneal strength. They did report a significant loss of inversion.

The surgical technique for the modified Brostrom–split Evans involves a posterior curvilinear incision extending from 4 to 5 cm proximal to the tip of the lateral malleolus along the course of the peroneal tendons to a point approximately 2 cm proximal to the base of the fifth metatarsal. The skin flaps are then elevated to expose the anterolateral ankle capsule, the anterior

distal fibula, and the peroneal tendons with care to avoid damage to branches of the superficial peroneal and sural nerves. The modified Brostrom portion of the procedure is carried out in identical fashion as described in the previous section with the sutures placed in the ATFL and CFL but not immediately tied. The peroneus brevis tendon is then exposed proximally and distally while maintaining the superficial peroneal retinaculum. The anterior one third of the peroneus brevis tendon is isolated distally and, using a no. 2 nylon suture, split from this distal point

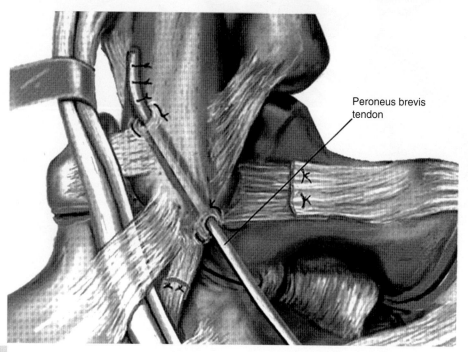

Peroneus brevis
tendon

Figure 66-3 Modified Brostrom–split Evans procedure. The end to end (shortening with imbrication) Brostrom repair of the anterior talofibular ligament and calcaneofibular ligament is performed with nonabsorbable suture. The anterior one third of the split peroneus brevis is then rerouted through the fibula and secured with either sutures at entrance and exit with suture (shown) or with a biotenodesis screw. (From Girard P, Anderson RB, Davis WH, et al: Clinical evaluation of the modified Brostrom-Evans procedure to restore ankle stability. Foot Ankle Int 1999;20:246–252.)

678

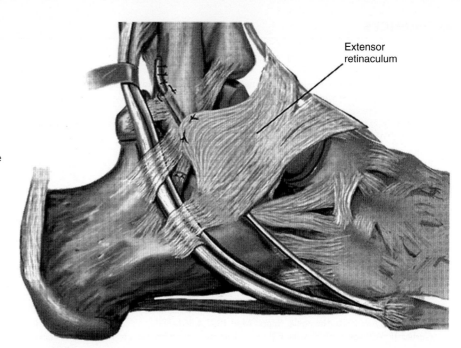

Extensor retinaculum

Figure 66-4 The Gould et al[35] modification augments the modified Brostrom-split Evans with the advancement of the extensor retinaculum to the distal fibula. This reinforces the repair, limits inversion, and helps to correct the subtalar component of instability. (Girard P, Anderson RB, Davis WH, et al: Clinical evaluation of the modified Brostrom-Evans procedure to restore ankle stability. Foot Ankle Int 1999;20:246–252.)

to its musculotendinous junction. The anterior one third is then transected proximally and brought into the distal aspect of the wound. Next, a drill hole is made in the tip of the lateral malleolus lateral to the articular surface between the insertions of the ATFL and CFL. The drill hole is directed posteriorly and proximally exiting approximately 2.5 cm proximal to the fibular tip. The split portion of the peroneus brevis is passed through the tunnel in a distal-to-proximal direction. Then the sutures of the CFL and ATFL are secured in the manner as described in the modified Brostrom. The peroneal transfer is tensioned with the foot in mild plantarflexion and eversion and secured either with a biotenodesis screw or sutures at its entrance and exit sites in the fibula.

Chrisman-Snook Reconstruction

The Elmslie[39] procedure is a nonanatomic reconstruction of the lateral ligaments that uses a strip of fascia lata passed through drill holes in the distal fibula and calcaneus. Chrisman and Snook[40] modified the Elmslie procedure using a split portion of the peroneus brevis and published their results in 1969. The course of the peroneus brevis graft is designed to recreate the vectors of both ATFL and CFL.

The surgical technique for the Chrisman-Snook reconstruction is performed through a posterior curvilinear incision along the course of the peroneal tendons in a manner similar to the modified Brostrom-Evans. The anterior half to the peroneus brevis tendon is identified distally and split from its insertion up to the musculotendinous junction. Next, the anterior half is transected proximally and left attached distally on the base of the fifth metatarsal.

In an attempt to replicate the course of the ATFL, the peroneus brevis graft must recreate the insertion of the ATFL on the talus. This can be done by either passing the graft through a small hole at the base of the ATFL's insertion on the talus or by creation of a bone tunnel. A fibular bone tunnel is then made to recreate the insertion of the ATFL and CFL on the distal

fibula. This is done by fashioning a tunnel that begins anteriorly at the level of the ankle joint and runs anterior to posterior at a 30-degree distal angle, taking great caution to not disrupt the articular surface. The calcaneal insertion of the CFL, a tubercle called the eminenta retrotrochlearis, is identified on the lateral wall of the calcaneus. Two drill holes (1.5 cm apart) are made anterior and posterior to the tubercle. These holes are then joined using curved curets.

The next task is passing the peroneus brevis graft. It is first passed from the base of the fifth metatarsal through the bone tunnel or soft tissue on the talus and then through the fibular tunnel in an anterior to posterior direction. With the ankle in neutral position and the hindfoot in gentle eversion, the graft is pulled taut and then sutured to both the periosteum at the anterior distal fibula and to the remaining stump of the ATFL. The graft is passed below the peroneus longus and remaining peroneus brevis tendons and taken in a posterior-to-anterior direction through the calcaneal drill holes. It is sutured back on itself with 2-0 nonabsorbable suture. Additional sutures are then placed at the entry/exit of all bone tunnels. This technique has been simplified (and perhaps improved) with the advent of the biotenodesis screw.

Postoperative Rehabilitation

The standard postoperative management consists of 2 weeks of non-weight bearing in a splint followed by 4 weeks weight bearing in a short-leg cast. After cast removal, the ankle is protected in a walker boot or an ankle brace (off-the-shelf), and a home program of range of motion and peroneal strengthening for an additional 4 weeks follows. At the 10-week postoperative mark, the patient's progress is reassessed and physical therapy initiated for more aggressive motion and strengthening. For the competitive athlete, we recommend that a protective brace be worn for practice and game situations for the first year after surgery.

REFERENCES

1. Colville MR: Surgical treatment of the unstable ankle. J Am Acad Orthop Surg 1998;6:368–377.
2. Garrick JG: The frequency of injury, mechanism of injury, and epidemiology of ankle sprains. Am J Sports Med 1977;5:241–242.
3. Ekstrand J: Soccer injuries and their mechanisms: A prospective study. Med Sci Sports Exerc 1983;15:267–270.
4. Jackson DW, Ashley RL, Powell JW: Ankle sprains in young athletes. Clin Orthop 1974;101:201–215.
5. Brand RL, Collins MD: Operative management of ligamentous injuries to the ankle. Clin Sports Med 1982;1:119–130.
6. Anderson ME: Reconstruction of lateral ligaments of the ankle using plantaris tendon. J Bone Joint Surg Am 1985;67:930–934.
7. Brostrom L, Sundelin P: Sprained ankles: IV. Histologic changes in recent and "chronic" ligament ruptures. Acta Chir Scand 1966;132:248–253.
8. Freeman MR: Instability of the foot after injuries to the lateral ligaments of the ankle. J Bone Joint Surg Br 1965;47:669–676.
9. Smith RW, Reischl SF: Treatment of ankle sprains in young athletes. Am J Sports Med 1986;14:465–471.
10. Balduini FC, Vegso JJ, Torg JS, et al: Management and rehabilitation of ligamentous injuries to the ankle. Sports Med 1987;4:364–380.
11. Gerber JP, Williams GN, Scoville CR, et al: Persistent disability associated with ankle sprains: A prospective examination of an athletic population. Foot Ankle Int 1998;19:653–660.
12. Stormant DM, Morrey BF, An K, et al: Stability of the loaded ankle. Am J Sports Med 1985;13:295–300.
13. Siegler S, Block J, Schneck CD: The mechanical characteristics of the collateral ligament of the human ankle joint. Foot Ankle 1988;8:234–242.
14. Brostrom L: Sprained ankles. I. Anatomic lesions in recent sprains. Acta Chir Scand 1964;128:483–495.
15. Renstrom P, Theis M: Biomechanics and function of ankle ligaments: Experimental results and clinical application. Sportverletzing Sportschaden 1993;7:29–35.
16. Hamilton WG: Sprained ankles in ballet dancers. Foot Ankle 1982; 3:99–102.
17. DiGiovanni BF, Partal G, Baumhauer JF: Acute ankle injury and chronic lateral instability in the athlete. Clin Sports Med 2004;23:1–19.
18. Stiell I, Greenberg G, McKnight R, et al: A study to develop clinical rules for the use of radiography in acute ankle injuries. Ann Emerg Med 1992;21:384–390.
19. Diamond JE: Rehabilitation of ankle sprains. Clin Sports Med 1989;8:877–891.
20. Kannus P, Renstrom P: Current concepts review: Treatment for acute tears of the lateral ligaments of the ankle. J Bone Joint Surg Am 1991;73:305–312.
21. Konradsen L, Holmer P, Sondergaard L: Early mobilizing treatment for grade III ankle ligament injuries. Foot Ankle 1992;12:69–73.
22. Eiff M, Smith A, Smith G: Early mobilization versus immobilization in the treatment of lateral ankle sprains. Am J Sports Med 1994;22:83–88.
23. Berlet GC, Anderson RB, Davis WH: Chronic lateral ankle instability. Foot Ankle Clin 1999;4:713–728.
24. Ahouvuo J, Kaartinen E, Slatis P: Diagnostic value of stress radiography in lesions of the lateral ligaments of the ankle. Acta Radiol 1988;29:711–714.
25. Karlsson J, Bergsten T, Lansinger O, et al: Surgical treatment of chronic lateral instability of the ankle joint. Am J Sports Med 1989;17:268–273.
26. Louwerens JK, Ginai AZ, Van Linge B, et al: Stress radiography of the talocrural joint and subtalar joints. Foot Ankle Int 1995;16:148–155.
27. Cox JS: Surgical and nonsurgical treatment of acute ankle sprains. Clin Orthop 1985;198:118–126.
28. Maki SE, Whitelaw RS: Influence of expectation and arousal on centre of pressure responses to transient postural perturbations. J Vestib Res 1993;3:25–39.
29. Fumich RM, Ellison AE, Guerin GJ: The measured effect of taping on combined ankle motion before and after exercise. Am J Sports Med 1981;9:165–170.
30. Rarick GL, Bigley G, Karst R: The measurable support of the ankle joint by conventional methods of taping. J Bone Joint Surg Am 1962;44:1183–1190.
31. Myburgh KH, Vaughan CL, Isaacs SK: The effects of ankle guards and taping on joint motion before, during and after a squash match. Am J Sports Med 1984;12:441–446.
32. DiGiovanni BF, Fraga CJ, Cohen BE, Shereff MJ: Associated injuries found in chronic lateral instability. Foot Ankle Int 2000;21:809–815.
33. Komenda GA, Ferkel RD: Arthroscopic findings associated with the unstable ankle. Foot Ankle Int 1999;20:708–713.
34. Taga I, Shino K, Inoue M, et al: Articular cartilage lesions in ankles with lateral ankle ligament injury: An arthroscopic study. Am J Sports Med 1993;21:120–127.
35. Gould N, Seligson D, Grassman J: Early and late repair of the lateral ligaments of the ankle. Foot Ankle Int 1980;1:84–89.
36. Evans DL: Recurrent dislocation of the ankle: A method of surgical treatment. Proc R Soc Med 1953;46:343–348.
37. Ottoson L: Lateral instability of the ankle treated by a modified Evans procedure. Acta Orthop Scand 1978;49:302–305.
38. Girard P, Anderson RB, Davis WH, et al: Clinical evaluation of the modified Brostrom-Evans procedure to restore ankle stability. Foot Ankle Int 1999;20:246–252.
39. Elmslie RC: Recurrent subluxations of the ankle joint. Ann Surg 1934;100:364–367.
40. Chrisman OD, Snook GA: Reconstruction of lateral ligament tears of the ankle: An experimental study and clinical evaluation of seven patients treated by a new modification of the Elmslie procedure. J Bone Joint Surg Am 1969;51:904–912.

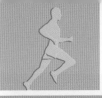

67 Ankle Intra-articular Injury

William I. Sterett and R. Matthew Dumigan

In This Chapter

Bony impingement
Soft tissue impingement
Chondral and osteochondral lesions
Surgery—ankle arthroscopy

INTRODUCTION

- Intra-articular injuries of the ankle encompass a wide variety of problems, including bony and soft-tissue impingement and osteochondral lesions of the talus.

- Bony anterior ankle impingement (footballer's ankle) is a common cause of chronic ankle pain and loss of dorsiflexion in athletes. Spur formation can occur with or without secondary degenerative changes in the joint.

- Persistent pain following an ankle sprain may be a sign of intra-articular soft-tissue impingement. Soft-tissue impingement lesions can occur in the anterolateral and posteromedial aspects of the joint.

- Osteochondral lesions of the talus are a well-known cause of chronic ankle pain and should be considered in patients who have persistent ankle pain following a sprain. Treatment of these lesions continues to evolve.

- Ankle arthroscopy provides excellent visualization of the joint with decreased operative morbidity and is gaining wider acceptance in the treatment of intra-articular lesions in the ankle.

CLINICAL FEATURES AND EVALUATION

Bony Impingement

Most patients with anterior bony impingement in the ankle will present with anterior ankle pain and loss of dorsiflexion. Soccer players seem to be particularly prone to this problem due to the repetitive trauma to the anterior capsule. Dancers and runners develop anterior bony impingement because of repetitive dorsiflexion. The pain and loss of motion may worsen slowly over time, but presentation to a physician is often precipitated by an acute injury.[1] The diagnosis can be confirmed with anteroposterior and lateral views of the ankle. Dorsiflexion stress radiographs can also be obtained to confirm contact between anterior osteophytes on the tibia and talus.[2] The features that should be carefully evaluated on plain radiographs include the location and size of osteophytes and the presence or absence of joint-space narrowing. Patients with spur formation, loss of dorsiflexion, and persistent pain who fail nonoperative management may be considered for operative treatment.

Soft-Tissue Impingement

Soft-tissue impingement lesions in the ankle should be part of the differential diagnosis in patients with persistent symptoms following an ankle sprain. Most patients with a routine ankle sprain demonstrate considerable improvement with 6 weeks of conservative therapy.[1] Patients without radiographic changes and symptoms of pain, catching, instability, swelling, stiffness, altered gait, or activity limitation should be carefully evaluated for soft-tissue impingement lesions. Soft-tissue impingement lesions can be classified based on the anatomic location. Most soft-tissue impingement lesions in the ankle occur in the anterolateral aspect of the ankle joint. The Bassett lesion represents impingement of the anterolateral talar body on the distal fascicle of the anteroinferior tibiofibular ligament[3,4] (Fig. 67-1). Patients with a Bassett lesion will have a history of an inversion ankle sprain and present with chronic anterolateral ankle pain with normal radiographs. Pain and or popping over the anterolateral ankle with forced dorsiflexion are the most consistent physical examination finding. Another type of anterolateral soft-tissue impingement can result from a tear of the anterior talofibular ligament. The torn soft-tissue becomes a mass of hyalinized connective tissue that impinges in the lateral gutter and has been termed the meniscoid lesion.[5] The physical examination for anterolateral impingement is usually nonspecific, but recently a new physical sign was described to aid in the diagnosis.[6] The test is performed by placing the foot in a plantarflexed position with direct pressure over the anterolateral ankle. The foot is then brought up to a maximally dorsiflexed position with continued pressure over the anterolateral ankle. Increased pain with this maneuver is caused by pinching of the hypertrophied synovium that is associated with anterolateral impingement lesions between the talus and tibia (Fig. 67-2). A positive test has been shown to be 95% sensitive and 88% specific for synovial impingement. Intra-articular injection of local anesthetic may be used as an adjunct to the physical examination to help differentiate intra-articular from extra-articular pathology. The addition of steroid to the injection may be considered for therapeutic purposes if synovial inflammation is suspected as the cause of the impingement. The diagnosis of anterolateral impingement is usually made based on the history and physical examination findings, but magnetic resonance imaging (MRI) can be considered if the diagnosis is unclear or other pathology is suspected.

Recently, a posteromedial impingement lesion was described following severe inversion ankle injury.[7] It has been hypothesized

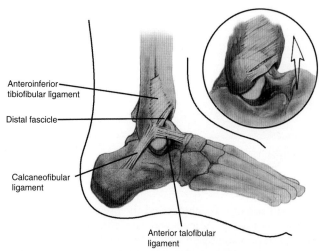

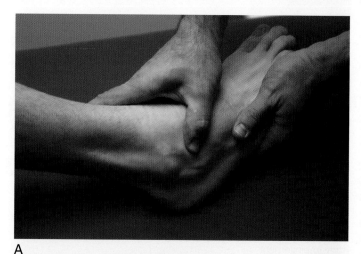

Figure 67-1 Diagram of the lateral aspect of the ankle joint. The distal fascicle of the anteroinferior tibiofibular ligament is parallel and distal to the anterior tibiofibular ligament proper and is separated by a fibrofatty septum. *Inset:* With dorsiflexion, the distal fascicle of the anteroinferior tibiofibular ligament may impinge on the anterolateral aspect of the talus. (From Bassett FH III, Gates HS III, Billys JB, et al: Talar impingement by the anteroinferior tibiofibular ligament. J Bone Joint Surg Am 1990;72:55–59.)

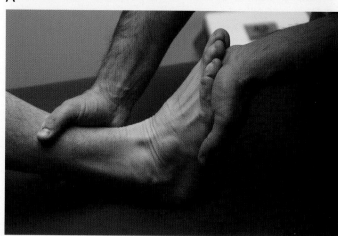

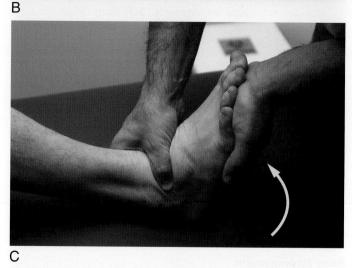

Figure 67-2 A, Ankle held in plantarflexion with pressure over anterolateral joint line. **B,** Ankle ranged from plantarflexed to dorsiflexed position. **C,** Ankle ranged from plantarflexed to dorsiflexed position with pressure over anterolateral joint line. Worsening pain over pressure alone is a positive test for anterolateral impingement.

that the deep fibers of the deltoid ligament become crushed between the posterior medial malleolus and the medial talar wall. While most of these lesions seem to resolve spontaneously, some develop chronic inflammation, hypertrophic fibrosis, and metaplasia of the damaged deltoid ligament. Patients will present with deep posteromedial ankle pain that is intensified with direct palpation, plantarflexion, and inversion of the ankle. Plain films and computed tomography are usually negative for this lesion, but bone scans have been useful in confirming the diagnosis.

Chondral and Osteochondral Lesions of the Talus

Like soft-tissue impingement lesions of the ankle, chondral and osteochondral lesions of the talus will usually present after failed conservative treatment of a presumed ankle sprain. The clinical presentation will be similar to soft-tissue impingement lesions and may include pain, swelling, instability, or catching.[8] The physical examination is usually nonspecific, and point tenderness over the lesion may be the only finding. A careful assessment of the lateral ligaments should be made since instability of these ligaments will have implications in the treatment of the talar lesion.[1,9] Radiographic examination includes anteroposterior, lateral, and mortise views of the ankle. Stress views can be obtained if lateral ligament laxity is detected on physical examination. Lateral lesions result from inversion and dorsiflexion of the ankle causing impaction between the anterolateral talus and the fibula. The lesions are typically thin, wafer-shaped osteochondral fragments located over the anterolateral talar dome, more likely to be symptomatic, and more closely associated with a history of trauma. Medial lesions result from combined plantarflexion, inversion, and external rotation. The lesions are usually located over the posteromedial talar dome and typically appear as a deep, cup-shaped defect. Unlike lateral lesions, many patients with medial lesions will have no history of trauma.[8] Historically, the classification system proposed by

Berndt and Harty[10] in 1959 has been used to classify osteochondral lesions of the talus: stage I, a small compression fracture; stage II, incomplete avulsion of the fragment; stage III, complete avulsion of the fragment without displacement; and stage IV, complete avulsion of the fragment with displacement. Although computed tomography scans and bone scans have been used to further evaluate osteochondral lesions seen on plain films, recent advancements in MRI have made it the preferred diagnostic tool. MRI allows visualization of the articular cartilage and can evaluate the location, size, and stability of a lesion. A recent report has shown that cartilage-sensitive pulse sequence MRI has correlated well with surgical findings and is useful in identifying patients who would benefit from operative versus nonoperative treatment.[11]

RELEVANT ANATOMY

Intra-articular lesions in the ankle can be treated with open or arthroscopic techniques. Knowledge of the local anatomy is important to avoid damage to vital structures. The medial and lateral malleoli, long extensor tendons, and the tibialis anterior are readily visualized and palpated over the anterior ankle and can serve as a guide to identifying neurovascular structures. The superficial peroneal nerve divides into the medial and intermediate dorsal cutaneous nerves approximately 6 to 7 cm above the tip of the fibula. The intermediate dorsal cutaneous nerve courses laterally and passes over the inferior extensor retinaculum near the level of the joint, then crosses the extensor digitorum longus tendons to the fourth and fifth toes distally. The medial dorsal cutaneous nerve is more centrally located and passes superficial to the common extensor digitorum longus tendon at or just distal to the joint line. These two nerves supply the bulk of the sensation to the dorsum of the foot and are at risk with placement of an anterolateral arthroscopic portal or with an anterolateral arthrotomy. The anterior tibial artery and deep peroneal nerve pass deep to the extensor retinaculum over

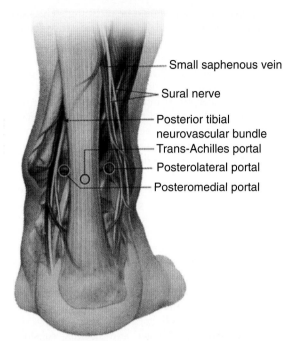

Small saphenous vein

Sural nerve

Posterior tibial neurovascular bundle

Trans-Achilles portal

Posterolateral portal

Posteromedial portal

Figure 67-4 Posterior portals. Posterolateral portal is most commonly used. Posteromedial portal should be used with caution; trans-Achilles portal is not recommended. (From Ferkel TD, Scranton PR: Current concepts review: Arthroscopy of the foot and ankle. J Bone Joint Surg Am 1993;75:1233–1242.)

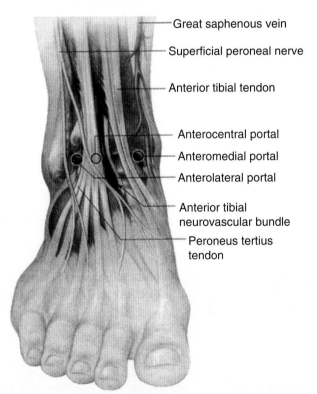

Great saphenous vein

Superficial peroneal nerve

Anterior tibial tendon

Anterocentral portal

Anteromedial portal

Anterolateral portal

Anterior tibial neurovascular bundle

Peroneus tertius tendon

Figure 67-3 Anterior portals. Use of anterocentral portal is not recommended. (From Ferkel RD, Scranton PE: Current concepts review: Arthroscopy of the foot and ankle. J Bone Joint Surg Am 1993;75:1233–1242.)

the central aspect of the anterior ankle. These structures usually run in the interval between the extensor hallucis longus and extensor digitorum longus tendons at the level of the ankle joint and should be palpated and marked prior to making a skin incision. The saphenous nerve and vein can have a variable course but usually cross the ankle just anterior to the medial malleolus. The saphenous nerve is a frequent site of neuroma formation when it is damaged and is at risk with placement of an anteromedial arthroscopic portal or with anteromedial arthrotomy (Fig. 67-3).

The posterior surface anatomy is defined by the posterior aspects of the medial and lateral malleoli and the Achilles tendon. The sural nerve and small saphenous vein travel over the posterolateral ankle and are at risk with posterolateral arthroscopic portal placement and posterolateral approaches to the ankle. The sural nerve is also a frequent site of neuroma formation when it is damaged. The tibialis posterior tendon, flexor digitorum longus tendon, posterior neurovascular bundle, and flexor hallucis longus tendon pass in sequential order from anterior to posterior behind the medial malleolus and are at risk with posteromedial arthroscopic portal placement and posteromedial approaches to the ankle. Damage to neurovascular structures in this area is particularly devastating due to significant loss of blood supply as well as the loss of protective sensation over the plantar aspect of the foot (Fig. 67-4).

TREATMENT OPTIONS

Anterior Bony Impingement
Anterior bony spurs often become symptomatic when synovial or scar-tissue impingement occurs following acute trauma. In the absence of loose bodies on radiographic evaluation, an initial trial

of nonoperative treatment should be instituted. This consists of a short course of nonsteroidal anti-inflammatory medications, heel lift, or a short period of immobilization in a weight-bearing cast or walking boot. Injection of local anesthetic with or without steroids can be used for diagnostic and therapeutic purposes.[2] Patients who have continued pain and loss of motion with dorsiflexion despite 6 months of nonoperative treatment may be considered for surgical treatment. Important considerations prior to surgery are (1) the duration of symptoms, (2) the size and location of osteophytes, and (3) the degree of joint space narrowing. Long-term follow-up studies have shown superior results in patients with symptoms less than 2 years, those without narrowing of the joint space, those with smaller osteophytes, and those who have removal of anteromedial versus anterolateral osteophytes.[12,13] Both open and arthroscopic techniques have been used to successfully treat this problem in selected patients. Arthroscopic treatment offers results similar to open techniques but has decreased operative morbidity, decreased pain, and quicker recovery time.

Soft-Tissue Impingement Lesions

Initial management of ankle sprains consists of rest, ice, compression, and elevation. As pain and swelling subside, active range of motion, strengthening, and proprioceptive training are advanced until the ankle regains normal function. Most ankle sprains improve significantly by 6 weeks. Ankle arthroscopy has become the treatment of choice for management of ankle sprains that continue to be symptomatic beyond 6 months.[1] Careful assessment of the articular cartilage should be made at the time of arthroscopy since approximately one in four patients will have an associated chondral lesion of the talus.

Posteromedial impingement lesions likely represent a small percentage of soft-tissue lesions following inversion ankle injuries but should be considered in the setting of a characteristic physical examination and a positive bone scan. Patients who fail to improve with a trial of conservative management should be considered for surgery. The lesion may be difficult to visualize with the arthroscope, and open excision of the lesion can be performed through a posteromedial approach with an arthrotomy through the base of the tibialis posterior tendon sheath.[7]

Chondral and Osteochondral Lesions of the Talus

Like soft-tissue impingement lesions, chondral lesions of the talus will often have nonspecific physical examination findings and normal radiographs. A high index of clinical suspicion will prompt an MRI confirming the diagnosis. Nonoperative management is similar to that of soft-tissue impingement lesions and should last for approximately 6 months before operative intervention is considered. Patients with continued pain or mechanical symptoms despite appropriate nonoperative treatment may be candidates for surgery. Lateral ligament instability may be present with a chondral lesion and is an important consideration prior to surgery.[9] Chondral lesions that are treated without addressing the overlying instability tend to have a worse outcome compared to lesions treated in stable ankles.[1]

Unless there is evidence of a loose body on plain radiographs or MRI, initial treatment of osteochondral lesions of the talus is nonoperative. Initial treatment can consist of a period of immobilization and limited weight bearing. There are no clear guidelines in the literature that quantify the duration of immobilization or protected weight bearing. The age of the patient and the location, size, and stability of the lesion are

factors that may contribute to decision making. Historically, lesions that are treated conservatively for up to 12 months still have a good outcome with appropriate surgical treatment.[8] Patients with loose bodies at presentation are treated with surgery from the onset, while patients with Berndt and Harty lesions stages I through III with persistent pain, swelling, or mechanical symptoms are considered for surgery after 3 to 6 months of failed nonoperative treatment.[14] With the improvements in MRI, the current trend is earlier diagnosis and treatment of osteochondral lesions. Surgical treatment of osteochondral lesions of the talus continues to rapidly evolve, and numerous techniques are available. The advantages and disadvantages of various arthroscopic and open procedures are discussed later in the chapter.

SURGERY

Diagnostic Arthroscopy of the Ankle

Patient positioning is usually based on surgeon preference. Patients can be placed in a supine position with the leg supported on the table or the leg can be placed in a leg holder and allowed to fall free. Some surgeons use the lateral decubitus position with the patient supported on a beanbag, and some surgeons recommend the prone position when the primary pathology is posterior and posterior portals are planned[15] (Fig. 67-5). A standard 4.0-mm 30-degree arthroscope is usually sufficient, but a 2.7-mm 30-degree arthroscope may allow easier maneuverability within the ankle joint. Prior to beginning an ankle arthroscopy, the surface landmarks should be delineated with a marking pen. The dorsalis pedis artery should be palpated and marked, and the saphenous vein and accompanying nerve can be marked just anterior to the medial malleolus. In some patients, the terminal branches of the superficial peroneal nerve can be visualized by grasping the fourth toe and bringing the foot into a plantarflexed and adducted position. Prior to starting the procedure, 10 to 15 mL of saline is injected into the ankle through the anteromedial side of the joint. Invasive or noninvasive distraction devices may be used to improve the visualization in the joint depending on the needs of the procedure. The anteromedial portal is more reproducible and usually established first. A vertical skin incision is made through the skin medial to the tibialis anterior tendon at or just above the joint line. A

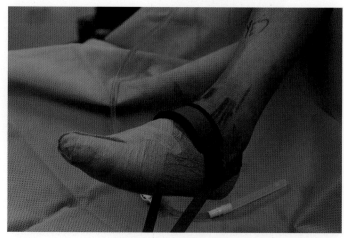

Figure 67-5 Patient position for ankle arthroscopy with external traction device.

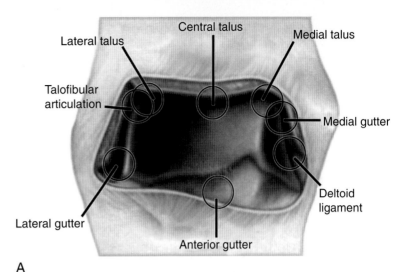

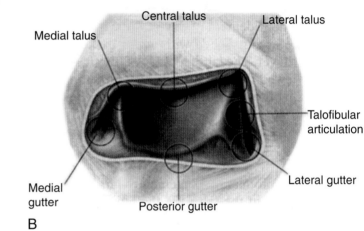

Figure 67-6 A, The eight-point anterior examination of the ankle through the arthroscope. **B,** The seven-point posterior examination of the ankle through the arthroscope. (From Ferkel TD, Scranton PR: Current concepts review: Arthroscopy of the foot and ankle. J Bone Joint Surg Am 1993;75:1233–1242.)

hemostat or blunt obturator is used to dissect through the capsule. The anterolateral portal is then established with the aid of the arthroscope. The skin is transilluminated to look for branches of the superficial peroneal nerve and traversing veins, and a skin incision is made just lateral to the peroneus tertius tendons at or just above the joint line. A central anterior portal has been described, but it engenders unnecessary risk to the anterior tibial artery and deep peroneal nerve and should be avoided.[2] Posterior portals include the posterolateral and posteromedial portals. The posterolateral portal is usually considered the "safe" portal and can be established with the use of the arthroscope through one of the anterior portals. The posterolateral portal is made just lateral to the Achilles tendon at the level of the joint line. An 18-gauge needle can be used to localize the correct placement under direct arthroscopic visualization, or alternatively a switching stick can be used through one of the anterior portals. Once this portal is established, it can be used for gravity inflow or as a working portal for posterior pathology.[2] The posteromedial portal has not gained wide acceptance due to the risk of damage to the nearby posterior neurovascular bundle. A recent anatomic study has described the safe use of posterolateral and posteromedial arthroscopic portals with the patient in the prone position.[15] This allows excellent visualization of the posterior half of the tibiotalar joint, the subtalar joint, and the flexor hallucis longus tendon if posterior ankle joint pathology is to be addressed. Once the portals

are established, a systematic diagnostic arthroscopy following an eight-point examination, as described by Ferkel and Scranton,[2] is performed to thoroughly evaluate the ankle (Fig. 67-6).

Arthroscopic Treatment of Anterior Bony Impingement

Open removal of anterior osteophytes has been performed in the past with good results. In the past several years, arthroscopy has been increasingly used to treat these lesions with equal effectiveness, but with the benefit of a much easier recovery. The surgery is performed with the patient in the supine position with the leg supported on the operating table, and standard anteromedial and anterolateral portals are established. Nearly all anterior osteophytes will be within the joint capsule and are best visualized without distraction with the ankle in maximal dorsiflexion[9,16] (Fig. 67-7). Small joint osteotomes and a 4.0-mm bur are used to take down the osteophytes off the anterior tibia and from the notch on the anterior talar neck. Any hypertrophic synovium or scar tissue in this area is carefully removed with a shaver.

Treatment of Soft-Tissue Impingement Lesions

After a thorough diagnostic arthroscopy, anterolateral impingement lesions can be removed with the aid of the arthroscope. Bassett lesions have been found in normal ankles but can become symptomatic in the setting of inversion ankle injuries. This distal

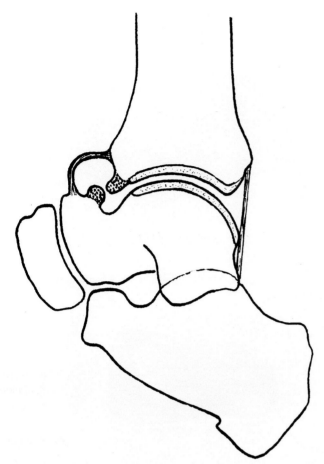

Figure 67-7 Ankle in maximal dorsiflexion without distraction. (From Van Dijk CN, Tol JL, Verheyen CC: A prospective study of the prognostic factors concerning the outcome of arthroscopic surgery for anterior ankle impingement. Am J Sports Med 1997;24:737–745. Copyright 1997 American Orthopaedic Society for Sports Medicine.)

fascicle will be separate from the anteroinferior tibiofibular ligament by a fibrofatty septum and can be removed without compromising the stability of the syndesmosis. The articular cartilage should be carefully evaluated once the accessory ligament is removed. All abnormal synovium and scar tissue should be removed, and any fraying of the anterior syndesmosis or anterior talofibular ligament should be débrided.

Posteromedial impingement lesions may be difficult to visualize and treat with arthroscopic techniques using standard anterior portals. Prone posterior ankle arthroscopy may have a role in treatment of this lesion but has not been described. An open technique has been described in which the tendon sheath of the tibialis posterior tendon is opened, the tendon is retracted anteriorly, and the bed of the tendon sheath is opened to gain access to the posteromedial aspect of the joint. The pathologic tissue tends to "erupt through this incision" and is removed. The incision in the bed of the tendon sheath is left open, and the superficial sheath incision and skin are closed.[7]

Arthroscopic Treatment of Chondral and Osteochondral Lesions of the Talus

Lesions confined to the cartilage alone can be treated arthroscopically with a simple chondroplasty to smooth the articular surface and débride back to normal healthy cartilage (Fig.

67-8). As stated earlier, strong consideration should be given to stabilizing ankles with lateral ligament instability in the setting of a chondral lesion.[1]

Treating osteochondral lesions with arthroscopic techniques requires a systematic approach based on the arthroscopic appearance of the lesion. There are numerous techniques available, and the surgeon should be familiar with the advantages and disadvantages of each type of treatment to optimize treatment of a given lesion. Arthroscopy provides excellent visualization of the joint, but some far posteromedial lesions may be difficult to visualize. Therefore, the surgeon should be prepared to convert to an open procedure if necessary.

Stage I lesions appear as an area of softened articular cartilage without a definable fragment. If this lesion is symptomatic, then the main treatment decision is whether the articular cartilage should be violated to try to stimulate the lesion to heal. Drilling of an intact lesion can be performed by drilling a 0.062-inch Kirschner wire through the intact cartilage and into the base of the lesion. It is believed that the drill holes stimulate revascularization of the avascular fragment. Anterolateral lesions can usually be easily drilled through the anterolateral portal. Posteromedial lesions can be more difficult to access because of their location. With the arthroscope in the anterolateral portal, the ankle is placed in maximal plantarflexion. If the area of softened cartilage can be visualized, then drilling can be performed through the anteromedial portal. If this is unsuccessful, then transmalleolar drilling can be considered. A small joint drill guide is placed over the lesion, and the Kirschner wire is drilled through the medial malleolus and into the lesion (Fig. 67-9).[2] These techniques have the advantage of decreased operative morbidity compared to open techniques but injure articular cartilage. An alternative approach allows grafting behind an intact lesion without violating the integrity of the articular cartilage. A small joint drill guide is placed over the lesion, and a guide wire is placed in the sinus tarsi. Retrograde transtalar drilling is then performed under direct arthroscopic visualization (Fig. 67-10).[2,8] The tunnel is expanded with a small reamer, and the lesion is grafted with local or distal tibia cancellous bone graft.

Stage II lesions have a breach in the articular cartilage, but the fragment is not displaceable. Once the overlying cartilage has been débrided, the underlying bone bed can be addressed. It is important to remove any sclerotic or nonviable bone until bleeding subchondral bone is seen at the base of the lesion.[14] Drilling can be performed as described for stage I lesions, or the microfracture technique may be used. The microfracture technique uses specialized awls, and multiple perforations are made in the subchondral plate approximately 3 mm apart.[17] Both drilling and microfracture stimulate the release of growth factors and mesenchymal stem cells, which result in filling of the defect with fibrocartilage.[16] The advantages of these techniques are decreased operative morbidity compared to open procedures and filling of the defects with fibrocartilage. Two of the potential shortcomings of these techniques are that they are not able to reconstitute significant loss of subchondral bone and long-term durability of fibrocartilage on the talus is not known.

Stage III lesions have a breach in the articular cartilage with a displaceable fragment. The size and viability of the fragment as well as the condition of the overlying articular cartilage should be carefully assessed. Some acute traumatic lesions may be candidates for internal fixation (discussed later in chapter). If the lesion is loose and not amenable to internal fixation, then it

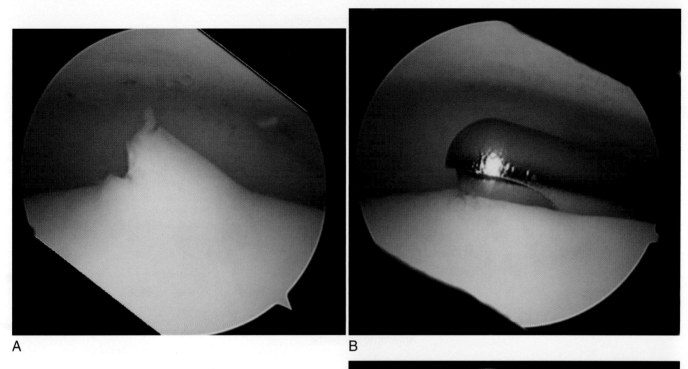

A

B

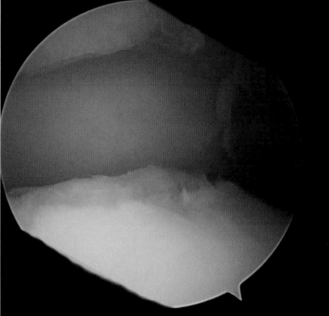

C

Figure 67-8 A, Partial-thickness chondral lesion of the talar dome viewed arthroscopically. **B,** Motorized shaver débriding the lesion. **C,** Articular surface of the talus after débridement.

should be removed and the subchondral bed treated as discussed for stage II lesions. Loose lesions will often have a flap of articular cartilage attached to the lesion. In the past, there has been some question about what to do with this cartilage. A recent report has shown that leaving this remaining cartilage in place may obstruct regeneration of healing tissue and that the removal of all degenerative cartilage improves results.[9]

Stage IV lesions are loose bodies in the ankle joint. Unlike stage I through III lesions, loose bodies are treated surgically as soon as the diagnosis is made. Once again, acute traumatic lesions can be assessed for internal fixation. If the lesion is chronic, nonviable, less than 1 cm in size, or has poor overlying articular cartilage, it is removed.[8,14] The site of loose body displacement is débrided, and the subchondral bone bed is treated like stage II and III lesions.

Open Treatment of Osteochondral Lesions
Open Débridement
Open débridement of osteochondral lesions can be performed through a variety of approaches.[18] Most lateral lesions are anterior and can be treated through a standard anterolateral arthrotomy. A skin incision is made just medial to the fibula about 2 cm proximal to the joint and extended 1 to 2 cm distal to the joint. Branches of the superficial peroneal nerve are carefully protected, and the extensor retinaculum is incised. The extensor digitorum longus tendons are retracted medially, and the joint capsule is incised in line with the skin incision. Visualization of the articular surface may be improved with plantarflexion of the ankle. In the rare occurrence of a posterolateral lesion, a fibular osteotomy and incision through the anterior syndesmosis can be performed.

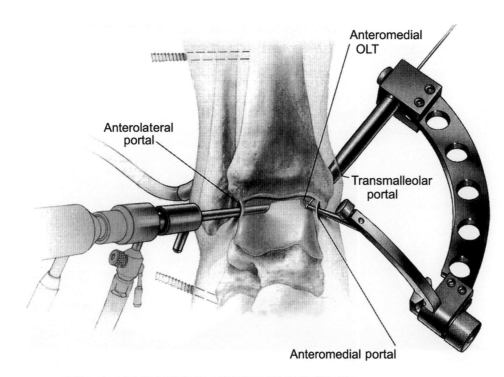

Figure 67-9 Transmalleolar drilling with a small-joint drill guide inserted through the anteromedial portal. Visualization is through the anterolateral portal. OLT, osteochondral lesion of the talus. (From Ferkel TD, Scranton PR: Current concepts review: Arthroscopy of the foot and ankle. J Bone Joint Surg Am 1993;75:1233–1242.)

Medial lesions may be difficult to visualize both arthroscopically or with a standard medial arthrotomy. In these cases, a medial malleolar osteotomy can be performed. Numerous techniques have been described in an attempt to minimize the complications associated with this procedure. Although this approach provides excellent visualization, there is a risk of malunion, nonunion, hardware complications, and articular cartilage injury.

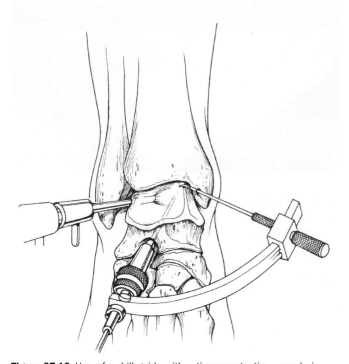

Figure 67-10 Use of a drill guide with a tissue-protective cannula in retrograde transtalar drilling of a posteromedial talar dome lesion. (From Stone JW: Osteochondral lesions of the talar dome. J Am Acad Orthop Surg 1996;4:63–73, with permission.)

Internal Fixation

Since there are no universally accepted guidelines in the literature, internal fixation of loose or displaced fragments remains somewhat controversial. In general, patients suitable for internal fixation are younger patients with acute traumatic lesions. The ideal type of fragment should be 1 cm or greater and have a large piece of attached subchondral bone, and the overlying articular cartilage should be in good condition.[8] The ideal type of fixation is also controversial. Metal implants provide good fixation with excellent biocompatibility but may require a second procedure for removal. This is a particularly difficult problem for posteromedial lesions that required a medial malleolar osteotomy. Bioabsorbable fixation devices are another alternative. These devices have the advantage of not requiring later removal, but bone resorption around the implants remains a concern.

Autologous Osteochondral Transplant

Autologous osteochondral grafts from the ipsilateral knee are transplanted to the talus using the mosaicplasty technique.[19] The procedure can be used as an initial procedure for larger lesions or for revisions that have failed previous arthroscopic procedures. Lesions should be over 1 cm in size, and the cartilage on the remainder of the tibia and talus should be normal. Specialized instruments are used to remove osteochondral plugs from the non-weight-bearing portion of the medial femoral condyle. The talar lesion is then prepared and the plugs are inserted perpendicular to the articular surface. Anterolateral arthrotomies are usually sufficient for lateral lesions, and medial lesions usually require a medial malleolar osteotomy. The procedure replaces the defect with hyaline cartilage and can replace lost subchondral bone stock. Disadvantages include potential donor site morbidity in the knee, and complications associated with open arthrotomies and osteotomies.

Autologous Chondrocyte Transplant

One of the newer techniques used to treat osteochondral lesions of the talus is autologous chondrocyte transplantation.[20,21] The exact indications for this procedure are still evolving but are similar to mosaicplasty. The procedure is performed in two stages. The first stage requires an arthroscopic cartilage biopsy either from the knee or from the non-weight-bearing portion of the anterior talus. The chondrocytes are then grown in culture for approximately 2 to 3 weeks. This is followed by the second procedure that uses an arthrotomy or osteotomy. The lesion is débrided back to normal cartilage with a bleeding subchondral bed. A 10 × 10-mm cortical window is then made in the distal tibia metaphysis, and cancellous bone graft is removed. This graft is packed into the base of the defect to restore subchondral bone stock. A periosteal flap is then harvested from the ipsilateral proximal tibia and is sewn over the defect with a 5-0 polydiaxone monofilament suture. The cultured chondrocytes are then injected under the periosteal flap, and then the flap is sealed with fibrin glue. The theoretical advantage of this procedure is that it replaces lost subchondral bone stock and hyaline cartilage is restored to the articular surface. The two main disadvantages are the high cost of the procedure and the need for two operations. Further research comparing autologous chondrocyte transplantation to other procedures are needed to determine whether the high cost of this procedure is justified in treating osteochondral lesions of the talus.

POSTOPERATIVE REHABILITATION

Anterior Bony Impingement
Following arthroscopic treatment of anterior bony impingement, patients are placed in a compressive dressing and are partial weight bearing for 3 to 5 days. Active dorsiflexion exercises are started immediately postoperatively and are continued several times daily within the confines of the patient's comfort. The patient then returns to progressive weight bearing as tolerated.[12,13]

Soft-Tissue Impingement Lesions
Arthroscopic removal of isolated soft-tissue impingement lesions is followed by early range of motion in a compressive dressing. Patients are instructed to weight bear as tolerated as soon as their comfort allows. Once pain and swelling have subsided, strengthening and proprioceptive training are started at 2 to 3 weeks.

Chondral and Osteochondral Lesions
The type of procedure and the size of the lesion determine the postoperative rehabilitation. Active and passive range-of-motion exercises are started early in the postoperative course and will precede weight bearing. Restrictions in weight bearing can range from 3 to 6 weeks, with drilling, microfracture, and grafting procedures having longer restrictions than simple débridement.

CRITERIA FOR RETURN TO SPORTS

Return to sport after treatment of these lesions is largely based on the patient's examination. Patients should be carefully assessed for pain, swelling, stiffness, instability, and mechanical symptoms. In the absence of these symptoms, those who undergo isolated removal of soft-tissue lesions or osteophytes can expect an early return to sport once the goals of the postoperative physical therapy regimen have been met. Patients with osteochondral lesions who are treated with drilling, microfracture, or grafting procedures should satisfy both the stated criteria in addition to having radiographic evidence of a stable or healed lesion. In general, these patients should be kept out of competitive sports for 4 to 6 months.

RESULTS AND OUTCOMES

Arthroscopic Treatment of Anterior Bony Impingement
At 5- to 8-year follow-up, patients who had removal of anterior osteophytes without preoperative narrowing of the joint space had 77% good to excellent results.[12] Radiographic recurrence of the osteophytes occurs in approximately two thirds of the patients, but this does not seem to correlate with recurrence of clinical symptoms.[13]

Arthroscopic Treatment of Soft-Tissue Impingement Lesions
Several small series have shown excellent results after removal of isolated soft-tissue impingement lesions. Good to excellent results can be expected in 80% to 90% of these patients with a high percentage of those being able to return to sport.[22]

Chondral and Osteochondral Lesions of the Talus
Débridement of chondral lesions in stable ankles had good results in 75% of cases, while treatment of similar lesions in unstable ankles showed only 33% good results.[1] This confirms the need to restore stability when treating articular cartilage injuries in the talus. Most reports on arthroscopic treatment of osteochondral lesions of the talus using débridement and drilling of the lesion have been favorable with good to excellent results reported in 85% to 90% of cases.[14] These results equal or surpass those of traditional open techniques. A recent report on the microfracture technique at 2-year follow-up has shown good to excellent results in 78%.[17] Mosaicplasty has also shown encouraging results in treating lesions over 1 cm in size. Good to excellent results have been reported in 94% of patients having this procedure with 2- to 7-year follow-up.[19] A few small series of patients treated with autologous chondrocyte transplantation have been reported with good results in most patients.[20,21]

COMPLICATIONS

Most complications that occur as a result of these procedures are related to complications associated with arthroscopy of the ankle. The overall complication rate with ankle arthroscopy is 10%. Most of these complications are neurologic (49%). Of the neurologic complications, 56% involve the branches of the superficial peroneal nerve, 24% involve the sural nerve, and 20% involve the saphenous nerve.[2] The use of the central anterior portal has been condemned due to the risk to the anterior tibial artery and deep peroneal nerve, and the posteromedial portal should be used with caution. A good understanding of the local anatomy will minimize complications.

CONCLUSIONS

Ankle symptoms that persist following an injury despite nonoperative treatment should be carefully assessed for intra-articular pathology. A high index of clinical suspicion in addition to a thorough history, physical examination, and radiographic studies will often lead to an accurate diagnosis. Arthroscopy is gaining wider acceptance in the treatment of the majority of these lesions, but those who treat these lesions in the ankle should be familiar with the advantages and disadvantages of all available options.

REFERENCES

1. Ogilvie-Harris DJ, Gilbart MK, Chorney K: Chronic pain following ankle sprains in athletes: The role of arthroscopic surgery. Arthroscopy 1997;13:564–574.

2. Ferkel RD, Scranton PE: Current concepts review: Arthroscopy of the foot and ankle. J Bone Joint Surg Am 1993;75:1233–1242.

3. Bassett FH 3rd, Gates HS 3rd, Billys JB, et al: Talar impingement by the anteroinferior tibiofibular ligament. J Bone Joint Surg Am 1990;72:55–59.

4. Nikolopoulos CE, Tsirikos AI, Sourmelis S, Papachristou G: The accessory anteroinferior tibiofibular ligament as a cause of talar impingement. Am J Sports Med 2004;32:389–395.

5. Lahm A, Erggelet C, Reichelt A: Ankle joint arthroscopy for meniscoid lesions in athletes. Arthroscopy 1998;14:572–575.

6. Molloy S, Solan MC, Bendall SP: Synovial impingement in the ankle. J Bone Joint Surg Br 2003;85:330–333.

7. Paterson RS, Brown JN: The posteromedial impingement lesion of the ankle: A series of six cases. Am J Sports Med 2001;29:550–557.

8. Stone JW: Osteochondral lesions of the talar dome. J Am Acad Orthop Surg 1996;4:63–73.

9. Takao M, Uchio Y, Kakimaru H, et al: Arthroscopic drilling with debridement of remaining cartilage for osteochondral lesions of the talar dome in unstable ankles. Am J Sports Med 2004;32:332–336.

10. Berndt AL, Harty M: Transchondral fractures (osteochondritis dissecans) of the talus. J Bone Joint Surg 1959;41:988–1020.

11. Mintz DN, Tashjian GS, Connell DA, et al: Osteochondral lesions of the talus: A new magnetic resonance grading system with arthroscopic correlation. Arthroscopy 2003;19:353–359.

12. Tol JL, Verhcycn CP, van Dijk CN: Arthroscopic treatment of anterior impingement in the ankle. J Bone Joint Surg Br 2001;83:9–13.

13. Van Dijk CN, Tol JL, Verheyen CC: A prospective study of the prognostic factors concerning the outcome of arthroscopic surgery for anterior ankle impingement. Am J Sports Med 1997;25:737–745.

14. Baker CL, Morales RW: Arthroscopic treatment of transchondral talar dome fractures: A long-term follow-up study. Arthroscopy 1999;15:197–202.

15. Sitler DF, Amendola A, Bailey CS, et al: Posterior ankle arthroscopy: An anatomic study. J Bone Joint Surg Am 2002;84:763–769.

16. Philbin TM, Lee TH, Berlet GC: Arthroscopy for athletic foot and ankle injuries. Clin Sports Med 2004;23:35–53.

17. Thermann H, Becher C: Microfracture technique for treatment of osteochondral and degenerative chondral lesions of the talus: Two year results of a prospective study. Unfallchirurg 2004;107:27–32.

18. Navid DO, Myerson MS: Approach alternatives for treatment of osteochondral lesions in the talus. Foot Ankle Clin 2002;7:635–649.

19. Hangody L: The mosaicplasty technique for osteochondral lesions of the talus. Foot Ankle Clin 2003;8:259–273.

20. Koulalis D, Schultz W, Psychogios B, Papagelopoulos PJ: Articular reconstruction of osteochondral defects of the talus through autologous chondrocyte transplantation. Orthopedics 2004;27:559–562.

21. Koulalis D, Schultz W, Heyden M: Autologous chondrocyte transplantation for osteochondral dissecans of the talus. CORE 2002;395:186–192.

22. DeBerardino TM, Arciero RA, Taylor DC: Arthroscopic treatment of soft tissue impingement of the ankle in athletes. Arthroscopy 1997;13:492–498.

Ankle Fractures and Syndesmosis Injuries

Jeffrey B. Selby

In This Chapter

INTRODUCTION

- Ankle fractures and syndesmosis injuries are a significant source of lost participation in sports.

- These injuries are the major differential diagnoses in the much more common ankle sprains and are also frequently missed injuries, when attributed to a simple sprain.

- This chapter focuses on the treatment of these more severe injuries that usually cause considerably more impairment and often require surgical fixation.

RELEVANT ANATOMY

The ankle is composed of a complex hinge with both bony and ligamentous structures playing a role in stability. This allows for adequate dorsiflexion and plantarflexion during normal gait and provides for stability throughout the hinge motion. The articular surface of the tibia is concave with large anterior and posterior prominences. The medial malleolus is the distal medial portion of tibia and provides for a medial buttress to the talus. The distal fibula or lateral malleolus is the lateral buttress to the talus. It fits into the incisura of the distal lateral tibia, which is concave 75% of the time and is a marker for injury to the syndesmosis. This bony architecture, called the ankle mortise, is not sufficient to keep the talus within the ankle joint despite its conformity with the distal tibia, medial malleolus, and lateral malleolus (Fig. 68-1).

The medial malleolus is covered with articular cartilage in contact with the talus except for the region of the deep deltoid ligament. This thick ligament is the primary medial stabilizer to the joint and runs from the posterior colliculus of the medial malleolus to the talus. It restrains external rotation of the talus within the mortise. The superficial deltoid ligament runs from the anterior aspect of the medial malleolus to the talus and is less important as a stabilizer as it is primarily a thickening of the joint capsule (Fig. 68-2).

The lateral ligamentous portion of the ankle has three major portions. The major ligamentous restraint to foot inversion and the most commonly injured ligament in sprains is the anterior talofibular ligament (ATFL). In plantarflexion, the ligament aligns with the fibula and resists inversion of the talus acting as a collateral ligament. In dorsiflexion or neutral position, it resists anterior translation of the tibia as tested in the anterior drawer test of the ankle. The calcaneofibular ligament (CFL) originates in the middle of the distal lateral fibula, traverses deep to the peroneal tendons, and inserts on the calcaneus. This ligament functions as the collateral ligament resisting inversion with the talus in a neutral or dorsiflexed position. There is a posterior talofibular ligament, which runs from the posterior distal fibula to the posterior process of the talus.

The syndesmosis has a separate ligamentous structure with three definable ligaments: (1) the anteroinferior tibiofibular ligament, (2) the posteroinferior tibiofibular ligament, and (3) the interosseous ligament. The tibia and fibula are connected throughout their length by the interosseous membrane, and the distal connection of this contributes to the syndesmotic complex. The anteroinferior tibiofibular ligament is the most frequently injured ligament in sprains and in frank diastasis of the syndesmosis.[1] It runs from the anterolateral tubercle of the tibia (Tillaux-Chaput tubercle) to the anterodistal fibular shaft and is approximately 20 mm wide and 20 to 30 mm long. The posteroinferior tibiofibular ligament has a deep portion and a superficial portion. The superficial portion originates on the posterolateral portion of the tibia, covers the back of the tibiotalar joint, and runs obliquely down to the posterior aspect of the distal part of the fibula. It is approximately 20 mm wide, 30 mm long, and 5 mm thick and is usually the last structure to tear in syndesmosis injury.[2,3] The interosseous ligament runs between the tibia and fibula approximately 1 to 2 cm above the plafond and is considered the primary bond between the tibia and the fibula. It is continuous with the interosseous membrane, which is often torn in syndesmotic injuries, but provides minimal additional strength to the stabilizing syndesmotic ligaments (Fig. 68-3).

BIOMECHANICS

The tibiotalar articulation averages about 3 degrees valgus at the plafond. The angle between the plafond and a line drawn from the tip of the medial malleolus to the tip of the lateral malleolus are called the talocrural angle and averages 83 ± 4 degrees.[4] The ankle hinge axis runs anterior to posterior from the tip of the medial malleolus to the tip of the lateral malleolus.[5] Because of this oblique axis, there is an obligatory internal and external rotation of the foot with plantarflexion and dorsiflexion, respectively. Normal gait requires 10 degrees of plantarflexion, and the normal ankle has mean dorsiflexion of 32 degrees and mean plantarflexion of 45 degrees when a load is applied.[6]

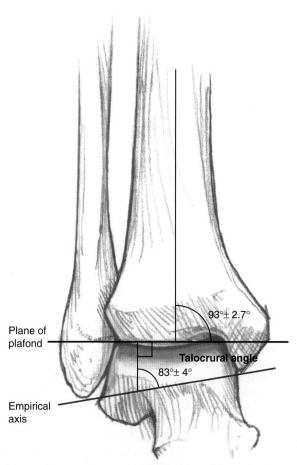

Plane of
plafond

$93° \pm 2.7°$

Talocrural angle

$83° \pm 4°$

Empirical
axis

Figure 68-1 Bony ankle anatomy. (From Pugh KJ: Fractures and soft-tissue injuries about the ankle. In Fitzgerald RH, Kaufer H, Malkami AL [eds]: Orthopaedics. St. Louis, Mosby, 2002, p 422.)

The intramalleolar distance increases an average of 1.5 mm when the ankle goes from full plantarflexion to full dorsiflexion. This motion as well as rotation is allowed by the mobile relationship of the tibia and fibula at the syndesmosis. The tibia can rotate 5 to 6 degrees on the talus in walking and almost half of this comes from the inferior tibiofibular joint.[7] There is only a 1- to 2-degree increase in external rotation of the fibula with isolated section of the anteroinferior tibiofibular ligament with no effect on frontal plane motion.[8] When all the ligaments are cut, there is a 10.2-degree increase in rotation.[9]

ANKLE FRACTURES

History

The mechanism of injury is an important aid in the diagnosis and treatment of ankle fractures. These are usually low-energy injuries in athletic events, and the fractures are usually not open. Medical history is important, and athletes with diabetes or peripheral neuropathies may pose different treatment scenarios. Also, a history of fracture and/or surgery may be helpful in interpreting radiographs and in preoperative planning. The direction of injury is important in treatment and diagnosis of fracture or ligament injury.

Examination

Rapidly identifying injuries that may require urgent treatment and those that keep a player from returning to play are usually obvious if there is gross deformity. Inspection of the skin and soft tissues is performed, dressings applied to open injuries, and deformities are grossly aligned. The neurovascular examination is very important and should be performed both before and after gross realignment of the ankle. A complete sensory examination is performed and motor function is evaluated, although often difficult because of pain limitations.

When the injury is not subtle, the extent of the fracture may be obvious, but when subtle, all bony prominences must be palpated. Local tenderness directly over the bone may indicate fracture rather than ligamentous injury. Defects or crepitus can often be palpated at a fracture site. Stability is tested and the ankle is put through a range of motion. It is imperative to palpate the proximal tibia and fibula to ensure that there is not a proximal injury, which is often present in syndesmotic injury.

Imaging

Standard views of the ankle should be obtained in any injury that is suspicious for fracture and include anteroposterior, lateral, and oblique internal rotation (mortise view) views. The mortise view is obtained by placing the leg in 15 degrees of internal rotation with the x-ray beam perpendicular to the flat surface of the table. Stress views are not normally obtained unless syndesmosis injury is suspected. Anteroposterior and lateral views of the entire tibia and fibula are imperative to ensure that there is not a proximal injury. The lateral view helps to rule out injuries to bones other than the mortise such as talus or calcaneus fractures. Computed tomography scans can be obtained as a secondary study if there is significant comminution or suspicion of intra-articular pathology.

Classification

The two main classification schemes used, Lauge-Hansen and Danis-Weber, are helpful in communicating about fractures and in determining the treatment of the fractures. The Lauge-Hansen classification scheme is most useful in describing the mechanism of injury, so that the forces across the ankle determine the direction and extent of injury. Knowledge of these patterns allows for anatomic reduction and maintenance of reduction with closed means in treating these fractures. The Danis-Weber classification solely describes the injury level of the fibula in relation to the plafond. This is a more simple classification scheme and aids mostly in determining the appropriate operative treatment of the ankle fracture. Both schemes are shown in Figures 68-4 and 68-5.

Goals of Treatment

Restoration and maintenance of normal anatomic relationships by the most expedient and least invasive means will lead to fastest rehabilitation and earliest return to sport. Ankle dislocations are grossly realigned on the field, and anatomic reduction is obtained and ensured with radiographs. Many of these injuries have neurovascular and skin compromise, and prompt reduction relieves tension on the skin, nerves, and vessels. Injuries that are stable are usually managed without surgery and unstable injuries are usually managed with anatomic reduction and fixation.

Nonoperative Treatment

Nonoperative treatment is indicated when the injury did not require a reduction maneuver and the mortise is not widened on standard radiographs. There is usually no medial tenderness to palpation. Subtle medial tenderness to palpation with fracture of the lateral malleolus and without fracture of the medial

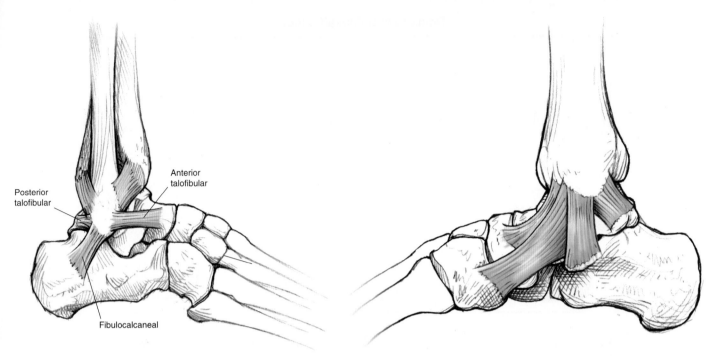

Figure 68-2 Lateral and medial ankle ligament anatomy. (From Pugh KJ: Fractures and soft-tissue injuries about the ankle. In Fitzgerald RH, Kaufer H, Malkami AL [eds]: Orthopaedics. St. Louis, Mosby, 2002, pp 420–421.)

malleolus may indicate injury to the deltoid ligament and may require stress radiographs to rule out an unstable fracture pattern more adequately treated with surgery. Weber C fractures are rarely stable and are almost always treated surgically. Bimalleolar ankle fractures are difficult to treat with closed means because of their instability. When closed management of bimalleolar ankle fractures is chosen, there must be anatomic alignment ensured with weekly serial radiographs for the first month, then biweekly until healed.

Nonoperative treatment usually consists of closed reduction and casting. With Weber A fractures, a removable boot can be applied, and weight bearing initiated as tolerated. For Weber B fractures treated nonoperatively, a short leg cast is applied and patients are non-weight bearing initially. The mechanism of injury as determined by the history and the Lauge-Hansen classification is reversed, the foot is placed in a plantigrade position, and the cast is molded to resist redisplacement. Maintenance of the normal mortise relationship must be ensured throughout

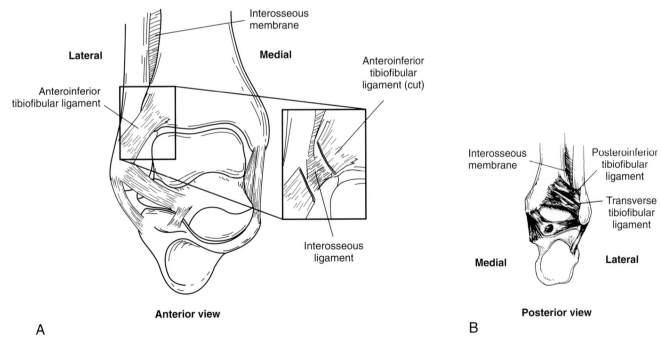

Figure 68-3 A and **B,** Syndesmosis anatomy. (From Coughlin MJ, Mann RA: Surgery of the Foot and Ankle, 7th ed. St. Louis, Mosby, 1999, p 1134.)

Danis-Weber Classification

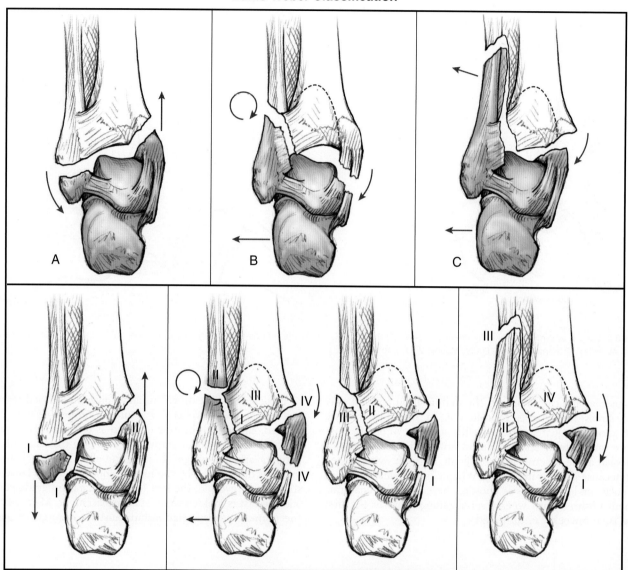

Lauge-Hansen Classification

Figure 68-4 Classification of ankle fractures. (From Pugh KJ: Fractures and soft-tissue injuries about the ankle. In Fitzgerald RH, Kaufer H, Malkami AL [eds]: Orthopaedics. St. Louis, Mosby, 2002, p 424.)

nonoperative treatment with serial radiographs. Bimalleolar ankle fractures require stabilization above the knee to manage rotatory deforming forces across the ankle (Fig. 68-6).

Operative Treatment
Surgery is usually indicated in those fractures that are initially unstable or have lost reduction with closed treatment. If the mortise is widened medially more than 4 mm on initial radiographs or there is a Weber C fracture or bimalleolar fracture, closed treatment is much more difficult and can lead to a poor result.[10] The detailed description of operative treatment can be found in other texts, and preoperative planning is imperative. The weight-bearing status after surgery is determined by the injury pattern, type of fixation used, and patient compliance. Immobilization is determined by the same factors and varies with different injuries or fixation. Usually patients are placed in a removable orthosis at 2 weeks and are weight bearing by 6 weeks.

SYNDESMOSIS INJURIES

Diagnosis
Syndesmosis injuries are a continuum of ankle injuries, but there is a more protracted course than both ankle sprains and ankle fractures. The diagnosis, therefore, is important to rule out in all ankle injuries because it determines the time away from sport and, if missed, can lead to chronic ankle pain and disability. Close attention to these injuries and their early diagnosis may alleviate time and discontent while the athlete wonders why he or she is still not playing after 6 weeks. With fractures, early attention to these injuries decreases the chance of a poor result. Traumatic diastases are usually diagnosed with radiographs, but history and examination are helpful.

History
In syndesmosis injury, the patient has well-localized pain located over the anterolateral aspect of the ankle. The patient will

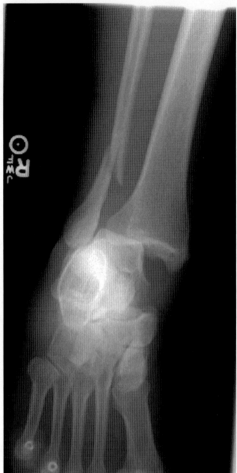

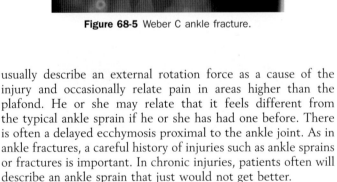

Figure 68-5 Weber C ankle fracture.

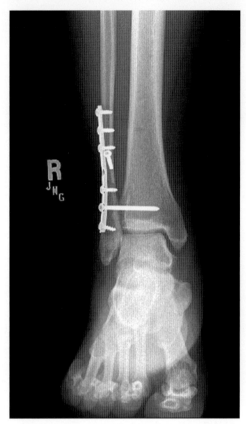

Figure 68-6 Weber C ankle fracture after open reduction with internal fixation.

usually describe an external rotation force as a cause of the injury and occasionally relate pain in areas higher than the plafond. He or she may relate that it feels different from the typical ankle sprain if he or she has had one before. There is often a delayed ecchymosis proximal to the ankle joint. As in ankle fractures, a careful history of injuries such as ankle sprains or fractures is important. In chronic injuries, patients often will describe an ankle sprain that just would not get better.

Examination
Swelling and tenderness are usually more precisely located than in a typical sprain. There is very little tenderness and swelling over the anterotalofibular or calcaneofibular ligaments, with tenderness more proximal than a usual ankle sprain. The lateral and medial malleolus must be palpated to rule out fracture, and the entire fibula must be palpated to rule out proximal fracture (Maisonneuve's fracture).

The squeeze test, popularized at West Point, is provocation of pain at the syndesmosis by squeezing the tibia and fibula at midcalf.[11] It is poorly studied as a sensitive or specific test but can heighten suspicion of this injury. The anterior drawer test is usually performed and usually negative, although there may be some varus-valgus instability. A more specific test is to hold the leg stabilized with the knee flexed at 90 degrees and apply external rotation stress to the ankle. This reproduces pain at the syndesmosis and should indicate syndesmosis injury unless ruled out by radiographs.

Imaging
Standard ankle radiographs may reveal a normal-appearing ankle but may also show subtle signs of injury such as a fleck of bone off the posterior tubercle of the tibia. Radiographs may also reveal chronic injury to the syndesmosis with calcification of the ligaments and interosseous membrane. Diastasis of the syndesmosis is indicated when there is no malleolus fracture and the mortise is widened medially more than 4 mm. This can be variable, and comparison radiographs may be necessary. Another method is to use the amount of overlap of the fibula and tibia of 5 mm on the anteroposterior view or 1 mm on the mortise view. The tibiofibular clear space is the distance between the fibula and the incisura of the tibia 1 cm proximal to the plafond. This normal distance has been found by several studies to be fairly consistent at about 4 mm.[12–14]

If there are clinical findings of syndesmosis injury and standard radiographs are negative, external rotation stress radiographs are indicated. These can be difficult to interpret and may be limited by patient pain, but if there is obvious widening, it is a useful test. A bone scan may be a way to diagnose injuries that are not diagnosed with stress radiographs limited by patient pain. Magnetic resonance imaging is also very sensitive in detecting ligamentous injury and is becoming more common in helping to determine return to play and prognosis in high-demand athletes. Certainly, if there is any widening of the mortise on any view, the entire fibula must be visualized on radiographs (Fig. 68-7).

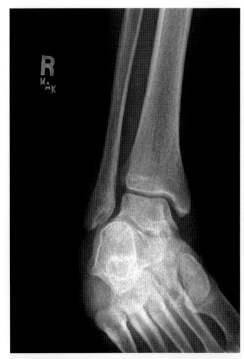

Figure 68-7 Syndesmosis injury.

Treatment of Syndesmosis Injury

Treatment of these injuries is based on whether there is diastasis on plain radiographs, diastasis on stress radiographs, or if fracture is present.

Sprain without Diastasis

These injuries are assumed to be stable, and treatment is generally weight bearing as tolerated with or without a high pneumatic brace. For more severe stable injuries, a period of non-weight bearing up to 4 weeks may be employed. Counseling the patient and coach is very important because these injuries have been shown to take an average of 43 days of recovery time.[11] This is almost double the recovery time of lateral ankle sprains. Reinjury is common, and return too early can result in a prolonged course. Eighty-six percent of these athletes can be expected to have a good to excellent result, but one third will have mild stiffness and one fourth will have mild activity-related pain.[15] A custom brace to limit rotation can be helpful on return to sports.

Sprain with Diastasis on Stress Radiographs

These patients do not require surgery as long as the syndesmosis is anatomic. This can be confirmed with computed tomography or magnetic resonance imaging. The patient should be placed in a non-weight-bearing cast or brace for 4 weeks followed by progressive weight bearing for 2 to 4 weeks. Maintenance of reduction should be confirmed during the course of 2 to 3 weeks to ensure proper anatomic healing.

Frank Diastasis with or without Proximal Fibula Fracture

There is little question that these patients require anatomic reduction of the syndesmosis with operative fixation. There is some discussion over the exact method with which to fix them. The standard teaching is to reduce the syndesmosis closed, using

a large clamp with the ankle dorsiflexed. This is viewed on anteroposterior and lateral projection to ensure anatomic reduction. After reduction, the screws are placed percutaneously from the fibula to the tibia at a 20-degree angle posteriorly to anteriorly to ensure placement of the screw into the tibia. The postoperative course is then non-weight bearing for 6 to 8 weeks, followed by weight bearing as tolerated for a few weeks, followed by screw removal at 10 to 12 weeks.

Some authors recommend open reduction with direct ligament repair of the syndesmosis. Certainly, if a significant amount of force is required or if the syndesmosis will not reduce, open reduction is indicated, but this is rarely necessary. There is controversy over the size of screws and how many to place. Most recommend either two 3.5-mm cortical screws 1 cm apart, with the inferior screw 1 cm above the plafond, or one 4.5-mm cortical screw. The length of the screw is also debated, with some recommending three cortices and others recommending four. Controversy also exists over whether to remove screws. Screws limit the ability of the fibula to rotate normally. The screws often eventually break, but broken screws rarely cause any sequelae. They are more difficult to remove after they have broken. Regardless of the fixation used, anatomic reduction and maintenance of fixation until the syndesmotic ligaments have healed are the mainstays of treatment.

Frank Diastasis with Weber B or Weber C Fibula Fracture

Surgery of the ankle fracture is usually indicated in this case, and stability of the syndesmosis can be assessed intraoperatively. The cotton test involves a towel clip on the fixed fibula and application of a lateral pull on the fibula. The external rotation

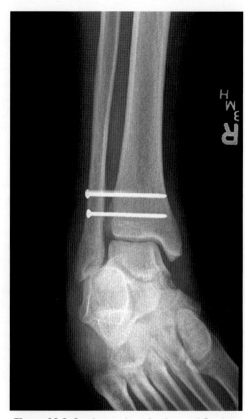

Figure 68-8 Syndesmosis reduction and fixation.

stress test can also be performed with a mortise view of the ankle and external stress applied. Any diastasis at the syndesmosis indicates instability and should be repaired with screws as described previously. The screws can go either through or around the plate so preoperative planning is a must to prepare for possible screw placement. In many bimalleolar ankle fractures, fixation of the medial malleolus restores the medial anatomy and ligamentous structure; thus, syndesmosis screws may not be required. Stress views can help determine whether they are needed (Fig. 68-8 and Table 68-1).

Results

Most follow-up studies of syndesmosis injuries have few patients. In Fritschy's report on 10 patients with syndesmotic injury, three were treated surgically and seven with walking casts. They all returned to World Cup skiing, with one having persistent pain.[16] Edwards and DeLee reported on six cases of frank diastasis; four patients had good results and two patients with mild ankle pain and restriction in ankle motion had fair results.[17] Syndesmosis injuries appear to add morbidity to ankle fractures and early diagnosis may lead to an improved result both clinically and emotionally because the expectations will be more appropriate.

Table 68-1 Treatment of Ankle Fractures

Nonoperative	Operative
Weber A	Weber C
Mortise displaced <4 mm	Mortise displaced >4 mm
Contraindications to surgery	Bimalleolar fracture
Serious comorbidity	Displaced Weber B
Soft tissue related	

REFERENCES

1. Bonnin JG: Injuries to the Ankle. Darien, CT, Hafner, 1970.
2. Shereff MJ: Radiographic analysis of the foot and ankle. In Jahss MH (ed): Disorders of the Foot and Ankle, 2nd ed. Philadelphia, WB Saunders, 1991.
3. Sarrafian SK: Anatomy of the Foot and Ankle: Descriptive, Topographic, Functional. Philadelphia, JB Lippincott, 1983.
4. Phillips WA, Schwartz HS, Keller CS, et al: A prospective randomized study of the management of severe ankle fractures. J Bone Joint Surg Am 1985;67:67–78.
5. Inman VT: The Joints of the Ankle. Baltimore, Williams & Wilkins, 1976.
6. Lindsjo U, Danckwardt-Lilliestrom G, Sahlstedt B: Measurement of the range of motion of the loaded ankle. Clin Orthop 1985;199:68–71.
7. Close JR: Some applications of the functional anatomy of the ankle joint. J Bone Joint Surg Am 1956;38:761–781.
8. Rasmussen O: Stability of the ankle joint: Analysis of the function and traumatology of the ankle ligaments. Acta Orthop Scand Suppl 1985;211:1–75.
9. Rasmussen O, Tovberg-Jensen I: Mobility of the ankle joint: Recording ankle movements in the talocrural joints in vitro with and without the lateral collateral ligaments of the ankle. Acta Orthop Scand 1982;53:155–160.
10. Mak KH, Chan KM, Leung PC: Ankle fracture treated with the AO principle—An experience with 116 cases. Injury 1985;16:265–272.
11. Hopkinson WJ, St. Pierre P, Ryan JB, et al: Syndesmosis sprains of the ankle. Foot Ankle 1990;10:325–330.
12. Leeds HC, Ehrlich MG: Instability of the distal tibiofibular syndesmosis after bimalleolar and trimalleolar ankle fractures. J Bone Joint Surg Am 1984;66:490–503.
13. Whiteside LA, Reynolds FC, Ellsasser JC: Tibiofibular synostosis and recurrent ankle sprains in high performance athletes. Am J Sports Med 1978;6:204–305.
14. Gabarino JL, Clancy M, Harcke T, et al: Congenital diastasis of the inferior tibiofibular joint: A review of the literature and report of two cases. J Pediatr Orthop 1985;5:225–228.
15. Taylor DC, Englehardt DL, Bassett FH: Syndesmosis sprains of the ankle and the influence of heterotopic ossification. Am J Sports Med 1992;20:146–150.
16. Fritschy D: An unusual ankle injury in top skiers. Am J Sports Med 1989;17:282–286.
17. Edwards GS Jr, DeLee JC: Ankle diastasis without fracture. Foot Ankle 1984;4:305–312.

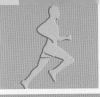

Ankle Tendon Disorders and Ruptures

Sharrona Williams and James Nunley

In This Chapter

INTRODUCTION

Peroneal Tendons

- Peroneal tendon injury must be considered any time a patient presents with lateral ankle pain.

- Acute injuries to the peroneal tendons usually present similar to a lateral ankle sprain and often these two injuries occur concomitantly. These injuries are common in the athletic population.

- Chronic peroneal conditions are frequently overlooked as a source of chronic lateral ankle pain.

- Peroneal tendonitis is usually successfully treated nonoperatively, although recalcitrant cases may respond to surgical débridement.

- Attritional tears of the peroneal tendons may do well with conservative treatment.

- Peroneal subluxation and dislocation may be managed nonoperatively, but rarely with good results. These injuries usually require surgical intervention.

- Surgical outcomes are generally good in cases of subluxation, dislocation, and longitudinal tearing of the peroneal tendons.

Achilles Tendon

- Achilles tendon overuse injuries are common in the athletic population, especially runners.

- Posterior heel pain is usually multifactorial and can include tendonitis, tendonosis, tendonosis with partial rupture, insertional tendonitis, retrocalcaneal bursitis, and subcutaneous tendo-Achilles bursitis.

- Most cases of posterior heel pain are successfully treated conservatively. However, if conservative treatment fails, operative treatment has been shown to be effective.[1,2]

- Achilles tendon ruptures are usually treated operatively in athletes. Operative treatment has shown an advantage over nonoperative treatments in isokinetic strength and return to preinjury activities.[3-6] Both percutaneous and open repair techniques are available.

PERONEAL TENDONS

Clinical Features and Evaluation

Tendonitis

Peroneal tenosynovitis commonly presents in athletes and is usually due to repetitive activities, but direct trauma such as ankle fracture, calcaneal fracture, and chronic lateral ankle instability can also be a source. Furthermore, there are anatomic considerations that may cause peroneal tendon inflammation, including crowding of the tendons in the fibro-osseous canal by a low-lying peroneus brevis muscle or the presence of a peroneus quartus muscle/tendon that can also cause overcrowding of the tendon sheath. Tendon irritation can occur at the retromalleolar sulcus, peroneal tubercle, and the os perineum, where the tendons sheaths can become stenosed. Patients may have malalignment at the knee and/or ankle contributing to overload of the peroneals. A cavovarus foot commonly causes more stress on the lateral aspect of the foot and may lead to tenosynovitis, recurrent ankle sprains, or longitudinal peroneal tears.

Patients with peroneal tenosynovitis usually complain of pain and swelling at the lateral aspect of the ankle over the peroneals. A palpable thickening over the tendons may be present. The subtalar joint range of motion may be limited secondary to peroneal spasm. The physical examination may reveal pain with passive inversion or resisted eversion and dorsiflexion of the foot. There may be a decrease in peroneal strength as well. If there is doubt about the source of lateral ankle pain, an injection of local anesthesia into the peroneal sheath can be diagnostic for pathology. Anteroposterior and lateral weight-bearing radiographs should be obtained to rule out bony injury.

Tendon Tears and Ruptures

Peroneal tendon tears commonly occur in athletes and have the same mechanism as lateral ankle sprains, plantarflexion, and inversion. These injuries often are combined and must be considered especially when, after sufficient time for an ankle sprain to heal, complaints of persistent lateral ankle pain and swelling still exist. Bassett and Speer,[7] in a cadaveric study, showed that peroneal tendon tears occur at between 25 and 15 degrees of plantarflexion as the peroneus longus impinges against the tip of the fibula and as the peroneus brevis impinges against the lateral wall of the fibula. Acute tendon tears can occur in both the peroneus longus and brevis, as shown in the above study.

Attritional or longitudinal tears in the peroneus brevis tendon may occur without any particular inciting event or in patients who have a history of recurrent lateral ankle sprains. These tears typically occur in the retromalleolar region. Sobel et al,[8] in an anatomic study of 124 fresh cadavers, found 11.3% with attritional tears of the peroneus brevis tendons centered over the tip of fibula and within the groove; these tears averaged 1.9 cm in length. These authors found no involvement of the peroneus longus tendon. The peroneus longus may act as a wedge and divide the peroneus brevis over the fibrocartilaginous ridge of the posterolateral aspect of the fibula. If the superior retinaculum is incompetent, the tendon is further stressed. Degenerative tears of the peroneus longus are rare, but when they occur, they are usually within the cuboid groove just distal to the os peroneum.

The clinical presentation of peroneal tendon tears is similar to peroneal tendonitis, except symptoms are prolonged with more pronounced pain and weakness. Magnetic resonance imaging (MRI) may be diagnostic and can identify tears, tendonitis, tendonopathy, or anomalous muscle, but MRI is less than 100% accurate.

Traumatic ruptures of the peroneal tendons, though unusual, do happen secondary to trauma or sports injury. Patients often complain of pre-existing pain or disability. Complete rupture usually occurs at areas where stenosis is present. There are case reports of both peroneal tendons rupturing, but typically only one tendon is involved.[9]

Dislocation and Subluxation

Acute dislocation or subluxation of the peroneal tendons is an uncommon injury that has a traumatic cause. Sport participation is responsible for about 92% of acute peroneal dislocations. Skiing has been reported to cause approximately 66% of the sports injuries.[10] Peroneal tendon dislocation may be difficult to distinguish from an acute ankle sprain, but it is rare for both to occur simultaneously. The acute dislocation is caused by a sudden forceful dorsiflexion with simultaneous "violent" reflex contraction of the peroneal muscles. With skiing injuries, the mechanism has been described as forceful peroneal contraction occurring with sudden deceleration and ankle dorsiflexion as the ski tips dig into the snow. Acute injuries frequently exhibit ecchymosis, tenderness, and swelling over the lateral aspect of the ankle and may look similar to a high ankle sprain. Most patients are unable to describe the mechanism of injury, as opposed to lateral ankle sprains, where most are able to describe an inversion injury. There are several findings on physical examination that help make a distinction between lateral ankle sprain and peroneal dislocation; typically, the tenderness is posterior to the fibula with acute dislocation versus anterior over the anterior talofibular ligament or anterior tibiofibular ligament with a sprain. Patients may complain of a painful "snapping" sensation and have apprehension on resisted dorsiflexion and eversion with dislocation. The anterior drawer sign should be negative in peroneal dislocation.

Eckert and Davis[11] described a classification of acute peroneal tendon dislocation after exploring 73 cases. In grade I injuries, the superior retinaculum and periosteum are stripped off the posterior lateral border of the fibula. The peroneus longus dislocates anteriorly, sitting between the periosteum and the fibula. In grade II injuries, the fibrous rim of the superior peroneal retinaculum is avulsed along with the periosteum of the fibula, mim-

icking a Bankart lesion in the shoulder. The peroneus longus dislocates anteriorly. In grade III injuries, a bony rim fracture involving the posterior lateral corner of the fibula along with the periosteum and fibrous rim are avulsed by the retinaculum. None of these 73 cases had an actual tear of the superior peroneal retinaculum.

In chronic peroneal tendon dislocation, the ankle may appear normal. This injury should be suspected when there is a history of pain with unusual "popping." A popping or snapping sensation is often reproducible with dorsiflexion and eversion of the foot. Slight swelling and tenderness are usually present posteriorly, and if more significant pain is noted, a tendon tear should be suspected. There may be a complaint of instability, yet the anterior drawer and talar tilt tests remain normal.

Standard weight-bearing anteroposterior, lateral, and mortise radiographs should be obtained and inspected for a flake or fibular cortex rim fracture. This finding on radiographs is pathognomonic of grade III tendon dislocation and is found in 10% to 30% of cases.

Tenography, computed tomography, and MRI have been used to diagnose peroneal tendon dislocations, with MRI currently the study of choice. MRI has the best ability to define soft-tissue structures including the peroneal tendons, superior retinaculum, and inferior retinaculum.

Relevant Anatomy

The peroneus longus and peroneus brevis muscles originate in the lateral compartment of the leg and run distally to course behind the lateral malleolus. The musculotendinous junctions are usually proximal to the superior peroneal retinaculum, but a low-lying brevis muscle can exist, contributing to stenosis within the sheath. The brevis runs deep to the longus and approximately 4 cm proximal to the lateral malleolus, both the brevis and longus pass through the common peroneal sheath. This sheath passes through a fibro-osseous tunnel that is stabilized by the superior peroneal retinaculum, posterior talofibular ligament, calcaneofibular ligament, posterior inferior tibiofibular ligament, and fibula. As the peroneals pass distal to the inferior border of the superior peroneal retinaculum, the synovial sheaths bifurcate into separate sheaths for each tendon. The tendons pass deep to the inferior peroneal retinaculum. The inferior peroneal retinaculum is 2 to 3 cm distal to the fibula and acts as a pulley over both tendons, but it has no significant role in peroneal tendon subluxation. The tendons then pass anterior to the peroneal tubercle of the calcaneus, which can be a source of irritation to the tendons as well. The brevis then crosses anterior to the longus and inserts on the base of the fifth metatarsal. The peroneus brevis is the primary evertor of the foot and has a negligible role in ankle and foot plantarflexion. The peroneal longus enters the deep sole of the foot through a groove in the inferolateral cuboid. This tunnel is another area where stenosis can occur. The os peroneum, an accessory bone located plantar to the cuboid, lateral to the cuboid, or at the calcaneocuboid articulation, is found within the substance of the tendon and ossified in approximately 20% of feet. The os peroneum can also be a cause of stenosing peroneus longus tenosynovitis in the cuboid tunnel. The longus lies directly under the cuneiforms and inserts into the plantar lateral aspect of the base of the first metatarsal. The longus is a weak evertor of the foot but functions primarily to plantarflex the first ray. Both the peroneus longus and brevis are innervated by the superficial peroneal nerve.

The peroneus quartus muscle exists in 6.6% of patients according to Zammit and Singh[12] and in 22% according to Sobel et al.[8] It usually arises from the peroneus brevis muscle and inserts into the retrotrochlear eminence of the calcaneus. The presence of this muscle has been associated with longitudinal tears in the brevis, prominent retrotrochlear eminence, and lax superior peroneal retinaculum.

The posterior aspect of the distal fibula is also called the retromalleolar sulcus. There is variability in its depth and width. Seventy percent of fibulas have a bony ridge that can add 2 to 4 mm of depth to the sulcus. The width of the sulcus usually ranges from 5 to 10 mm. Edwards[13] examined 178 cadaver fibulas but found that 82% had a substantial recess/groove in posterior fibula and 18% were flat or convex, a finding that can contribute to peroneal tendon instability.

The superior peroneal retinaculum maintains the peroneal tendons behind the fibula. It averages 10 to 20 mm in width and at least one band runs parallel to the calcaneofibular ligament. Variability exists in the width, thickness, and insertions of the superior peroneal retinaculum. The superior peroneal retinaculum is a condensation of the superficial fascia of the calf and the peroneal tendon sheath. Approximately 2 cm proximal to the tip of the distal fibula, the superior peroneal retinaculum originates from periosteum and is the principal structure injured in acute peroneal tendon dislocation. This structure is also a secondary restraint to ankle inversion. Beck[14] elucidated that division of the superior peroneal retinaculum alone is not sufficient to cause peroneal tendon dislocation and that additional fibular pathology is necessary. Laxity in the superior peroneal retinaculum can lead to subluxation and splitting of the tendons.

Treatment Options
Tendonitis

The conservative treatment modalities available for peroneal tenosynovitis include rest, ice, activity modification, nonsteroidal anti-inflammatory drugs, and orthotic management such as a lateral heel wedge. Occasionally, immobilization in a short-leg walking cast is required for a 4- to 6-week trial. Alternatively, an ankle-foot orthosis for 8 to 12 weeks can be used for immobilization. Steroid injections in the tendon sheath are controversial; if used, the risk of subsequent attrition or rupture must be considered.

Tear or Rupture

Attritional tendon tears can be managed similar to peroneal tenosynovitis depending on the severity of symptoms. With mild to moderate symptoms, rest, nonsteroidal anti-inflammatory drugs, activity modification, or orthotic management may help. If symptoms are more severe, then immobilization with a cast is necessary. Once again, localized intrasheath steroid injection has been advocated by some authors, but we recommend against this.[15]

Dislocation or Subluxation

Acute   Conservative measures for treating acute peroneal dislocation include a below-knee cast in slight plantarflexion and inversion. Non-weight bearing in the cast is generally maintained for 6 weeks; some authors advocate advancing weight bearing in the cast.

After discontinuation of the cast, range-of-motion exercises are initiated. A good result after nonoperative treatment of acute peroneal dislocation occurs in 50% to 57% of patients. Eventually, 44% of patients require surgery after nonoperative measures fail.

Chronic   There is little benefit of conservative treatment for symptomatic chronic peroneal tendon dislocation. Sammarco[16] states that conservative treatment does help reduce inflammation or pain, but chronic peroneal tendon dislocation frequently recurs after immobilization is discontinued. Observation is acceptable if subluxating or dislocating peroneal tendons are found incidentally, with an absence of symptoms and no athletic compromise.

Surgery
Tendonitis

If conservative treatment is unsuccessful for peroneal tendonitis, surgical treatment is considered. A curvilinear incision paralleling the posterior and inferior aspect of the fibula is used to allow for adequate tenosynovectomy. In addition, other pathology found intraoperatively should be addressed. The superior peroneal retinaculum should be maintained.

Tear or Rupture

When conservative treatment fails for longitudinal peroneal tears, surgical management is indicated. The same curvilinear incision described above following the course of the peroneals is used. The sural nerve is identified and protected. Tendon subluxation or dislocation is assessed. The sheath is opened longitudinally and the tendons are inspected. A tenosynovectomy is performed and the degenerative split débrided. Krause and Brodsky[15] proposed a clinical classification of peroneus brevis tears. They recommended that if 50% or more is viable after débridement (grade 1), then repair should be done using a running absorbable suture, tubularizing the tendon (Fig. 69-1). However, if less than 50% of the tendon is viable after débridement (grade 2), then a proximal and distal tenodesis of the brevis to the longus tendon should be performed using an absorbable suture. The tenodesis should be done approximately 3 to 4 cm proximal to the tip of the fibula and 5 to 6 cm below. Any associated pathology including tendon subluxation or chronic ankle instability should be addressed simultaneously. The superior peroneal retinaculum is repaired with suture or drill holes in the fibula.

Surgical exploration should be performed for acute peroneal tendon ruptures. A long curvilinear incision over the area of suspected rupture is made. The sural nerve is protected. The anterior talofibular and calcaneofibular ligaments are inspected. The peroneal sheath is incised with preservation of the superior peroneal retinaculum. The proximal and distal ends of the tendon are identified and débrided. The tendon can be repaired with Bunnell, Krackow, or Kessler sutures and an additional running epitenon stitch. The sheath and wound are closed in standard fashion.

Dislocation or Subluxation

Acute   Operative management is considered in the young athletic population. There is a high failure rate of conservative treatment and a better success rate with surgery. Superior peroneal retinacular repair will address acute subluxation or dislocation. The patient can be placed in a prone, lateral, or supine position; we use the lateral position. A 7-cm longitudinal incision, 1 cm posterior to the fibula and following the tendons, is used. The sural nerve is identified and protected. The superior peroneal retinaculum is identified and the defect located. Each tendon should be inspected for concomitant defects. The tendons are retracted and the fibular groove is inspected. If the groove is shallow, flat, or convex, the groove is deepened. The superior peroneal retinaculum is repaired by placing three to four drill holes in the posterolateral margin of the fibula. The sutures

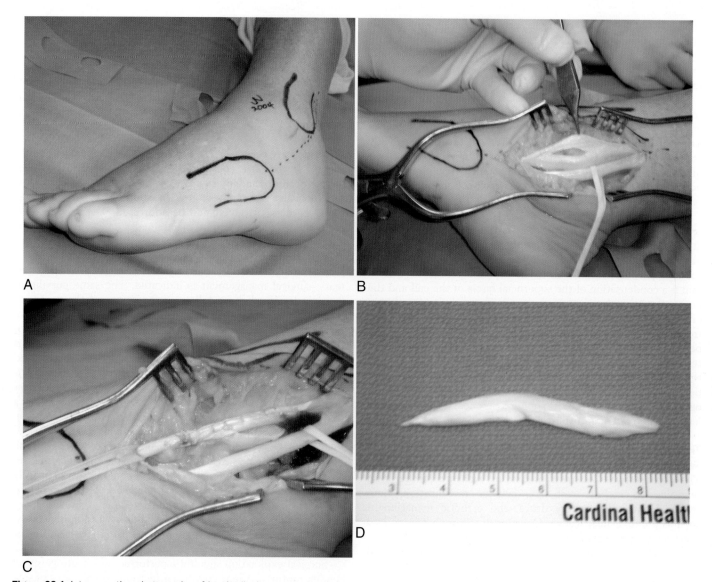

Figure 69-1 Intraoperative photographs of longitudinal peroneus brevis tear requiring tubularization. **A,** Planned incision along the course of the peroneal tendons; **B,** identified tear in the peroneus brevis; **C,** tubularized tendon; **D,** débrided portion.

through the superior peroneal retinaculum are advanced through the drill holes. Finally, the retinaculum is imbricated for reinforcement.

Chronic There is a multitude of surgical procedures described to address chronic peroneal dislocation: retinaculum reinforcement and repair, tissue transfer, tendon rerouting, bone block, and groove deepening are discussed here.

Superior peroneal retinaculum reinforcement entails the same technique as with acute repair. If a fibula avulsion fracture exists, then open reduction and internal fixation are recommended. The advantages of this repair include a small incision, anatomic approach, and avoidance of an osteotomy. The potential disadvantage of this procedure is the failure to correct predisposing anatomy, such as sulcus deformities and insufficient retinaculum.

Tissue transfers use tendons and periosteal flaps from other places to recreate or reinforce the superior retinaculum. The most common procedure was described by Jones using a distally attached slip of the Achilles tendon routed through the fibula.

This stabilizes the peroneals and reinforces the retinaculum. Modifications using the plantaris or peroneus brevis have also been reported.

Tendon rerouting relies on the calcaneofibular ligament to constrain the peroneal tendons. Four methods of tendon rerouting have been reported.

Platzgummer described dividing the calcaneofibular ligament near the fibular insertion and suturing it over the tendons.[10] A modification of this was described by Sarmiento and Wolf who transected the peroneal tendons, passed them below the calcaneofibular ligament, and then repaired them.[10]

Pozo and Jackson demonstrated another technique, taking the calcaneofibular ligament origin with a predrilled piece of distal fibula.[10] The tendons were replaced in the sulcus and the fibula reattached with screw fixation. Poll and Duijfjes reversed this procedure by detaching the insertion of the calcaneofibular ligament with a predrilled piece of the calcaneus.[10]

Bone Block Bone block procedures attempt to contain the peroneal tendons using the fibula. This procedure was first described by Kelly in 1920 by using a partial thickness osteotomy of the distal fibula rotated posteriorly to deepen the fibular groove. DuVries modified this technique by driving a wedge of fibula posteriorly to hold the dislocating peroneal tendons.[10]

Groove Deepening Groove deepening addresses the shallow or absent retromalleolar groove that often exists in cases of peroneal subluxation or dislocation. The classic groove deepening and newer methods are described. The patient is positioned in the lateral decubitus position. A curvilinear incision starting 5 to 6 cm proximal to the tip of the fibula is made, ending just distal to the fibula. The sural nerve is identified and protected throughout the entire procedure. The entire sheath and retinaculum are visualized prior to incising them just posterior to the border of the fibula. The peroneal tendons are inspected for any associated pathology. Some form of tendon pathology usually exists, primarily longitudinal tearing, and this must be addressed intraoperatively. The retromalleolar sulcus is exposed. Often the groove is shallow, ranging from flat to convex. A saw is used to create a 3-cm long × 1-cm trapdoor within the fibula that is hinged medially (Fig. 69-2). An osteotome is used to elevate the trapdoor. A curet is used to remove 7 to 9 mm of cancellous bone before reinserting the flap into the deepened bed. The retinaculum and periosteum are reattached to the posterolateral border using suture placed through drill holes. The superior peroneal retinaculum is reinforced simultaneously.

The more recently described groove-deepening technique is generally easier to perform. Once the retromalleolar sulcus is exposed, an incision just anterior to the origin of the calcaneofibular ligament is made. Care is taken not to incise the calcaneofibular ligament. A periosteal elevator is used to mobilize the soft tissue at the distal fibula. The medullary canal is then reamed using sequential drill bits. The drilling is started at the distal tip of the fibula and advanced proximally into the shaft. The drill bit size is sequentially increased at the most posterior portion of the fibula, being careful not to perforate the cortex.

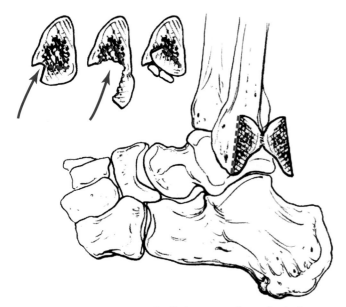

Figure 69-2 Classic technique for fibular groove deepening in the treatment of peroneal subluxation or dislocation.

Once the cortex has been weakened, a bone tamp is used to impact the posterior fibular cortex into the medullary canal. This can increase groove depth by 3 to 8 mm. The retinaculum is then closed in a pants-over-vest fashion.

Postoperative Rehabilitation
Tendonitis
After peroneal tenosynovectomy, the patient is immobilized until the wound heals. This is followed by range-of-motion exercises and sport-specific strengthening exercises. There is a gradual return to preinjury activities as tolerated.

Tear or Rupture
If simple débridement and repair or tubularization is performed, the patient is kept non-weight bearing for 2 weeks. This is followed by weight bearing in a short-leg cast for two additional weeks. A removable boot is used at 4 weeks, and range-of-motion exercises for dorsiflexion/plantarflexion are initiated. At 6 weeks, inversion/eversion and a progressive strengthening program is instituted. Patients are then gradually advanced to full activity. Some authors advocate non-weight bearing for up to 5 weeks and immobilization in a removable boot for up to 10 weeks, especially when a tenodesis is performed.[15]

After acute repair of the peroneal tendons, the patient is placed in a short-leg walking cast for 6 to 8 weeks. Weight bearing is allowed after 2 weeks. The rehabilitation program consists of range-of-motion, strengthening, and proprioception exercises. Return to competitive sports should be allowed at 5 to 6 months.

Dislocation or Subluxation (Acute and Chronic)
Patients are maintained non-weight bearing for 2 weeks in a short-leg cast. A walking boot or short-leg cast is used for 4 to 6 weeks. A stirrup brace may be used for several weeks after discontinuation of the boot. At this point, formal physical therapy is introduced to start range of motion and sport-specific strengthening, which is slowly advanced. It may take 4 to 6 months before full range of motion is obtained.

Criteria for Return to Sports
Range of motion and full strength must be recovered prior to resuming athletics. After a progressive rehabilitation program, most patients are able to return to athletic activities without limitations by 4 to 6 months.

Results and Outcomes
Some reported series combine all peroneal injuries when presenting outcomes. Overall, peroneal tendon disorders that require operative intervention have good to excellent outcomes. Alanen et al[17] reported a series of 38 patients treated for chronic peroneal tendonitis (five patients), peroneal tears (13 patients) and ruptures (six patients), peroneal subluxation/dislocation (nine patients), and peroneal anomalies (five patients). Eighty percent of the patients were competitive athletes, and 50% of the cases were associated with lateral ankle instability. Ninety percent of the patients had good to excellent outcomes.

The outcomes after tenosynovectomy for peroneal tenosynovitis are good to excellent. Peroneal tendon ruptures are uncommon, but of those reported, good to excellent outcomes are obtained. Athletes are able to return to competition without limitations. Bassett and Speer,[7] at our institution, reported on acute peroneal tears in athletes that were repaired surgically. The outcomes were generally excellent, with all ankles remaining asymptomatic while maintaining full athletic activity at follow-up of an average of 7.9 years. Good to excellent clinical results after surgical repair of longitudinal peroneal brevis tears were reported by Krause and Brodsky.[15] These authors found that return to maximal function is prolonged but achievable.

Surgical reconstruction after acute peroneal dislocation has a success rate of 96%. Patients are able to return to full athletic activities with no limitations. In chronic cases, with retinacular reinforcement and repair, the recurrence rate is about 3%. Of the Jones procedures reported, there have been no redislocations. The main reported complication is loss of motion, occurring in 15% of patients. This is thought to be secondary to the tenodesis effect.

There has been no reported recurrence of peroneal dislocation after surgical stabilization with tendon-rerouting procedures. Only minor complications have been reported, including sensory nerve injuries and minor discomfort. Bone block procedures for chronic peroneal tendons dislocation have a redislocation rate of 8%. The overall complication rate after this procedure is up to 30%. Screw-related problems, nonunion, and fracture are reported. With the classic groove-deepening procedure, there are no reported recurrences of subluxation, dislocation, or instability in the 28 reported cases.

Complications

In all procedures addressing peroneal pathology, the sural nerve is at risk of injury. The nerve must be identified and protected throughout the procedure. This is one of the most frequent minor complications. Loss of motion after stabilization of the peroneal tendons with rerouting procedures is another potential complication.

Conclusions

Peroneal tendonitis usually occurs in the athletic population secondary to overuse but can also occur after a traumatic event. Peroneal tendon disorders must be considered in the evaluation of lateral ankle pain. The mechanism for ankle sprains and peroneal tendon tears are the same, and these injuries often occur concomitantly. Peroneal tendonitis is usually successfully managed conservatively. An adequate trial of all modalities must be given before the option of surgery is considered. Longitudinal peroneal tears are also initially managed conservatively, but when symptoms persist, these tears are successfully managed surgically.

Acute peroneal subluxation or dislocation is uncommon and can be frequently difficult to diagnosis. A high index of suspicion must be maintained. There is a 50% success rate for non operative treatment in acute injury, and most believe that these injuries have a better outcome when treated surgically. Chronic peroneal dislocation most commonly occurs from misdiagnosed or nontreated acute dislocation. A deficient superior peroneal retinaculum and shallow fibular groove may increase the instability risk. If asymptomatic, conservative measures are employed, but operative intervention is necessary in symptomatic patients. There are multiple procedures with good outcomes available to stabilize the peroneal tendons. At the time of surgery, all pathology must be addressed.

ACHILLES TENDON

Clinical Features and Evaluation

When investigating the causes of posterior heel pain in the athlete, the history of recent change in duration, intensity, and frequency of training must be elicited, as these may be contributory factors. Also, the type of shoes and running surfaces should be noted. During physical examination, mechanical alignment of the entire extremity must be evaluated, checking for a cavus foot, supinated forefoot, hyperpronation, genu varum, or femoral anteversion, all of which have been linked to increased stresses on the Achilles tendon.

Paratendonitis

Acute paratendonitis occurs most commonly in marathon runners; it is also the result of repetitive stress from cutting, jumping, and pushing off and therefore seen in all types of running athletes. Generally, the area of pain is 4 cm proximal to the calcaneal insertion of the Achilles tendon and the patient exhibits diffuse swelling and discomfort along the tendon. In acute paratendonitis, pain with swelling, warmth, and tenderness are noted and crepitus and pain with ankle motion are consistent findings. The painful arc sign helps distinguish paratendonitis from tendonitis (Fig. 69-3). The spot of tenderness in paratendonitis does not change with range of motion of the ankle, while with tendonitis it does (Fig. 69-4). Palpable tenderness can be noted on both sides of the tendon, but the medial side is more commonly involved. Tender nodules can form within the paratenon. Abnormal biomechanics of the running gait or extrinsic pressure, such as tight shoes, can lead to paratendonitis. Symptoms are typically aggravated by activity and relieved by rest.

Retrocalcaneal Bursitis

The hallmark of retrocalcaneal bursitis is pain anterior to the Achilles tendon, just superior to its insertion. The bursa becomes hypertrophied, inflamed, and adherent to the tendon. The pain is aggravated with dorsiflexion of the ankle. A positive two-finger squeeze test results in pain with medial and lateral pressure applied anterior and superior to the insertion of the Achilles

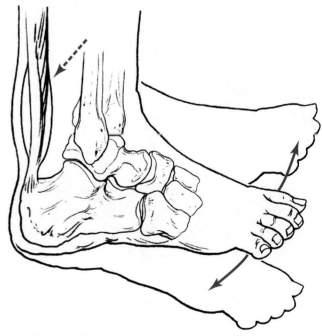

Figure 69-3 A positive physical examination sign for paratendonitis is described as the "painful arc sign." This occurs when the area of pain remains constant with ankle range of motion.

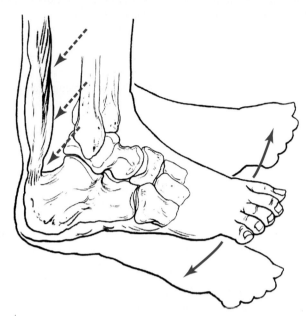

Figure 69-4 The area of pain moves with ankle range of motion if tendonitis exists.

tendon. This must be distinguished from inflammation of the subcutaneous tendo-Achilles bursa, which lies between the posterior aspect of the tendon and the skin and is usually the result of a harsh heel counter or high heels. If retrocalcaneal bursitis is present bilaterally, then the possibility of systemic disease must be considered.

Subcutaneous Tendo-Achilles Bursitis
This entity is commonly seen with retrocalcaneal bursitis, and frequently there is an element of insertional tendonitis as well. A prominence of the lateral aspect of the posterosuperior calcaneus causes irritation of the retrocalcaneal and subcutaneous bursa as a result of poorly fitting shoes. This has been called Haglund's deformity or "pump bump." The bump is usually asymptomatic until irritated by an abrasive heel counter. The prominence is classically present on the lateral side of the tendon at its insertion. This bump is common in women who wear high heels, but also common in hockey players and rock climbers who wear shoes with rigid heel counters. The patient population with this entity tends to be younger than those with isolated retrocalcaneal bursitis. It is not uncommon that these patients with tendo-Achilles bursitis have other features of retrocalcaneal bursitis and insertional tendonitis. Risk factors for Haglund's deformity include cavus foot, hindfoot varus, hindfoot equinus, and trauma to the apophysis in childhood.[18]

Insertional Tendonitis
True inflammation within the tendon occurs with insertional tendonitis. Patients present with pain over the insertion of the tendon, frequently associated with calcification or spurring seen within the tendon on a lateral radiograph. There is usually pain at the bone-tendon interface that worsens after exercise, and the pain may become constant. Symptoms are usually exacerbated by running up hills and on hard surfaces. A history of poor stretching and increased training are commonly elicited in patients with this problem. Insertional tendonitis has been asso-

ciated with retrocalcaneal bursitis or Haglund's deformity. The cavus foot is less efficient in absorbing shock and places more stress on the lateral side of the Achilles tendon and, thus, has been linked with insertional tendonitis.

The physical examination reveals tenderness directly posterior or posterolateral to the insertion of the Achilles tendon. Dorsiflexion of the ankle may be limited secondary to a tight Achilles. Pain is present with active or passive range of motion. Patients with insertional Achilles tendonitis are usually older than patients with paratendonitis or Haglund's deformity. The lateral heel radiograph may show ossification or spurring off the superior portion of the calcaneus. Ancillary imaging studies such as MRI and ultrasonography are not necessary to make the correct diagnosis.

When bilateral, causes of insertional enthesopathy must be considered, including seronegative spondyloarthropathy, gout, fluoroquinolone use, systemic corticosteroids, familial hyperlipidemia, sarcoidosis, and diffuse idiopathic skeletal hyperostosis.

Achilles Tendon Rupture
Achilles tendon ruptures occur most commonly during sports. There is a male predominance occurring in the third to fifth decades. The mechanism is frequently push-off occurring during sprinting and jumping sports resulting in violent ankle dorsiflexion. The patient often describes a sensation of "being kicked in the calf or heel."

The patient's calf and Achilles tendon should be palpated for continuity. Ecchymosis and swelling should be noted. The Thompson test should be done by placing the patient prone and squeezing the calf muscles. This should indirectly plantarflex the foot if the Achilles tendon is intact. The Thompson test is positive if the foot does not plantarflex. If the Thompson test is equivocal, then the O'Brien's test can also be done. This is done by placing a needle in the tendon proximal to the suspected area of rupture and passively ranging the ankle. If the needle hub moves in the opposite direction of ankle movement, this confirms an intact tendon distally. Finally, the hyperdorsiflexion sign should be noted. With the patient prone, both knees are flexed to 90 degrees while the examiner maximally dorsiflexes both ankles comparing the injured to the uninjured side.

Approximately 20% to 25% of Achilles tendon ruptures are initially misdiagnosed. MRI or ultrasonography are not routinely needed for diagnosis but can be helpful in surgical decision making.

Other disease-related factors that place people at greater risk of Achilles rupture include rheumatoid arthritis, lupus erythematosus, hypercholesterolemia, gout, dialysis, renal transplant, steroid therapy, endocrine dysfunction, infection, tumor, autoimmune disorders, diabetes mellitus, and the use of fluoroquinolones.

Relevant Anatomy
The medial and lateral gastrocnemius muscle originates from the posterior aspect of the distal femur while the soleus muscle originates from the posterior aspect of the tibia, fibula, and interosseous membrane. These two tendons from the respective muscles coalesce to form the Achilles tendon, which inserts into the posterior surface of the calcaneus, distal to the calcaneal tuberosity.[19] The Achilles tendon internally rotates 90 degrees onto itself, approximately 2 to 6 cm proximal to its insertion, where the posterior portion of the tendon becomes lateral. The area is also hypovascular according to angiographic studies done

by both Lagergren[20] and Carr and Norris,[21] and this hypovascular zone correlates with most noninsertional tendonitis, tendinosis, and ruptures. The Achilles tendon is not within a true synovial sheath but is covered by paratenon. The paratenon is penetrated anteriorly by the mesotenal arterioles that feed the tendon through vincula. Other sources of blood supply include the musculotendinous junction and osseous insertion. Deep to the tendon, the retrocalcaneal bursa sits superficial to the bone just proximal to the insertion. Another subcutaneous bursa between the tendon and the skin exists called the retrotendo-Achilles bursa or subcutaneous tendo-Achilles. These two areas can also be a source of irritation or inflammation.

During normal walking, at heel strike, the subtalar joint everts/pronates and the tibia internally rotates; simultaneously, passive knee extension causes external rotation through the tibia causing the Achilles tendon to absorb the stress. The Achilles is subjected to great stresses that may approach up to 10 times body weight depending on activity level.[22] Biomechanical malalignments of the foot including "functional" overpronation and cavus foot have been implicated as causing increased stress on the Achilles tendon, thus inciting tendonitis.[23]

Treatment Options: Posterior Heel Pain
Most cases of Achilles overuse injuries and posterior heel pain are managed conservatively. Kvist[23] has reported the most common cause as training errors. Modification of activity or complete rest should be the initial management. Depending on the severity of symptoms, an individualized program should be devised. The key is to allow cross-training, which will keep the athlete in shape; this includes activities such as stationary biking, water therapy, and aqua jogging. As symptoms are diminished, the athlete can advance to the elliptical machine, stair climber, and the NordicTrack as a stepping-stone before resuming running.

If symptoms are milder, then training adjustments are made, including a temporary termination of interval training and hill workouts. The training surface must be addressed as well. If the surface is hard or sloped, it must be changed to a softer and flatter surface. Nonsteroidal anti-inflammatory medications are helpful in acute cases of retrocalcaneal bursitis or paratendonitis. In addition, a course of physical therapy, addressing stretching and strengthening, can be advantageous. Stretching should be executed before and after exercises with the knees both flexed and extended. Other modalities that may be helpful include ice, massage, iontophoresis, and phonophoresis. Schepsis et al[18] noted that patients with chronic symptoms had limited passive dorsiflexion and benefited from passive static stretching exercises. They also found that in some cases a night splint to hold the foot and ankle dorsiflexed to neutral for 6 to 8 weeks was helpful to maintain passive dorsiflexion. Approximately 10% of patients with retrocalcaneal bursitis will fail conservative treatment.

Biomechanical or alignment problems that are causing excessive stress on the Achilles tendon must always be addressed. Orthotic devices may be useful in correcting malalignment problems to keep the foot and ankle in a neutral position. Gross et al[24] studied long-distance runners who were given orthotics for their lower extremity complaints. About 20% had a diagnosis of Achilles tendonitis, and of those patients, 75% had great improvement or cure with orthotic shoe inserts. Orthotic devices are most helpful in correcting hyperpronation and leg length discrepancies. Also, a one-fourth– to one-half–inch heel

pad built into the running shoe may be helpful in reducing stress on the tendon in patients with normal alignment.

Finally, after training errors and malalignment problems have been addressed, a program of calf strengthening should be instituted. Eccentric, heavy load calf exercises have been shown to be quite effective in chronic or resistant Achilles overuse syndromes.[25] Also, maintenance stretching should be continued.

Chronic paratendonitis occurs when symptoms are present for greater than 3 months duration. Nonoperative measures are less successful if there is a delay in treatment. Brisement or distention of the paratenon-tendon interface with lidocaine or other solution can be used in refractory paratendonitis. This is a mechanical lysis of adhesions between tendon and paratenon that occurs by the rapid infusion of 5 to 15 mL of local anesthetic or saline into the peritendinous space. Brisement can be done in the office and can possibly eliminate the need for surgical intervention. There is a 33% success rate with this procedure.

Surgery: Posterior Heel Pain
Most patients are successfully treated conservatively, but the ones who fail may benefit from surgical intervention. These patients may have coexisting retrocalcaneal bursitis and insertional Achilles tendonitis or paratendonitis and tendonosis. Schepsis et al[18] found that 15% of their surgical cases had a combination of these entities. Obtaining an MRI for preoperative planning may be helpful.

Paratendonitis
In addressing paratendonitis surgically, some authors advocate a J-shaped incision, starting medial to lateral distal to the Achilles tendon insertion, to turn back the skin for exposure. Others recommend the two-incision (medial and lateral) technique, keeping the skin bridge at least 4 cm wide. We recommend a medial incision. Dissection is carried down to the paratenon, which is freed from the superficial skin and subcutaneous tissue. The paratenon is usually hyperemic, fibrotic, and adherent to the underlying tendon. The affected paratenon is resected, but care is taken not to excise the anterior portion, where the critical blood supply enters the tendon. Complete excision of the paratenon could lead to severe postoperative fibrosis and is not recommended.

Insertional Tendonitis
Insertional tendonitis is usually seen in older athletes, and surgical exposure has been described with many different approaches. Some authors advocate a longitudinal incision placed either laterally or medially, or a combination of two incisions; however, we advocate the midline longitudinal incision. Full-thickness skin flaps are created until the paratenon is identified. The paratenon layer is then freed from the superficial tissues and split longitudinally, ensuring that a good closure can be obtained. The Achilles tendon is also longitudinally split and distally dissected medially and laterally off the calcaneus, being careful not to entirely detach the tendon. At this point, any degeneration of the tendon is excised along with the retrocalcaneal bursa and the prominence of the posterior os calcis. Two resorbable suture anchors are then used to enhance reattachment of the distal part of the tendon. A 2-0 Vicryl suture is used to reapproximate the Achilles tendon side to side and a 4-0 Vicryl suture is used to close the paratenon.

Retrocalcaneal Bursitis

Open For recalcitrant retrocalcaneal bursitis, the retrocalcaneal bursa should be completely excised. The exposure includes two longitudinal incisions medial and lateral. The bursa is usually hyperemic, thickened, and scarred down to the anterior portion of the tendon. The bursa can hold up to 1 to 2 mL of bursal fluid. There may also be fibrinous loose bodies found within the bursa. After excision of the entire bursa, the prominence of the posterior os calcis should be resected.

Endoscopic Endoscopic decompression of the retrocalcaneal space can be achieved as well. This is done with the patient either in the prone or supine position. If the patient is supine, the leg holder is applied to the calf, but if prone, the feet are positioned just over the edge of the operating table. The foot is plantarflexed using gravity, while the surgeon can control dorsiflexion of the foot with his or her body. The foot of the table is dropped.

A lateral portal is made first at the level of the superior aspect of the calcaneus. A blunt trocar is used to penetrate the retrocalcaneal space. A 30-degree 2.7- or 4-mm arthroscope is inserted, and the medial portal is made under direct visualization at the same level of the calcaneus. The motorized shaver is used to remove the bursa and the periosteal layer off the superior portion of the calcaneus. The foot is then placed in full plantarflexion and the posterior superior rim of the calcaneus removed with an abrader. The insertion of the Achilles tendon should now be visualized and protected. A bur is then inserted to resect the prominence of the os calcis under fluoroscopic guidance. Finally, the shaver is used to smooth the edges and clean debris. The skin is closed with nylon suture.

Treatment Options: Achilles Tendon Rupture

There is still debate over the best management for Achilles tendon ruptures. The treatment options include nonoperative (cast or brace) and operative treatment. Nonoperative treatment is usually reserved for individuals who are elderly and sedentary and have poor skin quality or other comorbidities that would preclude surgery. Immobilization is provided using a short-leg cast or brace in the equinus position for 4 weeks. The patient is then placed in a neutral walking short-leg cast for 4 more weeks with gradual weight bearing. At 8 weeks, a 2.5-cm heel lift in the shoe is used for another 4 weeks.

McComis et al[26] developed the concept of functional bracing as an alternative to casting for nonoperative management of Achilles tendon ruptures. Their technique has subsequently been modified and has gained popularity as an acceptable option for selected patients. Wallace et al[27] had 140 consecutive patients with acute Achilles ruptures that were treated with combined conservative orthotic management. Initial immobilization includes a non-weight bearing short-leg cast with the ankle in equinus for 4 weeks. At 2 weeks, a rigid polyethylene double-shell patellar tendon–bearing orthosis is fabricated and the cast changed. At 4 weeks after injury, the orthosis is then worn for an additional 4 weeks; during this time, it is removed for ankle and subtalar exercises. The patients are also given gait training and progressed to full weight bearing while wearing the orthotic device.

Operative treatment for Achilles tendon rupture is advocated by most surgeons because it allows direct repair, aggressive rehabilitation, and predictable results and has a lower rerupture rate compared to nonoperative treatment.[4–6,28,29] Proponents of nonoperative treatment maintain that overall complications from surgery including skin necrosis, wound infection, sural neuroma, and adhesions to the skin are high. Problems with wound healing remain the most common and significant problem associated with the operative technique. Achilles tendon ruptures are treated surgically in nearly all athletes, and we discuss both the open and percutaneous methods.

Surgery: Achilles Tendon Repair

Percutaneous Technique

In 1977, Ma and Griffith introduced percutaneous Achilles tendon repair in 18 patients, reporting no reruptures and only two suture complications.[30] Their technique has subsequently been modified and has gained popularity as an acceptable option for selected patients.

To successfully perform a percutaneous Achilles tendon repair, the tendon gap must be reducible with the ankle in plantarflexion. The patient is placed in a prone position. A solution composed of a 1:1 mix of 1% lidocaine and 0.5% Marcaine is used to locally anesthetize the skin and subcutaneous tissues. Intravenous medication may be given to sedate the patient. Medial and lateral stab wounds at the level of the tear and 2 cm above and below are made. The subcutaneous tissues are spread using a hemostat. Nylon suture (0 or 1) with Keith needles on both ends is passed transversely through the tendon at the proximal puncture. The needle is then advanced distally from both sides in a crisscross fashion through the tendon at 45-degree angles through the middle puncture hole. The suture is then passed through the tendon into the most distal puncture sites. Finally, the medial suture is passed laterally to meet the other strands where both are tied with the tendon gap closed. A hemostat is used to bury the knot. Nylon suture is used to approximate the skin and an adjustable boot locked in 30 degrees of equinus applied (Fig. 69-5). New devices are available that assist the surgeon in performing the percutaneous method, and early results are encouraging.

Open Technique

Open surgical repair of the tendon allows direct visualization and the ability to restore functional length of the musculotendinous unit. The longitudinal skin incision is placed medially to avoid the sural nerve (Fig. 69-6). The tissues are elevated with a full thickness flap until the paratenon is reached. The paratenon is incised and the tendon ends are identified. A minimal to no touch technique for the tendon is used, with a no. 5 nonabsorbable suture with application of simple modified Kessler, Bunnell, or Krackow interlocking stitch. Also an absorbable 2-0 interrupted or running epitendinous suture can be placed. A four-strand repair is advocated to increase strength and allow aggressive rehabilitation. Bulky knots or suture should not be placed directly beneath the incision. The paratenon should be closed over the repair to prevent skin adherence to the tendon. The appropriate tensioning of the repair is crucial, and draping out the contralateral uninjured extremity to allow comparison of ankle dorsiflexion is recommended. The appropriate tension is set with the knee in 90 degrees of flexion. Postoperatively, the patient is placed in a cast or splint with the foot at 30 degrees of equinus to minimize tension on the soft tissues and repair.

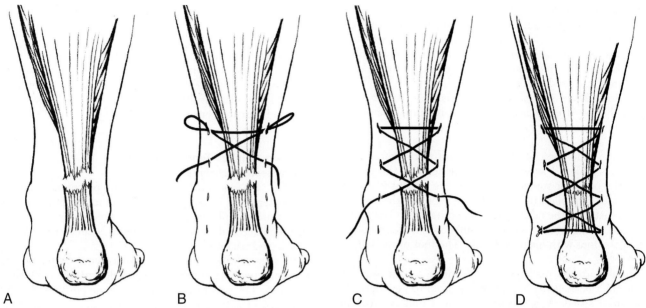

A   B   C   D

Figure 69-5 A–D, The surgical technique for percutaneous Achilles tendon repair.

Postoperative Rehabilitation: Posterior Heel Pain

Paratendonitis

The patient is placed in a removable boot walker and early motion is started immediately to prevent scarring and fibrosis. Weight bearing is limited until the wound is healed, and progressive weight bearing and strengthening should continue for 2 to 3 weeks. When ambulating without pain, the patient may begin closed-chain activities, such as biking or stair climbing. Running may begin at 6 to 10 weeks after surgery.

Insertional Achilles Tendonitis

Wound healing is a major concern after débridement of insertional Achilles tendonitis; therefore, the patient is placed in a short-leg splint for 2 weeks and kept non-weight bearing until the wound is healed. The patient is then placed in a removable boot, and range-of-motion exercises are started. There should be emphasis on active dorsiflexion and a progressive resistance exercise program instituted as tolerated. Sports-specific training is started at 3 months, and competition begins at 6 months.

Retrocalcaneal Bursitis

Open   The patients are placed in a boot walker for 2 weeks with protected weight bearing. Range-of-motion exercises can be started immediately. A heel lift is used after discontinuation of the boot walker. A progressive exercise program should be instituted.

Endoscopic   After endoscopic calcaneoplasty, the patient is non-weight bearing and splinted in comfortable equinus for 2 to 3 days. Weight bearing as tolerated is then initiated in a removable boot with a 1-inch heel lift. At this time, range-of-motion exercises are instituted, and the boot is discontinued after 4 weeks. A one-half–inch heel lift in the tennis shoe is then used for an additional 6 weeks. Athletics are not allowed until 3 months after the operation.

Postoperative Rehabilitation: Achilles Tendon Repair

Percutaneous Repair

The postoperative protocol includes 3 weeks in an adjustable boot locked in 30 degrees of plantarflexion with no weight bearing. During this time, gentle movement of the foot, straight leg raises, and knee range of motion is started. After week 3, the orthosis is adjusted up 5 degrees of dorsiflexion each week until 10 degrees of plantarflexion is achieved. Weight bearing is also increased from toe touch to partial, as tolerated. After 6 weeks, full weight bearing as tolerated is allowed, and at 8 weeks, shoe wear with heel lift is initiated for up to 12 weeks. Throughout this time, light active dorsiflexion of the ankle, muscle strengthening, proprioception exercises, stationary cycling (with heel push only), and soft-tissue treatments commence. Three months postoperatively, closed-chain exercises, cycling, and NordicTrack use should be instituted. Finally, at 6 months, running, jumping, and sports activities are permitted.

Open Repair

Earlier protocols for postoperative rehabilitation after Achilles repair advocated cast immobilization for periods of 6 to 8 weeks with the ankle in equinus. The ankle was placed in progressive dorsiflexion at 2-week intervals. After cast removal, the patient began range-of-motion exercises with a physical therapist. Some authors even advocated a long-leg cast; however, Sekiya et al[31] used a cadaveric study to disprove that knee position caused displacement of the Achilles tendon with the ankle plantarflexed. These results suggest that the nonoperative treatment of Achilles tendon ruptures requires immobilization in maximal ankle plantar flexion and that immobilization of the knee may not be necessary to achieve tendon-edge apposition.

The detrimental effects of immobilization on tendon and bone healing are well documented. The long-term immobilization of joints while tendons are healing slows the recovery of injured tendons. The remodeling of new collagen fibrils is impeded as well. The flexor tendon work of Gelberman et al[32]

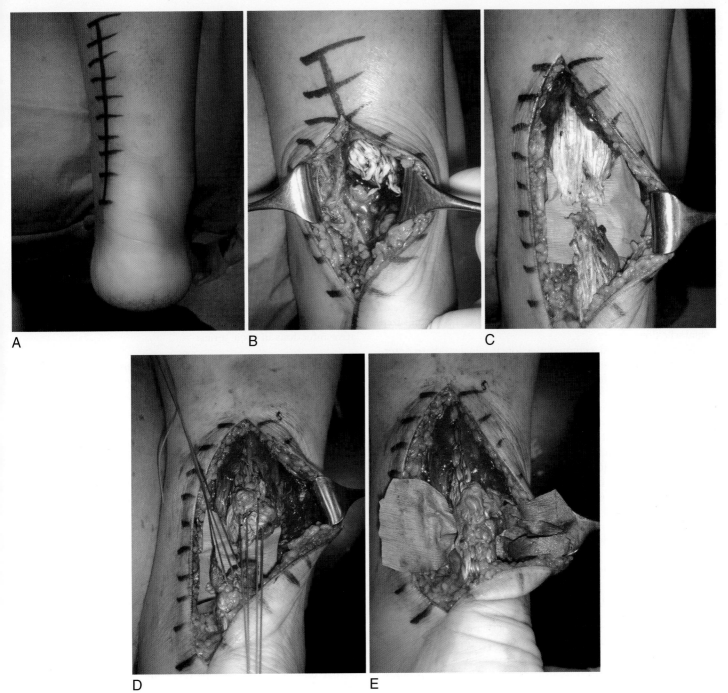

Figure 69-6 Open Achilles tendon repair. **A,** Planned incision medial to the Achilles tendon. **B,** Tendon rupture identified. **C,** Tendon edges prepared for repair. **D,** Nonabsorbable sutures placed. **E,** Completed repair.

showed that early mobilization leads to increased organization at the repair site and increases strength. Mobilization also decreases muscle atrophy and promotes collagen fiber polymerization.

There have now been more reports of favorable results with protocols of early motion after Achilles tendon repairs. Mandelbaum et al[33] treated 29 athletes with Achilles tendon rupture using Krackow repair and began range-of-motion exercises 72 hours after surgery, using a posterior splint for 2 weeks. Ambulation was started in a hinged orthosis at 2 weeks. The orthosis

was discontinued at 6 weeks and full weight bearing allowed. Progressive resistance exercises were also initiated. There were no reruptures. Isokinetic strength testing revealed a 2.9% deficit at 6 months and no deficit at 12 months. All patients returned to preinjury activity levels at a mean of 4 months.

More recently, authors have proposed early range of motion exercises and early weight bearing with a functional orthosis after surgical Achilles tendon repair. Speck and Klaue[34] proposed early mobilization with early full weight bearing after surgical repair of Achilles tendon ruptures. This was instituted to allow the tendon to experience tension during healing. Tension improves strength and orientation of collagen fibers as well as vascularity. Twenty patients were treated with a Kessler-type suture repair and plantigrade splint for 24 hours. The postoperative program included 6 weeks of full weight bearing in a removable walker. There were no reruptures. All patients reached their preinjury activity level and showed no statistically significant difference in isokinetic strength.

Aoki et al[35] reported early active motion and weight bearing after cross-stitch Achilles tendon repair in 22 patients. Twenty of the tendons (91%) healed without rerupture. Patients returned to full sports activity in 13.1 weeks. MRI studies were obtained at 4, 6, 8, 12, 16, and 20 weeks. Excellent healing was seen on the MRI at an average of 12.6 weeks. Akizuki et al[36] defined the relative stress on the Achilles tendon during weight bearing with immobilization in varying degrees of plantarflexion. They examined electromyographic activity during ambulation in 10 subjects in normal walking, immobilization with a walker boot in neutral plantarflexion, walker boot with a half-inch heel lift, and a walker boot with a 1-inch heel. They concluded that the stress of the Achilles tendon is determined by the degree of plantarflexion and that a 1-inch heel lift sufficiently minimized plantarflexion activity.

Maffulli et al[37] did a comparative longitudinal study to determine the effects of early weight bearing and ankle mobilization after repair of Achilles tendon rupture. One group, at 2 weeks, was mobilized with weight bearing as tolerated in the plantigrade position. An anterior below-the-knee slab was secured to the leg with Velcro straps, and patients were instructed by the physical therapist to perform concentric exercises against manual resistance and mobilization within the limits of the anterior slab. The anterior slab was discontinued at 6 weeks. The second group was initially casted in the equinus position and was non-weight bearing for 4 weeks. The patients were casted in the neutral position at 4 weeks and made weight bearing as tolerated. There were no differences found in isometric strength or thickness of the tendon. These results suggest that it is not deleterious to start early weight bearing and ankle mobilization after open repair of Achilles tendon ruptures.

Criteria for Return to Sports: Achilles Tendon Repair

Full painless range of motion and strength must be recovered prior to resuming athletics. The average time required before light jogging is 2 to 3 months. Competitive athletic activities are usually allowed by 4 to 6 months; however, decisions to allow the athlete to resume activities are made only if adequate strength gains are present.

Results and Outcomes
Paratendonitis

Generally, surgical results after resection of chronic paratendonitis are acceptable. The literature varies with reports of 72% to 100% good to excellent results. Schepsis et al[18] reported in a series of competitive and serious recreational athletes, 87% satisfactory results after surgical treatment of paratendonitis. The best surgical outcomes of the Achilles tendon disorders occur in paratendonitis. Nelen et al[38] reported an 89% satisfactory outcome in 92 cases.

Insertional Achilles Tendonitis

Maffulli et al[39] reported 75% good to excellent results in 21 patients treated surgically for insertional Achilles tendonitis, but 25% were unable to return to their normal level of sporting activities. Schepsis et al[18] achieved an 86% satisfactory result and Nelen et al[38] achieved a 73% outcome after surgical intervention for insertional Achilles tendonitis.

Retrocalcaneal Bursitis

Open Reports in the literature are variable, with success rates ranging from 50% to 90%. Paavola et al[1,2] achieved 76% good to excellent results. Schepsis et al[18] demonstrated a 71% satisfactory rate in their first series and an increase to 75% in their second series.

Endoscopic Leitze et al[40] performed a prospective study to compare the endoscopic technique with the standard open technique. They found that postoperative American Orthopaedic Foot and Ankle Society scores were not significantly better, but the endoscopic procedures were associated with fewer complications. The complications included infection (3% versus 12%), altered sensation (10% versus 18%), and scar tenderness (7% versus 18%), in endoscopic and open procedures, respectively. van Dijk et al[41] reported 75% excellent results, 20% good results, and 5% fair results, with no surgical complications or postoperative infections in their series.

Achilles Tendon Rupture: Nonoperative Treatment

In a prospective, randomized comparison between operative and nonoperative management of Achilles tendon ruptures by Moller et al,[6] the rerupture rate for the operative group was 1.6% and 20.7% for the nonoperative group. In the quantitative review of Wong et al[28] of 645 Achilles tendon ruptures, it was noted that conservative treatment had the highest rerupture rate at 10.7% and skin complications were lowest at 0.5%. In another systematic review of the literature by Kocher et al,[5] the probability of rerupture after conservative management was 12.1%, while after operative repair, it was 2.2%. However, the probability of wound complications with conservative treatment was 0.3% compared to 7.5% with operative repair.

Wallace et al[27] recently reported on 140 patients treated conservatively with combined casting and orthotic treatment. Using the scoring system of Leppilahti, the overall outcomes were 56% excellent, 30% good, 12% fair, and 2% poor. There was a 5.7% rerupture rate including two complete and five partial reruptures. There also was a significant difference in plantarflexion strength, but the authors state that 89% of the patients had no or minimal subjective symptoms of calf weakness. The key point is that only 33% returned to the same level of activity, 54% returned to a lower level of activity, and 9% were unable to return to sports.

Josey et al[42] reported on 32 patients with Achilles tendon rupture treated conservatively with full weight-bearing cast treatment and found a rerupture rate of 6.25%. These patients also had plantarflexion weakness but overall were satisfied with their treatment.

Achilles Tendon Repair

Percutaneous Bradley and Tibone[43] did a comparative study between percutaneous (1.8-year follow-up) and open surgical repairs (4.6-year follow-up) and found no statistically significant difference in strength, power, or endurance between groups at the 1.8-year follow up. There were two reruptures (13%) in the percutaneous group. FitzGibbons et al[44] found a significant difference of a 13% power loss after percutaneous Achilles repair at an average follow-up of 3.8 years. The patients who were recreational athletes returned to their preinjury activity level. In the Tomak and Fleming[45] study, a 21% power loss after percutaneous repair was found at an average of 34 months of follow-up. There were no reruptures or sural nerve complications. Despite the loss of plantarflexion power, patients were generally very satisfied with their treatment. There was one recreational athlete who reported weakness. These authors recommend that percutaneous repair be reserved for the recreational athlete only.

A cadaveric study comparing the biomechanics of percutaneous repair with that of open repair was done by Hockenbury and Johns,[46] who found that percutaneous repairs result in half the strength of open repairs. In the literature, percutaneous repairs have an increased rate of rerupture when compared to open repairs but a lower rerupture rate when compared to nonoperative treatment. The range of repeat rupture after percutaneous repair has been reported from as low as 2.8% to as high as 12%.

Haji et al[47] recently published a retrospective study of 108 patients comparing percutaneous (38 patients) versus open repair (70 patients) revealing a lower rerupture rate in the percutaneous group (2.6% versus 5.7%, respectively). The percutaneous group had no wound infections and 10.5% transient sural nerve lesions. No significant difference in power was found, but power was defined as normal if the subject was able to stand on his or her tiptoes. There was no mention of return to athletic activities.

Open Cetti et al[3] conducted a prospective, randomized study to compare operative and nonoperative treatment of Achilles tendon ruptures and also performed a review of the literature. They found that the operative group had a 5.4% rerupture rate compared to a 14.5% rerupture rate in those who received conservative treatment. Another important outcome reported was that 57% of patients returned to their preinjury level of athletics in the operative group. In contrast, in the conservative group, only 29% returned to their preinjury level of athletics. The authors' literature review revealed a rerupture rate of 13.4% versus 1.4% for nonoperative and operative treatment, respectively. There were fewer minor complications in the nonoperative group than in the operative group. Various methods were used to objectively evaluate functional recovery and mean plantarflexion strength after surgery. After surgical repair, there was an 87% functional recovery compared to 78% with conservative treatment. An increased return to preinjury athletic participation was also noted after surgical treatment.

Kellam et al[4] reported a retrospective series of 68 patients whose ruptured Achilles tendon were managed operatively. Of the 48 patients who were clinically evaluated, 92% returned to a preinjury level of activity. The rerupture rate in this operative series was 3%, and 13% had incisional complications.

Complications

The major complication after Achilles tendon surgery is skin necrosis or superficial infection. Paavola et al[2] analyzed complications of 432 consecutive patients after surgical treatment of chronic Achilles tendon overuse injuries. Eleven percent of the patients had complications, including skin edge necrosis in 14 patients, superficial wound infections in 11 patients, partial rupture in one patient, deep venous thrombosis in one patient, seroma formation in five patients, hematoma in five patients, fibrotic reaction in five patients, and sural nerve irritation in four patients. Most of the complications (54%) involved compromised wound healing. The skin envelope in this region is tenuous and excessive skin mobilization must be avoided.

Sural nerve injuries occur most commonly with percutaneous repair of Achilles tendon injuries but can occur with all Achilles tendon operative procedures. The nerve must be either avoided by going medial to the Achilles or visualized and uncompromisingly protected.

Reruptures are more common in Achilles tendon ruptures treated nonoperatively, followed by percutaneous repairs. Open repairs have a much smaller occurrence of rerupture. Another complication after treatment of Achilles rupture is lengthening of the tendon. This is more common in closed treatment and percutaneous treatment of Achilles tendon ruptures. Decreased plantarflexion power may result in difficulty with walking, running, or jumping.

Conclusions

Most of the Achilles tendon overuse injuries are successfully treated with nonoperative management. This usually consists of a brief period of rest, activity modification, and correction of malalignment with orthotics, and nonsteroidal anti-inflammatory drugs. Other modalities that are helpful include ionophoresis, stretching, eccentric calf strengthening exercises, and a heel lift. Steroid injections are not indicated because this places the Achilles tendon at higher risk of rupture. A gradual, progressive rehabilitation program should be instituted. Nonoperative measures are 90% to 95% successful for acute treatment; however, up to 29% require surgical treatment for chronic problems that fail conservative management.[1]

Surgical treatment of chronic Achilles tendon overuse injuries obtains approximately 80% satisfactory results. There are options in surgical technique; however, regardless of the approach, meticulous soft-tissue management must be maintained. The major complications of all surgical treatment in this anatomic area include skin edge necrosis, wound infection, sural nerve injury, and fibrotic scar formation. Once the soft-tissue envelope is healed, it is important to start mobilization.

Finally, there is still debate regarding the best way to manage Achilles tendon ruptures. Studies have shown that operative repair has the most reliable results, the lowest rate of rerupture, and greater recovery of push-off strength compared to nonoperative treatment. The operative options include open and percutaneous repair. Open repair allows better control of tendon tension and has a lower rerupture rate, but the rate of wound complications is higher. Percutaneous methods present fewer wound complications but sacrifice repair strength and push-off power and risk rerupture or elongation of the tendon. There is also a greater risk of sural nerve injury. We recommend open repair in the athletic population with percutaneous repair as an acceptable alternative in the older, sedentary individual who may be at risk of skin complications.

The trend of rehabilitation after Achilles tendon repair has been early mobilization and earlier weight bearing to facilitate healing, decrease atrophy, and shorten rehabilitation. Multiple clinical studies have shown that early weight bearing and mobilization are not deleterious after Achilles tendon repair.

Section VII Ankle and Foot

REFERENCES

1. Paavola M, Kannus P, Paakkala T, et al: Long-term prognosis of patients with Achilles tendinopathy: An observational 8-year follow-up study. Am J Sports Med 2000;28:634–642.

2. Paavola M, Orava S, Leppilahti J, et al: Chronic Achilles tendon overuse injury: Complications after surgical treatment. An analysis of 432 consecutive patients. Am J Sports Med 2000;28:77–82.

3. Cetti R, Christensen SE, Ejsted R, et al: Operative versus nonoperative treatment of Achilles tendon rupture. A prospective randomized study and review of the literature. Am J Sports Med 1993;21:791–799.

4. Kellam JF, Hunter GA, McElwain JP: Review of the operative treatment of Achilles tendon rupture. Clin Orthop 1985;201:80–83.

5. Kocher MS, Bishop J, Marshall R, et al: Operative versus nonoperative management of acute Achilles tendon rupture expected-value decision analysis. Am J Sports Med 2002;30:783–790.

6. Moller M, Movin T, Granhed H, et al: Acute rupture of tendo Achillis. A prospective, randomised study of comparison between surgical and non-surgical treatment. J Bone Joint Surg Br 2001;83:843–848.

7. Bassett FH III, Speer KP: Longitudinal rupture of the peroneal tendons. Am J Sports Med 1993;21:354–357.

8. Sobel M, Bohne WH, Levy ME: Longitudinal attrition of the brevis tendon in the fibula groove: An anatomic study. Foot Ankle Int 1990;11:124–128.

9. Pelet S, Saglini M, Garofalo R, et al: Traumatic rupture of both peroneal longus and brevis tendons. Foot Ankle Int 2003;24:721–723.

10. Mann RA, Coughlin MJ: Surgery of the Foot & Ankle, 7th ed. St. Louis, Mosby, 1999.

11. Eckert WR, Davis EA: Acute rupture of the peroneal retinaculum. J Bone Joint Surg Am 1976;58:670–673.

12. Zammit J, Singh D: The peroneus quartus muscle: Anatomy and clinical relevance. J Bone Joint Surg Br 2003;85:1134–1137.

13. Edwards ME: Relations of peroneal tendons to fibula, calcaneus, cuboideum. Am J Anat 1928;42:213–253.

14. Beck E: Operative treatment of recurrent dislocation of peroneal tendons. Arch Orthop Trauma Surg 1981;98:247–250.

15. Krause JO, Brodsky JW: Peroneus brevis tendon tears: Pathophysiology, surgical reconstruction, and clinical results. Foot Ankle Int 1998;19:271–279.

16. Sammarco GJ: Peroneal tendon injuries. Orthop Clin North Am 1994;25:135–145.

17. Alanen J, Orava S, Heinonen OJ, et al: Peroneal tendon injuries. Report of thirty-eight operated cases. Ann Chir Gynaecol 2001;90:43–46.

18. Schepsis A, Jones H, Haas A: Current concepts: Achilles tendon disorders in athletes. Am J Sports Med 2002;30:287–305.

19. Chao W, Deland JT, Bates JE, et al: Achilles tendon insertion: An in vitro anatomic study. Foot Ankle Int 1997;18:81–84.

20. Lagergren C, Lindholm A: Vascular distribution in the Achilles tendon. An angiographic and microangiograhic study. Acta Chir Scand 1958–1959;116:491–496.

21. Carr AJ, Norris SH: The blood supply of the calcaneal tendon. J Bone Joint Surg Br 1989;71:100–101.

22. Burdett RG: Forces predicted at ankle during running. Med Sci Sports 182;14:308–310.

23. Kvist M: Achilles tendon injuries in athletes. Sports Med 1994;18:173–201.

24. Gross ML, Dalvin L, Evanski PM: Effectiveness of orthotic shoe inserts in the long distance runner. Am J Sports Med 1991;19:409–412.

25. Alfredson H, Pietila T, Johnson P, et al: Heavy-load eccentric calf muscle training for the treatment of chronic Achilles tendonosis. Am J Sports Med 1998;26:360–366.

26. McComis GP, Nawoczenski DA, Dehaven KE: Functional bracing for rupture of the Achilles tendon. Clinical results and analysis of ground-reaction forces and temporal data. J Bone Joint Surg (Am) 1997;79:1799–1808.

27. Wallace RG, Traynor IE, Kernohan WG, et al: Combined conservative and orthotic management of acute ruptures of the Achilles tendon. J Bone Joint Surg Am 2004;86:1198–1202.

28. Wong J, Barrass V, Maffulli N: Quantitative review of operative and non-operative management of Achilles tendon ruptures. Am J Sports Med 2002;30:565–574.

29. Myerson MS: Achilles tendon ruptures. Instr Course Lect 1999;48:219–230.

30. Ma GW, Griffith TG: Percutaneous repair of acute closed ruptured Achilles tendon: A new technique. Clin Orthop 1977;128:247–255.

31. Sekiya JK, Evensen KE, Jebson PJL, et al: The effect of knee and ankle position on displacement of Achilles tendon ruptures in a cadaveric model implications for nonoperative management. Am J Sports Med 1999;27:632–635.

32. Gelberman RH, Woo SL-Y, Lothringer K, et al: Effects of early intermittent passive mobilization on healing canine flexor tendons. J Hand Surg 1982;7:170–175.

33. Mandelbaum BR, Myerson MS, Forster R: Achilles tendon ruptures. A new method of repair, early range of motion, and functional rehabilitation. Am J Sports Med 1995;23:392–395.

34. Speck M, Klaue K: Early full weightbearing and functional treatment after surgical repair of acute Achilles tendon rupture. Am J Sports Med 1998;26:789–793.

35. Aoki M, Ogiwara N, Ohta T, et al: Early active motion and weightbearing after cross-stitch Achilles tendon repair. Am J Sports Med 1998;26:794–800.

36. Akizuki KH, Gartman EJ, Nisonson B, et al: The relative stress on the Achilles tendon during ambulation in an ankle immobiliser: Implications for rehabilitation after Achilles tendon repair. Br J Sports Med 2001;35:329–333.

37. Maffulli N, Tallon C, Wong J, et al: Early weightbearing and ankle mobilization after open repair of acute midsubstance tears of the Achilles tendon. Am J Sports Med 2003;31:692–700.

38. Nelen G, Martens M, Burssens A: Surgical treatment of chronic Achilles tendonitis. Am J Sports Med 1989;17:754–759.

39. Maffulli N, Testa V, Capasso G, et al: Calcific insertional Achilles tendinopathy: Reattachment with bone anchors. Am J Sports Med 2004;32:174–182.

40. Leitze Z, Sella EJ, Aversa JM: Endoscopic decompression of the retrocalcaneal space. J Bone Joint Surg Am 2003;85:1488–1496.

41. van Dijk CN, van Dyk GE, Scholten PE, Kort NP: Endoscopic calcaneoplasty. Am J Sports Med 2001;29:185–189.

42. Josey RA, Marymont JV, Varner KE, et al: Immediate, full weightbearing cast treatment of acute Achilles tendon ruptures: A long-term follow-up study. Foot Ankle Int 2003;24:775–779.

43. Bradley JP, Tibone JE: Percutaneous and open surgical repairs of Achilles tendon ruptures. A comparative study. Am J Sports Med 1990;18:188–195.

44. FitzGibbons RE, Hefferon J, Hill J: Percutaneous Achilles tendon repair. Am J Sports Med 1993;21:724–727.

45. Tomak SL, Fleming LL: Achilles tendon rupture: An alternative treatment. Am J Orthop 2004;33:9–12.

46. Hockenbury RT, Johns JC: A biomechanical in vitro comparison of open versus percutaneous repair of tendon Achilles. Foot Ankle 1990;11:67–72.

47. Haji A, Sahai A, Symes A, et al: Percutaneous versus open tendo Achillis repair. Foot Ankle 2004;25:215–218.

Midfoot and Hindfoot

Steven J. Lawrence

In This Chapter

Peritalar dislocations
Os trigonum syndrome
Lisfranc injuries
Navicular stress fracture
Plantar fasciitis
Tibial nerve entrapment
Posterior tibial tendonitis

INTRODUCTION

- Sport-related foot injuries generally result from either acute or cumulative injuries.

- Most painful foot structures can be examined by direct palpation.

- A thorough patient history and physical examination facilitates the formulation of an appropriate differential diagnosis.

- The hindfoot and midfoot absorb tremendous torsional and shock-absorbing stresses during athletic endeavors. Hindfoot function and midfoot function are intimately interconnected.

- The hindfoot joint complex permits subtle adaptations to uneven terrain.

- The midfoot largely functions as a simple block, transmitting forces applied to and from the hindfoot and forefoot.

- Midfoot structures are integral components of the longitudinal and transverse arches.

RELEVANT ANATOMY AND BIOMECHANICS

Hindfoot and midfoot components are easily delineated. The former is largely composed of its two bony structures, the talus and calcaneus, while the latter is composed of the navicular, the three cuneiforms, and the cuboid. Anatomically, the boundaries of the hindfoot region begin at the subtalar joint and extend to the Chopart (or transverse-tarsal) joint; the midfoot begins at this joint and extends to the Lisfranc (or tarsometatarsal joint) complex. The subtalar articulation links the talus and calcaneus via three articular facets. The Chopart joint comprises the talonavicular and calcaneocuboid joints. The term subtalar joint complex refers to both the subtalar and Chopart joints. In addition to osseous and chondral injuries, soft-tissue structures such

as the capsule, tendon, ligament, nerve, and heel pad may be injured in isolation or combinations during competitive sport.

The biomechanics of the subtalar joint complex remain poorly understood; in fact, the joint complex is perhaps the most poorly understood articulation. Efficient locomotion requires alternating flexibility and rigidity of the foot. Flexibility is necessary for shock absorption, while rigidity is required for propulsive activities. The alternating inversion-eversion of the subtalar joint within the gait cycle is necessary for efficient locomotion.[1] Subtalar motion is intimately linked to the adduction/abduction and pronation/supination movements of the talonavicular joint.

Due to skeletal alignment, natural hindfoot alignment is valgus; therefore, normal hindfoot function is dependent on voluntary control of hindfoot inversion. A competent posterior tibial tendon is, therefore, essential for regulation of subtalar joint control.

Midfoot architecture comprises the longitudinal and transverse arches. Bone stability is enhanced by its unique structural design. The second metatarsal base insets into the adjacent cuneiforms in mortise-and-tenon fashion (Fig. 70-1). A dense network of stout, plantar ligaments secure the metatarsal bases to the cuneiforms. The plantar fascia supplies supplemental longitudinal arch support. If midfoot integrity is disrupted, force transmission from the hindfoot to the forefoot (and vice versa) is impaired. If injury is not diagnosed in a timely manner, continued weight bearing may result in midfoot collapse.[2]

Significant hindfoot or midfoot injury sustained during an athletic injury may result in considerable dysfunction. Overuse injury involving bone and tendon is commonly present in runners and dancers. Periarticular fractures are not infrequent; they are difficult to detect due to intricate three-dimensional foot anatomy. Injury sequelae, especially stiffness and pain, result in impairment in select abilities, such as jumping and ballistic motions, preventing return to elite competition. Therefore, prompt diagnosis, appropriate intervention, and aggressive rehabilitation are essential to optimize outcomes.

SELECT INJURIES

Peritalar Dislocations
Anatomy
Peritalar dislocations are acute hindfoot injuries. They result from an extreme rotational injury. The injury may also be termed a subtalar dislocation. However, since the initial event is a talonavicular dislocation with subsequent subluxation/dislocation of the subtalar joint, the term peritalar dislocation appears to be more anatomically accurate (Fig. 70-2). The condition, therefore, results in complete disruption of the talonavicular joint capsule with a variable interosseous ligament injury.

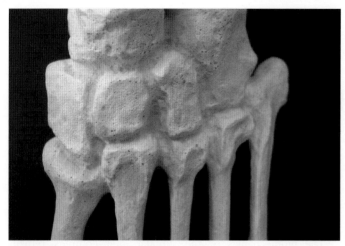

Figure 70-1 A schematic representation of the midfoot demonstrating the mortise and tenon-like configuration of the second metatarsal base and the adjacent cuneiforms.

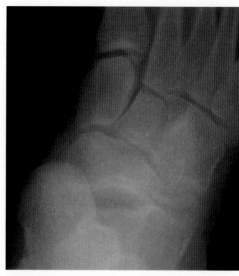

Figure 70-3 An anteroposterior radiograph of a lateral peritalar dislocation. The deformity is dramatic with the uncovered talar head noted medially in the subcutaneous tissues.

The posterior tibial tendon and a multitude of supporting ligaments including the spring, calcaneofibular, and/or deltoid may also be damaged. Articular injury is not infrequent.

The injury subtype is based on the forefoot's anatomic relationship to the talar head. Although four subtypes are possible, medial and lateral peritalar dislocations comprise the vast majority of injuries. The more common medial peritalar dislocation is thought to result from a forced inversion injury, while its counterpart results from a forced eversion injury.[3]

Most published series are relatively small with the mechanism of injury associated with high-energy trauma such as motor vehicle accidents, not athletic endeavors. Nonetheless, a peritalar dislocation is not an uncommon athletic injury, especially with basketball players landing on an irregular surface.

Clinical Findings

A dramatic deformity is typically present; the protruding talar head is palpable on either side of the ankle (Fig. 70-3). Palpation of the uncovered talar head should make the diagnosis evident by clinical means. A thorough neurovascular examina-

tion should be performed prior to and following joint reduction. In addition, open injuries occur due to wide displacement and tearing of thin subcutaneous tissues.

Differential Diagnosis
Ankle fracture-dislocation

Treatment Options

Joint reduction is accomplished in a timely fashion, typically after radiographs have been performed and assessed. Reduction is best performed with the patient under general anesthesia or deep conscious sedation. Suitable anesthesia facilitates relaxation while decreasing the incidence of iatrogenic chondral damage during reduction attempts. Reduction is performed with the knee flexed to 90 degrees to negate the effect of the gastrocnemius. The joint is reduced in steplike fashion. First, one accentuates the deformity. Next, joint distraction is accomplished with application of longitudinal traction. Finally, a reduction maneuver is performed in a direction opposite to that of the injury-producing force.[4,5]

Irreducible dislocations do occasionally occur, as reduction may be blocked by soft-tissue or bony impediments. Irreducible injuries are most commonly associated with lateral peritalar dislocations. Such instances necessitate an open procedure. This permits excision or reduction of the impediments to reduction. In the instance of a lateral dislocation, the posterior tibial tendon is the most commonly encountered impediment. It may become incarcerated into the joint, blocking reduction. In contrast, with medial peritalar dislocations, the talar head may become buttonholed through the extensor digitorum brevis or the peroneal tendons.[5]

Typically, once the talonavicular joint has been congruently reduced, the foot is stable. Recurrent dislocations are rare; however, on occasion, insertion of a Kirschner wire is necessary due to a persistent unstable foot.[3]

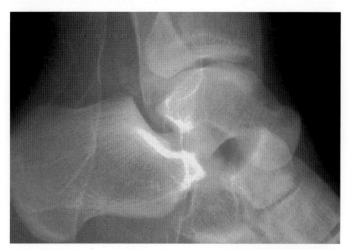

Figure 70-2 A lateral radiograph demonstrating a peritalar dislocation. The talonavicular joint is disrupted and the subtalar joint is subluxated.

As previously noted, medial peritalar dislocations are decidedly more common than lateral.[3,4,6,7] The rate of open injury is variable; Merchan,[3] in a series of 39 injuries, documented a 41% rate of open injuries. Compound injuries obviously represent orthopedic emergencies and are managed with urgent irrigation and débridement, reduction, and appropriate antibiotic coverage to prevent deep infection.

Peritalar injuries are commonly associated with osteochondral fractures involving the head and/or body of the talus as well as associated foot and ankle fractures, especially metatarsal and malleolar fractures. Multiple authors have highlighted an incidence of associated fractures in the range of 40% or more.[3,4,6] These concomitant injuries may adversely affect rehabilitation efforts. A computed tomography study of the hindfoot is recommended to rule out occult injuries not evident by conventional radiography.[5,6]

Overall, the prognosis following a peritalar dislocation is guarded. In their series of 17 patients, DeLee and Curtis[4] found only five patients with range of motion comparable to that of the contralateral, noninjured extremity. Specifically, the average arc of subtalar motion following a medial dislocation was 24 degrees, whereas with lateral dislocations a subtalar arc of 17 degrees was present.[4] Similarly, in a report of 18 peritalar dislocations, Garofalo et al[7] reported excellent results in only 56% at an average follow-up of 10 years. Subtalar arthrofibrosis and/or post-traumatic arthritis are thought to be primary deterrents to satisfactory outcomes. A subtalar fusion or triple arthrodesis may be considered as a salvage procedure for persistent subtalar dysfunction.

Rehabilitation

Institution of an aggressive rehabilitation program is vital to optimize outcome following this injury. The program should include foot intrinsic muscle strengthening, ankle and subtalar joint range-of-motion exercises, and proprioceptive training. Proprioception training enhances the ability of the central nervous system to monitor joint position. Closed-chain exercise and skill-specific training for the athlete's particular sport demands are essential components of rehabilitation prior to return to competition.

Long-term outcome has been associated with multiple factors including direction of the dislocation, concomitant fractures, compound injuries, and length of immobilization.[3] Most authors report fewer satisfactory outcomes with lateral peritalar dislocations.[3,4,6–8] Range of motion of the subtalar joint appears to directly correlate with the outcome. DeLee and Curtis[4] strongly recommend restricting the immobilization period to 3 weeks if possible; otherwise considerable stiffness results. Unfortunately, the presence of a concomitant, unstable fracture may make early mobilization impractical without risking fracture displacement. Aggressive stabilization of associated fractures using internal fixation may permit early rehabilitation, improved outcomes, and a more normal range of joint motion.[5]

These guarded outcomes must be cautiously viewed, as most series are composed of high-energy injuries rather than lower energy, sport-related injuries. The prognosis for the latter injuries may be more favorable, particularly if associated periarticular injuries are not present and aggressive, timely rehabilitation is instituted.

Os Trigonum Syndrome
Anatomic Features

The os trigonum is a small oval accessory bone found in less than 10% of the population[9] (Fig. 70-4). In 1955, McDougall high-

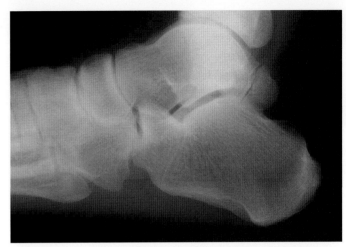

Figure 70-4 A lateral radiograph of the foot demonstrating a large os trigonum of the posterior aspect of the ankle and subtalar joints.

lighted the painful conditions associated with this accessory bone.[10] The ossicle represents an un-united secondary ossification center of the talus. Therefore, its presence alone is not an indication of pathology. However, if an ossicle is present in one foot, it is commonly found in both. The ossicle is located adjacent to the posterolateral talus.

Due to its periarticular position, the bone is vulnerable to impingement with ankle plantarflexion. Injury may result from either a single traumatic injury or from repetitive trauma. Furthermore, injury may involve the ossicle or its fibrous connection (synchondrosis) with the talus.

The os trigonum syndrome (OTS), therefore, is a painful condition of the posterior triangle of the ankle. The syndrome most commonly involves athletes that perform with the ankle positioned in extreme plantarflexion. Ballet dancers, particularly those who perform *en pointe*, appear to be the most commonly afflicted athletes. Such athletes may also develop tenosynovitis of the flexor hallucis longus tendon. This latter entity may masquerade as OTS; the two may coexist. Therefore, surgical decompression of the long flexor tendon may be necessary at the time of surgical ablation of the os.[11]

Clinical Findings

Athletes with OTS generally manifest discomfort within the posterior ankle; however, symptoms may be nonspecific. Pain is accentuated with the end range of both passive and active ankle plantarflexion. Resisted isometric ankle plantarflexion, however, should not elicit a painful response. Active or passive ankle dorsiflexion relieves discomfort. Retrocalcaneal bursitis must be distinguished from OTS; the "two-finger squeeze test" is positive with retrocalcaneal bursitis but is negative in OTS (Fig. 70-5). The painful condition may result from either bony or soft-tissue impingement.

Radiographic Findings

The presence of an os trigonum can be generally confirmed with plain radiographs. Lateral radiographs of the ankle in maximal plantarflexion may demonstrate impingement of the os between the distal tibia and the calcaneus. A bone scan will usually demonstrate intense and localized radionucleotide uptake over the posterior talus if significant injury has occurred (Fig. 70-6).

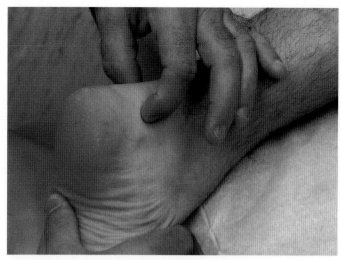

Figure 70-5 A photograph demonstrating the two-finger squeeze test. This is a sensitive clinical test for retrocalcaneal bursitis.

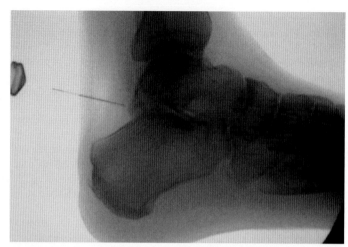

Figure 70-7 A fluoroscopic image of the hindfoot confirming appropriate needle location for injection of a symptomatic os trigonum.

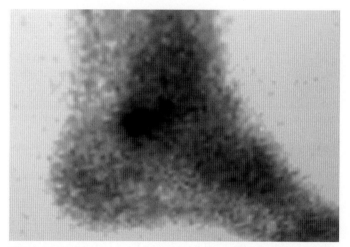

Figure 70-6 A bone scan representing localized radionucleotide uptake in the region of the os trigonum. In the proper clinical setting, this study is consistent with os trigonum syndrome.

A computed tomography study may demonstrate an acute fracture or irregular margins of the os trigonum, thereby suggesting the presence of pathology. In the event that diagnosis remains uncertain, OTS may be confirmed by a positive response to a fluoroscopically guided injection of approximately 0.5 mL of a short-acting anesthetic[12] (Fig. 70-7).

Differential Diagnosis
Achilles tendonitis
Retrocalcaneal bursitis
Flexor hallucis longus tenosynovitis
Subtalar arthritis
Calcaneal stress fracture
Painful accessory soleus

Treatment Options

Activity restrictions, short-term immobilization, and/or use of nonsteroidal anti-inflammatory medications are cornerstones of conservative management. Commonly, the correct diagnosis is missed or delayed. As previously described, if the diagnosis is uncertain, an injection with a local anesthetic may confirm the diagnosis; an injection with steroid preparation may be therapeutic.[12,13] In a series of 19 athletes with OTS, Mouhsine et al[13] reported a 84% success rate using one or two fluoroscopically guided steroid injections at 2-year follow-up. The recalcitrant cases were managed with surgical excision with complete relief of symptoms.

Abramowitz et al[11] reported the outcomes of open surgical resection in 41 symptomatic os trigona. Excellent pain relief and restoration of function was reported at 44-month follow-up; the patients scored an average of 87.6 points on the American Orthopaedic Foot and Ankle Society test (range, 0 to 100). Therefore, resection was recommended if symptoms persisted following 3 months of conservative management. Abramowitz et al observed a trend toward a lower success rate when symptoms had been present for more than 3 years. Finally, iatrogenic sural nerve injury was documented in nearly 20% of their series.[11]

Marrotta and Micheli[14] reported on 16 athletes who underwent open excision of a painful os trigonum. Their series included 12 ballet dancers. Surgical excision was undertaken following failure of conservative management. All patients undergoing excision noted significant improvement of impingement symptoms. All professional dancers returned to full activity; however, two thirds reported occasional discomfort with athletic endeavors.

In addition to open resection, an alternative form of ablation, arthroscopic resection, has been performed. In a series of 11 patients, Marumoto and Ferkel[15] reported on results following arthroscopic os trigonum excision. At mean follow-up of 35 months, the average American Orthopaedic Foot and Ankle Society score increased from 45 to 86 points. Therefore, this technique may produce superior outcomes due to minimization of scar tissue and shorter recovery times. However, this is a technically demanding procedure; therefore, only surgeons familiar with subtalar arthroscopic techniques should consider this form of minimally invasive excision.

Rehabilitation

Conservative management emphasizes means to reduce inflammation. Physical modalities are used. Cross-training techniques are invaluable in maintaining cardiovascular fitness while avoiding irritation of the posterior ankle.

Following surgical excision, postoperative rehabilitation programs focus on restoration of ankle and subtalar motion, while increasing strength, power, and endurance to the gastrocsoleus complex. Sural nerve desensitization may be beneficial if hypersensitivity is present. The os trigonum is closely associated with the flexor hallucis longus tendon; therefore, early tendon mobilization should decrease the potential of postoperative tendon-sheath scarring.

Lisfranc Injuries
Anatomy

The foot's mid-portion functions primarily as a simple block transmitting forces to and from the hindfoot and forefoot. Its composite range of motion is very limited. Midfoot injuries commonly affect the complex osseoligamentocapsular structures of the Lisfranc joint complex.

Injury pathomechanics result from either forefoot hyperdorsiflexion or hyperplantarflexion. Such injuries may be either ligamentous, bony, or mixed. Pure ligamentous injuries are commonly underdiagnosed or delayed in diagnosis due to minimal radiographic changes. Furthermore, the midfoot's inherent bony stability may mask the ligamentous disruption, unless weight-bearing radiographs are obtained or stress radiography is performed. Therefore, a high index of suspicion and specialized testing is often necessary to detect occult injuries.[2]

As previously discussed, the joint complex has unusual bony stability represented by the unique dovetail configuration of the second metatarsal base interlocking into the three cuneiforms. Extensive plantar ligaments connect the metatarsal bases to the cuneiforms and the cuboid. Intermetatarsal ligaments span each of the metatarsal bases except the first and second, where the obliquely oriented Lisfranc ligament is found. This ligament spans the second metatarsal base to the medial cuneiform, providing second metatarsal security.

In low-energy athletic injuries, the injury is primarily ligamentous and instability affects only the second metatarsal. However, more extensive injury may occur; the amount and direction of applied energy determine the extent and direction of the Lisfranc disruption. Football-related injuries are not uncommon, especially in linemen. Snowboarding- and windsurfing-related injuries may result as one falls away from the forefoot, which is secured by a foot sling.

Clinical Findings

Classically, an athlete presents with a painful midfoot and decreased ability to fully weight bear. Swelling and tenderness about the Lisfranc complex are typically present. With isolated stress applied to individual Lisfranc joints, painful clicking may be elicited. Ecchymosis may develop on the plantar aspect of the midfoot.[16] The athlete usually cannot stand on tiptoe secondary to pain. However, classic signs and symptoms may not be present due to the wide continuum of pathology.

Nunley and Vertullo[17] emphasize the uniqueness of athletics-related Lisfranc injuries compared to those of high-energy trauma. The radiographic findings are usually subtle. Fractures are rarely present. A sport midfoot injury classification system stratifies these injuries into three subclasses (Table 70-1). Stage I represents a true ligamentous strain; therefore, the ligament is

Table 70-1 Midfoot Sprain Classification	
Stage I	No diastasis or loss of arch height
Stage II	Diastasis of the I–II metatarsal bases is present with no loss of arch height
Stage III	Diastasis of the I–II metatarsal bases is present with loss of arch height

From Nunley JA, Vertullo CJ: Classification, investigation, and management of midfoot sprain. Lisfranc injuries in the athlete. Am J Sports Med 2002;30:871–878.

intact and competent with no diastasis between the first and second metatarsal bases. In stage II, dorsolateral subluxation of the second metatarsal is radiographically evident; however, despite the diastasis, no loss of arch height is present. Finally, in stage III, both diastasis and loss of longitudinal arch height is apparent on radiographs.[17]

Typically, midfoot disruption proceeds in steplike fashion. In these injuries, the second metatarsal base commonly subluxates as the initial event[18] (Fig. 70-8). The "clear space" between the first and second metatarsal bases should not exceed 2 mm.

Radiographs must be carefully scrutinized to ensure anatomic alignment of the metatarsal bases to the cuboid and respective cuneiforms in all projections. A small radiopacity (the fleck sign) in the one-two interspace may represent an avulsion fracture of the Lisfranc ligament, belying a midfoot ligamentous injury. Pathologic forces may propagate proximally between the cuneiforms rather than progressing laterally. Therefore, the soft-tissue disruption may be longitudinal rather than transverse. Moreover, metatarsophalangeal joint injuries or metatarsal fractures may also accompany midfoot injury.

Differential Diagnosis

Metatarsal and tarsal stress fractures

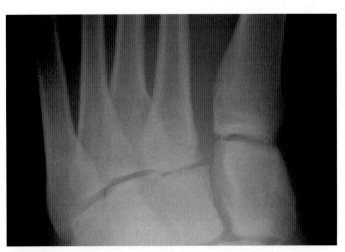

Figure 70-8 An anteroposterior radiograph of the Lisfranc complex demonstrating a widening of the first and second metatarsal bases.

Treatment Options

A continuum of injury occurs and varies from an isolated joint injury (typically the second tarsometatarsal joint) to more extensive joint complex injury. Treatment strategy varies from simple immobilization for simple ligamentous/capsular strains to complex reconstruction with internal fixation for extensive fracture/dislocations. The means to achieve the most suitable outcome remains controversial.

Faciszewski et al[19] retrospectively studied the long-term outcomes of 15 "subtle" injuries of the Lisfranc joint. "Subtle" injuries were defined as those with a 2- to 5-mm diastasis between the first and second metatarsal bases. Athletes comprised one third of the series. Thirteen of 15 injuries were treated with cast immobilization; the remaining two underwent open reduction and internal fixation. Five of the 13 patients treated with immobilization eventually underwent arthrodesis due to pain and deformity.

After review of their series, Faciszewski et al emphasized the value of weight-bearing radiographs. Long-term outcomes were noted to be dependent on an arch height assessment determined by a weight-bearing lateral radiograph. Surgical repair was recommended when significant arch loss was present. Moreover, the measurement of metatarsal diastasis (if <5 mm) documented by weight-bearing anteroposterior radiographs was thought to have little predictive value with regard to outcome.[19]

Treatment strategies continue to evolve. There is a growing consensus for anatomic, rigid fixation of any diastasis of the articular complex to permit ligamentous healing to occur[20,21] (Fig. 70-9). Nonetheless, anatomic repair does not ensure normal midfoot function.[20] Chronic pain and impairment of athletic performance are not uncommon sequelae following the more advanced injury subtypes. Furthermore, post-traumatic arthritis develops in approximately one fourth of patients.

Navicular Stress Fractures

Anatomic Features

The C-shaped navicular bone is nestled between the talar head and the three cuneiforms. The bone is subject to repetitive, high-level stresses of the medial column of the foot. Navicular stress reactions/fractures are located within the central one third of the bone, an area of stress concentration.[22–24] Abnormal foot morphology, such as a cavus and/or forefoot adductus, may concentrate additional forces to this region. Using a microangiographic technique to study bone perfusion, Torg et al[22] detailed a relative watershed area in the central portion of the navicular. Due to vast articular surfaces on the proximal and distal surfaces, vascular channels are restricted to the navicular's medial and lateral surfaces. Osseous perfusion is provided via the posterior tibial and the dorsal pedis arteries, respectively. The pathomechanical basis of this injury is the cumulative stresses applied to a region of decreased vascularity.

Clinical Findings

A high index of suspicion is necessary and should be heightened in athletes with persistent midfoot or medial arch discomfort. This injury is most commonly found in sprinters. On clinical examination, a specific area of discomfort may be difficult to localize. Weight-bearing activities should accentuate the discomfort. Discomfort may be elicited by direct bony palpation at the "N spot" (Fig. 70-10). The N spot is 2 inches distal to the ankle joint and just medial to the anterior tibialis tendon. Discomfort may also be reproduced with adduction/abduction of the forefoot or resisted inversion of the hindfoot.

To rule out alternate sources of pain emanating from adjacent structures, palpation of the anterior tibialis tendon and the talar neck aids in ruling out tendon tear and occult fracture, respectively. In addition, one should also consider anterior ankle impingement in the differential diagnosis of discomfort in this anatomic area.

Radiographic Findings

Correct diagnosis is difficult by clinical examination alone. Commonly the diagnosis is delayed for several months; therefore, clinical suspicion of a navicular stress fracture must be high. Plain radiographs are frequently negative.

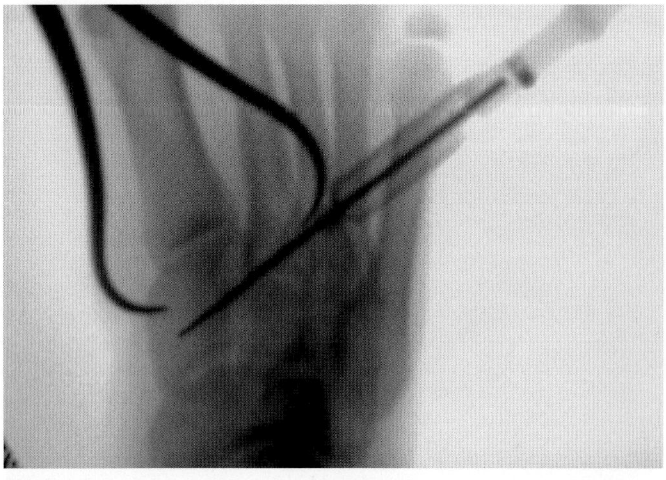

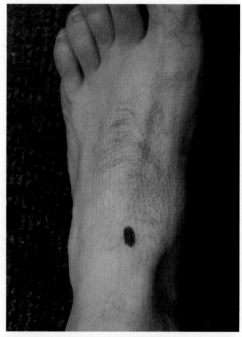

Figure 70-9 An anteroposterior radiograph demonstrating the surgical repair of an isolated Lisfranc injury. The clamp has reduced the first-second metatarsal gap. The depth gauge measures the length of an appropriate screw prior to insertion.

Figure 70-10 A clinical photograph demonstrating the location of the N spot. This is the area of maximal tenderness elicited in the presence of a navicular stress fracture.

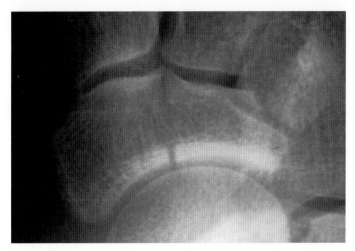

Figure 70-11 Anteroposterior foot radiograph demonstrating a navicular stress fracture. The fracture line is characteristically in the sagittal plane and within the central one third of the bone.

The fracture is commonly incomplete and nondisplaced. The fracture tends to propagate from the proximal/dorsal cortex of the navicular and extends distally and plantarly.[24] Again, the fracture line is characteristically in the sagittal plane and within the central one third of the bone (Fig. 70-11). A three-phase bone scan is helpful if the scan is positive; however, false-positive results are not uncommon (Fig. 70-12).

A thin-section computed tomography scan provides excellent fracture detail. In contrast, magnetic resonance imaging is a sensitive, but expensive, imaging modality with the added capability of detecting subtle soft-tissue pathology. T2-weighted images are extremely sensitive for detecting a stress reaction/fracture of bone. This modality can be extremely valuable, especially when the history and physical examination are suggestive with inconclusive radiographs.

Differential Diagnosis

Anterior ankle pain
Talonavicular joint sprain
Posterior tibial tendonitis
Saphenous neuritis
Anterior tibialis tendon rupture

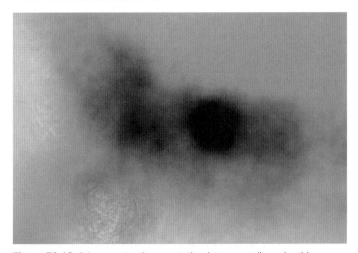

Figure 70-12 A bone scan demonstrating intense radionucleotide uptake in the region of the navicular.

Treatment Options

Again, the time from onset of symptoms to correct diagnosis may be considerable. Fracture management is determined by multiple factors. First, the fracture may be either complete or incomplete. Second, fracture chronicity may be either acute or delayed. The fracture zone is commonly sclerotic with delayed fracture healing subtypes. Finally, the athlete's expectations and level of competition may affect the practicality of conservative management; a prolonged period of immobilization may be unacceptable to both the coach and athlete.

Treatment is divided into nonoperative and operative treatment. Conservative management is most appropriate for nondisplaced and incomplete fractures. An initial period of 6 to 8 weeks of non-weight bearing is usually necessary for healing this fracture subtype.[23] Following immobilization, the athlete is re-examined. If the region is nontender and radiographic healing is present, progressive weight bearing is initiated.

Operative treatment primarily consists of internal fixation with or without bone grafting. Surgical repair may be open or with minimally invasive technique (see later). Fracture "personality" will often guide surgical selection. An open repair necessitates additional soft-tissue stripping of a poorly vascularized zone; however, it is a "necessary evil" when bone grafting of the fracture is necessary for union.

Author's Preferred Surgical Technique

The author's approach to nondisplaced navicular fractures is through a lateral surgical approach, either via a percutaneous or limited incision. Localization of the incision adjacent to the lateral navicular can be confirmed with intraoperative fluoroscopy (Fig. 70-13). Careful dissection is carefully performed through the subcutaneous tissues with care to avoid injury to branches of the superficial peroneal nerve. The extensor retinaculum is divided longitudinally. The long toe extensors are retracted, exposing the lateral aspect of the navicular. Since most stress fractures are nondisplaced, fracture reduction is usually unnecessary.

A guidewire is inserted in a lateral-to-medial direction. Appropriate orientation is confirmed with biplanar fluoroscopy. The guidewire is overdrilled with a cannulated drill, and a short-threaded cancellous screw is inserted over the guidewire. For a proper lag screw effect, all threads must pass beyond the frac-

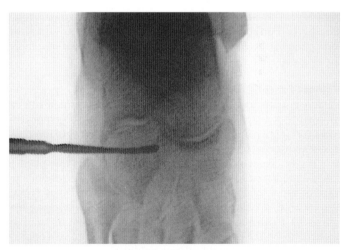

Figure 70-13 An intraoperative fluoroscopic radiograph demonstrating localization of the lateral aspect of the navicular. This facilitates the determination of the proper entry site for a lateral to medial–based screw for osteosynthesis of a navicular fracture.

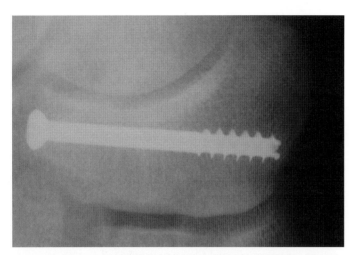

Figure 70-14 An anteroposterior foot radiograph demonstrating lag screw position for internal fixation of the central one third fracture of the navicular.

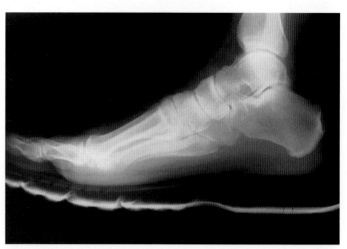

Figure 70-15 A lateral foot radiograph demonstrating the position of the foot within an athletic shoe. Appropriate shoewear performs the vital function of foot support and protection.

ture line into the medial fracture fragment; otherwise, the "near fragment" must be overdrilled. Although two parallel screws can be used, a single well-positioned lag screw has been quite successful in my experience (Fig. 70-14).

Rehabilitation

A comprehensive rehabilitation of the lower extremities is prescribed following this midfoot injury. Ambulation in a partial weight-bearing environment such as a pool may be an invaluable rehabilitation environment. Furthermore, the use of a bone stimulator may be a therapeutic adjunct to facilitate osseous healing.

Assessment and correction of biomechanical abnormalities are vital components of the rehabilitation program. A thorough lower extremity biomechanical examination is performed to assess for possible angular and rotational misalignment. The forefoot-hindfoot relationship is particularly important. Mechanical causes, such as improper shoe wear or training technique should be corrected (Fig. 70-15). Therefore, a custom foot orthosis may facilitate timely return to sport and prevent recurrences by accommodating for abnormal foot-ground relationships. Furthermore, athletes at risk of nutritional or endocrinologic causes of bone fragility should be thoroughly investigated.

Plantar Fasciitis

Plantar fasciitis, or painful heel syndrome, is a common source of medial heel pain that affects both athletes and nonathletes.[25-27] This painful hindfoot condition is conceptualized as either an overuse or degenerative phenomenon. Proximal plantar fasciitis is characterized as heel pain isolated to the plantar fascia's origin onto the plantar-medial calcaneus. It develops in all foot types, including both high- and low-arched foot types. It is a dense, fibrous cord consisting of three bands bridging the calcaneus to the five toes. The origin of the central band is thought to be the most symptomatic region due to its concentrated region of strain and relative rigidity.[25]

Classic symptoms include morning heel pain on the medial aspect of the heel and pain on arising from a recumbent position (or "start-up" pain). The plantar fascia serves as a bowstring,

a static longitudinal arch support structure, bridging the hindfoot and the forefoot. The plantar fascia's origin undergoes degenerative and inflammatory changes due to repetitive microtrauma; an Achilles tendon contracture is often a coexisting condition.

The differential diagnosis of heel pain is usually fairly straightforward. However, other hindfoot conditions may masquerade as plantar fasciitis and must be differentiated for diagnostic accuracy. These include calcaneal stress fractures, tarsal tunnel syndrome (and other nerve entrapments), and painful heel-pad syndrome. Careful physical examination assists in distinguishing pathology in adjacent hindfoot structures and confirming an accurate diagnosis. For instance, the medial and lateral walls of the calcaneus are tender to direct palpation if a calcaneal stress fracture is present. Percussion over the tibial nerve (a positive Tinel sign) reproduces symptoms of tarsal tunnel syndrome. In a somewhat similar condition, the first branch of the lateral plantar nerve (or Baxter's nerve) becomes entrapped and may coexist with plantar fasciitis. The nerve divides from the lateral plantar nerve and becomes entrapped as it courses to the abductor digiti minimi. This clinical scenario, therefore, combines symptoms of a painful heel with neurogenic pain. Finally, in painful heel-pad syndrome, the physical examination is notable for a tender heel pad to direct palpation.

Differential Diagnosis
Calcaneal stress fracture
Tarsal tunnel syndrome
Nerve entrapment
Painful heel-pad syndrome

Noninvasive Treatment

The condition is generally self-limiting with conservative means; however, improvement is often gradual and commonly prolonged. Daily plantar fascia and Achilles tendon stretching are cornerstones of management[25-27] (Fig. 70-16). Multifaceted con-

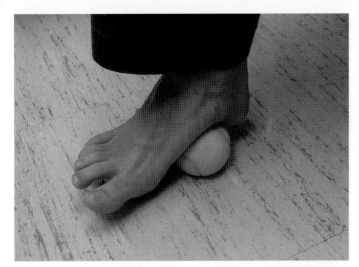

Figure 70-16 A clinical photograph demonstrating a stretching exercise for the plantar fascia. A tennis ball is placed under the heel. Downward pressure is applied to the ball. The ball is rolled back and forth, stretching the proximal plantar fascia.

servative treatment yields success rates in excess of 90%.[26] Adjunctive treatment such as orthotics devices, night splints, anti-inflammatory medications, and ultrasound therapy are other treatment modalities.

Activity modification with cessation of impact-loading activities and institution of cross-training activities are also helpful. A cortisone injection may be used with caution; its strong anti-inflammatory effect should be weighed against potential side effects (e.g., plantar fascia rupture or fat-pad atrophy).

Biomechanical assessment of lower extremity alignment is a vital component in treatment and to circumvent recurrence. Physical examination of the foot with the patient positioned in prone facilitates assessment of the hindfoot-forefoot alignment (Fig. 70-17). Semirigid shoe inserts may be prescribed to accom-

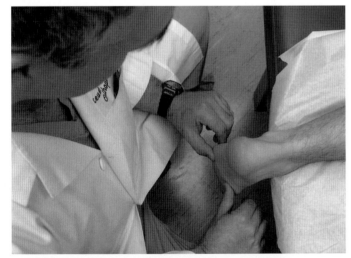

Figure 70-17 A clinical photograph of a biomechanical foot examination performed in a prone position. The "tripod" of the foot formed by the calcaneal tuberosity and head of the first and fifth metatarsals can be readily assessed.

modate abnormal foot structure. It remains an essential component of treatment, especially in running athletes.

Invasive Treatment

Recalcitrant plantar fasciitis is generally defined as persistent symptoms following 6 months of conservative management. Such failure may necessitate more aggressive treatment strategies. Partial surgical transection of the fascia's central band may be performed by either open or endoscopic techniques. In a series of open releases, Snider et al[28] reported excellent relief of symptoms in 10 of 11 patients at 25-month follow-up. Their series included nine long-distance runners. Similarly, Schepsis et al[25] reported satisfactory results in 24 of 27 open releases. At the time of open operative release, microscopic examination of the biopsy specimens revealed collagen necrosis, angiofibroblastic hyperplasia, chondroid metaplasia, and matrix calcification.

Endoscopic plantar facial release is an alternative means to resect the plantar fascia. As a minimally invasive technique, it is reported to hasten recuperation due to minimal scar formation. O'Malley et al[29] reported the surgical results in 16 individuals following 20 endoscopic plantar facial procedures. The patients reported an average duration of symptoms of 4 years. They reported improvement in 18 of 20 heels with complete relief in 45%.[29] The average American Orthopaedic Foot and Ankle Society score increased from 62 to 80. No surgical complications such as infection or nerve injury were reported. Therefore, based on their experience, this minimally invasive technique of plantar fascia release was recommended as a safe and effective method to treat recalcitrant plantar fasciitis.

Recently, the therapeutic application of high-energy shock waves to the plantar fascia has been used for recalcitrant cases. This noninvasive, but powerful treatment focuses high-energy acoustic forces to the plantar fascia's origin. This results in an apparent acute inflammatory reaction that promotes neovascularization and a natural healing response. The efficacy of this modality remains controversial, largely due to variations in technique, level of energy formation, and delivery.

Ogden et al[30] reported the results of high-energy treatment in a large randomized, double-blind study. Good or excellent results were achieved in 48% of patients in the series at 3- and 12-month follow-up. Moreover, the treatment resulted in no apparent side effects or complications. Future investigation into management of recalcitrant plantar fasciitis and other musculoskeletal pathologies is anticipated.

Tibial Nerve Entrapment
Anatomy

Tibial nerve entrapment was not recognized as a clinical entity until its description by both Keck and Lam in 1962.[31] This pathologic process is termed tarsal tunnel syndrome. The nerve entrapment involves the tibial nerve or one or more of its distal branches. The hallmark symptoms include neurogenic, lancinating pain about the medial ankle with radiation into the plantar foot.

The tibial nerve, a mixed motor and sensory nerve, supplies motor function to the intrinsic foot muscles, as well as sensation of the medial heel and plantar foot. The tarsal tunnel consists of a fibro-osseous space, located plantar and inferior to the medial malleolus. The most superficial border is the flexor retinaculum. Within this tunnel passes the tibial nerve and its terminal branches, the lateral and medial plantar and medial calcaneal nerves (Fig. 70-18). Impingement may occur anywhere from the proximal aspect of the tunnel to the plantar midfoot.

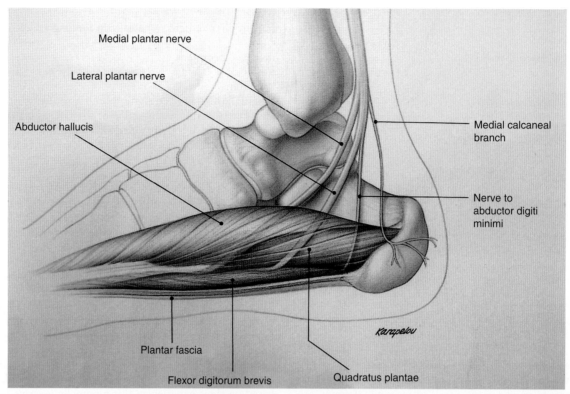

Medial plantar nerve

Lateral plantar nerve

Abductor hallucis

Medial calcaneal branch

Nerve to abductor digiti minimi

Plantar fascia

Flexor digitorum brevis

Quadratus plantae

Karapelou

Figure 70-18 Schematic of the anatomy of the tarsal tunnel. The four branches of the tibial nerve are demonstrated. The medial and lateral plantar nerves and the nerve to the abductor digiti minimi course deep to the abductor hallucis muscle. (From Beskin JL, Baxter DE: Tarsal tunnel and associated nerve entrapment. Op Tech Orthop 1992;2:162–166.)

Clinical Findings

The incidence of painful entity is likely not increasing; however, increased awareness in athletes has resulted in an increased rate of diagnosis. Symptoms generally include either shocklike sensations or numbness of the medial heel or all (or portions) of the plantar foot. Muscle weakness may also be present. A positive percussion test (Tinel's sign) over the tibial nerve is typically present with exacerbation of paresthetic symptoms. Abnormal foot alignment is reported to represent the most common cause of tarsal tunnel syndrome in athletes.[31] Excessive knee and/or hindfoot valgus with foot hyperpronation may create increased nerve tension.

This syndrome must be differentiated from an L5 radiculopathy, which may manifest similar symptoms. Neurodiagnostic studies can assist in differentiating the two entities. Electromyographic muscle sampling about and below the tarsal tunnel must be undertaken. Prolongation of distal motor and sensory latencies across the tarsal tunnel with diminished muscle amplitudes in the distribution of one or both plantar digital nerves confirms the diagnosis. Nerve entrapment may result for the presence of a space-occupying lesion (e.g., lipoma, ganglion, or neurilemoma) within the fibro-osseous tunnel.

Differential Diagnosis

Lumbar radiculopathy
Posterior tibial tendonitis

Treatment Options

Initial treatment is conservative. The nerve may become stretched or contused rather than entrapped. Immobilization or restriction of hindfoot motion, typically, eversion, may decrease symptoms. Correction of abnormal foot mechanics may be beneficial; hindfoot taping or orthotics may decrease nerve stretch. Vitamin B_6 may also assist in resolving nerve-related symptoms.

Surgical decompression is warranted if conservative treatment fails. The prognosis following surgery, however, is not uniformly successful. The presence of a space-occupying lesion increases the likelihood of success following surgery. In an outcome-analysis of 68 procedures performed on 60 patients, Gondring et al[32] observed a significant dichotomy between objective and subjective testing of postsurgical results following nerve decompression.

Author's Preferred Surgical Technique

The surgical release of the tarsal tunnel is performed with the patient in a side-lying position. Appropriate support is provided by a beanbag. A well-padded thigh tourniquet is applied. The limb is exsanguinated. A J-shaped incision is made along the course of the nerve with the superior aspect of the incision approximately 6 cm above and 1 cm posterior to the medial malleolus. The incision extends distal to the level of the midfoot. The procedure is performed with the assistance of loupe magnification.

Surgical dissection proceeds to the flexor retinaculum. The nerve is then located in the proximal aspect of the incision and traced distally into the tunnel. The retinaculum is incised carefully. The tibial nerve generally divides into its terminal branches under the cover of the retinaculum. The nerve trunk and its divisions are traced distally into the forefoot. Any restrictive structures are incised. Space-occupying lesions are removed, if present. The nerve is decompressed, but dissection is limited to preserve microvascular perfusion.

Following a thorough inspection of the tunnel, ensuring complete nerve decompression, the retinaculum is reapproximated. A suction drain is placed, and the limb splinted in a plantigrade position. Sutures are removed after 12 to 14 days in most instances. Range-of-motion exercises are initiated thereafter to prevent adhesion formation. Weight bearing is initiated when the incision is completely healed.

Rehabilitation
The initial conservative care has been already outlined. Following surgical decompression, early motion is desirable to maintain the gliding action of the nerve; otherwise, the nerve will become adherent to adjacent soft tissues and produce excessive traction during ankle and hindfoot motion.

Posterior Tibial Tendonitis
Anatomy
The posterior tibial tendon courses from its origin on the posterior tibial muscle, about the medial malleolus, to its insertion on the navicular and the first, second, and third metatarsal bases. It supports the longitudinal arch and serves as an ankle plantar flexor and hindfoot invertor. The tendon is the primary regulator of the talonavicular joint.

Maffulli et al recommend that the tendon injury be conceptualized on an anatomic basis.[33] Tendon pathology, therefore, has been stratified into subclasses dependent on the extent of tissue involvement (Table 70-2). In young athletes, paratendonopathy is a preferable descriptive term to tendonitis, when an inflammatory condition of the tendon sheath results due to overuse.

Abnormal foot type and arch height commonly produce increased tension within the posterior tibial tendon. For example, a hyperpronated foot with a contracted Achilles tendon will increase tensile stress within the posterior tibial tendon, resulting in a higher likelihood of structural failure over time.

Clinical Findings
Classic symptoms are local tenderness to palpation with swelling along the insertional or retromalleolar locations. Pain with resisted hindfoot inversion is typical. To isolate posterior tibial tendon function, the hindfoot is tested in dorsiflexion to neutralize the other invertor, the anterior tibial tendon.

As paratendonopathy advances to pantendonopathy, foot deformity occurs. The forefoot becomes abducted; the "too

many toes" sign is present. In addition, when performing a single-limb toe raise, hindfoot inversion is not possible due to the dysfunction of the posterior tibial tendon.

Differential Diagnosis
Tarsal tunnel syndrome
Painful accessory navicular

Radiography
Conventional radiography is typically normal; however, in advanced stages of dysfunction, dorsolateral peritalar subluxation is evident. Additional pathology may be evident if weight-bearing films are obtained. Radiographs may demonstrate a "break" in midfoot contour with forefoot abduction and elevation. Currently, magnetic resonance imaging is the most appropriate imaging modality to assess the posterior tibial tendon and the adjacent spring ligament. This permits assessment of the integrity of tendon and ligamentous structures.

Treatment Options
Inflammation involving the paratenon (paratendonopathy) may be treated with activity modification, physical modalities, and anti-inflammatory medications. Limb immobilization with a removable boot or cast is generally reserved for recalcitrant cases. A custom foot orthosis directly accommodates abnormal foot mechanics. Achilles tendon stretching and posterior tibialis muscle strengthening may also be helpful.

A steroid injection into the tendon sheath is not recommended. Recalcitrant paratendonopathy may respond to tendon sheath débridement. Moreover, longitudinal tears (or splits) are treated with débridement or repair. Central one third longitudinal tears may be repaired in side-to-side fashion with a running stitch; peripheral tears are generally débrided.

McCormack et al[34] reported on eight competitive athletes with an average age of 22 who underwent surgical débridement of their posterior tibial tendons following failure of conservative management. At an average follow-up period of 22 months, seven of the eight athletes were able to return to their previous level of competition. The eighth athlete was able to return to sport but had some intermittent symptoms.

Stage II and III posterior tibial tendon pathology is uncommon in young athletes. Tendonosis with elongation of the tendon occurs in Stage II. As the tendon lengthens, it becomes dysfunctional (Fig. 70-19). Diminution of posterior tibial tendon forces creates an unbalanced foot. The longitudinal arch collapses. The hindfoot shifts into valgus and the forefoot into abduction. These deformities remain flexible. Conservative management of Stage II pathology is bracing with an ankle-foot-orthosis or UCBL shoe inserts. Surgical treatment is most commonly undertaken in the form of a combined tendon transfer (usually the FDL) and medial-translation osteotomy of the calcaneus, or with lateral column lengthening procedures. Stage III disease develops when the deformities are no longer passively correctible. Arthrodesis is the most common form of operative intervention.

Table 70-2 Classification of Tendon Pathology	
Paratendonopathy	Inflammation of the paratenon
Tendonopathy	Inflammation involving the tendon
Pantendonopathy	Inflammation involving the tendon and its sheath

From Maffulli N, Khan KM, Puddu G: Overuse tendon conditions: Time to change a confusing terminology. Arthroscopy 1998;14:840–843.

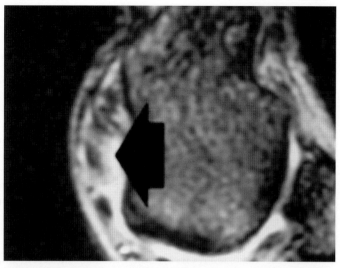

Figure 70-19 Magnetic resonance imaging of a posterior tibial tendon. The *arrow* demonstrates an abnormal intrasubstance signal of the posterior tibial tendon without tendon disruption. A normal tendon would be oval shaped and homogeneous. This magnetic resonance imaging study is pathology consistent with type II dysfunction.

CONCLUSIONS

The correct diagnosis of hindfoot pain and dysfunction in athletes can be challenging. In-depth knowledge of topographic anatomy, function, and foot biomechanics assists in the formulation of an appropriate differential diagnosis. The physical examination is aided by the foot's thin soft-tissue cover, permitting direct palpation of most painful structures. A rigorous history and physical examination should help pinpoint the appropriate diagnosis.

Injury types are commonly associated with specific sports or sport positions. Overuse syndromes, such as navicular fractures and posterior tibial tendonitis, are most commonly seen in long-distance runners. Midfoot ligamentous injuries are not uncommon in football players, especially linemen. Finally, posterior ankle injuries occur most commonly in dancers.

Imaging studies are used to confirm the physical examination so that appropriate and timely treatment can be implemented. Although complete recovery is not always possible, a prompt, accurate diagnosis with appropriate management facilitates timely return to sport.

REFERENCES

1. Perry J: Anatomy and biomechanics of the hindfoot. Clin Orthop 1983;177:9–15.
2. Lawrence, SJ: Midfoot trauma, bony and ligamentous: Evaluation and treatment. Curr Opin Orthop 2002;13:99–106.
3. Merchan ECR: Subtalar dislocations: Long-term follow-up of 39 cases. Injury 1992;23:97–100.
4. DeLee JC, Curtis R: Subtalar dislocations of the foot. J Bone Joint Surg Am 1982;64:433–437.
5. Bohay DR, Manoli A: Subtalar joint dislocations. Foot Ankle Int 1995;16:803–808.
6. Bibbo C, Anderson RB, Davis WH, et al: Injury characteristics and the clinical outcome of subtalar dislocations; a clinical and radiographic analysis of 25 cases. Foot Ankle Int 2003;242:158–163.
7. Garofalo R, Moretti B, Ortolano V, et al: Peritalar dislocations: A retrospective study of 18 cases. J Foot Ankle Surg 2004;43:166–172.
8. Tucker DJ, Burian G, Boylan JP: Lateral subtalar dislocation: Review of the literature and case presentation. J Foot Ankle Surg 1998;37:239–247.
9. Sarrafian SK: Osteology. In Sarrafian SK (ed): Anatomy of the Foot and Ankle: Descriptive, Topographic, Functional. Philadelphia, Lippincott, 1993, pp 51–55.
10. McDougall A: The os trigonum. J Bone Joint Surg Br 1955;37:257–265.
11. Abramowitz Y, Wollstein R, Barzilay Y, et al: Outcome of resection of a symptomatic os trigonum. J Bone Joint Surg Am 2003;85:1051–1057.
12. Jones DM, Saltzman CL, El-Khoury G: The diagnosis of the os trigonum syndrome with a fluoroscopically controlled injection of local anesthetic. Iowa Orthop J 1999;19:122–126.
13. Mouhsine E, Crevoisier X, Leyvraz PF, et al: Post-traumatic overload or acute syndrome of the os trigonum: Possible cause of posterior ankle impingement. Knee Surg Sports Traumatol Arthrosc 2004;12:250–253.
14. Marrotta JJ, Micheli LJ: Os trigonum impingement in dancers. Am J Sports Med 1992;20:533–536.
15. Marumoto JM, Ferkel RD: Arthroscopic excision of the os trigonum: A new technique with preliminary clinical results. Foot Ankle Int 1997;18:777–784.
16. Ross G, Cronin R, Hauzenblas J, et al: Plantar ecchymosis sign: A clinical aid to diagnosis of occult Lisfranc tarsometatarsal injuries. J Orthop Trauma 1996;10:119–122.
17. Nunley JA, Vertullo CJ: Classification, investigation, and management of midfoot sprain. Lisfranc injuries in the athlete. Am J Sports Med 2002;30:871–878.
18. Mantas JP, Burks RT: Lisfranc injuries in the athlete. Clin Sports Med 1994;13:719–730.
19. Faciszewski T, Burks RT, Manaster BJ: Subtle injuries of the Lisfranc joint. J Bone Joint Surg Am 1990;72:1519–1522.
20. Teng AL, Pinzur MS, Lomasney L, et al: Functional outcomes following anatomic restoration of the tarsal-metatarsal fracture-dislocation. Foot Ankle Int 2002;23:922–926.
21. Philbin T, Rosenberg G, Sferra JJ: Complications of missed or untreated Lisfranc injuries. Foot Ankle Clin N Am 2003;8:61–71.
22. Torg JS, Pavlov H, Coley HL, et al: Stress fractures of the tarsal navicular: A retrospective review of twenty-one cases. J Bone Joint Surg Am 1982;6:700–712.
23. Lee S, Anderson RB: Stress fractures of the tarsal navicular. Foot Ankle Clin 2004;9:85–104.
24. Coris EE, Kaeding CC, Marymont JV: Tarsal navicular stress injuries in athletes. Orthopedics 2003;26:733–737.
25. Schepsis AA, Leach RE, Gorzyca J: Plantar fasciitis. Clin Orthop 1991;266:185–196.
26. Dyck DD Jr, Boyajian-O'Neill LA: Plantar fasciitis. Clin J Sports Med 2004;14:305–309.
27. Leach RE, DiIorio E, Harney RA: Pathologic hindfoot conditions in the athlete. Clin Orthop 1983;177:166–121.
28. Snider MP, Clancy WG, McBeath AA: Plantar fascia release for chronic plantar fasciitis in runners. Am J Sports Med 1983;11:215–219.
29. O'Malley MJ, Page A, Cook R: Endoscopic plantar fasciotomy for chronic heel pain. Foot Ankle Int 2000;21:505–510.
30. Ogden JA, Alverez RG, Levitt RL, et al: Electrohydraulic high-energy shock-wave treatment for chronic plantar fasciitis. J Bone Joint Surg Am 2004;86:2216–2228.

31. Jackson DL, Haglund B: Tarsal tunnel syndrome in athletes. Case reports and literature review. Am J Sports Med 1991;19:61–65.

32. Gondring WH, Shields B, Wenger S: An outcomes analysis of surgical treatment of tarsal tunnel syndrome. Foot Ankle Int 2003;24:545–550.

33. Maffulli N, Khan KM, Puddu G: Overuse tendon conditions: Time to change a confusing terminology. Arthroscopy 1998;14:840–843.

34. McCormack AP, Varner KE, Marymont JV: Surgical treatment for posterior tibial tendonitis in young competitive athletes. Foot Ankle Int 2003;24:535–538.

Forefoot and Toes

Lisa T. DeGnore

In This Chapter

Fifth metatarsal fracture
Stress fracture
Turf toe
Metatarsalgia
Sesamoid problems
Nerve entrapments

INTRODUCTION

- Forefoot problems are varied and common in athletes of all ages.

- The majority of these problems are generally treated with conservative measures.

- Acute Jones fractures and fifth metatarsal stress fractures are commonly treated surgically in athletes.

- Return to sports is dependent on response to treatment.

FIFTH METATARSAL FRACTURES

Injuries to the base of the fifth metatarsal are common in athletes and are often due to an inversion force combined with the resistance of strong ligamentous structures.[1] These fractures are termed *avulsion fractures* and usually involve the proximal 1 to 1.5 cm of the fifth metatarsal metaphysis. This area of the bone has been termed the *tuberosity*. These are considered type 1 fractures.[2] Type 1 fractures are usually nondisplaced and are generally extra-articular.

Patients present with a history of an inversion injury, often reporting they hear a "pop." A complete physical examination of the foot and ankle should be performed to identify any other injuries. Patients with this fracture will have tenderness and ecchymosis over the lateral midfoot. Neurovascular status must be evaluated, as well as the integrity of the Lisfranc joint complex.

All patients should have weight-bearing (if at all possible) anteroposterior and lateral and non-weight-bearing oblique views of the foot. Additional ankle views should be included if there is any question of injury in the ankle area.

The vast majority of these type 1 fractures may be treated nonoperatively. In general, a firm-soled shoe and activity modification are all that is needed for the athlete. Occasionally, a more symptomatic patient may need a more supportive fracture brace. Healing is usually uneventful and can be expected in 6 to 8 weeks. Not all fractures will show complete radiographic union, but very rarely are these symptomatic. If a symptomatic nonunion occurs, simple excision is usually successful.[3] In the rare case of an intra-articular fracture that is displaced more than 2 to 3 mm, fixation with small lag screws is preferred.

As opposed to the fifth metatarsal tuberosity fracture, true Jones fractures involve the metatarsal in the area 2.5 cm distal to the tuberosity at the metaphyseal-diaphyseal junction. These are termed type 2 fractures. Acute injuries involve inversion, axial load, and adduction of the forefoot. Radiographs show a lucent line at the metaphyseal-diaphyseal junction of the bone and usually minimal displacement (Fig. 71-1). The presence of sclerosis around the fracture site and the history of a prodrome of vague pain in the area indicate a Jones stress fracture (Fig. 71-2) Stress fractures almost always require operative intervention and are discussed subsequently.

Physical examination of an acute Jones fracture finds pain to palpation over the lateral midfoot and varied amounts of swelling and ecchymosis. It is important to examine the foot and ankle fully in order to identify any associated injuries to the ankle, forefoot, and especially the Lisfranc complex.

Radiographs consisting of anteroposterior, lateral, and oblique views are necessary to fully evaluate the foot. Again, weight-bearing films are preferred if the patient is able. Rarely are any other studies indicated.

Treatment of a Jones fracture is significantly different from that of an avulsion fracture. The Jones fracture occurs in what has been described as a watershed area of blood flow and is associated with a relatively high rate of nonunion.[4] Symptomatic treatment, with a shoe or boot, is not acceptable. If nonoperative treatment is chosen, the patient should be immobilized in a non-weight-bearing fiberglass cast for 6 to 8 weeks (preferably 8 weeks) until radiographic union occurs and the fracture site is nontender. Because the rate of nonunion using a non-weight-bearing cast has been reported to be as high as 28%, surgical treatment is often preferred for the athletic patient.[5]

Surgical treatment is performed using a percutaneous technique. Under fluoroscopic guidance, a small incision is made laterally at the base of the metatarsal tuberosity and a drill or guidewire for a cannulated screw is inserted. The choice of screw size has been discussed fairly extensively, and discussion exists as to whether solid or cannulated screws should be used.[5,6] Various studies have examined techniques using 4.5-, 5.5-, and 6.5-mm screws.[4-9] It is the author's opinion that screw size should be based on the patient's anatomy. The canal is tapped as needed, and the appropriate length screw is inserted. Care must be taken to ensure that the screw threads cross the fracture site completely, yet the screw should not be so long as to

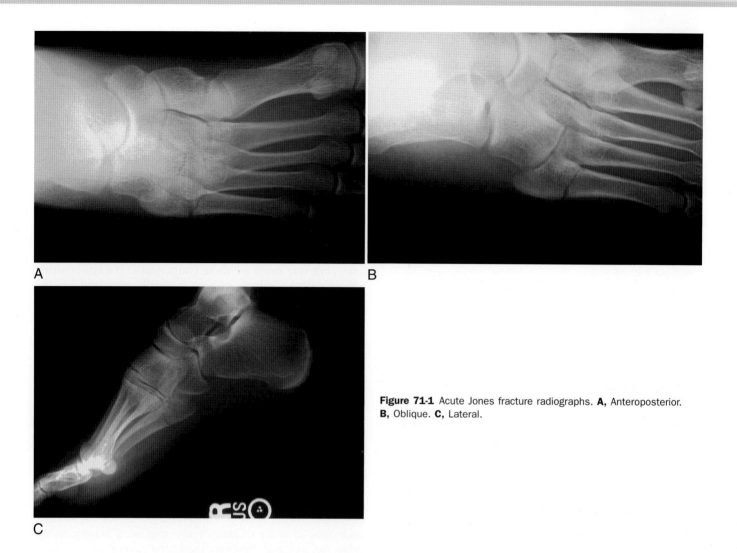

Figure 71-1 Acute Jones fracture radiographs. **A,** Anteroposterior. **B,** Oblique. **C,** Lateral.

straighten the normal curve of the bone and thus distract the fracture (Fig. 71-3). The author's preference is to use a 6.5-mm cannulated screw in most fractures with a 4.5-mm screw used in smaller bones. Initial discussion of screw fixation in athletes suggested that early weight bearing could be allowed; however, this has not been reliable.[7] The athlete must be protected from weight bearing until union is fully established, generally 6 to 8 weeks (Fig. 71-4A).

Jones stress fractures are commonly identified when a relatively minor acute injury occurs preceded by a prodrome of

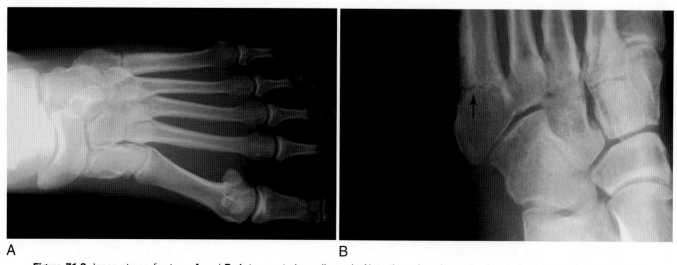

Figure 71-2 Jones stress fracture. **A** and **B,** Anteroposterior radiograph. Note the sclerosis proximal and distal to the fracture *(arrow)*.

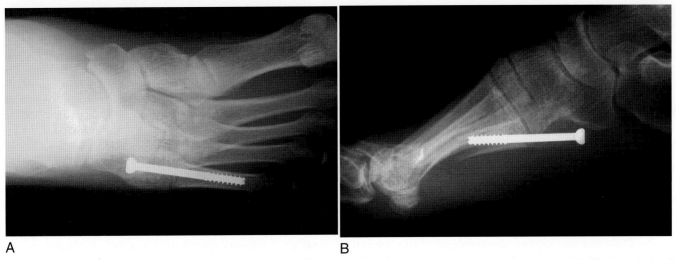

A   B

Figure 71-3 Operative treatment of an acute Jones fracture. **A** and **B**, Anteroposterior and lateral views of a properly positioned 4.5-mm cannulated screw.

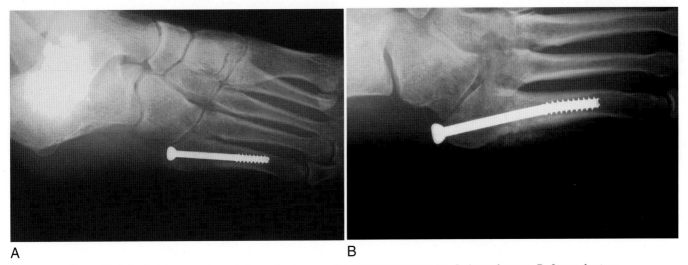

A   B

Figure 71-4 Healed Jones acute and stress fractures: anteroposterior radiographs. **A**, Acute fracture. **B**, Stress fracture.

lateral foot pain. They may occur in the classic Jones location or in the next 1 cm distal to this region. These are considered type 3 fractures. The radiographic appearance shows sclerosis in the canal at the fracture site and sometimes a lucent gap (see Fig. 71-2). Operative treatment is almost always indicated. Screw fixation as described previously, with or without onlay bone grafting has been described as successful.[6] It is the author's preference to use a bone graft in the well-established nonunions. Generally, an H-shaped trough across the fracture is made and bone graft packed into and around this trough. It is important to fully drill the sclerotic canal to encourage new vascular ingrowth. Weight bearing should be delayed until union occurs and may be prolonged in severe cases (see Fig. 71-4B). The addition of electrical and/or ultrasonic stimulation may be useful.

METATARSAL STRESS FRACTURES

Stress fractures in any population occur most commonly in the metatarsals, with the second and third metatarsals as the most common site. It has been suggested that fatigue and poor train-

ing play a role in the development of metatarsal stress fractures, and athletes involved in repetitive impact sports are at the most risk.[10–13] High arches, forefoot varus, and metatarsal adduction are risk factors. Stress fractures may occur in healthy players, but those with unusual or multiple injuries should be evaluated for structural or metabolic abnormalities. The most common metabolic abnormality associated with these fractures in female athletes is amenorrhea.[11]

The clinical presentation is usually one of an insidious onset of pain and swelling on the dorsum of the foot. Patients report more pain with increased activity that improves with rest. They will have a varied amount of swelling over the metatarsals but will be reproducibly tender over the affected bone.

In the first few weeks of symptoms, radiographs are commonly negative. An experienced clinician will proceed with treatment based on history and clinical examination. In questionable cases, a three-phase bone scan or magnetic resonance imaging may be performed.

In general, metatarsal stress fractures may be treated conservatively with a supportive shoe and rest. Rarely, a cast or fracture boot may be needed for more symptomatic injuries. Athletes should be encouraged to participate in nonimpact exercise to maintain condition while resting. Return to prior activity may proceed when clinically healed. Radiographic union may lag behind clinical healing. A nonunion is rare and should be treated with fixation and bone grafting.

In ballet dancers, an unusual stress fracture of the base of the second metatarsal has been reported. It occurs at the metaphyseal-diaphyseal junction and may generally be treated conservatively, although several reinjuries have been reported.[13]

TURF TOE INJURIES

Originally described as occurring on artificial turf surfaces, turf toe injuries involve a primarily hyperdorsiflexion force to the first metatarsal phalangeal joint.[14] Varus and valgus forces may also play a role and may increase the likelihood of late instability. These injuries occur in football, soccer, dance, and other sports that involve great toe dorsiflexion activity. The injury involves primarily the plantar plate; the sesamoid complex and the collateral ligaments are injured depending on the severity and direction of the forces involved.

Clinically, patients present with pain, swelling, ecchymosis, and a history consistent with the injury. Physical examination of the foot should be complete, with careful attention to neurovascular evaluation. Additionally, examination of the great toe should include an evaluation of range of motion and medial, lateral, and anteroposterior stress testing. The injury has been classified into three grades: grade 1, stretching of the capsule; grade 2, partial capsule tear; grade 3, complete tear.[15] The physical examination will show increasing swelling, ecchymosis, tenderness, and instability with each grade. In the most severe cases of irreducible dislocation, the metatarsal phalangeal joint is usually dorsiflexed, and the distal interphalangeal joint is plantar flexed in a "claw toe" position.

Radiographic evaluation is necessary in all injuries. Careful attention should be paid to the presence of fractures of the base of the phalanx, sesamoids, and symmetry of the joint. In severe injuries, the sesamoid complex may be disrupted, and there may be an irreducible dislocation (Fig. 71-5). Rarely, especially in late

presentations, magnetic resonance imaging may be useful to define injured structures.

In most injuries, conservative treatment is optimal. Patients with grade 1 and 2 injuries are treated with taping, activity modification, and a stiff orthotic support in their athletic shoe. They may return to play in 2 to 4 weeks when symptoms resolve. Grade 3 injuries involve instability of the joint and require cast immobilization with the hallux in a neutral position and prolonged rest. They may return to play at 6 to 8 weeks if the joint is stable. For an unstable or irreducible joint, surgery is indicated. There are no large series regarding acute operative treatment of severe turf toe injuries, but surgery should be directed toward the affected structures. Sesamoid fracture fixation or excision and collateral ligament and plantar plate repair are performed as indicated.[15]

Orthotic modification is often necessary for a prolonged duration if patients are to remain active. A simple over-the-counter turf toe insert is often sufficient. Alternatively, a steel plate may be inserted into the sole of the shoe or a custom insert made with steel or carbon fiber reinforcement under the hallux. Long-term sequelae of this injury may include hallux valgus, claw toe, stiffness, and degenerative arthritis. Late surgical treatment of these problems may involve osteotomy, chilectomy, or arthrodesis.

METATARSALGIA

Pain and overload of the metatarsal head region has been termed *metatarsalgia*. The etiology is often complex, with body habitus, foot deformity, muscular imbalance, training style, training surface, chosen sport, and shoe wear all contributing to the problem. The addition of heavy equipment to the player also increases risk of metatarsalgia.

By definition, metatarsalgia is pain under the metatarsal head, and for this discussion, we concentrate on the second through fifth metatarsals. Pain under the first metatarsal head is often a sesamoid problem and is discussed subsequently.

Generally, the patient will present with complaints of pain with ambulation. It is important to take a complete medical history from the patient, as rarely an underlying inflammatory

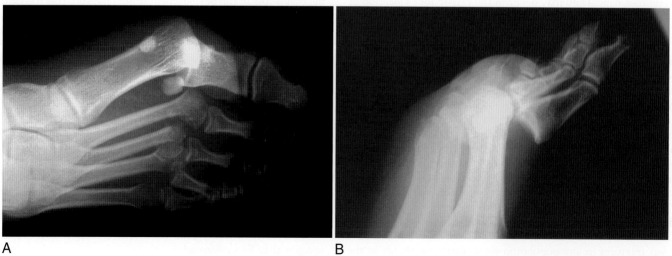

A   B

Figure 71-5 Turf toe injury with irreducible dislocation of the first metatarsophalangeal joint. Anteroposterior **(A)** and lateral **(B)** radiographs of a turf toe injury with an irreducible dislocation. The sesamoid complex is disrupted, and the metatarsal head is buttonholed through the plantar plate.

arthropathy (like rheumatoid arthritis) or neurologic abnormality (such as Charcot-Marie-Tooth syndrome) will present as metatarsalgia. It is also important to obtain a complete description of the pain and aggravating and alleviating factors. Some patients will have pain alone; others will present with pain, intermittent numbness, a burning sensation, and varying degrees of plantar callus making it very difficult in some cases to differentiate between metatarsalgia and nerve entrapment on physical examination alone, and the history often gives the best clues to the diagnosis. Most patients with metatarsalgia will describe an insidious onset of symptoms. It often starts as a feeling of a marble, pea, or a swollen feeling under the forefoot. Pain generally increases with activity, although some runners will describe that an area hurts initially, then goes "numb" after a certain point during their run, and then later hurts more. Almost universally, however, patients will report that the pain is worst barefoot on hard surfaces (in the shower, for example) and feels better in a padded shoe and/or on carpet. Often their good athletic shoes feel the best on the foot, and dress shoes (especially heels) make it worse. Unlike nerve entrapments, patients with metatarsalgia do not report that they remove their shoe and walk barefoot to relieve the pain.

All patients should have weight-bearing radiographs. On a weight-bearing radiograph, the functional position of the foot is most apparent. The angle of hallux varus, intermetatarsal angle, and presence of abnormalities can be most correctly identified.

Physical examination is directed toward identifying the source of the pain. Again, it may be difficult to differentiate metatarsalgia versus a nerve problem on examination alone. Patients with metatarsalgia will be tender directly under the metatarsal head, at the level of the metatarsal phalangeal joint. They are nontender, or minimally tender, in the web spaces associated with the joint. The joint may be swollen, and a Lachman's test to evaluate dorsal-plantar stability should be performed. The position of the toes should be noted. It is important to evaluate dorsiflexion, plantarflexion, lateral deviation, and the presence or absence of fixed angulation of the toe joints. There may be varying degrees of callus formation, from broad diffuse callus to small punctate keratoses. Often patients will have associated deformities causing the metatarsal overload. Hallux valgus and metatarsus primus varus lead to elevation of the first ray and commonly to an overload of the second metatarsal head. Patients with hammertoes and claw toes will have more metatarsalgia, as the metatarsal head is pushed plantarward in these deformities. Congenital deformities can also increase the risk of metatarsalgia, including metatarsus adductus and cavovarus feet.

An additional predisposing factor to metatarsalgia that may be overlooked is tightness in the gastrocsoleus complex and hamstrings. This inflexibility leads to increased forefoot pressures and often metatarsal pain.[16]

Treatment of metatarsalgia is initially conservative. As previously described, heel cord and hamstring stretching may be quite helpful. Shoe modification is essential. A simple felt pad that sticks to the liner of the shoe may be enough, or a more complex custom orthosis may be indicated (Fig. 71-6). Metatarsal bars are not useful in the athletic population. It is important to examine the athlete's training shoe. In cyclists and soccer players, the shoe may be too small or too stiff, contributing to the problem. These patients should be encouraged to choose wider shoes with better padding in the forefoot and deeper toe boxes. In addition, patients should be instructed to

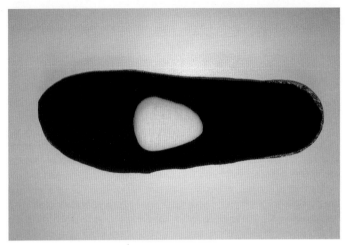

Figure 71-6 Metatarsal pad.

pumice or file their calluses frequently, as the thicker skin often increases pain.

Surgery is rarely indicated for metatarsalgia. When performed, it should be directed at the deformity causing the problem: correction of hallux valgus, hammertoe, claw toe, or plantar condyle prominence. Surgery to shorten or elevate the metatarsal alone is fraught with difficulty and has a high risk of transfer metatarsalgia or other problems.

SESAMOID PROBLEMS

In the vast majority of the population, there are two small sesamoid bones under the first metatarsal head. They are incorporated into the medial and lateral heads of the flexor hallucis brevis tendons and are termed the tibial and fibular sesamoids. Sesamoid problems are more common in women, possibly due to the greater degree of dorsiflexion present normally in their first metatarsophalangeal joints and more common in the tibial sesamoid. Up to 50% of body weight may be carried by the first metatarsal head, and the sesamoids receive even more stress. The sesamoids are involved in push off and serve as an integral part of forefoot function. The sesamoid complex includes the two sesamoids, the interosseous ligament, the flexor brevis tendons, the joint articulation, and the flexor hallucis longus. Problems may range from sesamoiditis to stress fracture, acute fracture, osteonecrosis, and fragmentation. In the older population, degenerative arthritis may involve the sesamoid-metatarsal articulation with loss of cartilage and overgrowth of the sesamoid. Sports that involve dorsiflexion of the first ray and repetitive impact such as dance, soccer, and running are most likely to produce problems.

Sesamoiditis is a fairly nebulous term. It does not necessarily mean that actual inflammatory tissue is present. Some patients will have true inflammation with swelling and joint effusion while others have only pain. It is generally a term used for sesamoid pain without apparent fracture or necrosis.

Clinically patients with sesamoid problems report the insidious onset of pain under the first metatarsal head, sometimes accompanied by swelling. Acute fractures are uncommon and usually associated with an acute dorsiflexion event. Again, harder surfaces generally increase the pain and softer surfaces improve it. Some patients will describe burning or lightning type pain, likely from local irritation of the digital nerves as they run close to the sesamoids.[17]

Physical examination should include range of motion of the great toe, identification of effusion, palpation, examination for calluses, and neurovascular status. Recently, a new provocative test was described for evaluation of sesamoid pain.[18] The test is performed by dorsiflexing the toe to its fullest extent, placing the thumb firmly against the proximal pole of the sesamoid and plantar flexing the toe. Reproduction of symptoms by this test indicates a sesamoid problem. Examination of the digital nerves should be performed; a Tinel's sign may indicate nerve injury or entrapment. In order to differentiate sesamoid pain from flexor hallucis longus tendonitis, this tendon should be tested by resisting active plantarflexion of the distal interphalangeal joint.

Radiographs and other studies are often helpful in identifying fracture, necrosis, arthritis, and fragmentation of the sesamoids. All patients should have radiographs including an axial view and weight-bearing anteroposterior and lateral views of the sesamoids (Fig. 71-7). They should be evaluated for location, size, contour, and presence of fractures. Bipartite sesamoids are relatively common, and should not be confused with fractures. Bipartite sesamoids fragments have rounded outlines. When in doubt, a radiograph of the opposite foot can be helpful as bipartite sesamoids are frequently (but not exclusively) bilateral. In the case in which a stress fracture or necrosis is suspected, a bone scan with pinhole collimation or magnetic resonance imaging can be very helpful, especially when plain radiographs are normal (Fig. 71-8). Rarely, computed tomography is needed to evaluate the sesamoid-metatarsal articulation for degenerative changes or bony overgrowth.[17]

Treatment of most sesamoid problems is conservative. Rest, activity modification, and shoe change are the first steps in treatment. A dancer's pad is very useful and inexpensive (Fig. 71-9). As sesamoid pain is common in dancers, these pads are designed to even fit into ballet slippers. The pads should be placed in the athlete's training shoes. For more prolonged symptoms, a durable custom orthotic can be constructed with this type of padding. In some cases, especially those with swelling or joint effusion, an intra-articular steroid injection may be very helpful. Physical therapy also plays an important role. Ultrasonography, heel cord stretching, taping, and strengthening of the flexor brevis muscles should be ordered.

For degenerative arthritis of the sesamoid, orthotic management is usually sufficient with the addition of steroid injection if needed. In cases in which overgrowth of one sesamoid leads to a prominence causing an intractable keratosis, shaving of the sesamoid is helpful.

In acute fractures or symptomatic stress fractures, 6 to 8 weeks of rest and cast (fiberglass or functional brace) followed by orthotic wear, taping, and physical therapy are often very successful. In the rare case of a symptomatic nonunion, the sesamoid should be preserved if possible. Bone grafting of the

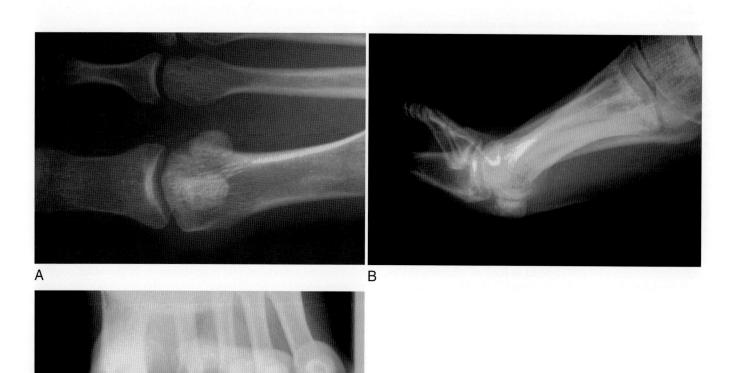

A

B

C

Figure 71-7 Sesamoid radiographs. **A,** Anteroposterior view. **B,** Lateral view. **C,** Axial view.

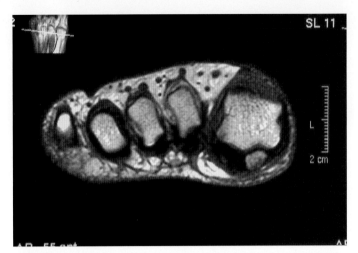

Figure 71-8 Magnetic resonance imaging shows avascular necrosis of fibular sesamoid; note the dark signal in the fibular sesamoid on this T1-weighted image.

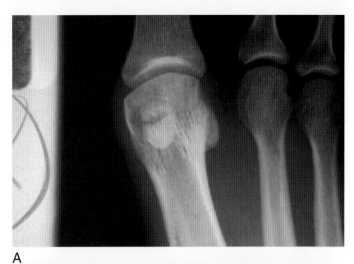

A

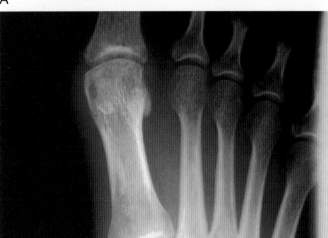

B

Figure 71-10 Sesamoid fracture nonunion that healed after bone graft. **A,** Anteroposterior radiograph of a tibial sesamoid fracture nonunion. **B,** Healed results after bone grafting.

tibial sesamoid has been described, and reports are encouraging.[19] The author has had three patients in the past several years who have improved with this procedure and returned to their work or sport (Fig. 71-10). If the proximal pole of the nonunion is small and bone grafting is not possible, then excision of this fragment with preservation of the tendon continuity is indicated. In even rarer cases of necrosis, fragmentation, or simply chronic unremitting pain, the sesamoid may be excised.[20] This surgery has a significant rate of complications including hallux valgus, hallux varus, clawing, and neurogenic pain. The sesamoids play a very important role in push off and should only be excised as a last resort.

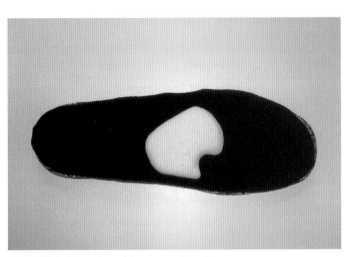

Figure 71-9 Dancer's pad for sesamoid pain.

NERVE ENTRAPMENTS

Nerve entrapment in the forefoot involves the digital nerves in the spaces between the metatarsal heads. This has been termed interdigital neuroma (IDN), more commonly known as Morton's neuroma. Classically, this neuroma is found in the third web space. More than 90% of all forefoot neuromas occur here, with the remaining 10% in the second web space.[21] Neuromas in the fourth or first web space are exceedingly rare and are usually associated with prior surgery. The IDN is not a true neuroma, but a pseudoneuroma. A true neuroma implies derangement of the actual nerve fibers, whereas IDN is a perineural fibrosis. IDN is thought to be due to repetitive trauma of the nerve against the tough intermetatarsal ligament joining the metatarsal heads as the toes dorsiflex. It is thought to be more common in the third web space due to the increased mobility in this area. As the trauma continues, fibrosis occurs around the nerve, and the larger nerve is thus more vulnerable to trauma. Thus, the cycle continues. It is probably aggravated by shoes that narrow the interval as well as repetitive activity.

Symptoms primarily involve pain. Patients will report a sharp, burning, lightning-like, or radiating pain. They may report feeling a fullness, "a wadded up sock" feeling, or a "click" in the web space. The click is often accompanied by pain relief. They reproducibly report that the pain is worse in shoes and often best barefoot. Most will relate a history of removing their shoe and massaging the foot to obtain relief. Narrow shoes will aggravate the problem. This history is one of the most reliable clues that IDN is involved and not metatarsalgia.

Radiographs should be routinely obtained. Weight-bearing anteroposterior, lateral, and non-weight-bearing oblique views of the foot are needed. In general, radiographs will be normal, but occasionally a bone abnormality causes the nerve compression. History and physical examination are the primary ways to identify the diagnosis; ultrasonography and magnetic resonance imaging are less useful but may be ordered in confusing cases or cases of recurrent neuroma.[6,22]

Physical examination procedures are similar to those for metatarsalgia. Patients will be tender in the web space as opposed to under the bone. Some will have an alteration in sensation, determined by subjective decrease to light touch, or objective decrease to a Semmes-Weinstein 5.07-mm fiber. Sometimes palpation of the web space will reproduce the radiating pain, but this is not common. A Mulder's sign has been described as an audible or palpable click occurring when the forefoot is compressed medial to lateral.[22] If pain is reproduced, it is thought to indicate a neuroma. However, painless clicks are common and do not indicate pathology, making this test not particularly useful.

A very useful diagnostic and therapeutic maneuver is the injection of 1 to 2 mL of long-acting local anesthetic and 1 mL of steroid around the nerve. In the office, I inject this mixture and have the patient put their shoes on and walk, climb stairs, run, or do the activity that usually produces pain. The absence of pain after injection helps confirm IDN.

Conservative treatment is usually successful. Wider shoes, having shoes stretched, simple metatarsal pads, and the injection described are often helpful. A custom insert with metatarsal padding is also helpful. Very occasionally a second or third injection 3 to 6 months apart may be needed. More injections should be avoided due to the potential for fat pad atrophy. One especially difficult patient to treat conservatively is the competitive cyclist, due to his or her shoe preference. Very stiff soled shoes increase the interdigital pressures, and the foot position in cycling puts increased stress on the metatarsal heads.[23]

For patients in whom conservative treatment is unsuccessful, surgery is indicated. Discussion of surgery for IDN has revolved around excision of the nerve (with or without transposition) with transection of the transverse metatarsal ligament, to neurolysis, to transection of the ligament without excision of the nerve. Dorsal and plantar approaches have been described. The author prefers the dorsal approach for all primary excisions and the plantar approach only for revision surgery. Excision of the nerve with transection of the ligament has the widest popularity, and reports indicate 85% success.[21] Care must be taken to excise the nerve very proximally and allow it to retract into the deep muscles of the foot. For the percentage of resections that have persistent pain due to a recurrent neuroma, repeat surgical resection is less successful, with a reported 60% improvement. With a primary neuroma excision, most highly competitive athletes may return to their sport within 4 to 6 weeks postoperatively.

CONCLUSIONS

In conclusion, forefoot problems are common in athletes. Most nonacute problems may be managed conservatively with good success. In the carefully chosen patient, various surgical procedures may be successful. Acute injuries such as severe turf toe injuries and fractures may more often require surgical intervention. Return to competitive or sporting activity must be based on each individual's response to treatment.

REFERENCES

1. Dameron TB: Fractures of the proximal fifth metatarsal: Selecting the best treatment option. J Am Acad Orthop Surg 1995;3:110–114.
2. Theodorou DJ, Theodorou SJ, Kakitsubata Y, et al: Fractures of proximal portion of fifth metatarsal bone: Anatomic and imaging evidence of a pathogenesis of avulsion of the plantar aponeurosis and the short peroneal muscle tendon. Radiology 2003;226:857–865.
3. Rosenberg GA, Sferra JJ: Treatment strategies for acute fractures and nonunions of the proximal fifth metatarsal. J Am Acad Orthop Surg 2000;8:332–338.
4. Portland G, Kelikian A, Kodros S: Acute surgical management of Jones fractures. Foot Ankle Int 2003;24:829–833.
5. Kelly IP, Glisson RR, Fink C, et al: Intramedullary screw fixation of Jones fractures. Foot Ankle Int 2001;22:585–589.
6. Shah SN, Knoblich GO, Lindsey DP, et al: Intramedullary screw fixation of proximal fifth metatarsal fractures: A biomechanical study. Foot Ankle Int 2001;22:581–584.
7. Larson CM, Almekinders LC, Taft TN, et al: Intramedullary screw fixation of Jones fractures: Analysis of failure. Am J Sports Med 2002;30:55–60.
8. Porter DA, Duncan M, Meyer SJ: Fifth metatarsal Jones fracture fixation with a 4.5-mm cannulated stainless steel screw in the competitive and recreational athlete: A clinical and radiographic evaluation. Am J Sports Med 2005;33:726–733.
9. Wiener BD, Linder JF, Giattini JF: Treatment of fractures of the fifth metatarsal: A prospective study. Foot Ankle Int 1997;18:267–269.
10. Gefen A: Biomechanical analysis of fatigue-related foot injury mechanisms in athletes and recruits during intensive marching. Med Biol Eng Comput 2002;40:302–210.
11. Korpelainen R, Orava S, Karpakka J, et al: Risk factors for recurrent stress fractures in athletes. Am J Sports Med 2001;29:304–310.
12. Milgrom C, Finestone A, Sharkey N, et al: Metatarsal strains are sufficient to cause fatigue fracture during cyclic overloading. Foot Ankle Int 2002;23:230–235.
13. O'Malley MJ, Hamilton WG, Munyak J, et al: Stress fractures at the base of the second metatarsal in ballet dancers. Foot Ankle Int 1996;17:89–94.
14. Bowers KD Jr, Martin RB: Turf-toe: A shoe-surface related football injury. Med Sci Sports 1976;8:81–83.
15. Watson TS, Anderson RB, Davis WH: Periarticular injuries to the hallux metatarsophalangeal joint in athletes. Foot Ankle Clin 2000;5:687–713.
16. DiGiovanni CW, Kuo R, Tejwani N, et al: Isolated gastrocnemius tightness. J Bone Joint Surg Am 2002;84:962–970.
17. Richardson EG: Hallucal sesamoid pain: Causes and surgical treatment. J Am Acad Orthop Surg 1999;7:270–278.

18. Allen MA, Casillas MM: The passive axial compression (PAC) test: A new adjunctive provocative maneuver for the clinical diagnosis of hallucal sesamoiditis. Foot Ankle Int 2001;22:345–346.

19. Anderson RB, McBryde AM: Autogenous bone grafting of hallux sesamoid non-unions. Foot Ankle Int 1997;18:293–296.

20. Saxena A, Krisdakumtorn T: Return to activity after sesamoidectomy in athletically active individuals. Foot Ankle Int 2003;24:415–419.

21. Kay D, Bennett GL: Morton's neuroma. Foot Ankle Clin 2003;8:49–59.

22. Ashman CJ, Klecker RJ, Yu JS: Forefoot pain involving the metatarsal region: Differential diagnosis with MR imaging. Radiographics 2001;21:1425–1440.

23. Jarboe NE, Quesada PM: The effects of cycling shoe stiffness on forefoot pressure. Foot Ankle Int 2003;24:784–788.

Foot and Ankle Rehabilitation

John Nyland

In This Chapter

Functional deficits
Mechanical and functional instability
Taping and bracing
Older, athletically active individuals
Performance testing

INTRODUCTION

- Whether an athletically active patient experiences disability due to foot or ankle impairments such as developmental tarsal coalition, accessory ossicle formation such as os trigonum, acute injuries such as fractures or sprains, tendon subluxations, enthesopathies, or overuse inflammatory reactions, successful rehabilitation outcomes ultimately depend on restoration of sufficient function for patients to return to their desired sports activity.

- Early intervention with therapeutic modalities intended to decrease pain, swelling, and inflammation and protection or realignment with taping, or orthoses may enable earlier, safe participation in a therapeutic exercise program designed to improve dynamic functional stability, neuromuscular responsiveness, and balance.

- Patient disability is minimized when they can return to the sports activities that they value without experiencing continued symptoms or increasing their risk of developing chronic conditions that may compromise their quality of life in the future.

FUNCTIONAL DEFICITS

Athletes who participate in running, jumping, and cutting sports are at risk of foot and ankle injuries, particularly lateral ankle sprains. Ankle injuries are responsible for more than 25% of time lost from sports participation, may develop into a chronic disability in up to 30% to 40% of cases, and have an injury recurrence rate as high as 80%.[1,2] Distal syndesmosis or high ankle sprains account for between 10% and 20% of all ankle sprains with considerably more disability and a greater loss of sports participation time than with lateral ankle sprains.[3]

Both capsuloligamentous and musculotendinous foot and ankle tissues have mechanoreceptors that send increasing afferent signals as tension increases during dynamic functional stability challenges, resulting in efferent neuromuscular responses.

Cutaneous and pressure receptors located in the plantar surface of the foot also have a significant influence over the protective activation of the lower leg muscles.[4] Reduced plantar fascia stiffness due to injury may create a more deformable longitudinal arch and a more pronated foot. Intensified stresses in the centralized metatarsals, dorsal calcaneocuboid joint junction, plantar ligaments, and their attachment bony areas after plantar fascia injury or surgical release may cause stress or fatigue failure and subsequent midfoot pain.[5,6] Foot impairments related to turf toe and/or heel conditions can also affect plantar fascia stiffness, thereby contributing to dysfunction both in the foot and proximally up the lower extremity kinetic chain.

Neural tissue heals much more slowly than other body tissues, conceivably leading to a mechanically stable foot or ankle prior to the re-establishment of a functionally stable ankle. Chronic symptoms following foot or ankle injury may include decreased proprioception, muscle weakness, delayed reflex and reaction times, and diminished postural control.[7]

MECHANICAL AND FUNCTIONAL INSTABILITY

Not all feet or ankles that are mechanically unstable are functionally unstable, and the cause-effect relationship between these variables is highly questionable. The anterior talofibular and calcaneofibular ligaments function in tandem to stabilize the ankle joint. The ankle is in its most stable osseous position when it is dorsiflexed and is in its most unstable position when it is plantar flexed. Sudden displacement of the foot and ankle activates a sequence of neuromuscular responses in which motor programs interact with peripheral reflexes. Afferent information is provided by proprioceptors in addition to the visual, vestibular, and auditory systems. In a plantar flexed, inverted ankle, the peroneal muscle activation provides a dynamic defense mechanism that is far more effective than any combination of footwear, taping, or bracing.[8] Fortunately, this dynamic defense mechanism is most effective when the ankle is in its most vulnerable position (plantar flexed, inverted) for lateral capsuloligamentous injury. When the ankle is in this position, the peroneal muscles create 63% to 73% more power than when the ankle is aligned in neutral.[8] Programmed foot and ankle muscle responses vary according to the direction of the perturbation, the phase of gait, and the alignment of the foot on the ground. When peripheral afferent input is compromised, there is an increased reliance on visual and vestibular cues. While protective peroneal muscle activation may occur in patients with chronic ankle instability, the response is delayed significantly. When the patient is at rest, normal peroneal muscle activation latency, in addition to electromechanical delay, is insufficient to protect the ankle during a sudden trip, fall, or landing on uneven terrain. Fortunately, when a person is hopping, jumping, or running, ankle and foot muscles are generally preactivated prior to foot-ground contact. This preactivation increases both segmental reflex activity and stretch velocity enabling muscles to produce significantly greater forces at touchdown without significant time delay.

TAPING AND BRACING

Athletic ankle taping can increase the ankle eversion moment (resistance to inversion); however, the protective benefits decrease over the initial 10 to 40 minutes following application.[9] The application of tape or braces may change the orientation of the talocrural, subtalar, transverse tarsal joints, and first metatarsophalangeal joint, thereby influencing neuromuscular responses. Combining ankle taping or bracing and high top shoes can enhance joint protection, but it may also reduce performance.[10] Use of a lace-up ankle brace with low top shoes may provide optimal protection without adversely affecting performance. Ankle or foot taping may have both mechanical and proprioceptive benefits; however, long-term use may lead to dependence and weakening of capsuloligamentous, musculotendinous, and osseous structures that are "protected" by the brace as the tissues may be shielded from both beneficial as well as injurious loads. Prescriptive taping for enhanced proprioception and restoration of distal fibula alignment may enable earlier participation in therapeutic exercise activities following an inversion ankle sprain (Fig. 72-1).

WALKING

In terminal stance, tibialis posterior activation assists in locking the transverse tarsal joints, creating a rigid foot necessary for normal heel rise as the body progresses forward during gait.

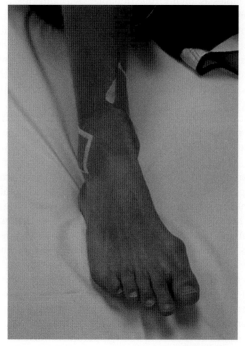

Figure 72-1 Proprioceptive ankle taping with fibula repositioning.

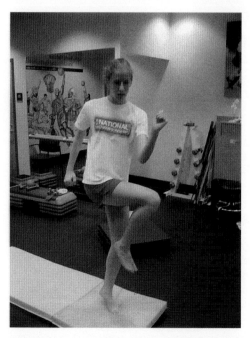

Figure 72-2 Form run simulation with exaggerated trunk rotation.

Kulig et al[11] reported that the tibialis posterior muscle was most selectively and effectively activated during therapeutic exercises that focused on foot adduction movements. During aquatic walking, lower extremity extensor moments display increased hip and decreased knee and ankle contributions compared to land walking, providing an opportunity to initiate early gait training with limited ankle joint forces.[12] Compared with heel-toe walking, toe walking produces greater plantar flexor moments during stance, higher peak plantar flexor moments during the loading response and midstance, lower mean plantar flexor moments during terminal stance, earlier soleus and gastrocnemius activity, and higher levels of mean soleus and gastrocnemius activity during stance.[13] During toe walking, the peak internal knee extensor moment is lower in midstance and the power absorption is reduced in the loading response. Toe walking can be incorporated into a form run simulation with exaggerated transverse plane trunk rotation to restore nonimpaired active mobility and improve dynamic functional foot, ankle, knee, and hip stability while minimizing impact forces prior to return to running (Fig. 72-2). Backward walking on a treadmill can be used to facilitate ankle dorsiflexion and eversion in synergy with knee flexion and hip flexion-extension (Fig. 72-3). To further increase the dynamic stability demands at the foot and ankle, functional tasks such as single leg standing with trunk twists (Fig. 72-4), punching with dumbbells during single leg stance (Fig. 72-5) and single leg step-ups with trunk twists (Fig. 72-6), each performed barefoot with exaggerated transverse plane rotation, are encouraged to challenge synergistic dynamic lower extremity functional stability from the foot to the hip.

UNSTEADY SURFACES

Eils and Rosenbaum[14] reported that patients with chronic ankle instability who performed a multistation therapeutic exercise program displayed improved joint position sense, postural sway,

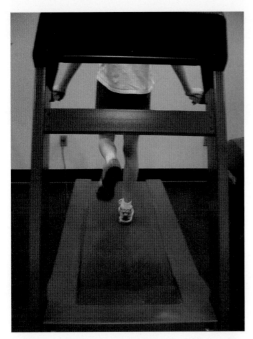

Figure 72-3 Backward walking on a treadmill.

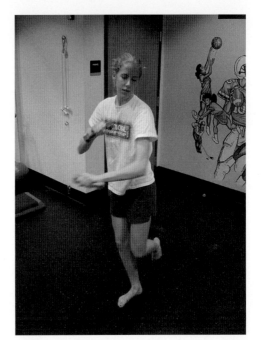

Figure 72-5 Punching with dumbbells during single leg stance.

and neuromuscular reaction times compared to a control group. Postural control through the ankle is of primary importance during relatively stationary single leg stance on firm, foam, and multiaxial surfaces.[15] Wobble board or soft disk training does more to improve neuromuscular responsiveness and balance than it does to improve proprioception. The benefit of this type of training is that the patient improves his or her ability to discriminate different degrees of active subtalar joint inversion and ankle plantar flexion moments.[16,17] Wobble board training

improves the foot and ankle motor control processes that occur below the level of conscious attention, but the effect is relatively short and may need to be performed daily for the effect to continue.[18]

Footwear may attenuate the deformation, shear, and mechanical transients that provide foot position information through mechanoreceptors during wobble board or soft disk training[4]; therefore, as previously mentioned, in a protected environment, barefoot training is recommended, particularly early during ther-

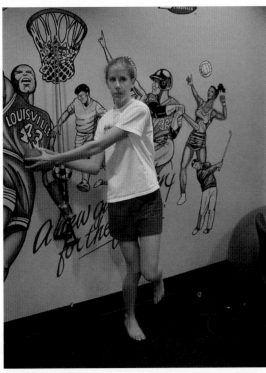

Figure 72-4 Single leg standing trunk twists with medicine ball.

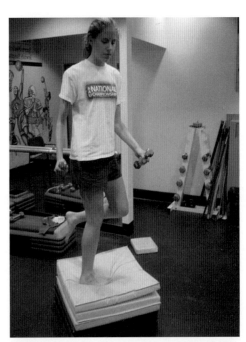

Figure 72-6 Single leg step-ups and trunk twists with dumbbell resistance.

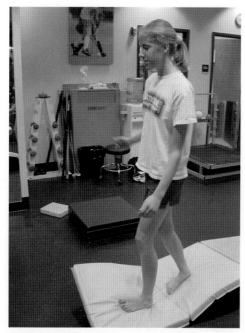

Figure 72-7 Forward stepping across an uneven matted surface.

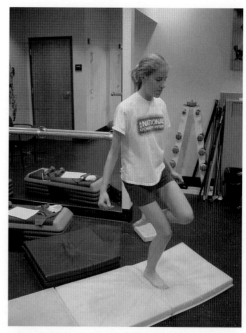

Figure 72-9 Single leg hop down and stabilize.

apeutic exercise performance.[4] Dynamic functional stability at the articulations of the foot can be emphasized to a greater extent when the patient is asked to perform these activities barefoot. Forward (Fig. 72-7) and lateral (Fig. 72-8) walking across an uneven obstacle course first with the eyes open and then closed can facilitate protective neuromuscular responses from foot and ankle musculature. The knee and hip joints have an increased postural control stability function under more challenging conditions such as hopping down to perform a stable, one-foot landing (Fig. 72-9) and should be eventually evaluated in synergy with the involved ankle and/or foot, particularly in regards to frontal plane knee position.

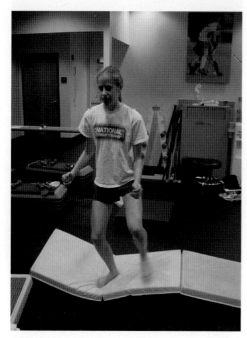

Figure 72-8 Lateral stepping across an uneven matted surface.

SENSORIMOTOR-ENRICHED REHABILITATION AND CONDITIONING ENVIRONMENT

Effective lower extremity function influences the patient's ability to be actively mobile and independent throughout his or her life, and this function largely depends on regular exercise or active use. Animal studies have indicated that exposure to an enriched rehabilitation or conditioning environment has a beneficial effect on compensational central nervous system plasticity following peripheral nerve injury.[19] An enriched environment seems to stimulate activity and enhances learning processes and compensational processes.[20] Neuroanatomic changes following exposure to an enriched environment persist the longer the exposure to the enriched environment lasts, but it is unknown whether a ceiling for this effect exists.[20]

OLDER, ATHLETICALLY ACTIVE PATIENTS

As with young, athletically active patients, older patients can show improvements with wobble board or soft-disk training. However, the ability to balance while barefoot appears to decrease with advancing years, compared with balancing while wearing shoes, particularly if the patient is accustomed to wearing shoes.[4] Several studies have established the role of lower extremity muscle strength (maximum force generating capacity) as a predictor of functional limitation in disabled and nondisabled older patients. The ankle plantar flexors and dorsiflexors serve important torque-generating roles in functional activities such as gait and rising from a chair. Also, low peak plantar flexor muscle torque production has been linked to increased falling risk in institutionalized older patients.[21] Ankle plantar flexor power is an independent predictor of chair rise performance, and ankle dorsiflexor power is an independent predictor of stair climb performance among older patients.[20] Peak muscle power (strength/time) may be a more critical factor than muscle strength in explaining physical function decrements in older patients because of its rapid decline with advancing age.[21,22]

Elderly patients who need to stop walking when they start talking show an increased falling risk indicating that enhanced cognitive capacity is required to combine walking and talking.[23] Elderly patients also show an increased dependency on vision, when experiencing reduced or conflicting sensory inputs, likely due to impaired proprioceptive mechanisms.[24] Although derived from upper limb studies, it appears that task performance is impaired in the elderly, but the acquisition of skill learning is not.[25-27] Analogous to motor control, it is suggested that sensorimotor adaptations seem to be associated with a higher computational load in the elderly.[26] van Hedel and Dietz[28] reported that healthy elderly subjects are able to perform the task of high precision obstacle stepping quite well when full visual information is provided. They can quickly adapt kinematics and muscle activity to the task and improve the accuracy of performance in a similar way to that of younger subjects. However, in contrast to younger subjects, they cannot improve their task accuracy when vision becomes restricted. This agrees with the observation that during locomotion, elderly subjects rely more on visual control due to impaired proprioceptive feedback mechanisms.[29,30] In addition, elderly subjects might be less able to use the available sensory information. Relearning adaptive locomotor control represents an important aspect of the rehabilitation process in many patient groups, in particular with older patients.

TESTING FUNCTIONAL FOOT AND ANKLE STABILITY

Performance testing for functional foot and ankle instability includes the modified Romberg test, a single leg hop test, and proficiency with single leg balance activities on a disk or wobble board.[10] During the modified Romberg test, the athlete assumes a single leg stance with the affected lower extremity with the other leg flexed at the knee (Fig. 72-10). The arms are crossed over the chest. The patient focuses their eyes straight ahead. Balance and stability are assessed with the eyes open and then

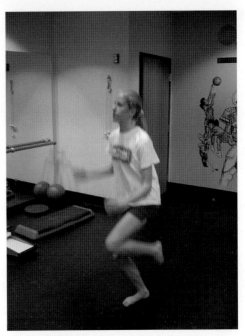

Figure 72-11 Single leg hop test.

closed. Patients with good functional foot and ankle stability should be able to stand for 30 seconds without falling out of position. By having the patient perform this task barefoot, dynamic foot and ankle stability can be assessed concurrently. This test may also be performed on a wobble board or soft disk.

The single leg hop is a modification of the Romberg test that evaluates strength, balance, and level of pain at the affected foot and ankle. During this test, the patient is asked to rise up on the forefoot of the same weight-bearing lower extremity and perform five single leg-hopping maneuvers onto the forefoot in succession (Fig. 72-11). The arms are outstretched to assist with balance. Pain, weakness, or poor balance may all contribute to impaired performance during this test.

CONCLUSIONS

Dynamic or functional stability at the foot and ankle joints is essential to the daily activities of athletically active patients, regardless of age. As part of a regular conditioning program or following management of a given foot or ankle impairment, it is essential that the athletically active patient perform prescribed therapeutic exercises in a sensorimotor-enriched environment that challenges neuromuscular responsiveness, balance, and postural awareness. Developing a series of functionally relevant sensorimotor "puzzles" that challenge the individual patient is essential to having a successful outcome. Ultimately, functional performance tests are used to determine readiness for return to recreational athletic or vocational activities, but assessing how the patient performs these tests (qualitative assessment of technique) is as important as how many repetitions or how long a duration they maintain a given posture (quantitative assessment). Last, no single functional performance test should be used as an indicator of functional readiness for return to increased activity. In addition to the previously discussed tests, one or two additional tasks deemed appropriate for the individual patient should be used as part of functional test battery with the patient displaying proficiency with each test prior to release to increased activities.

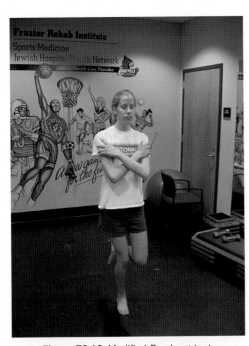

Figure 72-10 Modified Romberg test.

REFERENCES

1. Yeung MS, Chan CH, So CH: An epidemiological survey on ankle sprain. Br J Sports Med 1994;28:112–116.
2. Lynch SA, Renstrom PA: Treatment of acute lateral ankle ligament rupture in the athlete. Conservative versus surgical treatment. Sports Med 1999;27:61–71.
3. Title CI, Katchis SD: Traumatic foot and ankle injuries in the athlete. Orthop Clin N Am 2002;33:587–598.
4. Robbins S, Waked E, Allard P, et al: Foot position awareness in younger and older men: The influence of footwear sole properties. J Am Geriatr Soc 1997;45:61–66.
5. Bolgla LA, Malone TR: Plantar fasciitis and the windlass mechanism: A biomechanical link to clinical practice. J Athl Train 2004;39:77–82.
6. Cheung JTM, Zhang M, An KA: Effects of plantar fascia stiffness on the biomechanical responses of the ankle-foot complex. Clin Biomech 2004;19:839–846.
7. Hertel J: Functional instability following lateral ankle sprain. Sports Med 2000;29:361–371.
8. Ashton-Miller J, Wojtys E, Huston L, et al: Can proprioception really be improved by exercises? Knee Surg Sports Traumatol Arthrosc 2001;9:128–136.
9. Manfroy PP, Ashton-Miller JA, Wojtys EM: The effect of exercise, prewrap and athletic tape on the maximal active and passive ankle resistance to ankle inversion. Am J Sports Med 1997;25:156–163.
10. Richie DH Jr: Functional instability of the ankle and the role of neuromuscular control: A comprehensive review. J Foot Ankle Surg 2001;40:240–251.
11. Kulig K, Burnfield JM, Requejo SM, et al: Selective activation of tibialis posterior: Evaluation by magnetic resonance imaging. Med Sci Sports Exerc 2004;36:862–867.
12. Miyoshi T, Shirota T, Yamamoto S, et al: Lower limb joint moment during walking in water. Disabil Rehab 2003;25:1219–1223.
13. Perry J, Burnfield JM, Gronley JK, et al: Toe walking: Muscular demands at the ankle and knee. Arch Phys Med Rehabil 2003;84:7–16.
14. Eils E, Rosenbaum D: A multi-station proprioceptive exercise program in patients with ankle instability. Med Sci Sports Exerc 2001;33:1991–1998.
15. Riemann BL, Myers JB, Lephart SM: Comparison of ankle, knee, hip, and trunk corrective action shown during single-leg stance on firm, foam, and multiaxial surfaces. Arch Phys Med Rehabil 2003;84:90–95.
16. Waddington G, Adams R: Discrimination of active plantar flexion and inversion movements after ankle injury. Aust J Physiother 1999;45:7–13.
17. Waddington G, Adams R: Textured insole effects on ankle movement discrimination while wearing athletic shoes. Phys Ther Sport 2000;1:119–128.
18. Waddington GS, Adams RD: The effect of a 5-week wobble-board exercise intervention on ability to discriminate different degrees of ankle inversion, barefoot and wearing shoes: A study in healthy elderly. J Am Geriatr Soc 2004;52:573–576.
19. Strasberg SR, Watanabe O, Mackinnon SE, et al: Wire mesh as a postoperative physiotherapy assistive device following peripheral nerve graft repair in the rat. J Peripher Nerv Syst 1996;1:73–76.
20. Van Praag H, Kempermann G, Gage FH: Neural consequences of environmental enrichment. Nat Rev Neurosci 2000;1:191–198.
21. Suzuki T, Bean JF, Fielding RA: Muscle power of the ankle plantar flexors predicts functional performance in community-dwelling older women. J Am Geriatr Soc 2001;49:1161–1167.
22. Metter EJ, Conwit R, Tobin J, et al: Age-associated loss of power and strength in the upper extremities of women and men. J Gerontol A Biol Sci Med Sci 1997;52:B267–B276.
23. Lundin-Olsson L, Nyberg L, Gustafson Y: Stops walking when talking as a predictor of falls in elderly people. Lancet 1997;349:617 (letter).
24. Dietz V, Colombo G: Influence of body load on the gait pattern in Parkinson's disease. Mov Disord 1998;13:255–261.
25. Durkin M, Prescott L, Furchtgott E, et al: Performance but not acquisition of skill learning is severely impaired in the elderly. Arch Gerontol Geriatr 1995;20:167–183.
26. Bock O, Schneider S: Sensorimotor adaptation in young and elderly humans. Neurosci Biobehav Rev 2002;26:761–767.
27. McNay ED, Willingham DB: Deficit in learning of a motor skill requiring strategy, but not perceptuomotor recalibration, with aging. Learn Mem 1998;4:411–420.
28. van Hedel HJ, Dietz V: The influence of age on learning a locomotor task. Clin Neurophysiol 2004;115:2134–2143.
29. Mulder T, Zijlstra W, Geurts A: Assessment of motor recovery and decline. Gait Posture 2002;16:198–210.
30. Woollacott M, Shumway-Cook A: Attention and control of posture and gait: A review of an emerging area of research. Gait Posture 2002;16:1–14.

Index

Note: Page numbers by f indicate figures and those followed by t indicate tables.